W9-BOD-806

GLENBROOK PEDIATRICS, S.C.
2050 PFINGSTEN RD. STE. 150
GLENVIEW, ILLINOIS 60025
(847) 729-6445

Pediatric Otolaryngology:
Principles and Practice Pathways

Pediatric Otolaryngology:
Principles and Practice Pathways

Edited by

Ralph F. Wetmore, M.D.
Associate Professor
Department of Otorhinolaryngology—
Head and Neck Surgery
University of Pennsylvania School of Medicine
Children's Hospital of Philadelphia
Philadelphia, Pennsylvania

Harlan R. Muntz, M.D.
Associate Professor of Otolaryngology
Washington University School of Medicine
Department of Pediatric Otolaryngology
St. Louis Children's Hospital
St. Louis, Missouri

and

Trevor J. McGill, M.D.
Associate Professor of Otology and Laryngology
Harvard Medical School
Department of Otorhinolaryngology and Communication Disorders
The Children's Hospital Medical Center
Boston, Massachusetts

Contributing Editors
William P. Potsic, M.D.
Gerald B. Healy, M.D.
Rodney P. Lusk, M.D.

2000
Thieme
New York • Stuttgart

Thieme New York
333 Seventh Avenue
New York, NY 10001

Editorial Director: Avé McCracken
Editorial Assistant: Michelle Schmitt
Developmental Editor: Lucinda Houston
Developmental Manager: Kathleen P. Lyons
Director, Production & Manufacturing: Anne Vinnicombe
Production Editor: Janice G. Stangel
Marketing Director: Phyllis Gold
Sales Manager: Ross Lumpkin
Chief Financial Officer: Seth S. Fishman
President: Brian D. Scanlan
Medical Illustrator: Susan Brenman
Cover Designer: Michael Mendelsohn
Compositor: Maryland Composition
Printer: Maple-Vail Book Manufacturing Group

Library of Congress Cataloging-in-Publication Data

Pediatric otolaryngology: principles and practice pathways / edited
  by Ralph F. Wetmore. Harlan R. Muntz, and Trevor J. McGill.
       p.   cm.
     Includes bibliographical references and index.
     ISBN 0-86577-835-3
     1. Pediatric otolaryngology. 2. Children—Diseases. I. Wetmore.
  Ralph F.   II. Muntz, Harlan R.   III. McGill, Trevor J. I.
     [DNLM: 1. Otorhinolaryngologic Diseases—Child.
  2. Otorhinolaryngologic Diseases—Infant,   WV 140 P3715 1999]
  RF47.C4P399   1999
  618.92′09751—dc21
  DNLM/DLC
  for Library of Congress   99-39601
                                                    CIP

Important note: Medical knowledge is ever-changing. As new research and clinical experience broaden our knowledge, changes in treatment and drug therapy may be required. The authors and editors of the material herein have consulted sources believed to be reliable in their efforts to provide information that is complete and in accord with the standards accepted at the time of publication. However, in view of the possibility of human error by the authors, editors, or publisher of the work herein, or changes in medical knowledge, neither the authors, editors, publisher, nor any other party who has been involved in the preparation of this work, warrants that the information contained herein is in every respect accurate or complete, and they are not responsible for any errors or omissions or for the results obtained from use of such information. Readers are encouraged to confirm the information contained herein with other sources. For example, readers are advised to check the product information sheet included in the package of each drug they plan to administer to be certain that the information contained in this publication is accurate and that changes have not been made in the recommended dose or in the contraindications for administration. This recommendation is of particular importance in connection with new or infrequently used drugs.

Some of the product names, patents, and registered designs referred to in this book are in fact registered trademarks or proprietary names even though specific reference to this fact is not always made in the text. Therefore, the appearance of a name without designation as proprietary is not to be construed as a representation by the publisher that it is in the public domain.

Printed in the United States of America
Compositor: Maryland Composition   Printer: Maple-Vail Book Manufacturing Group

Contents

Contributors

Max M. April, MD, FAAP, FACS
Co-Director
Department of Pediatric Otolaryngology
Lenox Hill Hospital
New York, New York

John P. Bent, III, MD
Assistant Professor
Department of Otolaryngology
Albert Einstein University
New York, New York

Leigh A. Berry, PhD
Clinical Psychology Program Director
Department of Psychology
St. Louis Children's Hospital
St. Louis, Missouri

Patrick E. Brookhouser, MD
Boys Town National Research Hospital
Father Flanagan Professor and Chair
Department of Otolaryngology and Human
  Communication
Creighton University School of Medicine
Omaha, Nebraska

Dorothy M. Brown, MD
Early Childhood Specialist for Communication Disorders
The Children's Hospital Medical Center
Boston, Massachusetts

Orval E. Brown, MD
Professor
Department of Otolaryngology—
Head and Neck Surgery
Southwestern Medical Center at Dallas
Dallas, Texas

Randall A. Clary, MD
Assistant Professor
Department of Otolaryngology—Head and Neck Surgery
Washington University School of Medicine
St. Louis Children's Hospital
St. Louis, Missouri

Andrew T. Costarino, Jr., MD
Associate Professor
University of Philadelphia School of Medicine
Children's Hospital of Philadelphia
Philadelphia, Pennsylvania

Michael J. Cunningham, MD
Associate Professor of Otology and Laryngology
Department of Otolaryngology
Harvard Medical School
Massachusetts Eye & Ear Infirmary
Boston, Massachusetts

David H. Darrow, MD, DDS
Assistant Professor
Department of Otolaryngology and Pediatrics/Eastern
  Virginia Medical School
Norfolk, Virginia

Andrew L. de Jong, MD
Assistant Professor
Departments of Otolaryngology and Pediatrics
Baylor College of Medicine
Texas Children's Hospital
Houston, Texas

Craig S. Derkay, MD
Professor
Departments of Otolaryngology and Pediatrics
Eastern Virginia Medical School
Norfolk, Virginia

Ronald W. Deskin, MD
Paul E. Suchs Professor of Otolaryngology—Head and
  Neck Surgery
Departments of Otolaryngology and Pediatrics
University of Texas Medical Branch
Galveston, Texas

Hope E. Dickinson, MS
Speech Language Pathologist
Department of Otolaryngology and Communication
  Disorders
The Children's Hospital Medical Center
Boston, Massachusetts

Michael E. Dunham, MD
Professor
Department of Otolaryngology—Head and Neck Surgery
Children's Memorial Hospital
Northwestern University
Chicago, Illinois

Kara R. Fletcher, MS
Speech Language Pathologist
Department of Otolaryngology and Communication
  Disorders
The Children's Hospital Medical Center
Boston, Massachusetts

James W. Forsen, MD
Assistant Professor
Department of Otolaryngology
Washington University School of Medicine
St. Louis Children's Hospital
St. Louis, Missouri

Jacob Friedberg, MD
Associate Professor, Faculty of Medicine
Department of Otolaryngology
University of Toronto
Hospital for Sick Children
Toronto, Ontario
Canada

Ellen M. Friedman, MD, FAAP, FACS
Professor
Departments of Otolaryngology and Pediatrics
Baylor College of Medicine;
Chief of Service
Department of Otolaryngology
Texas Children's Hospital
Houston, Texas

Kenneth M. Grundfast, MD, FAAP, FACS
Interim Chairman
Department of Otolaryngology
Georgetown University School of Medicine
Washington, DC

Joseph Haddad, Jr., MD
Associate Professor
Department of Otolaryngology—Head and Neck Surgery
Columbia College of Physicians and Surgeons
Babies Hospital
New York, New York

Steven D. Handler, MD
Professor
Department of Otorhinolaryngology—Head and Neck
*   Surgery*
University of Pennsylvania School of Medicine
Children's Hospital of Philadelphia
Philadelphia, Pennsylvania

Geralyn Harvey-Woodnorth, MA
Speech Language Pathologist
Department of Otolaryngology and Communication
*   Disorders*
The Children's Hospital Medical Center
Boston, Massachusetts

Gerald B. Healy, MD
Professor of Otology and Laryngology
Department of Otolaryngology
Harvard Medical School
The Children's Hospital Medical Center
Boston, Massachusetts

Richard L. Hebert, MD
Fellow
Department of Pediatric Otolaryngology
Children's Memorial Hospital
Chicago, Illinois

Arden Hill, MS
Speech Language Pathologist
Department of Otolaryngology and Communication
*   Disorders*
The Children's Hospital Medical Center
Boston, Massachusetts

Philip T. Ho, MD
Chief Resident
Department of Otolaryngology—Head and Neck Surgery
Columbia-Presbyterian Medical Center
New York, New York

Robert S. Holzman, MD
Associate Professor of Anesthesia
Harvard Medical School;
Senior Associate in Anesthesia
The Children's Hospital Medical Center
Boston, Massachusetts

Donald V. Huebener, DDS, MA, MAEd
Professor of Surgery (Plastic and Reconstructive)
Division of Plastic Surgery
Washington University School of Medicine
St. Louis Children's Hospital
St. Louis, Missouri

C. Anthony Hughes, MD
Department of Pediatric Otolaryngology
Northwestern University
Children's Memorial Hospital
Chicago, Illinois

Jill V. Hunter, MBBS, MRCP, FRCR
Assistant Professor of Radiology
Department of Neuroradiology
University of Pennsylvania School of Medicine
Children's Hospital of Philadelphia
Philadelphia, Pennsylvania

Hani Z. Ibrahim, MD
Chief Resident
Department of Otolaryngology
University of Pennsylvania School of Medicine
Philadelphia, Pennsylvania

Glenn Isaacson, MD
Professor and Chairman
Department of Otolaryngology and Bronchoesophagology
Temple University School of Medicine
Philadelphia, Pennsylvania

Ian N. Jacobs, MD
Assistant Professor
Department of Otorhinolaryngology—Head and Neck
  Surgery
University of Pennsylvania School of Medicine
Children's Hospital of Philadelphia
Philadelphia, Pennsylvania

Dwight T. Jones, MD
Assistant Professor of Otology and Laryngology
Harvard Medical School
The Children's Hospital Medical Center
Boston, Massachusetts

Jeffrey L. Keller, MD
Assistant Professor
Department of Otolaryngology—Head and Neck Surgery
Division of Pediatric Otolaryngology
Columbia-Presbyterian Medical Center
New York, New York

Kara B. Kelley-Corley, BS, MS-SP
Speech Language Pathologist
Department of Otolaryngology and Communication
  Disorders
The Children's Hospital Medical Center
Boston, Massachusetts

Margaret A. Kenna, MD
Associate Professor of Otology and Laryngology
Harvard Medical School
The Children's Hospital Medical Center
Boston, Massachusetts

Daniel J. Kirse, MD
Assistant Professor
Department of Otolaryngology—Head and Neck Surgery
University of Kansas Medical Center
Staff Otolaryngologist
Children's Mercy Hospital
Kansas City, Kansas

Edward J. Krowiak, MD
Chief Resident
Department of Otolaryngology
Georgetown University Medical Center
Washington, DC

Jane M. Lavelle, MD
Assistant Professor
Department of Pediatrics
Division of Emergency Medicine
University of Pennsylvania School of Medicine
Children's Hospital of Philadelphia
Philadelphia, Pennsylvania

Benjamin C.P. Lee, MD
Associate Professor
Department of Radiology
Washington University Medical School
St. Louis Children's Hospital
St. Louis, Missouri

Rodney P. Lusk, MD
Associate Professor
Department of Otolaryngology
Washington University Medical School
St. Louis Children's Hospital
St. Louis, Missouri

Carol J. MacArthur, MD
Assistant Clinical Professor of Otolaryngology
Department of Otolaryngology—Head and Neck Surgery
University of California, Irvine
Orange, California

Trevor J. McGill, MD
Associate Professor of Otology and Laryngology
Harvard Medical School
Department of Otorhinolaryngology and Communication
  Disorders
The Children's Hospital Medical Center
Boston, Massachusetts

J. Scott McMurray, MD
Assistant Professor
Departments of Surgery and Pediatrics
Division of Otolaryngology
University of Wisconsin Medical School
Madison, Wisconsin

Marnie S. Millington, MS
Speech Language Pathologist
Department of Otolaryngology and Communication
  Disorders
The Children's Hospital Medical Center
Boston, Massachusetts

Harlan R. Muntz, MD
Associate Professor of Otolaryngology
Washington University School of Medicine
Department of Pediatric Otolaryngology
St. Louis Children's Hospital
St. Louis, Missouri

Charles M. Myer, III, MD
Professor
Department of Otolaryngology—
Head and Neck Surgery
Children's Hospital Medical Center
Cincinnati, Ohio

Marilyn W. Neault, PhD, CCC-A
Assistant Professor
Department of Otology and Laryngology
Harvard Medical School
Director of Audiology
The Children's Hospital Medical Center
Boston, Massachusetts

Richard J. Nissen, DDS, MS
Assistant Professor of Surgery
Department of Plastic and Reconstructive Surgery
Washington University School of Medicine
St. Louis Children's Hospital
St. Louis, Missouri

Roger C. Nuss, MD
Assistant Professor of Otology and Laryngology
Harvard Medical School
The Children's Hospital Medical Center
Boston, Massachusetts

Laurie A. Ohlms, MD
Assistant Professor of Otology and Laryngology
Harvard Medical School
The Children's Hospital Medical Center
Boston, Massachusetts

Blake C. Papsin, MD, MSc, FRCSC
Assistant Professor, Faculty of Medicine
Department of Otolaryngology
University of Toronto
Hospital for Sick Children
Toronto, Ontario
Canada

Christopher P. Poje, MD, FACS
Assistant Professor
Department of Pediatric Otolaryngology
Kaleida Health System
State University of New York at Buffalo
Buffalo, New York

J. Christopher Post, MD, PhD
Professor
Department of Pediatric Otolaryngology
Allegheny General Hospital
Pittsburgh, Pennsylvania

William P. Potsic, MD, MMM
E. Mortimer Newlin Professor of
  Otorhinolaryngology—Head and Neck Surgery
University of Pennsylvania School of Medicine;
Director
Department of Pediatric Otolaryngology
Children's Hospital of Philadelphia
Philadelphia, Pennsylvania

Sarah N. Quinn, MS
Speech Language Pathologist
Department of Otolaryngology and Communication
  Disorders
The Children's Hospital Medical Center
Boston, Massachusetts

Reza Rahbar, DMD, MD
Department of Otology and Laryngology
Harvard Medical School
The Children's Hospital
Boston, Massachusetts

Jay S. Rechtweg, MD
Senior Resident and Assistant Clinical Instructor
Department of Otolaryngology
State University of New York at Buffalo
Buffalo, New York

Mark A. Richardson, MD, MSc
Bordley Professor;
Deputy Director
Department of Otolaryngology—Head and Neck Surgery
The Johns Hopkins University
Baltimore, Maryland

David W. Roberson, MD
Instructor in Otolaryngology
Department of Otology and Laryngology
Harvard Medical School
The Children's Hospital Medical Center
Boston, Massachusetts

Craig W. Senders, MD
Professor of Otolaryngology—Head and Neck Surgery
University of California Davis Medical Center
Sacramento, California

Udayan K. Shah, MD
Assistant Professor
Department of Otorhinolaryngology—Head and Neck
  Surgery
University of Pennsylvania School of Medicine
Children's Hospital of Philadelphia
Philadelphia, Pennsylvania

Howard C. Shane, PhD
Associate Professor
Departments of Otolaryngology and Communication
  Disorders
Harvard Medical School
The Children's Hospital Medical Center
Boston, Massachusetts

James D. Sidman, MD
Minneapolis ENT Clinic
Minneapolis, Minnesota

Kathleen C.Y. Sie, MD
Associate Professor
Department of Otolaryngology—Head and Neck Surgery
University of Washington
Seattle, Washington

Andrew B. Silva, MD
Assistant Chief
Department of Otolaryngology—Head and Neck Surgery
Madigan Army Medical Center
Tacoma, Washington

Richard J.H. Smith, MD
Professor and Vice-Chairman
Department of Otolaryngology
University of Iowa Hospitals and Clinics
Iowa City, Iowa

Thomas F. Smith, MD
Chief
Allergy Section
The Austin Diagnostic Clinic
Austin, Texas

Alma J. Smitheringale, MD, FRCSC
Associate Professor of Pediatrics
Department of Pediatric Otolaryngology
University of Toronto School of Medicine
Toronto, Ontario
Canada

Thomas G. Takoudes, MD
Residency Fellow in Otolaryngology—Head and Neck
  Surgery
Columbia Presbyterian Medical Center
New York, New York

N. Wendell Todd, MD
Professor of Otolaryngology and Pediatrics
Emory University
Egleston Children's Hospital
Atlanta, Georgia

Lawrence W. C. Tom, MD
Associate Professor
Department of Otorhinolaryngology—Head and Neck
  Surgery
University of Pennsylvania School of Medicine
Children's Hospital of Philadelphia
Philadelphia, Pennsylvania

Robert F. Ward, MD, FACS
Associate Professor of Clinical Otolaryngology
Department of Otolaryngology
Weill Medical College of Cornell University
New York, New York

Ralph F. Wetmore, MD
Associate Professor
Department of Otorhinolaryngology—Head and Neck
  Surgery
University of Pennsylvania School of Medicine
Children's Hospital of Philadelphia
Philadelphia, Pennsylvania

Brian J. Wiatrak, MD
Associate Professor of Surgery and Pediatrics
Chief
Department of Pediatric Otolaryngology—Head and Neck
  Surgery
University of Alabama at Birmingham
Birmingham, Alabama

Audie L. Woolley, MD
Assistant Professor of Otolaryngology and Pediatrics
Medical Director of the Pediatric Cochlear Implant
  Program
Children's Hospital
Birmingham, Alabama

Joan K. Zawin, MD
Children's Memorial Hospital
Chicago, Illinois

To our families—
Mary, Rick, and Alicia Wetmore;
Faye, Emily, Miriam, Helen, and Jon-Marc Muntz;
and
Angela and Trevor St. John McGill—

Through their love and support,
we have found the inspiration to make this book possible.

Foreword

Pediatric otolaryngology has evolved from a specialty that had only a few devoted individuals to what is today a large, well-organized national and international group. The specialty of pediatric otolaryngology recognizes the differences that exist in the care of children as compared to adults, and its members are fully committed to improving the quality of life of their patients. The development of pediatric otolaryngology has been driven by the prevalence of head and neck disorders in children and the wisdom of the founders of the specialty who understood that a focused effort leads to excellence.

The care of children has undergone many changes over the last century. The introduction of antibiotics profoundly changed pediatric otolaryngology by curing what were previously potentially lethal infections and allowing successful surgical reconstruction of the head and neck. The development of vaccines against mumps, measles, rubella, and poliomyelitis had an equally profound effect on viral infections that had caused severe sequelae. Recently, bacterial vaccines have tamed some of the most feared and invasive infections. The HIB vaccine has nearly eliminated epiglottitis, and pneumococcal vaccines show great promise in preventing invasive infections from *Streptococcus pneumoniae.*

We believe that the next millennium holds similar challenges and discoveries that will make pediatric otolaryngology an exciting field of study. The development of molecular genetics has placed pediatric otolaryngology at the threshold of a whole new era of medicine, allowing treatment of diseases that were formerly considered incurable. Gene transfer in the head and neck has been accomplished using non-invasive viral vectors, and in the not-too-distant future, gene therapy will be an important part of the armamentarium in the practice pediatric of the otolaryngologist.

This textbook is timely—arriving at the dawn of the new millennium and at the threshold of the molecular era of medicine. It is comprehensive, but focused to provide a usable, practical, single volume text that will serve as the preferred reference for general otolaryngologists, pediatric otolaryngologists, pediatricians, and students at all levels. We fully expect this text to serve as an accessible reference for the busy practicing physician. It should also prove to be an excellent library resource for the student who wishes to study pediatric otolaryngology in depth.

The fund of knowledge assembled in this text by its distinguished contributors and editors is a tribute to the growth and development of the children they serve and hopefully will prepare us to experience the next century of inevitable discovery and change.

William P. Potsic, MD
Gerald B. Healy, MD
Rodney P. Lusk, MD

Preface

At the turn of the twentieth century, specialization within medicine was still in its infancy. In Chevalier Jackson's autobiography, he discussed the difficulty of specialization, even noting that "specialists were still regarded as on the borderline of quackery . . . ." As we approach the twenty-first century, the specialization of medicine is well into its adulthood. Much as the field of otolaryngology has developed to care for the disorders of the head and neck, pediatric otolaryngology has blossomed as a subspecialty to care for needs of children with head and neck disorders.

This book has been written to offer insights into the care of children with otolaryngological diseases. Although the pathophysiology of many childhood diseases is the same as that of adults, the response of the child to such processes may be different. Understanding the normal physiology of children and the pathophysiology of their diseases is essential to their care: A child is *not* a smaller version of an adult. The initial section of this book reviews the general care of the pediatric patient, presents the basics of molecular genetics, and examines several topics relevant to the pediatric population. The remainder of the book deals with the specific disorders of the head and neck in children and includes a systematic approach to treating these disorders. This text is not an attempt to legislate practice guidelines, but rather to encourage a thoughtful approach to the care of infants and children, knowing that each child must be considered as an individual with specific needs.

This book is aimed at clinicians with a wide range of training and expertise including pediatric otolaryngologists, general otolaryngologists, primary pediatricians, pediatric intensivists, and other pediatric medical and surgical specialists. It is not meant to be an exhaustive reference; instead the format includes practice pathways and summary boxes that distill the major points of care. The clinician can utilize this text as a ready reference or as a springboard to further investigation of a topic.

We would like to acknowledge the work of the authors who have devoted their time and expertise to the development of this book. They have not come by their understanding through mere reading of monographs and journals. Much of their experience has been gained by their care of children on a daily basis. The insights that they bring to this text are founded in historical thought, scientific advances, and practical experience. They have seen the delight of a child with a middle ear effusion whose hearing is restored with the insertion of tympanostomy tubes. The child, who has never heard the birds sing or the squeak of the bedroom door, can now appreciate life in a new way. These authors have also felt the pain and tears of a family of a child with cancer as they struggle with heartache and uncertainty of the future. They have worked alone through the night deciding on the safest and best options for a child who needs airway reconstruction. They have learned to distinguish the early symptoms and signs of disease processes that if left untreated, could quickly result in tragedy. Our profound gratitude is offered to the authors.

We would also like to acknowledge the administrative assistance of Beth McCullough of the Children's Hospital of Philadelphia and Kathy Lyons of the Children's Hospital Medical Center in Boston. Sue Brenman created many of the outstanding illustrations scattered throughout the text. Finally, this book was made possible by the vision, expertise, and diligence of Avé McCracken of Thieme Publishers and her colleagues Kathy Lyons, Michelle Schmitt and Janice Stangel. Without the assistance of all of these people, this book would have remained just a dream.

Ralph F. Wetmore, MD
Harlan R. Muntz, MD
Trevor J. McGill, MD

I

GENERAL CONSIDERATIONS

1 Care of the Pediatric Patient

Jane M. Lavelle and Andrew T. Costarino, Jr

Pediatrics is a primary care, medical specialty that is focused on the health and well being of neonates, infants, children, and adolescents. Together with other pediatric specialists, pediatricians strive to advance the science, clinical care, and public health initiatives that are directed toward children so that each child's growth, development, and safety is optimized, allowing each child to achieve his/her potential as an adult. During the last several decades, pediatricians' efforts have resulted in new strategies to treat many pediatric diseases; consequently, tremendous reductions in infant and childhood mortality have occurred. For example, immunization programs have changed the prevalence of many serious diseases: smallpox has been eradicated worldwide, and in western countries, diphtheria and tetanus are now rare.[1] Most recently, the successful development of a vaccination against *Hemophilus influenzae B* has reduced the occurrence of childhood bacterial meningitis and epiglottitis so drastically that these are now considered mostly diseases of adults.[1-4] National efforts to promote childhood safety also have had a similar impact; for example, the introduction of child-proof caps on medications and other products produced a dramatic reduction in the incidence of accidental poisoning.

Despite these advances much work remains to be done, and the successful treatment of many acute illnesses has had the unfortunate consequence of increasing the number of children living with special medical needs.[5] This group of children requires multidisciplinary care and more frequent hospitalization and relies on medications and technology such as tracheostomy, mechanical ventilation, long-term vascular catheters, and enteral feeding tubes. Evaluating and treating challenging pediatric problems, as well as the satisfaction derived from helping a patient regain the potential for many years of productive life and freedom from morbidity, make pediatric specialization stimulating and rewarding.

This chapter provides a short overview of selected aspects of the field of pediatrics for the non-pediatrician health-care specialist. We begin by outlining the typical approach to well-child care and include graphs and tables of normal vital signs, growth parameters, and common developmental markers. Then, we discuss considerations for the hospitalized child and finally, we give a brief outline of the issues relevant to the chronically-ill patient.

WELL-CHILD HEALTH CARE

Routine Visits

Provision of health supervision throughout infancy, childhood, and adolescence is the central role for the primary care pediatrician.[6] The regular and "well-child" office visit has three primary goals: (1) to assess for the presence of occult disease through evaluation of growth and development, a general physical exam, and other screening tests; (2) to prevent disease by anticipatory guidance, immunization, and education/counseling; and (3) to build a relationship between the physician and the patient/family by establishing a rapport with the child and parents, by gaining an understanding of the family background and the child's relationship with his/her parents, and by evaluating for the presence of family stress. A focus on these three broad goals allows the pediatrician to become the primary health-care provider for the child and to establish a therapeutic alliance with the family in order to promote health.

AT A GLANCE. . .

Goals of the Well-Child Office Visit

- Assessment for occult disease
- Prevention of disease
- Build relationship between physician and family

Pediatric Otolaryngology, Edited by R.F. Wetmore, H.R. Muntz, and T.J. McGill. Thieme Medical Publishers, Inc., New York © 2000.

This relationship typically begins toward the end of pregnancy with the prenatal visit. This visit provides an opportunity for the physician to gather information and to provide anticipatory guidance relating to birth, infant feeding (breast or bottle), common early health-care issues, infant safety, and the introduction of the newborn to any siblings.

The second visit typically occurs in the newborn nursery on the first or second day of life. Occasionally, the physician is called to attend the delivery of a child who is premature, potentially ill, stressed, or when complications of pregnancy or labor exist. In any case, a basic knowledge of normal gestation, labor, and neonatal medicine is essential. A normal singleton gestation lasts, on average, 40 ± 2 weeks and term birthweight ranges from 2.5 kg (5 lbs 8oz) to 4.6 kg (10 lbs, 2 oz). By definition, any newborn weighing <2.5 kg is low birth weight (LBW) and any baby >4.6 kg is macrosomic.[7] Newborns above or below the fifth weight percentiles for gestational age are large (LGA) or small (SGA) for gestational age, respectively, and are at a higher risk for congenital diseases and birth complications.[8,9] In addition to a thorough physical exam and growth measurements, all neonates should undergo blood screening tests for hemoglobinopathies, hypothyroidism, phenylketonuria (PKU), and galactosemia prior to discharge.

SPECIAL CONSIDERATION:

Newborns above or below the fifth weight percentiles for gestational age are at a higher risk for congenital disease and birth complications.

The schedule for subsequent well-child office visits for the first year of life includes visits at 2 and 4 weeks at 2, 4, 6, and 9 months, and at 1 year.[6] After the first year, it is recommended that well-child visits take place at age 15, 18, and 24 months and then annually through age 6 and every 2 years thereafter.[6] Salient features of these scheduled visits include interval history of illness/injury, elimination and sleep patterns, nutrition, development and school performance, and parent/child interactions. Blood pressure measurements and vision and hearing tests are recommended at 3 years of age and thereafter annually.[6] At 18 months of age, the child should begin regular dental care.[10] All children should be

screened for lead poisoning between 9 and 12 months of age; those at high risk should be screened yearly until age 6.[11] Lipid profile is recommended in children with a family history of coronary artery disease prior to age 55 years or whose parents have a cholesterol level >240 mg/dl. Lipid profile also should be considered if the family history is not obtainable in families with multiple risk factors such as obesity, hypertension, smoking, and diabetes.[12,13] A tuberculin skin test should be placed at 9 months and then annually in children at risk.[14] Pubertal development is monitored in the teenage patient, and those who are sexually active should be screened for sexually transmitted diseases annually and pregnancy when indicated.

Routine History and Physical Exam

A central portion of any well-child visit relates to the interval history and physical examination. Performing this in children varies considerably with the age of the child.

As in any focused history, the direction of the physician's questions to the patient and parent are first keyed to the presenting complaint. Subsequent questions related to present and past history should usually include inquiries about the birth and neonatal periods and about growth and development because clues to the cause of the presenting complaint, the direction for work-up, and the choices of management often lie in this early history and growth record.

Although the parent is usually the primary historian, even a young child can make meaningful contributions to the interview and care should be taken to include him/her. Adolescents always should be given the opportunity to have a portion of the interview conducted alone without their parents present.[15] The physician should take this opportunity to address the teen's specific concerns and ask open-ended questions in a nonjudgmental fashion because the teen may reveal sensitive information that can be related to the chief complaint.

Inspection is the most important part of the physical exam of an infant and young child. Observation of his/her color, posture, attention to environment and others in the room, and play often provides the best overall information about wellness or acute or chronic illness. Many children can be fully examined while sitting in the parent's lap, where they feel safer and in control. In order to establish rapport with the child during the interview, the physician should begin the examination with portions that require the child's participation—the physician should include the child, speak to him/her, and inquire about her preferences. If the physician enjoys the child's spontaneity and is patient and flexible, the examination usually can be accomplished successfully within minutes. The physician should always respect the privacy and consider the comfort of even the small child, leaving the disagreeable or painful portions (e.g., the otoscopic examination) to the end. The ease of the examining physician as well as distraction techniques are indispensable in completing a thorough exam in a short period of time.

Special Features of the Pediatric Physical Examination

Vital signs and body size

In children, body temperature most often is measured rectally until they can cooperate with oral placement of the thermometer. Axillary temperatures are preferred in immunocompromised patients when an oral temperature cannot be obtained. The pulse can be obtained from any convenient peripheral site. In children, the pulse rate is more labile and sensitive to the effects of

illness, emotion, and exercise. Similarly, the respiratory rate is more labile, and in infants, the respiratory pattern varies. For this reason, pulse and respirations should be counted over 30 to 60 seconds to determine the rate. Automated oscillometric blood pressure machines have made routine blood pressure measurement in small infants and children simple compared to 2 decades ago. As a result, good data of normative values is available,[16,17] but attention to the measurement technique is still necessary for accurate readings. The blood pressure cuff bladder should encircle the arm completely.[16,17] The width of the cuff should cover one-half to two-thirds of the upper extremity.[16-18] The most important feature of vital signs in pediatric medicine is how the values vary with patient age (Table 1-1).[16-19]

SPECIAL CONSIDERATION:

In children, the pulse rate and respiratory rate are more labile and sensitive to the effects of illness, emotion, and exercise.

TABLE 1-1: Vital Signs

Age (Years)	Respiratory Rate	Heart Rate	Systolic BP (Girls)	Diastolic BP (Girls)	Systolic BP (Boys)	Diastolic BP (Boys)
Newborn	35 ± 50	126 ± 10	65 ± 10	40 ± 10	65 ± 10	40 ± 10
0.25	33 ± 6	147 ± 23	66 ± 6	55 ± 8	71 ± 10	55 ± 8
0.50	30 ± 4	139 ± 25	91 ± 10	53 ± 8	91 ± 9	53 ± 9
1.00	27 ± 3	127 ± 27	90 ± 10	54 ± 9	90 ± 10	56 ± 9
2.00	25 ± 3	121 ± 20	90 ± 9	56 ± 8	91 ± 9	55 ± 9
3.00	24 ± 2	108 ± 15	91 ± 10	57 ± 8	93 ± 8	55 ± 9
4.00	22 ± 2	108 ± 15	93 ± 9	57 ± 8	94 ± 9	56 ± 9
5.00	21 ± 3	100 ± 16	95 ± 9	57 ± 8	95 ± 9	57 ± 9
6.00	21 ± 2	100 ± 16	97 ± 9	58 ± 8	96 ± 10	58 ± 9
7.00	20 ± 2	100 ± 16	98 ± 9	59 ± 8	98 ± 9	59 ± 9
8.00	20 ± 2	91 ± 20	100 ± 9	60 ± 8	100 ± 9	60 ± 9
9.00	19 ± 2	91 ± 20	101 ± 10	62 ± 8	102 ± 9	62 ± 8
10.00	19 ± 3	91 ± 20	102 ± 10	64 ± 8	103 ± 9	63 ± 8
11.00	19 ± 2	91 ± 20	105 ± 10	65 ± 8	105 ± 10	64 ± 9
12.00	19 ± 2	85 ± 17	107 ± 10	67 ± 9	108 ± 9	65 ± 9
13.00	18 ± 3	85 ± 17	108 ± 11	68 ± 9	110 ± 10	66 ± 9
14.00	18 ± 3	85 ± 17	110 ± 10	67 ± 9	112 ± 9	63 ± 10
15.00	18 ± 3	85 ± 17	112 ± 9	68 ± 9	115 ± 10	65 ± 10
16.00	17 ± 3	70 ± 15	113 ± 8	67 ± 10	117 ± 10	67 ± 10
17.00	17 ± 3	70 ± 15	113 ± 9	66 ± 10	120 ± 10	69 ± 9
18.00	17 ± 3	70 ± 15	114 ± 9	67 ± 9	124 ± 9	71 ± 9

Data derived from references 16, 17, 18, and 19.

Growth is an extremely important measure of a child's health. During the first 2 years of life tremendous change in body mass occurs. Easily-remembered rules of thumb include: (1) birth weight doubles by 6 months and triples by 12 months of age; (2) on average, a 2-year-old weighs approximately 20 lbs, a 3-year-old weighs 30lbs, and a 4-year-old weighs 40lbs; (3) after 2 years of age the child gains approximately 2 kg (4 lbs 6.5 oz) yearly and grows 6.35 cm (2.5 inches) in height yearly until the growth spurt that occurs during puberty;[7] and (4) head circumference grows at a rate of more than 1 cm per month for the first year of life then drastically slows. Measurement of head circumference is an important part of the physical examination during the first 2 years of life and thereafter only if any problem exists.[18] Length is measured in the supine position during the first 2 years of life and later in the erect position. Growth charts are presented in Figures 1–1 through 1–8. Importantly, the growth plotted over time is more helpful than a single set of parameters.

Head

The posterior fontanelle (1 × 2 cm) closes by 2 months of age and the anterior fontanel (4 × 6 cm) by 12 to 18 months of age.[18] Bulging of the anterior fontanelle may be seen when the intracranial pressure is elevated such as in meningitis, hydrocephalous, or swelling following trauma.

Eyes

In neonates, presence of the red reflex on fundoscopic exam rules out major congenital abnormalities of the retina. Strabismus can be detected by noting asymmetry of the position of the light reflection on the pupil from a distant light source. Any strabismus present after 6 months of age is abnormal and should be referred to a ophthalmologist for evaluation.[20]

Ears

In response to a sudden sound 12 inches away the infant will blink. This is a positive acoustic blink reflex, which indicates intact hearing. At 3 to 4 months of age,[18] the infant will begin to turn toward the noise. In older children, whispering at 8 feet may be used to detect hearing abnormalities. Formal audiometric testing is indicated if abnormalities are noted, and this is done routinely before the child begins school.

Lymph nodes

Growth of lymphoid tissue peaks at 12 years of age.[18] Many children, therefore, have prominent, palpable lymph nodes in the cervical chain, which have little clinical significance.

Chest exam

Auscultation to judge the quality of breath sounds is necessary, but often limited in infants and young children because the lung fields are small in size and the child cannot inhale and exhale on demand. Thus, simple observation and determination of respiratory rate and effort often provide the most information. In this younger population, diaphragmatic breathing predominates, and as a result chest wall excursion with respiration may be minimal.[18,21]

Auscultation of heart sounds frequently reveals nonpathologic murmurs that are especially common in infancy. These murmurs are usually systolic sounds of low intensity with musical or vibratory quality. They are heard best at the second left intercostal space.[18] If an abnormal murmur is detected, comparison of the femoral and lower extremity peripheral pulses to the upper extremity pulses by palpation and determination of four limb blood pressures (decreased lower extremity pressure and pulse with coarctation), respiratory effort, hepatic size, skin temperature, capillary refill, and edema are physical exam features that are of interest to the cardiology consultant.

Abdomen

It is not unusual to feel the liver edge or spleen tip when palpating the soft abdomen of healthy small children.[18]

Neurologic Exam and Developmental Assessment

In older children and adolescents, the neurologic exam is similar to that of adults, however, for infants, the exam is much different. Persistence of the primitive reflexes is useful in detecting neurologic damage in neonates and infants younger than 3 months. Similarly, for older infants and young chil-

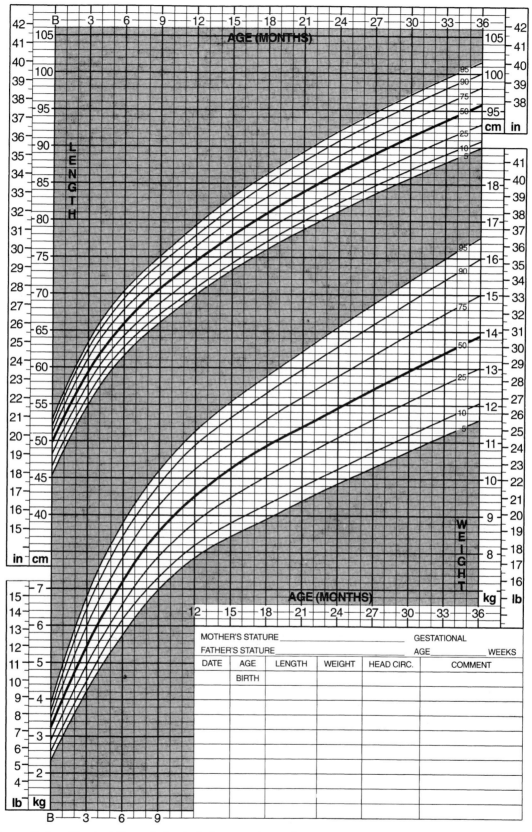

Figure 1–1: Physical Growth for Girls from Birth to 36 Months—I. (Adapted from Hamill PVV, Drizd TA, Johnson CL, et al. Physical growth: National Center for Health Statistics percentiles. Am J Clin Nutr 1979; 32:607–629. Data from the Fels Longitudinal Study, Wright State University School of Medicine, Yellow Springs, Ohio, with permission.)

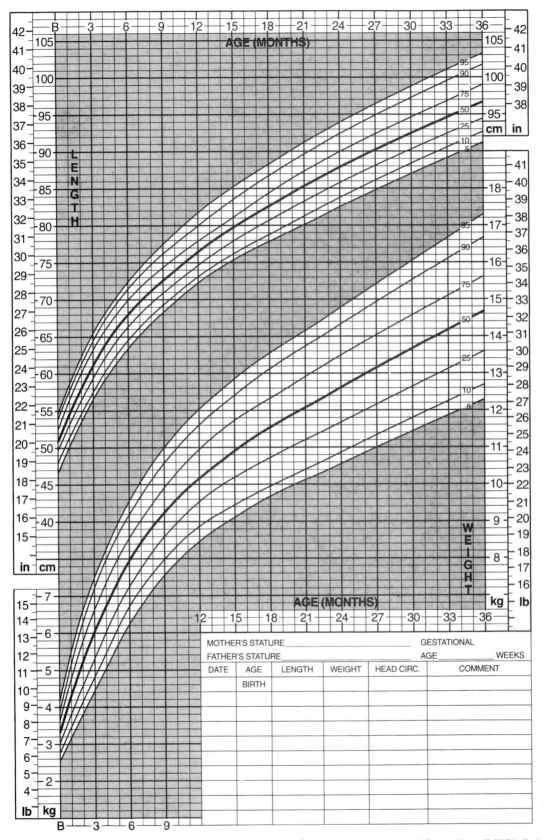

Figure 1–2: Physical Growth for Boys from Birth to 36 Months—I. (Adapted from Hamill PVV, Drizd TA, Johnson CL, et al. Physical growth: National Center for Health Statistics percentiles. Am J Clin Nutr 1979; 32:607–629. Data from the Fels Longitudinal Study, Wright State University School of Medicine, Yellow Springs, Ohio, with permission.)

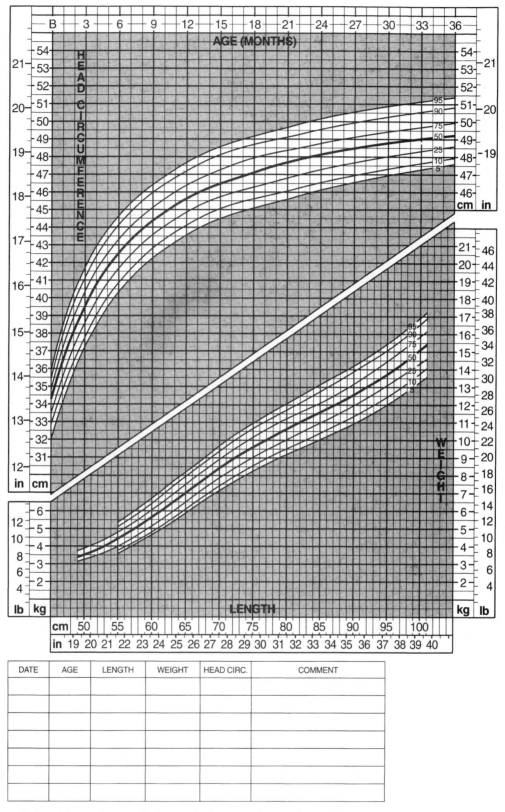

Figure 1–3: Physical Growth for Girls from Birth to 36 Months—II. (Adapted from Hamill PVV, Drizd TA, Johnson CL, et al. Physical growth: National Center for Health Statistics percentiles. Am J Clin Nutr 1979; 32:607–629. Data from the Fels Longitudinal Study, Wright State University School of Medicine, Yellow Springs, Ohio, with permission.)

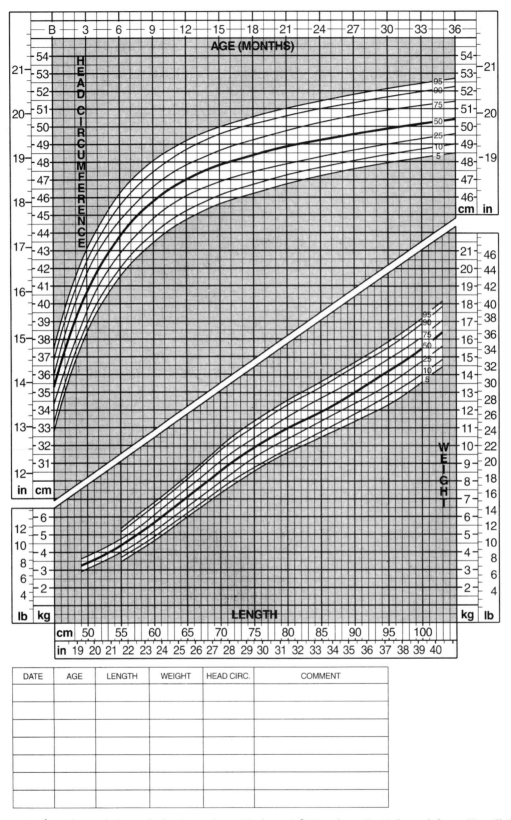

Figure 1–4: Physical Growth for Boys from Birth to 36 Months—II. (Adapted from Hamill PVV, Drizd TA, Johnson CL, et al. Physical growth: National Center for Health Statistics percentiles. Am J Clin Nutr 1979; 32:607–629. Data from the Fels Longitudinal Study, Wright State University School of Medicine, Yellow Springs, Ohio, with permission.)

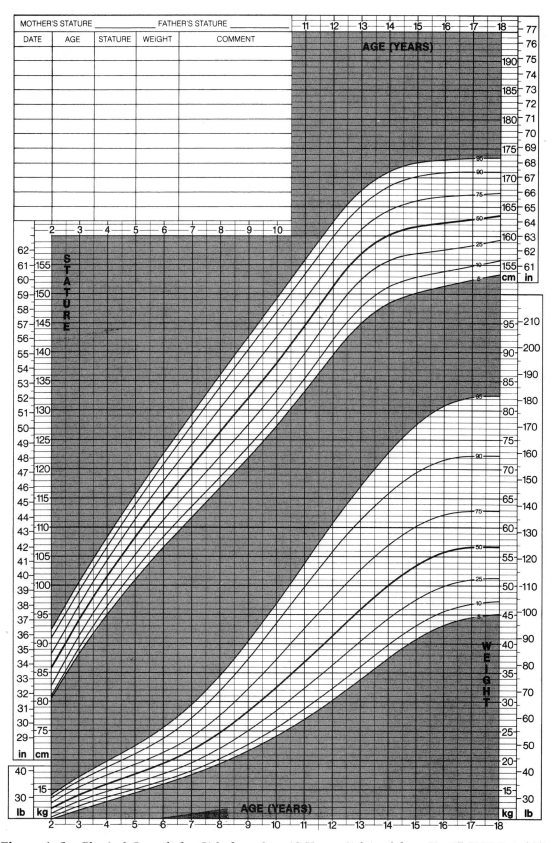

Figure 1–5: Physical Growth for Girls from 2 to 18 Years. (Adapted from Hamill PVV, Drizd TA, Johnson CL, et al. Physical growth: National Center for Health Statistics percentiles. Am J Clin Nutr 1979; 32:607–629. Data from the National Center for Health Statistics, Hyattsville, Maryland, with permission. From Ross Products Division, Abbott Laboratories, 1982, with permission.)

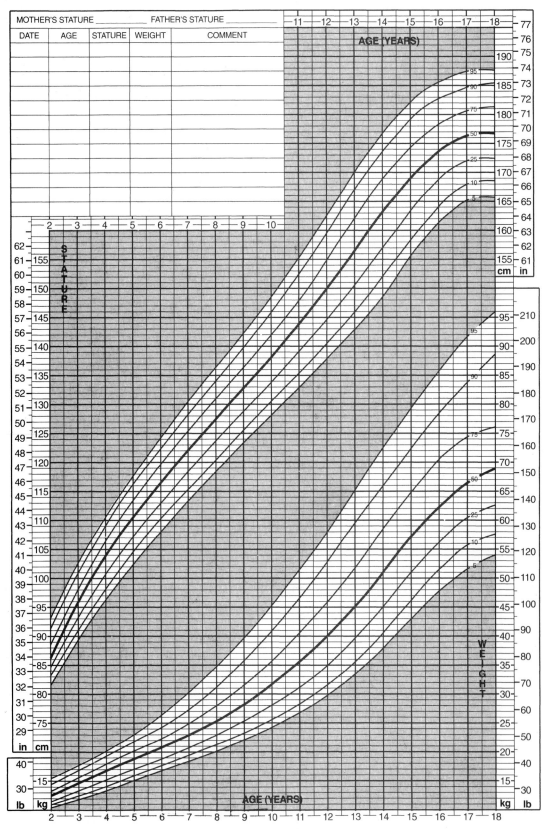

Figure 1–6:   Physical Growth for Boys 2 to 18 Years. (Adapted from Hamill PVV, Drizd TA, Johnson CL, et al. Physical growth: National Center for Health Statistics percentiles. Am J Clin Nutr 1979; 32: 607-629. Data from the National Center for Health Statistics, Hyattsville, Maryland, with permission.)

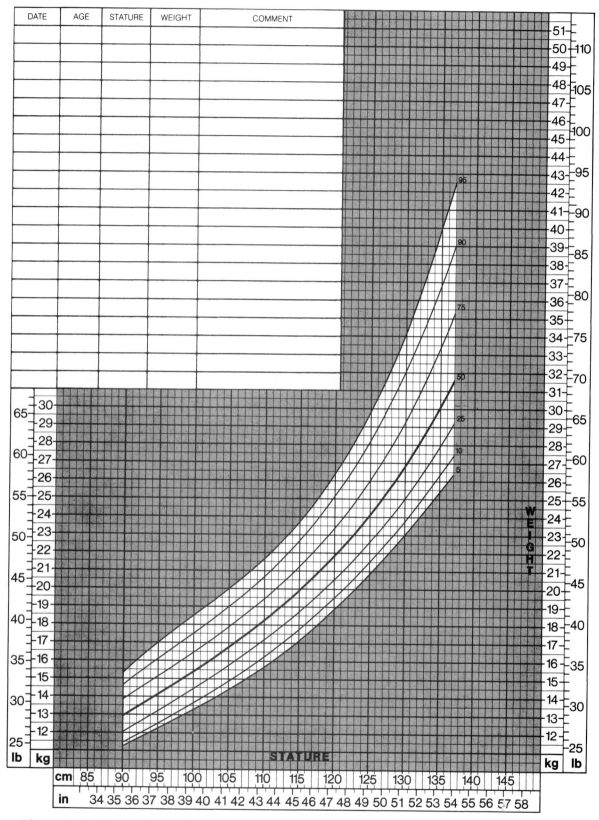

Figure 1–7:   Physical Growth for Prepubescent Girls. (Adapted from Hamill PVV, Drizd TA, Johnson CL, et al. Physical growth: National Center for Health Statistics percentiles. Am J Clin Nutr 1979; 32: 607–629. Data from the National Center for Health Statistics, Hyattsville, Maryland, with permission. From Ross Products Division, Abbott Laboratories, 1982, with permission.)

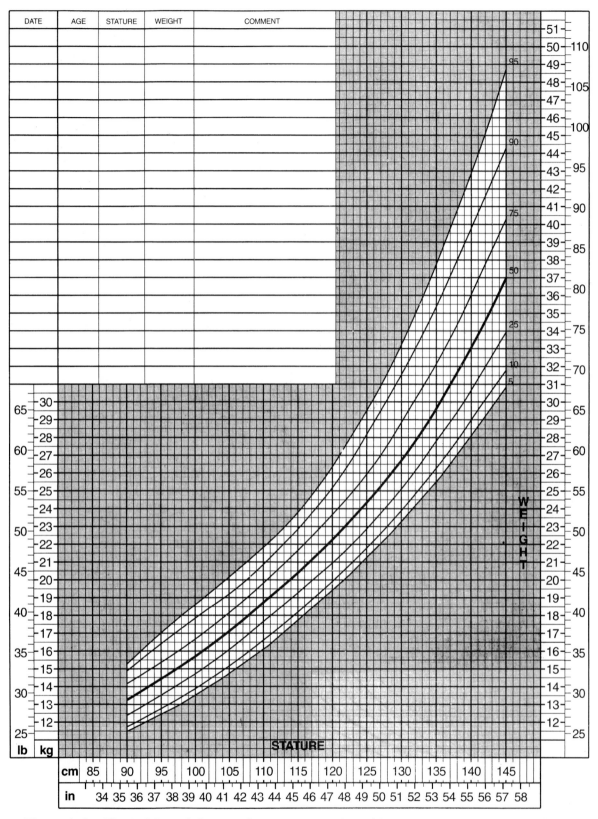

Figure 1–8: Physical Growth for Prepubescent Boys. (Adapted from Hamill PVV, Drizd TA, Johnson CL, et al. Physical growth: National Center for Health Statistics percentiles. Am J Clin Nutr 1979; 32: 607–629. Data from the National Center for Health Statistics, Hyattsville, Maryland, with permission.)

dren, behavioral and motor development gives significant information regarding cerebral function. Therefore, a general knowledge of the expected developmental milestones is necessary for the pediatric specialist.

Development occurs in an orderly, predictable sequence from head to toe and proximally to distally. The generalized reflexes of the infant gradually become specific and precise as the child becomes more independent. The development quotient (DQ) is a useful means of summarizing the child's developmental progress. This is calculated by dividing the child's developmental age by the chronologic age and multiplying by 100. DQs that are equal to 85% are within normal limits; those that are <70% are clearly abnormal. Table 1-2 lists some highlights of development in the first several years of life.[22-28] Similarly, the Denver Development Screening Test (DDST) is a useful reference tool to screen for social skills, fine and gross motor skills, and language skills from birth to 6 months of age (Fig. 1-9).[29] Each bar indicates when 25, 50, 75, and 90% of children reach that particular milestone.

When evaluating a child with an acute illness or a suspected neurologic injury, the Glasgow Coma Scale (GCS) or the GCS modified for infants is a useful and simple method to help the non-neurologist begin assessment of a child's cerebral function (Table 1-3).[30,31]

Nutritional Assessment

Assessment of nutrition is an essential part of well-child care because infants, young children, and pubescent adolescents have tremendous calorie and nutrient requirements for successful growth. The majority of infants will thrive during the first 6 months if they receive between 80 to 120 Kcal/kg/day or 150 to 200 ml of breastmilk or formula/kg/day. A simple method of calculating the daily caloric intake is to (1) multiply the first 10 kg of body weight by 100 Kcal; (2) then multiply each additional kg of body weight up to 20 kg by 50 Kcal; (3) then multiply each kg of body weight over 20 kg by 20 Kcal; and (4) finally, add to get the total daily caloric intake needed.[32] In the first year of life, the mainstay of nutrition is breastmilk or formula; the components and calorie content of human milk

TABLE 1-2:   Developmental Milestones

Age	Gross Motor	Fine Motor	Problem Solving	Language	Social
2 months	Holds head midline	Fisted hands	Follows past midline	Recognizes parent	Smiles socially
4 months	Rolls front to back	Holds rattle	Reaches for objects	Listens to speaker, responds	Laughs aloud
6 months	Sits leaning forward with support, rolls both ways, while prone pushes up on straight arms, primitive reflexes disappear, righting reflexes appear	Reaches, grasps object and transfers, mouths objects	Peek-a-boo, looks for dropped toy	Babbles, mimics speaker, raspberries	Stranger anxiety, understands different facial expressions
12 months	Crawls rapidly, Pulls to stand, cruises, first independent steps	Pincer grasp, holds, inspects objects, first words, associates meaning to words	Object permanence causality	Immature jargoning, first words, associates meaning to words	Cautious, assertive, concept of self-stranger anxiety
18 months	Crawls up stairs, runs	Builds tower of 3-4 blocks, scribbles	Matches objects to body parts	10-25 words, points, uses spoon and cup	Shyness, shame, guilt
2 years	Up/down steps, kicks ball, squats	Builds tower of 7-8 cubes, imitates vertical stroke	Two-step commands, matches objects to pictures	>50 words, 2-word combinations, pronouns	Socialization, assists in undressing
3 years	Alternates feet up steps, pedals tricycle, jumps from a step	Copies a circle, builds 9-10 block tower, Draws a head	Asks why, remembers rhymes, time	Sentences, tells stories	Shares toys, friendships begin, imaginary friends, impulse control
4 years	Alternates feet down steps	Copies a square, dresses, catches ball	Colors, sings song from memory, first and last name, draws person with 3 parts	Tells tales	
5 years	Skips, jumps over low object	Copies a triangle	Recognizes most letters, address, and phone number		Plays competitive games, dresses, plays make-believe

Data from references 22-28.

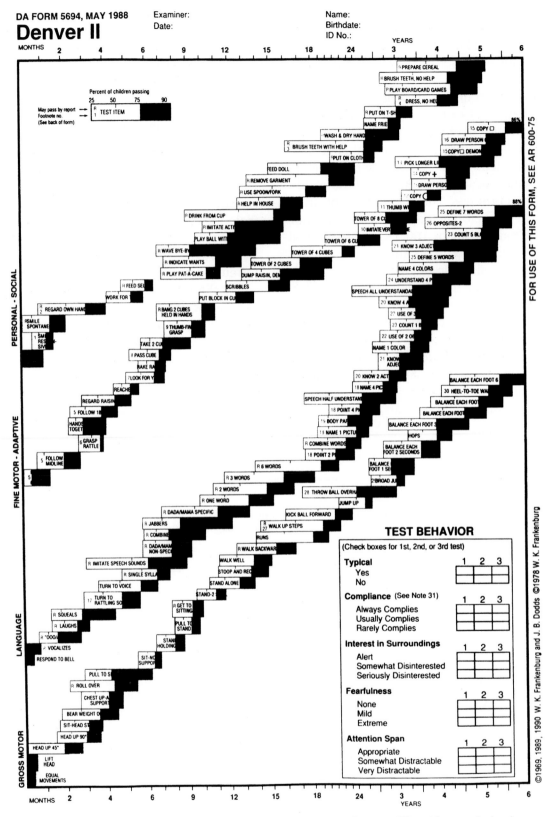

Figure 1–9: Denver Developmental Screening Test. (From reference 29, with permission.)

TABLE 1–3:   The Glasgow Coma Scale

Adult/Adolescent[30]		Infant/Child[31]
Eye Opening		*Eye Opening*
Spontaneous	4	Spontaneous
To voice	3	To voice
To pain	2	To pain
None	1	None
Verbal		*Verbal*
Oriented	5	Coos and Babbles
Confused	4	Irritable
Inappropriate words	3	Cries
Incomprehensible	2	Moaning
None	1	None
Motor		*Motor*
Follows commands	6	Spontaneous movement
Localizes	5	Withdraws to touch
Withdrawal	4	Withdraws to pain
Flexion	3	Abnormal flexion
Extension	2	Abnormal extension
None	1	None

From references 30 and 31, with permission.

and several commercially available formulas is listed in Table 1–4. During the first 2 months of life, most infants eat every 3 to 5 hours, accounting for approximately six feedings, and gain between 25 and 30 grams daily. Gradually, as the infant grows, there is less need for the night-time feedings, and by 6 months of age most infants eat four times a day and gain approximately 15 to 20 grams daily. Introduction of solid food is recommended between 4 and 6 months of age. Multivitamins are recommended if the mother's nourishment is a concern or if she has no exposure to sunlight. Fluoride (0.25 mg/day) should be given if the water is not supplemented (<0.3 ppm). Dietary iron is recommended in breastfed infants after the age of 6 months; most formulas are supplemented with the appropriate amount of iron. Water is also an essential nutrient and requirements can be determined from the caloric calculation outlined previously as 120 ml water/100 Kcal/day.[32]

Disease Prevention: Anticipatory Guidance and Immunization

The key component of disease prevention is anticipatory guidance related to the child's behavioral de-

velopment and immunization. Table 1–5 highlights the behaviors that should be discussed at various ages.[33] The current recommended schedule for immunizations is presented in Table 1–6.[34] The American Academy of Pediatrics Committee on Infectious Diseases provides an extensive set of recommendations and other resource information related to vaccines, dosing and administration, reimmunization, lapsed immunization, adverse effects, and special circumstances.[1]

THE HOSPITALIZED CHILD

Infectious disease and traumatic injury remain the most common reasons for medical encounters and hospitalization for children. This is reflected in Table 1–7, which lists the top causes of death by age group in the United States. Note that after the first year of life, injury is the leading cause of death in children.[35,36]

The needs of children who require hospital care are influenced by the functional maturity of the respiratory and circulatory systems. Clinical manifestations of illness and injury are greatly determined by these systems, and the characteristic changes in cardiorespiratory physiology and body fluids, as well as in behavior, that occur from birth through adolescence must be considered when evaluating and treating the hospitalized child. A brief overview of these systems is presented below, following an outline of resuscitation techniques. Finally, we discuss selected diagnostic entities.

> **SPECIAL CONSIDERATION:**
>
> The needs of children who require hospital care are influenced by the functional maturity of the respiratory and circulatory systems.

Resuscitation Techniques

Delivery room resuscitation

Pediatricians often are called to the delivery room to evaluate a neonate who is not tolerating the stress of labor (e.g., fetal heart rate decelerations, poor heart rate variability, and meconium staining of the

Table 1–4:   Components and Calorie Content of Common Formulas

Formula	kcal/oz	Protein gm/100 mL (% kcals)	Fat gm/100 mL (% kcals)	CHO gm/100 mL (% kcals)	Na+ (mEq/dL)	K+ (mEq/dL)	Ca++ (mg/dL)	PO++4 (mg/dL)	Source of CHO	Source of Protein
Human Milk	22.0	1.1(6.0)	4.5(55.5)	6.8(37.3)	0.7	1.3	34.0	121.0	Lactose	Human
Cow's Milk	20.0	3.5(21)	3.7(50)	4.9(29.4)	2.1	3.8	46.0	31.0	Lactose	Cow
Infant Formulas										
Human Milk Fortifier (per Packet)	4.5	0.2(18)	0.1(20)	0.7(62.2)	0.0	0.0	0.5	8.0	Corn Syrup	Whey, casein
Similac	20.0	1.5(9.0)	3.6(48.6)	7.2(43.2)	1.0	2.0	51.0	39.0	Lactose	Cow plus taurine and carnitine
Enfamil	20.0	1.5(9.0)	3.8(51.3)	6.9(41.4)	0.8	1.7	46.0	31.0	Lactose	Cow plus taurine and carnitine
SMA	20.0	1.5(9.0)	3.6(48.6)	7.2(43.2)	0.6	1.4	44.0	33.0	Lactose	Cow whey/lactalbumin (60/40 ratio)
Similac Special Care	24.0	2.2(11.0)	4.4 (49.5) [−50% as MCT]	8.6(43.)	1.7	2.8	144.0	72.0	Lactose 50%, polycose 50%	Cow plus taurine and carnitine (Whey/casein as 60/40 ratio)
Enfamil Premature	24	2.4(12.0)	4.0 (45) [40% as MCT]	8.9(44.5)	1.4	2.2	94.0	47.0	Corn syrup	Cow plus taurine
Isomil	20.0	2.0(12.0)	3.6(48.6)	6.8(41.0)	1.4	2.4	70.0	50.0	Corn syrup, sucrose	Soy, plus added methionine
I-Soyalac	20.0	2.1(12.6)	3.8(51.3)	6.7(40.2)	1.4	2.1	63.0	52.0	Sucrose, tapioca	Soy, plus added methionine
Pregestamil	20.0	1.9(11.4)	2.7(36.45)	9.1(54.6)	1.4	1.8	63.0	42.0	Corn syrup, tapioca	Casein hydrolysate, cystine, tyrosine, tryptophane
Nutramigen	20.0	2.2(13.2)	2.6(35.1)	8.8(52.8)	1.4	1.7	63.0	47.0	Corn syrup	Casein hydrolysate plus added cystine, tyrosine and tryptophan
Portagen	20.0	2.4(14.4)	3.2(43.2) [88% as MCT]	7.8(46.8)	1.4	2.0	63.0	47.0	Corn syrup, sucrose	Na casenate
Pediatric Formulas										
Vivonex	24.0	2.4(12)	5.0(25) [68% as MCT]	12.6(63)	1.7	3.1	97	80	Glucose, Oligosaccharides	L-aminoacids
Pediasure	30.0	4.9(12.0)	3.0(44.0)	11.0(44.0)	1.7	3.3	97.0	80	Sucrose, hydrolysed corn starch	Whey, Na Caseinate
Ensure	30.0	3.5(14.0)	3.56(32.0)	13.5(54.0)	3.6	4.0	52.0	52.0	Corn syrup, sucrose	Soy and Na and Ca caseinates
Isocal	32.0	3.25(13.0)	4.1(37.0)	12.5(50.0)	2.3	3.4	85.0	85.0	Maltodextrans	Soy and Na and Ca caseinates
Sustacal	45.6	6.1(16.0)	5.74(34.0)	19.0(50.0)	4.1	5.4	85.0	85.0	Sucrose, corn syrup	Soy and Na and Ca caseinates
Jevity	32.0	4.5(17.0)	3.6(30.0) [50% MCT oil]	14.1(53.0)	4.0	4.0	89.0	75.0	Hydrolysed corn starch, soy polysaccharide	Na and Ca caseinate
Peptamen Junior	30.0	3.0(12.0)	3.67(33) [60% MCT oil]	13.8(55)	2.0	3.9	100.0	80.0	Maltodextrin, starch	Hydrolysed whey
Tolerex	30.0	2.0(8.0)	0.11(1.0)	22.8(91.0)	2.0	3.1	56.0	56.0	Maltodextrin	Free amino acids
Nutrin 1.5	45	6.0(16.0)	5.5(33.0)	19.1(51.0)	5.1	4.8	100.0	100.0	Maltodextrin, corn syrup	Casein
Nutrin 2.0	60	8.0(16.0)	10.0(45.0)	19.5(39.0)	5.1	4.8	100.0	100.0	Maltodextrin, corn syrup, sucrose	Casein
Carnation instant breakfast	31.2	4.4(17.0)	3.12(27.0)	14.6(56.0)	3.9	6.3	185.0	111.0	Maltodextrin, sucrose, lactose	Whole and nonfat cow's milk
Pulmocare	45	6.38(17)	9.2(55.0)	10.5(28.0)	5.6	4.8	104	104	Hydrolysed corn syrup	Na and Ca caseinates

Data compiled from manufacturers' documentation

Abbreviations: CHO, carbohydrate; MCT, medium chain triglycerides

TABLE 1–5: Recommended Scheduled
Visits/Anticipatory Guidance

Age	Highlights of Anticipatory Guidance
Prenatal	Physical and emotional preparation for the new baby
Neonatal	Breast/bottle feeding and care of cord, circumcision, nails, and skin. Fever, signs of illness, car seat, crib safety, supine sleep position, smoke detectors, water temperature <120°C, smoke-free environment
1–2 weeks	Review feeding, check weight gain, temperment, and parent adjustment
1 month	Crying peaks at 6 weeks
2 months	Signs of illness, emergency procedures, daycare/childcare issues
4 months	Introduction of solid food, establish bedtime routine, begin to child-proof home
6 months	Further child-proofing, avoid walkers, syrup of ipecac, solids 2–3 times daily, avoid propping bottle, start cup use, assess need for supplemental flouride, brush teeth
12 months	Water safety, sunscreen, lower crib mattress, bike helmet, close supervision, eats meals with the family plus 2–3 snacks, start whole milk, limit sugar, limit TV, curiosity about genitalia
15 months	No hitting or biting
18 months	Eat with utensils, outings should be kept short, supervise closely
2 years	Supervise closely, toilet training when child is ready
3 years	Playground, stranger safety, limit TV, encourage reading
4 years	Consistency with rules, limits, school issues
5 years	Physical activity, sleep, prepare for school
6 years	Self-discipline, chores, family rules, sports, school
8 years	Nutrition, avoid tobacco, alcohol, drugs, reinforce helmet, water safety, issues of violence, encourage parents to know their child's friends
10 years	Prepare for puberty
11 years	Encourage nutrition, routine physical activity, drug, alcohol and violence avoidance, learn how to say no to peers, safe sex issues
12 years	same as 11 years
13 years	school performance, screen for mental health problems, especially depression
14 years	same as 13 years
15 years	same as 13 years

Modified from reference 33, with permission.

TABLE 1–6: Recommended Immunization Schedule for Children[1]

Birth	Hep B-1 (birth to 2 months)
1 month	Hep B-2 (1–4 months)
2 months	DTaP Hib IPV
4 months	DTaP Hib IPV
6 months	DTaP Hib IPV Hep B
12–15 months	Hib MMR*
12–18 months	OPV Varicella
15–18 months	DtaP
4–6 years	DTaP OPV MMR
11–12 years	Td MMR Hep B†

* The first dose is recommended ≥12 months; the second is usually given at 4–6 or 11–12 years, but may be given at any visit as long as 1 month as passed from the first dose.

† Older children/adolescents who have not been immunized during the first year of life should receive Hep B. The second dose should be given at least 1 month after the first, and the third at least 4 months after the first and 2 months after the second.

IPV, inactivated poliovirus vaccine; MMR, measle, mumps, and rubella vaccine; OPV, oral poliovirus vaccine.

environment. As in any resuscitation, attention is directed in a sequential fashion to the airway, breathing, circulation, and neurologic function (the ABCDE's), followed by helping the baby maintain body temperature. Clinical shorthand commonly used to express the physical exam characteristics that reflect the progress of the transition between environments and the response to resuscitative efforts is the time-honored Apgar score (Table 1–8).[37]

Most newborns who need delivery room resusci-

TABLE 1–7: The Most Common Causes of Childhood Mortality

All Trauma	136.7
Motor Vehicle	45.9
Homicide	35.5
Suicide	14.7
Other	40.9
Congenital Malformation	26.1
Heart	19.1
Other	7.0
Infection	29.1
Pneumonia/Other Respiratory	16.4
Sepsis	6.6
HIV	6.1
Malignancy	11.5
Other	25.6

Common causes of childhood mortality (ages 0–24 years) per 100,000 population.
Data from references 35 and 36.

amniotic fluid) or who demonstrates evidence of abnormal fetal growth or a structural malformation. In these circumstances, the initial goal of the physician is to assure that the newborn makes a successful transition from the in utero to the extrauterine

TABLE 1–8:   Apgar Score

Sign	Score		
	0	*1*	*2*
Heart rate	Absent	Slow (<100 BPM)	Normal (>100 BPM)
Respiratory effort	Absent	Irregular, weak cry	Regular, strong cry
Muscle tone	Flaccid	Some flexion of upper extremities	Well-flexed, active
Reflex irritability	No response	Grimace	Cough, sneeze
Color	Central cyanosis	Peripheral cyanosis	Pink

From reference 37, with permission.

tation can be successfully stabilized with clearing of the airway, supplemental oxygen, assisted ventilation, warming, and tactile stimulation with towel drying (which also serves to reduce evaporative heat loss and prevent cold stress).

Pediatric resuscitation

Emergency cardiorespiratory resuscitations of children after out-of-hospital and in-hospital arrests are generally more complicated than the usual delivery room resuscitation, and unfortunately, they run a greater risk of complication and poor outcome. Successful application of these techniques should always follow the same orderly sequence, which is divided nicely into the primary and secondary survey.

The *primary survey* focuses on the ABCDE's, or the rapid assessment of the airway patency, breathing, and circulation with determination of vital signs.[38] Pharyngeal suction, artificial airway placement, assisted ventilation, supplemental oxygen, and chest compressions are applied as needed. The D represents disability, dextrose, and decontamination, and acts as a reminder to assess briefly the child's level of consciousness, perform a bedside blood glucose determination, and consider the possibility of toxin exposure. The E refers to exposure; the patient is undressed in order to facilitate examination and treatment. During this initial phase, immediate life-saving interventions are performed as required by the patient's presenting condition before any specific diagnosis is made. Intravenous access is usually secured and monitors placed.

The *secondary survey* consists of a head to toe examination, diagnostic evaluation, consultation, and transfer of the child to the definitive area of care. Practice Pathway 1-1 reviews the American Heart Association's recommendations for treatment of the pulseless child,[39] and Table 1–9 lists the doses of the more common resuscitation medications.

The most common errors occurring during a resuscitation result from poor leadership, equipment failure, inattention to an orderly sequential approach to the "ABCDE's," or infrequent reassessment.[38] The Braselow tape is a useful tool to prevent equipment trouble, particularly for resuscitators who infrequently care for children.[40] The tape is used to measure the child's length, which is then used for estimation of weight; this aids in the selection of equipment size and recommended drug dosage.

By far the most common, acute, life-threatening events in childhood result from respiratory failure. In most instances, even cardiac arrest occurs as a secondary phenomenon following respiratory failure. Thus, it is important to recognize the signs and symptoms of respiratory failure and initiate early treatment correctly.[41]

> **SPECIAL CONSIDERATION:**
> The most common, acute, life-threatening events in childhood result from respiratory failure.

System Considerations

Recognition of respiratory failure

There are several reasons why illness and injury lead to respiratory manifestations in children. In comparison with the adult airway, the extrathoracic airway in children is smaller in relation to air flow require-

Practice Pathway 1-1   PROTOCOL FOR PULSELESS ARREST

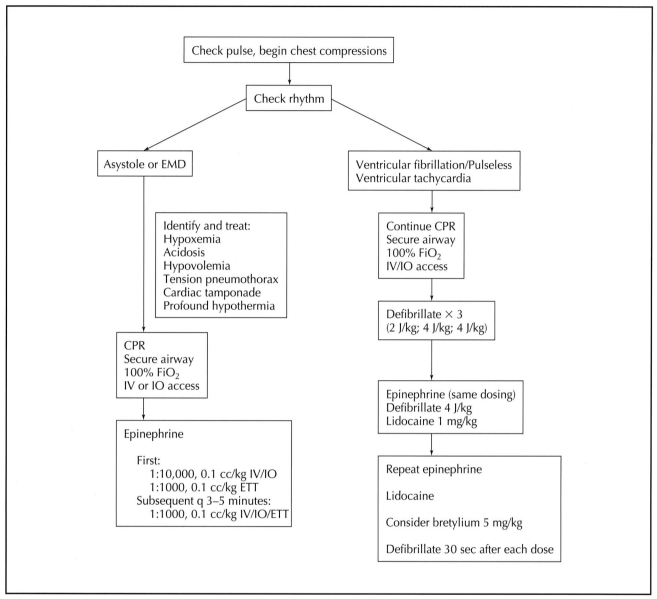

Abbreviations: EMD, electromechanical dissociation; CPR, cardiopulmonary resuscitation; IV, intravenous; IO, intraosseus; ETT, endotracheal tube.

ments because of the relative size of the tongue and oral cavity, the presence of hypertrophied tonsillar and adenoidal tissues, and the small lumenal caliber of the larynx and trachea.[18,21] These characteristics predispose the infant and child to extrathoracic airway obstruction. Similarly, a baby's intrathoracic airway is at a higher risk than an adult's for significant obstruction when any mucosal swelling is present. Additionally, at the level of the respiratory bronchiole and alveoli, the infant and young child have fewer intercommunications between adjacent lung units and thus fewer opportunities for collateral ventilation.[21] Before the age of 2 years, an infant's

soft-chest wall contributes to a smaller resting-lung volume.[21] In young children, the combination of these features contributes to the risk of ventilation/perfusion imbalance, mechanics abnormalities, low functional-residual capacity, and atelectasis. Finally, the respiratory control center in children under 1 year of age is immature and frequently performs unreliably (e.g., early fatigue and apnea) in the face of systemic illness.[21] Table 1-10 illustrates an approach for evaluation of respiratory disease in children by listing the physical findings, simple laboratory studies, and diagnosis in relation to the major anatomic site of the pathology.

TABLE 1–9: Emergency Medications for Children*

Drug	Dose	Supplied	Indications
Atropine	0.02 mg/kg IV	0.1 mg/ml	Symptomatic bradycardia. Minimum of 0.16 mg. Prophylaxis before intubation
Bretylium	5 mg/kg IV	50 mg/cc	V-tach unresponsive to lidocaine
Epinephrine	First dose 0.1 cc/kg IV (1:10,000)	1:10,000	Pulseless arrest
	0.1cc/kg IO,ETT (1:1000)	1:1000	Severe hypotension
	Subsequent 0.1 cc/kg any route	(1:1000)	Anaphylaxis
		0.01 cc/Kg to 0.35 cc SQ (1:1000)	Status asthmaticus
Diazepam	0.01 mg/kg IV, 0.5 mg/kg PR	5 mg/ml	Seizures
Glucose	0.25–0.5 gm/kg IV, 4–6 cc/kg D10, 2–3 cc/kg D25	10% (100 mg/cc), 25% (250 mg/cc)	Hypoglycemia
Lidocaine	1 mg/kg IV, q 3–5 mins × 3 (Maximum 100 mg)	1% and 2% solution	Ventricular tachycardia
Lorezapam	0.05–0.01 mg/kg, q 3–5 mins IV	5 mg/ml	Seizures
Phenytoin	20 mg/kg IV	50 mg/ml	Seizures
Phenobarbitol	20 mg/kg IV		Seizures
Morphine	0.1–0.2 mg/kg IV	2 mg/ml	Analgesia sedation
Fentanyl	1–2 mcg/kg IV (>12 yr, 50–100 mcg/1 g)	50 mcg/ml	Analgesia sedation
Midazolam	0.035 mg/kg IV 0.2–0.3 mg Intronasal	1 mg/ml	Amnesia, sedation
Ceftriaxone	50–75 mg/kg/24h (meningitis: 100 mg/1 g)		
Cefotaxime	100–120 mg/kg/l ÷ 3 dose (meningitis: 180 mg/1 g/1 d ÷ 4 doses)		
Vancomycin	10 mg/kg/d, q 8h (>2 mos)	15 mg/1 g 6 h (>1 mo, CNS infection)	
Solumedrol	1 mg/1 g, q 6h IV asthma 0.12–1.7 mg/kg/d anti-inflammatory ÷ q 6–12h		Asthma, Anti-inflammatory, Anaphylaxis
Racemic epinephrine	0.25–0.5 ml in 3 ml saline	2.25% solution	Croup
Albuterol	0.01–0.05 ml/kg in 3 ml saline	0.5% solution	
Calcium	30–60 mg/kg	10% saline	
Calcium gluconate	30–60 mg/kg	10% saline	
Sodium bicarbonate	1–2 mcg/kg		
Adenosine	100 mcg/1 g (double to 350 mcg/1 g)		SVT

Infusions

Dopamine	3–15 ug/kg/min		Septic Shock, myocardial dysfunction
Dobutamine	5–20 ug/kg/min		Shock states, myocardial dysfunction
Rule of 6's	6 × Body weight in kg equals the number of mg added to diluent to make a final volume of 100cc, 1 ml/h delivers 1 mcg/kg/min		

* Doses for neonates may differ, please refer to another text.

TABLE 1–10:   Recognition of Respiratory Failure

	Extrathoracic Airway	Central Respiratory Control Center	Neuromuscular Diseases	Thoracic Wall Disease	Intrathoracic Airway and Lung
Prominent physical exam findings	Stridor Snoring Mouth breathing Protruding tongue Drooling	Apnea Periodic breathing Decreased consciousness	Shallow or weak respiratory effort Paradoxical chest vs. abdominal movement with respiration Generalized decreased muscle tone	Asymmetric breath sounds Scoliosis Pectus excavatum Gibbus Other contractures	Tachypnea Wheezing Rale/rhonchus Suprasternal and subcostal retractions
Chest x-ray	Usually normal	Normal or Variable atelectasis	Bell-shaped thoracic shape High diaphragms Scoliosis Asymmetry	Small lung volumes High diaphragms Scoliosis Asymmetry	Hyperinflation Patchy atelectasis Diffuse radiodensity
$PaO_2/PaCO_2$	Early: normal Later: proportionally increased PCO_2 and decreased PO_2	Early: normal Later: proportionally increased PCO_2 and decreased PO_2	Proportionally increased PCO_2 and decreased PO_2	Early: normal Later: proportionally increased PCO_2 and decreased PO_2	Early: Mild to moderate hypoxemia with normal or decreased PCO_2 Later: Moderate to severe hypoxemia with normal or increased PCO_2
Pulse oximetry	Early: normal Later: desaturation corrected with small increases in FiO_2	Early: normal Later: paroxysms of desaturation corrected with small increases in FiO_2	Early: normal Later: paroxysms of desaturation corrected with small increases in FiO_2	Desaturation corrected with small increases in FiO_2	Early: mild desaturation treated with mildly increased FiO_2 Later: desaturation requires high FiO_2
Common diseases: Congenital Infection Trauma/Toxin	Congenital tracheal stenosis Laryngo-malacia Tonsillar/adenoidal hypertrophy Croup Epiglottitis Acquired tracheal stenosis	Apnea of prematurity Arnold-chiari malformation Post epilepsy CNS infection Systemic infection or sepsis Head trauma Sedative or narcotic effect	Wernig Hoffman Muscular dystrophy Guillain-Barré Infant botulism Spinal cord injury Steriod and neuromuscular blockade overdose	Congenital vertebral malformation Cerebral palsy Idiopathic scoliosis Other Flail chest Post thoracotomy Obesity	Hyaline membrane disease of the newborn BPD Asthma Bronchiolitis Aspiration pneumonia ARDS

AT A GLANCE. . .

Causes of Pediatric Respiratory Failure

- Extrathoracic obstruction
- Intrathoracic obstruction
- Problems with respiratory control

Circulatory failure

Circulatory failure that results from diseases and injuries significantly contributes to the need for hospitalization, and it has a disproportionately high morbidity and mortality rate. The classic system for categorizing clinical shock syndromes lists three types of circulatory failure: hypovolemic, cardiogenic, and distributive.[42,43] *Hypovolemic shock* is, by far, the most common type of shock in children, and it results from the depletion of some or all components of the blood so that blood flow and tissue perfusion cannot be maintained.[44] *Cardiogenic shock* results from pump failure (such as that seen in myocarditis), outflow obstruction (such as that in aortic stenosis or pericarditis), or dysrhythmias. *Distributive shock* is characterized by loss of vasomotor tone, as in anaphylaxis and spinal cord injury. Children with sepsis have clinical features of all three types of shock.[45]

AT A GLANCE. . .

Clinical Shock Syndromes

- Hypovolemic
- Cardiogenic
- Distributive

The child in shock will present with evidence of impaired oxygen delivery to multiple organ systems. Cutaneous manifestations of oxygen deprivation include circumoral pallor, grayish hue, cyanosis, diaphoresis, mottling, and poor capillary refill. Manifestations of central nervous system (CNS) hypoxia include irritability, confusion, delirium, seizures, and coma. The cardiovascular system itself is affected by inadequate oxygen delivery and manifests this with tachycardia, diaphoresis, bradycardia, and hypotension. Other manifestations include low urine output, ileus, hypoxemia, and nonrespiratory acidemia.

Because hypovolemia is the most common pediatric shock syndrome, initial therapy to improve cardiac output usually consists of administration of isotonic intravenous fluids. The crystalloid infusion should be administered rapidly in 10–20 ml/kg aliquots, followed by monitoring the improvement of the patient's condition (e.g., mental status, tachycardia, blood pressure, peripheral vasoconstriction, oliguria, and metabolic acidosis). If large-volume intravascular resuscitation (>60 ml/kg of fluid) fails to lead to clinical improvement, the addition of cardiotonic medications (e.g., dopamine or dobutamine) should be considered.[46,47]

Adjunctive measures that aid in the treatment of shock are correction of hypoxemia, acidosis, and electrolyte disturbances. Additionally, in the face of dysrythmias, specific medications, cardioversion, or defibrillation are indicated. Depending on the etiology of the shock, other interventions such as antibiotics may be necessary.

Body fluids

Water is the largest constituent of body mass. In adults, total body water (TBW) comprises 55 to 70% of body weight. The volumetric ratio of extracellular water (ECW): intracellular water (ICW) is 35:65% of the TBW, respectively.[47] The ECW compartment can be divided further into the interstitial water and the plasma water (which are approximately 28% and 7.5% of TBW, respectively). In infants, water comprises about 75% of body weight, and the ECW is 45% of the total.[47,48] Gradual changes in the proportion and the distribution of body water take place with maturation. Differences between adult body water and that of children result in infants and small children having a larger surface area:body mass ratio. These physiologic differences coupled with the general dependence of small children on adults for feeding and care put children at risk for dehydration and electrolyte ab-

normalities, making a general understanding of fluid management by pediatric specialists essential.

SPECIAL CONSIDERATION:

A general understanding of fluid management is essential to pediatric specialists because children's physiologic differences from adults put them at risk for dehydration and electrolyte abnormalities.

Maintenance fluid therapy is designed to replace normal body fluid losses, and is dependent upon metabolic rate in a predictable way.[32] As the nutrients necessary for growth and energy production are carried into the alimentary tract, the individual consumes water. Additionally, new tissue growth requires that water be incorporated into new cells. Lastly, elimination of waste (e.g., carbon dioxide, nitrogen waste, fixed acids, and heat) require water loss. Thus, for every 100 Kcal of daily energy requirement (calculated as in the Nutritional Assessment section on pg. 13) 110 to 120 ml of water are needed.[49,50] Fever increases maintenance requirements by about 12% for each degree increase in body temperature. Excessive losses due to disease and injury must be quantified and replaced accordingly.

In children with fluid and electrolyte problems, the prescription to correct the condition is based on the following: (1) estimation of the fluid deficit or excess; (2) the desired speed of correction; (3) addition of the ongoing standard maintenance fluid needs; and (4) determination if any ongoing losses exist (e.g., diarrhea) or if factors exist that modify usual maintenance needs (e.g., renal failure). Table 1–11 lists common pediatric dehydration syndromes and suggested fluid replacement regimens.[50]

AT A GLANCE. . .

Correction of Fluid and Electrolyte Problems

- Estimate fluid deficit or excess
- Decide on desired speed of correction
- Add ongoing standard maintenance fluids
- Determination of ongoing losses

TABLE 1–11:   Some Rules of Thumb for the Child with Dehydration

Type	Acute (<3 days)		Chronic (>3 days)	
	Replacement Fluid	*Rate*	*Replacement Fluid*	*Rate*
Isotonic (Normal serum Na)	D₅ 1/3 NS	1) Maintenance plus 1/2 the deficit in the first 8h 2) Maintenance plus the second 1/2 of deficit over the next 12h	D₅ 1/4 NS	1) Maintenance plus 1/2 the deficit in the first 12h 2) Maintenance plus the second 1/2 of deficit over the next 24h
Hypotonic (Na⁺ <130 meq/l)	D₅ 1/2 NS	1) Maintenance plus 1/2 the deficit in the first 8h 2) Maintenance plus the second 1/2 of deficit over the next 12h	D₅ 1/3 NS	1) Maintenance plus 1/2 the deficit in the first 12h 2) Maintenance plus the second 1/2 of deficit over the next 24h
Hypertonic (Na⁺ >150 meq/l)	D₅ 1/4 NS	1) Maintenance plus 1/2 the deficit in the first 12h 2) Maintenance plus the second 1/2 of deficit over the next 36h	D₅1 /5 NS	1) Maintenance plus 1/2 the deficit in the first 24h 2) Maintenance plus the second 1/2 of deficit over the next 48h

5% Dextrose in 1/3 normal saline solution
5% Dextrose in 1/2 normal saline solution etc.

Diagnoses

Infectious diseases

Infectious diseases account for the majority of acute illnesses in children.[35] The most common site of infection is in the respiratory tract and the second most common is the gastrointestinal tract.[35] Neonates and children during the first 2 years of life are at increased risk for invasive bacterial disease, which is manifested as upper and lower airway infections, pneumonia, meningitis, cellulitis, septic arthritis, osteomyelitis, and sepsis (Practice Pathway 1–2).[45] The physician should note that the presence of a fever (>38°C) in a child younger than 2 months requires a full evaluation.[51] Pediatric otolaryngologists play a significant role in controlling and improving the outcome of common respiratory infections. Table 1–12 lists common bacterial illnesses and recommended treatments.

Trauma

Injury is the leading cause of death in children beyond the first year of life. Trauma involving motor vehicles is the most common means of injury in children. Unfortunately, violence has seen an increase in recent years also Child abuse, a form of violence, deserves special consideration by the pediatric specialist.[52] No matter what the cause of trauma, head injury is relatively frequent in pediatrics because of children's relative large head size in relation to the body. The child with acute head trauma frequently needs emergency airway management, and may need extended treatment with an artificial airway when neurologic recovery is prolonged or if there is laryngeotracheal injury associated with the acute management. The otolaryngologist is often asked to participate in the airway management of these children.

> **SPECIAL CONSIDERATION:**
>
> The child with acute head trauma frequently needs emergency airway management, and may need extended treatment with an artificial airway when neurologic recovery is prolonged.

Child abuse

In 1994, over three million reports of suspected child abuse were made to Child Protective Services.[52] One third of these cases were substantiated and there were 1200 deaths. These statistics include cases of physical, sexual, and emotional abuse, as well as neglect. In most states health care professionals are mandated by law to report suspected child abuse or neglect. It is a criminal violation to

Practice Pathway 1–2   FEVER

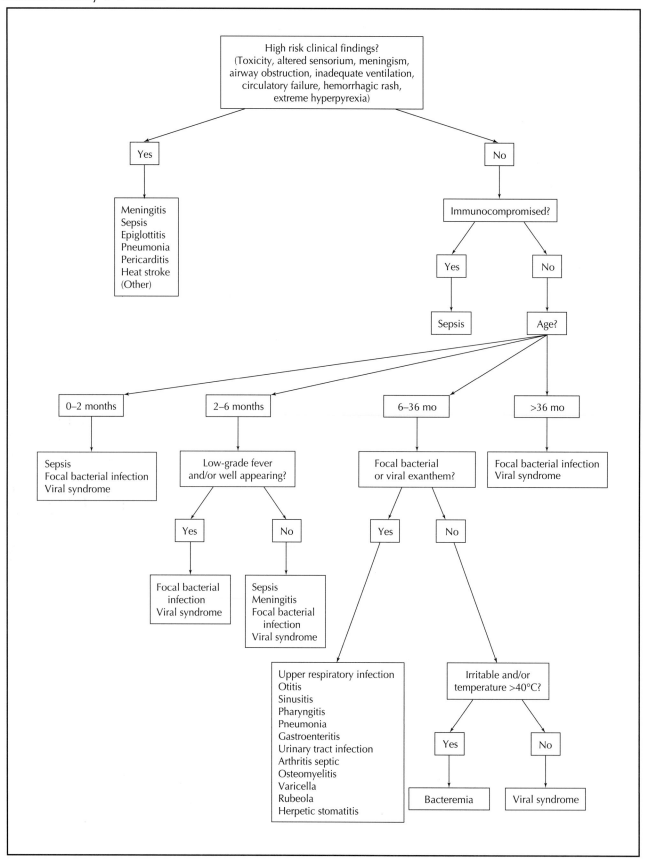

Modified from: Henretig FM. In: Fleisher GR, Ludwig S. *Textbook of Pediatric Emergency Medicine, 3rd ed.* Baltimore: Williams and Wilkins, 1993, pp. 202–209, with permission.

TABLE 1–12: Bacterial Illnesses and Recommended Antibiotics

Clinical Syndrome	Major Pathogens	Antibiotics

Bacterial Meningitis	Neonates (<1 month)
	  Group B streptococcus
	  Escherichia coli, other enterics
	  Listeria monocytogenes
		Ampicillin + gentamicin

	Children
	  Streptococcus pneumoniae
	  Neisseria meningitidis
	  Haemophilus influenzae type b
		Vancomycin + cefotaxime/ceftriaxone

Sepsis	Neonates
	  Group B streptococcus
	  E. coli
		ampicillin and gentamycin or cefotaxime

	Children
	  S. pneumococcus
	  N. meningitidis
	  H. influenzae
	  Staphylococcus aureus
	  Salmonella
	  Gram negative bacilli
		cefotaxime/ceftriaxone

Neonatal Fever (<2 mos)	Group B streptococcus Gram negative bacteria L. monocytogenes	ampicillin and gentamycin ampicillin and cefotxime/ceftriaxone (if CNS disease present)
Bacteremia (<24 mos)	S. pneumoniae	screen for invasive disease
Acute Otitis Media	S. pneumoniae H. influenzae (nontypeable) M. catarrhalis Group A streptococcus	**First line:** amoxicillin. **Second line:** βTrimethoprim-sulfasoxazole, erythromycin-sulfaoxazole. **Third line:** amoxicillin-clavulinate, cefuroxime, cefprozil, cefixime, azithromycin, clarithromycin
Pharyngitis Bacterial etiologies	Group A streptococcus Groups C, B, G, F streptococcus C. diptheriae Neisseria gonorrhoeae	Penicillin, erythromycin, cephalexin

Epiglottitis	All age groups
	  H. influenzae, type B
	  S. pneumoniae
	  Group A streptococcus
		Cefuroxime, cefotaxime, ceftriaxone

Pneumonia	Neonate Group B streptococcus, E. coli (other gram negatives), L. monocytogenes, S. pneumoniae	Ampicillin and cefotaxime
	Chlamydia trachomatis (2 weeks to 3 months) Ureaplasma urealyticum E. coli (other gram negatives)	Erythromycin

	Children
	  S. pneumoniae, S. aureus
	  M. pneumoniae
		Penicillin, ampicillin, cefuroxime
		Erythromycin

Urinary Tract Infection/Pyelonephritis	E. coli, K. pneumoniae, Enterococcus, Proteus mirabilis, Pseudomonas aeruginosa, S. epidermidis	Ampicillin and gentamicin, PO: amoxicillin, trimethoprim-sulfasoxazole, cephalexin
Cellulitis	Group A streptococcus, S. aureus H. influenzae	Cephalexin, dicloxacillin, clindamycin Cefotaxime, ceftriaxone
Cervical Adenitis	Group A streptoccocus, S. aureus Anaerobes Atypical mycobacterium	Cephalexin, dicloxacillin Clindamycin
Cat scratch disease	Rihensalae	Trimethoprim-sulfasoxazole

Osteomyelitis	Children
	  S. aureus
	  Group A streptococcus
	  H. influenzae
	  Salmonella
		Oxacillin, clindamycin, cefazolin
		
		Cefotaxime

Septic Arthritis	Neonates S. aureus, Group B streptococcus, Gram negatives	Cefotaxime

	Children
	  S. aureus, Group A streptococcus, S. pneumoniae
	  H. influenzae (rare)
		Cefuroxime, oxacillin

	Teen N. gonorrheae	Cefotaxime, ceftriaxone

fail to report such cases to child protective services and/or the police. Thus, it is important to be able to recognize child abuse if you are in the position of caring for children.[52]

The diagnosis of child abuse is made by history, physical examination, and observation of the child and caretaker interaction. Important findings in the evaluation of physical abuse include a history incompatible with the child's injury, a significant injury lacking any history, a history that changes over time with subsequent interviews, a delay in seeking care, or injuries attributed to a young sibling or playmate or to self-infliction that is inconsistent with the child's development. A complete physical examination is indicated.

The earliest and most common manifestations of physical abuse are found on the skin. A recent study by Johnson revealed that 80% of abused children had skin findings present.[53] Suspicious findings include bruising that is located centrally, multiple bruises of different ages, and patterned injuries (e.g., finger marks, cord marks, etc). As always, findings inconsistent with the history given should arouse suspicion. Visible color changes occur over time as the bruises heal; however, there is no accurate way of dating when the injury occurred by the appearance of the bruise.

A significant proportion of burns treated by physicians are also a result of abuse. Scald injury is by far the most common cause of injury. Suspicious injuries include immersion of the hands and feet (i.e., a stocking or glove distribution), immersion of the lower torso and proximal thighs, symmetric injury, and patterns.

In children less than 2 years of age, radiographs are recommended to identify the presence of old fractures. A skeletal survey includes views of the entire upper and lower extremities, the axial skeleton, and the skull, and should be read by an experienced radiographer. Fractures that are suspicious for abuse include fractures of the ribs, metaphyseal fractures, diaphyseal fractures, humeral fractures, and femoral fractures in children less than 1 year of age. Metaphyseal chip fractures that represent microfractures through the most immature portion of the metaphysis are highly specific for child abuse.

Head injury is the leading cause of morbidity in abused children.[54] Infants in the first year of life are most at risk. The mechanism is presumed to consist of an acceleration or deceleration force to the brain that is caused by shaking and followed by an impact.[54] Typical cranial computed tomography (CT) scan findings include subdural hemorrhage, loss of grey-white differentiation, and interhemispheric blood. Careful documentation of the history, physical examination, and suspicious findings is important, and will be of great assistance should the physician be called upon to testify regarding the medical evidence. Immediate referral to a pediatrician, child abuse specialist, or emergency department is indicated should the physician suspect abuse.[52]

Child sexual abuse is an exploitive sexual act imposed by an older dominant perpetrator on a child or adolescent who lacks emotional and cognitive maturity. Common themes in cases of sexual misuse include the use of power, age, and position in relation to the child; the inability of the child to consent, leading to helplessness; and an attempt on the part of the child to please the adult. This abuse incorporates a broad spectrum of acts that range from nontouching gestures, such as genital viewing, to fondling, kissing, masturbation, vulvar or gluteal coitus, and digital or genital penetration. *Incest* refers to the specific situation in which sexual abuse occurs between individuals who cannot marry and includes those having a family role regardless of blood relationship. The true incidence of sexual misuse is unknown and it remains largely underreported. It is estimated that 250,000 to 300,000 cases occur yearly in the United States, but that only 50,000 of these are reported. Girls are the victims twice as often as boys.

The diagnosis of sexual abuse or assault depends primarily upon what the patient tells the physician; the history is supplemented merely by physical and laboratory findings. The history obtained during the interview with the victim is the most important piece of evidence. The physical examination is a therapeutic as well as a diagnostic procedure, serving to provide further information and to document normalcy for the victim. It addresses three purposes: identification of pertinent physical findings and conditions that need treatment; collection of specimens for evidence; and most importantly, reassuring the patient that he/she is well or "undamaged." The presence of a normal physical examination is common (26–73% in children allegedly sexually abused) and *is consistent* with sexual abuse.

Every state requires physicians to report *suspected* sexual abuse to the appropriate agencies, including Child Protective Services and the police. Most cities have sites designated to evaluate the child with suspected sexual abuse. Be familiar with your local practice, laws, and referral site.

Chronic illness

Advances in medicine and technology have resulted in improved mortality,[5] but as a result, there are a larger number of children living with chronic illness who are dependent upon technology such as mechanical ventilation and enteral feedings. Although these children often require the care of multiple subspecialists, their overall health is managed best by a generalist who reviews all the medical problems and can coordinate necessary specialty care. Communication and discussion between the subspecialist and the generalist is imperative for good patient care. The generalist, in addition to organizing the care of the needed subspecialist, monitors overall health, plays a role in advocating appropriate educational and home care needs, and considers the child as a member of a family and a community.

REFERENCES

Section I: Active & Passive Immunization

1. American Academy of Pediatrics. In: Peter G, ed. *Redbook: Report of the Committee on Infectious Diseases, 24th ed.* Elk Grove Village, IL: American Academy of Pediatrics, 1997, pp. 1–71.
2. Bart KJ, Lin KF. Vaccine-preventable disease and immunization in the developing world. Pediatr Clin North Am 1990; 32:735–756.
3. Beck RA, Kambiss S, Bass JW. The retreat of Hemophilus influenzae type B invasive disease: Analysis of an immunization program and implications for OTO-HNS. Otolaryngol Head Neck Surg 1993; 109:712–721.
4. Senior BA, Radkowski D, MacArthur C, et al. Changing patterns in pediatric supraglottitis: A multi-institutional review, 1980 to 1992. Multicenter Study. Laryngoscope 1994; 104:1314–1322.
5. Cohen HJ, Pizzo P, Riley A, et al. Technical panel on children with special needs. In: *Caring for our Children. National Health and Safety Standards. Guidelines for Out-of-Home Child Care Programs.* Washington, DC: American Public Health Association and American Academy of Pediatrics, 1992, pp. 237–267.
6. Committee on Practice and Ambulatory Medicine. American Academy of Pediatrics. Recommendations for preventive medicine and pediatric healthcare. In: *Policy Reference Guide of the American Academy of Pediatrics.* Elk Grove Village, IL: American Academy of Pediatrics 1994; pp. 620.
7. Kliegman RM. The newborn infant. In: Behrman RE, Kliegman RM, Arvin AM, eds. *Nelson Textbook of Pediatrics, 15th ed.* Philadelphia: Saunders, 1996; pp. 433–440.
8. Copper RL, Goldenberg RL, Creasy RK, et al. A multicenter study of pre-term birth weight and gestational age-specific neonatal mortality. Am J Obstet Gynecol 1993; 168:78–84.
9. Phillip AGS, Little GA, Polivy DR, et al. Neonatal mortality risk for the Eighties: The importance of birth weight/gestational age groups. Pediatrics 1981; 60:122–130.
10. Johnsen DC. The preschool "passage." An overview of dental health. Dent Clin North Am 1995; 39:695–707.
11. Committee on the Environment. American Academy of Pediatrics. Lead poisoning from screening to primary prevention. Pediatrics 1993; 92:176–183.
12. Gutgesell HP, Atkins DL, Day RW. Common cardiovascular problems in the young: Part II. Hypertension, hypercholesterolemia and preparticipation screening of athletes. Am Fam Physician 1997; 56:1993–1998.
13. Benuck I. Cholesterol screening in children. Curr Probl Pediatr 1995; 25:254–260.
14. American Academy of Pediatrics. Tuberculosis In: Peter G, ed. *Redbook. Report of the Committee on Infectious Diseases, 24th ed.* Elk Grove Village, IL: American Academy of Pediatrics, 1997, 541–562.
15. Ehrman WG, Matson SC: The Approach to assessing adolescent on serious or sensitive issues. Pediatr Clin North Am. 1998; 45:189–204.
16. Report of the second task force on blood pressure control in children 1987. Pediatrics 1987; 79:1–25.
17. Update on the 1987 task force report on high blood pressure in children and adolescents: A working group report from the national high blood pressure education program. Pediatrics 1996; 98:649–658.
18. Hoekelman RA. The physical examination of infants and children. In: Bates B, ed. *A Guide to Physical Examination and History Taking, 5th ed.* Philadelphia: Lippincott, 1991, pp. 612–614.
19. Namin EP, Miller RA. The normal electrocardiogram and vectorcardiogram in infants and children. In: Cassels DE, Zeigler RF, eds. New York: Grune and Stratton, 1966, pp. 99–100.
20. Simons K. Preschool vision screening: Rationale, methodology and outcome. Surv Ophthalmol 1995; 41:3–30.
21. Watchko JF, Mayock DE, Standaert TA, et al. The ventilatory pump: Neonatal and developmental issues. Adv Pediatr 1991; 38:109–134.
22. Johnson CP, Blasco P. Infant growth and development. Pediatr Rev 1997; 18:224–242.

23. Olson ER, Dworkin PH. Toddler development. Pediatr Rev 1997; 18:255–259.

24. Barone MA, ed. Development *The Harriet Lane Book, 14th ed.* St Louis: Mosby, 1996, pp. 182–184.

25. Capute AJ, Biehl RF. Functional developmental evaluation. Prerequisite to habitation. Pediatr Clin North Am 1973; 20:3–26.

26. Capute AJ, Accardo PJ. Linguistic and auditory milestones during the first 2 years of life: A language inventory for the practitioner. Clin Pediatr 1978; 17: 847–853.

27. Capute AJ, Shapiro BK, Wachtel RC, et al. The clinical linguistic and auditory milestone scale (CLAMS). Identification of cognitive defects in motor-delayed children. Am J Dis Child 1986; 140:694–698.

28. Capute AJ, Palmer FB, Shapiro BK, et al. Clinical linguistic and auditory milestone scale: Prediction of cognition in infancy. Devel Med Child Neurol 1986; 28:762–771.

29. Frankenburg WK, Dodds JB. The Denver developmental screening test. J Pediatr 1967; 71:181–191.

30. Teasdale G, Jennett B. Assessment of coma and impaired consciousness: A practical scale. Lancet 1974; 2:81–84.

31. James HE, Trauner DA. The Glasgow coma scale. In: James HE, Anas NG, Perkin RM, eds. *Brain Insults in Infants and Children.* Orlando: Grune and Stratton, 1985, pp. 179–182.

32. Winters RW. Maintenance fluid therapy. In: Winters RW. *The Body Fluids in Pediatrics.* Boston: Little, Brown & Company, 1973, pp. 113–133.

33. Green M, ed. *Bright Futures: Guideline for Health Supervision of Infants, Children and Adolescents. Pocket Guide.* Arlington: National Center for Child and Maternal Health, 1996.

34. American Academy of Pediatric Committee on Infectious Diseases. Recommended childhood immunization schedule. Pediatrics 1998; 101:154–157.

35. Adams PF, Morano MA. Current estimates from the National Interview Survey, 1994. Hyattsville, MD: National Center for Health Statistics. Vital Health Statistics-101(193). 1995, pp. 1–141.

36. Singh Gk, Kochanek KD, MacDorman MF. Advance report of final mortality statistic, 1994. Monthly vital statistics report. Hyattsville, Md: National Center for Health Statistics 1996; 45(supplement 3):

37. Apgar V. Proposal for a new method of evaluation of the newborn infant. Anesth Anal 1952; 32:260–262.

38. Ludwig S, Kettrick RG. Resuscitation—pediatric basic and advanced life support. In: Fleisher G, Ludwig S, eds. *Textbook of Pediatric Emergency Medicine, 3rd ed.* Baltimore: Williams and Wilkins, 1993, pp. 1–31.

39. American Academy of Pediatrics and American Heart Association. Cardiac rhythm disturbances. In: Chameides L, Hazinski MF, eds. *Textbook of Pediatric Advances Life Support* Dallas: American Heart Association, 1994, pp. 7–9.

40. Lubitz DS, Seidel JF, Chameides L, et al. A rapid method for estimating weight and resuscitation drug dosage from length in the pediatric age group. Ann Emerg Med 1988; 17:576–581.

41. Ludwig S, Kettrick RG, Parker M. Pediatric cardiopulmonary resuscitation: A review of 130 cases. Clin Pediatr 1984; 23:71–76.

42. Perkin RN, Levin DL. Shock and the pediatric patient. J Pediatr 1982; 101:163–169.

43. Perkin RN, Levin DL. Shock and the pediatric patient-Part II. J Pediatr 1982; 101:319–332.

44. Carcillo JA, Davis AL, Zaritsky A. Role of early fluid resuscitation in pediatric septic shock. JAMA 1991; 266:1242–1245.

45. Parker MM. Pathophysiology of cardiovascular dysfunction in septic shock. New Horiz 1998; 6: 130–138.

46. Thomas NJ, Carcillo JA. Hypovolemic shock in pediatric patients. New Horiz 1998; 6:120–129.

47. Costarino AT, Baumgart S. Neonatal water metabolism. In: Cowett RM, ed. *Principles of Perinatal-Neonatal Metabolism.* New York: Springer-Verlag, 1991, p. 624.

48. Costarino AT, Brans YW. Fetal and neonatal body fluid composition with reference to growth and development. In: Polin RA, Fox WW, eds. *Fetal and Neonatal Physiology, 2nd ed.* Philadelphia: Saunders, 1998, pp. 1713–1721.

49. Food and Nutrition Board, National Academy of Sciences–National Research Council. Avery GB, ed. *Neonatology Pathophysiology and Management of the Newborn, 3rd ed.* Philadelphia: Lippincott, 1987 p. 1378.

50. Lewy JE, Boineau FG. Estimation of parental fluid requirements. Pediatr Clin North Am 1990; 37: 257–264.

51. Henretig FM, Fever. In: Fleisher GR, Ludwig S. Textbook of Pediatric Emergency Medicine, 3rd Ed. Baltimore: Williams and Wilkins, 1993, pp. 202–209.

52. Giardino AP, Christian CW, Giardino ER. *A Practical Guide to the Evaluation of Child Physical Abuse and Neglect.* Canada: Sage Publications, 1997, pp. 181–191.

53. Johnson CF. Inflicted versus accidental injury. Pediatr Clin North Am 1990; 37:791–814.

54. Duhaime AC, Alairo AJ, Lewander W, et al. Head injury in very young children: Mechanism, injury types, and opthalmologic changes in 100 patients less than 2 years of age. Pediatr 1992; vol 90 179–185.

Anesthesia in the Child and Adolescent

Robert S. Holzman

Few specialists consistently share a more intimate and vital working space than otolaryngologists and anesthesiologists. The goals of the pediatric otolaryngologic anesthesiologist are threefold: to understand the fundamental differences between children and adults; to know the anesthetic implications of otolaryngologic surgery broadly; and finally, to understand special situations and patient circumstances. This chapter focuses on salient features of anesthesia for pediatric otolaryngologic patients; it does not provide a complete discussion of pediatric anesthesia practice, for which there are already excellent textbooks.

FUNDAMENTAL DIFFERENCES BETWEEN CHILDREN AND ADULTS

Epidemiology of Anesthetic Risk

It has long been a perception that the risks of anesthetizing children are greater than those of adults. Mortality and morbidity are both inversely related to the patient's age and the anesthesiologist's experience, and directly related to overall health and fitness of the patient as assessed by the American Society of Anesthesiologists (ASA) Physical Status Category (Table 2-1).[1-4]

Of particular interest for the pediatric otolaryngologist are several longitudinal studies[5,6] that have shown that not only is the general incidence of laryngospasm and bronchospasm greater in children than adults, but that these adverse events occur more frequently during otolaryngologic procedures. Medical problems, such as concurrent upper respiratory infection, organic heart disease, and chronic lung disease, or prior anesthetic complications are also associated with an increased incidence of laryngospasm and bronchospasm (Fig. 2-1).

Psychological and Physiological Differences Between Children and Adults

Children are in a continual process of growth and development, and the essence of their anesthetic care flows from this basic fact. Stages of mastery of various psychosocial skills and emotional growth, including the child's response to the stress of anesthesia and surgery, have been described.[7-10] The induction of anesthesia should take these stages into account. In addition, parents need to be reassured about gentleness and care. For the youngest age groups (generally with the exception of babies aged less than 6 months), *separation* from parents who are a source of security is the overwhelming concern. The hallmark for preschoolers is their newly acquired *independence* through recent mastery of bodily functions, although they still lack independent social skills. School-age children, from about 5 years through early adolescence, are generally the

TABLE 2–1: American Society of Anesthesiologists Physical Status Categories

Category	Description
I	Healthy patient
II	Mild systemic disease*—no functional limitations
III	Severe systemic disease*—definite functional limitation
IV	Severe systemic disease* that is a constant threat to life
V	Moribund patient not expected to survive 24 hours with or without surgery

* Whether or not the disease is the one for which the patient is undergoing surgery.

Pediatric Otolaryngology, Edited by R.F. Wetmore, H.R. Muntz, and T.J. McGill. Thieme Medical Publishers, Inc., New York © 2000.

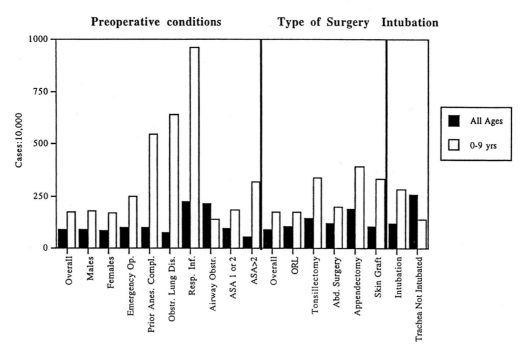

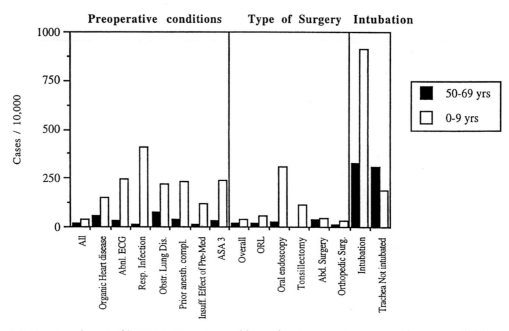

Figure 2–1: Incidence of laryngospasm (A) and bronchospasm (B) compared between children and adults in relation to preoperative conditions, type of surgery, and intubation of the trachea. (adapted from references 5 and 6, with permission.)

easiest group of patients because they are progressively acquiring *social and cognitive skills for coping* with threatening situations, they are capable of understanding the nature of what will happen to them and have a degree of faith that the end result will usually prove to be worthwhile. Teenagers, although cognitively capable, often have great fears about the procedure, the anesthetic, the potential for intraoperative awakening, and death. Operations that alter the body image in teenage years may

TABLE 2–2:   Premedication, Preinduction, and Induction Strategies

Technique	Onset	Recovery	Example
Premedication	Slow	Prolonged	Oral midazolam, diazepam, rectal methohexital or thiopental
Preinduction	Rapid	Variable	Nasal midazolam or sufentanil, sublingual midazolam, IM ketamine
Induction	Immediate	Prompt	Intravenous thiopental or propofol, inhalation sevoflurane or halothane

be a particular problem. Assuming that a preoperative visit has already provided information, as well as reassurance and trust, a variety of premedication or preinduction strategies are available (Table 2–2). No matter the age of the patient, the successful clinician should strive to be a good conversationalist who is prepared with age-appropriate patter for the patient, whether this is nursery rhymes, counting games, concrete questions, or thorough explanations focused on reassurance.

As a physiologic accompaniment to their growth, children have high metabolic rates, resulting in an elevated basal oxygen consumption (7–9 ml/kg/min) compared with adults (3 ml/kg/min) (Fig. 2–2). Because the production of carbon dioxide (CO_2) is directly related to the consumption of oxygen (O_2) (the *respiratory quotient* or RQ), during mechanical ventilation, children require a greater minute volume per kilogram weight than adults. The configuration of the thoracic cage differs between infants, small children, older children, and adults.[11] The ribs in younger children are more horizontal and therefore rise less during inspiration. The pliable rib cage of a newborn collapses with in-

creases in negative intrathoracic pressure, diminishing the efficacy of the infant's attempts to increase ventilation. Because of less anteroposterior movement during inspiration, the diaphragm takes on greater importance and is the infant's major muscle of ventilation. Histologically, an infant's diaphragm has only half the number of type 1 slow-twitch oxidative muscle fibers essential for sustained increased respiratory effort; thus the infant's diaphragm fatigues earlier than the diaphragm of adults.

The lungs of young children have high closing volumes, which fall within the lower range of the lungs' normal tidal volume. Below normal closing volume (e.g., during general anesthesia or sedation) alveolar collapse and shunting may occur. The elastic content of alveoli increases until maximal lung compliance is reached at approximately 18 years of age. With this greater amount of supporting elastic stroma in the small airways, the defense against early airway closure at low lung volumes is improved. Gravitational forces at small lung volumes cause collapse of small, noncartilaginous airways in infants and young children.

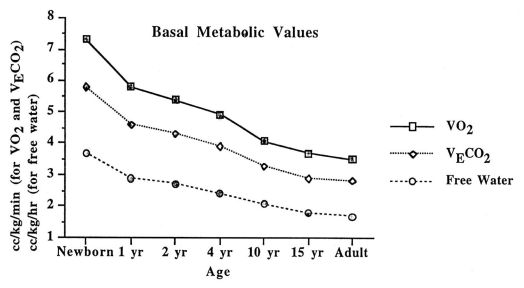

Figure 2–2:   Basal metabolic oxygen consumption (VO_2), carbon dioxide production (V_ECO_2) and free water requirements are greater for infants and young children than they are for adults. (From reference 66, with permission.)

One implication of these findings of a less compliant lung with a more compliant chest wall in children is a lower resting lung volume (lower *functional residual capacity* or FRC), leading to less oxygen reserve in the absence of ventilation. Children have a greater minute ventilation: FRC ratio, which results in a more rapid induction of anesthesia with inhalation agents than in adults. Encroachment on ventilation by abdominal distention is an important concern for children, and vigorous mask ventilation with gastric distention, particularly in the setting of airway obstruction, may lead to significant ventilatory restriction. In addition, intracardiac or extracardiac vascular shunts, including patent ductus arteriosus, patent foramen ovale, or atrial septal defects, may have increased flow with elevation of pulmonary artery pressure, particularly during hypoxia, hypoventilation, or excessively high-positive airway pressure. All of these characteristics conspire to produce rapid desaturation during apnea. Profound desaturation can occur, even with a properly positioned endotracheal tube, when an infant coughs or strains, resulting in alveolar collapse.

The cardiovascular system, likewise, has certain features that differ between children and adults. Cardiac output is 180 to 240 ml/kg/min in newborns, which is two to three times higher than in adults. This high cardiac output is necessary in order to meet the infant's higher metabolic demands. The ventricles have a smaller muscle mass in newborns and infants and are relatively noncompliant, with minimal compensatory reserve. There is a higher resting tone at end-diastole with a lower peak pressure achieved during systole. Although there is some limited ability to increase contractility, increases in cardiac output are rate-dependent for the most part. Likewise, baroreception and myocardial performance "mature" postnatally. Baroreflex sensitivity increases steadily within the first several weeks to months of life, with higher blood pressures causing greater bradycardia.[12-14] Inhalation anesthetics may aggravate the relative insensitivity in the neonate: halothane at 0.5 minimal anesthetic concentration minimum alveolar concentration (MAC) reduces the baroresponse of baby rabbits by 80%, whereas in adult rabbits it reduces the same response by only 54%.[15] Isoflurane also attenuates baroreflex control of the heart rate in neonates,[16] as does fentanyl.[17]

Current findings reveal a developmental basis for differences in excitation-contraction coupling due to altered calcium flux across the sarcolemma and adenosine 5'-triphosphate (ATP)-sensitive potassium channels in neonatal myocyte membranes.[18-21] Reduced ventricular compliance in less mature animal models supports the clinical observation of the young infant's limited ability to increase stroke volume. The important clinical principle is that because the infant has a relatively limited ability to increase cardiac output, other than by increasing heart rate or responding to massive doses of catecholamines, the anesthesiologist must be prepared to support the circulation, especially in the setting of frequent use of high doses of volatile anesthetics.

Compared to adults, infants and children have a greater surface: body weight ratio and therefore experience greater losses of body heat by radiation, evaporation, convection, and conduction. Infants less than 3 months of age cannot compensate for cold by shivering, but instead respond to cold stress by increasing norepinephrine production, which initiates the metabolism of brown fat. Norepinephrine produces pulmonary and peripheral vasoconstriction also, and may lead to right to left shunting, hypoxia, and metabolic acidosis. Particularly for patients with a history of chronic upper airway obstruction, hypoxemia, hypercarbia (or chronically-elevated, pulmonary artery pressures), cold stress, and acidosis may worsen apnea and should be avoided or addressed by the use of appropriate warming devices.

SPECIAL CONSIDERATION:

Children are not little adults: their higher metabolic rate and cardiac output as well as their greater surface: body weight ratio require a specialized anesthesia regimen.

SPECIAL CONSIDERATIONS FOR ADOLESCENTS

Superficially, considerations for the anesthetic care of adolescents would not appear to be very different than those of adults, aside from their recent onset of endocrine changes and accompanying explosive growth, and much less attention is devoted to this age group in the anesthesiology literature than to younger children. The first research findings, recently published from The National Longitudinal Study of Adolescent Health,[22] indicate that the main threats to the health of adolescents are the risk behaviors they choose, such as substance abuse (cigarettes, alcohol, and marijuana), sexual activity, and outlets for emotional distress (including violence, suicide, and eating disorders). Out-of-school adolescents are more likely to engage in behaviors with potentially severe adverse health outcomes (e.g., sexual intercourse and cigarette smoking) than are adolescents in school.[23] It is important for clinicians to understand that adolescents have high rates of preventable health problems that nevertheless may have significant implications for their perioperative anesthetic management. A recent Massachusetts survey of ninth through twelfth graders indicated that 53% of men and 47% of women reported having sexual intercourse; 58% used a condom, 30% used withdrawal or no method of birth control, and 25% used alcohol or other drugs at last intercourse. Thirty-five percent had 5 or more drinks in a row on one or more occasion in the 30 days preceding the survey, and among twelfth graders, 45% rode in a car with someone under the influence of alcohol in the preceding 30 days. Thirty-five percent of men and 19% of women drove under the influence. Sixty-two percent of women and 24% of men were trying to lose weight.[24]

SPECIAL CONSIDERATION:

Because adolescents may engage in behaviors that may result in severe adverse health outcomes, it is imperative that a thorough history is obtained before formulating an anesthetic regimen.

The implications are staggering and begin with a sensitive but thorough history taking. Information about anesthetic and surgical plans, including potential sequelae of treatment that require the disclosure of any risk-related behavior, must be shared with the patient. Pregnancy testing should be performed on every menarcheal female. Dietary risk behaviors such as high sodium, high fat, or recurrent crash diets may result in hypertension or accompany anorexia. Many adolescents do not consider "diet pills" to be part of the answer to an inquiry about any current medications. Likewise, adolescents should be asked about their use of alcohol and other abusable substances, as well as about their

use of over-the-counter or prescription drugs for nonmedical purposes, including anabolic steroids. The challenge for the clinician is to maintain sensitivity about the turbulence of the adolescent period and to preserve confidentiality while discussing the relevant issues and plans with parents (occasionally separately from the patient).

FUNDAMENTAL CONSIDERATIONS FOR ANESTHESIA FOR OTOLARYNGOLOGY

The skilled otolaryngologic anesthesiologist is easily recognizable to the cognoscenti, because he or she possesses knowledge about the surgical procedure, has a variety of technical skills for visualizing the airway, is knowledgeable about developmental anomalies of the head and neck and their anesthetic implications, and has an artist's ear and eye for titrating the depth of anesthesia. In otolaryngology, because many of the operations involve the airway, the anesthesiologist must provide good surgical access while preserving the ability to adequately ventilate and oxygenate the patient. More than in any other surgical specialty, alternate modalities of ventilation may be necessary, such as insufflation, apneic oxygenation, and jet ventilation.

Anesthesiologists know that almost all anesthetics decrease ventilation in a dose-dependent manner. Well understood but infrequently articulated, this principle is used daily to assess anesthetic depth in relation to surgical stimulation. In so doing, it becomes clear that whereas the volatile agents decrease tidal volume and minute ventilation and increase dead space, it is really the CO_2 level that clinicians manipulate to preserve spontaneous ventilation. The balance that ultimately exists between the depth of anesthesia, the level of CO_2, and the amount of surgical stimulation results in the spontaneous respiratory rate that the anesthesiologist orchestrates. Overly aggressive "assisting" of respiration may result in driving the CO_2 below apneic threshold* and the opportunity to truly understand the patient's response to stimulation may be lost. On the other hand, intentional hyperventilation below apneic threshold will often permit a quiet surgical field without the use of muscle relaxants.

---

* Apneic threshold is the $PaCO_2$ at which ventilation becomes zero (when spontaneous ventilatory effort ceases).[25]

Induced hyperpnea with doxapram may be particularly useful for stimulating respiration during a deep inhalation anesthetic.

Skill in understanding and controlling anesthetic depth is arguably the most important aspect of providing safe and expert anesthetic care for the otolaryngologic patient, it is critical to the success of spontaneous breathing techniques (for diagnostic examination of the native airway and dynamic changes such as extrinsic compression or tracheomalacia) and therapy (interventions such as a foreign body in the trachea). Aside from the assessment of heart rate, blood pressure, and patient movement, depth of anesthesia should be evaluated dynamically by continuous monitoring of the heart sounds and by repeated examination of muscle tone. The arms and legs should feel completely relaxed and the abdominal muscles should feel soft and easily compressible (like bread dough); the feel of the muscles should be distinct from the board-like rigidity of the excitement phase or the mild to moderate muscle tone of the awake or sedated state. Finally, the eye signs, as originally described for ether anesthesia, are useful in aiding clinical assessment of anesthetic depth. Disconjugate gaze and pupillary dilation shortly after inhalation induction support the assessment of light anesthesia, whereas mid-size pupils in mid-position, along with other physical findings of acceptable anesthetic depth, complete the clinician's assessment. All signs together should be used to form a composite so that, ideally, the anesthesiologist should be able to predict lack of patient movement in response to stimulation. Facility in determining anesthetic depth is also important for successful "deep" extubations, which is the removal of the endotracheal tube while the patient is deeply anesthetized and breathing spontaneously. The presumption is that the patient will have less coughing, bucking, and airway irritability during the emergence process without an endotracheal tube. In experienced hands, this technique is at least as safe as the more typical "awake" extubation.[26-28]

SPECIAL CONSIDERATION:

Skill in controlling anesthetic depth is arguably the most important aspect of providing safe and expert anesthesia care in children.

Laryngospasm occurs more frequently in conjunction with otolaryngologic patients and otolaryngologic procedures than in any other pediatric surgical specialty (Fig. 2–11). Multiple strategies for the prevention and treatment of laryngospasm have been sought. Continuous positive airway pressure (CPAP) is routinely used for treating laryngospasm, or other soft-tissue upper airway obstruction due to lymphoid hyperplasia, tissue inflammation from a localized infection such as supraglottitis, or cystic hygroma. Usually, 5 to 10 cm H_2O pressure, as measured on the pressure gauge at the top of the CO_2 absorber, will be effective; occasionally, higher pressures are required. Care should be exercised because lower esophageal sphincter-opening pressure may be as low as 10 to 12 cm H_2O, presenting the risk of gastric insufflation. In addition, although CPAP is effective for soft-tissue obstruction, it is not necessarily effective for tumors of the airway.

AT A GLANCE...

Anesthesia for Laryngospasm

Pathogenesis: excitement phase of anesthetic induction or emergence, light anesthesia relative to the surgical stimulus, mechanical irritants in the airway, gastroesophageal reflux, active upper respiratory tract infections

Adverse Effects: hypoxemia, hypercarbia, bradycardia, arrhythmias, cardiac arrest, pulmonary edema

Symptoms and Signs: stridor, hypoxemia, tachypnea, tachycardia, increase in pharyngeal secretions, retractions (sternal or intercostal), inability to ventilate with positive pressure, inability to phonate

Diagnosis: physical exam and findings during anesthetic administration

Treatment: CPAP with 100% oxygen using a bag and mask, attempt to improve airflow across the obstructed segment (employ standard airway maneuvers such as jaw thrust, oral or nasal airway insertion, apply CPAP), clear the airway of secretions, administer a small dose of succinylcholine IV or IM if no IV available, prepare to establish an airway by invasive means if oxygenation cannot be maintained

Even though the ready availability of a surgical airway exists in the otolaryngology room, all person-

Practice Pathway 2-1   MANAGING A DIFFICULT AIRWAY*

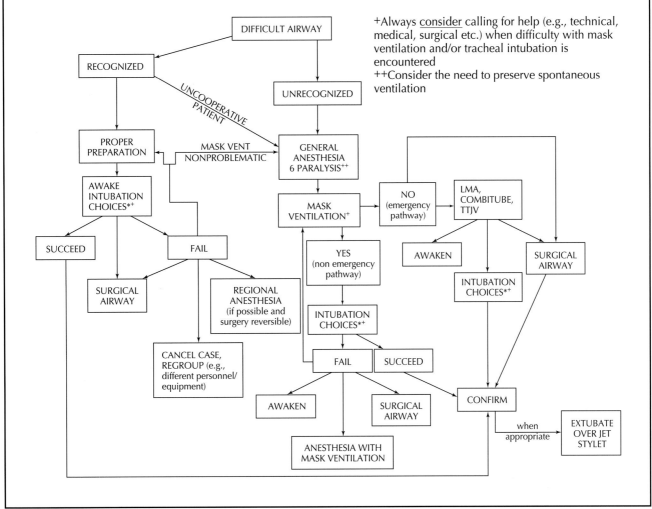

* LMA, laryngeal mask airway; TTJV, trans-tracheal jet ventilation.

nel should be familiar with the ASA Difficult Airway Algorithm (Practice Pathway 2-1). Modifications to the original algorithm now include the laryngeal mask airway (LMA) (Practice Pathway 2-2). Hopefully, an emergent situation may be averted and an uncontrolled situation converted to a semielective situation.

Children often have a typical constellation of medical problems accompanying their otolaryngologic disease. The child with a runny nose or chronic sinusitis, chronic lung disease (especially in association with an early history of prematurity, choanal atresia, tracheotomy, or reactive airway disease associated with chronic aspiration is not uncommon. Clinicians have to carefully distinguish the runny nose that is associated typically with myringotomy and adenoidectomy from pulmonary paren-

chymal disease as a result of a viral syndrome. Patients with the latter are clearly at higher risk, particularly when young (i.e., <5 years old).[29-33]

Stimulation of the oropharynx and aerodigestive tract often results in the elaboration of copious secretions; antisialagogues are very helpful in decreasing secretions for examination or intervention. Glycopyrrolate, a quarternary ammonium compound, does not cross the blood-brain barrier and will not result in a central anticholinergic syndrome, in comparison to tertiary ammonium compounds like atropine or scopolamine. We routinely administer glycopyrrolate for its antisialagogue effect following placement of an intravenous line.

Isolated masseter muscle spasm (MMS) after the administration of intravenous (IV) succinylcholine during volatile agent anesthetic induction in chil-

Practice Pathway 2–2   MANAGING A DIFFICULT AIRWAY WITH THE LARYNGEAL MASK AIRWAY*

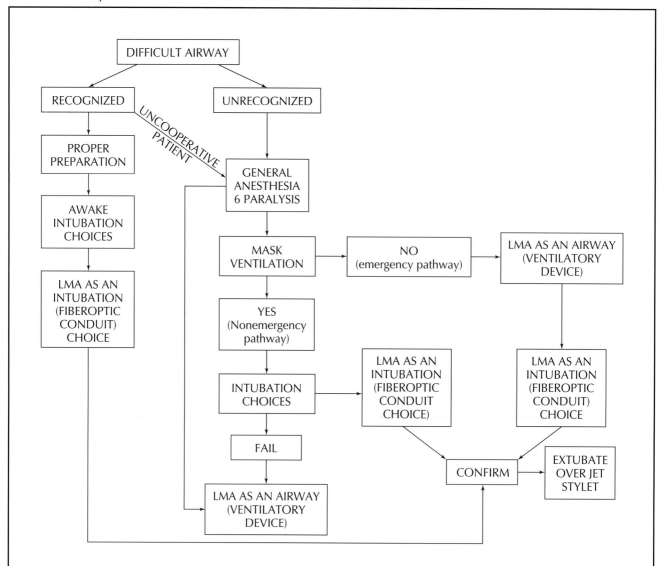

* LMA, laryngeal mask airway. The laryngeal mask airway fits into the ASA algorithm on the management of the difficult airway in five places. (From ref. 67, with permission).

dren may occur as frequently as 1:100 cases.[34-35] In the past, the usual approach was to assume that the patient was at imminent risk for developing malignant hyperthermia (MH) and to discontinue the anesthesia,[36] possibly administer dantrolene sodium, or modify the technique to exclude known triggering agents.[37] Failure of the masseter muscles to relax after administration of succinylcholine is not uncommon in children,[38,39] and it is suggested that anesthesia can be continued safely in cases of isolated MMS when careful monitoring accompanies diagnostic evaluation for hypercarbia, metabolic acidosis, elevation of serum creatine kinase, and myoglobinuria.[40] Moreover, it is recognized that

incomplete jaw relaxation is different from masseter muscle rigidity and trismus, and that it is not uncommon in children after a halothane-succinylcholine sequence. Incomplete jaw relaxation should be considered part of the range of normal responses that is in contrast to MMS or trismus, which should continue to be considered possible sentinel signs of MH susceptibility until proven otherwise.[41,42] This is of obvious importance in otolaryngologic surgery because the combination of general anesthesia with potent inhaled agents and the relatively common occurrence of airway emergencies, such as laryngospasm, may require more frequent use of succinylcholine than in other specialties (Practice Pathway 2-3).

Practice Pathway 2–3   DIAGNOSIS AND MANAGEMENT OF MALIGNANT HYPERTHERMIA

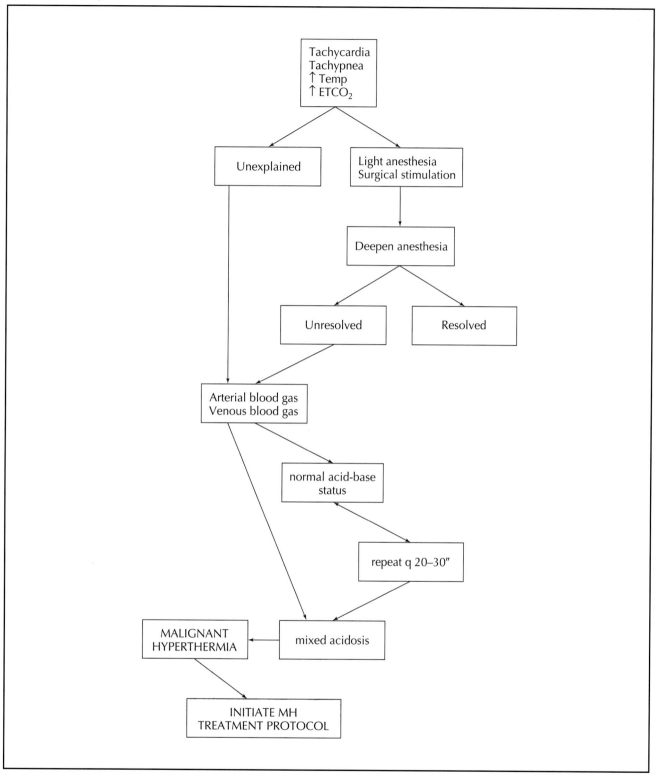

> ## SPECIAL CONSIDERATION:
>
> Laryngospasm is a frequent occurrence in the pediatric age group, especially in children undergoing otolaryngological procedures.

Finally, skilled nursing care in conjunction with a surgical and anesthesia team which is readily available in the postanesthesia care unit is essential because of the possibility of perioperative airway complications. High acuity observation for seemingly routine procedures is often indicated based on concerns about airway swelling or abnormal ventilatory control in the perioperative period.

> ## AT A GLANCE. . .
>
> Masseter Muscle Spasm
>
> **Pathogenesis:** following administration of succinylcholine during induction of anesthesia with a volatile anesthetic
>
> **Adverse Effects:** inability to intubate the trachea, difficulty in maintaining ventilation by mask, hypoxemia, myalgia and weakness may be present for as long as 36 hours after the acute episode, elevation of creatine kinase and myoglobinuria can follow within 24 hours, may be related in some cases to susceptibility to malignant hyperthermia
>
> **Symptoms and Signs:** subjective difficulty in opening the mouth, administration of additional succinylcholine does not result in relaxation of the masseter muscles, other skeletal muscles are typically relaxed although there may be contracture in other muscle groups as well
>
> **Diagnosis:** physical exam and findings during anesthetic administration, tea-colored urine, elevated creatine kinase, elevated end tidal CO_2, hypoxia, hypercarbia, tachycardia, arrhythmias
>
> **Treatment:** maintain positive pressure ventilation with bag and mask until the masseter muscles relax, intubate the trachea whenever it becomes feasible to do so, observe the patient carefully for signs of malignant hyperthermia (MH); if MH is developing or is strongly suspected, declare an MH emergency and treat accordingly; consider aborting surgery, continue anesthetizing with a nontriggering technique; if there is no evidence of MH, recent studies support continuing the anesthetic

ANESTHETIC CONSIDERATIONS FOR SPECIFIC OTOLARYNGOLOGIC PROCEDURES

Tonsillectomy alone or in conjunction with adenoidectomy, is one of the most common pediatric surgical procedures and is, at the same time, fraught with the potential for risk. Although recurrent tonsillitis and missed school days have commonly been reasons for tonsillectomy in school-age children, tonsillectomy at an earlier age for lymphoid hyperplasia and obstructive sleep apnea is becoming increasingly more common in pediatric cases.[43-45] Sequelae of chronic upper airway obstruction may include pulmonary hypertension, cardiomegaly, right ventricular hypertrophy, or right heart failure.[46-50] Such patients may experience daytime somnolence, behavioral problems, snoring, and frequent diaphoresis, and should be admitted to the intensive care unit postoperatively. Serious complications such as pulmonary edema and prolonged postoperative oxyhemoglobin desaturation have been found to occur following tonsillectomy and adenoidectomy in children with upper airway obstruction who were born prematurely and who have evidence of abnormal facial development or of respiratory distress preoperatively.[51] Anesthetic implications for patients with a significant history of chronic upper airway obstruction include airway irritability on induction; systemic and pulmonary hypertension, particularly in the setting of hypoxia and hypercarbia; delayed awakening; and abnormalities in ventilatory control. Difficult intubation should be anticipated for peritonsillar abscess, extreme lymphoid hyperplasia, or in the presence of a lingual tonsil. Finally, post-tonsillectomy bleeding may occur on the day of surgery or a week later anesthetic problems include a full stomach and hypovolemia.

Otologic conditions, both minor and major, form another large proportion of otolaryngologic procedures. Anesthetic considerations that are common to minor and major otologic procedures include the likelihood of multiple prior procedures and the potential for significant patient and family apprehension. Hearing may be impaired, thereby making communication and reassurance difficult. Parents can be extremely helpful in this circumstance, particularly if the child uses sign language for communication. Most patients undergoing myringotomy and tube procedures are anesthetized with an inhalation anesthetic, often with their parents present so that premedication can be avoided, and the anesthetic is usually accomplished without an IV line (which is nevertheless readily available). Most patients have stigmata of an upper respiratory infection, although parents typically report that this is the child's normal, baseline state. If the child's temperature is normal, if he or she is playful and active, and if he or she has a normal chest exam, then most anesthesiologists would proceed at this point. The anesthesiologist should be aware of patients who have congenital defects such as hemifacial microsomia, cleft palate, Pierre Robin anomaly, and Trisomy 21, which predispose them to recurrent otitis because they therefore return for multiple myringotomy and tube procedures. Such patients have additional special considerations for anesthetic management, including the potential for difficult airways or associated congenital heart disease.

SPECIAL CONSIDERATION:

Chronic upper airway congestion, the presence of congenital defects, and concerns about bleeding are all factors that must be considered when anesthetizing a child for an ear operation.

For major otologic procedures, such as tympanoplasty or tympanomastoidectomy, even a small amount of bleeding may interfere with surgery. The anesthesiologist may make a significant contribution to decreasing bleeding through the use of a spontaneous breathing technique, which will lower the mean airway pressure and thereby the venous pressure in the head and neck. In addition, hypotensive techniques that are directed toward lowering the mean arterial pressure by 15 to 20% from baseline may be helpful. Useful medications for this technique include labetalol in titrated doses of 50 to 100 μg/kg until the desired effect is produced. A modest (e.g., 15 degrees head-up position is helpful for lowering arterial and venous pressures and for promoting venous drainage. Because vasoconstrictor drugs such as epinephrine are often infiltrated in the surgi-

cal field, it is useful for the anesthesiologist to avoid halothane and use instead an agent less prone to ventricular ectopy, such as any of the methyl-ethyl ethers (enflurane, isoflurane, sevoflurane, desflurane). The procedures themselves can be lengthy, and concerns about the potential for alveolar collapse and worsening of shunting during prolonged spontaneous ventilation are legitimate; however, this does not appear to be a problem for healthy children, in whom it is easy to perform noninvasive monitoring with pulse oximetry and end tidal CO_2 analysis. In addition, we add 5 to 10 cm H_2O CPAP to the breathing circuit in an effort to minimize alveolar collapse. Oxygen saturation, as measured by pulse oximetry, is an excellent guide to shunting; occasionally, a "sigh" breath delivered manually may be required. Postoperative nausea and vomiting secondary to labyrinthine disturbance is common, and the preemptive use of medications and techniques that are known to have an antiemetic effect is indicated and should be addressed in the preoperative interview. Such medications and techniques include propofol as an intravenous (IV) induction agent or as a continuous infusion in low doses; ondansetron; metoclopramide; and IV droperidol; and the avoidance of nitrous oxide throughout the surgical procedure. Nitrous oxide is discontinued following the positioning of the graft during tympanoplasty because of its tendency to diffuse into gas-filled spaces. Deep extubation, as mentioned in the section on fundamental considerations is an effective strategy for avoiding coughing and bucking, particularly following tympanoplasty and graft placement.

Nasal surgery or transnasal surgery (e.g., *functional endoscopic sinus surgery* [FESS]) usually requires the application of topical vasoconstrictors, all of which may be associated with tachycardia, hypertension, and occasionally dysrhythmias. Physiologic consequences of systemic absorption of nasally-applied vasoconstrictors should be carefully monitored; occasionally, anesthetic agents or techniques have to be changed, or severe intraoperative hypertension has to be treated with vasodilators. Children with nasal polyps have blocked nasal airways, which may make them less comfortable with an inhalation induction of anesthesia. In addition, their nasal polyps may be associated with asthma or cystic fibrosis, so a careful history, physical exam, administration of their usual bronchodilators preoperatively, and the ready availability of bronchodilators intraoperatively is required. Transnasal FESS is frequently utilized in patients with recurrent sinusitis, immunoglobulin deficiencies, asthma, and cystic fibrosis.[52-55] All benefit from an anesthetic plan that addresses the need for perioperative antitussive and antiemetic medications. Frequently, patients require sedation for several hours after FESS to decrease struggling, lower venous pressure, and minimize bleeding.

Children with *choanal atresia* may experience respiratory distress immediately after birth because of their inability to breathe nasally. In addition, babies with the CHARGE association may have midface dysmorphism with other anomalies, including congenital heart disease, growth and mental retardation, ear anomalies, genitourinary abnormalities, and genital hypoplasia. If respiratory distress occurs, the mid-facial dysmorphism may make a mask difficult to fit as well as make tracheal intubation difficult. Additional anesthetic implications include the systemic consequences of chronic upper airway obstruction, the possibility of associated congenital heart disease, and the psychologic stress of frequent returns to the operating room for surgical procedures.

Aerodigestive tract *endoscopy* may be required for diagnostic or therapeutic purposes. *Laryngoscopy* may be required for evaluation of congenital or acquired disease of the laryngeal inlet, vocal cord dysfunction, hoarseness, or stridor. *Bronchoscopy* may be required for evaluation of functional or anatomic abnormalities of the tracheobronchial tree or as a follow-up to prior surgical intervention.

Esophagoscopy is most typically required for foreign body extraction in the toddler, although this problem may be encountered in any age group and is dependent on particular circumstances such as developmental delay, intrinsic esophageal disease, or accidental ingestion in an otherwise healthy patient. The child with chronic digestive tract problems may have undergone repeated esophagoscopies and thus be very apprehensive. In small infants, the passage of an esophagoscope may compress the trachea and obstruct ventilation, even when an endotracheal tube is in place. Coughing or other movements can result in esophageal perforation; therefore, patients must be adequately anesthetized to maintain complete immobility. A lower esophageal stricture or achalasia may result in esophageal dilation proximally; food and secretions accumulated in the dilated segment may be aspirated during anesthesia. Perioperatively, the operating team has to be alert for signs of esophageal perforation, especially if during the endoscopy difficulty was encountered.

Some patients scheduled for bronchoscopy and laryngoscopy will have chronic lung disease and a preexisting tracheotomy. Chronic lung disease is a significant risk factor for perioperative complications related to endoscopic procedures, and the anesthesiologist should anticipate shunting (impaired efficiency of oxygenation), alterations in normal dead space to tidal volume ratio (V_d/V_t), alterations in normal pulmonary mechanics (obstructive or restrictive lung disease), and bronchorrhea. Superimposed on these chronic problems may be difficulty in maintaining ventilation during airway endoscopy, which is a problem particularly in children with a very small airway and when an optical telescope is inserted through a bronchoscope, possibly making positive pressure ventilation, elimination of delivered breaths, and oxygenation far less effective. Spontaneous breathing in this circumstance may be advantageous because patients can breathe around as well as through the bronchoscope. Transpharyngeal oxygen insufflation and examination with only a telescope through the native airway may also permit improved oxygenation in a spontaneously breathing patient by allowing for the greater diameter of the natural airway. Adequate topical anesthesia is immensely helpful in deafferenting airway reflexes. Following induction of anesthesia we use lidocaine, 5 mg/kg (infants receive a 1%, children <12 years old a 2%, and children >12 years old a 4% concentration) delivered through a styletted topical anesthesia kit (Fig. 2–3) during direct laryn-

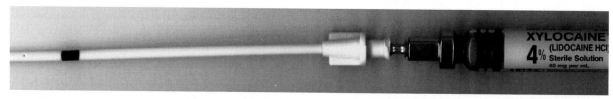

Figure 2–3:   Topical anesthesia kit (Duo-Trach,® Astra, Westborough, MA). The fenestrations along the delivery tube are more effective than a supraglottic atomizer in distributing the local anesthetic from the deep oropharynx through the laryngeal inlet to the subglottic space.

goscopy. The fenestrations along the delivery tube are more effective than a supraglottic atomizer in distributing the local anesthetic from the deep oropharynx through the laryngeal inlet to the subglottic space.

AT A GLANCE. . .

Anesthesia for Aspiration of A Foreign Body

Pathogenesis: food, beads, pins, tacks, coins, parts of toys found by a curious toddler, tooth dislodged during airway manipulation, surgical material left in the airway after a surgical procedure

Adverse Effects: pneumonia, airway rupture, hypoxemia, hypercarbia, hemoptysis, bronchospasm, pneumothorax

Symptoms and Signs: cough, dyspnea, cyanosis, decreased breath sounds, tachypnea, stridor, wheezing, hemoptysis, hoarseness, fever, aphonia, radiographic visualization of the foreign body or air trapping, infiltrates, or atelectasis

Diagnosis: physical examination looking for symmetry of breath sounds and bronchospasm; radiographic diagnosis looking for a foreign body, air trapping, atelectasis, pneumonia

Treatment: preoxygenation, immediate availability of rigid bronchoscope, inhalation induction with volatile anesthetic, 100% oxygen and spontaneous breathing, topical anesthesia to larynx, intubation of the trachea with a ventilating bronchoscope to remove the foreign body, facilitate passage of the foreign body through the laryngeal inlet using deep inhalation anesthesia or muscle relaxant, repeat bronchoscopy to evaluate for further trauma or mucosal damage, awaken via native airway or intubate and awaken

---

The possibility of complete airway obstruction during some procedures, such as foreign body removal, has to be anticipated. Procedural alternatives such as emergency rigid bronchoscopic intubation, advancement of a foreign body into a mainstem bronchus, instillation of intratracheal dilute epinephrine as a vasoconstrictor to try to extract the foreign body, tracheotomy to extract the foreign

body if it cannot be passed retrograde through the vocal cords, or thoracotomy and bronchotomy all have to be part of the plan to a greater or lesser extent. Identifying the laterality of the foreign body is crucial for anesthetic management, inasmuch as an endobronchial foreign body may be coughed into a more proximal position in the airway, and consideration should be given to anesthetic induction with the affected side dependent. Deep inhalation anesthesia with spontaneous breathing or a short-acting neuromuscular blocking agent may be necessary to extract a foreign body retrograde through the larynx. Both check-valve and ball-valve mechanisms may lead to postobstructive pulmonary edema due to transudation of lung fluid following removal of the intraluminal obstruction. (see Fig. 2–4) Often subtle in its presentation, postobstructive pulmonary edema may reveal itself subclinically as persistently low oxygen saturations in the setting of adequate patient efforts at spontaneous ventilation or seemingly adequate positive pressure ventilation.[56-59] Such postobstructive pulmonary edema in children is usually rapidly responsive to diuretics (e.g., furosemide), 100% oxygen, and CPAP by mask or positive pressure ventilation by endotracheal tube. Postoperative reduction in the airway lumen by subglottic edema as a result of multiple bronchoscopic exams is helped by the preemptive administration of decadron (0.25–1 mg/kg IV) and racemic epinephrine in the postanesthesia care unit, although patients should be watched carefully for recurrence.

Although it may be prudent to avoid preoperative sedation in children with obstruction of the aerodigestive tract, a very upset and frightened child may present an equally dangerous situation because of aerophagia, which may cause a stormy induction of anesthesia and an increased risk of laryngospasm or bronchospasm with attendant hypoxemia, hypercarbia, and dysrhythmias. Reassurance, a calm style, the presence of a parent, and a carefully titrated premedication may help to make the induction smoother. In anticipation of aerodigestive tract manipulation, administration of an antisialagogue such as glycopyrrolate is useful. The usual monitors are applied and spontaneous breathing, following an IV or inhalation induction, is typically maintained. Once the patient is asleep, nitrous oxide, if used, may be discontinued and the anesthetic continued with halothane or sevoflurane in 100% oxygen. It is possible to continue with enflurane or isoflurane, but in general, these inhalation anesthetics are more

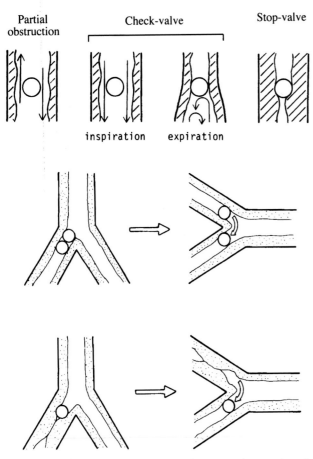

Figure 2–4: (A) Mechanisms of airway obstruction. In partial obstruction, air can enter and exit, but its passage may be delayed. In the check-valve, air is able to enter the lung during inspiration, but dynamic airway compression results in obstruction during expiration, producing obstructive emphysema. In the stop-valve, air cannot enter, and obstructive atelectasis results. (B) Mechanisms of bilateral bronchial obstruction following foreign body aspiration. If two objects are in the right mainstem bronchus, one of them can enter the opposite bronchus, if the patient assumes the left lateral decubitus position. If there is swelling distal to a foreign body, should that foreign body become dislodged and enter the opposite bronchus, total obstruction may result. (From reference 68, with permission.)

irritating to airways because of their greater pungency and are less well tolerated by children than halothane or sevoflurane.[60-62] After the patient is deeply anesthetized using the signs previously described, laryngoscopy and topical anesthesia via the supraglottic larynx is accomplished and the mask is replaced until the lidocaine becomes effective (2–3 minutes). During the endoscopy, oxygen and halothane or sevoflurane may be insufflated into the pharynx. Scavenging is performed with an open suction tube at the corner of the mouth.

AT A GLANCE...

Anesthesia for Stridor Evaluation

Pathogenesis: *Infantile Stridor:* congenital or acquired laryngeal, subglottic, or tracheal stenosis; edema; laryngomalacia or tacheomalacia; vocal cord paralysis; hereditary angioneurotic edema. *Noninfantile Stridor:* trauma, infection, laryngeal edema, tumor, foreign body

Adverse Effects: hypoxemia, hypercarbia, pneumothorax, pneumomediastinum, cardiac arrest

Symptoms and Signs: noisy respirations especially during inspiration, paradoxical inward chest wall movement during inspiration, decreased or low O_2 saturation, cyanosis, hypercarbia

Diagnosis: physical exam, chest x-ray

Treatment: administer 100% oxygen, attempt to improve airflow across the obstructed segment (employ standard airway maneuvers such as jaw thrust, oral or nasal airway insertion, apply CPAP), preserve spontaneous breathing if at all possible to enhance laminar flow, clear the airway of secretions, provide spontaneous breathing conditions to evaluate dynamic airway changes during negative inspiratory breaths, topical anesthesia to larynx, prepare to establish an airway by invasive means if oxygenation cannot be maintained, use steroids to decrease airway edema

---

Otolaryngological surgery with the *laser* requires specific knowledge about laser safety, airway requirements, and ventilation via the suspension laryngoscope. We most often use the CO_2 laser for childhood glottic lesions such as juvenile laryngeal papillomatosis, subglottic stenosis, subglottic hemangioma, glottic web, subglottic neoplasms, vocal cord nodules, or lymphangiomas.[63] Anesthetic induction techniques are dictated primarily by the patient's developmental needs, as long as respiratory distress is not a significant preoperative consideration. Symptomatic patients may still undergo an inhalation induction, but their induction time may be quite uncharacteristically prolonged. A variety of ventilatory options are available, broadly characterized into "no tube" and "tube" techniques. Spontaneous ventilation without an endotracheal tube fails to offer complete control of the airway or protection from apnea or laryngospasm, but is certainly done safely.[64] Venturi ventilation is an excellent alternative for us. An injection needle is secured to a straight blade laryngoscope and oxygen is forced through the needle by high pressure using through a variable pressure-reducing valve while entraining room air. Muscle relaxation provides the surgeon with an unobstructed view and a motionless field and the anesthesiologist with maximal chest wall compliance. The tracheas of infants and young children can be intubated with a standard polyvinyl-chloride tube in order to secure the airway while the operating table is turned and the suspension laryngoscope is placed. Following confirmation of laryngoscope placement and the aim of the injector, the trachea is extubated and insufflation pressure delivered through the injector is titrated incrementally with the variable pressure-reducing valve to clinical assessment of the adequacy of chest wall excursion by 2 psi per several breaths, beginning at 6 psi for infants, at about 12 psi for school-age children, and at 18 psi for teenagers. *It is critical to decompress the jet ventilation system and adjust the inflation pressure on the valve prior to mounting the injector on the suspension laryngoscope and delivering the first breath.* As an alternative, or when jet ventilation is not feasible, a red rubber, endotracheal tube wrapped with metal foil, nonmetal laser tubes, or metal endotracheal tubes may be employed. Tube techniques have the advantage of a secure airway and the disadvantage of a partially obstructed view for the endoscopist. If a jet ventilation technique is chosen, then total IV anesthesia is required; our typical choice is propofol at 150–250 μg/kg/min by continuous infusion, in order to avoid inhalation techniques in an unscavenged airway.

Precautions for working with the laser include eye protection for patient and staff and reduced concentrations of oxygen through the breathing circuit. Inasmuch as nitrous oxide also supports combustion, its addition is of no significant benefit in reducing the risk of oxygen use; air is a better choice. The risks of pneumothorax and pneumomediastinum during jet ventilation should be kept in mind, as well as the risks of airway fire while working with the medical laser.[65]

REFERENCES

1. Derrington M, Smith G. A review of studies of anaesthetic risk, morbidity and mortality. Br J Anaesth 1987; 59:815–833.
2. Tiret L, Nivoche Y, Hatton F, Desmonts JM, Vourc'h G. Complications related to anaesthesia in infants and children. A prospective survey of 40,240 anaesthetics. Br J Anaesth 1988; 61:263–269.
3. Holzman R. Morbidity and mortality in pediatric anesthesia. Pediatr Clin North Am 1994; 41:239–256.
4. Keenan RL, Shapiro JH, Dawson K. Frequency of anesthetic cardiac arrests in infants: Effect of pediatric anesthesiologists. J Clin Anesth 1991; 3:433–437.
5. Olsson GL, Hallen B. Laryngospasm during anaesthesia. A computer-aided incidence study in 136,929 patients. Acta Anaesth Scand 1984; 28:567–575.
6. Olsson GL. Bronchospasm during anaesthesia. A computer-aided incidence study of 136,929 patients. Acta Anaesth Scand 1987; 31:244–252.
7. Korsch B. The child and the operating room. Anesthesiology 1975; 43:251.
8. Greenspan S. Clinical assessment of emotional milestones in infancy and early childhood. Pediatr Clin North Am 1991; 38:1371–1385.
9. Licamele W, Goldberg R. Childhood reactions to illness and hospitalization. Am Fam Physician 1987; 36:227–232.
10. Perrin E, Perrin J. Clinicians' assessments of children's understanding of illness. Am J Dis Child 1983; 137:874–878.
11. Krahl V. *Anatomy of The Mammalian Lung.* Washington, DC: American Physiological Society, 1964, pp. 213–284.
12. Patton D, Hanna B. Postnatal maturation of baroreflex heart rate control in neonatal swine. Can J Cardiol 1994; 10:233–238.
13. Blanco C, Dawes G, Hanson M, McCooke H. Carotid baroreceptors in fetal and newborn sheep. Pediatr Res 1988; 24:342–346.
14. Holden K, Morgan J, Krauss A, and Auld P. Incomplete baroreceptor responses in newborn infants. Am J Perinatal 1985; 2:31–34.
15. Wear R, Robinson S, Gregory G. The effect of halothane on the baroresponse of adult and baby rabbits. Anesthesiology 1982; 56:188.
16. Murat I, Lapeyre G, Saint-Maurice C. Isoflurane attenuates baroreflex control of heart rate in human neonates. Anesthesiology 1989; 70:395–400.

17. Murat I, Levron J, Berg A, Saint Maurice C. Effects of fentanyl on baroreceptor reflex control of heart rate in newborn infants. Anesthesiology 1988; 68:717-722.

18. Klitzner T, Friedman W. Excitation-contraction coupling in developing mammalian myocardium: Evidence from voltage clamp studies. Pediatr Res 1988; 23:428-432.

19. Klitzner T, Friedman W. A diminished role for the sarcoplasmic reticulum in newborn myocardial contraction: Effects of ryanodine. Pediatr Res 1989; 26:98-101.

20. Chin T, Friedman W, Klitzner T. Developmental changes in cardiac myocyte calcium regulation. Circ Res 1990; 67:574-579.

21. Chen F, Wetzel G, Friedman W, and Klitzner. ATP-sensitive potassium channels in neonatal and adult rabbit ventricular myocytes. Pediatr Res 1992; 32:230-235.

22. Resnick MD, Bearman PS, Blum R, et al. Protecting adolescents from harm. Findings from the National Longitudinal Study on Adolescent Health. JAMA 1997; 278:823-832.

23. Anonymous. Health risk behaviors among adolescents who do and do not attend school—United States, 1992. MMWR 1994; 43:129-132.

24. Kann L, Warren W, Collins J, Ross J, Collins B, Kolbe L. Results from the national school-based 1991 Young Risk Behavior Survey and progress toward achieving related health objectives for the nation. Public Health Rep 1993; 108 (suppl):47-55.

25. Hanks E, Ngai S, Fink B. The respiratory threshold during halothane anesthesia. Anesthesiology 1961; 22:393-397.

26. Patel R, Hannallah R, Norden J, Casey W, Verghese S. Emergence airway complications in children: A comparison of tracheal extubation in awake and deeply anesthetized patients. Anesth Analg 1991; 73:266-270.

27. Karam R, Najm J, Kattar M, Raphael N. Respiratory complications in children emerging from halothane anesthesia-awake vs deep extubation. Mid East J Anesth 1995; 13:221-229.

28. Pounder D, Blackstock D, Steward D. Tracheal extubation in children: Halothane versus isoflurane, anesthetized versus awake. Anesthesiology 1991; 74:653-655.

29. Cohen M, Cameron C. Should you cancel the operation when a child has an upper respiratory tract infection? Anesth Analg 1991; 72:282-288.

30. Tait AR, Knight PR. The effects of general anesthesia on upper respiratory tract infections in children. Anesthesiology 1987; 67:930-935.

31. Empey D, Laitinen L, Jacobs L, Gold W, Nadel J. Mechanisms of bronchial hyperreactivity in normal subjects after upper respiratory tract infection. Am Rev Resp Dis 1976; 113:131-139.

32. Fryer A, Jacoby D. Parainfluenza virus infection damages inhibitory M2 muscarinic receptors on pulmonary parasympathetic nerves in the guinea-pig. Br J Pharm 1991; 102:267-271.

33. Jacoby D, Tamaoki J, Borson D, Nadel J. Influenza infection causes airway hyperresponsiveness by decreasing enkephalinase. J App Physiol 1988; 64:2653-2658.

34. Carroll J. Increased incidence of masseter spasm in children with strabismus anesthetized with halothane and succinylcholine. Anesthesiology 1987; 67:559-561.

35. Schwartz L, Rockoff MA, Koka BV. Masseter spasm with anesthesia: Incidence and implications. Anesthesiology 1984; 61:772-775.

36. Gronert GA. Management of patients in whom trismus occurs following succinylcholine. Anesthesiology 1988; 68:653-655.

37. Rosenberg H. Management of patients in whom trismus occurs following succinylcholine. Anesthesiology 1988; 68:654-655.

38. Van der Spek A, Fang W, Ashton-Miller J, Stohler C, Carlson D, Schork M. Increased masticatory muscle stiffness during limb muscle flaccidity associated with succinylcholine administration. Anesthesiology 1988; 69:11-16.

39. van der Spek A, Reynolds P, Fang W, Ashton Miller J, Stohler C, Schork M. Changes in resistance to mouth opening induced by depolarizing and non-depolarizing neuromuscular relaxants. Br J Anaesth 1990; 64:21-27.

40. Littleford JA, Patel LR, Bose D, Cameron CB, McKillop C. Masseter muscle spasm in children: Implications of continuing the triggering anesthetic. Anesth Analg 1991; 72:151.

41. Hannallah R, Kaplan R. Jaw relaxation after a halothane/succinylcholine sequence in children. Anesthesiology 1994; 81:99-103.

42. O'Flynn R, Shutack J, Rosenberg H, Fletcher J. Masseter muscle rigidity and malignant hyperthermia susceptibility in pediatric patients-an update on management and diagnosis. Anesthesiology 1994; 80:1228-1233.

43. Brodsky L. Modern assessment of tonsils and adenoids. Pediatr Clin North Am 1989; 36:1551-1569.

44. Berkowitz R, Zalzal G. Tonsillectomy in children under 3 years of age. Arch Otolaryngol Head Neck Surg 1990; 116:685-686.

45. Lieberman A, Tal A, Brama I, Sofer S. Obstructive sleep apnea in young infants. Int J Pediatr Otorhinolaryngol 1988; 16:39-44.

46. Theolade R, Seibert R, Goerlich E, et al. Obstructive sleep apnea syndrome and cardiovascular diseases. (French) Syndrome d'apnees obstructives du som-

meil (SAOS) et pathologies cardiovasculaires. Ann Cardiol Angeiol 1995; 44:507–516.

47. Schafer H, Koehler U, Hasper E, Ewig S, Luderitz B. Sleep apnea and cardiovascular risk. (German) Schlafapnoe und kardiovaskulares Risiko. Zeit Kardiol 1995; 84:871–884.

48. Wiegand L, Zwillich C. Obstructive sleep apnea. Disease A Month 1994; 40:197–252.

49. Hunt C, Brouillette R. Abnormalities of breathing control and airway maintenance in infants and children as a cause of cor pulmonale. Pediatr Cardiol 1982; 3:249–256.

50. Krieger J, Sforza E, Apprill M, Lampert E, Weitzenblum E, Ratomaharo S. Pulmonary hypertension, hypoxemia, and hypercapnia in obstructive sleep apnea patients. Chest 1989; 96:729–737.

51. McGowan F, Kenna M, Fleming J, O'Connor T. Adenotonsillectomy for upper airway obstruction carries increased risk in children with a history of prematurity. Pediatr Pulm 1992; 13:222–226.

52. Duplechain J, White J, Miller R. Pediatric sinusitis. The role of endoscopic sinus surgery in cystic fibrosis and other forms of sinonasal disease. Arch Otolaryngol Head Neck Surg 1991; 117:422–426.

53. Parsons D, Phillips S. Functional endoscopic surgery in children: A retrospective analysis of results. Laryngoscope 1993; 103:899–903.

54. Bolt R, de Vries N, Middelweerd R. Endoscopic sinus surgery for nasal polyps in children: Results. Rhinology 1995; 33:148–151.

55. Nishioka G, Barbero G, Konig P, Parsons D, Cook P, Davis W. Symptom outcome after functional endoscopic sinus surgery in patients with cystic fibrosis: A prospective study. Otolaryngol Head Neck Surg 1995; 113:440–445.

56. Galvis A, Stool S, Bluestone C. Pulmonary edema following relief of acute upper airway obstruction. Ann Otol Rhinol Laryngol 1980; 89:124–128.

57. Kanter R, Watchko J. Pulmonary edema associated with upper airway obstruction. Am J Dis Child 1984; 138:356–358.

58. Herrick I, Mahendran B, Penny F. Postobstructive pulmonary edema following anesthesia. J Clin Anesth 1990; 2:116–120.

59. Goldenberg J, Portugal L, Wenig B, Weingarten R. Negative-pressure pulmonary edema in the otolaryngology patient. Otolaryngol Head Neck Surg 1997; 117:62–66.

60. Fisher DM, Robinson S, Brett CM, Perin G, Gregory GA. Comparison of enflurane, halothane, and isoflurane for diagnostic and therapeutic procedures in children with malignancies. Anesthesiology 1985; 63:647–650.

61. Eger EI. New inhaled anesthetics. Anesthesiology 1994; 80:906.

62. Holzman R, van der Velde M, Kaus S, et al. Sevoflurane depresses myocardial contractility less than halothane during induction of anesthesia in children. Anesthesiology 1996; 85:1260–1267.

63. Holzman R. Anesthesia for pediatric subglottic laser surgery. Surv Anes 1991; 35:191.

64. Quintal M, Cunningham M, Ferrari L. Tubeless spontaneous respiration technique for pediatric microlaryngeal surgery. Arch Otolaryngol Head Neck Surg 1997; 123:209–214.

65. Sosis M. Anesthesia for airway laser surgery. In: Sosis M, ed. *Anesthesia Equipment Manual.* Philadelphia: Lippincott-Raven, 1997, pp. 279–291.

66. Holzman R. Pediatric anesthesia equipment. In: Sosis M, ed. *Anesthesia Equipment Manual.* Philadelphia: Lippincott-Raven, 1997, pp. 195–217.

67. Benumof J. Laryngeal mask airway and the ASA difficult airway algorithm. Anesthesiology 1996; 84:686–699.

68. Berry F. *Anesthetic Management of Difficult and Routine Pediatric Patients.* New York: Churchill Livingstone, 1986, pp. 221–222.

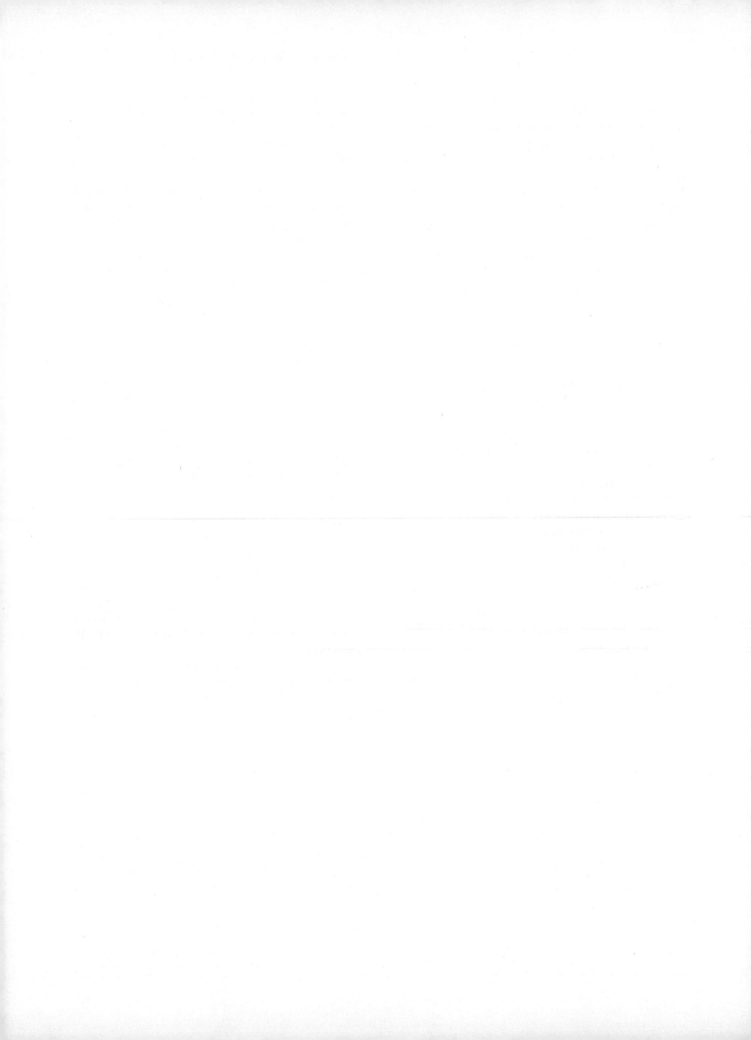

3 Role of Allergy and Immunologic Dysfunction in Upper Respiratory Diseases

Thomas F. Smith

Inflammation of the upper respiratory tract (URT) primarily denotes alteration in the mucosa lining one or more of the structures thereof, including the nasal cavity, paranasal sinuses, eustachian tube (ET), and middle-ear cleft. The alteration that occurs is dependent both on the cause of the inflammation and on host responsiveness. Common causes of URT inflammation include viral infections, exposure to airborne irritants such as chemicals and inert or organic particles in the air, and allergic reactions. Uncommon causes include drugs such as α-adrenergic antagonists or oral contraceptives, endocrine abnormalities such as hypothyroidism, and systemic immunologic diseases such as Wegener's granulomatosis (WG) or sarcoidosis. URT inflammation may occur in the absence of an identifiable cause, as occurs in eosinophilic nonallergic rhinitis and vasomotor rhinitis. Bacterial or fungal infection of the URT certainly may perpetuate mucosal inflammation, but these usually occur as a consequence of pre-existing inflammation from another cause. Immunodeficiency is an uncommon cause of persistent or recurrent URT infections in children. This chapter discusses the role of allergy in causing URT inflammation [e.g., rhinitis, sinusitis, or otitis media (OM)]. It also describes when and how to consider immunodeficiency in patients with URT diseases.

ALLERGY IN URT DISEASES

General Considerations

Allergic respiratory diseases are very common. The annual prevalence of seasonal allergic rhinitis in population studies varies from 5 to 22%.[1] It has been estimated that 9% of all visits to physicians' offices are for one of the common allergic diseases. Production of immunoglobulin E (IgE)-class antibodies is known to trigger the mechanism of the allergic response. There likely are multiple genetic determinants of total IgE levels and specific responses to allergens, and clinical phenotype may be due to the interaction between each of these genes and environmental exposures.[2] More than 90% of patients with a history of clinical symptoms and IgE-specific antibodies have an immediate response to allergen exposure.[3] Although IgE-specific antibodies occur in patients with asymptomatic sensitivity to common allergens, several studies indicate that such patients are likely to develop clinical symptoms from allergen exposure over time.[4,5] Also, generation of IgE-specific antibodies requires repeated exposure to significant amounts of allergen. Children are not sensitized before exposure to a given allergen unless they have been sensitized to a cross-reacting allergen. They are highly unlikely to become sensitized to low levels of outdoor aeroallergens, to high levels of outdoor aeroallergens during their first (or second) season of exposure, or to intermittent brief exposure to high levels of indoor aeroallergens.

> **SPECIAL CONSIDERATION:**
>
> More than 90% of patients with a history of clinical symptoms and IgE-specific antibodies have an immediate response to allergen exposure.

Pediatric Otolaryngology, Edited by R.F. Wetmore, H.R. Muntz, and T.J. McGill. Thieme Medical Publishers, Inc., New York © 2000.

It also should be noted that URT diseases cause significant morbidity in children beyond the obvious symptoms of acute illness. Rhinitis may cause sleep disturbance and daytime fatigue and may impair learning, school performance, skilled performance, and reaction time (which is essential in children on bicycles or roller blades); antihistamines may impair these even further.[6-10] Rhinitis and OM also may impact hearing and speech. Thus, adequate therapy of chronic or recurrent URT symptoms in children is crucial.

Pathophysiology

Allergenic particles that are inhaled into the airway are deposited on mucosal surfaces, where allergen elution and diffusion occur. Allergens that reach and are recognized by specific IgE antibodies bound to receptors on the surface of immunologic cells (primarily mast cells and basophils) cause cross-linking of adjacent IgE molecules. This in turn causes transduction of a signal that results in cell activation and release of mediators of inflammation. Human mast cells store histamine, neutral proteases, many acid hydrolases, cathepsin G, and carboxypeptidase along with heparin preformed in cytoplasmic granules, and these are released rapidly after cell activation. On appropriate stimulation, mast cells may produce lipid mediators such as prostaglandin D_2, leukotriene C_4 (LTC_4) and platelet-activating factor. They also produce a number of cytokines, including interleukin (IL)-4, IL-5, IL-6, IL-8, IL-13, and tumor necrosis factor (TNF)-α.[11] Certain mediators, such as histamine, are rapidly acting and cause immediate symptoms (i.e., the *immediate* or *early phase response*). Others, including some of the cytokines and other chemotactic factors, recruit additional inflammatory cells, which in turn may be activated and release proinflammatory mediators. These recruited cells are responsible for later onset of signs and symptoms of the allergic reaction (i.e., *late phase response*). Ongoing recruitment of inflammatory cells and their effects may result in subacute or chronic inflammation.

It should be noted that there are inflammatory cells other than mast cells present in the normal respiratory mucosa. These include CD1 + Langherans-like cells, Th2-lymphocytes, B-lymphocytes, macrophages, and eosinophils.[12] Allergen induces Th2-lymphocyte proliferation in persons with allergies with the release of their characteristic combination of cytokines, including IL-3, IL-4, IL-5, IL-9, IL-10, and IL-13. These substances promote IgE and mast cell production. Inflammatory mediators and cytokines upregulate endothelial cell adhesion markers, such as vascular cell adhesion molecule 1. Chemoattractants, including eotaxin, IL-5, and RANTES (regulated on activation normal T-cell expressed and secreted), lead to further infiltration by eosinophils, basophils, Th2-lymphocytes, and mast cells.[13]

AT A GLANCE . . .

Inflammatory Cells in the Respiratory Mucosa

- Mast cells
- CD1 + Langherans-like cells
- Th2-lymphocytes
- B-lymphocytes
- Macrophages
- Eosinophils

Eosinophils in particular are increased in the mucosa of allergic patients at baseline and are recruited into the sites of allergic inflammation. Eosinophils also store a number of preformed mediators in cytoplasmic granules; these mediators include major basic protein, eosinophil cationic protein, eosinophil-derived neurotoxin, eosinophil peroxidase, lysosomal hydrolases, and lysophospholipase. On activation, eosinophils may produce lipid mediators such as LTC_4 and lipoxins. They also may produce a large number of cytokines, including IL-1α, IL-2, IL-3, IL-4, IL-5, IL-6, IL-8, IL-10, IL-16, GM-CSF, TNF-α, RANTES, eotaxin, and T-cell growth factor (TGF)-α.[11]

These mediators have profound effects on the respiratory mucosa. Acutely, there may be disruption of the mucosal surface, activation of epithelial cells, increased mucous secretion, alteration of both sol and gel phases of mucus, ciliary dyskinesis or stasis, vascular and mucosal exudation of plasma, and pooling of blood in cavernous sinusoids in the mucosa. The latter is the primary cause of nasal congestion, whereas mucosal edema contributes to ET obstruction. Histamine and perhaps other mediators cause nasal pruritis and sneezing by activation of nerve endings located in epithelial tight junctions. Further mucosal swelling occurs as additional inflammatory cells are recruited. With mucosal injury and accumulation of inflammatory cells, the amount of allergen required to elicit symptoms decreases, which is a phenomenon termed *priming*.[14,15] With ongoing inflammation, there may be loss of surface epithelium, metaplasia or hyperplasia of mucus-producing cells, and thickening of the basement membrane. Chronic inflammation from allergy makes tissues responsive to irritants and other nonspecific stimuli, such as tobacco smoke, strong odors, and air pollution. Allergic inflammation decreases mucociliary clearance of particles,[16] including airborne and resident bacteria, and risk of secondary bacterial infection increases.

Common Allergens

The most common allergens to which children are sensitized are house dust mites. House dust mites are eight-legged, sightless members of the Acaridae subclass of Arachnida. They are microscopic (roughly 0.3 mm in length), feed on skin scales and other debris, and require both warmth and humidity to survive. Mites are found in high concentrations in carpets, mattresses and pillows, and upholstered furniture, where they can withdraw from the surface as humidity on the surface falls. Mite numbers in houses may decrease in the summer or winter when indoor humidity is decreased because of air conditioning, dry heating, and decreased outdoor humidity. Seasonal increases in mite numbers have been documented when houses are opened up in the spring or fall and outdoor humidity is increased. Large amounts of mite allergen are excreted and concentrated in fecal particles, which are roughly 20 μm in diameter. Airborne allergen levels are low in undisturbed rooms but rise immediately with activity in the room.

> ## SPECIAL CONSIDERATION:
> The most common allergens to which children are sensitized are house dust mites.

Children also are commonly sensitized to other allergens in house dust, and exposure to these depends on their home environment. They frequently become allergic to mammals kept indoors as pets, especially cats, but they also may become allergic

to indoor pests such as mice and rats. Children in urban environments frequently are sensitized to cockroaches. Children also may be sensitized to indoor molds, which may be found commonly in basements, around window moldings or plumbing fixtures, in food storage areas, garbage containers, soiled upholstery, and even in kapok and conventional wallpaper.

Children also may become sensitized to outdoor aeroallergens including pollens from trees, grasses, and weeds and outdoor molds. Sensitization to outdoor aeroallergens alone, without concomitant sensitization to indoor allergens, occurs commonly in patients with allergic rhinitis. In a given geographic area, patterns of exposure to these aeroallergens are reasonably predictable. It should be noted that only a minority of flowering plants shed windborne pollen, and of these, even fewer cause clinical symptoms.[17]

Rhinitis is a common symptom in food allergic patients, but rhinitis is rarely the only symptom[18]; it would be highly unusual for a child to have clinically-symptomatic hypersensitivity to a food and experience rhinitis without simultaneous cutaneous or gastrointestinal symptoms.[19-21] Complaints of nasal congestion without other symptoms from ingestion of cow's milk have been confirmed only infrequently by prospective challenge with milk.[19]

Clinical Presentation

Clinical history is important in the diagnosis of allergic disease (Practice Pathway 3-1). Details as to what symptoms are present, when and where symptoms occur, what allergen exposures the patient has, and what things appear to be causing symptoms provide the basis for allergy testing and environmental control measures. Symptoms of allergic rhinitis may include congestion, rhinorrhea, postnasal drip, sneezing, itchy nose, watery eyes, headache, and loss of smell and taste (Table 3-1); however, itching of mucous membranes and repeated

TABLE 3-1: Symptoms of Allergic Rhinitis

Nasal itching*	Watery eyes
Repeated sneezing*	Itchy eyes
Rhinorrhea	Headache
Nasal congestion	Loss of sense of smell
Post-nasal drip	Loss of sense of taste

* Most distinctive complaints associated with allergic rhinitis

Practice Pathway 3–1   DIAGNOSIS AND MANAGEMENT OF RHINITIS

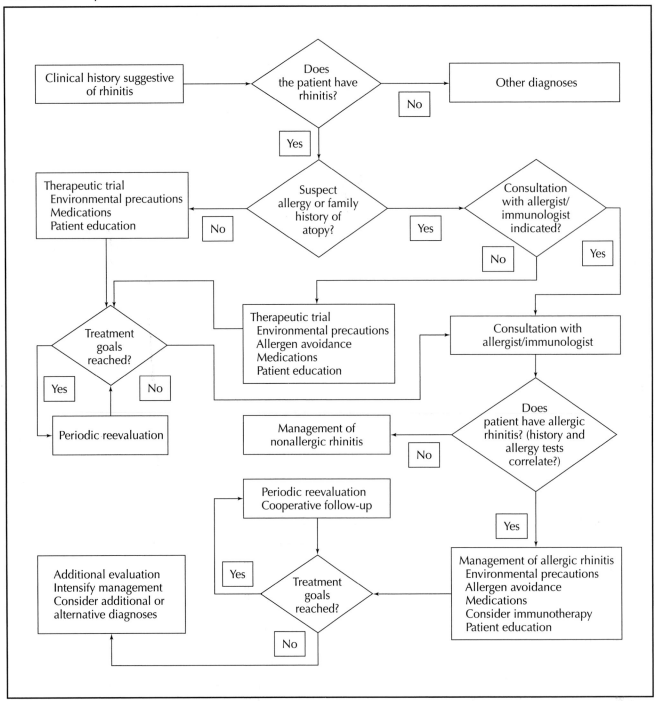

Modified from reference 47, with permission.

sneezing are the most distinctive complaints associated with allergic rhinitis.[17] Consistent symptoms during repeated seasons strongly suggests the presence of allergy as the basis for the symptoms, and the identity of the responsible allergens may be suggested by the season in which they occur. For example, in temperate climates, tree pollens usually are present only in the spring; grass pollen counts usually peak in late spring or early summer; and most weeds pollinate only in the fall until the first frost. Consistent symptoms on repeated exposure also suggest allergy. Symptoms that occur each time the child visits a certain house might be due to exposure to any of the indoor aeroallergens. Increased symptoms from cutting the grass often results from allergy to molds.

Clinical history is less useful in predicting presence of allergy in two circumstances. First, continual environmental allergen exposure may result in chronic, low-grade symptoms without obvious cause-and-effect. This is often seen in children who are allergic to indoor aeroallergens to which they have ongoing exposure, such as house dust mites, indoor pets, cockroaches, or molds. In these cases, identifying the cause of the child's symptoms requires a high level of suspicion, documentation of specific sensitivity, and some estimate of the child's exposure.[22] Careful history to inquire about exposures to indoor allergens is essential to the process. Second, allergy to outdoor molds is sometimes difficult to predict because an isolated "mold season" does not occur,[22] although many molds show distinctive annual trends. Family history of atopy, especially in parents or siblings, also increases the likelihood of current or future allergic sensitization.

Diagnosis of respiratory allergy by physical examination is unreliable. On physical examination, children with nasal allergy often develop dark discoloration beneath the lower eyelids (i.e., "allergic shiners") from chronic periorbital edema and venous stasis, a crease on the lower eyelid (i.e., *Dennie-Morgan line*), or a transnasal crease from an "allergic salute" (i.e., rubbing the nose upward with the palm of the hand).[23] Chronic nasal congestion in childhood and mouth-breathing is thought to contribute to abnormal facial modeling and dental overbite or crossbite. Classically, the nasal mucosa is a pale blue color and appears boggy. Secretions typically are clear, if present. Unfortunately, these physical findings may occur in rhinitis of any etiology and are not specific for allergy.

Allergy by Age of Patient

The likelihood of allergy causing URT symptoms increases with age, and which allergens are likely causes also are age-related. Infants under 6 months of age almost never are sensitized to aeroallergens. Their exposure to indoor aeroallergens usually is minimal, in that their bedding usually is Spartan, what they have usually is exceptionally clean, and they have little if any exposure to other reservoirs of indoor allergens. They have had insufficient exposure to outdoor aeroallergens to become sensitized. By 9 to 10 months of age most infants are crawling, usually on carpeting, with their noses at

or quite near the surface, and their exposure to allergens in the carpeting is considerable. Because of this exposure, crawling infants may become sensitized to mites, animal danders, or less commonly, cockroach or molds. Even so, the prevalence of positive skin tests in infants 1 year of age is quite low. By age 2 years, perhaps as many as 20% of children with chronic respiratory symptoms have developed positive allergy skin tests, which are still usually limited to indoor aeroallergens. By age 3 years, the rare child may have a positive skin test reaction to an outdoor aeroallergen, but in general, sensitization to these allergens occurs uncommonly in preschool children. Prevalence of allergy skin tests increases in school-aged children who have chronic respiratory symptoms and peaks in the second decade of life. School-aged children with recent onset of URT symptoms may have acquired positive skin tests to either indoor or outdoor aeroallergens or both.

SPECIAL CONSIDERATION:

The likelihood of allergy causing URT symptoms increases with age.

Allergy Testing

As noted above, identifying the cause of a child's symptoms requires a high level of suspicion, documentation of specific sensitivity, and some estimate of the child's exposure. Allergy testing in clinical practice has been reviewed previously.[24-26] The goal of allergy testing is to document the involvement of IgE-mediated degranulation of mast cells and basophils in causing or worsening a disease and to identify the allergens involved. No test by itself can replace the rational thinking and clinical acumen of the physician actually dealing with the patient. It is important to order tests and to interpret their results appropriately.

The most common reason allergy testing of children is undertaken probably is to satisfy the curiosity of their parents. In fact, allergy testing is done more appropriately for one or more of the following reasons. First, testing may be done to convince parents to institute specific environmental precautions. In particular, families with indoor warm-blooded pets sometimes may be more willing to remove the pets from the home if the child is found to be skin-test positive to the pet: Second, testing may help predict response to pharmacotherapy. For example, patients with eosinophilic nonallergic rhinitis are more likely to respond to antirhinitis medicines than are those with nonallergic rhinitis.[27] It is possible that this represents a fundamental difference in the pathogenesis of these entities. However, studies of medicine responsiveness rarely require that subjects strictly avoid allergen exposure, and it is the experience from practice that pharmacotherapy without allergen avoidance often produces a suboptimal result. Third, testing to identify a specific allergy is requisite if allergen immunotherapy is to be considered.

AT A GLANCE . . .

Reasons to Perform Allergy Testing

1. Convince parents to institute environmental precautions
2. May help to predict response to pharmacotherapy
3. Identify a specific allergy for immunotherapy

The only hazards of performing allergen testing prematurely are that parents often take negative test results as encouragement not to institute strict environmental control measures (in particular, measures to reduce exposure to house dust mites) or as permission to obtain or keep indoor warm-blooded pets. It is quite clear that indoor allergen exposure results in allergic sensitization in infants and children.[28,29] Strict avoidance measures also should be in place in atopic children before they are sensitized in order to attempt to decrease the chance of sensitization. Negative skin test results to potential pets should be accompanied by three important warnings. First, levels of allergen needed to cause sensitization are higher than those needed to provoke symptoms in someone already sensitized. These sensitizing levels are usually found only in homes with the particular pet, and allergen levels in homes without pets usually are not sufficient to result in sensitization. Thus, the risk of becoming sensitized is decreased by not having the pet indoors, where

allergen accumulates. Second, cat and dog allergens are readily transported on clothing, so that significant levels of both are found in schools, hospitals, homes without pets, and even allergists' offices.[30-32] These levels probably are high enough to cause perennial symptoms in sensitized patients.[33] Last, major cat and dog allergens share IgE epitopes, so that patients sensitized to the allergen from one species may experience symptoms on exposure to the other.[34]

AT A GLANCE . . .

Warnings about Pets

1. Levels of allergen needed to cause sensitization are higher than those needed to provoke symptoms and usually are found only in homes with pets.
2. Cat and dog allergens are found everywhere
3. Patients sensitized to allergen from one species may experience symptoms on exposure to another

---

If allergy testing is undertaken, either in vivo or in vitro, the following points apply. First, allergy testing with materials not shown to be allergenic is unlikely to produce clinically useful information. Availability of a test using a given substance does not necessarily mean that the substance has been shown ever to cause clinical symptoms, much less by IgE-mediated mechanisms. Although contact sensitivity to newsprint may be a rare manifestation of coal-tar allergy,[35] there is no data to suggest that IgE-mediated symptoms result from exposure to it, and this "allergen" is no longer marketed. Results of allergy testing with extracts that are prepared by a clinician or laboratory using materials not proven to be allergens or materials in which allergen content has not been assessed should be interpreted with great caution.

Second, degranulation of mast cells and basophils may be caused by mechanisms other than those that are IgE-dependent.[36] For example, codeine causes histamine release from skin mast cells directly without participation of IgE antibodies, and a positive response to skin testing indicates mast cell reactivity rather than allergy.[37] In the same way, production of a wheal-and-flare reaction by epicutaneous or intradermal application of a suspected allergen does not by itself demonstrate IgE-mediated hypersensitivity.

Third, tests that document the presence of IgE antibodies do not predict necessarily that these antibodies are involved in clinical illness. This is of particular importance, for two reasons. It is quite clear that allergy operates on a dose–response curve. A low level of IgE antibody (which is detected in vivo or in vitro) is less likely to predict a positive response to provocation testing and, presumably, clinical symptoms than is a high level. A test should have threshold criteria both for detection of the analyte and for prediction of clinical significance (a "positive" test). In the same way, it should be noted that exposure to a low level of an allergen (such as house dust mites) may not cause clinical symptoms in an allergic patient, whereas exposure to a high level of the allergen is likely to cause symptoms. Also, positive tests for IgE antibody (in vivo or in vitro) are not correlated necessarily with either current clinical symptoms or provocation test[38,39] and may be found in up to 30% of asymptomatic individuals.[40,41] These discrepancies might be explained by heterogeneity of IgE, in particular its ability to bind histamine-releasing factors.[42]

hood of finding a positive test in the absence of specific clinical evidence to incriminate a test agent. For example, skin testing with shrimp in infants (little chance of exposure), with chrysanthemum (not an aeroallergen) in anyone who does not handle flowers, or with watermelon (uncommon allergen) in anyone without a clearly obvious clinical history is unlikely to yield useful clinical information.

It should be kept in mind that the gold standard for diagnosis of clinically-relevant allergic reactions is double-blind challenge that duplicates natural exposure. No other in vivo test and no in vitro test by itself provides the same information (although either in vivo or in vitro tests may be part of provocation testing).

SPECIAL CONSIDERATION:

Gold standard for diagnosis of clinically-relevant allergic reactions is a double-blind challenge that duplicates natural exposure.

AT A GLANCE . . .

Points to Remember about Allergy Testing

1. Allergy testing with materials not shown to be allergenic is unlikely to produce clinically-useful information

2. Degranulation of mast cells and basophils may be caused by mechanisms other than those that are IgE-dependent

3. Tests that document IgE antibodies do not predict necessarily that these antibodies are involved in clinical illness

4. Testing using agents that are unlikely to cause IgE-mediated symptoms is unlikely to produce positive results

---

Fourth, testing using agents unlikely to cause IgE-mediated symptoms is unlikely to produce positive results. Likelihood of positive response is related both to the likelihood of exposure and the likeli-

Allergy testing of children is most commonly performed by skin testing. Allergy skin testing customarily is accomplished by introducing a small amount of an extract of an allergen into the skin of a patient with suspected allergic symptoms in an attempt to trigger skin mast cells and produce a wheal-and-flare reaction at the site of allergen administration. Skin testing can be accomplished more rapidly and at less cost than alternative methods of testing in vivo or in vitro. Percutaneous (i.e., prick or puncture) skin testing is recommended as the primary test for the diagnosis of IgE-mediated allergic diseases.[43,44] Prick–puncture tests are less sensitive and less reproducible than intradermal tests, but they also correlate better with symptoms and provocation test results.[24] Intradermal testing rarely is warranted for the diagnosis of clinical hypersensitivity to aeroallergens. Prick–puncture testing also is safe; although systemic reactions have been observed,[45] they occur less commonly than with intradermal testing.[46] Skin testing of course must be done with potent extracts, using appropriate allergens, careful technique, and positive and negative controls.

SPECIAL CONSIDERATION:

Prick–puncture tests are less sensitive and less reproducible than intradermal tests, but they correlate better with symptoms and provocation test results.

There has been a proliferation of in vitro tests to diagnose allergy, but the marketing of in vitro tests that are to be performed in physicians' offices and their availability to all physicians through commercial laboratories poses several challenges.[24] First, testing in both settings must be done with strict quality control to monitor precision and changes in bias. Physicians or laboratories who do not understand what is involved in internal quality control and external quality assessment should not be performing allergy testing, either in vivo or in vitro. Second, both in vivo and in vitro testing are readily available to physicians who may not be trained to order or perform these tests and to interpret their results appropriately. A third challenge with in vitro testing is that testing that is available in laboratories remote from the patient may be used inappropriately as the basis for recommendations concerning environmental control, pharmacotherapy, immunotherapy, and other therapeutic procedures. It is inappropriate when these recommendations are made by physicians or others who are not personally involved in the care of the patient.

Total serum level of IgE is correlated with allergy in only a general way. Routine measurement of serum IgE is not a useful screening test for allergy.

SPECIAL CONSIDERATION:

Routine measurement of serum IgE is not a useful screening test for allergy.

Therapy for Allergic URT Symptoms

Three interventions that have been shown to be useful in treating allergic URT symptoms are environmental precautions, pharmacotherapy, and immunotherapy.[47]

Environmental precautions

Environmental precautions should be instituted in all children with chronic respiratory complaints in order to reduce exposure to irritants, avoid exposure to specific allergens to which they are sensitized, and to decrease risk of future sensitization to allergens. Avoidance of indoor allergens is accomplished by removing warm-blooded animals from the home and by instituting control measures for house dust mites, cockroaches, and indoor molds. Outdoor aeroallergens should be kept out of the home by keeping windows closed and using air conditioning or heat to regulate indoor air temperature. There should be no smoking permitted in the child's home, daycare, or transportation.

Pharmacotherapy

For children who have persistent rhinitis in spite of environmental measures or while these measures are being put in place, pharmacotherapy with an antiinflammatory medicine should be considered. The two categories of medicines most commonly recommended for treatment of allergic rhinitis in children are nonsteroid antiallergy agents such as cromolyn sodium and corticosteroids. Cromolyn is considered a mast cell stabilizing agent because it blocks or decreases both immediate and late-phase mast cell-mediated reactions in acute allergen provocation testing. It often is recommended for children because almost no significant adverse reactions have been reported with its use. It is not as effective as intranasal corticosteroids, and the use of cromolyn as long-term therapy in addition to intranasal corticosteroids offers no advantage to use of corticosteroids alone. Cromolyn has a relatively short duration of action and usually requires dosing 4 times each day. However, it is particularly useful in anticipation of unavoidable allergen exposure, such as when a cat-allergic child is to visit a home in which there is a cat. In this circumstance it may be instituted immediately before exposure. Nedocromil sodium may have additional antiinflammatory properties and has clinical efficacy comparable with cromolyn. An intranasal form is not available in the United States yet.

Azelastine (Astelin®) is an antihistamine that also has antiinflammatory properties. It is available as an aqueous nasal spray. Clinical trials suggest that it is effective in treating allergic rhinitis, and some trials have suggested that it is as effective as are intranasal steroids. There is a low incidence of sedation associated with its use.

There is information to suggest that selective antagonists of cysteinyl leukotriene activity such as zafirlukast (Accolate®) and montelukast (Singulair®) may benefit allergic rhinitis.[48,49] At present, these are indicated only for treatment of asthma.

Intranasal corticosteroids most effectively control symptoms of allergic rhinitis.[23,50] A number of alternative preparations are available. There is no information to suggest that any one is clinically more effective than any of the others; rather, differences are related to delivery device, frequency of administration, and potential for systemic adverse effect. In children, intranasal metered dose inhalers often are preferred because of ease of administration. Patients who use aqueous nasal sprays should be instructed on proper technique in order to deliver the medicine into the nasal airway across the turbinates instead of upward into the nasal vestibule. Patients should be instructed that intranasal steroids must be used routinely rather than "as needed" to be effective. Potent preparations such as fluticasone (Flonase®) and mometasone (Nasonex®) that have been shown to be effective with once daily dosing might be preferred to improve adherence. At recommended doses, the risk of systemic adverse effect is negligible. Nonetheless, intranasal corticosteroids should be used initially in dosage that is sufficient to relieve symptoms and then, the dose should be reduced incrementally to see if symptom control can be maintained with less medication.

Oral or intramuscular corticosteroids usually are not indicated for allergic rhinitis. In particular, depot corticosteroids should be avoided in children because of their adverse effect on growth. Initially, a short course of high-dose oral corticosteroids may be useful in children with severe allergic rhinitis in order to achieve sufficient patency of the nasal airway to permit penetration by an intranasal corticosteroid, which should be instituted simultaneously.

SPECIAL CONSIDERATION:

Oral or intramuscular corticosteroids usually are not indicated for allergic rhinitis.

An antihistamine often is recommended as first-line therapy for allergic rhinitis or in addition to an intranasal corticosteroid. Comparisons of antihista-

mine with intranasal corticosteroids have suggested differences in spectrum of symptoms controlled by the two.[51] It is not clear that addition of antihistamine to intranasal corticosteroids results in any additional advantage over steroids alone.[52] If used, nonsedating antihistamines such as loratadine (Claritin®) or fexofenadine (Allegra®) or an antihistamine with low incidence of sedation such as cetirizine (Zyrtec®) should be considered.[53,54]

Other pharmacologic agents may be useful as adjunctive therapies. Patients with nasal congestion may benefit from concomitant dosing with a decongestant. Although effective, oral decongestants may interfere with sleep and potentially could elevate blood pressure. Intranasal decongestants such as oxymetazoline (Afrin®) also are effective, although patients should be warned about the possibility of rebound nasal congestion or rhinitis medicamentosa with prolonged, excessive use. An intranasal anticholinergic agent such as ipratropium bromide (Atrovent®) may benefit patients with rhinorrhea.

AT A GLANCE . . .

Allergy Pharmacotherapy

Anti-inflammatory Nasal Sprays: *Cromolyn sodium:* recommended for children because no adverse side effects have been reported, but it is not as effective as corticosteroids. *Corticosteroids:* most effective for symptoms of allergic rhinitis. Azelastine: Some trials have suggested that it is as effective as are costicosteroids

Antihistamines: used as the first-line therapy for allergic rhinitis or in conjunction with intranasal corticosteroids

Decongestants: an adjunctive therapy, but oral dosing may interfere with sleep and/or elevate blood pressure

Anticholinergic Agents: an adjunctive therapy that may benefit patients with rhinorrhea

---

Immunotherapy

Allergen immunotherapy also is called specific immunotherapy, hyposensitization, or "allergy shots." When used appropriately, immunotherapy is safe and effective for the treatment of allergic rhinitis.[55-58] Efficacy depends on dosage, duration of treatment, and allergen selection. Low initial doses are increased at a set rate until reaching a high dose that is expected to induce protective immunologic responses without significant reactions. Long-term treatment for 3 to 5 years results in a more sustained effect than short-term therapy. Patients should be much improved or symptom-free for 1 to 2 years before immunotherapy is discontinued. Immunotherapy using conventional, commercially-available extracts has been shown to be beneficial in childhood pollen allergy and for perennial allergy in dust mite-allergic and cat-allergic children. In addition, benefit from immunotherapy with several mold spore extracts has been documented in adults. It must be emphasized that environmental measures should precede and be continued during immunotherapy.

Relative indications for immunotherapy include inability to avoid the allergen and poor results or significant side effects from pharmacologic treatment. In practice, once-weekly injections may be a preferred alternative to daily medication. More importantly, a successful course of immunotherapy may result in prolonged benefit after the course is completed.[59] This is in contradistinction to pharmacotherapy, in which symptoms return promptly after therapy is stopped if there is ongoing allergen exposure.

There are three reasons in particular to consider immunotherapy early in the treatment of allergic rhinitis in childhood (Table 3–2). First, it has been demonstrated that immunotherapy is more effective in patients who are allergic to a single allergen than in those who are allergic to multiple allergens ("polysensitized").[60] This suggests that immunotherapy is best used in children when they first become allergic to a single allergen before they have had time (and exposure) to develop additional sensitizations. Second, information suggests that specific immunotherapy prevents the onset of additional sensitiza-

TABLE 3–2:   Reasons to Consider Immunotherapy Early in The Treatment of Allergic Rhinitis in Childhood

1. Immunotherapy is more effective in patients who are allergic to a single allergen than in those allergic to multiple allergens. Therefore, it is best used in children when they first become allergic to a single allergen before they have had time (and exposure) to develop additional sensitizations.
2. Specific immunotherapy may prevent the onset of additional sensitizations in children.
3. Immunotherapy may prevent acquisition of asthma in children with allergic rhinitis.

tions in children.[61] Third, early results from a large study of specific immunotherapy in children with allergic rhinitis indicate that immunotherapy may prevent acquisition of asthma in these children.[62]

Local nasal immunotherapy may represent an alternative route of allergen administration. Recent studies using freeze-dried allergens in powdered form have shown clinical efficacy and good tolerability in perennial (mite, cat) and seasonal (pollens) allergic rhinitis.[63] The development of better extracts for both injection immunotherapy and local immunotherapy continues, and techniques for the production of recombinant allergens and peptides will be important for future vaccines.

Specialist Referral for Allergy Consultation

Referral to an allergy specialist should be considered when there are questions about the diagnosis, when allergy testing is needed, when the patient is not responding to optimal therapy, when special counsel on environmental control is needed, or when allergy immunotherapy is being considered. Specialist referral also may be useful when difficult problems in adherence inhibit the partnership care between patients, parents, and physicians.

AT A GLANCE . . .

Reasons for Referral to an Allergy Specialist

1. When there are questions about diagnosis
2. When allergy testing is needed
3. When patient is not responding to therapy
4. When counsel is needed for environmental control
5. When immunotherapy is considered

Nasal Polyps, Sinusitis, and Otitis Media

The pathogenesis of nasal polyps is not known, but allergy does not appear to be an important factor. The possibility of cystic fibrosis (CF) should be considered when children younger than 10 years develop nasal polyps.[64]

Sinusitis, on the other hand, typically follows and is intimately associated with rhinitis, allergic or otherwise (hence the term *rhinosinusitis*).[64] It should be noted that sinusitis does not imply infection necessarily. The mucosa of the nose and sinuses are contiguous, and inflammation of the mucosa may occur at both sites. Because of this, therapy of rhinitis as described above is an essential component of the treatment of sinusitis. If bacterial superinfection is suspected, then antibiotic therapy is warranted. However, the need for antimicrobials in persistent sinusitis in children has been called into doubt by a prospective study that failed to find any benefit from antimicrobial therapy of subacute sinusitis.[65]

The role of allergy in OM with effusion (OME) is less clear. It has been estimated that 35 to 50% of children with chronic OME have allergic rhinitis, depending upon the age of the child.[66,67] Conversely, only about 21% of allergic children have OME.[67] There is evidence that ET function is altered by nasal allergy, with both nasal provocation and natural exposure in children during a normal allergy season.[66,68] Furthermore, allergy management has been shown to benefit refractory OME.[69] Evaluation for respiratory allergy seems reasonable in children with persistent or recurrent OME.

SPECIAL CONSIDERATION:

Approximately 35 to 50% of children with chronic OME have allergic rhinitis.

IMMUNOLOGIC DYSFUNCTION

General Considerations

Host defense of the respiratory tract against bacterial pathogens depends primarily on humoral immune responses. Patients with severe B-lymphocyte abnormalities commonly present with chronic or recurrent sinusitis, OM, and pneumonia, as well as bronchiectasis. These are caused by recurrent infections with encapsulated bacteria because of inadequate opsonization in the absence of antibody. Patients may experience hematogenous spread of infection causing meningitis, septicemia, osteomyelitis, and lymphadenitis with abcess formation. It

would be highly unusual for a child with severe B-cell abnormality to experience chronic or recurrent infections limited to the URT. The only exception to this might be patients with common variable immunodeficiency (CVID), in whom infections of the URT may occur several years before the appearance of lower respiratory tract infections.[70] CVID occurs uncommonly in childhood, however.

SPECIAL CONSIDERATION:

Patients with B-lymphocyte abnormalities commonly present with chronic or recurrent sinusitis, OM, pneumonia, and bronchiectasis.

On the other hand, patients with less profound deficiencies of antibody formation may experience URT symptoms only. For example, the 20 children with impaired antibody responses and immunoglobulin G (IgG) subclass deficiency reported by Umetsu et al. all had more than six episodes of otitis and at least two episodes of clinically-obvious sinusitis each year, but not all had experienced pneumonia.[71] It is not clear how many infectious illnesses suggest the presence of these deficiencies. Primary immunodeficiency diseases are quite rare.[72] On the other hand, children with normal immune systems have an average of six to eight URT infections each year for the first 10 years of life,[73] and children with small caliber ETs and small ostia to their paranasal sinuses commonly experience otitis and sinusitis as a complication of these URT infections. Last, as noted below, it is the impairment of antibody responses (i.e., ''selective antibody deficiency'') rather than the level of IgG subclasses that renders the patient susceptible to respiratory infections.

IgG Subclass Deficiency

There was initial interest in IgG subclass deficiency as a distinct entity. It is now clear that it is difficult to know the significance of deficiency of IgG subclasses in the absence of broader measurements of antibody function.[72,74] Levels of IgG2 similar to those in patients with recurrent infections have been reported in healthy children and adults. Furthermore, healthy individuals who have no IgG2 have been reported; in most cases, this was shown to be the result of deletions of the $\gamma2$ heavy chain constant region gene. Not unexpectedly, these patients have a skewed pattern of antipolysaccharide antibodies, with a shift to IgG1 and IgG3. Furthermore, finding a low level of an IgG subclass does not indicate necessarily that the patient has immunologic abnormalities related only to that subclass. Patients with recurrent infections who have low levels of a subclass often are unable to make antibodies in other subclasses. These observations suggest that IgG subclass deficiency is a marker of a more global defect rather than a primary abnormality. Also, finding a normal level of an IgG subclass does not indicate necessarily that the patient does not have immunologic abnormalities related to that subclass. Patients who have normal levels of an IgG subclass, but are unable to make antibodies of one or more specificity, have been described. These patients are classified as having selective antibody deficiency. Last, measuring the level of an IgG subclass in children does not predict the level of antibody that is supposed to be restricted to that subclass. These results are different from those found in adults by other investigators using identical assays.

SPECIAL CONSIDERATION:

It is difficult to know the significance of IgG subclass deficiency in the absence of broader measurements of antibody function.

Laboratory Diagnosis of Humoral Immunodeficiency

It is reasonable to quantify serum levels of IgG, IgA, IgM, and IgE in patients with suspected humoral immunodeficiency. Finding frank hypogammaglobulinemia would eliminate the need for additional measurements of humoral immunocompetency, but normal results should not deter further evaluation of patients with an appropriate clinical history. It should be noted that infections usually cause a rise in serum IgG; thus, finding a level in the lower range of normal in a patient who has been experiencing significant infections may suggest immunodeficiency.

It can be seen from the discussion above that the relationship between selective IgG subclass defi-

ciencies and susceptibility to bacterial infection is complex. Obviously, functional (antibody) deficiency is related more closely to occurrence of infections than is structural (subclass) deficiency.[45] Measuring IgG subclass levels may be useful in a research setting, but it is difficult to argue for the need to measure them in clinical practice.

On the other hand, measurement of antibody-forming capacity is clinically useful in defining those patients who might be candidates for antibody-replacement therapy. Clinical experience indicates that antibody concentrations to a panel of protein (e.g., diphtheria and tetanus) and polysaccharide [e.g., pneumococcal and *Hemophilus influenzae* type B (HIB)] antigens should be measured in serum obtained immediately preimmunization and again 4 weeks later. Although the use of the HIB vaccine alone has been suggested, reports of patients who are unable to make antibody to HIB vaccine but who respond normally to the polyvalent pneumococcal vaccine suggest that the opposite could occur, and this in fact has been our experience. Furthermore, no results have been presented yet to indicate that antibody response to a single pneumococcal capsular antigen predicts the ability to respond to the other pneumococcal antigens studied. Full antibody responses to all of the antigens in the polyvalent pneumococcal vaccine, such as those that occur in adults, may not be seen in immunologically-normal children until they are about 10 years of age. Thus, all 12 of the pneumococcal antibody measurements that are available routinely should be obtained.

Therapy for Antibody Deficiency Diseases

There have been few studies assessing therapeutic approaches to children with IgG subclass or selective antibody deficiencies. However, recommendations for their management can be derived from experience treating children with other chronic illnesses, including immunoglobulin deficiency syndrome.

As with other immunoglobulin deficiency diseases, the major goal of therapy for children with antibody deficiency should be to prevent the occurrence of bacterial infections, or at the least to minimize their frequency and severity. Antibiotic therapy should be instituted promptly to treat acute infection; the antibiotic should be chosen according to the sensitivity of the identified causative agent or according to the most likely identity and sensitivity of agents associated with infections of a particular site. Prophylactic antibiotic treatment also may be useful in some of these children.

> ## SPECIAL CONSIDERATION:
>
> The major goal of therapy for children with antibody deficiency should be to prevent the occurrence of bacterial infections.

Immunization with protein-conjugated capsular polysaccharide vaccines also may be useful in patients who are unable to make antibody responses to the native polysaccharide antigens. For example, antibody-deficient children who experience infections with HIB might be immunized successfully using a conjugated HIB vaccine, although they may require more than one dose. It should be noted that infections with nontypable *Hemophilus influenzae* will not be affected by immunization with the HIB vaccine. Protein-conjugate vaccines using pneumococcal capsular polysaccharides have been studied in adults and potentially also will be useful for patients with IgG subclass or selective antibody deficiencies who experience infections with pneumococci.

Antibody replacement using human gammaglobulin is essential in the treatment of patients with profound deficiency of immunoglobulin. Several groups of investigators have reported improvement of both adults and children with selective deficiency of antibody following treatment with intravenous gammaglobulin (IVIG). As noted previously, assessing efficacy of this (or any) form of therapy will be difficult until problems interpreting low levels of IgG subclasses and defining this syndrome have been resolved.

Although ongoing research may expand its role in the future, at present the decision to treat a patient with IVIG should be based on documentation of the inability to make appropriate amounts of antibodies in response to appropriate challenges in the context of significant clinical symptoms. The use of multiple protein and polysaccharide antigens for challenge of the immune system makes overestimating antibody-forming capacity unlikely; therefore, empiric trials of antibody replacement therapy for the most part are unwarranted.

Specialist Referral for Immunodeficiency

Referral to an immunology specialist should be considered when there are questions about the diagnosis, when specialized immunologic testing is needed, or when the patient is not responding to optimal therapy. As noted previously, specialist referral also may be useful when difficult problems in adherence to the medical regimen inhibit a partnership care.

> ### AT A GLANCE . . .
>
> Reasons for Referral to an Immunology Specialist
>
> 1. When there are questions about diagnosis
> 2. When specialized immunologic testing is needed
> 3. When the patient is not responding to therapy

REFERENCES

1. Smith JM. The epidemiology of allergic rhinitis. In: Settipane GA, ed. *Rhinitis. 2nd ed.* Providence, RI: Oceanside Publications, 1991, pp. 151–159.
2. Meyers DA, Bleecker ER. Genetics of allergic disease. In: Middleton EJ, Reed CE, Ellis EF, et al, eds. *Allergy: Principles and Practice.* St. Louis: Mosby, 1998, pp. 40–45.
3. Iliopoulos O, Proud D, Adkinson NFJ, et al. Relationship between the early, late and rechallenge reaction to nasal challenge with antigen: Observations on the role of inflammatory mediators and cells. J Allergy Clin Immunol 1990; 86:851–861.
4. Horak F. Manifestation of allergic rhinitis in latent-sensitized patients. Arch Otorhinolaryngol 1985; 242:239–245.
5. Hagy G, Settipane G. Prognosis of positive allergy skin tests in an asymptomatic population. A three year follow-up of college students. J Allergy 1971; 48:200–205.
6. McLoughlin JA, Nall M, Berla E. Effect of allergy medication on children's reading comprehension. Allergy Proc 1990; 11:225–228.
7. Vuurman EF, van Veggel LM, Uiterwijk MM, et al. Seasonal allergic rhinitis and antihistamine effects on children's learning. Ann Allergy 1993; 71:121–126.
8. Burns M, Shanaman JE, Shellenberger CH. A laboratory study of patients with chronic allergic rhinitis: Antihistamine effects on skilled performance. J Allergy Clin Immunol 1994; 93:716–724.

9. Nolen TM. Sedative effects of antihistamines: Safety, performance, learning, and quality of life. Clin Therapeutics 1997; 19:39-55.

10. Craig TJ, Teets S, Lehman EB, et al. Nasal congestion secondary to allergic rhinitis as a cause of sleep disturbance and daytime fatigue and the response to topical nasal corticosteroids. J Allergy Clin Immunol 1998; 101:633-637.

11. Costa JJ, Weller PF, Galli SJ. The cells of the allergic response: Mast cells, basophils, and eosinophils. J Amer Med Assoc 1997; 278:1815-1822.

12. Bousquet J, Vignola AM, Campbell AM, et al. Pathophysiology of allergic rhinitis. Int Arch Allergy Immunol 1996; 110:207-218.

13. Baraniuk JN. Pathogenesis of allergic rhinitis. J Allerg Clin Immunol 1997; 99:S763-S772.

14. Wachs M, Proud D, Lichtenstein LM, et al. Observations on the pathogenesis of nasal priming. J Allergy Clin Immunol 1989; 84:492-501.

15. Connell JT. Quantitative intranasal pollen challenges-III. The priming effect in allergic rhinitis. J Allergy 1969; 43:33-44.

16. Schuhl JF. Nasal mucociliary clearance in perennial rhinitis. J Invest Allergol Clin Immunol 1995; 5: 333-336.

17. Naclerio R, Solomon W. Rhinitis and inhalant allergens. J Amer Med Assoc 1997; 278:1842-1848.

18. Host A. Mechanisms in adverse reactions to food. The nose. Allergy 1995; 50:S56-S59.

19. Bock SA. Prospective appraisal of complaints of adverse reactions to foods in children during the first 3 years of life. Pediatr 1987; 79:683-688.

20. Kivity S, Dunner K, Marian Y. The pattern of food hypersensitivity in patients with onset after 10 years of age. Clin Exper Allergy 1994; 24:19-22.

21. Sampson HA. Adverse reactions to foods. In: Middleton EJ, Reed CE, Ellis EF, et al eds. *Allergy: Principles and Practice.* St. Louis: Mosby, 1998, 1162-1182.

22. Solomon WR, Platts-Mills TAE. Aerobiology and inhalant allergens. In: Middleton EJ, Reed CE, Ellis EF, et al eds. *Allergy: Principles and Practice.* St. Louis: Mosby, 1998, 367-403.

23. Druce HM. Allergic and nonallergic rhinitis. In: Middleton EJ, Reed CE, Ellis EF, et al, eds. *Allergy: Principles and Practice.* St. Louis: Mosby, 1998, 1005-1016.

24. Smith TF. Allergy testing in clinical practice. Ann Allergy 1992; 68:293-301.

25. Perlmutter LL. In vitro allergy testing. Past, present, and future. Clin Rev Allergy 1994; 12:151-165.

26. Nelson HS. Variables in allergy skin testing. Allergy Proc 1994; 15:265-268.

27. Mullarkey MF. Eosinophilic nonallergic rhinitis. J Allergy Clin Immunol 1988; 82:941-949.

28. Popp W, Rauscher H, Sertl K, et al. Risk factors for sensitization to furred pets. Allergy 1990; 45:75-79.

29. Wahn U, Lau S, Bergmann R, et al. Indoor allergen exposure is a risk factor for sensitization during the first three years of life. J Allergy Clin Immunol 1997; 99:763-769.

30. Enberg RN, Shamie SM, McCullough J, et al. Ubiquitous presence of cat allergen in cat-free buildings: Probably dispersal from human clothing. Ann Allergy 1993; 70:471-474.

31. Patchett K, Lewis S, Crane J, et al. Cat allergen (Fel d1) levels on school children's clothing and in primary school classrooms in Wellington, New Zealand. J Allergy Clin Immunol 1997; 100:755-759.

32. Berge M, Munir AK, Dreborg S. Concentrations of cat (Fel d1), dog (Can f1), and mite (Der f1 and Der p1) allergens in the clothing and school environment of Swedish school children with and without pets at home. Pediatr Allergy Immunol 1998; 9:25-30.

33. Munir AK, Einarsson R, Schou C, et al. Allergens in school dust—I. The amount of the major cat (Fel d1) and dog (Can f1) allergens in dust from Swedish schools is high enough to probably cause perennial symptoms in most children with asthma who are sensitized to cat and dog. J Allergy Clin Immunol 1993; 91:1067-1074.

34. Spitzauer S, Pandjaitan B, Muhl S, et al. Major cat and dog allergens share IgE epitopes. J Allergy Clin Immunol 1997; 99:100-106.

35. Illchyshyn A, Cartwright PH, Smith AG. Contact sensitivity to newsprint: A rare manifestation of coal tar allergy. Contact Dermatitis 1987; 17:52-53.

36. Smith TF, McKean LP. Activation and modulation of mediator release from mast cells and basophils. Immunol Allergy Clin 1987; 7:179-189.

37. Berther T, Conroy MC, de Weck AL. Urticarial skin reaction to codeine. A measure of mast cell reactivity. Schweiz Med Wochenschr 1980; 110:758-763.

38. Lindblad JH, Farr RS. The incidence of positive intradermal reactions and demonstration of skin sensitizing antibody to extracts of ragweed and dust in humans without history of rhinitis or asthma. J Allergy 1961; 32:392-401.

39. Halpern GM. Evaluation of in vitro IgE testing to diagnose atopic diseases. Clin Rev Allergy 1989; 7:23-48.

40. Haahtela T, Heiskala M, Suoniemi I. Allergic disorders and immediate skin test reactivity in Finnish adolescents. Allergy 1980; 35:433-441.

41. Adinoff AD, Rosloniec DM, McCall LL, et al. Immediate skin test reactivity to Food and Drug Administration-approved standardized extracts. J Allergy Clin Immunol 1990; 86:766-774.

42. Lichtenstein LM. Histamine-releasing factors and IgE heterogeneity. J Allergy Clin Immunol 1988; 81: 814-820.

43. The European Academy of Allergology and Clinical Immunology. Position paper: Allergen standardization and skin tests. Allergy 1993; 48:48-82.

44. Bernstein IL, Storms WW. Practice parameters for allergy diagnostic testing. Joint Task Force on Practice Parameters for the Diagnosis and Treatment of Asthma. The American Academy of Allergy, Asthma, and Immunology and the American College of Allergy, Asthma, and Immunology. Ann Allergy Asthma Immunol 1995; 75:543–625.

45. Novembre E, Bernardini R, Bertini G, et al. Skin-prick-test-induced anaphylaxis. Allergy 1995; 50:511–513.

46. Reid RJ, Lockey RF, Turkeltaub PC, et al. Survey of fatalities from skin testing and immunotherapy 1985–1989. J Allergy Clin Immunol 1993; 92:6–15.

47. Dykewicz MS, Fineman S, eds. *Diagnosis and Management of Rhinitis: Parameter Documents of the Joint Task Force on Practice Parameters in Allergy, Asthma, and Immunology.* Ann Allergy Asthma Immunol 1998; 81:463–518.

48. Rachelefsky G. Childhood asthma and allergic rhinitis: The role of leukotrienes. J Pediatr 1997; 131:348–355.

49. Aharony D. Pharmacology of leukotriene receptor antagonists. Amer J Respir Crit Care Med 1998; 157:S214–S218.

50. Meltzer EO. Treatment options for the child with allergic rhinitis. Clin Pediatr 1998; 37:1–10.

51. Frolund L. Efficacy of an oral antihistamine, loratadine, as compared with a nasal steroid spray, beclomethasone dipropionate, in seasonal allergic rhinitis. Clin Otolaryngol 1991; 16:527–531.

52. Jeal W, Faulds D. Triamcinolone acetonide. A review of its pharmacological properties and therapeutic efficacy in the management of allergic rhinitis. Drugs 1997; 53:257–280.

53. Barnett A, Kreutner W. Pharmacology of non-sedating H1 antihistamines. Agents & Actions—Supplements 1991; 33:181–196.

54. Shall L, Thompson DA, Barkley AS, et al. Comparative inhibition profiles of three non-sedating antihistamines assessed by an extended Lewis model. Clin Exp Allergy 1992; 22:711–716.

55. Evans Rd. Environmental control and immunotherapy for allergic disease (Part 2). J Allergy Clin Immunol 1992; 90:462–468.

56. Creticos PS. The role of immunotherapy in allergic rhinitis/allergic asthma. Allergy Proc 1995; 16:297–302.

57. Hedlin G. The role of immunotherapy in pediatric allergic disease. Curr Opin Pediatr 1995; 7:676–682.

58. Nelson HS. Immunotherapy for inhalant allergens. In: Middleton EJ, Reed CE, Ellis EF, et al., eds. *Allergy: Principles and Practice.* St. Louis: Mosby, 1998, pp. 1050–1062.

59. Des Roches A, Paradis L, Knani J, et al. Immunotherapy with a standardized Dermatophagoides pteronyssinus extract V. duration of the efficacy of immunotherapy after its cessation. Allergy 1996; 51:430–433.

60. Bousquet J, Becker WM, Hejjaoui A, et al. Differences in clinical and immunologic reactivity in patients allergic to grass pollens and to multiple-pollen species—II. Efficacy of a double-blind, placebo-controlled, specific immunotherapy with standardized extracts. J Allergy Clin Immunol 1991; 88:43–53.

61. Des Roches A, Paradis L, Menardo JL, et al. Immunotherapy with a standardized Dermatophagoides pteronyssinus extract—VI. Specific immunotherapy prevents the onset of new sensitizations in children. J Allergy Clin Immunol 1997; 99:450–453.

62. Valovirta E. Capacity of specific immunotherapy in prevention of allergic asthma in children: The Preventive Allergy Treatment Study (PAT). J Invest Allergol Clin Immunol 1997; 7:369–370.

63. Andri L, Senna GE, Dama AR. Clinical efficacy and safety of local nasal immunotherapy. Allergy 1997; 52(33 Supplement):36–39.

64. Slavin RG. Nasal polyps and sinusitis. In: Middleton EJ, Reed CE, Ellis EF, et al., eds. *Allergy: Principles and Practice.* St. Louis: Mosby, 1998, pp. 1024–1035.

65. Dohlman AW, Hemstreet MP, Odrezin GT, et al. Subacute sinusitis: Are antimicrobials necessary? J Allergy Clin Immunol 1993; 91:1015–1023.

66. Fireman P. Otitis media and eustachian tube dysfunction: Connection to allergic rhinitis. J Allergy Clin Immunol 1997; 99:S787–S797.

67. Spector SL. Overview of comorbid associations of allergic rhinitis. J Allergy Clin Immunol 1997; 99:S773–S780.

68. Bernstein JM. Role of allergy in eustachian tube blockage and otitis media with effusion: A review. Otolaryngol Head Neck Surg 1996; 114:562–568.

69. Hurst DS. Allergy management of refractory serous otitis media. Otolaryngol Head Neck Surg 1990; 102:664–669.

70. Karlsson G, Petruson B, Björkander J, et al. Infections of the nose and paranasal sinuses in adult patients with immunodeficiency. Arch Otolaryngol 1985; 111:290–293.

71. Umetsu DT, Ambrosino DM, Quinti I, et al. Recurrent sinopulmonary infection and impaired antibody response to bacterial capsular polysaccharide antigen in children with selective IgG-subclass deficiency. N Engl J Med 1985; 313:1247–1251.

72. Buckley RH. Primary immunodeficiency diseases. In: Middleton EJ, Reed CE, Ellis EF, et al, eds. *Allergy: Principles and Practice.* St. Louis: Mosby, 1998, pp. 713–734.

73. Puck JM. Primary immunodeficiency diseases. J Amer Med Assoc 1997; 278:1835–1848.

74. Smith TF. IgG subclasses. Adv Pediatr 1992; 39:101–126.

4 Genetics Principles

J. Christopher Post

The revolution in molecular genetics is changing the practice of medicine and biologic research. The ever increasing pace of disease gene discovery is dramatically expanding our understanding of the basic pathophysiology of disease. This fundamental knowledge offers the best hope for revolutionary new treatments for our patients. Just as advances in the basic science of infectious disease and in anesthesia and surgical techniques led to our clinical successes today, advances in molecular biology will lead to unimagined new therapies for our patients. Gene therapy, although currently in its infancy, will undoubtedly provide us with the tools to treat and ultimately prevent diseases that are now incurable.

Part of the challenge of providing comprehensive, genetics-based care is that many practitioners received their medical education during the period of time when genetics was limited to morphological classification, population analysis, gross chromosomal abnormalities, biochemical delineation of rare metabolic problems, and experiments in fruit flies. Even the basic, classic Mendelian understanding of genetics has been shown to be incorrect in many instances. For example, genomic imprinting is a process that modifies the genome differently in the male and the female germlines, thus leading to a differential expression of the parental genome in the offspring.[1] Stated another way, this means that, in some cases, it does matter whether you inherited a gene from your mother or from your father. Thus, this violates the Mendelian concept that both maternal and paternal genes contribute to the offspring equally. Linkage analysis, which is the basis of genetic mapping, takes advantage of a fundamental violation of Mendel's Law of Independent Assortment.

This chapter attempts to provide the pediatric otolaryngologist with a working knowledge of molecular genetics by discussing the basic science of

DNA, inheritance, and some of the molecular technologies that have so dramatically impacted the field. Advances in specific disease states that are of interest to the practitioner are reviewed. The importance of animal models, gene therapy, the Human Genome Project (HGP), and the significance of ethical issues are discussed. Finally, the role of the clinician in molecular medicine is emphasized. Given the pace of discovery, current information can only be disseminated by electronic methods; therefore, use of the World Wide Web is encouraged and electronic addresses are included throughout the text where appropriate.

WHAT IS A GENETIC DISEASE?

In concert with the molecular revolution, the concept of what constitutes a genetic disease has been greatly expanded. Traditionally, we thought of genetic disease in terms of single gene disorders that led to some sort of biochemical or somatic disorder, which was readily recognizable and which had an inheritance pattern that was clearly dominant or recessive. Chromosomal aberrations (such as trisomy 21 in Down syndrome) were recognized also as being genetic in origin. Although many diseases remain of interest to pediatric otolaryngology that are the result of a single gene mutation (Crouzon, Apert, and Treacher Collins syndromes, as well as most instances of inherited deafness) or a chromosomal abnormality (Down and Turner's syndromes), it is becoming increasingly evident that many of the diseases we deal with are due, at least in some part, to a genetic component. The course of many diseases is determined by multiple factors and is a combination of the interplay between the genetic predisposition of the patient and environmental factors. For example, the host response to infectious agents is clearly genetically influenced (see Modes of Inheritance later), and there is a definite

Pediatric Otolaryngology, Edited by R.F. Wetmore, H.R. Muntz, and T.J. McGill. Thieme Medical Publishers, Inc., New York © 2000.

inherited component in the development of otitis media.[2] Cancer can be the result of the inheritance of aberrant genes (Li-Fraumini families and p53 and familial breast cancer and the BRCA1 gene) or the end result of a series of somatic cell genetic mutations. Basic developmental processes, such as language development, are also, at least in part, under the influence of the genetic basis of the child.

DNA

Deoxyribonucleic acid (DNA) is the information storage system of most biologic organisms. DNA consists of a long molecule that is composed of a series of four nucleotide subunits covalently linked by phosphate bonds in an irregular but nonrandom pattern. Each nucleotide consists of a deoxyribose sugar molecule with an attached phosphate group and either a purine or a pyrimidine base that determines the identity of the nucleotide. These bases are adenine, guanine, cytosine, and thymine, abbreviated A, G, C, and T, respectively. The general structure of DNA is independent of the particular nucleotide sequence. The sequence of bases determines the protein that is encoded by utilizing a three-base pair code that is partially redundant. The structure and function of each protein are basically determined by the primary sequence of amino acids. Therefore, DNA can encode all the information needed to specify a specific protein. In addition to regions that encode for proteins, other regions of DNA contain sequences that are recognized by regulator molecules, which control the expression of certain genes. Of interest, only about 10% of our DNA encodes for proteins or is involved in gene regulation; the function of the remaining 90% is unclear. This DNA is often referred to as "junk" DNA or "parasitic" DNA, which is DNA that exists only to replicate itself. The human genome contains approximately three billion base pairs, which is enough information to fill 390,000 pages of *Scientific American*.[3]

SPECIAL CONSIDERATION:

Only 10% of our DNA encodes for proteins or is involved in gene regulation. The function of the remaining 90% is unclear.

DNA exists in two strands that are complementary to each other, and the base pairs of the two strands preferentially form hydrogen bonds with each other, such that A binds with T and that C binds with G. This preferential binding is the basis of almost all molecular technology, and is exploited in a variety of very clever ways. These complementary strands form the *double helix*. DNA replication occurs in a semi-conservative manner, such that the strands of DNA separate each acting as a template for the formation of a new strand. Thus, each daughter cell inherits one maternal strand and one new strand of DNA.

CHROMOSOMES

Each molecular unit of DNA is packaged in a *chromosome*. Chromosomes are so named because early studies revealed that they are dye-absorbing structures in the cell's nucleus derived from the Greek for *color*. The total genetic information of an organism constitutes its *genome*. The human genome consists of 22 pairs of chromosomes (known as the autosome), two sex chromosomes (the paternal Y and the maternal X), and a small amount of DNA in the mitochondria (see Modes of Inheritance, below). One member of the autosomal pain is maternal in origin and the other is paternal. Having a maternal and a paternal copy of each chromosome makes us diploid organisms.

Karyotyping is the process of examining chromosomes for structural abnormalities or variation from the standard number. Before the advent of molecular technology, karyotyping was the laboratory mainstay used to try to determine if a disease had a genetic component. To karyotype a patient, chromosomes are obtained from peripheral blood lymphocytes or other sources. The lymphocytes are stimulated to undergo mitosis with phytohemagglutinin and are then arrested in metaphase with a microtubule inhibitor such as colchicine. The cells are killed, placed in a hypotonic solution to disperse the chromosomes and separate them from one another, and then fixed on slides. The chromosomes are labeled with specific stains, examined microscopically, and photographed. The chromosomes are then assembled into homologous pairs (either electronically or by cutting them out of the photograph, and then arranged in order of decreasing size. With *Giemsa banding (G-banding)*, 350–550 light and dark bands are seen per chromosome set. Each band represents between five and ten million base pairs.

Each individual chromosome has its own unique staining pattern, which means that by using specific staining patterns and chromosomal size, the cytogeneticist can identify not only specific chromosomes but also any insertions, deletions, or structural rearrangements. Other types of stains are used to reveal different aspects of the chromosomes. *C-banding* is used to highlight the centromeres; *Q-banding*, which uses the fluorescent dye quinacrine mustard, is useful to identify the Y chromosome and polymorphisms not readily identifiable by G-banding; and *R-banding* results in a reversal of the G-banding pattern, which is particularly useful in examining terminal bands.

SPECIAL CONSIDERATION:

Karyotyping is the process of examining chromosomes for structural abnormalities or variations from the standard number.

Cytogenetics has undergone a revolution with the advent of *fluorescent in situ hybridization (FISH).* This technology has ushered in the era of molecular cytogenetics. With FISH, a much greater resolution is gained, making it possible to detect deletions or translocations of just a few kilobases; this is at least a 1000-fold increase in resolution over older techniques. FISH is based upon the complementary hybridization of a biotin-labeled single strand of DNA with the chromosome of interest, which is then detected by fluorochrome-linked avidin. Various dyes such as fluorescein or rhodamine are used, such that the chromosomes can be "painted" with various colored markers. Many such assays are now commercially available. Current cytogenetic technology still does not allow the detection of point mutations, which must be detected using molecular-based techniques.

INFORMATION FLOW IN THE CELL

The information of the DNA is contained in the nucleus of the cell, and the protein manufacturing systems are located in the cytoplasm. To transmit the encoded message regarding protein structure from the nucleus to the cytoplasm, cells use molecules

known as *messenger ribonucleic acid,* or mRNA. RNA differs from DNA in that it contains ribose instead of deoxyribose and in that instead of the thymine base of DNA, there is uracil. In a process known as *transcription,* a long stretch of RNA is transcribed from the entire length of the gene, including both DNA coding sequences known as *exons* and noncoding region known as *introns* (for introvening sequences). This primary transcript is then processed to remove all of the introns and attach the exons together. This splicing produces a molecule of RNA (mRNA) that is much shorter than the original transcript. The mRNA is further processed by the addition of a methylation cap to the 5 end and a 3 polyadenosine (polyA) tail. The mRNA then moves from the nucleus to the cytoplasm, where it provides the information encoded in the three-nucleotide code to produce a protein in a process known as *translation.* (The DNA/mRNA language is *translated* into the language of proteins.) Each triplet of nucleotides is called a *codon,* which specifies either a specific amino acid or a signal to start or stop protein synthesis. RNA is a linear molecule with only four different nucleotides, so there are 4^3 or 64 possible codon triplets. Since only 20 amino acids are commonly used, most amino acids are specified by several different codons. This degenerate code is highly conserved, as it is the same for organisms as diverse as bacteria and humans (with a few minor exceptions). Thus, the genetic code for serine is UCU, UCC, UCA, UCG, AGU, or AGC. Stop codons are UAA, UAG, or UGA.

GENES AND GENE EXPRESSION

A *gene* is the functional unit of heredity and is defined as an ordered sequence of nucleotides that code for a specific functional product, either a protein or a RNA molecule. In simple bacteria, an unbroken stretch of DNA encodes for a single protein product. Most eukaryotic genes are more complex, and contain exons broken up by introns. Humans have approximately 80,000 to 100,000 genes. The boundaries of exons and introns are delineated by specific nucleotide sequences; researchers exploit this characteristic in their search for new unknown genes in a process known as "exon trapping."[4]

Organisms go to great lengths to control gene expression, which is the generation of a protein product from a genetic sequence. Regulatory mechanisms that function to control gene expression include promoter regions, enhancer and repressor elements. Introns are spliced out of the transcriptional mRNA and exons can be arranged in a variety of ways, further increasing the diversity of protein products. Although every nucleated cell in the body contains the entire genome, gene expression is controlled both temporally and spatially, with certain genes being expressed only at certain times in the organism's life or in certain tissues of the body. For example, fetal tissue tends to heal with very little scar formation, whereas pediatric and adult tissue heals with scar formation. The genes that control fetal healing are still present in adult tissues, but are no longer expressed. The identification of fetal wound-healing genes and the delineation of the control mechanisms is an area of great interest to researchers. Once these genes and their control mechanisms have been characterized, it should be possible to induce pediatric and adult tissues to heal in scarless fashion. Such an advance has tremendous surgical implications.

As humans are diploid organisms, we inherit a copy of a gene from our mother and another copy from our father. Each copy of the gene is termed an *allele;* thus, we have a maternal allele and a paternal allele at each locus (or a specific point in the genome). The gene can be normal (i.e., "wild type") or abnormal (i.e., "mutated"). Mutations are either *point mutations* (changes in a single nucleotide), *deletions* (missing nucleotides), or *translocations* (nucleotides moved to another point in the genome). Not all mutations are necessarily harmful, as the nucleotide code is redundant; a change from one nucleotide to another may not have any effect on the protein encoded (i.e., *silent mutation*). The genetic constitution of an individual is referred to as the *genotype,* whereas the individual's *phenotype* is the observable characteristics that are determined by the interaction between the genotype and the environment.

SPECIAL CONSIDERATION:

Humans have approximately 80,000 to 100,000 genes. The genetic constitution of an individual is referred to as the genotype, whereas the phenotype is the observable characteristics determined by the interaction between the genotype and the environment.

MODES OF INHERITANCE

Classical Mendelian inheritance can be defined in terms of genes. Single gene inheritance can be either *autosomal, sex-linked* or *mitochondrial,* depending on the location of the inherited gene. The manifestation of a dominant trait in a person requires that only one mutant allele be inherited; manifestation of a recessive trait requires that both inherited alleles be mutated. The characteristics of *autosomal dominant inheritance* are: (1) each affected individual has an affected parent, thus the disease is present in every generation; (2) each child of an affected person will have a one in two chance of being affected; and (3) unaffected relatives of an affected person will have unaffected children. Since autosomal recessive traits require the presence of two mutated genes, a person having only one copy of the affected gene (i.e., an abnormal genotype) will have a normal phenotype. Such a person is known as a *carrier* for that trait. *Autosomal recessive inheritance* is characterized by: (1) the trait is rarely present in the carrier parent or in every generation; (2) each child of two carriers will have a one in four chance of being affected; (3) parents of affected children have a greater likelihood of being related to each other (consanguinity); and (4) in small families, there is likely to be only one affected child.

Genes on the X chromosome can be either dominant or recessive in effect, but since females have two X chromosomes and males only have one, pedigrees with X-linked inheritance have different patterns than do pedigrees of autosomal traits. *X-linked recessive inheritance* is characterized by: (1) the trait almost always appears in males; (2) there is never male to male transmission (as a son must receive a Y chromosome from his father); (3) all daughters of affected males will be carriers; and (4) sons of carrier females have a one in two chance of being affected, whereas daughters of carrier females have a one in two chance of being carriers. *X-linked dominant inheritance* is rare, and its chief characteristic is that all the daughters and none of the sons of an affected male will be affected.

Mitochondrial inheritance, although rare, is becoming of increasing interest to pediatric otolaryngologists (see Mitochondrial Disease later). Mitochondria are organelles in the cytoplasm that contain a small amount of DNA. As sperm do not carry paternal cytoplasm, mitochondrial inheritance is passed maternally. Therefore, a hallmark of mitochondrial inheritance is that although both males and females are affected, only affected females can transmit the trait in question.

Several factors arise to confound the orderly inheritance of traits as described above, including *expressivity, penetrance, phenocopies, genetic heterogeneity,* and *anticipation.* These factors can, singly or in combination, cause a great deal of confusion when analyzing inheritance patterns. *Expressivity* describes the degree of phenotypic severity that a mutant gene produces; a gene that is variably expressed may produce a severe phenotypic change in one person and a minimal change in another. *Penetrance* is an all-or-nothing phenomena, which means that a mutant gene that produces a change in phenotype in one patient may produce absolutely no detectable change in another person's phenotype. *Phenocopies* are the concept that phenotypes that appear identical can be caused by a mutant gene in one instance and by non-genetic causes in another. Congenital deafness is a ready example of this phenomena, in that the lack of hearing could be due to the inheritance of two copies of a recessive gene or to an intrauterine infection. *Genetic heterogeneity* is characterized by the same phenotype being caused by mutations in more than one gene. Again, hereditary deafness is an excellent example of this because the same phenotype, in this case deafness without any other abnormalities, can be caused by genes inherited in an autosomal dominant, autosomal recessive, X-linked, or mitochondrial fashion. *Anticipation* is the phenomenon in which the severity of a genetic disorder becomes either more severe or manifest at an earlier age with each subsequent generation.

Advances in molecular technologies now allow gene hunters to begin to identify the genes involved in multifactorial illnesses, which are illnesses that result from a combination of multiple genetic effects and environmental factors. Many such phenotypes are quantitative in nature, such as blood pressure levels in hypertension. Susceptibility loci that are related to a quantitative phenotype are known as *quantitative trait loci* (QTL). There are many such QTLs that are of interest to the pediatric otolaryngologist. Traits such as language development and susceptibility to otitis media clearly have environmental and hereditable components. Experimental design limitations and ethical concerns make it extremely difficult to determine the exact environmental contribution to the development of phe-

notype (i.e., "nature versus nurture"). The breakthroughs in molecular genetics now promise to shed light on the "nature" component by determining the relative contribution of genetics.

AT A GLANCE. . .

Inheritance Patterns

Characteristics of Autosomal Dominant Inheritance:
1. Each affected individual has an affected parent.
2. Each child of an affected person will have a one in two chance of being affected.
3. Unaffected relatives of an affected person will have unaffected children.

Characteristics of Autosomal Recessive Inheritance:
1. The trait is rarely present in parents or in every generation.
2. Each child of two carriers will have a one in four chance of being affected.
3. Parents of affected children have a greater likelihood of consanguinity.
4. In small families, only one child is likely to be affected.

Characteristics of X-linked Recessive Inheritance:
1. The trait almost always appears in males.
2. There is never male to male transmission.
3. All daughters of affected males will be carriers.
4. Sons of carrier females have a one in two chance of being affected; daughters of carrier females have a one in two chance of being carriers.

Characteristics of X-linked Dominant Inheritance:
1. All daughters of affected males will be affected.
2. None of the sons of affected males will be affected.

Characteristics of Mitochondrial Inheritance:
1. Since sperm do not carry paternal cytoplasm, mitochondrial inheritance is passed maternally; that is, only females may pass the trait in question.
2. Both males and females can be affected.

MITOCHONDRIAL DISEASE

Although the vast majority of DNA is located in the nucleus of the cell, a small percentage is contained in the mitochondria. Mitochondria are oval-shaped organelles in the cytoplasm of the cell that contain the protein subunits for oxidative phosphorylation, which is an energy-producing biochemical pathway. Mitochondria are enclosed by two membranous spaces; the inner membrane is folded into a series of projections known as *cristae.* Mitochondria most likely evolved from independent life forms that became endosymbiotically incorporated in the cell. Therefore, mitochondria have the capability to replicate, transcribe, and translate their own DNA in a semi-independent fashion from the nuclear DNA. Mitochondrial DNA (mtDNA) consists of a double-stranded circular molecule composed of 16,569 nucleotides. mtDNA has a mutation rate that is up to 10 times greater than nuclear DNA. Several factors that contribute to this high mutation rate are: (1) mtDNA contains no introns, so any nucleotide change will be in a functional portion of the DNA; (2) mitochondria have no effective DNA repair mechanisms; and (3) as mitochondria are the sites of oxidative phosphorylation in the cell, mtDNA is exposed to the oxygen free radicals. The proportion of mutated mitochondria can vary from tissue to tissue; therefore, the clinical expression of the disease can vary widely. Thus, there is a very poor correlation between genotype and phenotype in mitochondrial disease. The coexistence of normal and mutated mtDNA in the same cell is known as *heteroplasmy. Homoplasmy* is the presence of completely normal or completely abnormal mtDNA in a cell. As mtDNA does not undergo recombination, mutations will accumulate sequentially along maternal lines in the pedigree. Although mtDNA sequence can vary greatly among normal human populations, some mtDNA mutations are associated with disease, including such rare encephalomyopathies such as mitochondrial encephalomyopathy, lactic acidosis, and stroke-like episodes (MELAS); myoclonic epilepsy with ragged-red fibers (MERRF); Leber's hereditary optic neuropathy (LHON); and neuropathy, ataxia, and retinitis pigmentosa (NARP).

SPECIAL CONSIDERATION:

Mitochondrial DNA has a mutation rate up to 10 times greater than nuclear DNA.

Of interest to otolaryngologists is the increasing body of evidence that demonstrates that mitochondrial mutations are associated with hearing loss. A single point mutation in mtDNA has been associated with deafness and diabetes in several families.[5] Another point mutation is associated with nonsyndromic deafness in an Arab-Israeli pedigree, with the onset of deafness generally in infancy, but occasionally occurring in adulthood.[6] The same mutation also has been shown to predispose individuals to aminoglycoside-induced hearing loss.[7] Aminoglycoside-induced hearing loss is a major cause of hearing loss in those countries where aminoglycosides are used liberally. These findings raise two very interesting questions: (1) why should the same mutation cause early-onset hearing loss in one patient and adult-onset in another and; (2) why is the ear the only organ affected? Environmental epigenetic factors, other mitochondrial factors, and nuclear genome mutations are thought to contribute in a threshold fashion to the development of the deafness phenotype.[8] The high mutation rate and poor DNA repair mechanisms may contribute to the development of degenerative disorders that manifest themselves later in life.

The immediate clinical implication of the above findings is that the clinician should inquire as to any family history of aminoglycoside-induced hearing loss prior to the administration of aminoglycosides. It is also recommended that any patient with aminoglycoside-induced hearing loss is screened for mitochondrial mutations predisposing to this loss because effective family counseling may prevent future hearing loss in the maternal relatives.[8]

TEMPORAL BONE BANKS AND MOLECULAR GENETICS

The field of otolaryngology has been fortunate in that a great deal of effort has been expended to develop temporal bone libraries in the United States and abroad. The National Institute on Deafness and Other Communicative Disorders (NIDCD), which is part of the National Institutes of Health (NIH) sponsored National Temporal Bone, Hearing, and Balance Pathology Resource Registry, encourages donation of temporal bones, and serves the research community by maintaining a database of over 12,000 specimens.[9] Many of these bones are accompanied by the medical histories and audiograms of the patients that donated them. Recently, it has been shown that DNA from archived temporal bones can be amplified by the polymerase chain reaction (PCR) with recovery rates sufficient to allow some very interesting research questions to be asked.[10] Preliminary application of molecular technology to this resource demonstrates that, in a small sample of temporal bones, mtDNA mutations associated with the aging process appear to be more common in patients with presbycusis compared to age-matched controls without a history of presbycusis.[11] Investigators using molecular techniques have demonstrated the presence of DNA from herpes simplex virus in the geniculate ganglion of a patient with Bell's palsy.[12]

MOLECULAR TECHNOLOGY

PCR is an automated technique that can make a billion copies of a DNA segment of interest, and it is the basis for a wide variety of gene analysis technologies. PCR utilizes two short, oligonucleotide primers, each of which is complementary to one end of the segment of interest, and a heat-stable DNA polymerase that is isolated from a bacteria known as *Thermus aquaticus (Taq),* which adapted to life in hot springs by developing enzymes that function at high temperatures. PCR is a successive, repetitive process of: (1) denaturation, in which the hydrogen bonds of the template DNA are broken in order to separate the two target strands; (2) annealing, in which the reaction mixture is cooled, allowing the first primer to bind in a complementary fashion to one end of one target strand and the second primer to bind to the other end of the second strand; and (3) elongation, where the *Taq* polymerase adds nucleotides in a complementary fashion to each dissociated strand of the target DNA. Thus, at the end of the first cycle, two copies of the DNA segment of interest are present. The second cycle utilizes each of the two copies as templates to produce four copies. Repeated cycles result in an exponential increase in the number of copies, such that after approximately 30 cycles, one billion copies of the target DNA are present. The amplified DNA then can be subjected to a wide variety of analytical techniques. Major strengths of PCR are that: (1) its high degree of sensitivity and specificity allow correctly-designed primers to amplify only the DNA segment of interest and no other; (2)

it does not require isolation of the DNA segment of interest prior to amplification, and thus individual DNA segments can be amplified out of a sea of DNA; (3) DNA is a stable molecule and can be amplified from almost any type of specimen; and (4) the heat-stable nature of *Taq* means that the PCR process can be automated, producing a billion copies of DNA in just a few hours. PCR can also be used to amplify RNA, but requires an enzyme known as reverse transcriptase (RT) to transform the RNA segment into a segment of DNA (RT-PCR) that can then act as the template for the PCR reaction as described above.

Differences in nucleotide sequences between two DNA segments of interest (such as a normal allele and a mutant allele) can be detected by a variety of techniques. Direct sequencing of the DNA can be accomplished, but it is a resource-intensive and relatively slow process. *Single-strand conformation polymorphism* (SSCP) is a rapid technique that can reliably detect sequence differences between two DNA fragments.[13] SSCP is based upon the fact that the speed of migration of DNA fragments through gels is a function not only of their length (i.e., short fragments move faster) but also of their nucleotide sequence. The DNA fragments will assume different shapes (i.e., secondary structure) based upon the nucleotide sequence. This difference in shape affects migratory speed.

SPECIAL CONSIDERATION:

Single-strand conformation polymorphism (SSCP) is a rapid technique that can reliably detect sequence differences between two DNA fragments.

To date, most DNA sequencing has been accomplished using gel-based technologies. Despite remarkable advances in automation in sample preparation, specimen handling, and data interpretation, future sequencing will be accomplished using chip-based technologies. These chips are silicon-based with dense arrays of specific oligonucleotides fused to them, and represent an unparalleled advance in sequencing speed and accuracy. Chip technology will be used to genotype, sequence DNA, evaluate samples for mutations, and perhaps most importantly, examine the changes in RNA expression over time (the *expresome*).

Just as cells have developed chromosomes to be the packaging and handling systems for genomic DNA, researchers have developed systems for the handling and propagation of smaller portions of DNA. These systems should be easy to manipulate, and should be able to maintain the clones of DNA with a high degree of fidelity. There is a large variety of artificial chromosomes, which are distinguished by the size of the DNA fragment and the machinery associated with the fragment. Yeast artificial chromosomes (YAC) can generally handle a DNA insert size up to 1,000,000 base pairs (1000kb). Several cloning systems have been designed based upon *Escherichia coli.* These systems, which allow for the propagation of intermediate-sized clones, include the *bacteriophage P1 cloning system,* the *bacterial artificial chromosome* (BAC), and the *P1-derived artificial chromosome* (PAC). The P1 cloning system can carry DNA fragments up to 70–100kb, the BAC carries up to 300kb, and the PAC carries insert sizes between 100–300kb. *Cosmids* (40kb) carry much smaller fragments of DNA.

AT A GLANCE...

The Process of Polymerase Chain Reaction

1. **Denaturation:** the hydrogen bonds of the template DNA are broken to separate the two target strands.

2. **Annealing:** the reaction mixture is cooled, allowing the first primer to bind in a complementary fashion to one end of one target strand and the second primer to bind to the other end of the second strand.

3. **Elongation:** the *Taq* polymerase adds nucleotides in a complementary fashion to each dissociated strand of the target DNA.

An important resource for gene mappers is a tissue-specific library of *complementary DNAs* (cDNA). cDNA sequences are derived from the mRNA that is expressed in a certain tissue. Since the mRNA expressed in a tissue is derived from the processed exons and introns, mRNAs do not necessarily correspond to the exact sequence of the entire gene, but rather only to the exonic sequence.

Nonetheless, mRNA sequence data provide powerful clues as to the actual gene sequence information. *Sequence tagged sites* (STS) are short DNA sequences that occur only once in the human genome and have a known location. *Expressed sequence tags* (ESTs) are STSs that are derived from cDNAs. The importance of this is that, for example, if a research team has mapped a hearing gene to a small area of a chromosome and an EST derived from the cochlea also has been mapped to the same region, then that EST becomes a strong candidate for containing a portion of the DNA sequence of the entire gene.

GENE MAPPING AND CLONING

Two types of maps have been developed to represent the genome: physical maps and genetic or linkage maps. *Physical maps* show the location of identifiable landmarks along individual chromosome lengths, with the distances between landmarks measured in base pairs. This is analogous to mile markers along a road. The lowest resolution map is the banding patterns on chromosomes; the highest resolution is achieved with the complete delineation of the entire nucleotide sequence. STSs serve as useful landmarks for physical maps. A major goal of the HGP (see The Human Genome Project, below) is to produce a physical map of the human genome with an STS every 100,000 bases. Genetic maps, on the other hand, describe the relative position of loci on a chromosome as a function of how frequently the loci are inherited together. Distances between these loci is measured in centimorgans, which is a measure of recombination frequency. For the human genome, a centimorgan is approximately equal to one million base pairs.

A major thrust of the molecular revolution has been the identification of disease genes. This task is similar in magnitude to finding an individual person who is living somewhere in the world. Genes are identified by first mapping the gene to a particular chromosome (localizing a person to a particular continent and country), refining the mapping to a region of the chromosome (localizing to a state or province), placing the gene within a YAC (city), narrowing the focus to a cosmid (neighborhood), and then identifying the gene (street address).

Genes can be identified by using several different strategies, including functional and positional cloning or linkage analysis. *Functional cloning* involves isolating the gene based upon an understanding of the basic pathophysiology of a disorder. Thus, the gene for insulin was discovered after the protein deficiency of diabetes was known. This process is very limited, as the basic protein defect of most disease states is simply unknown. A far more powerful technology is *positional cloning,* which analyzes the coinheritance of the trait of interest and markers throughout the genome. A trait and marker that are inherited more frequently than would be noted by chance alone must be closely linked together on the same chromosome. The power of this approach is that absolutely nothing needs to be known about the gene's function. A variety of naturally occurring DNA sequence variations, including microsatellite repeats, provide a source of markers that are amenable to the PCR amplification.

Linkage analysis methods are parametric, meaning that certain assumptions must be made concerning mode of inheritance (dominant or recessive) and degree of penetrance.[14] The statistical analysis of a parametric model involves comparing the fit of the proposed model with the observed data, with the null hypothesis of no linkage. This is expressed as the logarithm of the odds (LOD) score. When the LOD score is three or greater (1000:1), it is generally accepted that linkage has been demonstrated.

While these techniques work well for simple Mendelian traits, parametric models do not work well for the isolation of genes that are associated with more complex traits. Nonparametric models, which assume no models for the inheritance of a trait, involve determining how frequently a chromosomal region is shared between affected sibs and is inherited from a common ancestor (identical by descent).

AT A GLANCE. . .

Types of Genome Mapping

1. **Physical Mapping:** show the location of identifiable landmarks along individual chromosome lengths; distances are measured in base pairs.

2. **Genetic or Linkage Mapping:** show the relative position of loci on a chromosome as a function of how frequently the loci are inherited together; measured in centimorgans.

GENETIC OTOLARYNGOLOGIC DISORDERS

Nonsyndromic Hearing Loss

Profound early-onset (prelingual) deafness affects 4–11 per 10,000 children in the United States. As recognized by Politzer, over half of those children affected have a genetic predisposition to hearing loss.[15] Coinherited anomalies are present in approximately 30% of affected patients (i.e., *syndromic hearing loss* [SHL]), and the remaining 70% have no other discernable associated findings (i.e., *nonsyndromic hearing loss* [NSHL]). Approximately 80% of cases of NSHL are autosomal recessive in nature; 15–20% are autosomal dominant; 2% are X-linked; and less than 1% is mitochondrial.[16] Congenital hearing loss is hearing loss that is present at birth, and it can be hereditary, infectious, or traumatic in origin. Conversely, inherited hearing loss does not necessarily present at birth, but can present later in life after language development has occurred (i.e., *postlingual hearing loss*). By convention, autosomal dominant genes are abbreviated as DFNA1, DFNA2, etc., autosomal recessive genes are DFNB1, DFNB2, etc., and X-linked genes are DFN1, DFN2, etc.

SPECIAL CONSIDERATION:

Approximately 80% of nonsyndromic hearing loss is autosomal recessive, 15 to 20% is autosomal dominant, 2% is X-linked, and less than 1% is mitochondrial.

Several challenges combine to make the mapping and cloning of NSHL nonsyndromic deafness genes a formidable task: (1) most deafness genes are autosomal recessive, making the identification of large families with multiple affected individuals difficult; (2) members of the Deaf community tend to marry and have children with other Deaf partners, a phenomenon known as assortative matings, which tends to introduce several deafness genes into a single pedigree; and (3) considerable genetic heterogeneity exists in the deafness phenotype, making the pooling of multiple small families problematic.[17] To further facilitate research into the molecular basis of hearing loss, the NIDCD recently established the Hereditary Hearing Impairment Resource Registry (HHIRR) (Http://www.boystown.org/hhirr/). This registry provides a mechanism whereby interested families can participate in genetic research.[9]

Despite these challenges, a great deal of progress has been made in the mapping and cloning of deafness genes. Whereas prior to 1994 only three loci had been identified for NSHL, as of this writing, over 30 chromosomal loci for NSHL have been identified. An updated listing of genetic information regarding NSHL is maintained on the Hereditary Hearing Loss Homepage (http://dnalab-www.uia.ac.be/dnalab/hhh) by Dr. Guy Van Camp and Dr. Richard J. H. Smith.

A handful of nuclear genes have been identified, including POU3F4, which is responsible for DFN3,[18] and myosin VIIA, which is an unconventional myosin associated with DFNB2 and Usher syndrome type 1B.[19] Mutations in myosin VIIA have also been found in families with DFNB1 and DFNB5.[20] The gene responsible for the first autosomal dominant syndrome mapped, DFNA1, was discovered recently.[21] This gene encodes for a protein that regulates the polymerization of actin, which is a major component of the cytoskeleton of hair cells. DFNA1 is characterized by a progressive sensorineural hearing loss (SNHL) that begins at around age 10 years and progresses to a profound deafness at age 30 years. DFNA1 was first mapped using DNA from a large Costa Rican family, who were descended from a common ancestor from the early 1700s. Linkage analysis refined the interval on chromosome 5 to an area of approximately one centimorgan, and then a BAC was constructed of the region and sequenced. Computer programs matched sequence information to databases, and a human gene homologous to the *Drosophila* gene *diaphanous* was identified. Using mouse genetic information, the human gene was characterized further, and affected and unaffected members of the Costa Rican family were screened for mutations. A guanine to thymine substitution in a splice donor site was identified, which led to a four-base pair insertion in mRNA, a frameshift, and a resultant protein truncation.

Syndromic Hearing Loss

Several genes associated with SHL have been identified. Usher syndrome, which is an autosomal recessive disorder, is characterized by retinitis pigmentosa (RP) and SNHL, and is the most common cause of deafness and blindness. Approximately 5% of deaf children have Usher syndrome. Usher syndrome exists in at least three clinically recognizable forms; type 1, type 2, and type 3. Type 1 is characterized by profound deafness, absent vestibular responses, and onset of RP by age 10 years; type 2 has a lesser degree of hearing loss, normal vestibular responses, and a later onset of RP; and type 3 is associated with progressive audiovestibular dysfunction and variable onset of RP. There are at least eight different loci associated with Usher syndrome: five different genes for type 1 (USH1A, USH1B, USH1C, USH1D,[22] USH1E);[23] two loci for type 2 (USH2A, USH2B), and one for type 3 (USH).[24,25]

USH1B was shown to map to a chromosomal region that was syntenic to the mouse region containing the mouse deafness gene shaker-1, which encoded for an unconventional myosin. Although the mouse phenotype did not include retinal degeneration, shaker-1 became an excellent candidate gene for USH1B, and as noted, mutations in the human myosin VIIA gene were shown to be responsible for USH1B.[26] Unconventional myosins are motor molecules that move along actin filaments and are important components of a cell's cytoskeleton. Myosin VIIA is expressed in the pigment epithelium, the photoreceptor cells of the retina, and the cochlear and vestibular neuroepithelia. Thus, the deafness associated with the syndrome may well result from defects in the morphogenesis of the stereocilia of the inner ear[27] and may suggest that mutations in additional cytoskeletal genes may be responsible for the other variants of Usher syndrome.

Waardenburg syndrome is another deafness syndrome that is characterized by SNHL, pigmentary abnormalities, and dystopia canthorum, which is the lateral displacement of the inner canthi of the eyes and should be distinguished from hypertelorism, which is the lateral displacement of the orbits. Three subtypes of Waardenburg syndrome have been distinguished on clinical grounds: type 1 is characterized by dystopia canthorum, congenital SNHL, and pigmentary abnormalities such as heterochromia irides (irises of different colors), patchy skin hypopigmentation, or a white forelock; type 2 has absence of dystopia canthorum; and type 3 is characterized by mental retardation, microcephaly, and skeletal abnormalities in addition to the characteristics of type 1. The hearing loss associated with Waardenburg syndrome shows a high degree of variable expression. Waardenburg syndrome type 1 and type 3 are caused by mutations in PAX3 a gene that encodes a transcription factor that controls the expression of other genes.[28-30] PAX3 was identified after a mouse model of Waardenburg syndrome (i.e., splotch) was shown to be caused by a mutation in the murine pax3 gene. A large number of different pax3 mutations have been identified in various patients with Waardenburg's type 1 with no correlation between mutations and phenotype severity shown.[16] Type 2 was shown to be secondary to mutations in the human microphthalmi (MITF) gene, after the identifications of mutations in the mitf gene were shown to be responsible for the microphthalmic mouse (a murine model of Waardenburg's type 2).[31]

The Jervell and Lange-Nielsen syndrome is characterized by congenital SNHL and a prolonged QT interval on electrocardiogram. It is important to attempt to identify patients with this syndrome because affected patients have a high incidence of sudden death. A variety of mutations that encode cardiac ion channels have been identified as causing the long QT syndrome, and a patient with the Jervell and Lange-Nielsen syndrome has been described with a homozygous mutation of the cardiac potassium channel gene, KVLQT1.[32]

Neurofibromatosis

Neurofibromatosis type 1 (NF1) is a common autosomal dominant disorder that is characterized by multiple neurofibromas, "cafe au lait" spots, and Lisch nodules of the iris, which are hamartomas. NF1 varies widely in its clinical expression, and the same mutation in a given family can produce widely variant phenotypes, which are possibly due to the influence of unknown modifying genes. The gene responsible for NF1 has been mapped and cloned,[33-35] and has been shown to produce a protein termed neurofibromin, which has been widely expressed in many different tissues, including brain, skin and Schwann cells of peripheral nerves. On the subcellular level, neurofibromin has been localized with cytoplasmic microtubules. Further studies suggest that NF1 may be a tumor-suppressor gene as it has shown homology to genes involved in the control of cell growth and differentiation. Although prenatal diagnosis for NF1 is possible in most affected

families, current demand for it is low for several reasons: the variable expression of the disease makes it impossible to predict the clinical severity based upon the molecular information available, the clinical diagnosis is not difficult, and no effective medical treatment exists to ameliorate the course of the disease.[36]

Neurofibromatosis type 2 (NF2) is an inherited disorder that is distinct from the more common NF1. NF2 is an autosomal dominant disease that affects approximately one of 40,000 individuals. There is a negative family history in approximately 50% of patients, thus the disease represents new mutations. The hallmark of NF2 is the development of bilateral, vestibular schwannomas and tumor growth causing functional impairment, such as hearing loss and vestibular disturbances. Patients can also develop meningiomas, spinal schwannomas, and posterior capsular lens opacities. Genetic linkage studies and a candidate gene search discovered that the gene associated with NF2 was a tumor suppressor gene belonging to a family of genes that encoded for proteins linking elements of the cytoskeleton with the cell membrane. This gene was named merlin (for moesin-ezrin-radixin-like protein).[37,38] *Merlin* is composed of 16 exons and one alternatively spliced exon that span 110 kb. Highly conserved throughout evolution, the merlin protein exists in at least two isoforms. Most of the mutations associated with merlin result in the loss of function, which is supportive of the tumor suppressor concept. Merlin appears to be localized at the cell membrane, and could play a role in conveying information between the cell membrane, cytoskeleton, and nucleus. Merlin is the first structural gene that appears to play a tumor suppressor role.[39] Normal tumor suppressor genes act to prevent uncontrolled cell growth. Knudson has advanced the "two-hit" model of tumorigenesis.[40] Both maternal and paternal copies of the gene must be inactivated for the cell to escape this control and begin to form tumors. Thus, in a person inheriting a defective copy of the tumor suppressor gene, only a single mutation in a somatic cell results in the inactivation of both copies, with the cell escaping from growth control and a tumor developing. In contrast, in sporadic (i.e., noninherited) cases, two mutations are required in the same somatic cell for uncontrolled cell growth to begin. The likelihood of two mutations inactivating both copies of the tumor suppressor gene occurring in one cell is, of course, much less likely than one mutational event occurring. The loss of function of tumor suppressor genes appears to be a fundamental mechanism in the development of solid tumors.[41]

Infectious Disease

It is well-known that the host response to infectious agents can be varied. A pathogen may produce relatively asymptomatic illness in one person and a life-threatening illness in another. Pandemics, such as the Black Death in the Middle Ages, the influenza epidemic of 1918, and acquired immune deficiency syndrome (AIDS) are remarkable not only for the number of people that succumb, but also for the number of people that, although exposed, do not develop the disease. Infectious mononucleosis in a toddler is relatively innocuous, whereas the same disease in a young adult can be debilitating. While age and overall health status both play a role, the genetic background of the host clearly is important in disease resistance, as demonstrated by recent reports of individuals highly resistant to infection by human immunodeficiency virus type I (HIV-1). These individuals are homozygous for mutant alleles of the macrophage receptor for HIV. The mutant allele produces a nonfunctional receptor; thus, the virus cannot bind to and subsequently infect the macrophage.

The genetics of virus resistance in mice are better understood than in humans, as inbred mouse strains that vary in their susceptibility to viruses are available. A series of murine virus-resistant genes has been cloned, with products ranging from virus receptors with decreased affinity to natural killer cell receptors. These insights are being used to identify candidate virus-resistant genes in humans.[42]

There is also a genetic component controlling the susceptibility of humans to parasitic disease. A parasitic disease of interest to otolaryngologists is leishmaniasis. Occurring after a bite from sandflies infected with *Leishmania braziliensis,* the disease occurs in two stages: a primary cutaneous lesion that is occasionally followed by secondary involvement of the nasal, buccal, pharyngeal, and laryngeal mucosa, which can result in severe facial deformities. A recent analysis of susceptibility to *Leishmania braziliensis* in a Bolivian population revealed that there is evidence for a recessive major gene that controls the onset of the primary cutaneous lesion.[43] Young patients are genetically more susceptible than older subjects, suggesting that the gene is involved in childhood development of individual protection.

Craniofacial Syndromes

Children with craniofacial syndromes have many problems that fall within the purview of the pediatric otolaryngologist. Challenged with hearing loss, obstructive sleep apnea, and voice and language development problems, these patients often require long-term management. Until very recently, the molecular basis of these problems was completely unknown. A rapid succession of discoveries have begun to allow a fundamental understanding of craniofacial syndromes and have shed light on the complex process of human development, thereby offering potential for improved therapies for these patients.

Closely following the mapping of Crouzon syndrome to 10q25–26,[44] mutations in a family of proteins known as fibroblast growth factor receptors (FGFRs) were shown to be associated with four craniosynostotic syndromes: Crouzon; Apert; Jackson-Weiss, and Pfeiffer.[45,46] FGFRs are members of a large family of receptors that bind fibroblast growth factors (FGFs). These growth factors play key roles in a multitude of functions that are central to growth and development, including cell proliferation and development, morphogenesis, chemotaxis, cell survival, and angiogenesis. FGFRs are present in all germ layers and in a wide variety of eukaryotic systems. In mammals, there are four FGFRs and nine FGFs that are expressed in specific temporal spatial patterns in the developing embryo. Alternative RNA splicing produces an even larger number of functional polypeptides. Although each is genetically distinct, there is a certain amount of overlap and redundancy in function. The FGFRs have several features in common. There is an extracellular immunoglobulin (Ig)-like domain that consists of three separate regions, IgI, IgII, and IgIII. These loop-like domains are held together by a disulfide bond between two highly-conserved cysteines. A transmembrane domain connects the extracellular domain with the intracellular tyrosine kinase domain. FGFRs function by binding FGF with resultant receptor dimerization, and subsequent phosphorylation of the intracellular tyrosine, and initiation of downstream signaling pathways that lead to activation of intranuclear transcription pathways.[47] One of the fascinating (and puzzling) discoveries has been that identical point mutations in the FGFRs can lead to clinically different syndromes. For example, Crouzon syndrome (ocular proptosis, maxillary hypoplasia, and normal hands and feet) and Pfeiffer's syndrome (abnormal thumbs and large toes) can be caused by identical mutations[48] in FGFR2. Crouzon syndrome and Jackson-Weiss syndrome (craniosynostosis and abnormal feet) are also allelic.[46] Conversely, Pfeiffer syndrome can be caused by mutations in FGFR1 and in FGFR2.[49] To date, only mutations in FGFR1 and FGFR2 have been associated with craniosynostotic syndromes. Mutations in FGFR3 have been associated with achondroplasia, the most common form of human dwarfism, and with two types of thanatophoric dysplasia, a lethal form of dwarfism.[50,51]

ANIMAL MODELS IN GENETIC RESEARCH

Work in less complex organisms continues to illustrate that strategies and functions that have developed in lower animals are often very similar to those used by human cells. Understanding the information systems of lower organisms continues to shed important insights into fundamental human functions. Genomes that are of interest include bacteria (*Hemophilus influenzae*), yeast (*Saccharomyces cerevisiae*), roundworms (*Caenorhabditis elegans*), flies (*Drosophila melanogaster*), and mice. These systems can be useful not only in identifying the location of genes, but can also provide models to test intervention strategies, evaluate the potential of gene therapy, and identify modifier genes. However, at some level, the utility of these models will break down, as the interactions of the environment and the increased complexities of the human genome will not be able to be modeled in less complex organisms.[52] At the DNA sequence level, humans and chimpanzees are between 98 and 99% identical, thus the main differences between humans and other primates may not be in the actual genes themselves, but rather in the sequence and timing of expression during development.

The zebrafish has recently emerged as an animal that holds great potential as a model system for the study of vertebrate development in general and inner ear development in particular.[53] Several features of the zebrafish are attractive to researchers: zebrafish have a rapid life cycle and can easily and inexpensively be maintained by the thousands; large genetic mutations and point mutations can be induced readily, and the resulting phenotype (e.g., a mutation in the inner ear) can be ascertained easily because the developing embryos are transparent; and once a phenotype of interest has been identified, the mutant locus can be mapped quickly. As inner ear development is a continuous, dynamic process that depends upon sequential interactions with a variety of surrounding tissues, such a model system may be very helpful in not only providing new information, but also allowing the integration of information derived from mouse and human studies.

An organism of potential interest to otolaryngologists is *Deinococcus radiodurans,* which is a bacteria that can withstand up to 1,500,000 Rads of radiation. Sequencing this genome will provide insights into the strategies that the bacteria uses to maintain the functional integrity of its DNA, and this will have obvious implications for the radiation-based treatment of humans.

Mice have long been a workhorse in biologic experimentation, but have achieved new prominence in the era of genetic research, particularly in the identification of deafness genes. As most deafness genes in humans are autosomal recessive, human families that are large enough to provide adequate statistical power for positional cloning are very rare. Combining multiple small families to generate adequate power for mapping is almost impossible because so many genes are involved in human deafness and no other phenotypic distinctions to allow rationale grouping exist. On the other hand, mice do not share these limitations as it is relatively easy to generate large populations of mice with the same mutant gene. Thus, a powerful approach for identifying human deafness genes is to map the mutant mouse gene, clone the gene, identify the human homologue, and look for mutations in affected families. Central to this is the development of a comparative map, which identifies areas of the human and mouse genome that have nearly identical gene content. With this, identification of the mouse gene predicts the location of the human gene.[54] By convention, mouse genes are denoted by lower-case type and human genes are capitalized.

An example of this strategy is the isolation of the gene for Usher 1B. The mouse deafness mutation shaker 1 and human Usher 1B were mapped to homologous areas of the respective genomes. Thus, when the mouse phenotype was shown to be caused by a mutation in the gene known as myosin VIIa the human gene myosin VIIA was quickly shown to be mutated in patients with Usher syndrome. Spontaneous mouse mutations were generally first identified by other phenotypic abnormalities that were more obvious, such as vestibular dysfunction (in the Japanese dancing mice) or pigmentation defects in the animals coat.[55] The recently identified murine deafness gene *Snell's waltzer* encodes for another unconventional myosin (myo VI) and is an additional candidate gene for human deafness.[56] Other mutations have been induced using a variety of means, such as radiation, or chemical mutagenics such as, N-ethyl, N-nitrosourea (ENU), or chlorambucil. Mouse genes can be identified by microinjecting transgenes, which then randomly insert into the murine genome. Occasionally, this random insertion will disrupt a gene, generating an observable phenotypic change. The transgene can be identified and thus becomes a probe for the identification of the disrupted gene. Specific mutations can be induced into the murine germ line by homologous recombination or by "knockout" strategies, in which specific genes are rendered nonfunctional, and these can provide insight into in vivo gene function.

Genetic defects resulting in hearing loss can affect structures from the external and middle ear through the inner ear to the central auditory system. Grouping the mutations into categories based upon the abnormal pathologic features observed provides a useful strategy for categorizing the mutations. A recent grouping strategy provides for seven groups: middle ear defects, morphogenetic inner ear defects, central auditory system defects, peripheral neural defects, neuroepithelial defects, cochleo-saccular defects, and late-onset hearing loss.[55] Neuroepithelial defects are associated with abnormalities of the sensory neuroepithelium (the cochlear organ of Corti, and the vestibular saccular, utricular maculae, and cristae) and appear to be a very common form of human inner ear pathology. Cochleo-saccular defects are associated with a primary abnormality in the stria vascularis, which is the structure responsible for generating the endocochlear potential in the endolymph. Of interest, melanocytes in the stria play a key role in generating the endocochlear potential, therefore a lack of melanocytes in the stria results in an absent endocochlear potential. This melanocyte deficiency occurs in other organ systems, including the integumentary system. This explains the association of hearing loss and coat color defects in mammals such as the Dalmatian dog and the splotch mouse (a model for Waardenburg's syndrome). Conversely, albino animals have normal hearing, which means that the defect in melanocytes associated with endocochlear potential generation is distinct from the defect associated with pigment production.

GENE THERAPY

Advances in molecular medicine have provided new insights into the molecular mechanisms of health and disease and have begun to provide rational biochemical targets for therapy. New pharmaceutic agents and biologic products are being developed based upon a molecular understanding of specific pathophysiologies. *Gene therapy* refers to the concept that manipulation of the genes themselves may be of therapeutic benefit to the patient. While gene therapy can be conceptualized in several different ways, one common distinction made is between somatic and germline therapies.

Germline therapy refers to technologies that are designed to alter the genetic makeup of the reproductive cells of an individual with the goal of changing the genes that are inherited by that individual's offspring. Germline therapies are currently considered ethically unacceptable. Indeed, the Recombinant DNA Advisory Committee (RAC) of the NIH, which is the group that oversees human gene therapy studies, will not consider proposals for germline alteration. *Somatic therapies* are those that are designed to integrate new genes or change mutated genes in the somatic cells of the individual patient. Somatic therapies are currently divided into ex vivo therapies, in which cells are genetically altered outside of the patient's body and then introduced into the patient, and in vivo therapies, in which genes are directly introduced into patients either by various sorts of vectors or as the DNA itself. Once inside the patient, the new DNA can be involved in the production of therapeutic protein products and in the replacement or repair of defective genes.

Genes can be delivered by a vector to cells within a patient's body, where the gene would then produce a therapeutic protein product. For example, genes expressing insulin could be introduced into patients with diabetes or genes encoding viral proteins could be introduced for the purpose of vaccination. This approach does not necessarily require integration of the new gene into the host genome. Rather, the gene could exist for a period of time as an extrachromosomal piece of DNA. Gene integration could be manipulated so that short-term or long-term protein production is obtained. Thus, therapy could be optimized and adjusted to reflect patient growth, development, or intercurrent disease, and maximum therapeutic benefit could be achieved. Other proposed forms of gene therapy include the delivery of antisense molecules, cytotoxic genes, immunostimulatory genes, and chemoprotective genes.[57]

Although gene therapy has had several successes, there remain several formidable technical obstacles. Our basic understanding of the molecular basis of most diseases is limited, and relatively few genes have been identified. Effective vector systems are still in the developmental process, and adequate animal models for most disease processes are lacking. When first introduced, the concept of gene therapy immediately captured the imagination of clinicians, scientists, policy makers, the media, and the general public. Gene therapy was widely regarded as the answer to most of humankind's ailments. When major therapeutic advances did not quickly follow, there was a general disappointment at the relatively slow pace of clinical success. A more realistic set of expectations along with the realization that the best way to make progress is through a complete and thorough understanding of the basic molecular biology have supplanted the initial enthusiasm for gene therapy.

Several different vector systems have been developed over the years, each with its own advantages and disadvantages. Commonly used vector systems include retroviruses, adenovirus, adeno-associated virus (AAV), and nonviral methods such as plasmid-liposome complexes and electroporation. Retroviruses have a RNA-based genome that is complexed with the enzyme called RT, which converts RNA into single-stranded, or proviral, DNA (ssDNA). This proviral DNA is transported to the nucleus of the target cell where it is converted into double-stranded DNA (dsDNA) and randomly integrated into the genome. To use a retrovirus as a vector, viral genes are deleted to make the virus "defec-

tive," that is, the retrovirus cannot reproduce inside the host cell or produce undesirable viral proteins. Advantages of retroviral gene transfer include high-efficiency gene transfer, stable integration of the delivered gene, and a wide variety of target cells.

Although retroviruses are biologic systems that seem tailor made for gene transfer, several problems exist that currently limit their use as vectors: random insertion of the vectored gene into the target genome carries the risk of disrupting a gene already in place (i.e., random insertional mutagenesis); if insertion disrupts a tumor suppressor gene or activates an oncogene, uncontrolled cell growth could occur; since the integration is theoretically permanent, chronic overexpression of the gene product could be potentially deleterious; and retroviruses can integrate only into dividing cells, and can carry only about 7 kB of inserted DNA.

Adenovirus vectors also are characterized by high-efficiency gene transfer and a wide variety of target cells, but have the advantage of not requiring the division of target cells. Disadvantages include a lack of stable gene integration with transient gene expression and host inflammatory reactions. AAVs are vector systems that show promise because they can integrate into dividing and nondividing cells as well as into the host genome. However, AAVs can carry only 5 kB of inserted DNA, and have lower efficiencies than retroviruses and adenoviruses. Nonviral methods of gene transfer include the use of plasmid-liposome complexes, electroporation, and a variety of chemical techniques. These methodologies suffer from low-efficiency gene transfer and the transient nature of gene expression.

Additional barriers to gene therapy include ensuring the delivery of genes to specific tissues, that the insertion of genes does not result in a mutagenic process and subsequent development of malignancy, controlling the administered dose, and avoiding immunologic reactions by the host to engineered proteins or cells.[58] Gene therapy for complex genetic diseases (such as cancer) and the regulation of temporal and spatial gene expression for other complex diseases remain future goals.

Another example of a gene-based therapy is the recent birth of two genetically identical lambs, Polly and Molly, that carry the human gene that encodes for Factor IX, which is the clotting factor deficient in patients with hemophilia B. When these lambs mature they will produce Factor IX in their milk, allowing for ready purification of the protein for administration to humans.

AT A GLANCE. . .

Advantages and Disadvantages of the Vectors for Gene Therapy

1. **Retroviruses:** advantages include high-efficiency gene transfer, stable integration of the delivered gene, and a wide variety of target cells; disadvantages include random insertional mutagenesis, inability to integrate into nondividing cells, and limited (7 kB) capacity for carrying inserted DNA.

2. **Adenoviruses:** advantages include high-efficiency gene transfer, a wide variety of target cells, and ability to integrate into nondividing target cells; disadvantages include unstable gene integration and host inflammatory reactions.

3. **Adeno-associated viruses:** advantages include the ability to integrate into dividing and nondividing cells and integration into the host genome; disadvantages include limited (5 kB) capacity for inserted DNA and low-efficiency gene transfer.

4. **Plasmid-liposome complexes:** advantages include its nonviral state; disadvantages include low-efficiency gene transfer and the transient nature of gene expression.

5. **Electroporation:** advantages include its nonviral state; disadvantages include low-efficiency gene transfer and the transient nature of gene expression.

THE HUMAN GENOME PROJECT

The HGP is a research effort to determine the complete DNA sequence of the human. The project is a joint initiative between the NIH and the Department of Energy (DOE), and is coordinated by the National Center for Human Genome Research (now the National Human Genome Research Institute) at the NIH and the Office of Health and Environmental Research at the DOE. Whereas the role of the NIH is easy to understand, the role of the DOE is more complex. The DOE and its predecessor agencies have long been interested in the detection of genetic changes that are induced by ionizing radiation and the health effects thereof.[59] The concept that knowing the entire sequence of the genome would lead to the detection of mutations, even point mutations, more easily arose from the DOE. DOE laboratories had a great deal of experience in creating multidisciplinary, large-scale scientific projects; they possessed engineering expertise; and they worked with high-performance computing centers. Information on the DOE projects and links to Los Alamos, Lawrence Berkeley, and Lawrence Livermore National Laboratories are available at http://www.er.doe.gov/.

The long-term goals of the HGP are to construct a series of high-resolution physical and genetic maps of the human genome, to construct various model systems, to sequence completely the human and animal model DNAs, and to develop the information technologies necessary to handle the immense amount of data generated. To accomplish these goals, a series of short-term goals have been established. These goals are to assemble a genetic and physical map of the human genome, to begin work on a series of model organisms, to improve DNA sequencing technologies and the information systems required and to develop training programs and other programs to consider the ethical, legal, and social issues associated with the research. The HGP has assigned the mapping and sequencing responsibilities of the various chromosomes to a number of laboratories. Issues of sequencing strategy, methods to determine data quality in the various databases, and timing of data are important aspects of the HGP that are continually reviewed.

The Human Genome Organization (HUGO) is an international effort affiliated with the HGP. The principal countries associated with HUGO are Great Britain, France, Japan, and Russia.[60] These international research efforts have generated an incredible amount of information, and new technologies for information handling have been an important part of the HGP. The information is being accumulated in a variety of databases, and a number of tools for the efficient storage, analysis, and display of this information are being developed. Foremost has been the integration of the Internet and the World Wide Web into daily research activity. Not only have national and international collaborative efforts been strengthened by the use of e-mail, but the relative ease of retrieval, the continuous updating, and the interrelated nature of databases from organisms that span the evolutionary spectrum (from bacteria to humans) have made electronic access to data the major information methodology of genetics. Now, databases exist that contain physical maps (including STSs, cytogenetic YAC, BAC, and cosmid), genetic linkage maps, and mouse (normal, transgenic, and knockout) and human phenotypes. Numerous academic and governmental institutions, as well as commercial businesses, maintain databases. Problems with the databases include the tasks of organizing the sheer amount of information, maintaining the accuracy and integrity of the data, and integrating the information derived from the different methodologies. In addition, proprietary databases exist and not all databases are accessible to the general public. As the information available is expanding so rapidly, any attempt to catalogue the various data bases will be quickly out of date. However, a partial list of the major data bases is included (Table 4–1). Starting at one of these sites and then linking to other sites, or using a search engine to look for key words, are strategies that will give the interested reader the most current information.

Although not associated with the HGP, the Human Genome Diversity Project (HGDP) is a proposal to sample and preserve the genetic diversity of human populations around the world. Although various sampling strategies have been proposed and issues such as funding and confidentiality remain to be resolved, most anthropologists agree that this collection would be a tremendous resource to allow

TABLE 4–1: A Partial List of Databases Containing Information Generated by The Human Genome Project

Online Mendelian Inheritance in Man (OMIM) is a comprehensive catalogue of human genes and genetic disorders that describes the phenotype and the clinical management. It also gives genotype information such as the mode of inheritance, mapping information, and the state of the molecular genetics. A clinical synopsis is also included. http://www.ncbi.nlm.nih.gov/omim/

National Center for Biotechnology Information (NCBI) is responsible for GenBank, which is a NIH-sponsored effort that collects all known DNA sequences. http://www.ncbi.nlm.nih.gov/

Genome Data Base (GDB) is the major human genetic data repository. Maintained as a relational database, the information in GDB is linked to the OMIM data. http://gdbwww.gdb.org/

Cooperative Human Linkage Center (CHLC) contains genetic maps of the human genome showing the position of well-defined microsatellite markers with a high degree of heterozygosity. http://www.chlc.org/

investigators to study human diversity in whatever gene or segment of DNA that was of interest.[61] The Human Population Genetics Laboratory at Stanford is a center for analyzing the genetics of human population movements (http://lotka.stanford.edu/).

SPECIAL CONSIDERATION:

The long-term goals of the Human Genome Project are to construct a series of high-resolution physical and genetic maps of the human genome, to construct various model systems, to sequence completely the human and animal model DNAs, and to develop the information technologies necessary to handle the data generated.

Molecular anthropology is defined as the use of molecular genetics to address questions concerning human evolution and diversity.[61] By analyzing specific areas of the mtDNA genome and the nuclear genome (which has areas of hypervariability and areas that are highly conserved), molecular anthropologists can select areas of the genomes with mutational rates that are most informative. These investigations provide insights into human origins and migration patterns, the origin and spread of disease-causing mutations, and a genetic basis for understanding normal human variation; these investigations provide a "molecular physical anthropology."

ETHICS OF GENETICS

The advances in molecular genetics are accompanied by a concern for the rights and welfare of patients and individuals who participate in genetic research. Technological advances now make it possible to perform genetic analysis on a wide variety of biologic specimens that were not considered amenable to such analysis previously. In addition, evaluation of consenting family members generates information concerning other family members, including those that specifically may not have granted consent to the research project. The American Society of Human Genetics recently has issued a Statement on Informed Consent for Genetic Research.[62]

This statement recognizes that the ethics of biomedical research evolves as technological advances are achieved. A particular area of change is the prospective collection of specimens for genetic research purposes. It is now considered inappropriate for subjects to be asked to grant blanket consent for any future genetic project. Informed consent should be obtained for the study proposed, and the confidentiality of subjects should be maintained. Information should not be shared with other family members, employers, insurance companies, or other parties without written consent. Subjects should understand that information regarding identification of medical risk, carrier status, or risk to offspring may result. Misidentified parentage, adverse psychological sequelae, disruption of family dynamics, social stigmatization, and adverse financial consequences, such as employment refusal and difficulties obtaining insurance, are all potential outcomes of genetic research. The need for informed consent varies by study design and by the degree of anonymity of the subjects. Informed consent clearly needs to be obtained for research utilizing identified specimens, whereas the use of "anonymized" specimens (specimens that were initially identified but have been stripped of all identifiers) does not. Anonymous specimens (material originally collected without identifying information) obviously do not require consent.

The importance of ethical issues in genomic research is illustrated by the inclusion of funding for the study of Ethical, Legal and Social Issues (ELSI) within the funding for the HGP. Approximately 3% of the budget for the HGP is devoted to investigating these issues. Thus, the HGP is the first scientific project to study systematically such issues from its inception.[63] Overarching issues studied under the ELSI mandate include how to use the tremendous amount of information generated, how to identify the limits of genetic manipulations that should be undertaken, and how to respond to the upcoming changes in self-understanding.[63] Issues of privacy of genetic information, effective and fair use of genetic information, and professional and public education need to be addressed. Genetic screening, genetic privacy, employment and insurance concerns, and the implications of patenting genomic sequences are examples of some of the current ELSI's areas of interest. Educational initiatives such as workshops for judges to help them better understand forensic genetics and the inclusion of genetics in the curricula for high school biology students are examples

of the fundamental importance of educating the citizenry so that informed decisions can be made.

Many other areas of the federal government are involved in the genetic revolution. The National Bioethics Advisory Committee (formed by Executive Order 12975 on October 3, 1995) is a panel of scientists and citizens responsible for advising the President and other members of government about the ethical concerns posed by the new technology, including the advisability of cloning human beings. The Department of Defense has begun to store the DNA of aircrews, special operations forces, and other members of the armed forces who are at high risk, with a view toward the identification of remains unidentifiable by other technologies, the so-called "DNA dog tags." The Americans with Disabilities Act of 1990 (ADA) is a federal civil rights law that addresses employment discrimination. Using genetic information to deny employment opportunities or limit health care coverage is a potential violation of this act.[64] In addition, state and federal governments have proposed various genetic privacy bills to prevent abuses of genetic information, with a particular focus on health insurance accessibility, employment, and health care practices. Indeed, the notion has been advanced that once the genetic susceptibilities of all of us can be determined, the only way to ensure equitable access to health care will be through a socialized form of medicine.

Commercialization of the products of the genetic revolution is an area of intense activity, and attempts to profit from the basic information of the human has generated a great deal of controversy. The U.S. Patent and Trademark Office rejected a proposal (by the NIH) to patent a large number of genetic sequences, even though the discoverers had no knowledge of the sequences' function.[65] The proposal was rejected on the grounds that not knowing the function of the sequences meant that the inventors could not demonstrate the "utility" of their invention; demonstration of utility, inability of previous workers to anticipate their meaning, and their importance being nonobvious are criteria that inventions must meet to be patentable.

It is almost inescapable that a genetic profile of ever-increasing complexity will be compiled on each of us. One of the potential dangers of this is the concept of genetic determinism, which is the assumption that just because a person has a gene for a particular trait then he or she will definitely develop that trait. The presence of genetic alterations must be interpreted with care, as identifying the presence of a disease gene is not the same as actually having the disease. The converse of this is that, for example, if a person does not possess the genes for high intelligence or some other desirable trait, then that person will not exert effort to achieve his or her best. These issues are particularly important when the patient is a child.[66]

ROLE OF THE PEDIATRIC OTOLARYNGOLOGIST

Whereas it is not difficult to identify children with gross dysmorphology, many other syndromes present with more subtle abnormalities of the head, neck, and organs of communication. The pediatric otolaryngologist is often called upon to evaluate children with hearing loss or delayed speech and language acquisition. Constellations of subtle findings, such as slightly dysmorphic facial appearance, anatomic abnormalities of the external auditory canals, ossicular malformations, or cochlear radiographic abnormalities, may suggest a genetic basis for a child's problems. Chromosomal abnormalities should be suspected when craniofacial dysmorphology presents with developmental delay, speech or language developmental delay, growth retardation, or mental retardation. It is important to note that many of the clues to a genetic diagnosis may not be apparent in the newborn period and only become more obvious as the child matures. Therefore, repeated evaluations may be in order. As advances in karyotyping occur, higher resolution analysis becomes possible. Chromosomes that were interpreted as normal in the past may reveal abnormalities on repeat evaluation with higher resolution technology. Thus, children who underwent genetic screening with karyotyping as infants with no specific diagnosis being reached may benefit from repeat examinations later in life. The pediatric otolaryngologist is in a unique position to recognize subtle abnormalities of the ears, head, and neck, and developmental delay may be more apparent to a clinician with special training and a special interest in the area.

As surgeons who care for children, pediatric otolaryngologists have unique opportunities to fully participate in the molecular revolution.[67] Indeed, surgeons possess skill sets and clinical opportunities that make their participation mandatory. One of the most fundamental contributions a clinician can make is to pose a clinically relevant question. Patients suffering from disease do not come to laboratories seeking care, they come to clinicians. An attuned physician can recognize that a molecular-based research inquiry may benefit a particular patient population. Surgeons, in particular, have immediate access to tissue specimens, both normal and pathologic. This is not a trivial matter, and collection of useful clinical material requires a conscious and committed effort from an informed surgeon who already focuses so much energy on the surgical procedure at hand. Surgeons have a detailed understanding of wound healing, the inflammatory process, the relationships of physiology to pathology, and the reaction of the body to trauma, which are all fundamentally important questions that are amenable to molecular-based inquiries.

> **SPECIAL CONSIDERATION:**
> Constellations of subtle findings, such as slightly dysmorphic facial appearance, anatomic abnormalities of the external auditory canals, ossicular malformations, or cochlear radiographic abnormalities, may suggest a genetic basis.

Clinicians are attuned by training and temperament to the protection of the individual. This trait will stand subjects of genetic research in good stead, if informed attentive clinicians are actively involved in genetics research. Pediatric otolaryngologists must be attuned to the concept that hearing loss can involve cultural and linguistic differences, and that members of the Deaf community do not necessarily view research directed at mitigating hearing loss in the same light as members of the hearing community.[68,69] Surgeons who routinely operate on children are familiar with issues of informed assent and concerns about fairness and potential benefit, which are important issues when considering gene therapy in children.[70]

It is inescapable that molecular-based discoveries, technologies, and therapies will increasingly drive biomedical research and the clinical practice of medicine.[71] Determining a patient's risk of developing or transmitting a disease will become an increasingly important role for the clinician. Testing for breast and colon cancer susceptibility, hereditary hemochromatosis, and carrier status of cystic fibrosis are already possible. Interpreting these results for patients will become an integral part of preventative health care. Unfortunately, most physicians are not prepared to integrate fully modern genetics into their clinical practices. To address this, intensive education efforts are underway. The National Coalition for Health Professional Education in Genetics has been formed and now includes over one hundred organizations focused on providing an integrated educational approach to educating health care professionals. License and board examinations and medical school curricula are being revised to reflect the new knowledge. Importantly, the courts are already holding physicians to a higher standard in terms of providing genetic counseling. In Pate v Threlkel, the Florida Supreme Court determined that a physician caring for a patient with a hereditary disease owes a duty of care to the children of the patient and should warn the patient of the potential risk to the children. This ruling arose from a malpractice suit in which a surgeon caring for a woman with a medullary thyroid cancer did not tell the woman of the hereditary nature of the disease. The woman's daughter then developed medullary cancer three years later and sued her mother's physician for failing to inform her mother of the daughter's risk, thus preventing the daughter from obtaining earlier diagnosis and treatment of her disease.[72]

As predictive genetic testing and gene-based therapies become part of our armamentarium, we are beholdened to understand these changes and to be able to communicate them to our patients. Traditional genetic counselors and medical geneticists will continue to play an important role, but there will simply be too few of these highly-qualified specialists to adequately manage all the patients. Counseling patients as to the appropriateness of obtaining genetic testing to determine disease susceptibility, interpretation of genetic test results, and offering gene-based therapies increasingly will become part of the way we care for our patients. Pediatric otolaryngologists must have a working knowledge of genetic principles in order to provide state-of-the-art care for our patients.

REFERENCES

1. Nakao M, Sassaki H. Genomic imprinting: Significance in development and diseases and the molecular mechanisms. J Biochem 1996; 120:467–473.
2. Casselbrant ML. The heritability of otitis media: A twin study. Presented at the II Congress of the Interamerican Association of Pediatric Otorhinolaryngology and the III Brazilian Congress of Pediatric Otorhinolaryngology, Sao Paulo, Brazil, September 23, 1997.
3. Beardsley T. Vital data. Sci Am 1996: 100–105.
4. Church DM, Stotler CJ, Rutter JL, et al. Isolation of genes from complex sources of mammalian genomic DNA using exon amplification. Nat Genet 1994; 6:98–105.
5. Reardon W, Ross RJM, Sweeney MG, et al. Diabetes mellitus associated with a pathogenic point mutation in mitochondrial DNA. Lancet 1992; 340:1376–1379.
6. Jaber L, Shohat M, Bu X, et al. Sensorineural deafness inherited as a tissue specific mitochondrial disorder. J Med Genet 1992; 29:86–90.
7. Prezant TR, Agapian JV, Bohlman MC, et al. Mitochondrial ribosomal RNA mutation associated with both antibiotic-induced and non-syndromic deafness. Nat Genet 1993; 4:289–294.
8. Fischel-Ghodsian N. Mitochondrial mutations and hearing loss: Paradigm for mitochondrial genetics. Am J Hum Genet 1998; 62:15–19.
9. Snow JB. News from the National Institute on Deafness and Other Communication Disorders. Am J Otol 1995; 16:253–256.
10. Wackym PA, Simpson TA, Gantz BJ. Polymerase chain reaction amplification of DNA from archival celloidin-embedded human temporal bone sections. Laryngoscope 1993; 103:583–588.
11. Seidman MD, Bai U, Khan MJ, et al. Association of mitochondrial DNA deletions and cochlear pathology: A molecular biologic tool. Laryngoscope 1996; 106:777–783.
12. Burgess RC, Michaels L, Bale JF Jr, et al. Polymerase chain reaction amplification of herpes simplex viral DNA from the geniculate ganglion of a patient with Bell's palsy. Ann Otol Rhinol Laryngol 1994; 103:775–779.
13. Orita M, Suzuki Y, Sekiya T, et al. Rapid and sensitive detection of point mutations and DNA polymorphisms using the polymerase chain reaction. Genomics 1989; 5:874–879.
14. Lander ES, Schork N. Genetic dissection of complex traits. Science 1994; 265:2037–2048.
15. Politzer A. Lehrbuch der ohrenheilkunde für praktische Ärzte und Studierende. II Band. Stuttgart: Ferdinand Enke, 1882.
16. Mhatre AN, Lalwani AK. Molecular genetics of deafness. Otolaryngol Clin North Am 1996; 29:421–435.
17. Camp GV, Willems PJ, Smith RJH. Nonsyndromic hearing impairment: Unparalleled heterogeneity. Am J Hum Genet 1997; 60:758–764.
18. de Kok YJM, van der Maarel SM, Bitner-Glindzicz M, et al. Association between X-linked mixed deafness

and mutations in the POU domain gene POU3F4. Science 1995; 267:685–688.

19. Weil D, Küssel P, Blanchard S, et al. The autosomal recessive isolated deafness, DFNB2, and the Usher 1B syndrome are allelic defects of the myosin-VIIA gene. Nat Genet 1997; 16:191–193.

20. Liu XZ, Walsh J, Mburu P, et al. Mutations in the myosin VIIA gene cause non-syndromic recessive deafness. Nat Genet 1997; 16:188–199.

21. Lynch ED, Lee MK, Morrow JE, et al. Nonsyndromic deafness DFNA1 associated with mutation of a human homolog of the *drosophila* gene *diaphanous*. Science 1997; 278:1315–1318.

22. Wayne S, Kaloustian VMD, Schloss M, et al. Localization of the Usher syndrome type ID gene USHID to chromosome 10. Hum Mol Genet 1996; 5:1689–1692.

23. Chaïb H, Kaplan J, Gerber S, et al. A newly identified locus for Usher syndrome type I, USH1E, maps to chromosome 21q21. Hum Mol Genet 1997; 6:27–31.

24. Joensuu T, Blanco G, Pakarinen L, et al. Refined mapping of the Usher syndrome Type III locus on chromosome 3, exclusion of candidate genes, and identification of the putative mouse homologous region. Genomics 1996; 38:255–263.

25. Kimberling WJ, Möller C. Clinical and molecular genetics of Usher syndrome. J Am Acad Audiol 1995; 6:63–72.

26. Weil D, Blanchard S, Kaplan J, et al. Defective myosin VIIA gene responsible for Usher syndrome type 1B. Nature 1995; 374:60–61.

27. Weil D, Lévy G, Sahly I, et al. Human myosin VIIA responsible for the Usher 1B syndrome: A predicted membrane-associated motor protein expressed in developing sensory epithelia. Proc Natl Acad Sci 1996; 93:3232–3237.

28. Baldwin CT, Hoth CF, Amos JA, et al. An exonic mutation in the Hup2 paired domain gene causes Waardenburg's syndrome. Nature 1992; 355:637–638.

29. Tassabehji M, Read AP, Newton VE, et al. Waardenburg's syndrome patients have mutations in the human homologue of the Pax-3 paired box gene. Nature 1992; 355:635–636.

30. Hoth CF, Milunsky A, Lipsky N, et al. Mutations in the paired domain of the human PAX3 gene cause Klein-Waardenburg syndrome (WS-III) as well as Waardenburg syndrome type 1 (WS-I). Am J Hum Genet 1993; 52:455–462.

31. Tassabehji M, Newton VE, Read AP. Waardenburg syndrome type 2 caused by mutations in the human microphthalmia (MITF) gene. Nat Genet 1994; 8:251–255.

32. Splawski I, Timothy KW, Vincent GM, et al. Molecular basis of the long-QT syndrome associated with deafness. N Engl J Med 1997; 1562–1567.

33. Cawthon RM, Weiss R, Xu G, et al. A major segment of the neurofibromatosis type 1 gene: cDNA se-

quence, genomic structure, and point mutations. Cell 1990; 62:193–201.

34. Viskochil D, Buchberg AM, Xu G, et al. Deletions and a translocation interrupt a cloned gene at the neurofibromatosis type 1 locus. Cell 1990; 62:187–192.

35. Wallace MR, Marchuk DA, Anderson LB, et al. Type 1 neurofibromatosis gene: Identification of a large transcript disrupted in three NF1 patients. Science 1990; 249:181–186.

36. Shen MH, Harper PS, Upadhyaya M. Molecular genetics of neurofibromatosis type 1 (NF1). J Med Genet 1996; 33:2–17.

37. Trofatter JA, MacCollin M, Rutter JL, et al. A novel moesin-, ezrin-, radixin-like gene is a candidate for the neurofibromatosis 2 tumor suppressor. Cell 1993; 72:791–800.

38. Rouleau GA, Merel P, Lutchman M, et al. Alteration in a new gene encoding a putative membrane-organizing protein causes neurofibromatosis type 2. Nature 1993; 363:515–521.

39. Lutchman M, Rouleau GA. Neurofibromatosis type 2: A new mechanism of tumor suppression. Trends Neurosci 1996; 19:373–377.

40. Knudson AG: Mutation and cancer. Statistical study of retinoblastoma. Proc Natl Acad Sci 1971; 68:820–825.

41. Kley N, Seizinger BR. The neurofibromatosis 2 (NF2) tumour suppressor gene: Implications beyond the hereditary tumour syndrome? Cancer Surv 1995; 25:207–218.

42. Brownstein DG. Comparative genetics of resistance to viruses. Am J Hum Genet 1998; 62:211–214.

43. Alcaïs A, Abel L, David C, et al. Evidence for a major gene controlling susceptibility to tegumentary leishmaniasis in a recently exposed Bolivian population. Am J Hum Genet 1997; 61:968–979.

44. Preston RA, Post JC, Keats BJB, et al. A gene for Crouzon craniofacial dysostosis maps to the long arm of chromosome 10. Nat Genet 1994; 7:149–153.

45. Wilkie AOM, Slaney SF, Oldridge M, et al. Apert syndrome results from localized mutations of FGFR2 and allelic with Crouzon syndrome. Nat Genet 1995; 9:165–172.

46. Jabs EW, Li X, Scott AF, et al. Jackson-Weiss and Crouzon syndromes are allelic with mutations in the fibroblast growth factor receptor. Nat Genet 1994; 8:275–279.

47. Mason IJ. The ins and outs of fibroblast growth factors. Cell 1994; 78:547–552.

48. Rutland P, Pulleyn LJ, Reardon W, et al. Identical mutations in the FGFR2 gene cause both Pfeiffer and Crouzon syndrome phenotypes. Nat Genet 1995; 9:173–176.

49. Schell U, Hehr A, Feldman GJ, et al. Mutations in FGFR1 and FGFR2 cause familial and sporadic Pfeiffer syndrome. Hum Mol Genet 1995; 4:323–328.

50. Shiang R, Thompson LM, Zhu Y-Z, et al. Mutations in the transmembrane domain of FGFR3 cause the most common genetic form of dwarfism, achondroplasia. Cell 1994; 78:335-342.

51. Tarvormina PL, Shiang R, Thompson LM, et al. Mutations affecting distinct functional domains of FGFR3 cause different types of thanatophoric dysplasia. Nat Genet 1995; 9:321-328.

52. Hoffman EP. The evolving genome project: Current and future impact. Am J Hum Genet 1994; 54:129-136.

53. Riley BB, Grunwald DJ. A mutation in zebrafish affecting a localized cellular function required for normal ear development. Dev Biol 1996; 179:427-435.

54. Meisler MH. The role of the laboratory mouse in the human genome project. Am J Hum Genet 1996; 59:764-771.

55. Steel KP. Inherited hearing defects in mice. Annu Rev Genetics 1995; 29:675-701.

56. Avraham KB, Hasson T, Steel KP, et al. The mouse Snell's waltzer deafness gene encodes an unconventional myosin required for structural integrity of inner ear hair cells. Nat Genet 1995; 11:369-375.

57. Vile RC. Gene therapy for cancer—In the dock, blown off course or full speed ahead? Can Metastasis Rev 1996; 15:283-286.

58. Khavari PA, Krueger GG. Cutaneous gene therapy. Dermatol Clin 1997; 15:27-35.

59. Patrinos A, Drell DW. The human genome project: View from the Department of Energy. J Am Med Womens Assoc 1997; 52:8-10.

60. Dizikes GJ. Update on the human genome project. Clin Lab Med 1995; 15:973-988.

61. Stoneking M. The human genome project and molecular anthropology. Genome Res 1997; 7:87-91.

62. Statement on Informed Consent for Genetic Research (ASHG Report). Am J Hum Genet 1996; 59:471-474.

63. Murray TH, Livny E. The human genome project: Ethical and social implications. Bull Med Libr Assoc 1995; 83:14-21.

64. Blanck PD, Marti MW. Genetic discrimination and the employment provisions of the Americans with disabilities act: Emerging legal, empirical, and policy implications. Behav Sci Law 1996; 14:411-432.

65. Davis MH. Patents and the human genome project. Biotechnol 1993; 11:736-737.

66. Williams JK, Lessick M. Genome research: Implications for children. Pediatr Nurs 1996; 2:40-46.

67. Tzeng E, Shears LL, Lotze MT, et al. Gene therapy. Curr Probl Surg 1996: 969-1041.

68. Arnos KS, Israel J, Cunningham M. Genetic counseling of the deaf. NY Acad Sci 1992: 212-222.

69. Arnos KS. Hereditary hearing loss. N Engl J Med 1994; 331:469-470.

70. Fletcher JC, Richter G. Ethical issues of perinatal human gene therapy. J Maternal-Fetal Med 1996; 5:232-241.

71. Collins FS. Preparing health professionals for the genetic revolution. JAMA 1997; 278:1285-1286.

72. Makowski DR. The human genome project and the clinician. J Fla Med Assoc 1996; 83:307-314.

5 Vascular Anomalies of the Head and Neck

Trevor J. McGill

Standard classification of vascular anomalies offers an array of popular descriptive and pathologic terms. Unfortunately, the same word has been used to describe entirely disparate vascular lesions. *Hemangioma* has been used as a generic term for vascular lesions with distinctive natural histories. Thus, the most common tumor of infancy is known as a "strawberry," "capillary," or "cellular" hemangioma. This lesion undergoes rapid proliferation during infancy followed by involution. Port-wine stains, which never regress, also are classified as "capillary hemangiomas." Thus, our understanding of vascular anomalies has been greatly impeded by contradictory nomenclature. This antiquated nosology should be abandoned in favor of more biologically correct terminology.

In 1992, Mulliken and Glowacki[1] proposed a classification scheme based on the cellular features of vascular anomalies as correlated with clinical characteristics and natural history. They demonstrated that there are two major characteristics of vascular anomalies in infancy and childhood: (1) *hemangioma* is a distinctive lesion that is not present at birth, but grows rapidly in early infancy, is characterized by endothelial proliferation, and invariably undergoes slow involution and (2) *vascular malformation* is present at birth, is characterized by a normal rate of endothelial cell turnover, and grows commensurately with the child. Malformations are structural anomalies; that is, they are errors of vascular morphogenesis. These malformations are comprised of dysplastic vessels that are lined by quiescent endothelium. Vascular malformations are subcategorized according to vessel morphology. Slow-flow lesions can be divided into capillary (CM), lymphatic (LM), and venous (VM) malformations.

Fast-flow lesions include arterial (AM) and arteriovenous (AVM) malformations. Accurate diagnosis of a vascular anomaly is possible by correlating a clinical history and physical examination (Fig. 5-1).

SPECIAL CONSIDERATION:

Hemangiomas are vascular lesions with high endothelial cell turnover that always display a rapid post-natal phase of proliferation followed by a slow phase of involution. Vascular malformations are congenital lesions with normal endothelial cell turnover that growth commensurately with the child. They may be subdivided into slow-flow and high-flow lesions.

CHARACTERISTICS THAT DISTINGUISH HEMANGIOMA FROM VASCULAR MALFORMATION

Clinical

Hemangiomas are typically not seen at birth. However, approximately one-third, will present in the nursery as a reddish macule or telangiectasia. This lesion occurs more commonly in females, with a ratio of 3:1.[2] This tumor also occurs more frequently in whites than in blacks. Clinically, hemangioma is characterized by a rapid postnatal growth (the proliferative phase; Fig. 5-2A) for the first 8 to 12 months, followed by a slow regression over 5 to 8 years (involutive phase; Fig. 5-2B). A deep hemangioma may not manifest itself until 3 months of age.

Pediatric Otolaryngology, Edited by R.F. Wetmore, H.R. Muntz, and T.J. McGill. Thieme Medical Publishers, Inc., New York © 2000.

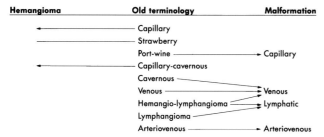

Hemangioma	Old terminology	Malformation
	Capillary	
	Strawberry	
	Port-wine	Capillary
	Capillary-cavernous	
	Cavernous	
	Venous	Venous
	Hemangio-lymphangioma	Lymphatic
	Lymphangioma	
	Arteriovenous	Arteriovenous

Figure 5–1: Old terminology and new classification for hemangioma and vascular malformations.

The skin over a deep hemangioma may be only slightly raised with a bluish hue. The terms *cavernous* for a deep hemangioma and *capillary* for a superficial lesion are confusing and should be discarded. As a hemangioma grows into the dermis, the skin becomes raised and bosselated and has a vivid red color. During the involution phase, the lesion shrinks and softens as the color fades. The signs seem to progress centrifugally (Fig. 5–3).

Vascular malformations, by definition, are present at birth. Many, but not all, present in the nursery. Most LMs and many VMs appear during infancy. AVMs more often manifest later in childhood. A vascular malformation grows proportionately with the child, although the lesion may expand secondary to trauma, infection, hormonal changes, or embolic or surgical intervention.

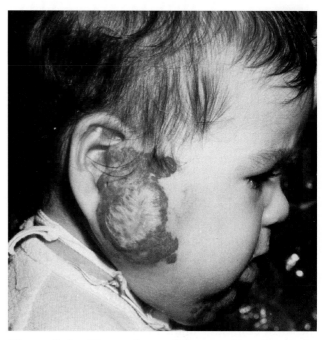

Figure 5–3: Hemangioma of the parotid region in the involutive phase. The shrinkage progresses is noted centrifugally.

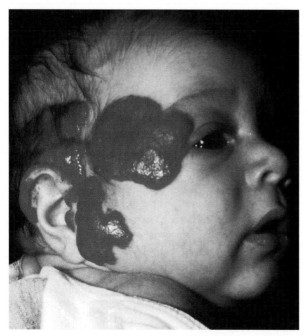

A

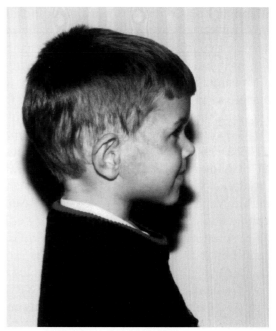

B

Figure 5–2: (A) A 6-month-old infant with extensive hemangioma involving the parotid auricle and temporal region (proliferating phase). (B) Same patient following complete involution of the hemangioma when the patient was $4\frac{1}{2}$ years of age (involution phase).

AT A GLANCE . . .

Clinical Characteristics

Hemangioma: not present at birth, proliferates rapidly in postnatal period, complete involution by age 5 to 8 years

Vascular malformation: present at birth, grows slowly with patient, no spontaneous regressions

SPECIAL CONSIDERATION:

Basic fibroblast growth factor (bFGF) is an angiogenic peptide that is elevated in the serum and urine of patients with proliferating hemangiomas. Its level is normal in patients with vascular malformations.

Cellular

Hemangioma in its proliferating phase is composed of rapidly dividing endothelial cells that form syncytial masses with and without lumens (Fig. 5–4). The concept that tumors are angiogenesis-dependent shines some light on the life cycle of hemangiomas. Angiogenic peptides act on endothelial cells and pericytes to initiate the formation of capillary networks.[3] This process is strictly regulated by inhibitors of endothelial cell growth that maintain a normal microvasculature in a quiescent state. Hemangioma is a model of pure unopposed angiogenesis. Hemangioma may result from the local absence of normal angiogenesis inhibition. Spontaneous regression of a hemangioma may be mediated by an increase in angiogenic inhibitors or a decrease in stimulators. Preliminary studies indicate that angiogenic peptide basic fibroblast growth factor (bFGF) is elevated in the serum and urine of infants with proliferating hemangiomas.[4] The peptide level is normal in patients with vascular malformations.

In contrast, histologic evaluation of vascular malformations shows no evidence of cellular proliferation, but rather a progressive dilatation of vessels of abnormal structure. Vascular malformations are lined by flat, quiescent endothelium that lay on a thin single laminar basement membrane. CM is comprised of ectatic, thin-walled, capillary-like vessels that are located in the papillary and upper reticular dermis. The walls of LMs and VMs are of variable thickness. The walls of LMs contain both striated and smooth muscle elements. Nodular clusters of lymphocytes are often seen in the connective tissues stroma of a LM. VMs are typically thin walled with sparse irregular islands of smooth muscle. Pale acidophilic fluid is typically seen within the cystic structure of a LM, whereas blood, thrombi, and phleboliths typically are seen in a VM. This dysplastic venous anomaly drains to adjacent veins, many of which are varicose. Clinically and histopathologically combined lymphatic and venous malformations (LVM) can occur. The vessels of an AVM are dysplastic and consist of thickened walls with hyperplastic smooth muscle fibers within the media. The veins in an immature AVM appear arterialized. The etiology of vascular malformations remains unclear.

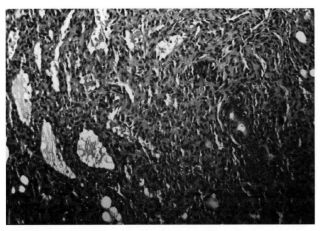

Figure 5–4: Microscopic section of a proliferative-phase hemangioma showing endothelial cells forming synctial masses with and without lumina.

AT A GLANCE . . .

Cellular Characteristics

Hemangioma: plump, proliferating endothelium (high turnover), multi-laminated basement membrane

Vascular malformation: flat, quiescent endothelium (low turnover), normal thin basement membrane

Hematologic

Large or extensive hemangiomas may cause platelet trapping, called the Kasabach-Merritt syndrome.[5] Neonates with this syndrome present with purpura and life-threatening bleeding into the pharynx, gastrointestinal (GI) tract, and/or brain. Although Kasabach-Merritt thrombocytopenic coagulopathy occurs in only 1% of infants with hemangiomas, it is associated with death in 30 to 40% of those affected despite therapy.[6]

In contrast, patients with AMs or LMs usually have normal bleeding studies. However, large or extensive VMs may be associated with localized or disseminated intravascular coagulopathy (DIC).

Imaging

Imaging studies show that a hemangioma is a well organized mass that is arranged in a lobular configuration. Magnetic resonance imaging (MRI) may reveal fast flow in a proliferative-phase hemangioma; this finding may be confused with an AVM. Vascular malformations consist entirely of vessels of a different caliber without intervening parenchyma.[7] Capillary, lymphatic, venous, and combined channel lesions have slow-flow characteristics that are apparent using ultrasonography, MRI, or computed tomography (CT).

SPECIAL CONSIDERATION:

When radiologic information is necessary for evaluation of a suspected hemangioma, MRI is the procedure of choice. Contrast and gradient studies should be included.

Skeletal

Hemangiomas only rarely cause bone or cartilaginous hypertrophy. They may obstruct the cartilaginous ear canal or distort the nasal bony-cartilaginous pyramid. Slow-flow vascular anomalies, specifically lymphatic, venous, or lymphatovenous types, can cause significant hypertrophy and distortion of the craniofacial skeleton. Fast-flow anomalies typically cause interosseus destruction.[8]

AT A GLANCE . . .
Skeletal Effects

Hemangioma: no effect
Vascular malformation: low-flow (bone hypertrophy or hypoplasia) or high-flow (bone destruction or hypertrophy)

Summary

This simplified classification of vascular anomalies of childhood as hemangioma or malformation can be called "biologic" because it is based on cellular and clinical behavior. It is a practical system, one that does not necessitate diagnostic studies such as MRI or biopsy. Obtaining an accurate history and clinical examination allows the clinician to distinguish between a hemangioma and vascular malformation in most patients.[9] Once a diagnosis is made, appropriate therapy can be planned (Practice Pathway 5–1).

HEMANGIOMA

Diagnosis and Natural History

There is an equal incidence of hemangioma in premature (1500 to 2500 g) and full-term white infants of 10 to 12% by 1 year of age. There is, however, a 23% incidence of hemangiomas in premature children weighing less than 1000 g.[10] A majority of hemangiomas appear during the first 6 weeks of life. The first sign of a hemangioma is a macular patch, blanched spot, or localized area of telangiectasia surrounded by a halo.[11] Hemangiomas undergo rapid proliferation in the early months of life as a localized tumor in a single area or in several sites throughout the body. Eighty percent of hemangiomas occur as an isolated lesion; 20% are multiple.[12] The head and neck region is most commonly involved, followed by the trunk and extremities.[9] Cervicofacial cutaneous lesions may be associated with laryngeal and tracheal lesions.[13]

When a hemangioma begins or extends into the superficial dermis, the cellular proliferation causes the skin to become raised with a vivid bright red color. Most lesions remain well circumscribed, measuring 0.5 to 5.0 cm in diameter, whereas some

Practice Pathway 5–1 MANAGEMENT OF VASCULAR ANOMALIES

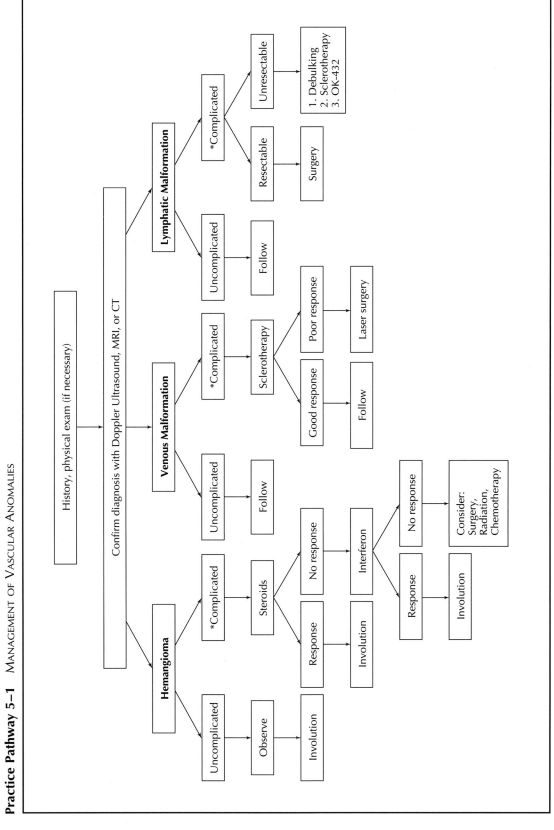

spread in a geographic fashion. Some hemangiomas proliferate in the lower dermis or subcutaneous tissue with little involvement of the superficial or capillary dermis. These lesions may be slightly raised. The overlying skin is smooth with a bluish hue; enlarged, radially-draining veins are often a clue. In the past, these deeper lesions were erroneously called cavernous hemangiomas. Likewise, when a hemangioma involves both deep and superficial skin layers, it was called a mixed, or capillary-cavernous, hemangioma. In fact, histologic examination of hemangiomas with these morphologic appearances show that the proliferating endothelial cell pattern is remarkably consistent throughout the depth of the tumor.[7] Therefore, the microscopic terms capillary and cavernous are confusing and should be discarded. Cavernous hemangiomas do not exist; the anomaly is either a deep hemangioma or a misdiagnosed VM.

A hemangioma feels firm and rubbery and is difficult to compress compared with a readily compressible VM. In certain instances in the head and neck region, it may be difficult to differentiate a deep hemangioma from a LM or VM, particularly in the preauricular or cervical areas.

Radiologic Imaging

Notwithstanding the accuracy of clinical findings in head and neck vascular anomalies, there are times when imaging technology is needed for a precise diagnosis. The following techniques should be considered in this order: ultrasonography (with Doppler flow study), MRI, CT, and angiography. Ultrasonography is highly operator-dependent; however, in experienced hands, it will differentiate slow-flow malformations (specifically venous or lymphatic anomalies) from hemangioma. MRI is more expensive but provides more information and is highly sensitive and specific.[7] MRI shows the extent of involvement within tissue planes and flow characteristics.

Complications

Obstruction

Visual. Obstruction of the visual axis by a hemangioma can result in deprivation amblyopia and failure to develop binocular vision. Even a small hemangioma of the upper eyelid may cause distortion of the growing cornea, producing refractive error that

may lead to astigmatic amblyopia.[14] Any infant diagnosed with a hemangioma in the periorbital region should have a prompt ophthalmologic examination.

Subglottic Hemangioma. Subglottic hemangioma is a potentially life-threatening lesion that usually presents after the first 6 weeks of life.[13,15,16] More than half of these infants have an associated cervicofacial cutaneous hemangioma.

Clinically, these patients, who are otherwise healthy, present with the onset of biphasic stridor. As the size of the hemangioma increases, there is reduction in the subglottic airway and subsequent insidious onset of respiratory distress. On other occasions, the child may present with a protracted episode of laryngotracheobronchitis. The child may be diagnosed with failure to thrive because of continued respiratory distress.

A lateral radiograph of the neck or a fluoroscopic study of the upper airway shows a smooth, usually posteriorly based, round swelling in the immediate subglottic space. Diagnosis requires direct laryngoscopy, which demonstrates the hemangioma as a smooth, easily compressible mass in the subglottic space (Fig. 5–5). The subglottic hemangioma may occupy 20 to 80% of the subglottic space. On rare occasions, it may extend circumferentially around the subglottic space. Biopsy of this lesion is *not* necessary to make the diagnosis. Further evaluation of the distal airway is important to rule out other hemangiomas.

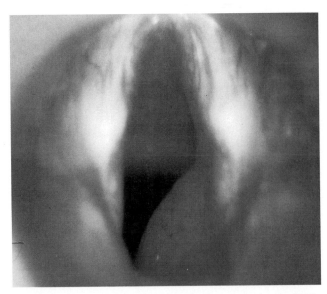

Figure 5–5: Endoscopic view of a typical subglottic hemangioma on the posterolateral wall of the subglottic space.

Ulceration and bleeding

Local complications such as ulceration and bleeding during the proliferative phase in infancy may necessitate active treatment. When a hemangioma penetrates the epidermal basement membrane, ulceration or bleeding may occur. Bleeding is often sudden, punctate, and frightening. Parents should be taught how to compress the area with a clean pad, applying pressure for 10 minutes. Repeated bleeding is rare. If it occurs, a mattress suture may be indicated. Localized bleeding is usually not a manifestation of platelet-trapping coagulopathy (i.e., Kasabach-Merritt syndrome).

Ulceration is particularly common in hemangiomas of the lips. Secondary infection invariably accompanies ulceration. Superficial ulceration usually responds to daily cleansing and application of a topical antibiotic ointment. Deeper ulceration may require dressings; these lesions often take several weeks to heal. Recurrent ulceration after healing is rare. Pharmacologic therapy may be indicated for extensive and/or refractory ulceration.

Alarming complications

Congestive Heart Failure.   Congestive heart failure is a life-threatening complication that is typically seen with multiple cutaneous hemangiomas and with hemangiomatous proliferation within the viscera, typically the liver. High-output congestive heart failure can also occur with large cervicofacial hemangioma. Despite multimodality treatment, the overall mortality rate is reported to be as high as 54%.[17]

Platelet-Trapping Coagulopathy.   Platelet-trapping coagulopathy, or Kasabach-Merritt syndrome, is the hematologic complication of hemangioma, first documented in 1940 by Kasabach and Merritt.[5] It occurs early in the postnatal rapid-growth phase. Characteristically, the involved skin is deep red-purple, tense, and shiny. In large lesions, there may be central areas of softness, which suggest intralesional bleeding. Petechiae and ecchymoses are seen overlying and adjacent to the hemangioma. Hematologic evaluation reveals profound thrombocytopenia (2000 to 40,000/mm^3). Early in the course of the syndrome, the fibrinogen level is slightly low. In time, fibrinogen falls to trace levels, and prothrombin time (PT) and thromboplastin time (PTT) become dangerously prolonged. There is a risk of acute hemorrhage in the GI tract or the pleural, peritoneal, pulmonic, or central nervous systems. In addition, rapid expansion of the hemangioma secondary to intralesional bleeding may cause compression of a vital structure.

Treatment

Most hemangiomas in the head and neck region grow as small tumors and invariably regress, leaving inconsequential skin changes. Clinical studies confirm that complete resolution of hemangiomas occurs in over 50% of children by age 5 years and in over 70% by 7 years, with continued improvement in the remaining children until ages 10 to 12 years. Typically, the skin after involution exhibits mild atrophy, or it may have a wrinkled quality or a few telangiectatic vessels. The skin may be slightly more pale than normal skin. Therefore, for the small hemangioma in an inconspicuous location, treatment is not necessary.

Laser excision for subglottic hemangioma

Not all infants with a subglottic hemangioma require treatment, especially those with a small lesion that occupies less than 20% of the subglottic airway. The treatment of choice is watchful waiting until involution. However, an adequate airway must be established if respiratory distress ensues. In the past, a tracheotomy was left in place for approximately 2 years until there was sufficient involution of the hemangioma. Systemic corticosteroid therapy is now an option; 60% of subglottic hemangiomas respond to steroids. The usual dose is prednisone 2 to 3 mg/kg/day.[18] A lower dosage or an alternate-day treatment of steroids may be continued for 4 to 6 weeks or longer.

The carbon dioxide (CO_2) laser is a therapeutic option for infants who fail to respond to steroids. Under general anesthesia, suspension microlaryngoscopy is used to expose the subglottic hemangioma. The operating microscope is coupled to a CO_2 laser. Jet ventilation with a Venturi apparatus is used to maintain oxygenation while the infant is paralyzed. The depth of injury is minimized by using the laser in the pulsed mode at 0.03 seconds and 2 to 5 watts, which delivers a short burst of laser energy to the target, allowing for minimal injury of the tissue. The CO_2 laser is ideally suited for treating eccentrically placed subglottic hemangiomas or when such a lesion can be removed with one operative procedure.[13] To prevent subglottic stenosis, circumferential subglottic hemangiomas should be removed in stages. Tracheotomy is reserved for patients with circumferential lesions, significant airway obstruction despite debulking with laser, multiple tracheal hemangiomas, or any other concomitant causes of airway obstruction such as vascular rings or tracheomalacia.

SPECIAL CONSIDERATION:

Hemangiomas are benign lesions, and most require no treatment. Watchful waiting and parental reassurance usually suffice. Hemangiomas that require treatment are those that cause significant cosmetic deformity, functional compromise (periorbital and subglottic), high-output cardiac failure, platelet-trapping thrombocytopenia (Kasalbach-Merritt syndrome), or other major system compromises.

Pharmacologic therapy for alarming complications

Since the first report appeared in 1967, high-dose corticosteroids remain the premier pharmacologic agent for control of endangering hemangiomas.[19] The decision to proceed with pharmacologic therapy should be made early. There is empirical evidence that a proliferating hemangioma in a very young infant is far more responsive to corticosteroid therapy than is a lesion in an older infant. The usual dosage is oral prednisone 2 to 3 mg/kg/day. Intravenous corticosteroids may be used in an infant with respiratory complications. However, there is no evidence that the response is more likely or profound with intravenous than with oral administration.

A hemangioma that is responding to corticosteroids exhibits signs of accelerated regression within several hours to days after therapy is initiated. The signs are usually obvious: lightening of color, softening, and diminished growth. If there is no evidence of accelerated regression on prednisone 2 to 3 mg/kg/day for 7 days, then the hemangioma must be termed unresponsive. Such a lesion will not respond to a higher dose, and therefore, the drug should be discontinued. If the lesion does respond,

the dosage can be lowered slowly over several weeks, or the patient can be switched to alternate-day therapy. The duration and dosage of corticosteroid therapy depend on the tumor's location and maturity. Rebound growth may occur in a proliferative-phase hemangioma at a low steroid level. To minimize regrowth, the corticosteroid must be continued until the hemangioma is well into the involuting phase, which usually occurs when the infant is 8 to 10 months old.

Intralesional corticosteroids should be considered for small protuberant hemangiomas in the face, particularly for upper eyelid and nasal tip lesions. The dosage is based on the size of the lesion and the infant's weight. No more than 40 mg triamcinolone acetate or 6 mg betamethasone is given at each injection.[20] Usually several injections (one to five) are necessary, spaced 4 to 6 weeks apart, to control the hemangioma.

SPECIAL CONSIDERATION:

Corticosteroids are the first line of therapy for all hemangiomas requiring treatment. They can be delivered orally, intravenously, or intralesionally. Subglottic hemangiomas that do not respond to corticosteroids can be treated with the CO_2 laser. Care should be taken to avoid creation of subglottic stenosis.

Inteferon therapy

Interferon α-2a is an effective treatment for life-threatening hemangiomas even after failure of steroid therapy. The dosage is 2 to 3 million U/m^2 subcutaneously daily. Interferon α-2a appears to be particularly effective in the treatment of large, cutaneous hemangiomas with associated Kasabach-Merrit syndrome.[21] Most children given interferon α-2a experience fever in the first 3 weeks of therapy. In addition, there may be transient neutropenia and anemia. The neutropenia is due to margination, not suppression of bone marrow, and resolves spontaneously. Spastic diplegia has also been reported.

Surgical therapy

Surgical excision during childhood is usually indicated for removal of the fibrofatty residuum or skin laxity that remains after complete regression of a hemangioma. There are, however, indications for earlier operative intervention. If a hemangioma is causing visual problems and is unresponsive to corticosteroid therapy, subtotal excision may relieve pressure on the developing cornea. Another example is early excision of an obstructing subglottic hemangioma using the CO_2 laser, as previously discussed. In instances in which the hemangioma is pedunculated and ulcerated, the lesion should be removed rather than waiting for involution.

As the child with hemangioma reaches age $2\frac{1}{2}$ to 3 years, he or she may evidence psychosocial problems. Problems are more likely to develop during the first grade, when the child is exposed to older classmates. This is a time to consider subtotal or possibly total excision of an involuting-phase hemangioma. Excision for psychological indications must be carefully discussed, and often a psychologist can help with the decision. Excision is also a consideration when it is obvious that skin removal will be necessary in the future, either because of color, quality, or contour, notwithstanding the final result of involution. Hemangiomas of the lip and nasal tip are psychologically sensitive foci. Subtotal or contour excision during early childhood may be of benefit. As a general rule, subtotal or staged excision is the best approach. Caution should be taken fear of causing late-contour deficiency or deformity. Residual fibrofatty tissue and skin can be removed, often with local anesthesia, when the child is older.

VASCULAR MALFORMATIONS

Vascular malformations usually grow commensurately with the child. Each channel type, however, may change because of different pathophysiologic influences. Venous anomalies often expand because of hormonal changes such as puberty, pregnancy, antiovulants, or secondary to trauma. LMs typically enlarge with infection or intralesional bleeding. AVMs may enlarge in association with trauma, puberty or other hormonal changes, or incomplete surgical excision. It is essential not to confuse these nonproliferative enlargements of vascular malformations with the proliferating phase of hemangioma.

Capillary Malformation

Histology

The skin or mucosa of a port-wine stain contains abnormally dilatated capillaries or venule-sized vessels in the superficial dermis.[22] The anomaly is present at birth and changes slowly with growth to a purple color in adulthood. The lesion also may become raised and nodular with progressive vascular ectasia.

Clinical features

Patients with port-wine stain within the V1 area alone or extending into the maxillary and mandibular region are at serious risk for choroidal and intracranial vascular anomalies (i.e., the Sturge-Weber syndrome).[23] Children with dermal staining of the V2 and/or V3 general areas alone are not at increased risk. The capillary malformation in Sturge-Weber syndrome may involve the entire face and neck or the trunk and distal extremities. The soft tissue is often hypertrophic, and frequently skeletal overgrowth occurs in the maxilla, particularly in the alveolar region. Skeletal overgrowth may not be obvious at birth, but it progresses throughout adolescence. Characteristic CT and MRI findings in Sturge-Webber syndrome include focal cerebral atrophy and superficial cortical calcification, diffuse leptomeningeal enhancement of the affected area, and enlargement of the ipsilateral choroid plexis.

Treatment

Laser Therapy. The flashlamp pulsed dye laser is used extensively for treatment of capillary malformation in infancy and children. Significant lightening of the lesion is achieved in 80% of patients, with the best results in younger children.[24]

Surgical Excision.   In selective cases, it may be possible to surgically excise the port-wine stain and obtain primary closure by skin advancement or skin grafting. There are serious potential problems after excision and grafting, including scarred hypertrophy at the junction of the graft and normal skin and unpredictable pigmentation of the skin graft itself. Tissue expansion techniques also may be considered for removing a port-wine stain. Contour excision of a hypertrophied lip is often necessary.

Venous Malformation

In the past, venous anomalies were erroneously termed "varicose" or "cavernous" hemangiomas or "lymphangiohemangiomas." These lesions are not hemangiomas, but rather are developmental anomalies of veins. VMs usually occur in pure form but may be combined as capillary venous malformations (CVM) or LVMs.

Histology

Histologic examination shows dilatated or ectatic vascular channels lined by normal endothelium. Thrombosis is common and is associated with dystrophic calcification, which is clinically and radiologically manifested as a phlebolith.

Clinical features

Various presentations of VM can occur and range from an isolated skin varicosity or localized spongy mass to complex lesions that infiltrate various tissue planes. The overlying skin may be normal, or it may exhibit a bluish tinge caused by involvement of the dermis. The combined venolymphatic lesions often exhibit dermal lymphatic vesicles overlying the deep venous anomaly.

Venous anomalies are common in the skin and subcutaneous tissue of the head and neck region, particularly the lips and cheeks. They also may form in skeletal muscle; intramasseteric lesions are most common. The clinical characteristic of VMs is a soft, compressible nonpulsatile mass with rapid refilling. Expansion occurs on compression of the jugular vein, with the Valsalva maneuver, or with the head in a dependent position. These lesions grow proportionately with the child and tend to expand following puberty, trauma, or attempted subtotal excision. Sluggish flow and stasis lead to phlebothrombosis, which presents clinically as recurrent pain and tenderness. Characteristic phleboliths can be palpated and seen on radiographic examination. Venous anomalies may also occur in the craniofacial skeleton and are most common in the mandible, less common in the maxilla, and rare in the nasal and cranial bones and zygomas. Mandibular venous anomalies may present with increased mobility of the teeth, expansion of the buccal cortex, or spontaneous bleeding.[25] The radiographic appearance of an intraosseous VM is consistent—plain films demonstrate a localized hypolucency with a honeycombed or soap bubble appearance. Profile or tangenital films show spicules of bone radiating in a sun-burst pattern.

Treatment

Most VMs do not require any specific treatment apart from reassurance and an explanation of the natural history of the lesion.

Sclerotherapy.   Direct injection of a sclerosing agent into the center of the soft-tissue VM is an accepted mode of treatment. Sclerosing agents such as 95% ethanol or sodium tetradecyl sulfate (1 or 2%) are injected into the epicenter of the venous anomaly during occlusion of the arterial inflow and venous outflow. Injection of a sclerosing agent can be dangerous and should be done under general anesthesia with fluoroscopic monitoring by an experienced interventional radiologist. Local complications such as edema, full-thickness necrosis, or nephrotoxicity have been reported. Multiple injections are usually required, often at several month intervals. Unfortunately, venous malformations have a propensity to recur.

Surgery.   Surgical resection is indicated for large or symptomatic venous anomalies. Often it is advisable to first shrink the VM with sclerotherapy. Under most circumstances, total surgical extirpation is impossible, and a subtotal resection is indicated to reduce bulk and improve contour and function or relieve pain. Lesions of the jaw, nasal bones, and zygoma are managed by curettage and packing with a hemostatic agent.

Lymphatic Malformation

Our understanding of lymphatic anomalies has been hampered by confusing terminology. Cystic hygroma is a term frequently used, which literally means watery tumor of the neck, a definition with no pathologic basis. Lymphangioma is a term that correctly defines an acquired lesion that is proliferative and hypercellular and increases in size by mitosis. However, these are not characteristics of lymphatic anomalies. Therefore, the term *lymphatic malformation* seems most appropriate. LMs are not proliferative and increase in size by distinction rather than by mitosis. The cellular constituents of LMs are quiescent.

LMs are congenital and are either evident at birth or detected before 2 years of age. They may occur throughout the body, although the head and neck region is the most common site. They expand or contract with the ebb and flow of lymphatic fluid through dysplastic valves and the presence of inflammation or intralesional bleeding. Symptoms are related to the anatomic location of the malformation and the extent of involvement.

Histology

The classic LM consists of multiple dilated lymphatic channels that are lined by a single layer of flattened endothelium. The vessel walls are of variable thickness with both striated-muscle and smooth-muscle components. Collections of lymphocytes frequently are found throughout the contained connective tissue. Hemorrhage within the cystic spaces is common. The lesion may be a combined capillary-lymphatic malformation (CLM) or LVM.

Clinical features

LM presents in various forms. Lymphatic infiltration of the tongue causes macroglossia in which the

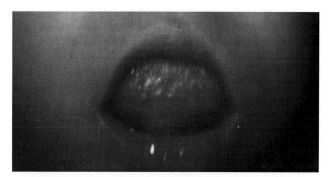

Figure 5–6: Lymphatic infiltration of the tongue.

tongue is typically covered with vesicles, and speech is impaired. Macroglossia is complicated by recurrent infection, swelling, bleeding, and poor dental hygiene and caries (Fig. 5-6). LM is also a common basis for macrocheilia, macroglossia, macrotia, and macrodontia. Macrocystic LM, formerly called a cystic hygroma, occurs in the anterior and posterior triangles of the neck. This lesion consists of large, thick-walled cysts, with less infiltration of surrounding tissue. The more severe forms of LM (microcystic) extensively infiltrate the head and neck, producing extensive deformities. This variety commonly involves the oral cavity, oropharynx, and pre-epiglottic space. Isolated supraglottic malformations are rare and are associated with these extensively infiltrative lesions.

LMs are associated with hypertrophy of bone and soft tissue. This is frequently seen as progressive distortion of the mandibular body, which causes prognathism (Fig. 5-7). LMs grow commensurately with the patient; however, spontaneous, sudden, and rapid increases in size associated with infection or intralesional bleeding may occur. Spontaneous decompression or shrinkage of LM is extremely uncommon but may occur in cystic lesions of the lower neck.

LMs can be divided into two treatment categories based on anatomic distribution, computerized imaging, and histologic findings. Type I LMs are located below the level of the mylohyoid muscle and involve the anterior and posterior cervical triangles. CT reveals ring-like margin enhancement with sharp demarcation of the cystic areas, which appear to be well circumscribed and discrete. Histologically, type I malformations have macrocystic structures without infiltration of surrounding soft tissue. These malformations correlate most closely with the lesions previously called cystic hygromas.

Type II LMs are found above the level of the mylo-

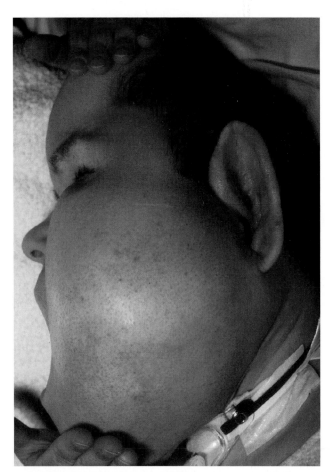

Figure 5–7: Lymphatic malformation with extensive involvement of the soft tissues of the face, auricle, and mandible.

hyoid muscle and involve the cheek, oral cavity, lip, and tongue. CT scans of type II lesions reveal isodense masses that are poorly defined and show obscured muscle and fatty planes. These lesions do not appear well circumscribed or discrete, and the ring-like enhancement seen in type I lesions is notably absent. Histologic examination of type II lesions reveals microcystic channels with infiltration of muscle and surrounding tissue. LMs are low-flow vascular anomalies. Their size often changes because of infection or bleeding. MRI shows a large, high-intensity mass with low-intensity septations and some fluid levels.

Treatment

Therapeutic modalities such as repeated incision and drainage, aspiration, radiotherapy, and injection of sclerosing agents should be avoided. Surgical resection is the treatment of choice for control of this vascular anomaly. Appropriate surgical planning

should be based on an understanding of the two forms of LM and realistic expectations for each patient.

> ## SPECIAL CONSIDERATIONS:
>
> LMs are primarily treated by surgical excision. Multiple resections may be necessary.

Physical examination of the patient and preoperative imaging results are extremely important, bearing in mind the clinical significance of the typical infiltrative disease above the mylohyoid muscle. Photographic documentation is important because the care of many of these patients spans several years. It is helpful to the surgeon and the family to document the initial condition as well as interval results.

The clinician should recall that LMs are benign; therefore, complete and total resection of the lesion is not necessary and sometimes not possible. Aggressive resection is not warranted, nor is an excessively conservative approach to be condoned. The long-term psychological and social ramifications of these malformations should not be underestimated.

Cold knife dissection is frequently the modality of choice for excision of LMs. Type I lesions are ideally removed in one procedure. Surgical intervention of type I lesions can be safely carried out within the first 9 to 12 months of life.

Type II lesions are more difficult to manage because no distinct tissue planes exist between the malformation and the normal structures. Because these lesions are not curable, the timing of intervention is less critical. Repeated procedures are necessary, and complete removal is almost impossible. Resection of a LM before the age of 5 or 6 years is recommended. In planning such a procedure, restrictions should be set for the extent of dissection, duration of procedure, and acceptable blood loss.

Meticulous dissection is necessary because anatomic structures frequently are not in their normal position. Magnification and the use of the nerve simulator are essential. The disruption of the abnormal lymphatic channels frequently leads to prolonged wound drainage. Suction drains should remain in position for an adequate period to avoid re-accumulation of lymphatic drainage under the skin flaps.

The use of the laser is reserved for disease that is not readily resectable by sharp dissection. Lesions that involve the oral cavity and tongue are particularly amenable to CO_2 laser resection, as is involvement of the supraglottic larynx. The CO_2 laser may be helpful in localized lesions in the lip and buccal area. The Nd-YAG laser has been relatively successful in controlling the vesicular lesions that are commonly found in the tongue.

Japanese researchers have recently described intralesional injection of OK-432, which is a lyophilized incubation mixture of group A *Streptococcus pyogenes,* both as primary and secondary treatments for LM.[26]

Special considerations

Airway Obstruction.   Airway obstruction caused by a cervical lymphatic anomaly and requiring intervention occurs primarily within the first 12 months of life. The lesion is usually an infiltrative LM that involves the tongue, floor of the mouth, and pre-epiglottic space. A sudden increase in size demands immediate attention. Progressive respiratory distress evidenced by tachypnea and increasing chest retractions requires orotracheal intubation. This procedure should be performed under general anesthesia, which provides an opportunity for detailed examination of the oropharynx, hypopharynx, and supraglottic larynx. If extensive involvement of the supraglottic airway exists, tracheotomy is indicated.

Hemorrhage.   Hemorrhage into a cystic LM in the anterior triangle is sometimes associated with the sudden onset of acute respiratory distress. The airway should be secured with endotracheal intubation, and intravenous antibiotics should be started. If there is a discreet mass, it may be removed, significantly improving the airway.

Sepsis.   A rapid increase in the size of a LM on the floor of the mouth or the tongue is usually secondary to cellulitis. In addition, there are systemic signs of infection. These clinical situations necessitate admission to the hospital, monitoring of the airway, and often prolonged intravenous antibiotics. If there is recurrent cellulitis, prophylactic antibiotics may be required. Dental hygiene should be stressed in these children.

Arteriovenous Malformation

High-flow vascular anomalies in the head and neck are AVMs or, less commonly, arteriovenous fistulae (AVF). These fast-flow lesions are relatively uncommon compared with slow-flow vascular anomalies. In contrast, AVMs are 20-fold more common in the intracranial vasculature than in branches of the external carotid artery.[27]

Histology

Histopathologic examination using serial sectioning may demonstrate the arteriovenous shunts. The dysmorphic arteries are thick-walled and of irregular caliber. Under high-power magnification, the arteries exhibit fragmentation of the internal elastic lamina and highly disorganized smooth muscle in the media. Secondary changes including progressive reactive hypertrophy, intimal thickening, and sclerosis caused by increased blood occur within the veins.

Clinical findings

AVMs in the head and neck are rarely symptomatic in the neonatal period. They manifest during late childhood, adolescence, or early adulthood. Many lesions exhibit either a warm, erythematous blush or a true port-wine stain in the overlying skin. Distressing symptoms of AVMs or AVF in children are throbbing pain or pulsatile tinnitus, which may prevent sleeping.[28,29] The involved skin has an elevated temperature, and a thrill may be felt. Arteriovenous shunting is confirmed by the presence of a bruit on auscultation or Doppler examination. These anomalies remain stable for years, only to enlarge following minimal trauma, infection, or hormonal changes. Shunting of blood diminishes nutritive flow, which may result in skin necrosis, ulceration, and bleeding. Slow destruction of facial bones may occur; these patients seek treatment for swelling, pain, or sudden hemorrhage.

Treatment

If an AVM or AVF is asymptomatic, no treatment is necessary. However, when complications such as pain, ulceration, bleeding, or heart failure are present, therapy is necessary. There *is no place for proximal ligation* of the feeding arterial system.

MRI and angiography are essential for evaluating symptomatic malformations. MRI best demonstrates the extent of involvement within tissue planes and the flow characteristics. Angiography is usually reserved until treatment planning is complete and is used for superselective embolization before surgical extirpation. Superselective embolization may have a role in palliation (i.e., for control of pain, tinnitus, or hemorrhage) or it may be used as primary therapy for surgically inaccessible AVMs or AVF.

SPECIAL CONSIDERATIONS:

AVMs are treated by embolization and surgical excision.

The only therapy that holds any hope for long-term success is total resection of the tissue involved with the arteriovenous anomaly. Leaving behind residual and dormant anomalous channels only invites further collateral formation, shunting, and expansion.[2] Preoperative superselective embolization will not diminish the extent of the resection. It will, however, minimize intraoperative bleeding. Preoperative embolization of proximal feeding vessels only complicates the problem. Embolization must be directed at the nidus, or epicenter, of the AVM. Often a two-team approach (for resection and reconstruction) is applicable for surgical management of these lesions. The critical decision is to what extent the resection must be done to include all of the pathologic vasculature. Reconstruction often necessitates closure and soft-tissue replacement using microvascular tissue transfer. Given proper indications and with careful planning, extensive resection is curative and justified.

REFERENCES

1. Mulliken JB, Glowacki J. Hemangiomas and vascular malformations in infants and children: A classification based on endothelial characteristics. Plast Reconstr Surgery 1982; 69:412-422.
2. Mulliken JB, Young AE. *Vascular Birthmarks: Hemangiomas and Malformations.* Philadelphia; WB Saunders, 1988.
3. Folkman J, Klagsbrun M. Angiogenic factors. Science 1987; 235:242-247.
4. Takahaski K, Mulliken JB, Kozakewich HP, et al: Cellular markers that distinguish the phases of hemangioma during infancy and childhood. J Clin Invest 1994; 93:2357-2364.
5. Kasabach HH, Merritt KK. Capillary hemangioma with extensive purpura. Am J Dis Child 1940; 50: 1063-1070.
6. el-Dessouky M, Azmy AF, Raine PA, et al. Kasabach-Merritt syndrome. J Pediatr Surg 1988; 23:109-111.
7. Meyer JS, Hoffer FA, Barnes PD, et al. MR correlation of the biological classification of soft tissue vascular anomalies. AJR 1991; 157:559-564.
8. Boyd JB, Mulliken JB, Kaban LB, et al: Skeletal changes associated with vascular malformations. Plast Reconstr Surg 1984; 74:789-797.
9. Finn MC, Glowacki J, Mulliken JB. Congenital vascular lesions: Clinical application of a new classification. J Pediatr Surg 1983; 18:894-899.
10. Amir J, Metzker A, Krikler R, et al. Strawberry hemangioma in preterm infants. Pediatr Dermatol 1986; 3: 331-332.
11. Hidano A, Nakajima S. Earliest features of the strawberry mark in the newborn. Br J Dermatol 1972; 87: 138-144.
12. Margileth AM, Museles M. Cutaneous hemangioma in children: Diagnosis and conservative management. JAMA 1965; 194:523-526.
13. Healy GB, McGill T, Friedman EM. Carbon dioxide laser in subglottic hemangioma: An update. Ann Otol Rhinol Laryngol 1984; 93:370-373.
14. Robb RM. Refractive errors associated with hemangiomas of the eyelids and orbit in infancy. Am J Ophthalmol 1977; 83:52-58.
15. Brodsky L, Yoshpe N, Rubin RJ. Clinical pathological correlation of congenital subglottic hemangiomas. Ann Otol Rhinol Laryngol 1983; 92(suppl 105):4-18.
16. Ferguson CF, Flake CG. Subglottic hemangioma as a cause of respiratory obstruction in infants. Ann Otol Rhinol Laryngol 1961; 70:1095-1112.
17. Berman B, Lim H. Concurrent cutaneous and hepatic hemangiomata in infancy: Report of a case and a review of the literature. J Dermatol Surg Obstet 1978; 4:869-873.
18. Cohen SR, Wang C. Steroid treatment of hemangioma of the head and neck in children. Ann Otol Rhinol Laryngol 1972; 81:584-590.
19. Zarem HA, Edgerton MT. Induced reduction of cavernous hemangiomas following prednisone therapy. Plast Reconstr Surg 1967; 38:76-83.
20. Sloan GM, Reinisch JF, Nichter LS, et al. Intralesional corticosteroid for infantile hemangioma. Plast Reconstr Surg 1989; 83:459-467.
21. White CW, Wolf SJ, Korones DN, et al. Treatment of childhood angiomatous diseases with recombinant interferon alfa-2a. J Pediatr 1991; 118:59-66.
22. Noe JM, Barsky SH, Geer DE, et al. Port-wine stains and the response to argon laser therapy: Successful treatment and the predictive role of color, age and biopsy. Plast Reconstr Surg 1980; 65:130-136.

23. Enjolras O, Riche MC, Merland JJ. Facial port-wine stains and Sturge-Weber syndrome. Pediatrics 1985; 76:48–51.

24. Tan OT, Sherwood K, Gilchrest BA. Treatment of children with port-wine stains using the flashlamp-pulsed tunable dye laser. N Engl J Med 1989; 320: 416–421.

25. Kaban LB, Mulliken JB. Vascular anomalies of the maxillofacial region. J Oral Maxillofac Surg 1986; 44: 203–213.

26. Ogita S, Tsuto T, Nakamura K, et al. OK-432 therapy in 64 patients with lymphangioma. J Pediatr Surg 1994; 29:784–785.

27. Olivecrona H, Ladenhein J. *Congenital Arterio-venous Aneurysms of the Carotid and Vertebral Arterial Systems.* Berlin: Springer-Verlag; 1957.

28. Coleman CC Jr. Diagnosis and treatment of congenital arteriovenous fistulas of the head and neck. Am J Surg 1973; 126:557–565.

29. Malan E, Azzolini A. Congenital arteriovenous malformations of the face and scalp. J Cardiovasc Surg 1968; 9:109–140.

6 Soft Tissue Sarcomas in Children

Trevor J. McGill

Children suffer from a variety of malignancies of the head and neck. Fortunately, their occurrence is uncommon. Lymphoma (Hodgkin's and non-Hodgkin's) is the most common malignancy in the pediatric age group. Soft tissue sarcomas, especially rhabdomyosarcoma, deserve special mention because they occur more frequently in childhood. Salivary gland and thyroid malignancies are rare in childhood, as is nasopharyngeal carcinoma, which is typically of epithelial origin.

Soft tissue sarcomas constitute 7% of all malignant tumors in children under 15 years of age.[1] Rhabdomyosarcoma accounts for 50% of all soft tissue sarcomas in children. Other soft tissue sarcomas include fibrosarcoma, synovial sarcoma, primitive neuroectodermol tumor (PNET), and alveolar soft tissue sarcoma.

Because soft tissue sarcomas are unique to the pediatric population, an understanding of their diagnosis, tumor biology, and management is essential for the physician caring for children who suffer from neoplasia.

AT A GLANCE . . .

Soft Tissue Sarcomas

- Rhabdomyosarcoma
- Synovial sarcoma
- Fibrosarcoma
- Malignant peripheral nerve sheath tumor (MPNST)
- Ewing's sarcoma
- Primitive neuroectodermal tumor (PNET)

Pediatric Otolaryngology, Edited by R.F. Wetmore, H.R. Muntz, and T.J. McGill. Thieme Medical Publishers, Inc., New York © 2000.

RHABDOMYOSARCOMA

Rhabdomyosarcoma is more common in males than females. There are two peak age groups: 4 to 8 years and 12 to 15 years. Head and neck tumors are more common in the younger group and are typically of the embryonal type, which have a good prognosis, whereas tumors in the adolescent group are of the alveolar type and have a poorer prognosis.[2] Rhabdomyosarcomas usually occur in isolation but may be associated with neurofibromatosis, Li-Fraumeni syndrome, or Beckwith-Wiedemann syndrome.[3]

SPECIAL CONSIDERATION:

Head and neck rhabdomyosarcomas are more common in the younger age group and are typically of the embryonal type and have a good prognosis, whereas tumors in the adolescent group are of the alveolar type and have a poorer prognosis.

Head and neck rhabdomyosarcomas account for 40% of rhabdomyosarcomas in children. Orbital tumors are usually embryonal and have a favorable prognosis. The remaining head and neck tumors are divided into parameningeal and nonparameningeal tumors. Parameningeal rhabdomyosarcomas arise in sites adjacent to the meninges including the nasal cavity, nasopharynx, paranasal sinuses, pterygopalatine and infratemporal fossae, middle ear, and mastoid (Fig. 6–1A). There is a high incidence of local recurrence in patients with parameningeal rhabdomyosarcoma.[4] This is related to the presence of extensive bony erosion of the skull base, cranial nerve neuropathy, and meningeal involvement. Parameningeal rhabdomyosarcoma is associated with a particularly poor prognosis if it is alveolar.

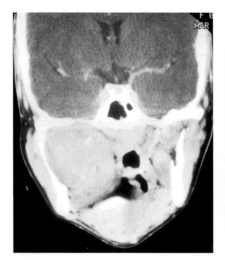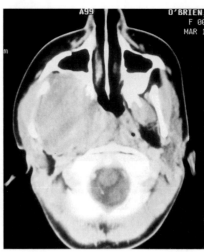

Figure 6–1: **(A, B)** Rhabdomyo-masarcoma of the right infratemporal fossa with erosion of the skull base and pterygoid plates.

A,B

Various inter-group studies have resulted in a significant increase in cure rates for rhabdomyosarcomas; however, there is concern that intensive multimodality treatment protocols are associated with an increase in long-term sequelae.

Histopathology

The classification of soft tissue sarcomas is based on the histopathologic resemblance of the tumor in question to one of the component mesenchymal tissues. Thus, the histopathologic diagnosis of embryonal rhabdomyosarcoma is predicted by the identification of crossed striations characteristic of skeletal muscle.

Rhabdomyosarcomas are divided into three histologic types: embryonal, alveolar, and undifferentiated.[5] The latter two are usually grouped together. Embryonal tumors are the most common variety in the head and neck. Histopathologically, the main cell type is a small round or spindle-shaped cell with a hyperchromatic nucleus. Sparsely cellular areas with loose myxoid stroma alternate with densely cellular areas, creating an alternating light and dark pattern.

Alveolar tumors show poorly differentiated small round cells with a dense appearance arranged along spaces resembling pulmonary alveoli. This histopathologic type is usually associated with a worse prognosis than the embryonal type. There is a greater propensity for lymphatic and systemic metastases. The alveolar type seems to indicate a better prognosis when diagnosed before the child is 10

years of age. Table 6-1 correlates location, age, and histology.

Immunohistochemistry

Light microscopic appearance of rhabdomyosarcoma may not be sufficient to permit a straightforward categorization into either the embryonal or alveolar/undifferentiated groups. Thus, if the light microscopy studies are equivocal, immunohistochemical studies may be helpful in confirming the diagnosis.

Immunohistochemical staining is a useful and reliable means of identifying skeletal muscle and muscle-specific proteins or genes. Muscle-specific proteins include α/actin, myosin, desmin, myoglobin, Z-ban/protein, and MYO-d.[6-8] Thus, for example, positive staining with antibodies directed against muscle, specifically actin and desmin, is considered sufficient for the diagnosis of embryonal rhabdomyosarcoma without the need to identify crossed striations by light microscopy or thick and thin filaments by electron microscopy. The immunohistochemical techniques can be useful in evaluating architectural changes in tissue that has been fixed in Formalin and embedded in paraffin. These tests are

TABLE 6-1: Location, Age Group and Pathology

Location	%	Age Group	Pathologic Type
Orbit	9%	4–8 years	Embryonal
Head and neck	33%	4–8 years	Both
Gen/Urinary	33%	<4 years	Embryonal
Trunk/extremities	25%	12–21 years	Alveolar

TABLE 6-2: 2;13 Translocations and Alveolar Rhabdomyosarcoma

1. Fusion between gene pax 3 and FKHR
2. Pax 3 appears important in transcription contact
3. New gene retains pax 3 DNA binding
4. Bisects FKHR DNA binding domain; incorporates FKHR activation domain
5. Between 67% and >90% of alveolar rhabdomyosarcomas contain translocation

also helpful in differentiating rhabdomyosarcoma from non-Hodgkin's lymphoma, neuroblastoma, PNET, and melanoma.

Tumor Biology

Cytogenetic studies have shown that many round-cell tumors have specific chromosome abnormalities that can aid in confirming the diagnosis. For example, alveolar and embryonal rhabdomyosarcomas have distinct genetic alterations that have important diagnostic and prognostic implications. Alveolar rhabdomyosarcoma has a characteristic balanced reciprocal translocation between the long arm of chromosome 2 and the long arm of chromosome 13 T(2;13)(q35;14)[9-11] (Table 6-2). This reciprocal translocation fuses the PAX 3 gene in band 2 q35 and the FKHR gene in band 13 q14. PAX 3 is a transcription regulatory protein that is important in neuromuscular development. The FKHR gene is a member of the forkhead family of transcription factors. The result of this fusion of PAX 3 and FKHR is still unknown. Polymerase chain reaction assays are now available that confirm the diagnosis of alveolar rhabdomyosarcoma.

Recently a different translocation—T(1;13)(p36;q14)—has been identified that fuses the PAX 7 on chromosome Ip36 and FKHR on chromosome 13 q14.

The gene fusion of T(2:13) and T(1;13) seen in alveolar rhabdomyosarcoma has important consequences[12] (Table 6-3).

TABLE 6-3: Alveolar Biology: Alternative 1;13 Fusion Pax 7 and FKHR Comparison 1;13 and 2;13

	Pax 3(2;13)	Pax 7(1;13)
Age	Adolescent	Younger
Sites	Multiple	Extremities
Status	Metastases	Localized
Prognosis	Bad	Good

In contrast, embryonal rhabdomyosarcoma lacks specific translocations but shows a consistent loss of heterozygosity at the chromosome 11 p15 site.

Changes in DNA content or ploidy of a cell is another genetic marker that impacts significantly on survival. Embryonal tumors have a DNA content between diploid and hyperdiploid. Hyperdiploidy tumors have a more favorable prognosis than diploidy tumors.

Thus, embryonal and alveolar tumors have distinct sets of genetic alterations that have important diagnostic, prognostic, and possibly therapeutic implications. In the future, rhabdomyosarcoma may be described by its unique cytogenetic abnormality.

Clinical Presentation

The clinical presentation of rhabdomyosarcoma of the head and neck is usually nonspecific and is related to the appearance of a painless mass lesion. Orbital tumors present with the rapid onset of proptosis.[13] Lesions that involve the nasopharynx and paranasal sinuses present with nasal obstruction and increasing upper airway obstructive symptoms, particularly at night. Parameningeal tumors may present with cranial nerve neuropathies, which may be subtle such as Horner's syndrome. Rhabdomyosarcomas of the external ear canal or middle ear present with persistent blood-stained otorrhea and otalgia despite appropriate medical treatment.[14] Examination of the external canal and middle ear usually shows a large, friable polypoid mass associated with some destruction of the bony external canal.[15] Rhabdomyosarcoma of the temporal bone has a high incidence of cranial nerve involvement at the time of presentation. Regional lymph node involvement is rare; approximately 7% of patients with head and neck tumors have regional lymph node involvement.[16] The most common sites of hematogenous spread are lung, bone, and bone marrow.

Clinical Evaluation

If rhabdomyosarcoma is suspected, additional radiologic evaluation may reveal metastatic disease that is more accessible for tissue diagnosis and may obviate the need for open surgical biopsy. A complete examination of the head and neck includes the ears, nose, oral cavity, nasopharynx, pharynx, larynx, and neck. This examination determines the location and size of this mass relative to surrounding tissues.

Surgical biopsy requires that an incision is made over the tumor, and a generous sample of non-crushed tumor is obtained for diagnosis. A frozen section is obtained at this time to allow the pathologist to determine if this specimen is adequate for a diagnostic evaluation. If the preoperative imaging and frozen section suggest a soft tissue sarcoma, a bone marrow aspiration biopsy should be performed under the same general anesthetic. Special stains, flow cytometry, including light and electron microscopy, and cytogenetic and molecular analysis may be necessary depending on the morphologic pattern. Once the histopathologic diagnosis has been made, a thorough search for metastatic disease can be undertaken as outlined below.

Imaging studies that are used in the search for metastases are computed tomography (CT) and magnetic resonance imaging (MRI) of the primary disease site, chest CT, bone scan, and liver/spleen scan.

Laboratory studies that are performed are a complete blood count (CBC), platelet count, liver enzymes, blood urea nitrogen (BUN), creatinine, serum electrolytes, calcium, phosphate, serum protein analysis, and cerebrospinal fluid (CSF) cytology.

Staging

Once the histopathologic diagnosis has been established, additional staging is necessary to determine the extent of dissemination beyond the primary site. Head and neck rhabdomyosarcomas are unlikely to be associated with lymph node involvement. The lungs are the most common site for distant metastases, followed by the bone marrow, liver, and central nervous system (CNS). The Intergroup Rhabdomyosarcoma Study (IRS) staging system, which is based on surgical staging at the time of the original biopsy, is the most frequently used system (Table 6–4).

Most tumors of the head and neck present as Stage III disease (Fig. 6–1B). Outcome generally correlates well with the IRS group system; however, any staging system that is based on the treatment of the primary tumor can be somewhat misleading. A TNM staging system is available, which takes into account the location, tumor size, node involvement, and distant metastases[17] (Table 6–5).

Treatment

Patients with rhabdomyosarcoma are presumed to have microscopic metastases at diagnosis. Treat-

TABLE 6-4: Intergroup Rhabdomyosarcoma Study Staging System

Group	Appearance
I	Localized disease completely resected (regional nodes not involved)
II	Grossly resected
A	No regional disease; microscopic residual at primary site
B	Regional disease, completely resected
C	Regional disease, involved nodes, microscopic residual
III	Incompletely resected or gross residual/biopsy
IV	Any primary tumor with or without regional disease with distant metastases irrespective of surgical approach to primary tumor

ment should focus on achieving both local control and eradication of metastases.

Successful management of rhabdomyosarcoma requires a multidisciplinary approach that begins with the correct histopathologic diagnosis of the primary tumor. Once the diagnosis is established, clinical staging is necessary to determine the exact extent of the disease. Surgery, radiation, and chemotherapy are the main options for managing these tumors. The optimal treatment of choice is the therapeutic regime that gives the best option for local, regional, and systemic control, without compromising functional or cosmetic outcome. Surgery and radiation are the principle options for managing the primary site.

Surgery

The role of surgery in the treatment of rhabdomyosarcoma has changed dramatically over the past 30

TABLE 6-5: TNM Staging

Stage	Site	Size	Node	Mets
1	Orbit, nonparameningeal head and neck, genitourinary, not bladder or prostate	Any	+/−	−
2	Bladder or prostate, extremity, parameningeal head and neck, other	<5 cm	−	−
3	Bladder or prostate, extremity, parameningeal head and neck, other	>5 cm, or any with node +	+/−	−
4	Any	Any	+/−	+

years. Prior to the introduction of multimodal treatment, radical surgery without reconstruction, followed by radiation therapy to the primary site, was the only therapeutic option for these patients. This resulted in a high incidence of regional and distant metastases and a 5 to 10% 5-year survival rate. Surgical excision of parameningeal tumors rarely included resection of the skull base, which resulted in a high incidence of local failure. With the advent of advanced radiation and sophisticated chemotherapy protocols, surgery has assumed a different role.

> ## Special Consideration:
> When possible, complete surgical excision is preferable because it decreases the incidence of local failure and eliminates the need for postoperative irradiation.

The primary role of the surgeon is to evaluate the primary tumor and to obtain a biopsy specimen for histopathologic examination (Fig. 6–2). When possible, complete surgical excision without removal of vital structures, such as the eye, is preferable because complete excision decreases the incidence of local failure and eliminates the need for postopera-

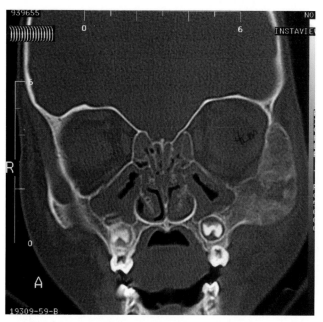

Figure 6–2: Rhabdomyosarcoma of the left maxilla and lateral wall of the orbit in a 4-year-old child.

tive irradiation. Tumor in sites other than parameningeal foci is more ideal for complete surgical excision; such locations include the auricle, zygoma, soft palate, tongue, and supraglottic larynx.[18] Patients with parameningeal rhabdomyosarcomas are best treated with a combination chemotherapy and local irradiation.

> ## Special Consideration:
> Patients with parameningeal rhabdomysarcomas are best treated with combination chemotherapy and local irradiation.

Because 50% of failures occur at the primary tumor site, there has been renewed interest in surgical excision as the primary mode of control. In addition, avoidance of complications such as arrest in facial growth and development of second malignancies within the radiation field has become a consideration in the management of these patients. These complications, in combination with the advent of new surgical techniques including craniofacial and skull base surgery, microvascular techniques, and nerve grafting procedures, raise the possibility that surgery should be considered for eradicating both the primary tumor and residual disease.[19] A combined intracranial/extracranial approach with a block removal of tumors is now possible (Fig. 6–3). Immediate reconstruction with free tissue transfer using microvascular techniques is useful to minimize functional and cosmetic deformities (Fig. 6–4). The infratemporal approach for lateral skull base lesions allows the surgical control of major neurovascular structures. It also permits removal of the contents of the infratemporal fossa and resection of the skull base, meninges, and if necessary, brain.[20]

Radiation Therapy

Radiation therapy plays a vital role in the management of rhabdomyosarcoma of the head and neck because the primary resection of most tumors is incomplete. Radiation therapy requires extensive pretreatment planning for optimal local control. This is particularly important for the treatment of parameningeal sites. High-risk patients are those with cranial nerve paresis, bony skull base erosion,

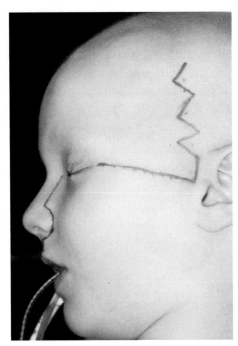

Figure 6–3: The facial translocation approach.

cytologically positive CSF, and direct intercranial extension. Pretreatment MRI is essential for defining tumor volume.

The standard approach for low-risk patients is to begin radiation therapy 6 to 9 weeks after induction

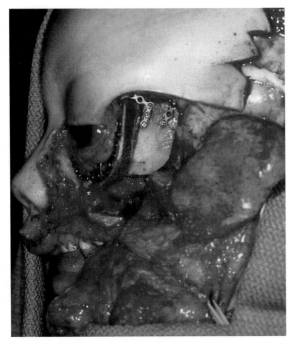

Figure 6–4: Final resection defect required bone and temporalis muscle to reconstruct inferior orbital rim, floor, and lateral wall of the orbit.

chemotherapy. Radiation should be delivered to the initial tumor volume with a 2-cm margin and in minimal tumor doses of 50 Gy. In high-risk patients, the approach is to be more aggressive, using wide margins around the tumor and starting radiation at the beginning of the treatment protocol.[21]

The potential complications of radiation therapy such as arrest in facial growth, radiation-induced tumors, and chronic irreversible CNS dysfunction continue to be real concerns. We must continue to explore new ways of administering radiation therapy including the use of hyper-fractionation and/or accelerated fractionation of radiation.[22]

Chemotherapy

The efficacy of chemotherapy can be augmented by the concurrent administration of several agents; that is, combination chemotherapy that involves the use of drugs with different mechanisms of action and minimal overlapping toxicity. Treatment protocols include vincristine plus actinomycin D plus cyclophosphamide (VAC), VAC plus adriamycin (Adr), VAC plus Adr plus cis-platinum (CDDP), and VAC plus Adr plus CDDP plus etoposide (VP16).[23] Actinomycin D potentiates the action of radiation therapy and should be carefully integrated with radiation therapy. Vincristine is administered at weekly intervals for 10 weeks if tolerated. Actinomycin D is given for 10 days every 12 weeks. Cyclophosphamide is given for 10 days every 6 weeks. Current protocols dictate that the timing of radiation therapy depends on the presence of high-risk factors such as extensive bony erosion of the skull base and cranial nerve involvement.[24] In high-risk groups, radiation therapy is started at the beginning of the treatment protocol. In patients without these high-risk factors, radiation therapy can begin 9 weeks after induction of chemotherapy.

AT A GLANCE . . .

Chemotherapy for Rhabdomyosarcoma

- Vincristine, actinomycin, cyclophosphamide (VAC)
- VAC plus adriamycin (Adr)
- VAC plus Adr plus cis-platinum
- VAC plus Adr plus cis-platinum plus etoposide

CT and MRI are frequently used to follow patients treated for rhabdomyosarcoma of the head and neck. These studies should be repeated every 3 months. Posttherapeutic residues are abnormalities on imaging studies that remain stable for at least 3 months. It is often difficult to determine whether viable tumor is present in these residues. Repeat biopsy of this tissue may be necessary to confirm the presence or absence of viable tumor.

> ### SPECIAL CONSIDERATION:
>
> Post-therapeutic residues are abnormalities on imaging studies that remain stable for at least three months. Repeat biopsy of this tissue may be necessary to demonstrate the presence or absence of viable tumor.

Controversies in Treatment

The main issues in the treatment of patients with rhabdomyosarcoma of the head and neck center on therapeutic options. Opinions regarding the timing and the extent of primary surgery for residual disease continue to evolve. Clearly, for accessible lesions, surgery is an important therapeutic option. The treatment of patients with postradiation residual lesions is controversial. It may be difficult to determine whether this tissue contains viable tumor. There is increasing evidence that these patients have an unfavorable prognosis and would benefit from wide-field surgical excision and immediate reconstruction.

Surgical extirpation of rhabdomyosarcoma may require skull base surgery with a team of surgeons that includes members of the otolaryngology, neurosurgery, oral and maxillofacial surgery, and microvascular surgery departments. This surgical team should work closely with the medical and radiation oncologists to provide optimal care for these patients.

In the most recent IRS core study, conducted between 1991 and 1997, there were 221 patients with parameningeal rhabdomyosarcomas. Over 50% of these children presented with tumors larger than 5 cm. Ninety-five percent of these were group III tumors, and 75% were embryonal rhabdomyosarcoma. The overall 5-year survival rate for embryonal rhabdomyosarcoma was 85 to 90%, and the overall 5-year survival rate for alveolar rhabdomyosarcoma was 55 to 60%.

Recent advances in histopathologic diagnosis, cytogenetics, and DNA analysis may allow us to better predict the biological behavior of these tumors in the future.

OTHER SOFT TISSUE SARCOMAS

Non-rhabdomyosarcoma soft tissue sarcomas are a complex and heterogeneous group of tumors with multiple morphologies, tissues of origin, and anatomic locations. These tumors comprise a large number of relatively uncommon tumors including synovial sarcoma, fibrosarcoma, malignant peripheral nerve sheath tumor (MPNST), Ewing's sarcoma, and PNET.[25] Ewing's sarcoma and PNET probably account for 20 to 25% of all soft tissue sarcomas in children. An unexplained observation is that the PNET has a predilection for soft tissues, and Ewing's sarcoma has a predilection for the skeletal system.[26]

The diagnostic evaluation of patients with suspected non-rhabdomyosarcoma soft tissue sarcoma is essentially the same as that for patients with rhabdomyosarcoma, because it is impossible to determine on clinical grounds alone whether the mass is a rhabdomyosarcoma or a non-rhabdomyosarcoma tumor. Several grading systems have evaluated factors such as the degree of mitosis, differentiation, cellularity, degree of matrix formation, and pleomorphism. More recently, ploidy and cytogenetic and molecular genetic abnormalities assume greater importance in providing biological information about these tumors.

Synovial Sarcoma

Synovial sarcoma is very rare in children and may occur in the head and neck at sites with no normal synovial structures (Fig. 6-5). The most common presentation in the neck is a slowly enlarging parapharyngeal mass.[27] It is unusual for these slow-growing tumors to present with distant metastases. A specific chromosomal translocation between chromosome X and 18,t(X;18)(p11;q11) has been described in 90% of these tumors.[28]

The typical pathologic appearance is biphasic with both spindle cell fibrous stroma and distinct glandular components. These biphasic tumors stain with antibodies to both cytokeratin and vimentin.

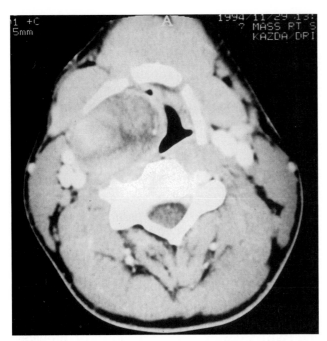

Figure 6–5: Axial computed tomographic imaging of a synovial cell sarcoma of the right parapharyngeal space.

Local control is the sine qua non of therapy because these tumors are very locally invasive. Wide surgical resection followed by radiation treatment is the optimal treatment. Synovial sarcomas are generally considered to be unresponsive to chemotherapy.

Fibrosarcoma

Fibrosarcoma may be seen in infants and older children. Histologically these tumors consist of malignant fibroblasts that are associated with variable collagen or reticulin production. Congenital fibrosarcoma has been well described in newborn infants and is considered a histologically low-grade tumor. Surgical excision is the treatment of choice and is associated with a good outcome. These tumors are associated with trisomies on chromosomes 8, 11, 17, and 20. Fibrosarcoma in children older than 10 years of age has a worse prognosis. Fibrosarcomas are commonly seen as radiation-induced secondary tumors.

Primitive Neuroectodermal Tumor

In the past decade, PNET has been recognized as an important soft tissue sarcoma in children.[29] PNET and Ewing's sarcoma are a family of neoplasms that shares cytogenetic abnormalities involving chromosome 22. PNET is a tumor found in children and young adults.

The typical presentation is that of a nonspecific mass that may be painful. Pathologically, it is seen as a trabecular arrangement of round hyperchromatic cells with minimal cytoplasm fibrovascular stroma. The balanced translocation T(11;22)(q24;q12) is characteristic of PNET and is the most widely recognized translocation occurring in soft tissue tumors.

The clinical course of PNET is highly aggressive, and the most effective treatment is local control by radiation or surgery and combination chemotherapy as described for rhabdomyosarcoma. PNET has a tendency of local recurrence followed by metastases to bone, bone marrow, lymph nodes, lung, and liver.

REFERENCES

1. Robinson LL. General principles of the epidemiology of childhood cancer. In: Pizzo PA, Poplack DG, eds. *Principles and Practices of Pediatric Otolaryngology,* 2nd ed. Philadelphia: JB Lippincott, 1993.
2. Cunningham MJ, Myers EN, Bluestone CD. Malignant tumors of the head and neck in children: A twenty-year review. Int J Pediatr Otorhinolaryngol 1987; 13: 279–292.
3. Li FP, Fraumeni JF Jr., Mulvihill JJ, et al. A cancer family syndrome in twenty-four kindreds. Cancer Res 1988; 48:5358–5362.
4. Triche TJ. Pathology of pediatric malignancies. In: Pizzo PA, Poplack PG, eds. *Principles and Practices of Pediatric Oncology,* 2nd ed. Philadelphia: JB Lippincott, 1993, pp. 115–152.
5. Raney RB, Hays DM, Tefft M, Triche TJ. Rhabdomyosarcoma and the undifferentiated sarcomas. In: Pizzo PA, Poplack PG, eds. *Principles and Practices of Pediatric Oncology,* 2nd ed. Philadelphia: JB Lippincott, 1993, pp. 769–794.
6. Parham DM, Webber B, Holt H, et al. Immunohistochemical study of childhood rhabdomyosarcomas and related neoplasms: Results of an Intergroup Rhabdomyosarcoma Study Project. Cancer 1991; 67: 3072–3080.
7. Dodd S, Malone M, McCulloch W. Rhabdomyosarcoma in children: A histological and immunohistochemical study of 59 cases. J Pathol 1989; 158: 13–18.
8. Dias P, Parham DM, Shapiro DN, et al. Myogenic regulatory protein (MyoD1) expression in childhood solid tumors: Diagnostic utility in rhabdomyosarcoma. Am J Pathol 1990; 137:1283–1291.
9. Turc-Carel C, Lizard-Nacol S, Justrabo E, et al. Consis-

tent chromosomal translocation in alveolar rhabdo-myosarcoma. Cancer Genet Cytogenet 1986; 19: 361–362.

10. Douglas EC, Valentine M, Etcubanas E, et al. A specific chromosomal abnormality in rhabdomyosarcoma. Cytogenet Cell Genet 1987; 45:148–155.

11. Barr FG, Galili N, Holick J, et al. Rearrangement of the PAX3 paired box gene in the paediatric solid tumour alveolar rhabdomyosarcoma. Nat Genet 1993; 3:113–117.

12. Davis RJ, D'Cruz CM, Lovell MA, et al. Fusion of PAX7 in FKHR by the variant t(1;13)(p36;q14) translocation in alveolar rhabdomyosarcoma. Cancer Res 1994; 54:2869–2872.

13. Wharam M, Beltangady M, Hays D, et al. Localized orbital rhabdomyosarcoma. An interim report of the Intergroup Rhabdomyosarcoma Study Committee. Ophthalmology 1987; 94:251–254.

14. Dehner L, Chen K. Primary tumors of the external and middle ear. A clinicopathologic study of embryonal rhabdomyosarcoma. Arch Otolaryngol 1978; 104:399–405.

15. Wiatrak BJ, Pensak ML. Rhabdomyosarcoma of the ear and temporal bone. Laryngoscope 1989; 99: 1188–1192.

16. Wharam MD, Beltangady MS, Heyn RM, et al. Pediatric orofacial and laryngopharyngeal rhabdomyosarcoma. An Intergroup Rhabdomyosarcoma Study report. Arch Otolaryngol Head Neck Surg 1987; 113: 1225–1227.

17. Rodary C, Flamant F, Donaldson SS. An attempt to use a common staging system in rhabdomyosarcoma: A report of an international workshop initiated by the International Society of Pediatric Oncology. Med Pediatr Oncol 1989; 17:210–215.

18. Ohlms LA, McGill T, Healy GB. Malignant laryngeal tumors in children: A 15-year experience with four patients. Annals of Otol Rhinol Laryn 1994; 103: 686–692.

19. McGill T. Rhabdomyosarcoma of the head and neck: An update. Otolaryngol Clin North Am 1989; 22: 631–636.

20. Healy GB, Upton L, Black PM, et al. The role of surgery in rhabdomyosarcoma of the head and neck in children. Arch Otolaryngol Head Neck Surg 1991; 117:1185–1187.

21. Crist W, Gehan E, Ragab A, et al. The third Intergroup Rhabdomyosarcoma Study. J Clin Oncol 1995; 13: 610–630.

22. Donaldson S, Asmar L, Breneman J, et al. Hyperfractionated radiation in children with rhabdomyosarcoma. Results of an Intergroup Rhabdomyosarcoma pilot study. Int J Radiat Oncol Biol Phys 1995; 32: 903–911.

23. Sutow WW, Lindberg RD, Gehan EA, et al. Three-year relapse-free survival rates in childhood rhabdomyosarcoma of the head and neck: Report from the Intergroup Rhabdomyosarcoma Study. Cancer 1982; 49:2217–2221.

24. Koscielniak E, Rodary C, Flamant F, et al. Metastatic rhabdomyosarcoma and histologically similar tumors in childhood: A retrospective European multi-center analysis. Med Pediatr Oncol 1992; 20:209–214.

25. Harms D, Schmidt D, Treuner J. Soft-tissue sarcomas in childhood. A study of 262 cases including 169 cases of rhabdomyosarcoma. Z Kinderchir 1985; 40: 140–145.

26. Angervall L, Enzinger FM. Extraskeletal neoplasm resembling Ewing's sarcoma. Cancer 1975; 36: 240–251.

27. Schmidt D, Thum P, Harms D, et al. Synovial sarcoma in children and adolescents. A report from the Kiel Pediatric Tumor Registry. Cancer 1991; 67: 1667–1692.

28. Ladanyi M. The emerging molecular genetics of sarcoma translocations. Diagn Mol Pathol 1995; 4: 162–173.

29. Schmidt D. Malignant peripheral neuroectodermal tumor. Curr Top Pathol 1995; 89:297–312.

7 Psychological Considerations for Pediatric Otolaryngologists

Leigh A. Berry

In day-to-day practice, pediatric otolaryngologists often will encounter children who present with otolaryngologic conditions, but who have or develop comorbid psychologic difficulties. When working with these children and their families, it is essential that the otolaryngologist be familiar with "normal" or nonpathologic child development and with commonly occurring psychologic difficulties during periods of high stress; they should also have a basic awareness of common childhood psychiatric conditions and psychologic issues that are often associated with specific medical conditions.

Individual differences in normal development exist, and a thorough understanding of normal child development, as well as the impact of the family system on the child, is essential for evaluating the presenting psychologic symptoms. When addressing these symptoms, professionals must consider what is developmentally appropriate for a child's age. Furthermore, if a child's development is delayed, the determination of "appropriate" behavior must be based on the child's level of development or mental age. Although formal psychometric testing can provide information about a child's level of development, parents often are able to provide a general estimate of a child's level of functioning. It is important to keep in mind that, at any age, there is a wide range of individual differences that are considered to be appropriate or "within normal developmental limits." Furthermore, parents, teachers, babysitters, and other professionals who work with a child often can provide valuable insight into a child's functioning across a variety of settings. Particularly, in the school setting, there is a built-in comparison group of same age peers against which a child's difficulties can be evaluated. Simply looking at a child's symptoms does not provide sufficient information for understanding these difficulties. It is vital to consider the family as a whole and the child as part of the bigger system. Each family member's functioning directly impacts both positively and negatively on the functioning of other family members. There is a wide range of "individual differences" within families, and individual families may cope with stressors in dramatically different, but equally functional or dysfunctional, ways.

Coping styles vary and it is important to distinguish those families who are experiencing some difficulties coping with the child's condition from those who are experiencing psychopathologic behavior. Children and families who are faced with an acute or chronic medical condition often experience a high level of stress and emotional distress. Throughout the course of any medical illness, there are crisis points when stress is most likely to impact on functioning. The more chronic or serious the condition, the more crisis points are encountered. The period of the initial diagnosis, the initiation of therapy, and the failure of treatment or the recurrence of the condition are commonly recognized crisis points. Families often are able to anticipate these periods of crisis and successfully mobilize social supports and resources to handle them. Other periods of crisis, which are often unanticipated, include: when the child or family members see other same-age children participating in an activity that is "off-limits" for the medically involved child; periods of hospitalizations or surgeries; or major events (e.g., birthdays, holidays) that mark the chronicity of the medical condition. Chronic medical conditions present the additional stress of coping with an on-going strain after the initial "rallying of support" has died down. Often, it is several years after the initial diagnosis of a chronic condition before the family and child truly face the knowledge that this condition is not going away. They may go through another period of grieving, which is similar to that which occurred at diagnosis. During this

Pediatric Otolaryngology, Edited by R.F. Wetmore, H.R. Muntz, and T.J. McGill. Thieme Medical Publishers, Inc., New York © 2000.

later stage, the family and child are often left to deal with these feelings of grief, anger, and hopelessness by themselves because family, friends, and even professionals assume they have "gotten over it."

> ## SPECIAL CONSIDERATION:
>
> Children and families who are faced with an acute or chronic medical condition often experience a high level of stress and emotional distress.

During any period of intense stress, some reduced level of functioning is likely to occur. Increased emotional lability is commonly seen and often will stabilize without significant intervention once the crisis period has passed. Children often show a decreased level of autonomy when under significant stress, and some children, particularly young children, may show some mild, usually temporary, regression in their skills. Furthermore, the stress of an illness often prompts parents to assume a more protective role with the child, thereby further inhibiting age-appropriate independence. Finally, the child's medical symptoms may also contribute to increasing his dependence on parents or medical staff. Together, these factors often combine to inhibit the child from developing autonomy. Although the child's delayed autonomy may be temporary, these factors can have a lasting impact on the child and family. Maladaptive coping in any family member may prompt other family members to take on additional responsibilities to compensate for the poorly functioning member, but this can also serve to impact negatively on the coping abilities of the family as a whole.

Many symptoms of emotional distress may be evident while the family is adjusting to the condition. If these symptoms persist for a long period of time or are severe enough to interfere with the child's treatment or the family's understanding of the child's condition, a more thorough evaluation of the family's adjustment and possible psychopathology is indicated. At times, a maladaptive coping style progresses into more traditional psychopathology, such as depression, anxiety, or behavioral disorders. Certainly, any pre-existing psychologic disorder in a family member impacts on coping, and the disorder

may be exacerbated by the current stress. In a sense, these crisis periods shine a spotlight on pre-existing tensions, conflicts, or dysfunctions in the family or individuals. Thus, the presence of a previously diagnosed or undiagnosed psychiatric condition in the child or parent is very likely to impact on the family's adjustment to the medical condition, on cooperation with the necessary treatments, and on interactions with the medical staff. Whereas the impact of some psychiatric conditions may be reduced in a relatively short period of time through increased support, psychotherapy, and/or psychotropic medications, other conditions are more pervasive and inflexible. These other conditions, particularly personality disorders, can have a strong impact on the family's adjustment and ability to work cooperatively with the medical staff. With these families, it is often helpful to solicit the input of mental health providers (e.g., psychologists, psychiatrists, and social workers) to develop a plan for how to manage these difficulties.

PSYCHOLOGICAL CONSIDERATIONS IN CHILDREN WITH CHRONIC ILLNESSES

Unfortunately, much of the psychological research involving children with medical conditions focuses on comparing differences between medically involved and noninvolved children, which often excludes those identifying factors that lead to adaptive adjustment within a given medical population.[2] Research suggests that having a chronic illness is a life stressor that *in interaction with other variables* may lead to an increased risk of adjustment difficulties, but it also suggests that a chronic illness is not the sole cause of adjustment problems.[3] Research also suggests that the personality strengths of chronically ill children outweigh the deficits and that no single personality pattern is associated with a given illness.[4,5]

Impact of Illness on Autonomy and Sense of Self

Having a chronic illness can impact significantly on a child's view of herself and on her sense of autonomy and competence in the world. Depending on the nature of the illness, children are often forced to rely heavily on others for basic tasks such as self-care and monitoring of the condition, and for decisions about treatment. Parents often assume an overly protective role with children who have medical conditions and this tendency to "protect" can conflict with the child's need for age-appropriate exploration and autonomy. The sense of needing to be cared for and to be protected by others can exacerbate the child's own sense of feeling like "damaged goods" or of feeling "not normal" due to the illness. Children whose daily lives are impacted by a medical condition often develop a sense of vulnerability, which is in marked contrast to the feelings of invulnerability and the often unstated belief that "nothing bad can happen to me" that typify childhood and adolescence. Although research on children with chronic illnesses has focused largely on those children who develop more significant or extreme psychological difficulties, there is some indication that many children with chronic illness, even those who do not develop extreme psychological difficulties, experience a sense of being stigmatized by their condition and often hesitate to share information about it with peers because they perceive that their peers have many misconceptions and apprehensions about the disease.[2] The impact of the condition on a person's sense of self in relationships with others also seems to continue into later life, as many children expect the disease to negatively affect the development of intimate personal relationships.[2]

> **SPECIAL CONSIDERATION:**
>
> Having a chronic illness can impact significantly on a child's view of herself and on her sense of autonomy and competence in the world.

Compliance with Treatment and Coping with Procedures

Children with chronic illnesses often develop issues that are related to treatment adherence/compliance as well as difficulty coping with specific procedures. With acute conditions, increased information given to the child, more precise instructions about

the treatment, and increased parental and medical supervision are often sufficient to ensure compliance.[6] With chronic illnesses, issues of compliance often present a more serious challenge. Research suggests that intervention programs that combine intensive education, self and parental involvement in the treatment and monitoring, and reinforcement procedures to reward compliance tend to be most effective.[7] A thorough understanding of the child's developmental level, family dynamics, and environmental factors that might support or undermine adherence are essential to developing an effective intervention program.

> **SPECIAL CONSIDERATION:**
>
> A thorough understanding of the child's developmental level, family dynamics, and environmental factors that might support or undermine adherence are essential to developing an effective intervention program.

Although noncompliance with treatment can be due simply to a lack of understanding or environmental factors (e.g., lack of money to buy the medication), it can also be related to psychological factors. For example, treatment adherence is often most difficult with adolescents who use their compliance/noncompliance with treatment to work through issues of independence and rebellion, which are hallmarks of this life stage. Equally, depression in a child or parent can significantly impact on compliance. In situations such as these, simply providing more specific information about the need for compliance is insufficient if the underlying psychologic issues are not recognized and treated.

Noncompliance with treatment can also be due to a child's difficulty in tolerating a certain procedure, such as swallowing pills, receiving injections, having bone marrow aspirations, etc. Pediatric psychologists are often helpful in addressing the child's fears and helping the child and family develop strategies for coping with these procedures. By combining education about the procedure, training in relaxation techniques, and cognitive-behavioral strategies with a reinforcement program, children often are able to improve their ability to cope with these procedures. When the child begins to develop a fear, early intervention is essential to reduce the fear quickly and allow the child to develop a sense of mastery that comes with coping well with the procedures. Fears, or phobias that are more long-standing can be addressed also but often require more intensive intervention to reduce the child's level of anxiety. As with many areas of psychological intervention, earlier is better!

In extreme situations, noncompliance may require legal intervention to protect the child. Legal intervention in the parent-child relationship is seen most commonly in situations of physical, sexual, and/or emotional abuse. However, family situations involving neglect of the child's needs, including noncompliance with necessary medical treatments, also warrant legal interventions. Clearly, the legal and child protection systems will intervene in situations of medical neglect when the risk of noncompliance has life-threatening consequences. In situations where the noncompliance may have permanent, but not life-threatening, consequences for the child's health, these child protection systems also may become involved, although their involvement is more controversial.[8] Efforts to protect the child through mandating treatment and/or providing support systems to assist the family with compliance should be pursued initially. When these options are unsuccessful, the child may be removed from the home for a period of time. However, even temporary removal of the child from the family can have a lasting negative impact on the parent-child relationship. Clearly, society and legal and child protection systems must intervene while respecting parental and familial rights fully and remaining cognizant that "harm is inherent in every violation of family integrity."[8] Therefore, decisions to pursue legal intervention should be weighed carefully by medical and mental health providers only after other, less intrusive options, have been exhausted (Practice Pathway 7-1).

> **SPECIAL CONSIDERATION:**
> Legal intervention in the parent-child relationship is seen most commonly in situations of physical, sexual, and/or emotional abuse.

PSYCHOLOGICAL ASSESSMENT

Often in the course of treating a child for a chronic or an acute illness, the pediatric otolaryngologist becomes concerned about a child's cognitive, academic, or social functioning. It is therefore important to have a general understanding of psychological assessment measures and the type of information that can be provided by such assessments.

Evaluation of Cognitive, Academic, and Personality Functioning

Psychologists, including those practicing in medical settings or in schools, often perform evaluations to assess a child's level of cognitive development, academic achievement, and personality characteristics, including emotional and behavioral difficulties. If the concerns about the child's functioning are impacting on school performance, many parents begin the assessment process through their school district. Through the child's public school district, public laws 94-142 and 99-457 ensure appropriate assessment and intervention services for all children with a "handicap" who are age 3 years and older. If a child is deemed eligible for intervention services because of his/her difficulties, an Individualized Educational Program (IEP) must be developed to specify which services will be offered and what specific goals will be achieved. The IEP is reviewed and revised on a yearly basis, with both school officials and parents providing approval. In addition, reevaluation of the child's functional level through formalized assessment measures is required every three years.[9] Often, parents start the assessment process through their school district and then, if needed, contact outside psychologists for more specialized assessment of personality and emotional factors or for neuropsychological assessment of specific cognitive processes, as well as diagnosis of psychiatric conditions.

Understanding the child's level of cognitive functioning, memory and language skills, and social-emotional development is essential to involving the child in her treatment process. Information that is shared with the child about her condition, prognosis, and treatment regimen must be presented at a level that matches the child's development. Often medical staff become frustrated when a child appears to be noncompliant with requests because

Practice Pathway 7–1   ASSESSING AND MANAGING THE CHILD WITH A PSYCHIATRIC ILLNESS

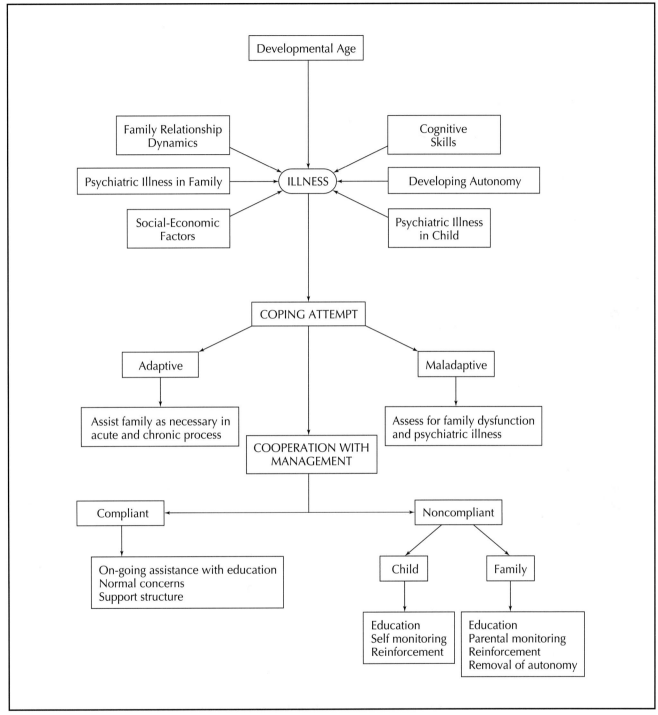

they are unaware that the child's significant cognitive delays are the "cause" of the noncompliance. In a highly structured setting, such as an office visit or hospitalization, a child's borderline intellectual functioning or mild mental retardation easily can go unrecognized if the child has good social skills or is cooperative with staff.

Conditions that Impact on Academic and Social Functioning

Psychological assessment measures often are used to evaluate difficulties that are first recognized in the school setting. Below average cognitive functioning or mild to moderate mental retardation often go undetected or at least unacknowledged by families until school officials raise concerns. Similarly, emotional difficulties such as depression and anxiety can have a significant impact on school performance. Children who have significant depression or anxiety often perform poorly on measures of cognitive functioning and academic achievement. In these situations, it is necessary to treat the underlying emotional condition with psychotherapy and/or medications before psychological assessments can be useful in gaining an accurate estimate of the child's abilities. Learning disabilities often are not diagnosed fully until first or second grade. A learning disability is considered to be a disorder in "... one or more of the basic psychological processes involved in understanding or in using language, spoken or written, which may manifest itself in an imperfect ability to listen, think, speak, read, write, spell, or to do mathematical calculations ..." (Federal Register, December 29, 1977, p. 65083, 121a.5). Generally, a diagnosis of a learning disability is based on a discrepancy between academic achievement (in one or more areas) and intellectual abilities, with the child having had sufficient opportunity to master the academic material.[9]

> **SPECIAL CONSIDERATION:**
>
> Generally, a diagnosis of a learning disability is based on a discrepancy between academic achievement and intellectual abilities.

Auditory processing difficulties and attentional difficulties can impact significantly on school performance and often are recognized first in the school setting. Although these two conditions have some different characteristics, there appears to be a fairly large overlap between the children who meet the criteria for each condition; as well, there is as an overlap between children who are diagnosed with one or both of these conditions and who have learning disabilities.[10] A central auditory processing deficit or disorder (CAPD) is diagnosed most frequently by an audiologist, but problems with concentration, understanding verbal information, and acquisition and use of language are warning signs that are often exhibited in schools. Psychological assessments are often useful when working with children who have CAPD to gain a broader understanding of the child's abilities and to rule out possible comorbid conditions. Classroom modifications that include preferential seating, use of an FM amplification system, and increased structure, as well as speech and language services, are often helpful for children with CAPD. Furthermore, some research suggests that stimulant medications that commonly are used with children who have attentional difficulties also can be useful in treating symptoms of CAPD.[11]

SOME PSYCHIATRIC CONDITIONS ENCOUNTERED BY PEDIATRIC OTOLARYNGOLOGISTS

Attention Deficit/Hyperactivity Disorder

Children with behavioral disorders present a variety of challenges to parents, teachers, and medical professionals. Of these behavioral disorders, the general public is most familiar with and medical professionals most frequently encounter children with attention deficit/hyperactivity disorder (AD/HD). This condition, which has previously been referred to as minimal brain dysfunction, hyperactivity, and attention deficit disorder, encompasses symptoms of inattention, hyperactivity, and impulsivity. Whereas most children with this diagnosis have symptoms in all three categories, some children only have symptoms of inattention and others only have symptoms of hyperactivity and impulsivity.[12] Generally, children with hyperactivity and impulsivity are identified at a young age, whereas children who solely have symptoms of inattention often go undiagnosed until later in their elementary school or junior high school years. Treatment of AD/HD often combines medications (primarily stimulants), increased structure in the classroom, parental psychotherapy focusing on behavioral management issues, and/or individual psychotherapy focusing on social skills and self-esteem issues.[13]

Autism and Other Pervasive Developmental Disorders

The category of pervasive developmental disorders (PDD) encompasses disorders that are characterized by severe and pervasive impairments in the areas of reciprocal social relationships and communication skills and by the presence of stereotyped behaviors, interests, or activities.[12] Within this category, there is a wide range of severity of symptoms and impairment of daily functioning. However, the conditions in this category share many qualitative features that are primarily related to the child's interest and/or ability to engage in emotionally connected, reciprocal relationships, and these are conditions that tend to be diagnosed early in childhood.

The most commonly known condition and often the most severe condition within this category is autism. This condition is marked by gross and sustained impairments in social relationships; these children often have no clear interest in interacting with others. Children with autism are often described as being "in their own world," seeming not to even recognize the presence of others. Approximately 75% of children with autism are functioning within the mentally retarded range, however they may exhibit unusual, highly-developed splinter skills or abilities. These children often have severe impairments in language, occasionally with more significant impairments in receptive language than in expressive language. Behavioral difficulties are often problematic and include hyperactivity, aggressiveness, self-injurious behaviors, volitional vomiting, and impulsivity. Unusual responses to sensory stimulations are seen and these children often engage in frequent self-stimulatory behaviors, such as flapping their fingers or hands, rocking, or spinning.

Rett's disorder and childhood disintegrative disorder are conditions within the PDD category that are marked by a period of normal development, ranging from 5 months to 2 years of age, followed by significant loss of previously acquired skills and development of social deficits. Asperger's disorder is marked by severe social impairments and highly-restricted interests or behaviors in a child who has normal language, cognitive, and self-help abilities. These children tend to be the highest functioning children within the PDD category, and due to their normal cognitive and language abilities may not be identified until school age or even adolescence. Finally, pervasive developmental disorder not otherwise specified is the diagnosis that is used to classify children who exhibit many of the characteristic symptoms of this category of disorders, but who do not fully meet the criteria for any one disorder.[12]

A diagnosis of autism or another condition within the PDD category can be emotionally devastating for a family. In general, these are life-long conditions with no clear etiology, and these conditions, particularly autism, tend to have a very poor prognosis. Although psychological theories previously postulated environmental and family-relationship factors as possible etiologies, these theories have proved to be unfounded. There is considerable evidence that central nervous system (CNS) abnormalities play a primary role in these conditions, but no single etiologic cause is known for these conditions.[14] Treatments tend to focus on promoting the development of social, communicative, and self-help skills, while reducing self-injurious, aggressive, and/or stereotyped behaviors. Although medications are often helpful in addressing the maladaptive behaviors, educational and behavioral treatments remain the core treatments for these conditions. With improvements in educational and behavioral treatments, as well as with increased opportunities for assisted living and sheltered employment, the prognosis for children and adults with these conditions is improving.[15] More positive outcomes clearly have been associated with higher intellectual abilities and the presence of useful speech by 5 years of age.[16]

Munchausen Syndrome by Proxy

Munchausen's syndrome by proxy is a relatively rare and complicated form of child abuse. This condition involves a parent, usually the mother, directly causing or simulating a child's physical symptoms, seeking treatment for the child, and then denying any knowledge of the etiology of these symptoms. The most common symptoms are bleeding, seizures, CNS depression, apnea, diarrhea, vomiting, fevers, and/or rashes.[17] Usually these symptoms present as an acute illness, although some cases have involved symptoms of more chronic conditions.[18] This condition should not be confused with situations in which a parent may exaggerate the child's symptoms because of concern for the child's safety, personal anxiety, psychological issues that make it difficult for the parent to accurately assess the child's condition, or a sense of being disregarded by the medical staff when they express concerns.

Currently, our understanding of the dynamics of this complicated condition is limited. However, there is some suggestion that these parents tend to have a greater than average understanding of medical information either through formal education or experience with medical conditions, tend to have a history of psychosomatic or factitious disorders themselves, and come from highly enmeshed, authoritarian families that have a history of child abuse or exploitation within the extended family system.[19] Often the parent believes that parenting a sick child will be socially rewarding or will help resolve personal conflicts. The parent may have had personal experiences of feeling more "loved" when physically ill themselves.[20] When Munchausen's syndrome by proxy or any form of child maltreat-

ment is suspected, it is essential to involve a range of medical and mental health professionals to evaluate the situation aggressively and to protect the child. Often involvement of social workers, psychologists, and/or psychiatrists are needed to assess the child's knowledge of the etiology of his symptoms adequately and to assess the parental behaviors in light of a broader understanding of the psychopathology that may contribute to child maltreatment.[21] When beginning the investigation process, it is important to elicit the help of various family members, including the mother, in solving this "puzzle" and to encourage the mother to work as part of a team to address her child's needs. Alienating the mother and family without clear evidence of maltreatment will only serve to make gaining the necessary information more difficult and will place the child at greater risk. Using techniques, such as a therapeutic double-bind or inexact interpretation of psychologic dynamics or defenses that the person then "corrects," are often difficult to accomplish, but will allow the parent and child to provide information about the factitious symptoms and etiology without "losing face."[22]

PSYCHOLOGICAL CONSIDERATIONS IN SPECIFIC MEDICAL CONDITIONS

Craniofacial Conditions

Children who have a variety of craniofacial conditions, including cleft lip and palate, encounter many difficult experiences due to their condition. These experiences include frequent medical appointments, multiple surgeries, curiosity or questions from others, and teasing. Even with these difficulties, research has not shown that these children are at increased risk for major emotional or behavioral disturbances.[23] Instead, research has shown consistently that these children are at risk for developing a variety of relatively mild psychological disturbances, which tend to be related to social difficulties and poor self-concept.[24,25] Although most of these conditions do not pose an increased risk for mental retardation, children with cleft lip and palate and some other craniofacial conditions are at increased risk for developing learning disabilities, particularly verbal or language-based learning disabilities.[26] It is not yet clear whether children with craniofacial conditions are at increased risk for developing AD/HD, but given the frequent co-occurrence of learning disabilities with AD/HD, an increased risk is likely.

Multidisciplinary treatment of children with craniofacial conditions is essential to address the many needs of these children and their families adequately. Treatment teams often include cleft/craniofacial surgeons, otolaryngologists, audiologists, speech/language pathologists, psychologists, dentists/orthodontists, opthamologists, and nurses. A psychologist's role focuses primarily on issues of facilitating appropriate placement and special education services in the schools; assessing the child's emotional and behavioral functioning; and addressing issues related to peer relationships, self-concept, and body image. At times, psychological preparation for surgery as well as addressing realistic and unrealistic expectations of changes that may occur with surgery may be needed also. Whereas direct delivery of psychological assessment and psychotherapy services may be provided, often the long distances families travel to reach the treatment team tend to prohibit direct provision of on-going services. As with many professionals on a craniofacial treatment team, the psychologist often serves as a resource for the family by identifying areas that need intervention and assisting the family with finding the appropriate intervention services within their local area.

Psychosomatic Conditions

Generally, psychosomatic disorders refer to any problem that has both physical and psychological components. Whereas more traditional views of mind-body separation suggest that conditions have either a physical or psychological cause, most professionals now acknowledge a variety of conditions that combine effects of biological, psychologic, and social influences in these illnesses.[27] Adding to this understanding is the discovery of "physical" causes for illnesses that previously were assumed to be largely psychologically related, such as some cases of asthma and ulcers. An integrative model of psychosomatic disorders (often referred to as a biopsychosocial model) has been developed, and it has emphasized the reciprocal causality with and across levels of the model.[28] Psychological factors include understanding the child's develop-

mental level and the impact of development on conceptualizations of illness, treatment adherence, and coping skills. The most widely researched social factors relate to the relationship between stress and illness, factors of family dynamics, and familial patterns of psychosomatic disorders. Social factors that often are considered to be "necessary" for the development of a severe psychosomatic disorder are family dysfunction and the role of the "sick child" in reducing family conflict. However, these social factors must occur within the context of a specific physical disorder or "organ vulnerability" in order for a psychosomatic disorder to develop.[29] Finally, research on biologic factors has focused largely on physiological responses to stress and understanding of disease heritability.[27]

Given a biopsychosocial model, the need for multidisciplinary assessment and treatment is clear. Psychologists are often included in order to conduct interviews and administer psychometric measures that explore issues of personality characteristics, family dynamics, and how the "illness" impacts both positively and negatively on individual and family functioning. In addition, determination of the presence or absence of psychiatric disorders in the various family members is necessary. The psychological component of the treatment often focuses on decreasing the "secondary gains" received from the illness and directly addressing the function of the illness within the family dynamics. The secondary gains that the "sick child" may receive include increased attention, decreased expectations, and a sense of power within the family because of being "sick." Furthermore, having a "sick child" also may meet needs within the family system by reducing conflict, keeping parents from divorcing, providing an outlet for parental needs to nurture and be "needed," and deflecting attention away from behavioral or emotional difficulties in other family members. Thus, family therapy is often a central component of the psychological intervention. Other components may focus more directly on addressing the psychosomatic symptoms through the use of relaxation training, biofeedback, behavioral reinforcement programs to encourage difficult activities, and cognitive-behavioral techniques to address issues of distorted thoughts and beliefs.[27]

Vocal Cord Dysfunction

Vocal cord dysfunction (VCD), or psychogenic stridor as it is sometimes called is a condition that often presents as asthma or other forms of respiratory difficulties. Paradoxical cord motion is seen on endoscopy. Most research suggests that this condition is best diagnosed and treated by a multidisciplinary team involving an otolaryngologist and/or pulmonologist, a speech pathologist, and a psychologist and/or psychiatrist. A multidisciplinary approach to diagnosis and treatment can often avoid repeated emergency room visits and inappropriate medications and/or surgical procedures.[30] Although previous literature has suggested a strong association with sexual abuse and/or significant psychiatric conditions, this literature has consisted largely of single case studies or research with a relatively small number of patients.[31,32] There is an increasing belief that although personality characteristics such as perfectionism, being "high-strung or driven," and having a strong need for control are often associated with the development VCD, these characteristics are neither necessary nor sufficient to explain this condition.[33] Although there is still the need for a greater understanding of possible psychological and/or physical factors associated with this condition, interventions combining short-term psychotherapy and speech therapy seem to be quite effective and are currently considered to be the treatment of choice. Psychotherapy interventions tend to focus on relaxation techniques such as diaphragmatic breathing, muscle relaxation, and imagery combined with cognitive strategies to combat the negative beliefs and "self-talk" the child may be using. In some cases, biofeedback and/or hypnosis may be helpful.[34] Family therapy that addresses the need to support the child while facilitating autonomy and setting realistic goals is often needed.[35]

CONCLUSIONS

Psychological issues, including both normal developmental patterns and psychopathology, can significantly impact the presentation of a child's symptoms, the family's and child's ability to cope with illness, and the family's ability to successfully interact with medical professionals. Although many medical professionals have some awareness and understanding of these issues, input from mental health professionals is often needed to gain a broader appreciation of these dynamics. Furthermore, due to the variety of issues associated with many medical conditions, a multidisciplinary approach to evaluation and intervention is often indicated. Thus, working to develop a cooperative, on-going professional relationship with a psychologist or other mental health professional can be beneficial.

REFERENCES

1. Sroufe LA, Cooper RG. *Child Development: Its Nature and Course.* New York: Albert A. Knopf, 1988.
2. Drotar D. Psychological perspectives in chronic childhood illness. In: Roberts MC, Koocher GP, Routh DK, et al. eds *Readings in Pediatric Psychology.* New York: Plenum, 1993, pp. 95–113.
3. Pless IB, Roghmann K, Haggerty RF. Chronic illness, family functioning, and psychological adjustment: A model for the allocation of preventive mental health services. Int J Epidemiol 1972; 11:403–410.
4. Drotar D, Owens R, Gotthold J. Personality adjustment of children and adolescents with hypopituitarism. Child Psychiatry Hum Dev 1980; 11:59–66.
5. Tavormina JB, Kastner LS, Slater PM, et al. Chronically ill children: A psychologically and emotionally deviant population? J Abnorm Child Psychol 1976; 4:99–110.
6. LaGreca AM, Schuman WB. Adherence to prescribed medical regimens. In: Roberts MC, ed. *Handbook of Pediatric Psychology.* New York: Guilford, 1995, pp. 55–85.
7. Baum D, Creer T. Medication compliance in children with asthma. J Asthma 1986; 23:49–59.
8. Goldstein J, Freud A, Solnit AJ. *Before the Best Interests of the Child.* New York: The Free Press, 1979, p. 136.
9. Sattler JM. *Assessment of Children,* 3rd ed. San Diego: Jerome M. Sattler, 1988.
10. Riccio CA, Hynd GW, Cohen MJ, et al. Comorbidity of central auditory processing disorder and attention-deficit hyperactivity disorder. J Am Acad Child Adolesc Psychiatry 1994; 33:849–857.
11. Cook JR, Mausbach T, Burd L, et al. A preliminary study of the relationship between central auditory processing disorder and attention deficit disorder. J Psychiatry Neurosci 1993; 18:130–137.
12. American Psychiatric Association. Diagnostic and Statistical Manual of Mental Disorders 4th ed. Washington: American Psychiatric Association, 1994, p.
13. Barkley RA. *Attention-Deficit Hyperactivity Disorder: A Handbook for Diagnosis and Treatment.* New York: Guilford, 1990.
14. Dawson G, Castelloe P. Autism. In: Walker CE, Roberts MC, eds. *Handbook of Clinical Child Psychology,* 2nd ed. New York: John Wiley, 1992, p. 375.
15. Stone WL, MacLean WE, Hogan KL. Autism and mental retardation. In: Roberts MC, ed. *Handbook of Pe-*

diatric Psychology. New York: Guilford, 1995, p. 655.

16. Lotter V. Follow-up studies. In: Rutter M, Schopler E, eds. Autism: A Reappraisal of Concepts and Treatment. New York: Plenum, 1978, p. 475.

17. Rosenberg DA. Web of deceit: A literature review of Munchausen syndrome by proxy. Child Abuse Negl 1987; 11:547-563.

18. Kahn G, Goldman E. Munchausen syndrome by proxy: Mother fabricates infant's hearing impairment. J Speech Hear Res 1991; 34:957-959.

19. Griffith JL. The family systems of Munchausen syndrome by proxy. Fam Process 1988; 27:423-437.

20. Sheridan MS. Munchausen syndrome by proxy. Health Soc Work 1989; 14:53-58.

21. Rosenberg DA. Recent issues in child maltreatment. In: Bross DC, Krugman RD, Lenherr MR, et al, eds. The New Child Protection Team Handbook. New York: Garland, 1988, p. 113.

22. Eisendrath SJ. Factitious physical disorders: Treatment without confrontation. Psychosomatics 1989; 30:383-387.

23. Richman L, Eliason M. Psychological characteristics of children with cleft lip and palate: Intellectual, achievement, behavioral, and personality variables. Cleft Palate J 1982; 19:249-257.

24. Broder H, Strauss RP. Self-concept of early primary school age children with visible or invisible defects. Cleft Palate J 1989; 26:114-117.

25. Kapp K. Self-concept of the cleft lip or palate child. Cleft Palate J 1979; 16:171-176.

26. Richman L, Eliason, M. Type of reading disability related to cleft type and neuropsychological patterns. Cleft Palate J 1984; 21:1-6.

27. Kager VA, Arndt EK, Kenny TJ. Psychosomatic problems of children. In: Walker CE, Roberts MC, eds. Handbook of Clinical Child Psychology. New York: John Wiley, 1992, p. 303.

28. Fabrega H, VanEgeren LA. A behavioral framework for the study of human disease. Ann Int Med 1976; 84:200-208.

29. Minuchin S, Baker L, Rosman BL, et al. A conceptual model of psychosomatic illness in children: Family organization and family therapy. Arch Gen Psychiatry 1975; 32:1031-1038.

30. Lacy TJ, McManis SE. Psychogenic stridor. Gen Hosp Psychiatry 1994; 16:213-223.

31. Tajchman UW, Gitterman B. Vocal cord dysfunction associated with sexual abuse. Clin Pediatr 1996; 35:105-108.

32. Freedman MR, Rosenberg SJ, Schmaling KB. Childhood sexual abuse in patients with paradoxical vocal cord dysfunction. J Nerv Ment Dis 1991; 179:295-298.

33. Thompson S. Personal Communication, 1997.

34. Smith MS. Acute psychogenic stridor in an adolescent athlete treated with hypnosis. Pediatrics 1983; 72:247-248.

35. Freedman MR, Rosenberg SJ, Schmaling KB. Transgenerational psychosomatic respiratory symptoms: A case illustration. J Fam Psychotherapy 1991; 2:17.

II

THE EAR

8 Structure and Function of the Temporal Bone

Christopher P. Poje and Jay S. Rechtweg

To have a formal understanding of the temporal bone (TB), its pathology, and treatment of disease therein, it is essential to have a firm understanding of the TB's anatomy and physiology. The TB is complex with five developmentally-different regions: the squamosa, the petrous, the tympanic, the mastoid, and the styloid. In the most general sense, the primary structure of the temporal bone is the *ear*. From medial to lateral, the ear is divided into the *inner ear* (which includes the cochlea and vestibular apparatus), the *middle ear* [which includes the ossicles, the eustachian tube (ET) and the nerves, muscles and tendons lying within the tympanic space], and the *external ear* [which includes the external auditory canal (EAC) and the pinna]. Also of prime importance are the relationships of the facial nerve, the internal auditory canal (IAC), and the mastoid air-cells to the sensory structures.

The inner ear has the distinct responsibility of being the source of hearing (i.e., the cochlea) and balance (i.e., the vestibular apparatus). If any anatomic structure is altered adversely or if the physiologic mechanisms of hearing and/or balance are disturbed, a disease state ensues.

Complete texts are written on each of these subjects. The purpose of this chapter is to provide a basic knowledge of the TB's anatomy and physiology so that the reader may understand the pathologic alterations that are discussed in later chapters. In addition, a detailed outline of the development of the TB is essential for understanding congenital or genetic disease states.

Pediatric Otolaryngology, Edited by R.F. Wetmore, H.R. Muntz, and T.J. McGill. Thieme Medical Publishers, Inc., New York © 2000.

ANATOMY AND PHYSIOLOGY OF THE TEMPORAL BONE

The External Ear

The auricle

The *auricle* is an irregular, vaguely funnel-shaped conglomerate of elastic cartilage.[1] The *perichondrium* of the anterior auricle tends to be tightly adherent to the skin, but is loosely connected to the cartilage. The posterior auricle has a thin layer of loose connective tissue and is without firm attachments of skin to cartilage. It attaches to the EAC by three extrinsic ligaments and muscles. Any intrinsic musculature is poorly developed in humans.

The auricle is located in a plane such that the anterior helical-cranial junction is at the same level as the lateral canthi. Furthermore, the angle of the ear should be no greater than 15 degrees off vertical. Alterations in the plane or slope of the auricle may be indicative of a congenital craniofacial syndrome.

> ### SPECIAL CONSIDERATION:
>
> Alterations in the plane or slope of the auricle may be indicative of a congenital craniofacial syndrome.

Innervation to the outer ear is rather complex, with multiple cranial and cervical nerves contributing branches. The innervation is derived from the fifth, seventh, and tenth cranial nerves, as well as the second cervical nerve (via the greater auricular nerve) and the second and third cervical nerves (via the lesser occipital nerve).

The shape of the outer ear allows for the concentration and funneling of sound from the external environment to the EAC. The auricular cartilage also plays a role in helping one locate the direction of sounds in space.

The external auditory canal

The *external auditory canal* is a 2.5 cm conduit that travels through the TB to the tympanic membrane (TM).[2] As the EAC courses through the TB, its medial portion comes to lie anterior to its lateral portion, forming a horizontal "s". Pulling the auricle superiorly and posteriorly during an exam straightens the canal so that otoscopy may be performed more simply.

The lateral third of the EAC is composed of skin with a thin layer of loose connective tissue overlying fibrocartilage. Skin in this region possesses adnexal appendages, including hair follicles, ceruminous glands, and sebaceous glands. *Ceruminous glands* are modified apocrine sweat glands that secrete a milky substance that becomes brown and waxy upon exposure to air. These secretions mix with the triglycerides and fatty esters secreted by the sebaceous glands to form cerumen or "ear wax". Thus cerumen normally should be present only in this region. Natural lateral migration of skin from the TM's umbo out of the EAC allows for cleansing of accumulated debris and cerumen.

The medial two-thirds of the EAC are composed of skin in direct apposition to periosteum and bone. The isthmus (i.e., the narrowest point) occurs at the bony-cartilaginous junction. The canal is innervated by the seventh and ninth cranial nerves.

The EAC acts as a resonance chamber, conducting sound to the TM. It has a *resonance frequency* (i.e., the natural frequency at which the physical properties of the structure allow maximal amplification of sound) of 3000 Hz.[3,4] Table 8-1 delineates resonance frequencies for several sound-conducting structures. It should be remembered that speech frequencies in humans are largely between 500 to 2000 Hz.

The Tympanic Membrane

The *tympanic membrane* is a curtain of tissue that forms the medial border of the EAC and the lateral border of the tympanic cavity.[2] It is a four-layered, 9 mm (the anterior-posterior axis) by 10 mm (the superior-inferior axis) sheet of tissue. From lateral to medial, the four layers are: skin, the radial fibrous tissue, the circumferential fibrous tissue, and the mucosa. The TM attaches to the wall of the EAC via a fibrous band known as the *annulus.*

Although the TM has an overall area of 70 to 80 mm,[2] its functional area is approximately 55 mm.[2] The TM has a resonance frequency of 800 to 1600 Hz.[3,4] The surface is divided by the attachment of the manubrium and lateral process of the malleus to the medial surface. It is firmly adherent to the fibrous layer at the lateral process, and at the distal most part of the manubrium it is adherent to the umbo. The rest of the manubrium is attached by mucosa known as *plica mallearis.*

Superior to the lateral process of the malleus is the *pars flaccida,* or Shrapnell's membrane. The majority of the TM (the *pars tensa*) is inferior to the lateral process of the malleus. The pars flaccida is thicker than the pars tensa and lacks an organized fibrous layer. Medial to the pars flaccida, in the middle ear, is a region known as *Prussack's space* (Table 8-2). Prussack's space is further bounded by the lateral malleal ligament anterosuperiorly and the anterior and posterior malleal folds inferiorly. It opens into the epitympanium posteriorly. This region is significant as it is the most common site for development of retraction pockets and cholesteatoma.

TABLE 8–1:   The Resonance Frequency of Temporal Bone Structures

Structure	Resonance Frequency
External Auditory Canal	3000 Hz
Middle Ear	800 Hz
Tympanic Membrane	800–1600 Hz
Ossicular Chain	500–2000 Hz

TABLE 8–2:   The Boundaries of Prussack's Space

Lateral	Tympanic membrane
Anterior/Superior	Lateral malleal ligament
Inferior	Anterior malleal fold
	Posterior malleal fold
Posterior	Opens into epitympanium

The Middle Ear and Tympanic Cavity

When referring to the middle ear, several different regions are defined (Figs. 8–1 and 8–2). The *epitympanum* is the space between the superior most TM and the tegmen (i.e., the roof of the middle ear and the floor of the middle cranial fossa). It opens into the mastoid antrum posteriorly, and is bounded laterally by the scutum. The *hypotympanum* extends from the inferior portion of the TM to the floor of the middle ear (primarily to the bone overlying the jugular bulb). The *mesotympanum* is the portion of the middle ear that is directly visible behind the TM. The *protympanum* lies anterior to the TM and contains the ET orifice. Posterior to the TM lie the facial recess, the incudal fossa, and the aditus ad antrum, as well as the mastoid air-cell system.

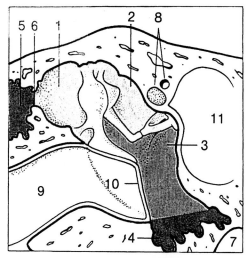

Figure 8–1: Anatomy of the middle ear cavity: 1 and 2, epitympanum; 3, mesotympanum; 4, hypotympanum; 5, mastoid antrum; 6, entrance to the antrum; 7, internal jugular vein. The lower part of the attic (2) is markedly narrowed by the facial nerve and the horizontal semicircular canal (8). 9, external meatus; 10, tympanic membrane; and 11, inner ear. (From Becker W, Naumann HH, Pfaltz CR. Ear: Applied anatomy and physiology. In: Buckingham RA, ed. *Ear, Nose and Throat Diseases. A Pocket Reference.* New York: Thieme, 1989, with permission.)

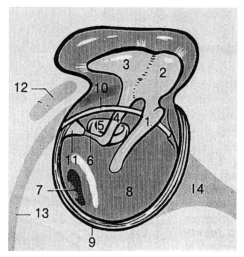

Figure 8–2: Medial wall of the middle ear: promontory (8) at the basal turn of the cochlea. Above is the oval window niche with the stapes (5) whose footplate is held loosely in the oval window by the annular ligament. The long process of the incus (4) forms a joint by its lenticular process with the head of the stapes. The body of the incus (3) forms the joint surface for the head of the malleus (2). The malleus and incus vibrate as one body in the middle part of the frequency range. The round window (7) lies below the pyramidal eminence (11) with the stapedius muscle whose tendon (6) runs to the head of the stapes. The bony facial canal (13) runs inferior to the horizontal semicircular canal (12). The handle and short process of the malleus (1) lie lateral to the chorda tympani (10). The pars tensa is anchored by the anulus fibrosus (9) in the bony niche of the anulus tympanicus. The middle ear cavity is aerated via the eustachian tube (14). (From Becker W, Naumann HH, Pfaltz CR. Ear: Applied anatomy and physiology. In: Buckingham RA, ed. *Ear, Nose and Throat Diseases. A Pocket Reference.* New York: Thieme, 1989, with permission.)

The ossicles

Three ossicles, two muscles, several nerves, and multiple bony landmarks are found in the middle ear. The three ossicles span the gap between the TM and the oval window/inner ear. The range of their resonance frequency is 500 to 2000 Hz. From lateral to medial lie the malleus, the incus, and the stapes.[2] As previously described, the *malleus* is adherent to the TM's medial surface. Its neck and head occupy part of the epitympanum. Attached to the medial surface of the neck and manubrium is the tensor tympani tendon. The tensor tympani muscle is a 2 cm long muscle that runs in the TB parallel to the ET. It enters the middle ear as a tendon emanating from the cochleariform process. The *cochle-*

ariform process is on the medial surface of the tympanic cavity and is adjacent to the orifice of the ET. The tendon emerges, makes a right angle turn, and inserts on the malleus. The muscle is innervated by the motor portion of the trigeminal nerve and acts to keep a tonic contraction upon the TM. Reflexive contraction of the tensor tympani pulls the malleus medially and increases the tension upon the TM.

The head of the malleus articulates with the body of the incus via a diarthrodial, moveable joint (i.e., the incudomalleolar joint). The *incus* is the largest of the ossicles and possesses the greatest mass. The short process of the incus is stabilized relative to the lateral wall by the posterior incudal ligament. The long process of the incus travels inferiorly, parallel to the manubrium, to terminate as the *lenticular process*. The lenticular process articulates with the head of the stapes via a diarthrodial joint. The distal portion of the long process of the incus and the incudostapedial joint are a vascular watershed area,[2] and are hence the portions of the ossicular chain most susceptible to trauma and infection.

The *stapes* is the most variably shaped of the ossicles. Its head is attached to the footplate via two crura, the anterior and posterior. The stapedial tendon attaches to the superior portion of the posterior crus and the head of the stapes. The stapedius muscle originates in the posterior temporal bone and travels in a reverse direction to the mastoid portion of the facial nerve. The stapedius muscle enters the tympanic cavity from the pyramidal eminence as a tendon. This muscle is innervated by the facial nerve.

The footplate of the stapes sits upon the oval window of the inner ear. The stapediovestibular joint is a fibrous joint known as the annular ligament. The foot plate is 1.5 by 3 mm in size,[2] whereas the surface area of the oval window is approximately 3 mm^2. Thus, sound is funneled from the 55 mm^2 effective surface area of the TM to the 3 mm^2 surface area of the oval window, resulting in a 17:1 increase in sound energy. Furthermore, the three ossicles act in unison as levers to give a mechanical advantage via exploitation of the lever arm ratio. As the manubrium of the malleus is approximately 1.3 times longer than the long process of the incus, there is a 1.3:1 increase in the energy conducted through the ossicles. Due to the mechanical advantage of the middle ear the net increase of sound energy that reaches the middle ear versus that which reaches the TM is 22:1 (17 × 1.3). This translates into approximately a 25 dB amplification, which is very close to the energy that is normally lost as sound crosses an air-water interface.

AT A GLANCE . . .

Mechanical Increase in Sound Energy due to Middle Ear Mechanics

TM/Oval Window Advantage:
Functional area of the TM = 55 mm^2
Functional area of the oval window = 3 mm^2
The gain of sound energy! 55/3 = 17 times increase in sound energy

Lever Ratio Advantage of the Ossicles:
The length of the malleus' manubrium is 1.3 times longer than the long process of the incus, giving a 1.3 times increase in sound energy.

Net Increase in Sound Energy: 1.3 × 17 = 22 times increase in sound energy, or a 22:1 ratio of sound energy reaching the inner ear vs. reaching the TM.

The oval and round windows

The *oval window* is one of two membranous partitions between the middle ear and the inner ear. It lies on the medial portion of the tympanic cavity, upon the bulge of bone overlying the cochlea known as the *promontory*. The *round window*, the second membranous partition between the inner ear and the middle ear, lies inferior to the oval window on the promontory. A ridge of bone known as the subiculum may drape itself over the anterior-superior portion of the round window niche.

The wall of the lateral epitympanum along the annulus forms a bony ridge known as the *scutum*, which often obscures direct visualization of the oval window. Part of the scutum might need to be removed for visualization of the oval window during middle-ear surgery. Furthermore, there is a tendency of the scutum to be eroded by middle-ear infectious processes, especially cholesteatoma.

The eustachian tube

The *eustachian tube* is the medial drainage and ventilatory path for the middle ear. Its middle ear ostium is on the anterosuperior wall of the tympanic cavity. Its lumen has been described as a shepherd's crook. The anteromedial two-thirds is composed of fibrocartilage, and the posterolateral one-third is composed of bone. It averages 35 mm in length.

The nasopharyngeal orifice is located approximately 10 mm above the nasopharyngeal floor. It is defined inferiorly by a cartilaginous rim, the *torus tubaris*. The dilatator tubae portion of the tensor veli palatini is the muscle primarily responsible for ET function. This muscle is innervated by the motor division of the trigeminal nerve. In children with a cleft palate, the dilatator functions poorly, resulting in ET dysfunction. In adults, the levator veli palatini also is believed to act synergistically with an intact dilatator tubae to open the ET. In children, the levator is too far from the nasopharyngeal orifice to be an effective adjunct.

During childhood, the ET is relatively short and lies in a primarily horizontal plane. With growth, the tube assumes a more vertical position, allowing for improved middle-ear aeration and drainage of middle-ear secretions. The elongation of the tube combined with its more vertical position and its muscular maturation is responsible for the decreased incidence of otitis media and middle-ear effusions in adults.

SPECIAL CONSIDERATION:

Because the ET in children is relatively short and lies in a primarily horizontal plane, children experience more incidences of otitis media and middle-ear effusions than adults.

For air flow between the middle ear and the nasopharynx to be produced, a pressure difference of 200 to 300 mm H_2O needs to be overcome. It is easier for air to egress from the middle ear than to enter.

Nerves of the middle ear

Coursing through the middle ear are several nerves. The facial nerve is the most important nerve associated with the tympanic cavity; however, frank exposure of this nerve in the tympanic cavity is not necessarily desired. The facial nerve's anatomy is discussed below in more detail.

The *chorda tympani,* which is a branch of the facial nerve that has parasympathetic preganglionic fibers to the submandibular and sublingual glands and sensory fibers for taste from the anterior two thirds of the tongue, is the most recognizable nerve in the middle ear. It emerges from the posterior wall of the cavity through the iter chordae posterius, travels through the tympanic cavity between the incus and the malleus, and exits the cavity via the iter chordae anterius. As the chorda tympani emerges in the temporal bone after leaving the facial nerve, a "V" of bone develops between the two structures. This "V" of bone, known as the *facial recess,* forms a portion of the posterior wall of the tympanic cavity, and it is a relatively safe area from which to enter the tympanic cavity during mastoid surgery.

Jacobson's nerve or the tympanic nerve is a branch of the glossopharyngeal nerve that travels on the medial wall of the middle ear. It is the primary source of sensory fibers for the middle ear mucosa and the ET. It consolidates with the sympathetic plexus (entering the middle ear with the carotid artery) to form the lesser superficial *petrosal nerve.* This nerve provides autonomic innervation for the parotid gland via the otic ganglion.

Arnold's nerve is a branch of the vagus that includes some glossopharyngeal nerve fibers and that courses over the dome of the jugular bulb. The superior fibers join with the facial nerve. Inferior fibers carry sensory information from the posterior surface of the EAC.

Table 8–3 reviews middle-ear structures and landmarks.

The facial nerve

The *facial nerve* is intimately associated with the mastoid and the middle ear (Fig. 8–3). The facial nerve is a complex nerve with five types of nerve fibers that are responsible for the innervation of derivatives of the second branchial arch. The visceral efferent fibers supply motor innervation to the muscles of facial expression, the stapedius muscle, the stylohyoid muscle, and the posterior belly of the digastric muscle. Parasympathetic fibers that supply the sublingual and submandibular glands, the lacrimal gland, and the mucinous glands of the nasal

TABLE 8–3: Tympanic Cavity Structures and Landmarks

Roof	Tegmen tympani (floor of the middle cranial fossa)
Floor	Jugular bulb
	Arnold's nerve
Posterior	Aditus ad antrum
	Pyramidal eminence
	Facial recess
	Sinus tympani
Anterior	Tensor tympani muscle
	Wall of the carotid canal
	Eustachian tube orifice
Medial	Promontory
	Oval window
	Round window
	Fallopian canal
	Cochleariform process
	Jacobson's nerve
Lateral	Tympanic membrane
	Annulus
	Scutum

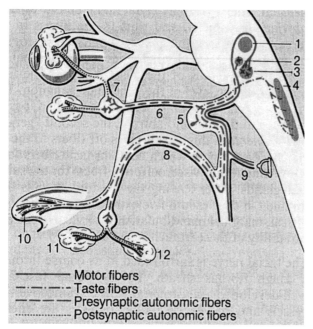

——— Motor fibers
—·—·—· Taste fibers
– – – – Presynaptic autonomic fibers
············ Postsynaptic autonomic fibers

Figure 8–3: Course of fibers in the facial nerve: 1, abducens nucleus; 2, secretory nucleus of the nervus intermedius; 3, motornuclei of the facial nerve; 4, nucleus of the solitary tract; 5, geniculate ganglion; 6, greater superficial petrosal nerve; 7, pterygopalatine ganglion with the lacrimal anastomosis; 8, chorda tympani; 9, stapedius nerve; 10, taste fibers to the anterior two thirds of the tongue; 11, sublingual gland; 12, submandibular gland. (From Becker W, Naumann HH, Pfaltz CR. Ear: Applied anatomy and physiology. In: Buckingham RA, ed. *Ear, Nose and Throat Diseases. A Pocket Reference.* New York: Thieme, 1989, with permission.)

cavity run with the nerve. Somatic afferent fibers receive sensation from portions of the auricle and the EAC, whereas visceral afferent fibers receive stimuli from the nose, pharynx, and the palate. Special sensory fibers are responsible for taste from the anterior two-thirds of the tongue, the tonsillar fossae, and the posterior palate.

The course of the facial nerve is complex and can be divided into six segments (Table 8–4). The intracranial segment originates at the pons and travels about 24 mm to the IAC. Just prior to entering the IAC, the nerve is joined by the nervus intermedius. The nervus intermedius possesses the sensory fibers for taste to the anterior two-thirds of the tongue. The intracanalicular component of the facial nerve runs the full 8-mm course of the IAC. It generally assumes an anterosuperior position within the canal.

After exiting the IAC, the nerve travels within the temporal bone. Its course in the TB is through a conduit called the *fallopian canal.* In most instances, the canal completely covers the nerve, although there may be dehiscences of the bony canal within the middle ear. Furthermore, in certain malformations of the TB, the nerve may be displaced into a more anterior course.

The labyrinthine segment of the facial nerve begins at the IAC apex and extends to the geniculate ganglion. Besides being the shortest segment at 3 to 5 mm, this segment is found within the narrowest portion of the fallopian canal. In addition, the first genu, or turn, for the nerve occurs here. The greater superficial petrosal nerve, which supplies parasympathetic innervation to the nasal, lacrimal, and palatine glands, begins in this region. In the distal portion of this segment is the *geniculate ganglion,* the site that contains the nerve cell bodies for taste. The region of the geniculate ganglion and the start of the greater superficial petrosal nerve serves to tether the facial nerve. Due to this tethering, the facial nerve that is just proximal and distal to this region is most prone to injury in skull-base trauma.

The tympanic segment extends from the geniculate ganglion to the pyramidal eminence. This is the region of the facial nerve where the canal is most often dehiscent. Furthermore, it is in this region that the second genu, a 40- to 80-degree turn, of the facial nerve occurs.

The mastoid or vertical segment forms the longest of the intramastoid segments at 10 to 14 mm, and it runs from the pyramidal eminence to the stylomastoid foramen. At this point in its course, the

TABLE 8–4:   Facial Nerve Segments

Segment	Anatomic Boundaries	Length	Branches & Landmarks
Intracranial	Brain stem to the IAC	23–24 mm	
Meatal	Fundus of the IAC to the meatal foramen	8–10 mm	
Labyrinthine	Meatal foramen to the geniculate ganglion	3–5 mm	Greater superficial petrosal nerve 1st Genu
Tympanic	Geniculate ganglion to the pyramidal eminence	8–11 mm	2nd Genu
Mastoid (Vertical)	Pyramidal eminence to the stylomastoid foramen	10–14 mm	Chorda tympani nerve to the stapedius muscle
Extratemporal	Stylomastoid foramen to the muscles of facial expression	Variable depending on the branch	Posterior auricular branch Temporal (frontal) branch Zygomatic branch Buccal branch Mandibular branch Cervical branch

Abbreviations: IAC, Internal Auditory Canal.

facial nerve assumes a fascicular arrangement of its nerve fibers. Furthermore, this is the region where branches to the stapedius and the chorda tympani divide. The course of the chorda tympani relative to the facial nerve defines the facial recess between them.

The facial nerve emerges from the stylomastoid foramen to run on the posterior belly of the digastric. Its main trunk enters the body of the parotid gland before splitting into six primary branches for innervation of the muscles of facial expression. This portion of the facial nerve is beyond the scope of this chapter.

The Inner Ear

The *inner ear* is the sensory-end organ for the ear and is directly responsible for hearing and balance. The *bony labyrinth,* which is the osseous architecture of the inner ear, includes the vestibule, the semicircular canals, and the cochlea.[2] The *membranous labyrinth* is composed of sensory epithelium and supporting tissues and is housed within the bony labyrinth. Included in the membranous labyrinth are the organ of Corti, the cristae of the three semicircular canals, and the maculae of the utricle and saccule.

Two types of extracellular fluid bathe portions of the inner ear. *Perilymph* essentially is equivalent to extracellular fluid with its high-sodium and low-potassium content. Indeed, it is most akin to cerebrospinal fluid (CSF). It is present in the scala tympani and the scala vestibuli of the cochlea, as well

as in those portions of the vestibule and semicircular canals that are external to the membranous labyrinth. *Endolymph* is a unique extracellular fluid. It is high in potassium and low in sodium, making it a biochemical analog of intracellular fluid. It is present within the vestibular organs, as well as the scala media of the cochlea. Ionic properties of these fluids are outlined in Table 8-5.

The inner ear may be divided further into an auditory and a vestibular component. Each component is addressed individually.

The auditory inner ear

The bony cochlea and its associated membranous labyrinth make up the auditory portion of the inner ear (Figs. 8-4 to 8-6). The *cochlea* lies within the most anterior portion of the bony labyrinth, and consists of a bony tube, known as the *cochlear duct,* that spiral along an axis from the anterolateral portion of the EAC to an apex that lies even more anterolaterally and extends inferiorly. A bony bulge, the promontory, is visible in the tympanic space as the cochlea's basilar end. The axis is composed of a 5 mm long bony spur called the *modiolus.* Along its

TABLE 8–5:   Labyrinthine Fluid Contents

	Perilymph	Endolymph
Sodium (mEq/L)	142–157	6–29
Potassium (mEq/L)	7–10.5	155–171
Protein (mg/dl)	160–223	125–216

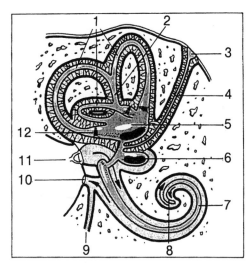

Figure 8–4:   Diagram of the inner ear: 1, membranous semicircular canals (horizontal, superior, and posterior); 2, crus commune of the posterior and superior canal; 3, saccus endolymphaticus on the posterior surface of the pyramid: 4, ductus endolymphaticus; 5, utricle; 6, saccule; 7, cochlear duct; 8, helicotrema; 9, perilymphatic duct; 10, round window; 11, oval window; 12, ampulla of the posterior semicircular canal with a cupula. (From Becker W, Naumann HH, Pfaltz CR. Ear: Applied anatomy and physiology. In: Buckingham RA, ed. *Ear, Nose and Throat Diseases. A Pocket Reference.* New York: Thieme, 1989, with permission.)

spiral course, the cochlea is 31 to 33 mm in length and makes 2.5 turns.

Traveling the length of the cochlea, in an axis perpendicular to the modiolus, are Reissner's membrane and the basilar membrane. These two partitions define three spaces within the cochlea. The *scala vestibuli* and the *scala tympani* are the two outer chambers, both of which contain perilymph. They unite at the cochlear apex in a region called the *scala communis* or the *helicotrema.* Sound, as mechanical energy, is transmitted from the stapedial footplate at the oval window into the scala vestibuli. The mechanical energy is propagated as a wave through the perilymph, causing deflection of a frequency-specific portion of the basilar membrane. As the basilar membrane spirals up the cochlea, the width and stiffness of the membrane varies, enabling it to generate a frequency-specific vibratory pattern for an individual stimulus (the lower the frequency, the more apical the stimulated basilar membrane). The organ of Corti, which rests upon the basilar membrane, is deflected as the wave energy is transmitted through the *scala media,* or the central chamber, into the scala tympani. The scala

tympani communicates with the round window, and energy from the fluid wave is dissipated in round window displacement.

The scala media is an endolymph-containing space. It is separated from the scala vestibuli by *Reissner's membrane,* which is a thin sheet of squamous epithelium and connective tissue that originates from the central wall of the cochlear duct and obliquely spans the duct and inserts into the *osseous spiral lamina* (which is the firm central attachment for this membrane and the basilar membrane). Along the peripheral wall of the cochlear duct between Reissner's membrane and the basilar membrane, lies the *stria vascularis,* which is the metabolically-active tissue that is responsible for endolymph production by active-ion transport processes.

The *basilar membrane* separates the scala media from the scala vestibuli. It spans the cochlear duct from the spiral ligament to the osseous spiral lamina. Sitting upon the basilar membrane is a complex structure with many features, including the *organ of Corti,* or the actual sensory organ for hearing. The majority of cells in the organ of corti (e.g., border cells, Deiter's cells, Hensen's cells, inner sulcus cells, inner pillar cells, inner phalangeal cells, etc.) primarily have a supportive function. The individual characteristics of each cell type have been described well in other texts, but are beyond the scope of this one.

Cochlear hair cells comprise the sensory cells for hearing (Table 8–6).[5] There are three rows of cylindrical *outer hair cells* (OHC) (12,000 total). The apical portion of each cell has a series of 48 to 150 stereocilia arranged in a "W" pattern. The stereocilia are arranged by height, with the shortest cilia being central and the tallest being lateral. OHCs possess the additional property of being contractile. Perturbations of the basilar membrane secondary to contraction of the OHCs are the source of otoacoustic emissions (i.e., actual sounds generated by the healthy cochlea and detectible by a microphone in the EAC). The aforementioned Deiter's cells act as their supporting cells.

There is one row of flask-shaped *inner hair cells* (IHC) on the basilar membrane (3500 total). The distal ends of each IHC contain about 120 stereocilia in three or four parallel rows. These cilia possess the same arrangement of height as found in the OHCs. Inner and outer pillar cells, as well as border cells, function to support the IHCs.

The IHCs and OHCs are separated by a space called the *tunnel of Corti.* The tunnel of Corti and

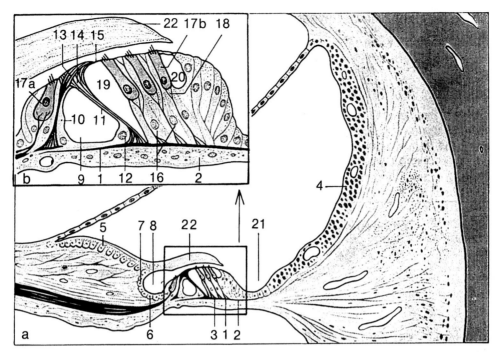

Figure 8–5: (A) Schematic representation of ductus cochlearis and (B) the organ of Corti. The organ of Corti (B) rests on the basilar membrane (1 and 2) in the cochlear duct. Medially, at the free edge of the lamina spiralis ossea, is the limbus spiralis (5) with two labia (6 and 7) enclosing the sulcus spiralis internus (8). The highly vascularized stria vascularis (4) with intraepithelial capillaries lies laterally. The organ of Corti (B) consists of inner (10) and outer (11 and 12) supporting or pillar cells constituting the borders of the inner tunnel (perilymph - 9). Above (13 to 15) is the top part of the supporting structure, the tonofibrils, and below are the supporting bodies (18) of the phalangeal cells (16) carrying the sensory cells (17). Between the outer pillars (11, 12) and Deiter's or outer phalangeal cells (16), acting as supporting cells of the organ of Corti, is Nuel's space with perilymph (19). In the extreme lateral position, we have the outer tunnel (20), which borders on the sulcus spiralis externus (21) and the stria vascularis (4), respectively. Above the hair cells (inner and outer, 17a and 17b) is the membrana tectoria (22), a gelatinous mass extending from the limbus spiralis (5). The intercellular spaces of the organum spirale (9, 19, 20) contain perilymph also known as cortilymph. (From Becker W, Naumann HH, Pfaltz CR. Ear: Applied anatomy and physiology. In: Buckingham RA, ed. *Ear, Nose and Throat Diseases. A Pocket Reference.* New York: Thieme, 1989, with permission.)

a second space known as the *inner spiral tunnel* are bridged by a gelatinous and filamentous acellular structure known as the *tectorial membrane.* The longest stereocilia of the OHCs are embedded in this membrane, whereas the stereocilia of the IHCs are attached loosely to the membrane. Thus, the stimuli for stereocilia deflection is different for each cell type. The OHC stereocilia move due to the shearing effect of tectorial membrane movement, and the IHC stereocilia move with motion of the endolymph in the tunnel of Corti.

The basal attachment of the stereocilia into the hair cells is associated with gated ion channels. Deflections toward the tallest of the stereocilia results in opening of the ion channel gates and depolarization of the cell. The high concentration of potassium in endolymph allows for the development of

an especially-high potential difference across the apical hair cell membrane, which is the driving force for depolarization.

Each hair cell is coupled to nerve fibers emanating from the spiral ganglion. The spiral ganglion possesses approximately 30,000 cells, 95% of which are type I cells. These type I cells are large bipolar neurons with an associated myelin sheath. Approximately 20 type I cells innervate each IHC. The remaining 5% of spiral ganglion cells are type II cells, which are pseudo-monopolar neurons with scant myelination. Each type II cell sends a branch to approximately ten OHCs. Therefore, IHCs, although lower in number, possess a much greater degree of sensory innervation than OHCs.

Experimentally-produced pure OHC lesions in animals will fail to produce deafness. Conversely, pure

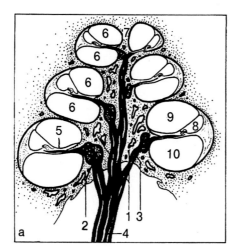
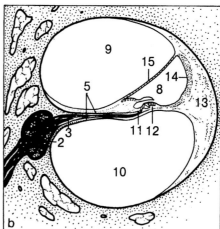

Figure 8–6:   Axial cross-section through the cochlea (A) and cochlear duct (B) The cochlea is spirally wound (2.5 windings) around the central modiolus (1) lying horizontally. Its base lies against the lateral end of the internal acoustic meatus and its apex is directed anterolaterally toward the medial wall of the middle ear. The spiral ganglion, [i.e., the ganglion of the cochlear nerve (2)] is located within the modiolus and its nerve fibers (3) join to form the stem of the cochlear nerve, the pars cochlearis nervi vestibulocochlearis (4). The lamina spiralis ossea, called also bony spiral lamina or spiral plate (5) is a bony plate running spirally from the base to the apex (7). Nerve fibers pass through the channels of the spiral lamina to the organum spirale, or organ of Corti (12). The cochlear duct (B) contains the ductus cochlearis (8) which is filled with endolymph, and lies between the scala vestibuli (9) above and the scala tympani (10) below, both of which contain perilymph. The lamina spiralis ossea (5) and the lamina basilaris (11) form the separating wall between the scala tympani on the one hand and the scala vestibuli as well as ductus cochlearis on the other. Reissner's membrane (15) separates the scala vestibuli and the ductus cochlearis. The stria vascularis (14) forms the lateral wall of the ductus cochlearis and has numerous vessels. This layer of fibrous vascular tissue is the site of production of the endolymph. Laterally, it borders on the ligamentum spirale cochleae (13). The perilymphatic spaces of the cochlea, the scala tympani and scala vestibuli, communicate with each other at the apex of the cochlea (A, 7) and at the helicotrema (see Fig. 8-3, 8), and also are connected with the perilymphatic space of the membranous labyrinth of the vestibule, which contains both the utriculus and the sacculus (see Fig. 8-3, 5 and 6). (From Becker W, Naumann HH, Pfaltz CR. Ear: Applied anatomy and physiology. In: Buckingham RA, ed. *Ear, Nose and Throat Diseases. A Pocket Reference.* New York: Thieme, 1989, with permission.)

TABLE 8–6:   Outer versus Inner Hair Cells

		Outer Hair Cells	Inner Hair Cells
Number		12,000	3500
Shape		Cylindrical	Flask or pear
Stereocilia	Number	48–148	120
	Arrangement	"V" or "W" pattern	Parallel Rows
	Contractibility	Yes	No
Support Cells		Deiter's cells	Inner and outer pillar cells Border cells
Innervation	Cell Type	Type II cells	Type I Cells
	Synapses	10 OHCs/Type II cells	1 IHC/20 Type I Cells
Function		Modulation of sound	Hearing

IHC lesions produce deafness. IHCs are the primary receptors, transducers, and conveyors of sound-energy information to the brain, and thus receive the majority of the innervation. The OHCs are believed to modulate the frequency specificity of nearby IHCs to an extremely fine degree. This is reputed to be secondary to the contractile properties of OHCs, which are elicited by local basilar membrane deflections and influenced by efferent stimulation from the brainstem. Type I cells form the afferent innervation from the cochlea, and type II cells form the efferent innervation.

As previously mentioned, the spiral ganglion is the locus of the hair cell innervation. The spiral ganglion coils along the axis of the cochlea within the modiolus and possesses about 30,000 cells in total. The cochlear nerve then arises from the spiral ganglion and travels down the modiolus to the IAC.

The vestibular inner ear

The vestibular portion of the inner ear is composed of two otolithic organs, the saccule and the utricle, and the three semicircular canals (Figs. 8–7 to 8–10).[2] The *saccule* makes up the medial wall of the bony labyrinth's vestibule. It is a vaguely-spherically-shaped sac that connects to the cochlea by a thin conduit known as the *ductus reuniens* and to the endolymphatic duct by the saccular duct. The *endo-*

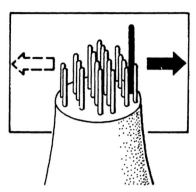

Figure 8–8: Diagram of polarization of a vestibular sensory cell in the cupula. Each sensory cell possesses one kinocilia (black fingerlike shape) and about 60 stereocilia (light). Displacement of the cupula, and with it the cilia, toward the kinocilia causes a nerve stimulation by an increase of receptor potential. Each displacement in the opposite direction inhibits the spontaneous receptor potential. In the horizontal semicircular canal, polarization is toward the utricle, but in the vertical canal, polarization is in the opposite direction toward the semicircular canal. (From Becker W, Naumann HH, Pfaltz CR. Ear: Applied anatomy and physiology. In: Buckingham RA, ed. *Ear, Nose and Throat Diseases. A Pocket Reference.* New York: Thieme, 1989, with permission.)

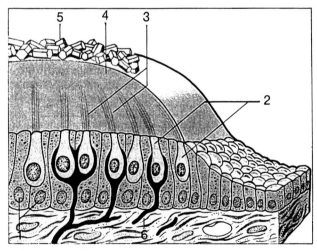

Figure 8–7: Diagram of a static macula: 1, supporting cells; 2, sensory cells; 3, cilia; 4, statolith membrane; 5, statoliths: 6, afferent nerve fibers. (From Becker W, Naumann HH, Pfaltz CR. Ear: Applied anatomy and physiology. In: Buckingham RA, ed. *Ear, Nose and Throat Diseases. A Pocket Reference.* New York: Thieme, 1989, with permission.)

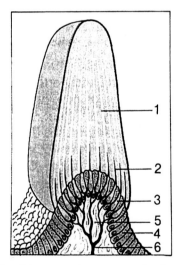

Figure 8–9: Diagram of a receptor in the semicircular canal: 1, cupula; 2, cilia; 3, sensory cells; 4, supporting cells; 5, crista ampullaris; 6, afferent nerve fibers. (From Becker W, Naumann HH, Pfaltz CR. Ear: Applied anatomy and physiology. In: Buckingham RA, ed. *Ear, Nose and Throat Diseases. A Pocket Reference.* New York: Thieme, 1989, with permission.)

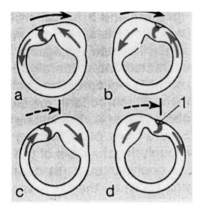

Figure 8–10: The principle of function of the mechanoreceptors of the horizontal semicircular canal. Positive acceleration in a clockwise direction causes endolymph flow in the opposite direction due to inertia, and utriculopetal deflection of the cupula in the right horizontal semicircular canal (b) and utriculofugal deflection in the left horizontal semicircular canal (a). The receptor potential thus increases on the right side and falls on the left side. Deceleration in a clockwise direction induces the opposite reaction: utriculopetal deflection on the left side (c) and utriculofugal deflection on the right side (d) with corresponding change in the receptor potentials (1 = Cupula). (From Becker W, Naumann HH, Pfaltz CR. Ear: Applied anatomy and physiology. In: Buckingham RA, ed. *Ear, Nose and Throat Diseases. A Pocket Reference.* New York: Thieme, 1989, with permission.)

lymphatic duct originates in the endolymphatic sac and terminates in the utricle. It is near the utricular end that the saccular duct joins with it. The endolymphatic sac and duct function to reabsorb water from the endolymph and to keep the endolymph content stable (i.e., ionic exchange and the removal of metabolic or cellular debris). They are also the site for immunologic monitoring of the inner ear.

The *utricle* is a flat ovoid sac that arises from the distal end of the endolymphatic duct. From the utricle, the three *semicircular canals* (SCC) arise. The arms of the SCCs, as they arise from the utricle, are called *crura.* Each SCC lies at a 90 degree angle to the other two. The horizontal SCC lies in a plane 30 degrees off the horizontal for the head and is coplanar with the contralateral horizontal SCC. The posterior and superior SCCs each lie in a vertical plane 45 degrees off the sagittal for the head. A posterior SCC is coplanar with the contralateral superior SCC, and vise versa. Each SCC has a dilated, ampulated end and an undilated, nonampulated end. The nonampulated ends of the posterior and superior SCCs fuse to form the *crus communis.*

The vestibular end organs are the maculae (in the saccule and the utricle) and the cristae (in the SCCs). The saccule is specialized in the detection of motion relative to gravity (i.e., vertical acceleration). Its macula is located in a plane that is perpendicular to the macula of the utricle. The utricle specializes in the detection of linear acceleration. The SCCs are responsible for the detection of rotational or angular acceleration. As in the cochlea, the vestibular sensory cells are hair cells, although they differ from the IHCs and OHCs significantly.

Vestibular hair cells are divided into two types. *Type I hair cells* are flask shaped and have a chalice-shaped nerve that ends at the base of the cell. These cells tend to be more sensitive, and occupy limited portions of the sensory epithelium. *Type II hair cells* are cylindrical and are coupled with a bouton-shaped nerve ending. These cells are less sensitive and are more diffusely distributed throughout the sensory epithelium. The stereocilia of the hair cells are embedded within a cuticular body. There are anywhere from 30 to 100 stereocilia in a hexagonal pattern on each hair cell, with a progression from shortest to tallest stereocilia. The tallest stereocilia are adjacent to a specialized individual stereocilium, the *kinocilium.* The kinocilium is not attached to the cuticular plate and is flexible when compared to stereocilia. The location of the kinocilium indicates the direction of polarization for that individual hair cell. The stereocilia and the kinocilia again are associated with gated ion channels at their base. When the kinocilium is deflected toward the other stereocilia, the gated ion channels close and the baseline discharge rate for that cell decreases. Deflection of the kinocilium away from the stereocilia results in an increased discharged rate for that hair cell.

The SCC's *crista* is located in its ampulla. The crista has a superstructure know as the cupula. The *cupula* is composed of a gelatinous cone-shaped mass that envelops the stereocilia. The cupula is deflected with the motion of the endolymph within the SCCs. The cupular deflection forms the mechanism for the stereocilia deflection. Flow toward the ampulla (i.e., *ampullopetal flow*) results in depolarization of the horizontal canal and hyperpolarization of the posterior and superior canals. Flow away from the ampulla (i.e., *ampullofugal flow*) causes the reverse to be true.

The otolithic organs' maculae have a superstructure known as the *otolithic membrane.* The otolithic membrane is composed of a gelatinous substance in which the calcium carbonate crystals (i.e., otoliths or otoconia) that envelop the stereocilia are embedded. Within the maculae is a central raised ridge known as the *striola*. Hair cells are oriented so that those on opposing sides of the striola are oriented opposite one another. The otoconia have a greater specific gravity than endolymph, so they have a greater inertia and tend to be displaced by linear acceleration (including gravity).

Miscellaneous Structures

The IAC lies on the medial TB, admitting the facial, cochlear, and vestibular nerves as well as the labyrinthine artery into the bone. The nerves are oriented such that the facial nerve is anterosuperior, the cochlear nerve is anteroinferior, and the superior and inferior vestibular nerves are posterior.

The *petrous pyramid* is the most anteromedial portion of the TB. Occasionally pneumatized, it often contains marrow. Inflammatory processes in the petrous pyramid can affect adjacent cranial nerves (i.e., the trigeminal and abducens).

Vascular relationships of the TB are outlined in the box below and in Figure 8–11.

AT A GLANCE . . .

Major Vasculature Associated with the Temporal Bone

Internal Carotid Artery: travels through the petrous apex in the carotid canal

Middle Meningeal Artery: a branch of the external carotid artery; travels on the dural surface of the squamous TB

Anterior Inferior Cerebellar Artery: a branch of the basilar artery; frequently loops into the IAC; gives off the Labyrinthine Artery (the blood supply to the inner ear)

Sigmoid Sinus: defines the posterior wall of the mastoid cavity

Jugular Bulb: defines the floor of the hypotympanum

Superior Petrosal Sinus: travels along the petrosal ridge of the TB; enters the sigmoid sinus

Inferior Petrosal Sinus: travels along the posterior inferior TB; enters the jugular bulb

---

The *vestibular aqueduct* lies on the posterior aspect of the TB. Normally very narrow, it is often seen on computed tomography (CT) as a lucent line that represents the endolymphatic sac covered by a cap of bone (i.e., the operculum). Widening of the vestibular aqueduct is associated with fluctuating hearing loss and perilymph fistulae.

EMBRYOLOGY OF THE TEMPORAL BONE

Each of the anatomic units of the ear (e.g., the cochlea, the vestibular apparatus, the middle ear, and the external ear) develops independently and is covered in sequence.[6]

The Inner Ear

The otic vesicle

The *otic vesicle,* or the otocyst, is the fundamental embryonic structure for the inner ear.[7] It gives rise to the utricle, the SCCs, the endolymphatic duct, the saccule, and the cochlea (Figure 8–12).

The vesicle's anlage first appears in the embryo at day 22 of development as a thickening of surface ectoderm upon both lateral surfaces of the rhombencephalon. At this point, it is known as the *ectodermal auditory placode.* By day 28 of development the placode will invaginate to form the *otic pit.* The pit further enlarges to form the *auditory vesicle.*

Day 31 of development is significant for the division of the otic vesicle into a superior and inferior portion. The anatomically superior or dorsal component (called the *pars inferior* due to its phylogenically older origin) differentiates into the utricle, the SCCs, and the endolymphatic duct. The anatomically inferior or ventral component of the otocyst, the *pars superior,* differentiates into the saccule and cochlear duct.

At the time the vesicle separates into two components, a conglomeration of ganglion cells separates from the vesicle. These ganglion cells migrate toward the medial wall of the vesicle and form the *acousticofacial ganglion.* The facial ganglion separates from the acousticofacial ganglion during the third week of development while the acoustic ganglion remains associated with the auditory vesicle.

The acoustic ganglion divides in conjunction with auditory vesicle division, forming a superior and in-

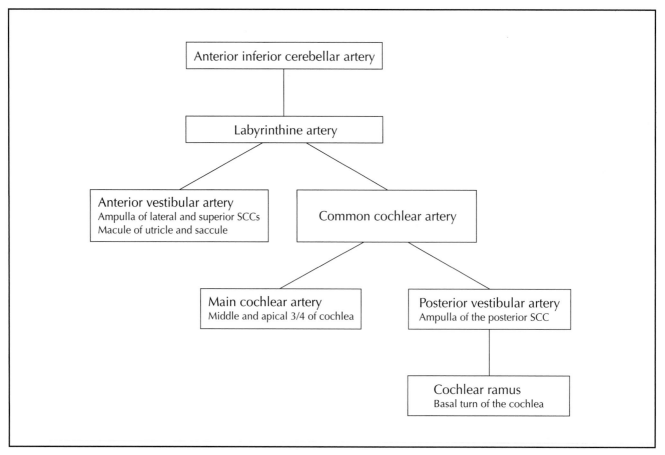

Figure 8–11: Blood supply to the inner ear. SCC, semicircular canals. (From Becker W, Naumann HH, Pfaltz CR. Ear: Applied anatomy and physiology. In: Buckingham RA, ed. *Ear, Nose and Throat Diseases. A Pocket Reference.* New York: Thieme, 1989, with permission.)

ferior portion. The superior branch innervates the majority of the neuroepithelium of the superior component of the otic vesicle, including the utricle and the superior and lateral SCC ampullae. The exception to this is the innervation of the ampulla of the posterior SCC. The posterior SCC is innervated by the inferior branch of the acoustic ganglion, which also innervates the saccule. An additional portion of the inferior branch becomes the spiral ganglion, which is eventually situated on the concave side of the nascent cochlear duct.

Concurrent with the acoustic ganglion differentiation, the facial nerve fibers extend from their neural tube to innervate derivatives of the second branchial arch.[8] The chorda tympani arises from peripheral fibers of the geniculate (formerly facial) ganglion and runs with the developing facial nerve for a short distance. By the fifth week of development, the chorda unites with the third branch of the trigeminal nerve to innervate the submandibular and sublingual gland (parasympathetic) and the

taste buds (special sensory) for the anterior two-thirds of the tongue.

Cochlea and the organ of corti

Nerve fibers are present in the otic capsule as early as 4.5 weeks in utero. Their synaptic connections are not present until just prior to cochlear function at 6 to 7 months of development. When the nerve fibers are absent, organ of Corti development is arrested. Therefore, it appears that these ganglion cells are necessary for the differentiation of the organ of Corti.

The cochlea derives from the inferior portion of the otocyst as a tubular evagination (cochlear duct) from the lower pole of the saccule.[7] The sensory end organs of the cochlea, the spiral ligament and its associated basilar membrane, develop from the epithelium along the posterior wall of this tube. At this point, the fibers from the inferior portion of the auditory ganglion enter the cochlear duct.

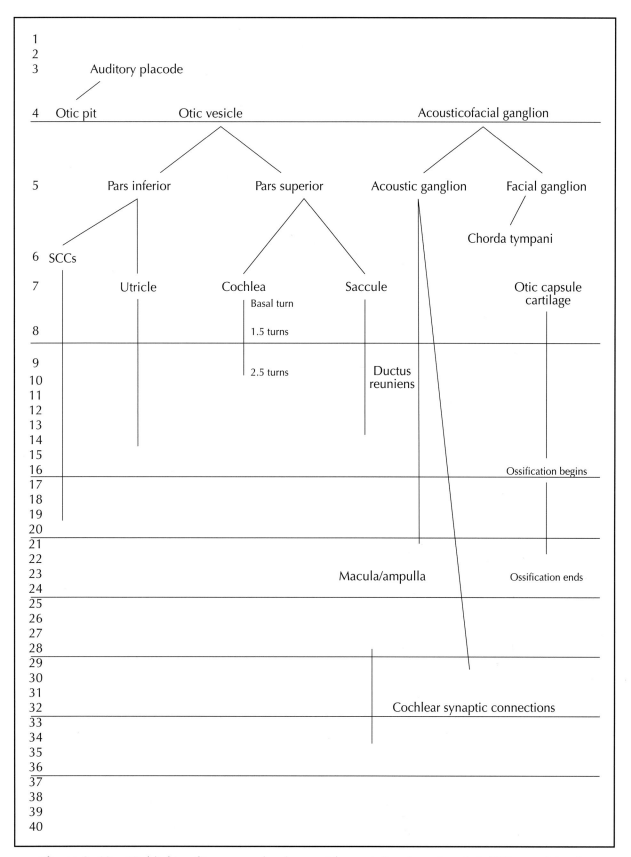

Figure 8–12: Highlights of inner ear development by gestational age (weeks). SCCs, semicircular canals.

With development, the cochlear duct continues to penetrate surrounding mesenchyme. By the seventh week of development, the first or basal turn of the cochlea is complete. By the eighth week 1.5 turns are present. Arrest of development at this stage is associated with a *Mondini's deformity,* one of the more common bony abnormalities of the inner ear that is associated with congenital sensorineural hearing loss (SNHL). The full complement of 2.5 turns is completed by the tenth week of development. By this time, the only endolymphatic connection left between the saccule and the cochlea is a narrow passage known as the *ductus reuniens.*

The mesenchyme surrounding the primordial cochlea differentiates into a cartilaginous shell. The cartilage undergoes programmed vacuolation to form two adjacent perilymphatic spaces, the *scala vestibuli* and the *scala tympani.* The *cochlear duct,* an endolymphatic space, is separated from the scala vestibuli by the vestibular or Reissner's membrane and from the scala tympani by the basilar membrane. The lateral wall of the cochlear duct attaches to the surrounding cartilage by the spiral ligament. The medial angle of the cochlear duct connects to a long process, the osseous spiral lamina of the modiolus, which is the future axis of the bony cochlea.

The epithelium of the cochlear duct begins as undifferentiated, stratified cells. During the eleventh week of development, the cells along the anterior wall of the duct (which become the future Reissner's membrane) lose their stratification and become simple columnar cells. The epithelium along the duct's outer wall assumes a more glandular appearance. This glandular tissue covers a vascular connective tissue, the *stria vascularis,* and the stria rests upon the spiral ligament.

The cochlear duct's posterior wall epithelium further differentiates into the *organ of Corti,* which is the functional component of the membranous labyrinth. The first cells to develop are the supporting cells, which bear microvilli, and then the hair cells develop with their stereocilia. This epithelium forms into two ridges. The inner ridge becomes the future *spiral limbus.* The outer ridge forms into one row of IHCs and three rows of OHC. Supporting cells proceed to secrete a gelatinous substance that forms a membrane that extends from the spiral limbus to rest upon the tips of the hair cells. Improper development of the membranous labyrinth results in a *Scheibe deformity,* the most-common congenital-development abnormality of the cochlear duct to result in SNHL.

> ## SPECIAL CONSIDERATION:
> Improper development of the membranous labyrinth results in Scheibe deformity, causing sensorineural hearing loss.

Although the formation of the membranous labyrinth begins during the fourth week of development, it is already surrounded by mesenchyme. After the seventh week of development, this mesenchyme is transformed into the cartilaginous precursor of the bony otic capsule. Ossification of the labyrinthine capsule begins at the sixteenth week (when the membranous labyrinth reaches adult form) and continues to the twenty-third week. It begins adjacent to the round window and ends in the oval window at the fissula ante fenestram. The bone of the otic capsule is endochondral bone, which is the hardest, densest bone in the body.

Utricle, saccule and semicircular canals

The SCCs first appear at the sixth week as flattened outpocketings of the utricular portion of the superior part of the otic vesicle.[6] The central portions of the walls of evagination become apposed to one another, disappear, and give rise to the three SCCs. The sensory neuroepithelium forms in the dilated end known as the *crus ampullarae.* Two of the nonampullare ends fuse, and only five crura enter the utricle.

The medial and lateral walls of otocyst ectodermal epithelium form the vestibular sensory structures. The maculae of the utricle and saccule arise from the anterior middle-third of the otocyst. Differentiation occurs at the seventh to eighth week and is completed by the fourteenth to sixteenth week. Cells in the ampullae form crests, the *cristae ampullaris,* that contain sensory cells for maintenance of equilibrium and attain adult size by the twenty-third week.

The Middle Ear and The Surrounding Temporal Bone (Fig. 8–13)

Figure 8–14 outlines the development of the middle and external ear.

During the third week of development and simultaneous with the formation of the auditory vesicle,

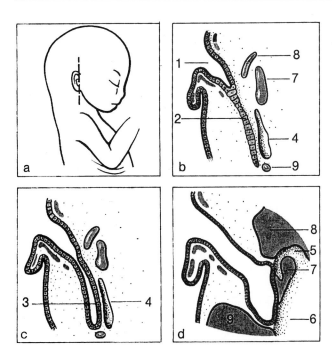

Figure 8–13: Diagram of development of the middle ear. The first ectodermal branchial arch forms the primary anlage of the cartilaginous part of the external auditory meatus. The funnel-shaped tube is shown by b1. A string of epithelial cells grows mediocaudally toward the pharyngeal pouch (b2). The tympanic membrane (c3), the bony part of the external auditory meatus, the primitive middle ear cavity (b4 and c4), and the anlage of the tympanic plate (b9 and d9) develop later. The parts of the middle ear then begin to develop: the epitympanum (d5), the mesotympanum (d6), the malleus (b7 and d7), and the squamous part of the temporal bone (b8 and d8). (Modified from Nager.) (From Becker W, Naumann HH, Pfaltz CR. Ear: Applied anatomy and physiology. In: Buckingham RA, ed. *Ear, Nose and Throat Diseases. A Pocket Reference.* New York: Thieme, 1989, with permission.)

an outpocketing of the foregut develops into the first pharyngeal pouch. The proximal portion of the pouch develops into the ET. The distal extension becomes the tubotypanic recess, the future antrum, and the tympanic cavity (Table 8-7).

The *tubotypanic recess* extends distally until it abuts the developing otic capsule. At about the same time, the six paired branchial arches develop; each has a major artery and nerve, a cartilage bar, and mesenchyme. The cartilage bar of the first branchial arch, *Meckel's Cartilage,* comes to lie anterior to the tubotypanic recess; the cartilage bar of the second branchial arch, *Reichert's Cartilage,* comes to lie posterior to the recess. The two cartilage bars are joined by condensation of the roof processes above the tubotypanic recess. The roof processes come to lie essentially between the recess and the otic capsule.

The *tegmen tympani,* which is the future floor of the middle cranial fossa, is formed as a flange-like outgrowth of the otic capsule and passes above and anterior to the tubotypanic recess. Concurrently, Meckel's cartilage, which is destined to guide development of the mandible, passes under the anterior free edge of the tegmen via the foramen of Huschke to enter the lower jaw. A sheet of membranous bone grows overlying the otic capsule and the tegmen tympani laterally to become the squamous portion of the TB.

By the sixth week of development, proximal portions of both Meckel's and Reichert's cartilages begin to develop into the malleus, incus, and the stapes superstructure. Meckel's cartilage becomes the malleus' head and neck and the incus' body and short process. Reichert's cartilage becomes the manubrium of the malleus, the long process of the incus, the lenticular process, and the stapes superstructure. By week 8, the incudomalleolar and incudostapedial joints are established. This is also the time when chondrification occurs.

AT A GLANCE . . .
Origin of the Ossicles

Malleus: *First Branchial Arch:* Meckel's cartilage forms head and neck; *Second Branchial Arch:* Reichert's cartilage forms manubrium

Incus: *First Branchial Arch:* Meckel's cartilage forms body and short process; *Second Branchial Arch:* Reichert's cartilage forms long process and lenticular process

Stapes: *Second Branchial Arch:* Reichert's cartilage forms lenticular process and the superstructure; *Otic Capsule:* footplate and annular ligament

---

The stapedial footplate is derived from the otic capsule and fuses with the superstructure derived from Reichert's cartilage. The annular ligament develops during the tenth to thirteenth weeks by dedifferentiation of cartilaginous stapedial lamina first into mesenchyme and then into fibrous tissue. Failure of the annular ligament to form completely is

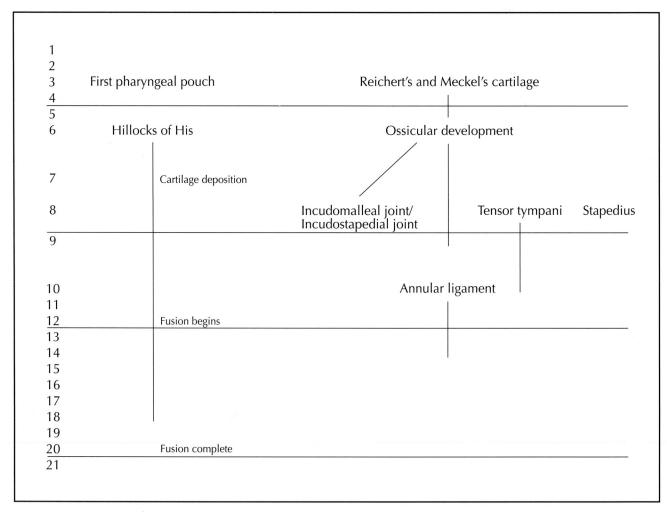

Figure 8–14:   Highlights of middle and external ear development by gestational age (weeks).

associated with a conductive hearing loss due to congenital fixation of the stapedial footplate. This is a disorder that must be distinguished from the more common otosclerosis. The developing ossicles remain embedded in mesenchyme until the eighth month of development when this tissue dissolves and the tympanic cavity forms. From the eighth to eleventh week of development, the tensor tympani develops from the first branchial arch mesenchyme. The second branchial arch forms the stapedius muscle at 8.5 weeks.

A portion of Reichert's cartilage envelops the facial nerve to form the *fallopian canal*. As the fallopian canal matures, the nerve moves posteriorly into the TB. Malformation of any portion of the fallopian canal may result in an aberrant course of the facial nerve, usually causing it to be displaced anteriorly. This is most commonly associated with congenital syndromes, and is of clinical significance when middle-ear or mastoid surgery is required.

TABLE 8–7:   First Pharyngeal Pouch Derivatives

Proximal	Eustachian Tube
Distal	Tubotympanic recess
	Antrum
	Tympanic cavity

SPECIAL CONSIDERATION:

Malformation of the fallopian canal may result in an aberrant course of the facial nerve, which is of clinical significance when middle-ear or mastoid surgery is required.

TABLE 8–8:   Branchial Arches Associated with The Ear and Their Temporal Bone Derivatives

Arch Number	Cartilage	Mesoderm	Artery	Nerve
1	Meckel's Malleus—head and neck Incus—body and short process Anterior Malleal ligament	Tensor tympani		Mandibular portion of the trigeminal nerve (V_3)
2	Reichert's Malleus—manubrium Incus—long process Lenticular process Stapes superstructure Styloid process Pyramidal eminence Lower half of the fallopian canal	Stapedius muscle	Stapedial artery (degenerates before birth)	Facial nerve (CN VII); Including the geniculate ganglion, chorda tympani, and greater superficial petrosal nerve
3			Internal carotid artery	Glossopharyngeal nerve (CN IX); Jacobson's nerve

Furthermore, the fallopian canal may form incompletely resultin in dehiscences.

The third branchial arch forms the posterior boundary of the ET. In the adult, this arch's artery, the internal carotid artery, eventually will lie posteromedial to the ET. In rare instances, the bony partition between the middle ear and the carotid artery may be incompletely developed, allowing the carotid artery to course aberrantly through the middle ear. See Table 8-8 for a summary of branchial derivatives.

The EAC is derived from the TB's tympanic ring. This is a distinct bony structure that begins to ossify at approximately the tenth week in utero. It is an incomplete ring that is open superiorly, forming the *notch of Rivinus.* At birth, the EAC is present but shallow compared to a mature canal. The TM spans the ring, including the notch of Rivinus. In the newborn, the TM lies in a more horizontal plane compared to the adult ear. Due to the shallow EAC, it can be injured easily by careless examination and the insertion of an instrument into the ear. Further intramembraneous ossification of the tympanic ring occurs after birth, resulting in the lateral growth of the EAC with the TM assuming a more vertical position.

SPECIAL CONSIDERATION:

The shallow EAC of the newborn can be injured easily by careless examination.

External Ear (Fig. 8-15)

During the sixth week of development, the first and second branchial arch's mesoderm condenses into the six hillocks of His (Table 8-9). Each of these hillocks is programmed to become a specific portion of the external ear. The first hillock becomes the *tragus.* The second hillock becomes the *helical crus,* and the third hillock becomes the *helix proper.* The fourth hillock is the *nascent antihelix,* and the fifth hillock becomes the *antitragus.* The sixth hillock becomes the *lobule* and the lower portion of the helix. The individual portions of the auricle do not assume their proper adult shape until the twelfth week when fusion begins, and by the

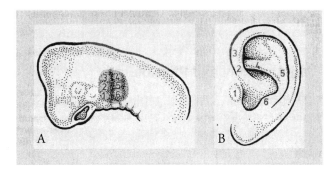

Figure 8–15:   (A) Development of the external ear 11 mm embryo, from the side. Outer ear development from 6 hillocks arising from the 1st and 2nd branchial arches. (B) 1, tragus, 2 crus helicis; 3, helix; 4, crus anthelicis; 5, anthelix; 6, antitragus. (From Becker W, Naumann HH, Pfaltz CR. Ear: Applied anatomy and physiology. In: Buckingham RA, ed. *Ear, Nose and Throat Diseases. A Pocket Reference.* New York: Thieme, 1989, with permission.)

TABLE 8–9: The Hillocks of His and Associated Derivatives

Hillock	Origin	Derivative
1	1ST brachial arch	Tragus
2	1ST brachial arch	Helical crus
3	1ST brachial arch	Helix
4	2nd brachial arch	Antihelix
5	2nd brachial arch	Antitragus
6	2nd brachial arch	Lobule and lower helix

twentieth week the fusion is complete. Cartilage formation occurs during the seventh week.

As development of the external ear is independent of the inner and middle ear, pinna abnormalities do not necessarily indicate other abnormalities of the ear. Because the timing of development of the external ear coincides with that of the inner and middle ear, outer ear anomalies do provide a clue to possible insults to the fetus during this period that also may contribute to further anomalies. The most common external ear anomalies include pits and reduplications.

POSTNATAL DEVELOPMENT

At birth, four-fifths of the elements of the TB are recognized: petrous, squamous, the tympanic ring, and the styloid process. The mastoid antrum, the fifth element, is present but the mastoid process is incompletely developed. The facial nerve exits the stylomastoid foramen and lies more superficially than in the adult due to the poorly-developed mastoid process. From birth until the end of the second year of life, the facial nerve gradually assumes a more adult-like position relative to the EAC, the mastoid tip, and the parotid gland.

Progressive expansion of the tympanic cavity, which originates as a void left as mesenchyme degenerates, results in its aeration and the development of a complex labyrinth of mucosal spaces and recesses, thereby creating the air cell tracts of the TB. This process is expressed most fully in the mastoid air cells.

The ET is 17 to 18 mm long and is 10 degrees off the horizontal plane in the newborn. An adult length of 35 mm and a 45 degree angulation off the horizontal plane occurs with continued maturation. The differences in the ET geometry play a role in the higher incidence of otitis media in children as opposed to adults.

CONCLUSION

This discussion of the anatomy, function, and development of the TB and the structures housed therein is not meant to be comprehensive. Rather, the relationships described above are meant to facilitate an understanding of the clinical entities and their management that are described in subsequent chapters. It is hoped that this brief foray into the workings of the TB stimulates readers' interest in derangements of form and function and how these relate to the symptomatology and treatment of disease.

REFERENCES

1. Brown MC. Auditory physiology. In: English GM, ed. *Otolaryngology.* Philadelphia: Lippincott, Williams, & Wilkins, 1997, pp. 1–54.
2. Schuknecht HF. *Pathology of the Ear, 2nd ed.* Philadelphia: Lea and Feibinger, 1993, pp. 31–75
3. Rosowski JJ. Outer and Middle ear. In: Fay RR, Popper AN, eds. *Comparative Hearing: Mammals.* New York: Springer-Verlag, 1994, pp. 172–274.
4. Pickles JD. *An Introduction to the Physiology of Hearing, 2nd ed.* London: Academic Press, 1988, pp.
5. Hudspeth AJ. How the ears works work. Nature 1989; 341:397–404.
6. Williams GH. Developmental anatomy of the ear. In: English GM, ed. *Otolaryngology.* Philadelphia: Lippincott, Williams, & Wilkins, 1990, pp. 1–68.
7. Pujol R, Lavigne Rebillard M, Uziel A. Development of the human cochlea. Acta Otolaryngol Suppl (Stockh) 1992; 482:7–12.
8. Gasser RF, Shigihara S, Shimada K. Three dimensional development of the facial nerve path through the ear region in human embryos. Ann Otol Rhinol Laryngol 1994; 103:395–403.

9 Radiologic Evaluation of the Temporal Bone

Jill V. Hunter

TECHNICAL CONSIDERATIONS

The mainstay of imaging the anatomy and pathology of the temporal bone (TB) is computed tomography (CT). Based on the properties of conventional X-ray technology, the higher the atomic number of any structure through which the X-ray beam passes the greater the attenuation of that beam. This leads to whitening of the exposed and developed film in areas where fewer high-energy photons strike the photographic plate/screen-film combination. As a result of the inherent contrast, CT is excellent at revealing bony detail.

Magnetic resonance imaging (MRI) results from the signal produced as a result of the interaction between hydrogen nuclei or protons within a high magnetic field and radiofrequency pulses. The signal intensity obtained from different tissues is proportional to the number of free protons within that tissue. The structure of bone matrix is such that few free protons are present; therefore only a weak signal is returned. Fat and water, however, produce high signal intensity that is either bright or dark depending on the sequence parameters used. Therefore, MRI is used increasingly to demonstrate fluid (e.g., fluid within a branchial cleft tract or the endolymphatic system). Different projections may be obtained simply by altering the angle of the radiofrequency gradients, rather than by repositioning the patient.

In order to understand a three-dimensional (3D) structure, such as the TB, imaging is required in at least two, preferably orthogonal, planes. Conventionally, CT of the TB is performed using thin (1–2 mm thick), contiguous sections in axial (i.e., trans-verse) and coronal planes. One of the advantages of MRI is the capability to acquire images in any plane. Additionally, utilizing a 3D volumetric sequence, postprocessing in software can be performed to reformat the information from a single MRI data set into any plane desired. This produces high-quality images, especially if the original acquisition contains *isovoxels* (i.e., individual imaging data cubes with the same dimensions in all three planes). There are, however, caveats to the use of both CT and MRI as imaging modalities.[1-3] CT does not cope well with the presence of very dense material or air-bone interfaces. This problem can be circumvented to some extent by the use of so-called "bone algorithms" that reduce the amount of "streak" or "beam-hardening" artifact, but at the expense of loss of soft-tissue detail. In general, MRI cannot be used in patients with pacemakers or other metal, such as cochlear implants or arterial clips, that may have the potential to move or torque within the child's body when placed in a magnetic field. Even dental braces can lead to severe degradation of image quality on both CT and, less predictably, MRI.

PROTOCOLS

Plain Film Radiography

In the evaluation of the TB, there is now little place for the plain radiograph, except perhaps to obtain an overview of a cochlear implant to check for a break in the electrodes. Tomography of the TB, including multiplanar and hypocycloidal techniques, has been superseded by CT and MRI. The orthopantomogram still has a role in assessing the mandible and temporomandibular joints (TMJ).

Pediatric Otolaryngology, Edited by R.F. Wetmore, H.R. Muntz, and T.J. McGill. Thieme Medical Publishers, Inc., New York © 2000.

CT Scanning

The *gantry,* which is the bank of X-ray tubes and detectors that rotates around the patient, is angled parallel to the canthomeatal anatomic baseline, and a series of 1-mm contiguous images of the TB is acquired, centered on the external auditory meatus. An unenhanced whole brain scan may be performed at the same sitting, if this is the first time that the child has been examined radiographically. The head is then gently lowered back into a head support to extend the neck, and the angle of the gantry is reversed to achieve imaging through the TB in the coronal plane, at approximately 60 degrees to the previous axial stack. (Especially in young and sedated children it is often easier and more acceptable to leave the patient supine rather than attempt to place him prone.)

The individual images are "zoomed" (magnified) separately for each ear and displayed on soft-tissue (400/60 window width/window center) and bony (3600/400) windows. The latter follows postprocessing with a bone "kernel" or edge-detection algorithm. Intravenous, iodinated, water-soluble contrast is given only to enhance the CT scan in the presence of soft-tissue swelling, pain, or fever, which suggests concern about tumor or abscess formation. Use of iodinated water-soluble contrast is contraindicated with an appropriate history of allergy or in the presence of significant renal impairment.

MRI

MRI, in general, follows the same radiographic baselines as CT, with sequences performed in at least two orthogonal planes. However, MRI can be tailored to any angle depending on the child's pathology and without moving the patient. Gadolinium (Gd) chelates may be given to enhance the scan and may be useful not only in ruling out abscess formation or venous sinus thrombosis, but for demonstrating pathologic enhancement of the facial nerve and for distinguishing between cholesteatoma (nonenhancing) and granulomatous (enhancing) tissue.

Sedation

In order to perform a biplanar CT examination successfully, most children under the age of 5 or 6 years require some form of sedation. For MRI, this age rises to 8 to 10 years because of the longer time taken to complete the test and the need for immobility during the course of the exam. Oral chloral hydrate may be used for infants up to 18 months old, whereas intravenous Nembutal® and/or morphine are used more effectively to sedate the older child. These "rules of thumb" do not apply to cognitively-impaired children or those with severe respiratory or cardiac difficulties. Particular care must be exercised in those children with micrognathism whose airways must be especially protected. In these children, it may be safer to perform electively any investigation requiring sedation under general anesthesia, because of the inherent difficulties in intubating such a child emergently.

Special Techniques

MRI with Gd enhancement is now the industry standard for examination of the internal auditory canal (IAC) to look for evidence of an acoustic neurinoma. Air meatography is no longer justifiable. MRI is also the modality of choice for the investigation of cochleovestibular disorders, such as the various causes of labyrinthitis, labyrinthine hemorrhage, intralabyrinthine schwannoma, invasive cholesteatoma, and labyrinthitis ossificans. Imaging of the inner ear is performed currently utilizing a 3D Fourier transform constructive interference in steady state (3DFTCISS, Siemens, Eurlagen, Germany) sequence, which acquires a stack of 46×0.75 mm contiguous slices with no gap that can be reformatted in any plane. Gd enhancement of the MRI scan always is performed when there is a history of sudden onset of sensorineural hearing loss (SNHL) or vertigo that is unexplained by vestibular aqueduct enlargement or labyrinthine fistula.

CT cisternography remains the current investigation of choice for the demonstration of cerebrospinal fluid (CSF) leak/recurrent meningitis (Fig. 9–1). This always should be preceded by a high-resolution unenhanced CT examination in axial and coronal planes that extends from the paranasal sinuses back through the petrous TB, so that acquired fistulation of the semicircular canals (SCCs) or congenital anomalies of the inner ear, which can lead to "gushers," are not missed. Although instillation of radionuclide rather than water-soluble nonionic iodinated contrast media has been used to detect CSF leaks, the spatial resolution is poor and, at best, any leak identified only may be resolved to a general

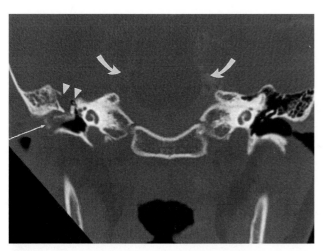

Figure 9–1: Coronal CT following nonionic water-soluble contrast cisternogram demonstrates a tegmental defect (arrowheads) with iodine-containing CSF (arrow) leaking out through the right-sided external auditory canal. There was also herniation of brain through the fracture site and persistent CSF otorrhea. Note contrast-containing CSF in the basal cisterns (curved arrows).

location within the head. All studies are best performed during the course of an active leak in order to get a definitive result.

SPECIAL CONSIDERATION:

CT cisternography remains the current investigation of choice for the demonstration of CSF leak with recurrent meningitis.

Any mass of the head, neck, or face that presents in a child and that may have a congenital etiology is investigated using a half Fourier turbo spin echo (HASTE) sequence, in addition to the conventional multiplane imaging, because this is exquisitely sensitive to water and identifies even very narrow fluid-filled tracks that may be missed on other sequences.

NORMAL ANATOMY

The normal adult TB is made up of five parts—the squamous, mastoid, petrous, and tympanic por-

tions, and the styloid process. Mastoid air-cell development is highly variable and the degree of pneumatization, in part, is familial but altered by pathology (e.g., sclerosis secondary to chronic otitis media). At birth, the mastoid is not completely developed, leading to the risk of facial nerve damage at the time of delivery. In the first few weeks of life it may be normal to see fluid in the middle ear cleft, but this should clear by age 1 month.

Embryologically, the ear develops as three separate regions: (1) the external and middle ear are derived from the first and second branchial arch apparatus; (2) the inner ear is derived from the otic cyst; and (3) the IAC.

Because the external and middle ear develop separately from the inner ear, deformities of these two areas generally are separate from one another as well.[4,5] Combined external, middle, and inner ear deformities are rare and seen only in conditions such as craniofacial dysplasias and trisomies 13, 18, and 21.[6,7]

Table 9-1 lists anatomic factors of the pediatric TB that may be of concern to the otolaryngologist. Figures 9-2 through 9-12 demonstrate the normal axial anatomy of the left TB in 1-mm-thick slices over a distance of 15 mm from the base of the skull

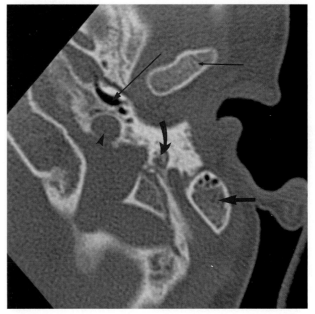

Figure 9–2: Axial CT, 1-mm-thick slice towards base of skull (table position 273 mm). Long thin black arrow = air in the eustachian tube; short thin black arrow = ramus of mandible; curved black arrow = descending or mastoid portion of the facial nerve; arrowhead = carotid artery; short thick arrow = mastoid process.

TABLE 9-1: Important Anatomic Factors of the Pediatric Temporal Bone

1. the thickness of a bony plate in external auditory canal atresia (see Figs. 9-27-9-29)
2. the size of the middle ear cavity
3. the status of the ossicles
4. the position of the facial nerve
5. the status of the oval and round windows
6. abnormalities of the inner ear structures
7. the position of vascular structures, namely the internal carotid artery and jugular bulb, in relation to the middle ear.

upwards in a plane parallel to the canthomeatal anatomic baseline.[8,9] Figure 9-13 demonstrates the setup for the direct coronal imaging of the TB. Figures 9-14 through 9-19 demonstrate the normal coronal anatomy of the left TB in 1-mm-thick slices over a distance of 14 mm from posterior to anterior.

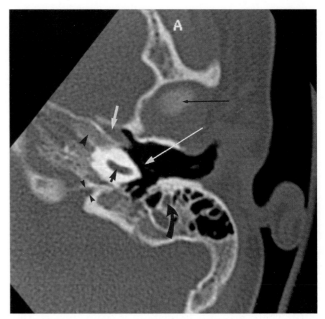

Figure 9-4: Axial CT, 1-mm-thick slice (table position 279 mm). Paired black arrowheads = cochlear aqueduct CA; short thin black arrow = condyle at top of TMJ; curved black arrow = beginning of the descending portion of VII; single arrowhead = petrous ICA; very short thick black arrow = basal turn cochlea; long white arrow = TM; short white arrow = TTM.

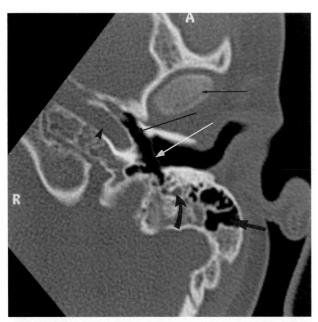

Figure 9-3: Axial CT, 1-mm-thick slice (table position 277 mm). Long thin black arrow = air in the eustachian tube and soft-tissue density of the tensor tympani muscle TTM; short thin black arrow = condyle in TMJ; curved black arrow = descending portion of the facial nerve (VII); arrowhead = ICA, petrous portion in carotid canal; short thick arrow = air in mastoid air cells; white arrow = normal tympanic membrane (TM).

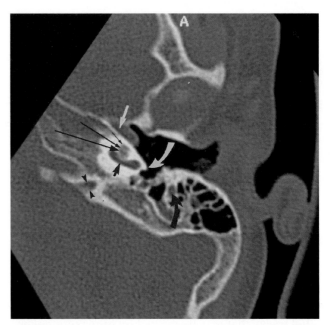

Figure 9-5: Axial CT, 1-mm-thick slice (table position 280 mm). Paired black arrowheads = CA; curved white arrow = promontory over the basal turn of the cochlea; curved black arrow = descending portion of VII; 3 thin black arrows outlining the bony spiral lamina separating the superior from the middle turns of the cochlea; short thick black arrow = basal turn cochlea; short white arrow = TTM.

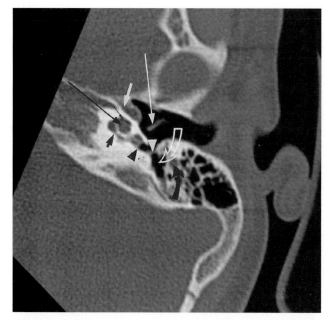

Figure 9–6: Axial CT, 1-mm-thick slice (table position 281 mm). Black arrowhead = round window at basal turn cochlea; curved hollow white arrow = sinus tympani; curved black arrow = descending portion VII; thin black arrows = middle and superior turns of cochlea; short straight black arrow = basal turn of cochlea; long thin white arrow = manubrium of the malleus; short white arrow = TTM; white arrowhead = tendon of stapedius.

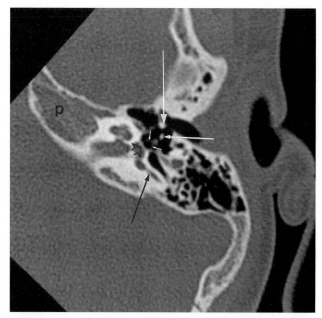

Figure 9–8: Axial CT, 1-mm-thick slice (table position 283 mm). **p** = petrous apex (nonpneumatized); long white arrow = malleus neck; thin white arrow = incus; open black arrow = oval window; pair of short white arrows = crura of the stapes—anterior and posterior; long black arrow = posterior semicircular canal (PSCC).

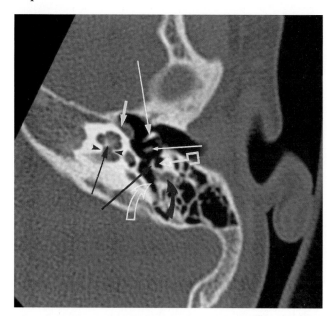

Figure 9–7: Axial CT, 1-mm-thick slice (table position 282 mm). Black arrowheads = osseous spiral lamina; curved black arrow = 2nd genu VII; short thin black arrow = modiolus; short thin white arrow = lenticular process incus; short thick white arrow = TTM; long thin white arrow = neck of manubrium, open curved white arrow = sinus tympani; square-ended white arrow = facial nerve recess; long black arrow = pyramidal eminence.

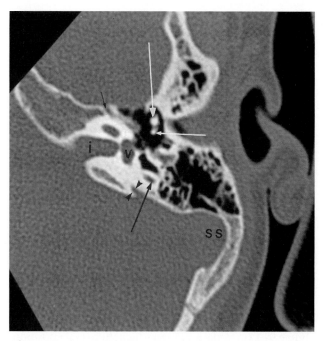

Figure 9–9: Axial CT, 1-mm-thick slice (table position 284 mm). **i** = IAC; **v** = vestibule; black arrowheads = vestibular aqueduct (VA); long white arrow = malleus; thin white arrow = incus; short black arrow = horizontal portion of VII; long black arrow = PSCC; **ss** = sigmoid sinus.

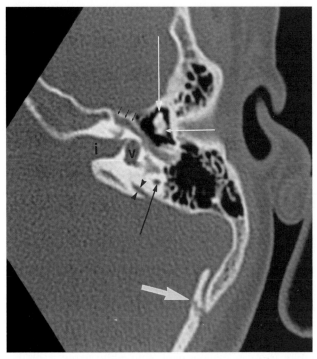

Figure 9–10: Axial CT, 1-mm-thick slice (table position 285 mm). **i** = IAC; **v** = vestibule; long white arrow = head of malleus; short white arrow = body and short process of incus; black arrowheads = VA; long black arrow = PSCC; short black arrows = tympanic and labyrinthine segments of VII; thick white arrow = occipito-mastoid suture.

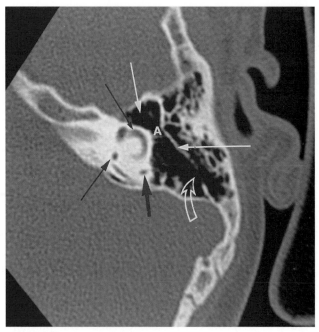

Figure 9–12: Axial CT, 1-mm-thick slice (table position 287 mm). **A** = aditus ad antrum; long black arrow = superior semicircular canal (SSCC); thin black arrow = lateral semicircular canal (LSCC); short white arrow = posterior epitympanic recess; short thick black arrow = PSCC; curved open white arrow = mastoid antrum; long white arrow = Koerner's septum.

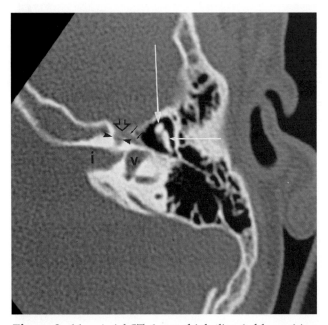

Figure 9–11: Axial CT, 1-mm-thick slice (table position 286 mm). Long white arrow = malleus head ("ice-cream in cone"); short white arrow = incus body and short process ("cone"); open black arrow = geniculate ganglion; arrowheads = labyrinthine segment of the facial canal; short black arrows = anterior tympanic segment of facial canal; **v** = vestibule; **i** = IAC.

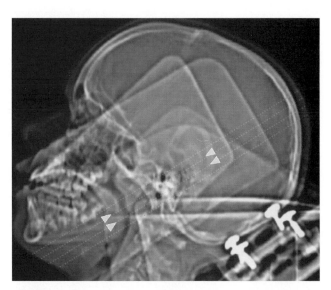

Figure 9–13: Lateral scanogram posted (arrowheads) with the coronal scout with the head in extension.

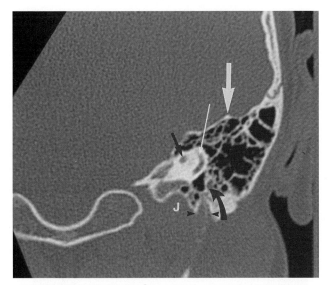

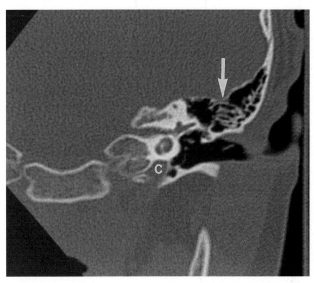

Figure 9–14:   Coronal CT, 1-mm-thick slice (table position 183 mm). Short black arrow = VA; white arrow = PSCC; **j** = internal jugular vein; black arrowheads = stylomastoid foramen; curved black arrow = descending portion VII; big white arrow = tegmen mastoideum.

Figure 9–16:   Coronal CT, 1-mm-thick slice (table position 192 mm). Big white arrow = tegmen mastoideum; **c** = carotid.

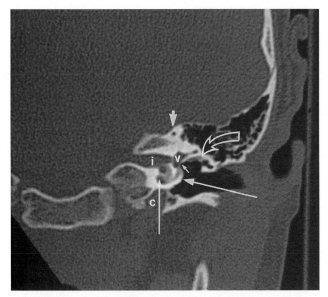

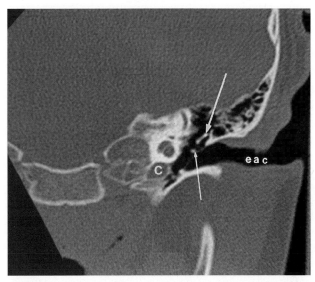

Figure 9–15:   Coronal CT, 1-mm-thick slice (table position 191 mm). **v** = vestibule; **i** = IAC; **c** = internal carotid artery; thin white arrow = basal turn cochlea; large white arrow = promontory; short white arrow = arcuate eminence overlying SSCC; curved open arrow = tympanic or horizontal VII; tiny arrow = oval window.

Figure 9–17:   Coronal CT, 1-mm-thick slice (table position 194 mm). Long white arrow = malleus; thin white arrow = incus; **c** = carotid; **eac** = external auditory canal (EAC).

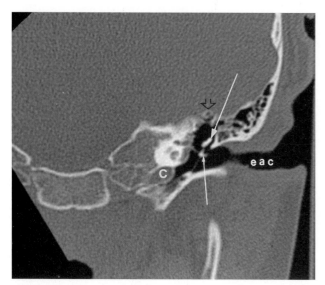

Figure 9–18: Coronal CT, 1-mm-thick slice (table position 195 mm). Open black arrow = geniculate ganglion; long white arrow = malleus, short white arrow = incus; **c** = carotid; eac = EAC.

BONY DYSTROPHIES

There are a number of inherited and congenital diseases that can lead to TB abnormalities.[10] These include *achondroplasia* (Fig. 9–20) with a short cranial base, small foramen magnum, basilar invagination, and short eustachian tubes (ET) that predispose to middle-ear disease. *Treacher Collins syndrome* (Fig. 9–21) is remarkable for hypoplastic

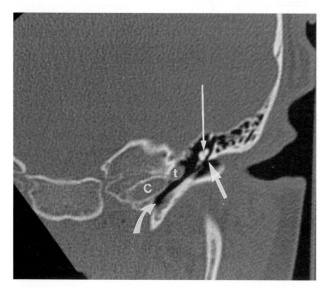

Figure 9–19: Coronal CT, 1-mm-thick slice (table position 197 mm). Long white arrow = incudomalleal joint; **t** = TTM; **c** = carotid; short white arrow = scutum.

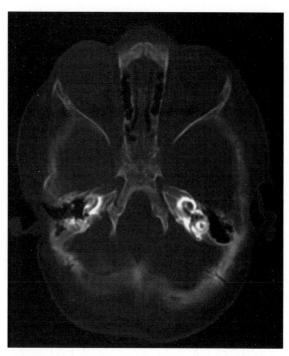

Figure 9–20: Axial CT through skull base in an 8-month-old infant with a history of achondroplasia, demonstrating small ETs with a somewhat acute angulation to the petrous TB (PTBs).

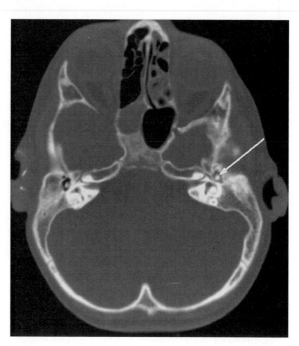

Figure 9–21: 8-year-old female with typical features of Treacher Collins. Note absence of EACs with deformed ossicular chains and soft-tissue density material within the left mesotympanum (arrow). The inner ear structures appear normal but note the lack of pneumatization of the mastoid air-cells. There is incidental left ethmoid and right sphenoid air-cell disease. Note previous surgery to right pinna.

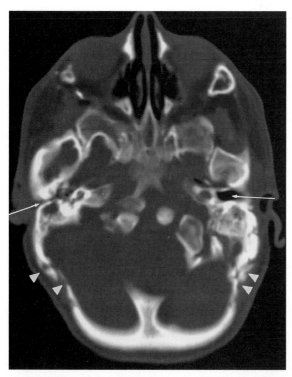

Figure 9–22: Axial CT skull base in a 16-year-old female with persistent patency of the skull sutures and Wormian bones (arrowheads). Stenotic right EAC is more than on the left (arrows). This child has CHL and Hadju-Cheney disease.

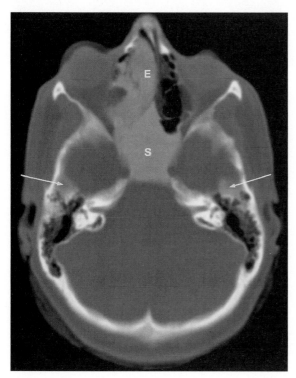

Figure 9–23: 12-year-old female with sphenoid (S), ethmoid (E), and to a lesser extent bilateral PTB involvement (arrows) by fibrous dysplasia, giving a typical "ground glass" appearance.

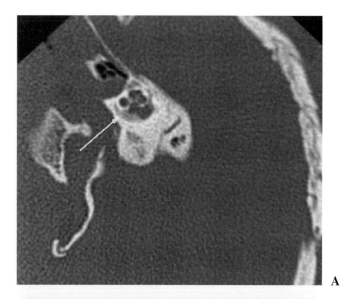

A

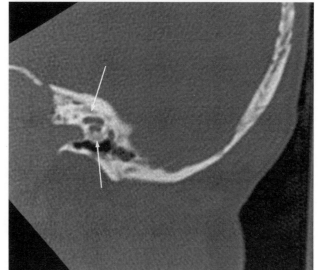

B

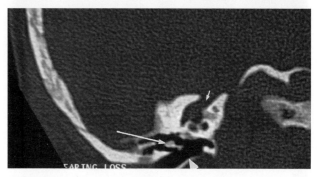

C

Figure 9–24: Axial (A) and coronal (B) CT views of the left PTB in an 18-year-old female demonstrate "otospongiotic" appearance to the otic capsule (arrows), mimicking otosclerosis. Note Wormian bones at the skull base. There is platybasia secondary to bone softening in this patient with osteogenesis imperfecta (OI). (C) Note on the right horizontal orientation of apparently-abnormally-formed ossicular chain (long arrow) with truncated, patulous, vertically-orientated IAC (short arrow) and abnormal horizontal course to EAC (arrowhead).

acellular mastoids, absent external auditory canals (EAC) and conductive deafness, on the basis of ossicular chain abnormalities and a hypoplastic tympanic cavity. Rarely, there is associated deficiency of the cochlea and vestibular apparatus. *Hadju-Cheney* is another, rarer, inherited disorder leading to stenotic EACs and conductive hearing loss (CHL) (Fig. 9–22).

Fibrous dysplasia is a bony dystrophy that not uncommonly affects the facial bones to give rise to the so-called "leonine facies." The TB is affected less commonly when compared with the remainder of the skull base, but gives a typical "ground-glass" appearance on CT (Fig. 9–23).

Osteogenesis imperfecta (OI) has a CT appearance identical to the spongiosa phase of otosclerosis (not normally seen in a strictly pediatric population) with low-density outlining the otic capsule (Fig. 9–24).

Other lytic processes affecting the petrous TB (PTB) include *Langerhans' cell histiocytosis,* specifically eosinophilic granuloma (Fig. 9–25): and *rhabdomyosarcoma* (Fig. 9–26). The TB is less commonly a site for metastatic disease; however, a TB

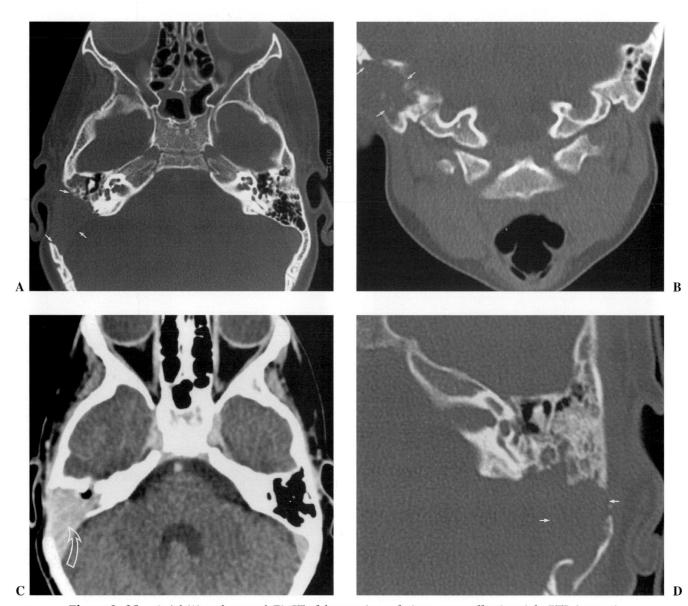

Figure 9–25:   Axial (A) and coronal (B) CT of destructive soft-tissue mass affecting right PTB (arrows) with a clean cut-off and uniform enhancement after contrast (C) (curved arrow) in a 10-year-old male with Langerhans' cell histiocytosis. Five years later after steroid therapy (D), there is recurrent disease with a destructive lesion affecting the left PTB (arrows).

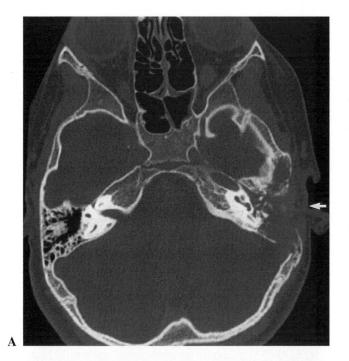

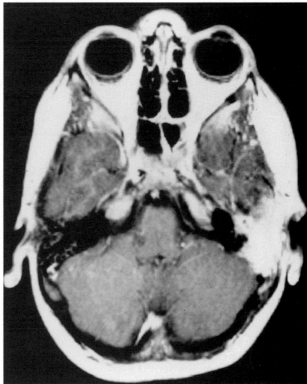

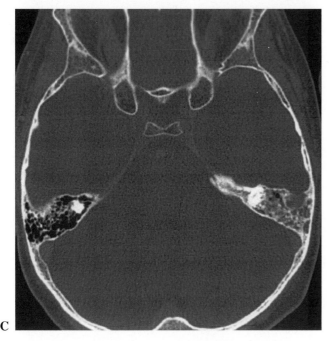

Figure 9–26: (A) Unenhanced axial CT in a 12-year-old female with rhabdomyosarcoma of the left ear. Note the destruction of the left temporal bone with sparing of the inner ear and associated soft-tissue swelling (arrow), which on MRI after gadolinium (Gd) (B) shows marked enhancement without evidence for intracranial extension. One year later following successful chemotherapy (C), there has been some reconstitution of previously-destroyed bone.

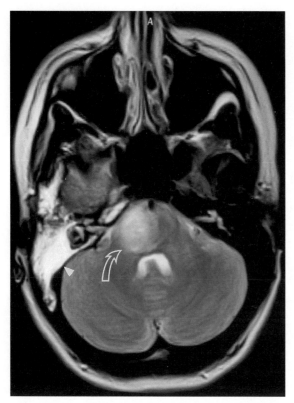

Figure 9–27: Axial T1-weighted post-Gd MRI demonstrating enhancement in the right side of the pons (curved arrow) from a brainstem glioma, with increased signal returned from opacified right mastoid air-cells (arrowhead) secondary to radiation therapy.

chloroma has been documented at our institution. Primary tumors of the PTB include benign lesions such as invaginating polyps and chondromas.

Abnormalities of the PTB that result from the presence of a tumor at the level of the nasopharynx include mastoid air-cell disease secondary to obstruction of the ET as well as mastoiditis/mucositis secondary to radiation therapy (Fig. 9–27).

AT A GLANCE . . .

Bone Dystrophies and Lytic Lesions

- Achondroplasia
- Treacher Collins syndrome
- Hadju-Cheney disorder
- Fibrous dysplasia
- Osteogenesis imperfecta
- Langerhans cell histiocytosis
- Rhabdomyosarcoma
- Metastatic lesions

CONGENITAL MALFORMATIONS OF THE EAR

Associations with microtia include cervical spine anomalies (Fig. 9–28), hemifacial microsomia (Fig. 9–29), and most commonly, varying degrees of atresia of the external auditory canal with or without anomalies of the ossicular chain (Fig. 9–30) and a variable abnormality of the soft tissue of the pinna.

Congenital anomalies of the inner ear can be divided into: (1) abnormalities of the SCCs; (2) malformations of the cochlea; (3) large vestibular aqueducts (Fig. 9–31); and (4) complete labyrinthine aplasia (*Michel deformity*) (Fig. 9–32). The SCCs develop from the sixth to the twenty-second gestational weeks, with the superior SCC (SSCC) developing first and the lateral SCC (LSCC) last. Developmental anomalies of the LSCC are the most common (Fig. 9–33) and may be associated with mild hearing loss. Malformations of the cochlea occur following insults during the first 8 weeks of gestation and

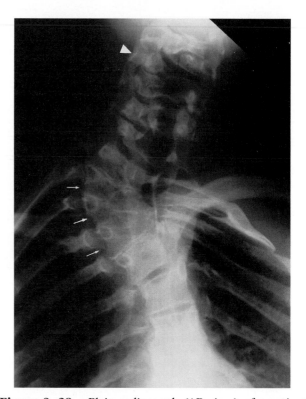

Figure 9–28: Plain radiograph (AP view) of a patient with typical clinical features of Klippel-Feil demonstrating cervical hemivertebrae (arrowhead) and block fusion of the upper thoracic vertebral bodies (arrows) in association with bilateral congenital external and middle ear anomalies (not illustrated) and conductive hearing loss.

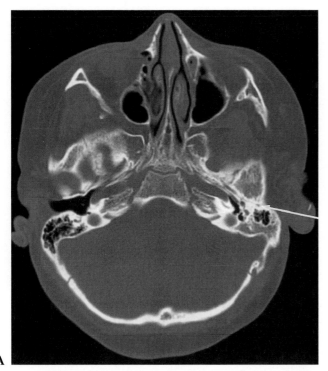

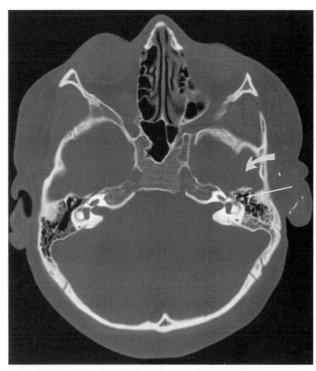

A   B

Figure 9–29: (A, B) Two axial CT slices through PTBs demonstrating left-sided microtia and hypoplastic pinna in a patient with left hemifacial microsomia. Note smaller left middle cranial fossa (curved arrow) and tympanic cavity (thin arrow) with absence of the left EAC (long arrow) in this 12-year-old male. The inner ear structures appear preserved.

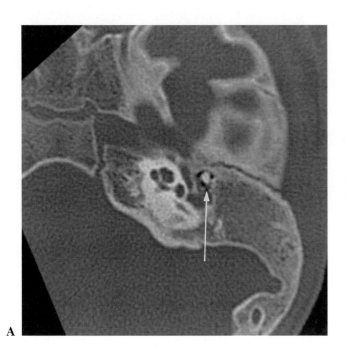

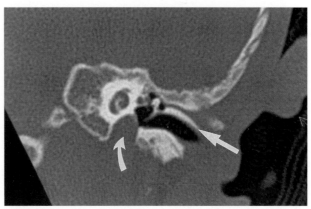

B

Figure 9–30: Axial (A) and coronal (B) CTs in an 11-year-old male with left EAC stenosis, showing an atretic bony plate (thick arrow) with malformed ossicles and small tympanic cavity containing soft tissue density material (thin arrow), some of which may represent the facial nerve. The mastoid air cells are hypoplastic, and there is a laterally-placed left ICA (curved arrow) separated from the middle ear by a thin segment of bone.

A

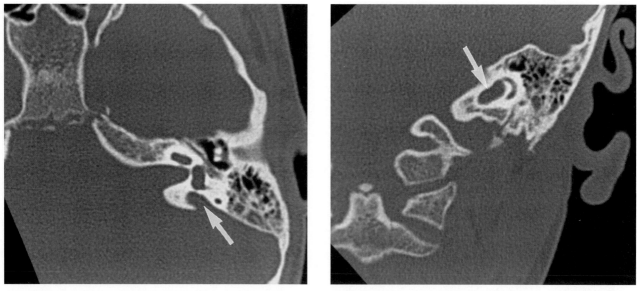

A   B

Figure 9–31:   Axial (A) and coronal (B) CT of a boy with bilateral large vestibular aqueducts (arrows) and SNI1L. The remainder of the inner ear structures appear normal.

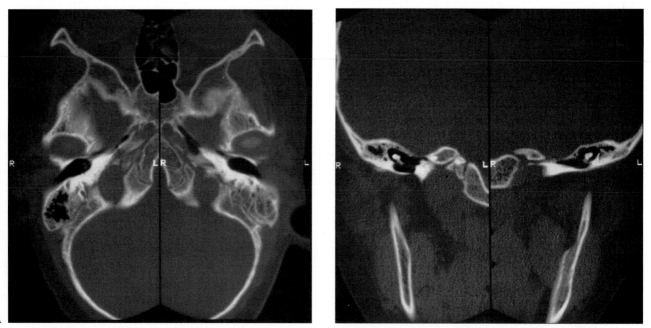

A   B

Figure 9–32:   Composite axial (A) and coronal (B) CT slices in this profoundly-deaf child following an insult to the otic placode during the third gestational week, leading to the Michel deformity seen here with complete absence of the otic cyst structures. (Images provided courtesy of Susan Blaser M.D., Hospital for Sick Children, Toronto, Canada).

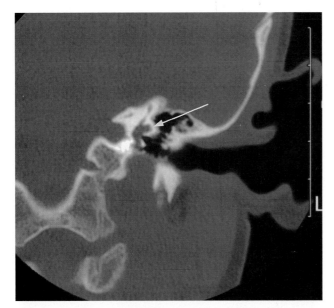

Figure 9–33: Coronal CT of the left ear in a young boy with an anomaly of the LSCC (arrow) with an associated hearing deficit.

range from a common cavity (cochlea and vestibule) (Figs. 9–34 and 9–35), to *cochlea aplasia* (normal vestibule and semicircular canal), *cochlear hypoplasia,* and *Mondini deformity.*[11-13] A true Mondini deformity is a specific entity resulting from an insult during the seventh week of gestation. The cochlea

develops only 1.5 turns and lacks an interscalar septum and osseous spiral lamina (Fig. 9–36). By definition the basal turn is normal. Vestibular, SCC, and endolymphatic duct/sac deformities occur in 20 percent of cases. In Michel deformity (see Fig. 9–32), there is complete absence of the inner ear structures.

AT A GLANCE . . .

Congenital Lesions of the Inner Ear

- Abnormalities of the semicircular canals
- Malformations of the cochlea
- Large vestibular aqueducts
- Complete labyrinthine aplasia

COCHLEAR IMPLANTATION

Before cochlear implantation is performed CT is the study of choice for assessing the osseous structures of the TB and MRI is the imaging modality of choice for the evaluation of the membranous labyrinth, the facial and acoustic nerves, the cerebellopontine angle (CPA) region, and the central cochlear and vestibular pathways.[14]

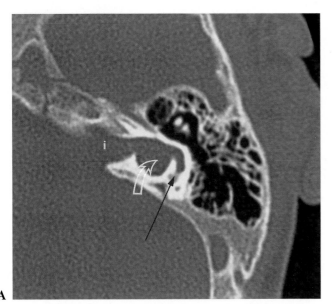

A

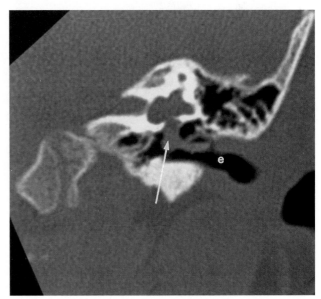

B

Figure 9–34: Axial (A) and coronal (B) CT images from a 3-year-old boy with a past history of pneumococcal meningitis and subdural empyema, resulting in a SNHL. There is a congenital anomaly involving the left cochlea and vestibule (curved arrow) with free communication to the IAC **(i).** Soft-tissue density within the common cavity is bone wax (white arrow), secondary to an operative procedure to stop the CSF otorrhea. The SCCs appear dysmorphic (black arrow). **e** = EAC.

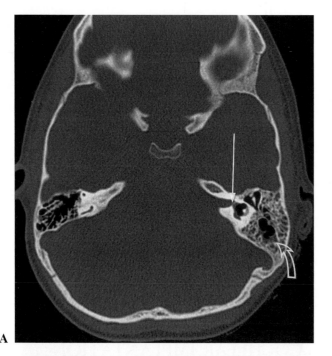

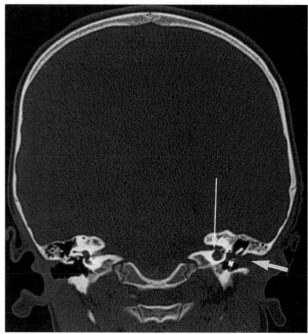

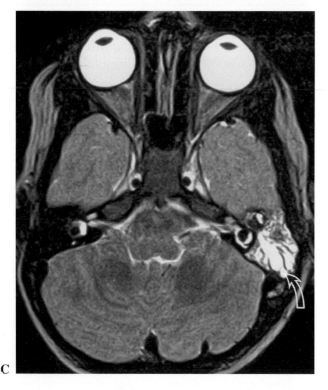

Figure 9–35: Axial (A) and coronal (B) HRCT and axial (C) T2-weighted MRI in an 8-year-old female with a history of CSF leak during left-sided myringotomy tube placement. Note the abnormally-formed inner ear with fluid filling the middle-ear cavity and EAC (short arrow). The left IAC and cochlear cavity are joined by a wide channel (long arrow). Air is present within the inner ear structures. Findings are consistent with a common cavity defect in a child who presented with left SNHL. Note the fluid within the mastoid air-cells (curved arrows).

The axial plane is best for assessing: (1) mastoid pneumatization; (2) the ET; (3) the middle-ear cavity; (4) the ossicular chain; (5) the round window niche and membrane; (6) the petrous segment of the facial nerve canal; (7) the carotid canal; (8) the jugular fossa; (9) the structures of the inner ear; (10) the petrous apex; and (11) the position of the lateral and sigmoid sinus plates.

Direct coronal imaging is best for visualizing: (1) the oval window; (2) the SCCs; (3) the facial nerve canal; (4) the tegmen tympani; (5) the position of the middle cranial fossa dura; (6) the floor of the hypotympanum; (7) the jugular fossa; (8) the carotid canal; and (9) the floor and roof of the EAC.

Following insertion of the implant, if the expected functioning is not achieved, plain radiogra-

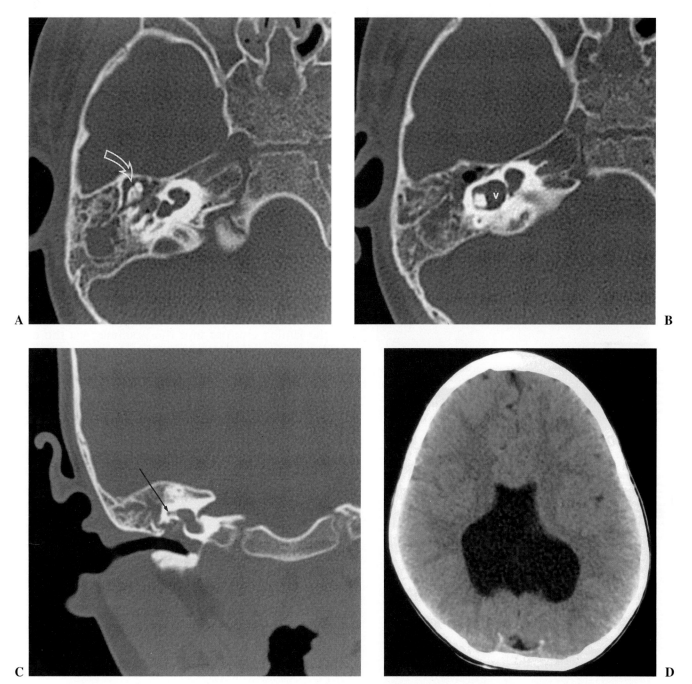

Figure 9–36:   A 3-year-old boy with bilateral hearing impairment being assessed for cochlear implant. Axial (A and B) and coronal (C) CT of right PTB demonstrate a Mondini deformity with abnormal cochlear turns and accompanying large vestibule (V) with a patulous IAC and stenotic EAC. There is fluid (curved arrow) within the middle-ear cavity (mesotympanum). Incidental note is made of accompanying semilobar holoprosencephaly (D) in this child with normal appearing SCCs. Black arrow = LSCC.

phy (Fig. 9–37) or even CT (Fig. 9–38) may be performed.[15] With certain implant devices, MRI with functional activation even may be possible.[16,17]

The various segments of the facial nerve canal can be evaluated by a combination of axial and coronal imaging. In the case of glomus or other tumors the

relationship between the intratemporal, extracranial, and intracranial components of tumor are better appreciated on coronal rather than axial sections. 3D T2-weighted MRI (such as 3DCISS, Siemens) can be performed at 1.5 Tesla to obtain volumetric studies with submillimeter cuts that can

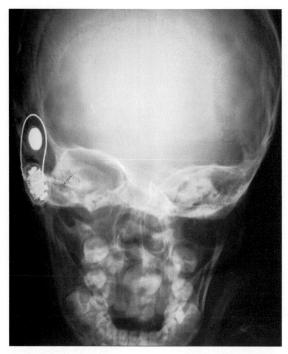

Figure 9–37: Anteroposterior radiograph demonstrating correct positioning without break of multiple electrodes following right-sided cochlear implantation.

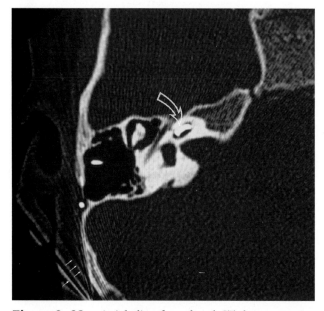

Figure 9–38: Axial slice from head CT demonstrating the path of the electrode from the squamomastoid through the antrum and Koerner's septum to lie within the basal coil of the cochlea (curved arrow). Note the streak artifact (small arrows) generated by the air/metal interface.

be reconstructed with high resolution (typically in the coronal and oblique parasagittal planes) to examine the endolymphatic system.[18,19]

ACQUIRED DISORDERS OF MEMBRANOUS LABYRINTH

Figure 9–39 demonstrates normal axial CT of the CPA and IAC. Figure 9–40 illustrates a normal 3DCISS MRI of the IAC and inner ear acquired in the axial plane with coronal and oblique parasagittal reconstructions.

Labyrinthitis may be classified according to etiology. It can be: (1) *tympanogenic*, secondary to middle-ear disease and therefore typically unilateral; (2) *meningogenic*, most commonly bacterial and bilateral by spread from the fundus of the IAC through the lamina cribrosa into the vestibule, via the cochlear nerve foramen into the cochlear apex, or by propagation of suppurative material through the cochlear aqueduct into the basal turn of the cochlea. (This is the most common cause of acquired childhood deafness.); (3) *hematogenic*, including rare viral causes such as mumps and measles; (4) *posttraumatic* due to fracture or perilymph fistula with superadded infection; and (5) *autoimmune*. Labyrinthitis results in varying degrees of ossification (best assessed by CT) and fibrosis (better assessed by MRI) (Fig. 9–41) of the membranous labyrinth.[20,21]

AT A GLANCE . . .
Etiology of Labyrinthitis

- Tympanogenic
- Meningogenic
- Hematogenic
- Posttraumatic
- Autoimmune

ASSESSMENT OF THE FACIAL (SEVENTH CRANIAL) AND VESTIBULOCOCHLEAR (EIGHTH CRANIAL) NERVES

The facial nerve runs in the anterosuperior portion of the IAC. A labyrinthine segment in the fallopian

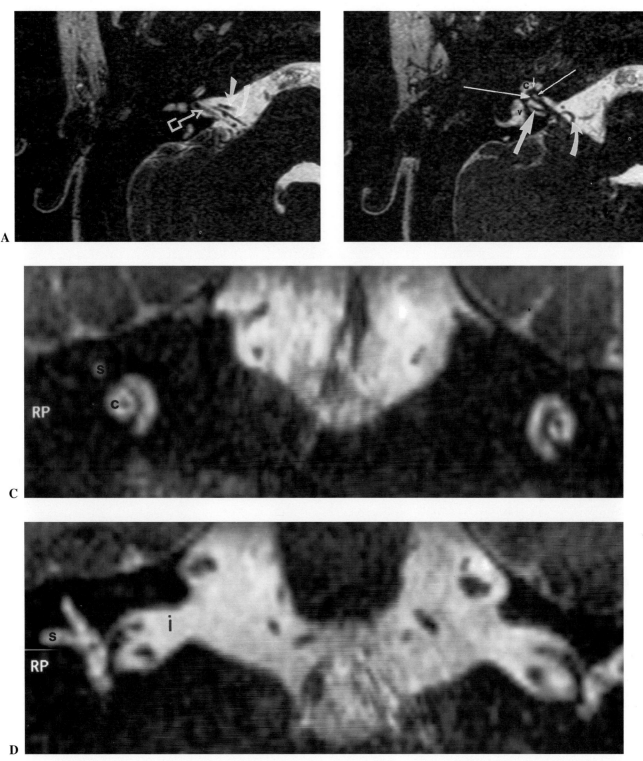

Figure 9–39: (A) Axial 0.7 mm MRI 3DFTCISS through the superior aspect of the right IAC in a newborn that demonstrates normal anatomy. Open arrow = vestibulocochlear nerve (VCN) (VIII); short arrow = superior fascicle (VII); curved arrow = middle fascicle (VII). (B) Axial 0.7 mm MRI 3DFTCISS through the middle of the right IAC. Short arrow = modiolus/osseous spiral lamina; thick arrow = superior vestibular nerve (SVN); thin arrow = inferior vestibular nerve (IVN); long arrow = cochlear nerve (CN); curved arrow = vascular loop; **c** = cochlea; **v** = vestibule. Note the sharp angulation between CN and IVN. (C) Coronal anterior multiplanar reconstruction (MPR) from 3DFTCISS. **c** = cochlea; **s** = semicircular canal. (D) Posterior coronal MPR that demonstrates IAC **(i)** and semicircular canal **(s).** VIII = eighth cranial nerve; VII = seventh cranial nerve.

166   The Ear

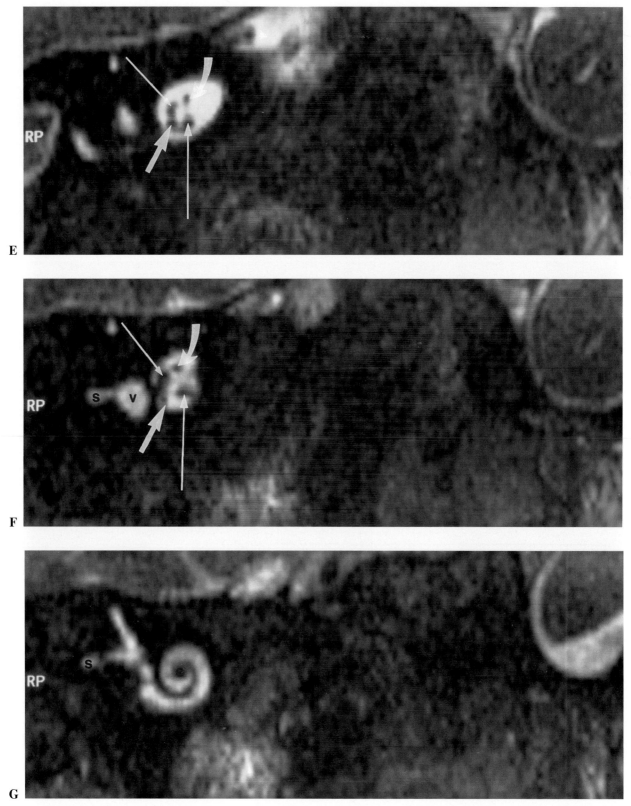

Figure 9–39: *(continued)* (E) Parasagittal oblique reconstruction from 3DCISS at midportion IAC demonstrates all four nerves with the appearance of a buttonhole. RP = right posterior; curved arrow = facial nerve ("7 Up"); long arrow = cochlear nerve ("Coke" down); thin arrow = SVN; short arrow = IVN. (F) Further lateral parasagittal oblique reconstruction again demonstrates all four nerves (see E). **s** = LSCC; **v** = vestibule. (G) Further lateral parasagittal oblique reconstruction. Note the snail-shaped appearance of the cochlea **(c)** seen in its entirety. **s** = LSCC.

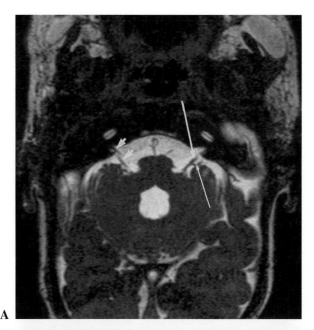

Figure 9–40: (A) Axial 3DCISS 0.7 mm thick MRI slice through IACs in a 14-month-old with CHARGE syndrome and left facial palsy. Note the short IACs. Long arrow = cochlear nerve; thin arrow = IVN; arrowheads = right facial and vestibulocochlear nerves. (B) Same patient with a parasagittal oblique reconstruction through the midportion of the left IAC. AR = anterior right; curved arrow = posteriorly-placed SVN; long arrow = IVN; short arrow = cochlear nerve. Note the absence of any left facial nerve.

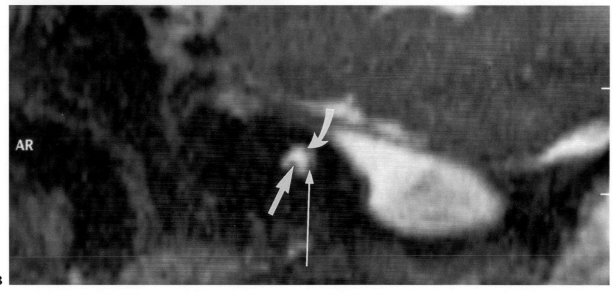

canal courses anterosuperiorly and laterally from the IAC to the geniculate ganglion, superior to the cochlea. In this region it gives off the greater petrosal nerve that supplies parasympathetic fibers for the lacrimal, nasal, and palatine glands. At the geniculate ganglion, the facial nerve forms its first turn or genu and then runs posteroinferiolaterally on the undersurface of the LSCC and above the oval window niche as its horizontal or tympanic portion. It makes a second turn to run inferiorly through the mastoid to exit at the stylomastoid foramen. The intramastoid portion provides innervation to the stapedius and, just above the stylomastoid foramen,

gives off the chorda tympani that supplies taste to the anterior two-thirds of the tongue.

The facial nerve normally may show some enhancement at the level of the geniculate ganglion and in its horizontal and descending portions. It is said that 76 percent of facial nerves enhance in one or more portions, and asymmetry may be present in 69 percent of cases.[22] Enhancement in the IAC (Figs. 9-42 and 9-43) and parotid gland is always abnormal. Swelling of the facial nerve may be seen in patients with Bell's palsy, which is thought to account for 80 percent of facial nerve paralyses. The differential diagnosis of facial nerve enhancement

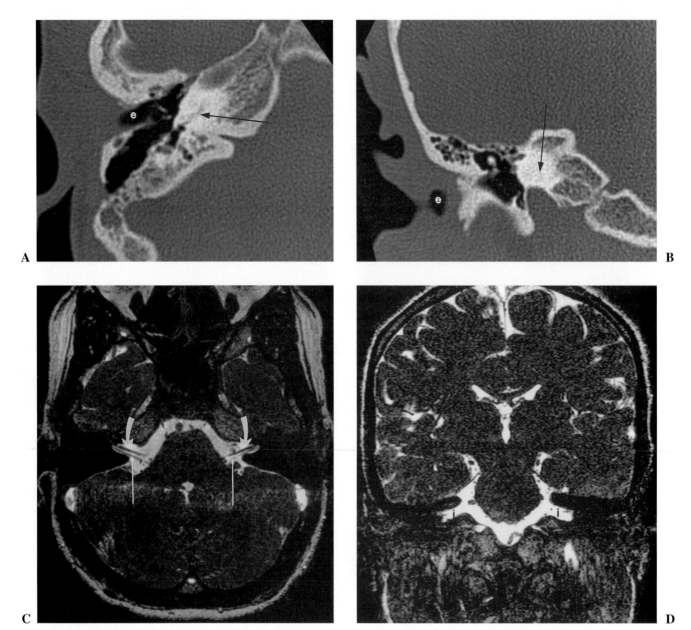

A

B

C

D

Figure 9–41: (A and B) Axial and coronal 1-mm CT slices demonstrating "ghost" of basal turn cochlea (black arrow) seen within a sclerotic petrous apex. **e** = EAC. (C) Same patient (axial 0.7 mm 3DCISS) at the expected level of inner ear structures. Curved arrow = facial nerve; straight arrow = VCN. No normal labyrinthine structures are visible on this T2-weighted image. (D) Coronal MPR through the expected level of the cochlea. **i** = IAC. No normal endolymphatic structures seen. Taken in conjunction with the CT, the appearance is consistent with bilateral ossifying labyrinthitis. This information is important in the evaluation for cochlear implantation.

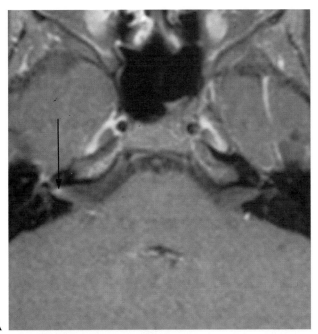

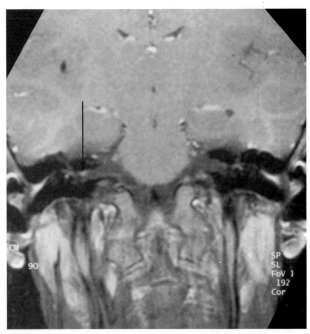

A   B

Figure 9–42:   (A and B) Axial and direct coronal post : Gd MR through the IACs. Note the abnormal intracanalicular enhancement involving the right facial nerve (arrow) in a child presenting with right-sided Bell's palsy.

includes schwannoma, Lyme disease, lymphoma, hemangioma, sarcoidosis (see Fig. 9-43), viral neuritis, and perineural tumor spread (Fig. 9-44). Facial nerve hemangiomas occur most frequently at the level of the geniculate ganglion, followed by the IAC, and least commonly at the posterior genu. They can demonstrate marked enhancement and may ossify. The latter is an important distinction from facial nerve schwannomas.

> ## SPECIAL CONSIDERATION:
>
> Enhancement of the facial nerve in the IAC or parotid gland is always abnormal.

The cochlear portion of the eighth cranial nerve runs in the anteroinferior portion of the IAC, whereas the superior and inferior vestibular nerves run in the upper and lower posterior aspects of the canal respectively.[23] SNHL may be divided into *sensory* (cochlear) and *neural* (retrocochlear, arising from the cochlear nerve or cochlear nuclei) types.[24] *Acoustic schwannomas,* typically bilateral in neurofibromatosis type 2 (NF2), arise from the cochlear

(Fig. 9-45) and not the vestibular branch of the eighth cranial nerve. Gd-enhanced MRI is important in defining early intracanalicular lesions[25] and the occasional intralabyrinthine schwannoma, usually situated close to the round window niche. Rarely metastatic disease is seen.

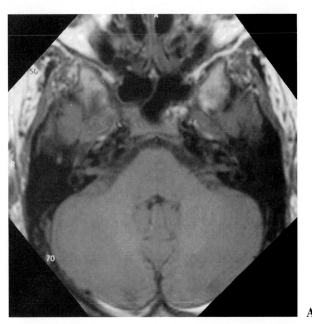

A

Figure 9–43:   (A) Axial T1-weighted unenhanced MRI through IACs in a patient with bilateral facial nerve palsies.

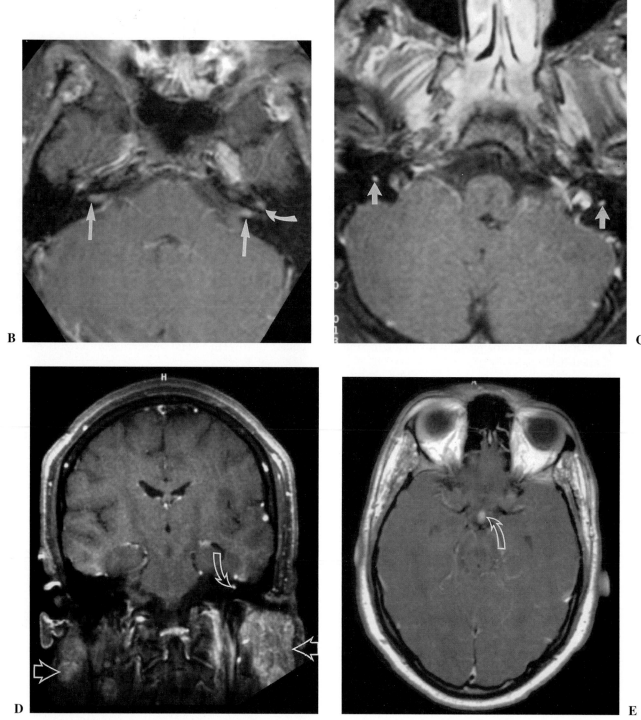

Figure 9–43: *(continued)* (B) Post-Gd T1-weighted axial MRI demonstrates bilateral intracanalicular (straight arrows) enhancement and also left anterior genu (curved arrow) facial nerve. (C) Inferior axial T1-weighted post-Gd MRI demonstrates enhancement in the descending portions (mastoid segments) of both facial nerves (arrows). (D) Coronal T1-weighted fat-suppressed post-Gd image shows enhancement of the posterior genu of the left facial nerve (curved arrow) and enhancement of bilateral enlarged parotid glands (short arrows). (E) Axial T1-weighted post-Gd image at the level of the midbrain shows a thickened pituitary infundibulum (curved arrow). Clinical history and imaging consistent with a diagnosis of sarcoidosis.

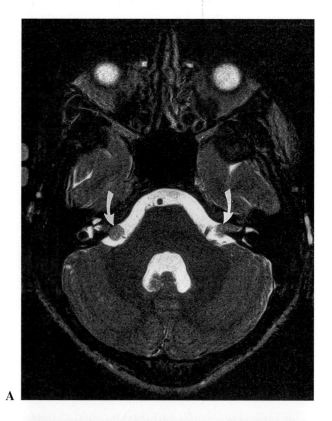

A

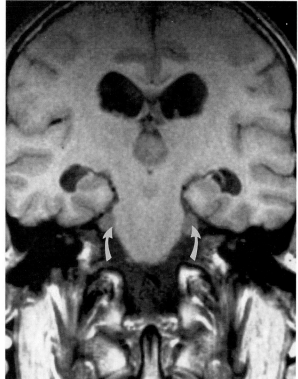

B

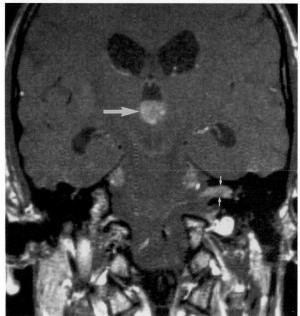

C

Figure 9–44: (A) Axial T2-weighted image demonstrating bilateral enlargement of the vestibulocochlear nerve complex (curved arrow) at the level of the CPA, mimicking acoustic neurinomas. (B) Coronal T1-weighted image confirms enlargement of the eighth cranial nerve (curved arrow) at the level of the brainstem. (C) Post-Gd more posterior coronal T1-weighted image demonstrates multiple areas of abnormal enhancement including third ventricle (arrow), confirmed as perineural spread from a previously-undiagnosed CNS primary in a child with obstructive hydrocephalus. Note the enhancement within the left IAC (small arrows).

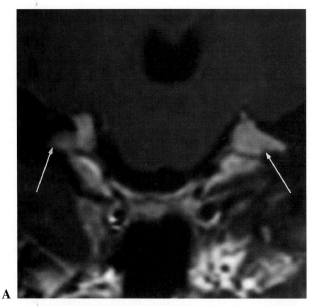
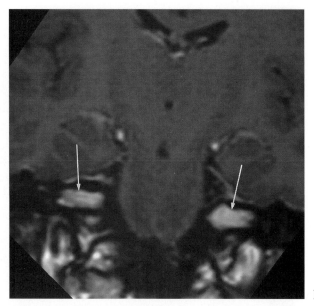

Figure 9–45: (A and B) Anterior and more posterior coronal T1-weighted post-Gd images, at the levels of the CPAs and IACs respectively. Imaging shows bilateral cochlear schwannomas (arrows), pathognmonic of NF2.

Trigeminal nerve schwannomas also may occur along the petrous apex. These lesions begin in an extraosseous location but may erode the medial petrous bone near the trigeminal impression.

AT A GLANCE . . .

Differential Diagnosis of Facial Nerve Enhancement

- Schwannoma
- Lyme disease
- Lymphoma
- Hemangioma
- Sarcoidosis
- Viral neuritis
- Perineural tumor spread

VASCULAR ANOMALIES

Vascular anomalies fall into two main groups—*venous* and *arterial*. The high-riding jugular vein is a normal variant. The more important dehiscent jugu-

lar bulb (Fig. 9-46) and the so-called ''aberrant carotid artery'' (Fig. 9-47) can both present at otoscopy as a bluish retrotympanic bulge. The latter condition is a misnomer and is thought to result from atresia or regression of the cervical portion of the internal carotid artery. In this case, what appears to be the internal carotid artery is actually an enlarged inferior tympanic branch of the ascending pharyngeal artery. This normally tiny vessel enters

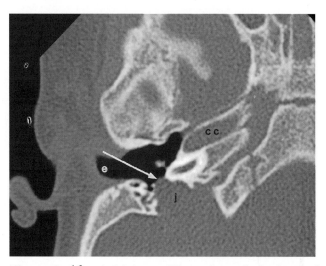

Figure 9–46: Axial 1-mm CT cut through the level of the right EAC (**e**) and cochlea demonstrates the jugular bulb (**j**) protruding into the mesotympanum or middle-ear cavity (arrow) due to dehiscence or loss of the normal intervening bony septum. **cc** = normal carotid canal.

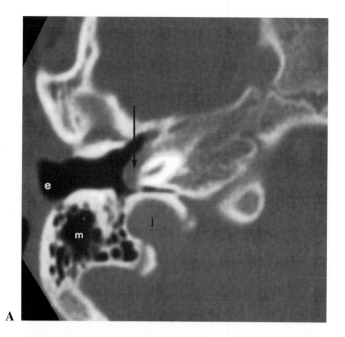

A

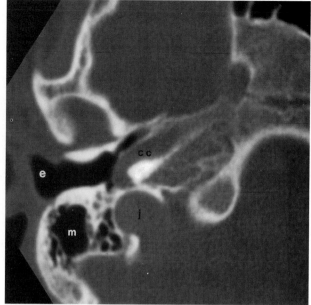

B

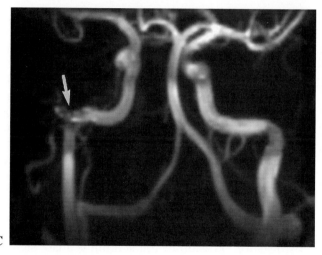

C

Figure 9–47: (A and B) CT cuts through the base of skull demonstrate an "aberrant" carotid artery (black arrow) presenting as a bluish retrotympanic mass. **cc** = right petrous carotid artery in carotid canal; **j** = jugular bulb without dehiscence; **e** = EAC; **m** = mastoid air-cells. (C) Coronal MRA of the same patient demonstrates a typical angiographic appearance of posterolaterally displaced and narrowed (arrow) reconstitution of petrous carotid by intratympanic anastamoses of the right ascending pharyngeal artery. Normal left side.

the tympanic cavity through the inferior tympanic canaliculus, which it shares with Jacobson's tympanic branch of the glossopharyngeal nerve. With reconstitution of the petrous portion of the internal carotid artery through this route, the vessel has a more lateral and posterior location than the usual carotid canal. Inadvertent biopsy of this vessel may result in uncontrollable bleeding or later development of pseudoaneurysm.

INFECTION/INFLAMMATORY CONDITIONS OF THE TEMPORAL BONE

Working from lateral to medial, many conditions affecting the EAC can be diagnosed using an oto-scope. *External otitis media* (Fig. 9–48) (rarely in a malignant form) may be imaged in children who present with severe pain. Imaging (CT and/or MRI with or without contrast) is helpful in identifying the sequelae of recurrent ear infections and otitis media with effusion (OME) (Fig. 9–49) and in excluding other conditions.[26]

The tympanic membrane (TM) separates the EAC from the mesotympanum. It is attached to the scutum superiorly and the floor of the EAC inferiorly, sloping at an angle of approximately 140 degrees with respect to the superior aspect of the canal. The TM has a thin anterosuperior portion, the *pars flaccida,* and a thick posteroinferior portion, the *pars tensa.* The TM routinely is imaged by high-resolution 1 mm CT. Thickening and retraction of the TM are appreciated easily, although perforation is more reliably diagnosed by direct visualization.

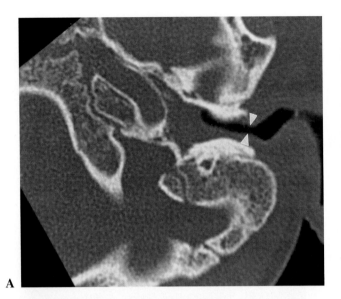

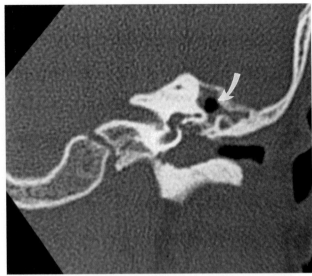

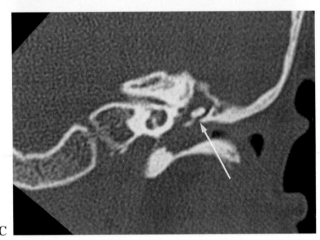

Figure 9–48: (A) Axial 1 mm unenhanced CT through the EAC demonstrates evidence of otitis externa (arrowheads) with mucosal thickening and relative narrowing of the meatus. (B and C) Direct coronal 1 mm unenhanced CT at the level of the EAC demonstrates soft-tissue density material within the middle-ear cleft and attic consistent with the presence of some fluid as suggested by an air pocket (curved arrow). Note the intact scutum (arrow) and normal mineralization of the ossicular chain that speak against an established cholesteatoma in this child with chronic otitis media (COM). The tympanic membrane TM cannot be identified.

SPACES AND RECESSES IMPORTANT IN CHRONIC INFECTION

Prussak's space, bordered laterally by the pars flaccida, inferiorly by the lateral (short) process of the malleus, superiorly by the lateral mallear ligament, and medially by the neck of the malleus, is a site of predilection for the development of cholesteatoma. *Cholesteatoma,* or keratoma, is essentially skin in the wrong place, and it may be congenital (Fig. 9–50) or acquired (Figs. 9–51 and 9–52). Cholesteatoma involves the pars flaccida 82 percent of the time (usually primary), and the pars tensa 18 percent of the time (usually secondary). Prussak's space opens posteriorly into the epitympanum or attic. Extension of cholesteatoma may lead to erosion of bone overlying the LSCC, resulting in labyrinthine fistulization. Erosion of the scutum is a late sign of disease.[27]

Immediately medial to the pyramidal eminence (PE), from which the stapedius tendon originates, lies the sinus tympani bordered medially by cortical bone overlying the posterior SCC. Lateral to the PE lies the facial nerve recess. Both of these recesses are important to examine radiographically because they are difficult to visualize directly and may harbor chronic granulation tissue or cholesteatoma. Gd-enhanced MRI may be helpful in distinguishing between these two entities.

MASTOID AIR-CELLS

Chronic infection of the mastoid air-cell system results in *mastoiditis* and *osteomyelitis* if this extends

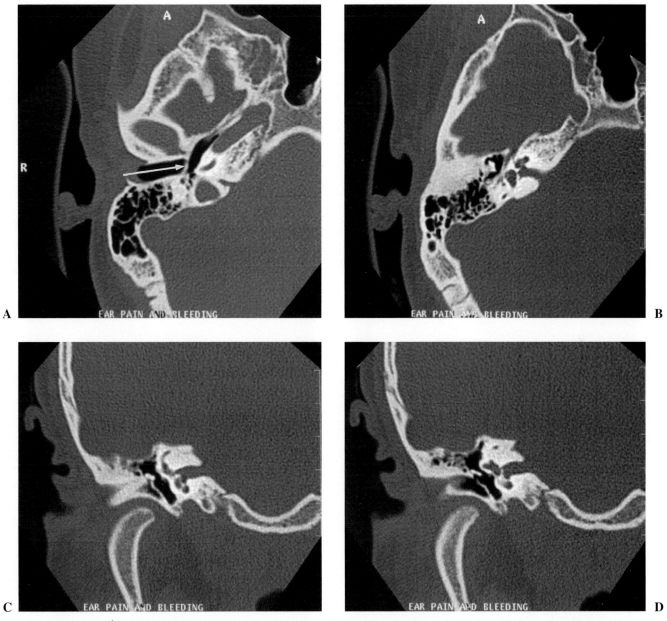

Figure 9–49: (A and B) Axial 1 mm unenhanced CT through the right EAC and mesotympanum shows generalized increased density of the mastoid with calcification of the TM (long arrow) and adherence of the ossicular chain in this child with a history of COM. The child now presents with right ear pain, bleeding, and a CHL. (C and D) Coronal 1 mm unenhanced CT in the same child confirms the presence of tympanosclerosis.

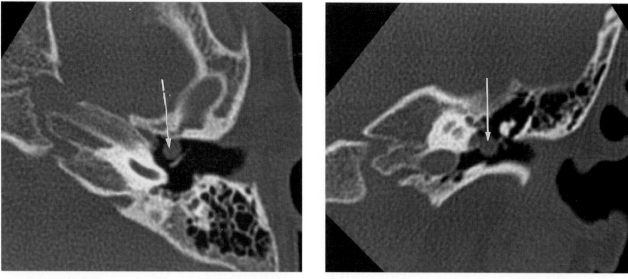

A   B

Figure 9–50: (A and B) Axial and coronal images of primary cholesteatoma (arrows) involving the pars tensa and adjacent to the long arm of the malleus.

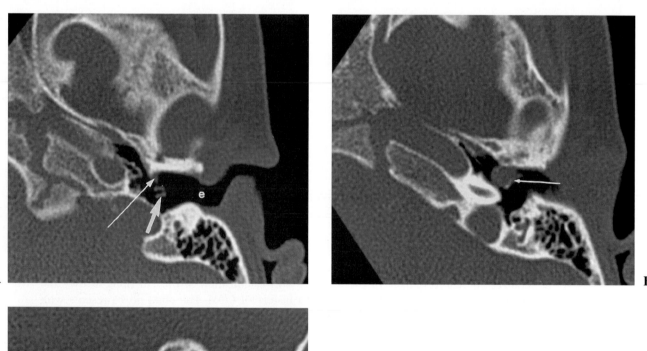

A   B

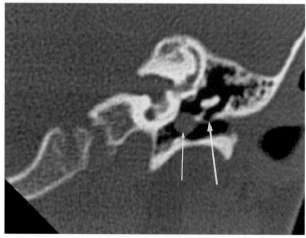

C

Figure 9–51: (A) Axial high-resolution CT demonstrates a myringotomy tube (short arrow) in TM. Note the soft-tissue thickening on the lateral surface of the pars flaccida (long arrow). **e** = EAC. (B) Axial high-resolution CT of the same patient demonstrates a proven secondary cholesteatomatous mass abutting the incus (arrow). (C) Coronal high-resolution CT confirms a thickened pars flaccida (long arrow) with secondary cholesteatoma involving the pars tensa (thin arrow).

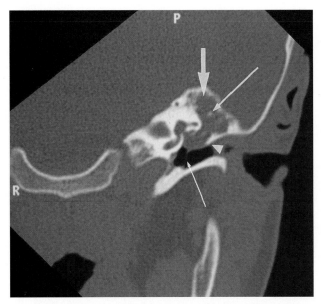

Figure 9–52: Coronal high-resolution CT shows a normal thin pars tensa (thin arrow) with secondary cholesteatoma arising from the pars flaccida and Prussak's space and extending posteriorly into the attic (short arrow) with destruction of the ossicular chain (long arrow) and early erosion of the scutum (arrowhead).

infection include venous sinus thrombosis and compression (Fig. 9-54) secondary to epidural abscess (Fig. 9-55) formation.

PETROUS APEX

The petrous apex is frequently nonpneumatized and shows evidence of soft-tissue density material by CT. On MRI it may appear dark or isointense on T1-weighted imaging and bright on T2-weighted imaging. The findings should not be confused with cholesterol granulomas (epidermoids) of the petrous apex that contain extracellular methemoglobin and tend to appear bright on both T1-weighted and T2-weighted imaging, often with expansion of the petrous apex and impingement on the CPA.

Petrous apicitis may lead to involvement of the sixth cranial nerve and clinical presentation with a lateral rectus palsy, known as *Gradenigo's syndrome* (Fig. 9-56).

into the bone (Fig. 9-53). A Bezold's abscess may point over the mastoid process. If infection is chronic, an automastoidectomy may occur giving the radiographic appearance of postsurgical changes on CT. Complications of mastoid air-cell

TEMPORAL BONE TRAUMA/FRACTURES

Due to its superior bony detail, CT is the technique of choice in assessing traumatic TB injury. On MRI,

A 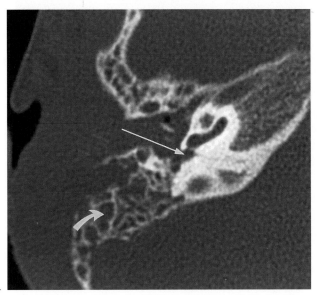   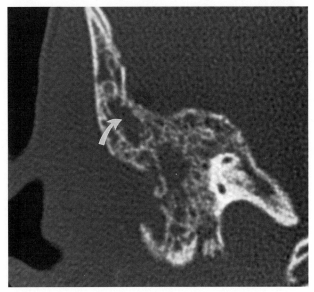 B

Figure 9–53: (A and B) Axial and coronal unenhanced CT through the right TB in a child with mastoiditis following a partial mastoidectomy. Note the bone thinning and destruction extending to the round window (long arrow) and the soft-tissue density material within the mastoid air-cells (curved arrow).

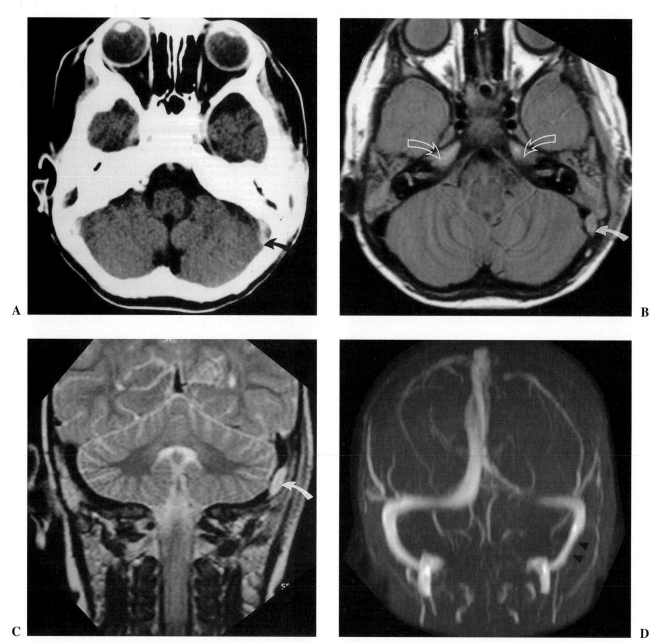

Figure 9–54: (A) Axial postcontrast CT shows an enhancing collection (arrow) around the left sigmoid sinus mimicking a venous sinus thrombosis. (B) Axial pre-Gd and (C) coronal post-Gd MRI confirm epidural collection (arrow) compressing the left sigmoid sinus that is patent on MRV (magnetic resonance venogram). (D) (arrowheads) in a child with bilateral mastoid air-cell disease. Note the isointense T1 signal returned from bilateral nonpneumatized petrous apices (open arrows B)

detail may be obscured due to the presence of blood. Special areas of concern when evaluating trauma of the TB include (from medial to lateral): (1) the carotid canal; (2) the bony labyrinth; (3) the facial nerve canal; (4) the ossicles; (5) the tegmen tympani; and (6) the medial wall mastoid air-cells.

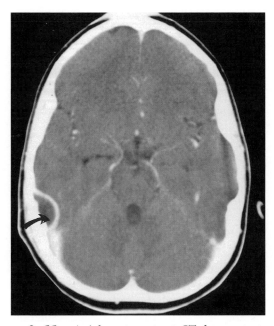

Figure 9–55: Axial post-contrast CT demonstrates extension of an epidural abscess into the middle cranial fossa (arrow) in a child with right-sided mastoiditis.

> ## SPECIAL CONSIDERATION:
>
> Due to its superior bony detail, CT is the technique of choice in assessing a traumatic TB injury.

A longitudinal (horizontal) fracture (Fig. 9–57) along the long axis of the TB is most common (70–80 percent), and usually presents with CHL from ossicular disruption and bloody CSF otorrhea from fracture through the tegmen (see Fig. 9–1). A transverse (vertical) fracture (Fig. 9–58) orthogonal

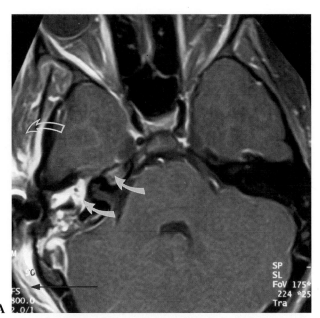
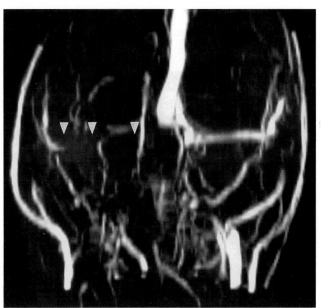

Figure 9–56:   (A) Axial T1-weighted post-Gd MRI with soft-tissue swelling and enhancement overlying the right mastoid (black arrow) and infratemporal fossa (open arrow) in a case of Gradenigo's syndrome with petrous apicitis (curved arrows), sixth nerve palsy, and venous sinus thrombosis. (B) Coronal reconstruction MRV of the same patient reveals the extent of the right-sided venous thombosis that involves the right transverse (arrowheads) and sigmoid sinuses down to the level of the right internal jugular vein, all of which are missing on the image.

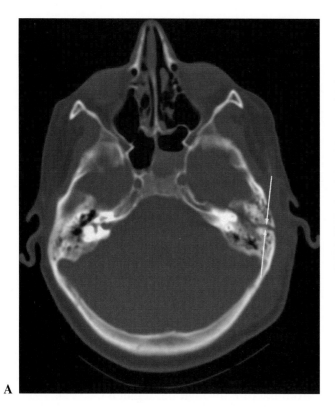

A

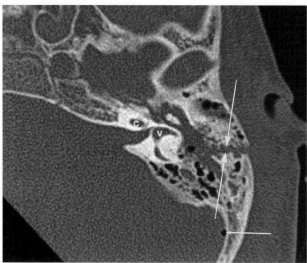

B

Figure 9–57: (A) Axial CT slice of the whole head demonstrates a longitudinal (horizontal) fracture (arrows) through the left PTB. (B) Axial high-resolution CT through the same longitudinal fracture of the left PTB (long arrows), sparing the vestibule (**v**) and cochlea (**c**), but with air and fluid surrounding the ossicular chain. Note the spot of air (short arrow) in the posterior cranial fossa from a fracture through the mastoid.

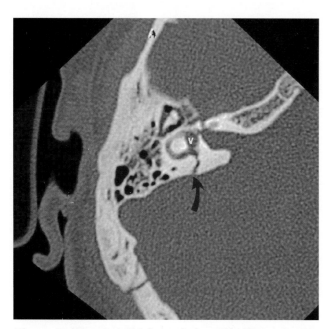

Figure 9–58: Axial high-resolution CT of the right PTB shows a vertical (transverse) fracture (arrow), extending into the vestibule (**v**).

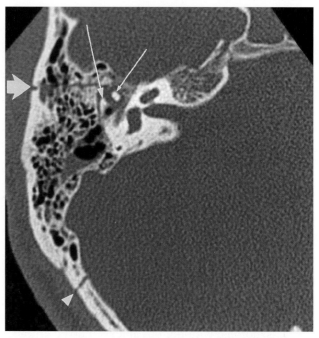

A

Figure 9–59: (A) Axial high-resolution CT shows a complex fracture (arrowheads) through the right PTB with a longitudinal component causing ossicular chain disruption. Note the head of the malleus (thin arrow) dislocated from the body of the incus (long arrow).

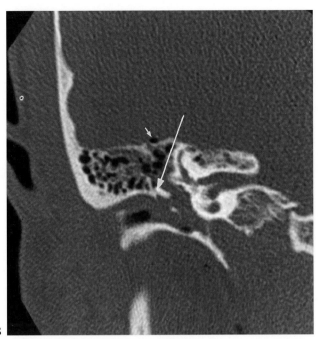

B

Figure 9–59: *(continued)* (B) Coronal CT of the same patient confirms air and fluid in the EAC with a vertical fracture through the roof of the meatus (long arrow). Note the dot of air (small arrow) that represents pneumocephalus resulting from a fracture through the tegmen.

to the long axis of the TB (20 percent) usually presents with anacusis (from SNHL): vertigo, and facial nerve injury (in the horizontal portion). Complex or mixed fractures are seen frequently (Fig. 9–59).

AT A GLANCE . . .

Temporal Bone Injury: Areas of Concern

- Carotid canal
- Bony labyrinth
- Facial nerve canal
- Ossicles
- Tegmen tympani
- Medial wall mastoid air-cells

REFERENCES

1. Valvassori GE, Buckingham RA. Imaging of the temporal bone (Part I). In: Valvassori GE, Mafee MF, Carter BL, eds. *Imaging of the Head and Neck.* New York: Thieme, 1995, pp. 2–154.

2. Som PM, Curtin HD. *Head and Neck Imaging, vol. 2, 3rd ed.* St. Louis: Mosby-Year Book, 1996, pp. 1300–1534.

3. Swartz JD, Harnsberger HR, eds. *Imaging of the Temporal Bone, 3rd ed.* New York: Thieme 1998, pp. 16–489.

4. Sandler TW, ed. *Langman's Medical Embryology, 6th ed.* Baltimore: Williams and Wilkins, 1990, pp. 142–143; 302–304.

5. Williams PL, ed. *Gray's Anatomy, 38th ed.* New York: Churchill Livingstone, 1995, pp. 262–263; 589–593.

6. *Radiology of Syndromes, Metabolic Disorders and Skeletal Dysplasia, 3rd ed.* Taybi & Lachman, Yearbook Publishers, 1990, pp. 460–461; 91–99; 676–681; 206–207.

7. Jones KL, ed. *Smith's Recognizable Patterns of Human Malformation, 4th ed.* Philadelphia: Saunders, 1988, pp. 10–25.

8. The Ear. In: Hollinshead WH, ed. *Anatomy for Surgeons, 3rd ed.* Hagerstown, MD: Harper and Row, 1982, pp. 159–221.

9. Chakeres DW, Spiegel RK. A systematic technique for comprehensive evaluation of the temporal bone by CT. Radiology 1983; 146:97–106.

10. Vignaud J, Jardin C, Rosen L, eds. *The Ear, Diagnostic Imaging.* NY Masson Publishing, 1986, pp. 112–119.

11. Streeter GL. On the development of the membranous labyrinth and the acoustic and facial nerves in the human embryo. Am J Anat 1906; 6:140–167.

12. Jackler RK, Luxford WM, House WF. Congenital malformations of the inner ear: A classification based on embryogenesis. Laryngoscope 1987; 97(supplement 40):2–14.

13. Nemzek WR, Brodie HA, Chong BW, et al. Imaging findings of the developing temporal bone in fetal specimens. AJNR 1996; 17:1467–1477.

14. Pappas DG, Simpson LC, McKenzie RA, et al. High resolution computed tomography determination of the cause of pediatric sensorineural hearing loss. Laryngoscope 1990; 100:564–569.

15. Shpizner BA, Holliday RA, Roland JT, et al. Post-operative imaging of the multichannel cochlear implant. AJNR 1995; 16:1517–1524.

16. Lo WWM. Imaging of cochlear and auditory brain stem implantation. AJNR 1998; 19:1147–1154.

17. Melcher JR, Eddington DK, Garcia N, et al. Electrically-evoked cortical activity in cochlear implant subjects can be mapped using MRI. Neuroimage 1998; 7:4 s385.

18. Oehler MC, Chakeres DW, Schmalbrock P. Reformatted planar "Christmas tree" MR appearance of the endolymphatic sac. AJNR 1995; 16:1525–1528.

19. Daniels DL, Swartz JD, Harnsberger HR, et al. Hearing I: The cochlea. AJNR 1996; 17:1237–1241.

20. Phelps PD, Lloyd GAS, ed. *Diagnostic Imaging of the Ear, 2nd ed.* London: Springer-Verlag, 1990, pp. 149–159.

21. Casselman JW, Kuhweide R, Ampe W, et al. Pathology of the membranous labyrinth: Comparison of T1- and T2-weighted and Gadolinium-enhanced spin-echo and 3DFT-CISS imaging. AJNR 1993; 14:59–69.

22. Grossman RI, Yousem DM. Temporal bone. In: Grossman RI, Yousem DM, eds. *Neuroradiology: The Requisites.* St. Louis: Mosby-Year Book, 1994, pp. 335–338.

23. Kim H-S, Kim D-I, Chung I-H. Topographical relationship of the facial and vestibulocochlear nerves in the subarachnoid space and internal auditory canal. AJNR 1998; 19:1479–1481.

24. Swartz JD, Daniels DL, Harnsberger HR, et al. Hearing II: The retrocochlear auditory pathway. AJNR 1996; 17:1479–1481.

25. Curtin HD. Rule out eighth nerve tumor: Contrast-enhanced T1-weighted or high-resolution T2-weighted MR? AJNR 1997; 18:1834–1838.

26. Weissman JL. A pain in the ear: The radiology of otalgia. AJNR 1997; 18:1641–1652.

27. Swartz JD. Cholesteatomas of the middle ear. Symposium on CT on the ear, nose and throat. Radiol Clin North Am 1984; 22:15–35.

10 Pediatric Audiology

Marilyn W. Neault

A child's hearing status can neither be seen nor palpated by physical examination. While findings such as otoscopic visualization of middle ear effusion or radiologic evidence of severe cochlear dysplasia may predict hearing loss, the otoscopically and radiologically normal ear may have normal hearing or no hearing at all. The parents' impressions and the child's behaviors in the office may offer clues, but other factors may masquerade as hearing loss or mask it. Only audiological measurements, coupled with careful history, elucidate hearing loss which otherwise is invisible. Evaluation of hearing loss in a child requires compassionate partnership and communication between the audiologist, otolaryngologist, pediatrician, and parents.

BEHAVIORAL AUDIOMETRY

Looking at Ear-Specific and Sound Field Audiograms

Regardless of advances in physiologic measures which are necessary to assess the function of portions of the auditory system, the pure tone audiogram remains, at this time, the standard measure of hearing function. The audiogram, obtained under carefully controlled conditions, plots the weakest intensity at which the child shows behavioral awareness of the presence of sound, as a function of stimulus frequency. Though the term "behavioral audiogram" suggests a less-than-gold standard of measurement, in fact one goal of physiological measures is to help estimate the behaviorally-elicited pure tone audiogram.

Figure 1 shows examples of pure tone audiograms. On the horizontal axis, frequency is plotted in octave intervals, an octave being a doubling of frequency in Hertz (Hz). The audiogram generally covers the range 125 to 8000 Hz or 250 to 8000 Hz. Measurement of acuity for frequencies higher than 8000 Hz is of interest for certain purposes such as early ototoxicity, but of less value for estimating functional auditory ability in daily life. Measurement of acuity for intermediate frequencies within an octave is advised when the audiometric curve rises or falls 20 dB or more in adjacent octaves. On the vertical axis, hearing thresholds are plotted in decibels hearing level (dB HL), with the 0 dB HL line representing average thresholds for the normally hearing young adult ear with a negative otologic history. Thus, 0 dB HL does not represent absence of sound, but rather the normal reference for perfect hearing at the frequency being measured, corrected for the normal human auditory sensitivity curve which detects sounds of 1000 to 4000 Hz at weaker intensities than lower or higher frequencies. Most clinical audiograms allow thresholds of −10 dB HL through 120 dB HL to be plotted, although the audiometer being used may not produce sounds as high as 120 dB HL at all test frequencies. The audiogram is measured in a sound-treated test suite. Low-frequency thresholds are elevated significantly if measured in a typical quiet room that is not an audiometric test suite.

The audiometric symbols key shown with Figure 1 displays symbols recommended by the American Speech-Language-Hearing Association.[1] Air conduction audiograms may be measured for separate ears using supra-aural earphones or insert earphones. The audiogram also should be obtained through a bone conduction oscillator for any frequency in the 250–4000 Hz range at which hearing thresholds exceed 15–20 dB HL. If the child does not accept the wearing of headgear for audiometric measurement, the air conduction audiogram may be obtained by delivering sounds through loudspeakers in a calibrated "sound field." It is important to note that

Pediatric Otolaryngology, Edited by R.F. Wetmore, H.R. Muntz, and T.J. McGill. Thieme Medical Publishers, Inc., New York © 2000.

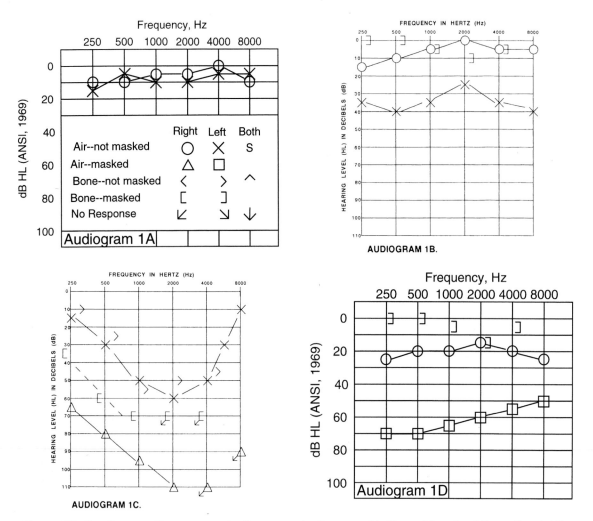

Figure 10–1:   Ear-specific pure tone audiograms. *Audiogram 1A:* Normal hearing bilaterally. *Audiogram 1B:* Normal hearing in the right ear; mild conductive hearing loss in the left ear. *Audiogram 1C:* Moderate sensorineural hearing loss with saucer-shaped audiometric contour in the left ear; profound sensorineural hearing loss in the right ear. *Audiogram 1D:* Minimal hearing loss in the right ear; maximal conductive hearing loss in the left ear.

the sound field audiogram reflects the hearing sensitivity of the better-hearing ear, if an ear difference should happen to exist, no matter whether the left or right speaker is used to deliver stimuli.

Audiogram 1A (Fig. 10-1) shows normal hearing bilaterally, from the standpoint of threshold sensitivity; one measures the clarity of speech perception separately as it may vary even with a normal audiogram. If the child had not tolerated earphones and the audiogram had been obtained in the sound field, the resulting audiogram might be that depicted in Figure 10-2A, assuming that the child was able to attend to threshold-level stimuli. Audiogram 1B shows normal hearing in the right ear and a mild conductive hearing loss in the left ear. Note, however, that a sound field audiogram for the same child

(Audiogram 2B in Fig. 10-2) would have shown only the better-ear thresholds. The amount of hearing loss present in the left ear in Audiogram 2B is slightly greater than the average 23-25 dB conductive hearing loss seen in the presence of asymptomatic middle ear effusion,[2] but the configuration is typical of the audiogram seen with middle ear effusion, with best hearing at 2000 Hz.

SPECIAL CONSIDERATION:

It is important to note that the sound field audiogram reflects the hearing sensitivity of the better-hearing ear.

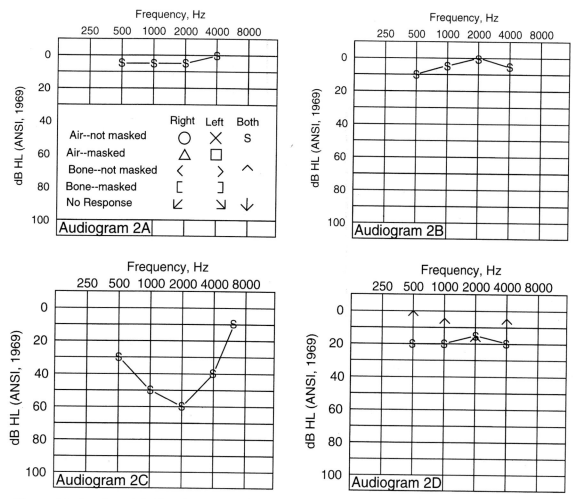

Figure 10–2: Sound field audiograms, which are not ear-specific and represent better-ear response thresholds when an ear difference does happen to exist. Audiograms 2A through 2D are the sound field audiograms one could expect corresponding to ear-specific audiograms 1A through 1D. *Audiogram 2A:* Normal hearing for the better ear. *Audiogram 2B:* Normal hearing for the better ear. *Audiogram 2C:* Moderate hearing loss with a saucer-shaped audiometric contour for the better ear. *Audiogram 2D:* Minimal hearing loss with normal cochlear sensitivity for the better ear.

When frequency-specific stimuli are presented in the sound field, conventional pure tones are not used because standing waves may render their calibration inaccurate in a closed room. Therefore, pulsed tones, warbled tones, or narrow band noise stimuli are presented for sound field testing.

While a sound field audiogram may include frequencies from 250–6000 Hz (but not 8000 Hz due to inaccuracy of calibration in the presence of standing waves in a room), often only 500–4000 Hz stimuli are presented in the sound field. Such a practice can miss valuable information. For example, Audiogram 1C in Figure 10–1 shows a moderate sensorineural hearing loss with a deep saucer-shaped contour. The right ear shows a profound sensorineural hearing loss. Note that the corresponding sound

field audiogram (2C in Fig. 10–2) captures the better-ear thresholds. Testing 6000 Hz helped to define the saucer-shaped contour, but adding 250 Hz would have provided even better definition and would have explained why this child is able to detect that speech is present at ''normal'' threshold levels despite a very significant hearing loss. The right ear (Audiogram 1C) was tested by air and bone conduction while a masking noise was presented to the left ear to preclude its participation by crossover of the stimulus to the nontest ear. Note that bone conduction thresholds are recorded for low frequencies in the right ear which reflect only vibrotactile sensation and not hearing, and a conductive component is not suspected. Bone conducted signals can be detected by vibration rather than hearing beginning at approximately these levels: 25 dB HL at 250 Hz; 55 dB HL at 500 Hz; and 70 dB HL at 1000 Hz. The frequencies 2000 and 4000 Hz cannot be detected by tactile sensation at 70 dB HL, which usually is the upper limit that the bone conduction oscillator produces at those frequencies.

Audiogram 1D in Figure 10–1 shows a very mild hearing loss in the right ear and a moderately severe conductive hearing loss in the left ear. The audiogram for the left ear is the maximum degree of conductive hearing loss possible, and is typical of an ear with atresia of the external auditory meatus. The corresponding sound field audiogram (2D in Fig. 10–2) shows only the nearly normal thresholds for the better ear. The bone conduction audiogram, obtained without masking, is not ear-specific and could be misconstrued as showing the cochlear sensitivity of the right ear, which indeed has not been measured and may or may not be better than the right air conduction audiogram.

Test Methods

Behavioral audiometry requires that the child's responses be brought under the control of the stimulus. In other words, some response within the child's spontaneous or taught repertoire is structured in such a way that it occurs reliably when and only when the child hears the stimulus. To engage the child in such a listening task and to judge whether a definitive behavioral response has occurred requires the skill of an audiologist experienced in testing children, particularly in the case of children younger than 4 or 5 years of age.

Conventional audiometry (age 4 or 5 years and older)

The child is asked to raise her hand or push a button every time she hears a tone. The audiogram is obtained for separate ears through earphones, and also using a bone conduction oscillator at any frequency exhibiting hearing loss. A masking noise is introduced into the non-test ear whenever bone conduction thresholds are more than 10 dB better than air conduction thresholds, and whenever a difference of 40 dB or more exists between the air conduction thresholds of the test ear and the bone conduction thresholds of the non-test ear.

Conditioned play audiometry (developmental age 2 to 4 or 5 years)

The child is shown, nonverbally, how to wait, listen, and perform a repetitive play task such as placing a peg in a pegboard every time he hears a tone. The audiogram usually is obtained through earphones and (if appropriate) a bone conduction oscillator, but it may be necessary to use sound field audiometry for some 2-year-olds, who do not always accept earphones. When conditioned play audiometry is performed for a child wearing earphones, a single-audiologist test paradigm (with the audiologist operating the audiometer at a small table in the same room with the child) succeeds. When this test is performed in the sound field, a second audiologist helps to keep the child on task. Thresholds obtained using conditioned play audiometry are as reliable as those obtained using conventional audiometry.

> ## SPECIAL CONSIDERATION:
> Thresholds obtained using conditioned play audiometry are as reliable as those obtained using conventional audiometry.

Visual reinforcement audiometry (VRA; developmental age 6 months to 2 years)

A typical arrangement of the audiometric suite for VRA is shown in Figure 10–3. A second audiologist who is a highly trained observer faces the child, who may be on a parent's lap or in a special positioning chair with a tray. Earphones, bone conduction oscillator, or loudspeakers may be used to deliver stimuli. If the child looks up or to the side on hearing the stimulus, the child is rewarded by activation of a lighted toy. Although it is not always possible (nor necessary) to demonstrate hearing better than 20 dB HL for all frequencies in a normally hearing toddler using VRA, response thresholds obtained by VRA for a normally developing child age 9 or 10 months and older with hearing loss typically match the true audiogram very closely, but are likely to be suprathreshold for 6-to-8 month old babies tested by VRA. The audiologist's impression of test reliability is helpful in judging whether the obtained response thresholds represent true thresholds of hearing sensitivity.

If a second audiologist is not available as the observer, necessitating that the parent be trained to attract the child's visual attention to the midline and

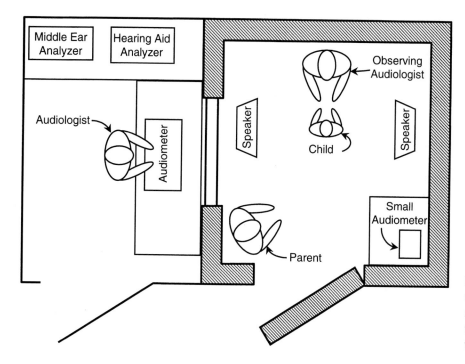

Figure 10-3: Typical setup of sound-treated audiology suite, arranged for behavioral audiometric testing of the infant or toddler using two audiologists.

down between responses but not to give any clues as to when a stimulus has been presented, the results will vary in reliability depending upon the parent's acumen. In a single-audiologist test paradigm, one may obtain instrumentation which allows the audiologist both to present the test stimuli and to activate the visual reinforcer from the same room as the child, to allow the audiologist to structure the child's attention and act as the observer as well as the tester. For a sound field audiogram using VRA, presenting stimuli from each side of the child is not necessary. It is possible to present all stimuli from the same loudspeaker, removing the overlaying task of localization which may give clues to ear differences in hearing but does not measure them.

Behavioral Observation Audiometry (BOA; developmental age 0 to 5 months)

BOA requires the same room arrangement as VRA. BOA may be employed for infants or developmentally delayed children who are not able to turn their head or eyes reliably toward the anticipated visual reinforcer during VRA. Any response on the part of the child, such as cessation of sucking on a pacifier, eye widening, or momentary breath-holding on presentation of a sound, may be accepted if repeatable and if it does not also occur randomly between stimuli. An audiogram obtained by BOA is likely to be suprathreshold by an indeterminate amount and should serve as an adjunctive measure

to physiological (evoked potential and/or otoacoustic emissions) test results. The use of "normative" values for the decibel level at which a baby under 6 months of age is likely to show responses to sound can be dangerously misleading, as a normally hearing baby age 4 months may react to speech at 40 dB HL but a baby the same age with a 30 dB sensory hearing loss also may react to speech at 40 dB HL.

Speech Audiometry

Measures of a child's responses to speech stimuli not only corroborate the pure tone audiogram, but also may provide information about the clarity of sound received and perceived. Speech audiometric tests may be presented through earphones for separate ears, through a bone conduction oscillator, or in a calibrated sound field. When speech audiometry is performed in the sound field, it may be for the purpose of assessing unaided function or for assessing the benefit of hearing aids or a cochlear implant speech processor.

The *speech awareness threshold (SAT)* or *speech detection threshold (SDT)* is the weakest intensity at which the child indicates awareness of the presence of sound, when a speech stimulus is presented through the audiometer using a developmentally appropriate test method (conventional audiometry, conditioned play audiometry, visual reinforcement audiometry, or behavioral observation audiometry). The SDT may be obtained for separate ears, via bone conduction, or in the sound field. When the child is responding reliably, the SDT in decibels agrees closely with the best pure tone threshold in the range of 250 to 4000 Hz. Thus, if a child clearly detects speech presented at 30 dB HL but does not respond to any frequency-specific stimuli until they reach 50 dB HL, the response thresholds for the frequency-specific stimuli are likely to be inaccurate in that they are suprathreshold. The SDT can be estimated by presenting music through the audiometric transducer so that its average intensity level is calibrated.

The *speech reception threshold (SRT)* is the weakest intensity at which the child can identify 50% of spondee words from a closed set of familiar items. A spondee word has two syllables with equal stress, such as "baseball" or "toothbrush." The child's response may be to repeat the words or to point to pictures representing the words. The SRT lies within 5 dB of the three-frequency pure tone average hearing level (the averaged pure tone thresholds at the frequencies 500, 1000, and 2000 Hz). In the case of a downward-sloping audiogram with a high frequency loss, the SRT agrees with the averaged threshold at 500 and 1000 Hz. It is possible to perform well on the SRT test by identifying only the vowels of the words and guessing at the words, when a closed set such as "baseball," "toothbrush," "hotdog," "cowboy," "ice cream," "pancake" is used. It is a common clinical observation that children can hear "ice cream" 5 dB weaker than other words. An SRT more than 10 dB better than the pure tone audiogram suggests that the pure tone audiogram may be wrong; the child either was not listening well for the audiogram or was malingering. Likewise, an SRT significantly poorer than the pure tone audiogram suggests that the audiologist may have been accepting some false positive responses on the audiogram.

SPECIAL CONSIDERATION:

An SRT more than 10 dB better than the pure tone audiogram suggests that the pure tone audiogram may be wrong.

Measures of *speech recognition,* more commonly called "speech discrimination" in the past, estimate the child's ability to hear speech clearly when it is presented at a comfortable listening level, 30 to 50 dB above the SRT. Alternatively, speech recognition tests may be given at a level of 50 dB HL even in the presence of partial hearing loss, to estimate the child's ability to perceive speech at a conversational intensity. The tests may be administered by calibrated live voice through the audiometer, or using recorded materials presented through the audiometer. Speech recognition tests fall into various categories. "Closed set" tests give the child a preset group of choices from which the stimulus items are chosen. Closed-set tests usually involve pointing to one of a set of pictures when the item is named. "Open set" tests give no range of choices, so that any response is possible. The scoring of open-set tests can be complicated when the child's speech articulation ability is not normal. If the child repeats a word erroneously, he may have heard it correctly but not have been able to reproduce all the sounds because of his developing speech patterns. When a hearing impaired child is seen for repeated monitoring of unaided and aided hearing over time, and when the child "graduates" from a relatively easy closed-set picture-pointing test of speech recognition such as the Word Intelligibility by Picture Identification (WIPI) test[3] or the NU-CHIPS Test[4] to a more difficult open-set test requiring word repetition without clues, such as the Lexical Neighborhood Test (LNT)[5] or the Phonetically Balanced Kindergarten (PBK) word lists,[6] the child's speech recognition score appears to drop, but the reason is the use of a more difficult test rather than a genuine decline in speech perception ability.

The need to evaluate candidacy and benefit for cochlear implants in children has spurred the development and more widespread use of speech perception tests for children with minimal auditory capabilities. Pediatric speech perception tests now exist which measure the ability to hear the syllabic pattern of a word even though the phonemic content is unclear, and the ability to perceive both predictable, overlearned multiword utterances and novel sentences.

Tests of speech recognition (speech discrimination) in children should be chosen carefully to suit the intended purpose. The patient's age, language level, and hearing status should place him within the population of individuals for whom the test was designed and the population for whom normative data are reported. Only tests with clearly established validity and reliability should be chosen. The test should be administered in the manner in which it was normed, in order for the results to be interpretable. If more than one word list is available for the test, equivalency of difficulty of the various word lists must be assured, if performance under two conditions (such as using Brand X vs. Brand Y hearing aids, or after 3 vs. 6 months of cochlear implant use) is to be compared. The reader is referred to Mendel and Danhauer's thorough discussion of speech perception tests.[7]

Speech perception tests for the assessment of *central auditory processing disorders (CAPD)* are designed to test the abilities of school-aged children who have normal pure tone audiograms but have difficulty perceiving speech that is degraded in any way by background noise, competing signals in the contralateral ear, rapid rate of presentation, or filtering. CAPD tests also address abilities such as binaural integration, auditory memory, and retrieval of auditorily presented information. The child appropriate for CAPD evaluation may present with recurrent complaints from teachers of "not listening," although the child passes school hearing screening tests. He may be having difficulty following directions or reading. Because many tests designed to tax the ability of the central auditory nervous system to process complex speech[8] require presentation of recorded materials at predetermined levels in a sound-treated suite, the evaluation of CAPD involves the audiologist; however, audiological CAPD testing must not be done in isolation. One may discover central auditory processing abilities that are below age level, and yet not be aware that those very abilities are the highest skills in that child's overall cognitive and perceptual profile. CAPD testing requires a team approach including careful observation by the teacher and parent, speech and language evaluation, and usually reading and cognitive evaluations as well, to obtain a profile of the child's use of audition for information gathering, storage and retrieval. Without a team evaluation, CAPD may not be distinguishable from attention deficit disorder, or may be felt to be a single-modality deficit when a multimodal information processing deficit exists.[9]

SPECIAL CONSIDERATION:

Without a team evaluation, central auditory processing disorders may not be distinguishable from attention deficit disorder, or may be felt to be a single-modality deficit when a multimodal information processing deficit exists.

Children with sensorineural or conductive hearing loss may have central auditory processing deficits as well, but these deficits are more difficult to separate from the effects of early auditory-based language deprivation, and an accepted assessment protocol has yet to emerge.

ASSESSMENT OF MIDDLE EAR FUNCTION

Tympanometry and acoustic (stapedial) reflex testing fall in the category of measurements called middle ear immittance (impedance and admittance) measures, and are obtained using a middle ear analyzer. Immittance measures assess middle ear function, not hearing. A child with no hearing whatsoever will have normal tympanograms if the middle ears are clear. Conversely, a child with normal-range hearing may have abnormal tympanograms if any middle ear effusion is present.

Tympanometry is performed by placing a metal probe surrounded by a soft tip in the ear canal, in such a way as to obtain an air-tight seal. Through the probe, these functions are performed: a probe tone of predetermined sound pressure is introduced into the ear canal; the sound pressure level in the ear canal is measured; and varying amounts of positive and negative air pressure are created in the sealed ear canal. If the acoustic energy of the probe tone readily travels through the tympanic membrane and middle ear, the resultant sound pressure level measured in the ear canal will be low. If, however, the middle ear is resistant to the flow of acoustic energy because of middle ear effusion or ossicular fixation, then the sound pressure level measured in the ear canal will be higher. In the normally functioning ear, the middle ear system shows its highest admittance (i.e., is most compliant or most efficient in transmitting acoustic energy) when atmospheric pressure is present in the ear canal, as shown in the normal tympanogram in Figure 10-4. If a negative middle ear pressure exists in the middle ear, then the introduction of a negative pressure (partial vacuum) into the sealed ear canal brings the retracted tympanic membrane into a normal position and allows it to move and transmit energy most efficiently. In this case, the peak of the tympanogram would be shifted to the left, in accordance with the amount of pressure in decaPascals (daPa) needed in order for maximal admittance to be achieved. A negative middle ear pressure may be quite variable and may

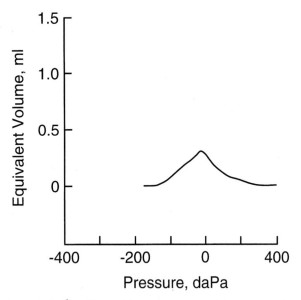

Figure 10–4: Normal tympanogram, obtained on a two year old child. Equivalent ear canal volume, the pressure at which peak admittance is observed, and static admittance are recorded.

be created, for example, by sniffing or by holding the nose while swallowing. A positive pressure may be seen on occasion in acute otitis media but also may be seen in a normal ear immediately upon awakening from sleep. A flat tympanogram with no peak, in the absence of complete cerumen impaction, correlates highly with the presence of middle ear effusion but does not predict its viscosity nor the degree of hearing loss associated with it. On rare occasion, a flat tympanogram may be seen in the presence of ossicular anomalies without middle ear effusion; however, an ear with ossicular fixation may show a normal tympanogram because it is the function of the most peripheral portion of the middle ear (the tympanic membrane) which is being measured by the tympanogram.

The values recorded for a tympanogram include the equivalent ear canal volume (which includes the middle ear if the tympanic membrane is not intact); peak pressure (the pressure at which maximal admittance of acoustic energy occurs); static admittance (the difference in admittance between the peak and the value recorded when the tympanic membrane is stiffened by creating a positive pressure of +200 daPa or more in the canal); and the gradient or tympanometric width.

The ear canal volume measure is extremely useful in assessing patency of pressure-equalization (PE)

tubes or presence of tympanic membrane perforation, when either happens to be difficult to visualize. For children age 1 to 7 years, equivalent ear canal volumes measured during tympanometry with intact tympanic membranes are 0.3 to 0.9 cc (5th to 95th percentile) but 1.0 to 5.5 cc in the presence of patent PE tubes[10]. Thus, the ear canal volume reading in the presence of patent PE tubes is more than double the volume seen when the tympanic membrane is intact or when the tube is blocked. A large volume reading in itself does not distinguish between a patent PE tube and a tympanic membrane perforation. In either case, the tympanogram for a non-intact tympanic membrane will be flat, with a high canal volume. When a PE tube is blocked, a normal tympanogram may be obtained if the middle ear is well aerated, or a flat tympanogram if there is middle ear effusion.

Tympanograms may be spuriously normal for infants under 6 months of age. While a flat tympanogram with a patent ear canal under 6 months of age does suggest middle ear effusion, a normal tympanogram may reflect a compliant ear canal wall in the presence of middle ear effusion. The use of a probe tone higher than the usual 226 Hz may reveal a flat curve in a young infant with middle ear effusion.

SPECIAL CONSIDERATION:

Tympanograms may be spuriously normal for infants under 6 months of age.

Infants under one year of age have abnormal tympanograms if their static admittance (height of the peak) is less than 0.2 ml or their tympanometric width greater than 235 daPa.[11] Children one year to school age have abnormal tympanograms if the static admittance is less than 0.3 ml or the tympanometric width greater than 200 daPa.[12,13]

Middle ear immittance also is used to measure the acoustic reflex, or the contraction of stapedius and tensor tympani muscles in response to tones that are 70 to 95 dB above threshold in the normal ear, and are approximately 10 dB better when recorded ipsilaterally to the reflex-eliciting stimulus than when recorded contralaterally.[14] The reflex is absent or not measurable in the presence of middle ear effusion, non-intact tympanic membrane, cerumen impaction, cochlear hearing loss greater than about 80 dB, or some hearing losses of retrocochlear origin. The reflex threshold may be normal in an ear with a partial hearing loss of cochlear origin. Because the acoustic reflex may happen to be absent in some individuals when there is no otologic abnormality, absence of the reflex is not a reliable flag for hearing abnormalities. However, the presence of the reflex confirms both the intact nature of the neural reflex arc and also the absence of significant middle ear effusion in the ear from which the reflex is being recorded

---

AT A GLANCE . . .

Values Recorded by the Tympanogram

1. Equivalent ear canal volume: includes the middle ear if the tympanic membrane is not intact
2. Peak pressure: the pressure at which maximal admittance of acoustic energy occurs
3. Static admittance: the difference in admittance between the peak and the value recorded when the tympanic membrane is stiffened by creating a positive pressure of +200 daPa or more in the canal
4. Gradient or tympanometric width: distance in data between the sides of the tympanogram at half the height of the peak

---

PHYSIOLOGICAL MEASURES OF HEARING

Several techniques exist for measuring the sound-evoked physiologic response of the auditory system. Of these, the measure most frequently used for testing infants and for children with developmental delay is the *Auditory Brainstem Response (ABR)*. The ABR represents changes in electrical activity from the auditory nerve to midbrain level, in the first 15 to 20 msec after the onset of a sound. These changes are recorded by 3 or 4 surface scalp electrodes and are time-locked to the onset of a repetitive sound such as a mixed-frequency click or a tone burst with rapid onset. The ABR waveform in re-

sponse to high-intensity clicks consists of a predictable series of vertex-positive waves. Wave I represents discharge of the auditory nerve, while subsequent waves may have multiple contributors. Wave V, most identifiable by the downslope which follows it, is the most robust and is the only wave which may be tracked down to audiometric threshold levels.

The ABR test may be used in adults or older children who are awake but resting quietly, if the only measure needed is that of peak and interpeak latencies of the response to high-intensity signals, for the purpose of assessing neural conduction times in brainstem auditory pathways. When the ABR is used for threshold estimation, however, the patient must be sleeping, with or without sedation. ABR thresholds reported for children who were awake or restless during the test are not to be trusted. Typically, babies under 6 months of age can be tested in an unsedated sleep after a feeding. Children age 6 months and older usually are sedated with chloral hydrate for the ABR test.

Auditory stimuli for the ABR test may be delivered by air conduction, usually with insert earphones, or by bone conduction, with masking as needed. A broad-spectrum, single-polarity (rarefaction or condensation) repetitive click signal 100 microseconds in duration is the stimulus most commonly used to elicit the ABR. Clicks of alternating polarity are not recommended because Wave V may have a slightly different latency in response to each polarity, making the averaged response less sharp, and because cochlear microphonic responses may average themselves out to a flat line if alternating polarity is used.[15] The response pattern to clicks is well understood for infants of different preterm and post-term ages.[16-18] The ABR response threshold to clicks alone best estimates hearing sensitivity (within 5 to 10 dB) in the frequency range 1000 Hz and above. It is quite possible for an infant to have a click-evoked ABR response of 20 to 25 dB HL and yet to have a significant frequency-specific loss of hearing at 4000 Hz, at 250 to 1000 Hz, or even a deep saucer-shaped audiogram which yields a near-normal click-evoked ABR threshold if hearing is normal at 8000 Hz. The click-evoked threshold reflects the best threshold for audiometric frequencies 1000 Hz and above. To obtain frequency-specific thresholds helpful in the differential diagnosis of the hearing loss and for the purpose of hearing aid fitting, three methods are available: (1) tone bursts presented in quiet, (2) derived-band technique, and (3) notched noise technique, any of which can provide a reasonable estimate of the audiometric contour.[19] Wave V latency is longer in response to low-frequency than high-frequency stimuli, consistent with longer basilar membrane travel time to the point of maximal excitation for lower frequency stimuli. Because the tone bursts must have a sharp onset in order to elicit synchronous discharge of auditory neurons, the tone bursts used for ABR testing are not as frequency-specific as those used for behavioral audiometry. Thus, a steeply sloping high frequency hearing loss (more than 20 dB drop in thresholds for adjacent octaves) will be predicted by ABR to be more shallow in contour than it actually is.

SPECIAL CONSIDERATION:

Definitive assessment of outer and middle ear status on the day of a threshold ABR evaluation is critical.

Figure 10–5A shows normal ABR waveforms of a 4-month-old. Figure 10–5B shows a click threshold series for a 10-month-old baby with a 55 dB sensorineural hearing loss. As is typical in a mild or moderate hearing loss of cochlear origin, peak latencies of the various waves at a high intensity (80 dB HL) fall within normal limits, so that a normal ABR waveform at a high intensity by no means rules in normal hearing. In a conductive hearing loss (Fig. 10–5C), wave latencies are delayed such that the response mimics that of the normal ear at a decibel level higher by the amount of conductive loss (i.e., the response to 60 dB HL clicks in the presence of a 40 dB conductive loss is similar to the response to 20 dB HL clicks in the ear with an audiometric threshold of 0 dB HL). A steeply sloping high frequency sensorineural loss, however, can yield click-evoked ABR responses with delayed Wave I latency that could masquerade as a conductive loss, if only air-conducted clicks are used. The addition of frequency-specific and of bone-conducted signals (Fig. 10–5D) in such a case differentiates between conductive and sensorineural loss.

The acoustic stimulus used to elicit the ABR response by air conduction does pass through the outer and middle ear, and thus cerumen impaction and middle ear effusion elevate the ABR thresholds. Definitive assessment of outer and middle ear status

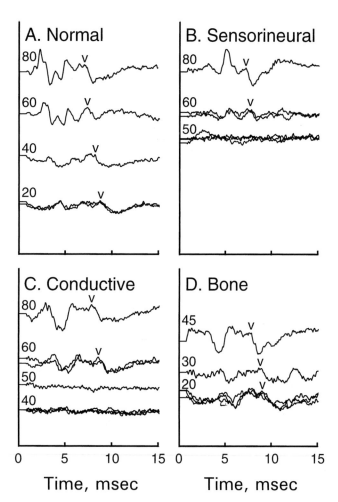

Figure 10–5: Auditory brainstem response (ABR) waveforms. *A:* Threshold series recorded to clicks from a four-month old female with normal hearing. *B:* Responses of a 10-month-old with sensorineual hearing loss. Note that the 80-dB response, just 20 decibels above threshold, has normal latency. *C:* Responses in conductive hearing loss. The type of hearing impairment is not always evident from the waveforms and latencies. *D:* Responses to bone-conducted clicks in the same infant. The normal bone-conduction thresholds confirm the loss in 5C as conductive.

on the day of a threshold ABR evaluation is critical. Cerumen should be removed, the ears examined, and tympanometry performed prior to rather than following the ABR test.

ABR waveforms in infants may be abnormal either by virtue of elevated threshold or absence of response, or by virtue of abnormal waveform configuration. Absence of a response is most often associated with profound sensorineural hearing loss, but a similar finding may be seen in "auditory neuropathy," in which outer hair cell function is normal as indicated by normal otoacoustic emissions. Such results—absence of an ABR with normal otoacoustic emissions—suggests a lack of synchronous firing of the auditory nerve, but does not tell us whether this lack of synchronous activity is due to peripheral abnormality at the level of the cochlea, for example absence of inner hair cells, or to a neural abnormality. This pattern of test results has been termed "auditory neuropathy" but does not suggest a particular underlying pathology. The ABR test itself may suggest auditory neuropathy. If single-polarity click stimuli are used, a cochlear microphonic potential may be seen in the first milliseconds of the display, confirming a cochlear response; this potential is reversed if stimulus polarity is reversed. The examiner must take care not to mistake this potential for a neural response. If tone-burst stimuli are employed, a similar waveform maybe seen, but here the early "waves" represent the electrical stimulus being delivered to the earphone but picked up by scalp electrodes as though it were physiological activity. Because the tone burst stimuli are longer in duration with lower stimulus frequency, the stimulus artifact to tone bursts may give the appearance of an abnormal cochlear response, but indeed the stimulus artifact ends at the termination of the stimulus and does not indicate a physiological response of the auditory system.

Otoacoustic emissions (OAEs) were described by Kemp[20] as tiny sounds present in the ear canal that are generated by the cochlea. OAEs are measured using a probe in the ear canal. Unlike ABR, the measurement of OAEs does not require scalp electrodes. OAEs may be spontaneous or evoked. Evoked OAEs have demonstrated significant clinical utility for assessing the function of outer hair cells, which are felt to generate their emissions by mechanical activity in response to the presentation of sounds. The understanding of OAEs and their application is expanding rapidly. OAEs are absent in ears having greater than 30 to 50 dB of hearing loss, and so the presence of normal OAEs strongly suggests normal cochlear sensitivity. OAEs are generated entirely preneurally and thus do not predict the ability of the child to perceive sound using the entire auditory system.

SPECIAL CONSIDERATION:

OAEs are generated entirely preneurally and do not predict the ability of the child to perceive sound using the entire auditory system.

Evoked OAEs fall into two categories. Transient evoked OAEs (TEOAEs) are evoked using a brief transient signal such as a click. A train of clicks is presented with stimulus inversion such that the stimulus cancels itself out in the ear canal, allowing the cochlear emission to be recorded. The broadband spectrum of the stimulus is mimicked by a broad-band emission which continues after stimulus termination, recorded from the normal ear. The response must not only be reproducible, but also must exceed the noise floor in the ear canal. In TEOAEs, the stimulus is not frequency-specific but the spectrum of the emission provides clues to the function of different frequency regions of the cochlea.

Distortion product OAEs (DPOAEs) are generated not by a transient click but rather by two pure tones that lie close to one another in frequency and intensity. The emission is a nonlinear response of the cochlea and is measurable at the frequency $(2f_1-f_2)$, where f_1 is the frequency of the lower tone and f_2 is the frequency of the higher tone. In Figure 10–6, for example, f_1 and f_2 are 2000 and 2400 Hz, respectively. The emission frequency is $(2 \times 2000-2400)$ or 1600 Hz. Other distortion products also may be present, but $(2f_1-f_2)$ has the highest amplitude and thus the greatest clinical utility. The effective stimulus frequency is felt to be f_2 or just apical to it.

Figure 10–7 shows screening OAEs recorded from a newborn, showing robust OAEs for the left ear and absent OAEs on the right. A clear outer and middle ear is necessary for OAEs to be recorded. The absence of OAEs may indicate a non-patent ear canal, non-aerated middle ear, or lack of normal outer hair cell function. DPOAEs are recordable in individuals with slightly greater degree of hearing loss than TEOAEs may be recorded, but DPOAEs are absent when the cochlear hearing loss exceeds 40 or 50 dB.[21,22] Thus, absence of OAEs, even in the presence of clear outer and middle ears, cannot distinguish between mild-to-moderate and profound hearing loss.

Because of the relative simplicity of administration of OAE measurement, with no electrode application required, OAEs already have established their clinical utility in several areas including newborn hearing screening (Fig. 10–8), evaluation of malingerers, and monitoring of hearing during repeated or extended courses of ototoxic medications. In these cases, the primary function of the OAE measurement is to confirm normal hair cell function as a place-holder for behavioral or ABR threshold estimation. However, the more basic contribution of

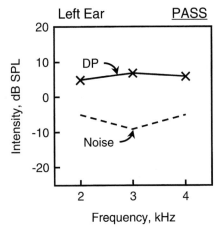

Figure 10–6: Distortion product otoacoustic emissions (DPOAE). In the normal ear, interactions between the probe tones, f_1 and f_2, give rise to distortion. The distortion product radiates from the cochlea through the middle ear to the ear canal, where it can be detected by spectral analysis.

OAEs to the measurement of auditory function, from the standpoint of historical novelty, is the ability to separate the measurement of cochlear function from the measurement of the function of the entire auditory pathway.

AT A GLANCE . . .

Audiological Test Methods

1. Conventional audiometry
2. Conditioned play audiometry
3. Visual reinforcement audiometry (VRA)
4. Behavioral observation audiometry (BOA)
5. Speech audiometry
6. Speech perception tests
7. Central auditory processing (CAP) tests
8. Tympanometry
9. Acoustic reflex testing
10. Auditory brainstem response (ABR)
11. Otoacoustic emissions (OAEs)

NEWBORN HEARING SCREENING

Prior to 1993, few hospitals provided newborn hearing screening tests except perhaps for those infants identified as having risk factors (indicators) for hearing loss. Such an approach identifies at best 50% of infants with hearing loss, as the others have no indicators apparent at birth. The average age of diagnosis of permanent hearing impairment at that time was felt to be 30 months, although documentation is lacking for this estimate. In 1993, the National Institutes of Health held a Consensus Conference. The result of this discussion[23] was to recommend that all newborns receive a hearing screening test within the first 3 months of life, with awareness that the practical means of accomplishing such universal screening in the US would be to screen all babies prior to discharge from the newborn nursery. In 1994, the Joint Committee on Infant Hearing,[24] a multiagency group, supported identification of all

Figure 10–7: Distortion Product Otoacoustic Emissions (DPOAE) screening results. The commonly used response detection criteria require that the emission itself exceed some value, and that the signal-to-noise ratio—the distance between the emission and the noise floor—be great enough that a false negative is unlikely. This infant passed on the left, with robust emissions at all frequencies, but not on the right.

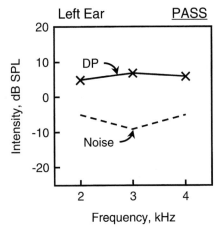

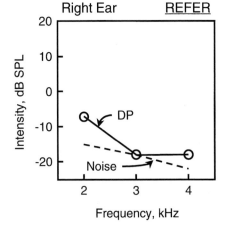

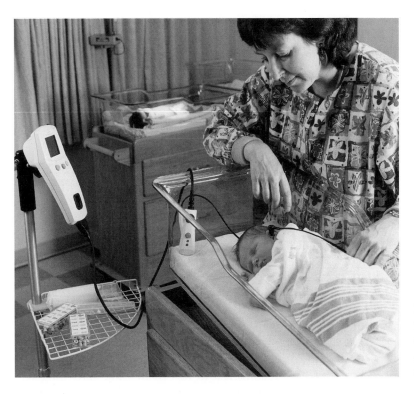

Figure 10–8: Instrument for distortion product otoacoustic emissions (DPOAE) screening which can be hand-held or mounted on a stand. (Courtesy of Grason-Stadler, Inc.)

infants with hearing impairment by 3 months of age and onset of habilitative programming by 6 months of age. The Joint Committee added a list of indicators associated with late-onset hearing loss and a recommendation for monitoring them.

Despite the inevitable wrangling over program costs, unnecessary aggravation for parents of newborns with false positive results on their screening test, and potential disruption of parental bonding with the infant, several states (16 as of this writing) have passed legislation intended to mandate or support the screening of all newborns prior to hospital discharge. The work of Christine Yoshinaga-Itano et al.[25] helped bolster the newborn screening effort by demonstrating that children with normal cognition whose hearing losses were identified before 6 months of age demonstrated significantly better receptive and expressive language scores than children with normal cognition whose hearing losses were identified after 6 months of age, regardless of degree of hearing loss or several demographic variables.

Methods available for universal newborn hearing screening include both transient-evoked otoacoustic emissions (TEOAEs) and distortion product OAEs (DPOAEs) in either diagnostic or automated form, and auditory brainstem response (ABR) in diagnostic or automated form. Automated versions of these tests compare the newborn's response to an internal criterion and read "pass" or "refer," whereas diagnostic versions of the test require waveform interpretation. Automated screening test methods clearly have advantages for the newborn nursery setting because a larger number of nursery staff or technicians can be trained to perform the screenings. While OAE screens have a lower cost of disposables and less set-up time because no scalp electrodes are needed, ABR screens have a lower initial failure rate and fewer babies need rescreens. Although OAE is a viable alternative to automated ABR in the well baby nursery, a combination of OAE and ABR screens is helpful in the NICU to unveil cases of normal cochlear function but abnormal auditory nerve activation. A failure to pass an OAE screen is likely to be unimportant if the ABR result is normal, but a failure to pass the ABR screen requires attention even if the OAE screen was normal. Regardless of the initial test method, rescreen to achieve a referral rate no higher than 3% from a well baby nursery is advised, because a high refer rate leads to a low follow-up rate. Given an incidence of permanent hearing loss detectable in newborns of 4 per 1000, then the following holds true: for every 1000 babies screened, 30 do not pass the test. Of those 30, 4 have permanent hearing loss, of which 1 is profoundly deaf, 2 have partial bilateral hearing loss, and 1 has unilateral loss. Of the 26 false positives, perhaps 2 will have important but treatable conductive hearing loss worth finding early, and the remainder may not have passed the screen for technical or transient causes. Bilateral "refers" are the most urgent to follow up quickly and are less likely to have been false positive results than unilateral "refers."

The appropriate follow-up for a baby referred from a newborn hearing screening program, following rescreen, is a diagnostic ABR evaluation, which should occur within one month for a bilateral "refer." If results are not within normal limits, OAE measures should be performed. Multifrequency tympanometry may help to uncover cases of middle ear effusion which may be difficult to visualize. Close communication with the pediatrician and referral to an otolaryngologist should take place. If the hearing loss is bilateral and not amenable to medical or surgical treatment, hearing aids should be fitted without significant delay, unless the hearing loss is profound and the family already communicates fluently in American Sign Language which does not require hearing aid use. The parents are urged to learn about the various options available to them for specialized early intervention services and communication modalities and should not be forced to choose a program or method before they have solid, unbiased information about various approaches. Parents who have discovered their child's hearing

loss via universal newborn screening receive a diagnosis they had neither suspected nor sought, at a time when they are still exhausted from childbirth and learning to feed and diaper the baby. They need time to understand what the diagnosis means, but usually are thankful that the child's hearing loss was found at birth.

> ## SPECIAL CONSIDERATION:
>
> As soon as a bilateral hearing loss has been documented and is not felt to be transient, there is no reason for delay in fitting hearing aids, even if the baby is only one or two months old.

The result on a newborn hearing screening test can be a valuable diagnostic aid for the otolaryngologist. If the baby passed the newborn screen but later presents with hearing loss, an etiology typical of progressive loss may be suspected. Table 10-1 de-

TABLE 10-1:   Possible Long-Term Outcomes From Four Newborn Screening Results, Showing Bases for False Positives and False Negatives, and Possible Reasons for Future Changes in Hearing Status

Permanent hearing loss at time of test?	Pass	Refer—Did Not Pass
	True Negative	*False Positive*
Yes	***Stable normal hearing may acquire hearing loss:*** With newborn indicators • Congenital CMV • Familial progressive loss • Prolonged ventilation, PPHN, ECMO No newborn indicators • Asymptomatic CMV • Later meningitis • Chemotherapy/radiation • Autoimmune hearing loss	Failure to detect response • Inadequate technique • Poor test conditions • Response does not meet instrument's criteria for "pass" Transient impairment • Debris in ear canal • Middle ear not aerated Poor or absent ABR not due to hearing loss • "Auditory neuropathy" • Hydrocephalus • Ischemia • Hyperbilirubinemia
	False Negative	*True Positive*
No	***Stable or progressive hearing loss*** Response absent but read as "present" • instrument error Response present with hearing loss • Very mild loss; passes ABR screen • Rising or saucer-shaped audiogram may pass ABR • Neural asynchrony causing auditory impairment; passes OAE	***Stable hearing loss*** ***Progressive hearing loss*** • Hereditary • CMV • Prolonged ventilation, PPHN, ECMO • Cochlear dysplasia, enlarged vestibular aqueduct • Over-amplification • Unknown etiology

picts the various ways in which a baby's hearing status may shift from its original category at the time of newborn screening. False positive results will normalize. True negative results (passed test and had normal hearing) may remain normal or hearing loss may develop; up to 10% of childhood hearing loss is acquired after birth and falls within this group. True positive hearing losses at birth may remain stable or may worsen. A very small number of false negative results may occur from newborn hearing screening. Some of these may be slight hearing losses which are milder than the screening criterion, hearing loss only in the low frequency range which may pass an ABR screen, or babies screened only by OAE who would have been found to have asynchronous ABR responses if they had been screened by ABR.

Congenital Cytomegalovirus (CMV) and Hearing Loss

Congenital CMV is important enough statistically as an etiology for hearing loss in infants to warrant separate discussion. A large-scale study involving universal screening for congenital CMV[26] showed that of all infants born with congenital CMV, only 10% are symptomatic, of which 44% have hearing loss by the age of 3 years. Of the remaining 90% of infants with congenital CMV, who are asymptomatic and would not have been suspected to have CMV without screening for it, 7.4% have hearing loss by the age of 3 years. Of hearing losses associated with congenital CMV, 21% have delayed onset in the symptomatic group and 33% have delayed onset in the asymptomatic group. Approximately 50% of each group showed progressive losses. Because congenital CMV involves 0.5 to 2.4% of all live births,[27] the incidence of sensorineural hearing loss associated with asymptomatic or undiagnosed symptomatic CMV undoubtedly accounts for a significant proportion of hearing losses of "unknown" etiology, after genetic factors have been accounted. The likely incidence of congenital CMV, coupled with the availability of antiviral therapies if initiated early, raises the question of whether a screen for CMV should be considered immediately after failure to pass a newborn hearing screening test. Practice Pathway 10-1 proposes a practice pathway for following newborns who are identified as having congenital CMV and therefore are at risk for progressive hearing loss and other sequelae.

NICU Graduates at Risk for Progressive Hearing Loss

Newborns with a history of persistent pulmonary hypertension of the newborn (PPHN)[28] or extracorporeal membrane oxygenation (ECMO) therapy are at high risk for late-onset or progressive hearing loss, with similar incidences of approximately 20-25% in the two groups. Figure 10-9 depicts a hearing loss acquired after the neonatal course in a child who underwent ECMO therapy for congenital diaphragmatic hernia. Out of 100 children seen for audiological monitoring following ECMO therapy, we found 23 with bilateral sensorineural hearing loss,

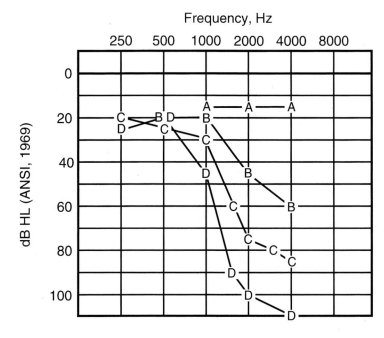

Figure 10–9: Progressive sensorineural hearing loss in a congenital diaphragmatic hernia patient status post extracorporeal membrane oxygenation (ECMO) therapy. Hearing loss was symmetrical between ears. Sequential audiograms A (obtained at age six months) through D (obtained at age 37 months) are shown.

Practice Pathway 10–1   Audiological Assessment and Management of Infants with Congenital CMV

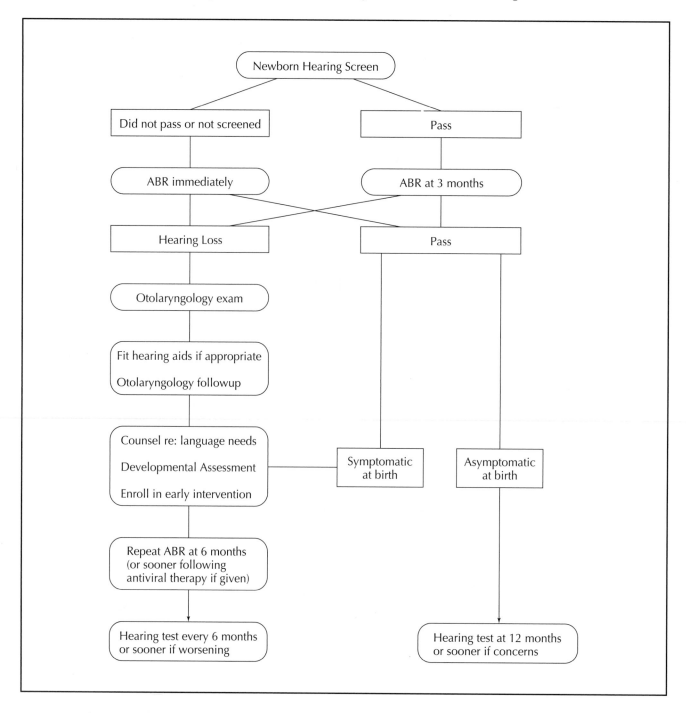

of whom 12 had progressive hearing loss, 5 of which were late in onset.[29] Therefore, infants with histories of PPHN or ECMO, regardless of newborn hearing screening results, should receive an ABR evaluation at age 6 months, behavioral audiometry at 1 year and annually thereafter to age 3 years. The Joint Committee on Infant Hearing[24] recommends follow-up for infants with a history of prolonged

mechanical ventilation and those with multiple courses of diuretics and aminoglycosides as well.

Ototoxicity of Chemotherapy and Radiation

Audiology departments in pediatric hospitals may follow significant numbers of children undergoing treatment for malignancies. Approximately 50% of

TABLE 10-2: Hearing Losses Associated with Chemotherapy and Cranial Irradiation

	Hearing Loss from Cisplatin or Carboplatin	Hearing Loss from Cranial Irradiation
Type of loss	Sensorineural (SNL)	Sensorineural, conductive (CHL) or mixed
Onset	Within hours after treatment	SNL develops months or years after treatment. CHL from middle ear changes may occur soon after treatment
Site of lesion	Damaged outer hair cells in basal turn	SNL: Damaged hair cells, support cells, and/or neurons CHL: Eustachian tube dysfunction, inflammation of middle ear mucosa, necrosis of ossicles
Other symptoms	Tinnitus in first week; resolves	Loudness intolerance during treatment; resolves
Symmetry	Symmetric	Asymmetric; depends on treatment field
Configuration	Predictable audiometric contour; high-frequency loss	Less predictable, though greatest loss is in high frequencies
Interaction	Prior or concurrent radiation exacerbates SNL from platinum compounds	

children treated with platinum compounds develop some degree of bilaterally symmetrical high frequency sensorineural hearing loss, and one-fifth to one-fourth of those 50% benefit from hearing aid use.[30] Hearing loss following cranial irradiation is less predictable in course and configuration and is seen as a late rather than immediate effect.[31] Characteristics of hearing loss associated with chemotherapy and radiation are summarized in Table 10-2.

FUNCTIONAL EFFECTS OF PERMANENT HEARING LOSS AND HABILITATION

Unilateral hearing loss does not cause delay in speech and language development but renders the child unable to localize the direction from which a sound is coming. The child with unilateral hearing loss has difficulty hearing a weak voice on the affected side and difficulty focusing on one voice in the presence of competing noises. Even with preferential classroom seating near the teacher and acoustic treatment of the classroom to reduce reverbation of background noise, academic progress should be monitored closely and supports initiated if listening-related difficulties emerge. A hearing aid in the poorer ear is rarely preferred by individuals with unilateral hearing loss. However, in school a low-power FM system with a Walkman™-style receiver and headset, or a sound field FM speaker, may be used to improve the amount by which the teacher's voice exceeds the background noise.

Children with bilateral hearing loss may experience significant psychosocial impact and educational needs, particularly in the case of late diagnosis and the resultant early language deprivation. The audiogram depicted in Figure 10-10 shows the approximate energy concentrations of speech sounds as they fall on an audiogram. If a child's audiogram falls above those sounds, they are detectable to him; if the child's audiogram falls below those sounds, they are not accessible to him at the intensities at which they occur in running speech.

As soon as a bilateral hearing loss has been documented and is not felt to be transient, there is no reason for delay in fitting hearing aids, even if the baby is only one or two months old. The process of obtaining funding for hearing aids and the necessity of earmold remakes to achieve an optimal fit tend to delay the process for a few weeks, and so prompt initiation of hearing aid fitting is advisable as soon as the family feels ready to proceed. Though newborns with severe to profound hearing loss may need to use a loaned body-level hearing aid for a few weeks or months until the fitting of power behind-the-ear aids without excessive feedback becomes feasible (usually around the time that the baby is sitting up independently), babies with mild to severe hearing loss usually can be fitted immediately with behind-the-ear hearing aids. Some young children use FM amplification even during infancy to provide distance hearing, and some instruments have FM receivers built into their hearing aid cases or into boots that fit onto the bottom of the instruments, bringing the voice of their parent or teacher transmitted by FM radio waves to their ears. In-the-ear hearing aids are not feasible for young children because of the need for frequent remakes with

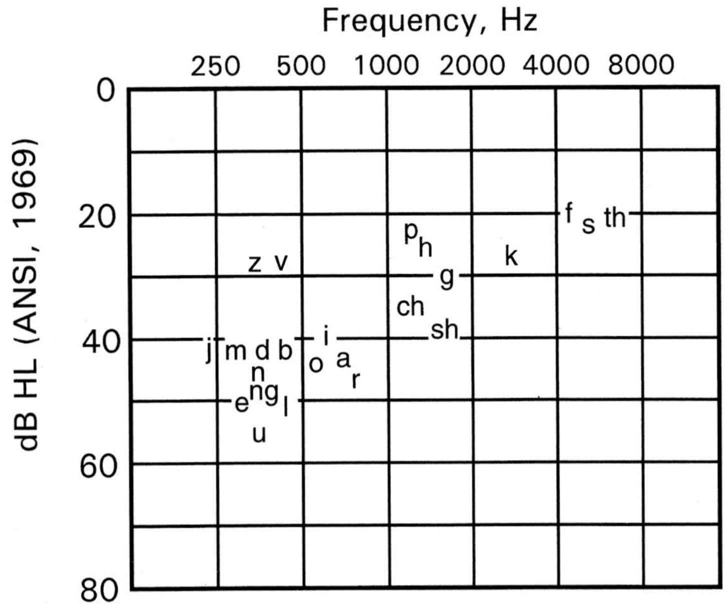

Frequency, Hz

Figure 10–10: Speech sounds. The major spectral component of each sound is plotted on audiometric coordinates. If the child's hearing is worse than the value for a given sound, the child will be unable to recognize that sound. Even mild hearing losses can affect speech recognition. Adapted from *Hearing in Children (4ᵗʰ ed)*, by Northern and Downs, Williams and Wilkins, 1991.

growth, but may be appropriate for some school-aged children with mild to moderate hearing loss.

The explosion of technology in the area of digitally programmable hearing aids, digital hearing aids, and multimicrophone directional hearing aids, all in small cases, enables infants to benefit from the same improvement in the ability to hear speech clearly that their elders are experiencing. The most consistent benefit of digital hearing aids, and of aids that are not digital but have one of the variants of wide dynamic range compression (WDRC), is that soft speech is amplified to a comfortable listening range without concomitantly amplifying loud speech to the point of distortion. Parents and audiologists face choices in hearing aid technology that may have significant financial implications, as digital hearing aids cost more than most state-supported programs for children's hearing aids can provide, and not all individuals hear better with them than with conventional hearing aids. Hearing aids for infants must be fitted with careful adjustments to the small size of their ear canals, which can result in 10–20 dB more amplification than the same instrument fitted in an adult's ear canal.

Children with mild (21 to 40 dB HL average hearing levels across the 500 to 2000 Hz range), moderate (41 to 55 dB HL), or moderately severe (56 to 70 dB HL) bilateral hearing loss benefit from the use of hearing aids and personal or sound field FM systems in the classroom, as well as speech and language therapy. With early diagnosis and prompt initiation of speech and language therapy, their speech and language may develop within normal or near

normal limits. However, with late diagnosis or concomitant conditions, speech and language may be significantly affected. The educational plan should include not only speech and language therapy but also educational supports in the form of acoustical treatment of the classroom, FM amplification, individual tutoring and teacher inservice training as needed by a teacher of the hearing impaired, and attention to social and emotional needs as well as ability to function in extracurricular activities.

SPECIAL CONSIDERATION:

The educational plan for a child with hearing loss should include not only speech and language therapy, but also educational supports and attention to emotional needs.

Children with severe (71 to 90 dB HL) and profound (greater than 90 dB HL) bilateral hearing loss generally have delayed language development, unless language has been made accessible and habilitation well under way by 6 months of age. These children vary in their ability to acquire spoken language and may need or benefit from the use of one of the several forms of visual communication (American Sign Language, total communication using both signed and spoken English, or Cued Speech). Each child and family presents an individual situation in terms of choice of communication modality and educational setting that ranges all the way from mainstreamed in regular classes with support services to residential placement at a school for the deaf. Children with profound bilateral hearing loss may be candidates for cochlear implantation if spoken language is a goal for the family and a reasonable expectation within the abilities of the child.

Regardless of choice of method and of educational placement, the audiologist, otolaryngologist, speech-language pathologist, teacher of the deaf, and parents work as a team to ensure that the child uses a language to which he has access, that the people in his environment use it effectively with him, that he is making demonstrable progress in that language sufficient to establish a basis for literacy, and that he is developing self-esteem as a successful communicator with his peers as well as with his family. The audiologist and otolaryngologist have an opportunity to monitor the child's progress, support the parents, and cheer them on in their good work through routine monitoring of hearing and ear health.

REFERENCES

1. American Speech-Language-Hearing Association: Guidelines for audiometric symbols. ASHA 1990; 32 (Suppl. 2):25-30.
2. Fria TJ, Cantekin EI, Eichler JA. Hearing acuity of children with otitis media with effusion. Arch Otolaryngol 1985; 111:10-16.
3. Ross M, Lerman J. A picture identification test for hearing impaired children. J Speech Hear Res 1979; 13:44-53.
4. Elliott LL, Katz D. Development of a new children's test of speech discrimination (Technical Manual). 1980; St. Louis, Mo., Auditec.
5. Kirk KI, Pisoni DB, Osberger MJ. Lexical effects on spoken word recognition by pediatric cochlear implant users. Ear Hear 1995; 16:470-481.
6. Haskins Ha. A phonetically balanced test of speech discrimination for children. 1949; unpublished master's thesis, Northwestern University, Evanston, IL.
7. Mendel LL, Danhauer JL. Audiologic Evaluation and Management and Speech Perception Assessment. San Diego, Singular Publishing Group, 1997.
8. Baran JA. Speech perception test materials for central auditory processing assessment. In LL Mendel and JL Danhauer (eds.): Audiologic Evaluation and Management and Speech Perception Assessment. San Diego: Singular Publishing Group, 1997, 149-168.
9. Cacace AT, McFarland DJ. Central auditory processing disorder in school-aged children: A critical review. J Speech Hear Res 1998; 41(2):355-373.
10. Shanks JE, Stelmachowicz PG, Beauchaine KL, et al. Equivalent ear canal volumes in children pre- and post-tympanostomy tube insertion. J Speech Hear Res 1992; 35:936-941.
11. Roush J, Bryant K, Mundy M, et al. Developmental changes in static admittance and tympanometric width in infants and toddlers. J Am Acad Audiol 1995; 6:334-338.
12. Nozza RJ, Bluestone CD, Kardatzke D, et al. Toward the validation of aural acoustic immittance measures for diagnosis of middle ear effusion in children. Ear Hear 1992; 13(6):442-453.
13. Nozza RJ, Bluestone CD, Kardatzke D, et al. Identification of middle ear effusion by aural acoustic admittance and otoscopy. Ear Hear 1994; 15:310-323.
14. Fria TJ, Leblanc J, Kristensen R. Ipsilateral acoustic reflex stimulation in normal and sensorineural impaired ears: A preliminary report. Can J Otolaryngol 1975; 4:695.
15. Berlin CI, Bordelon J, St. John P, et al. Reversing click polarity may uncover auditory neuropathy in infants. Ear Hear 1998; 19(1):37-47.
16. Hall JW III. Handbook of auditory evoked responses. Needham, MA: Allyn & Bacon, 1992.
17. Eggermont JJ, Salamy A. Development of ABR parameters in preterm and term born population. Ear Hear 1988; 9:283-291.
18. Cox LC, Martin RJ, Carlo WA, et al. Early ABRs in infants undergoing assisted ventilation. J Am Acad Audiol 1993; 4:13-17.
19. Gorga MP. Predicting auditory sensitivity from auditory brainstem response measurements. Semin Hear 1999; 20:29-42.
20. Kemp DT. Stimulated acoustic emissions from within the human auditory system. J Acoust Soc Am 1978; 64:1386-1391.
21. Hussain DM, Gorga MP, Neely ST, et al. Transient evoked otoacoustic emissions in patients with normal hearing and in patients with hearing loss. Ear Hear 1998; 19:434-449.
22. Gorga MP, Neely ST, Ohlrich B, et al. From laboratory to clinic: A large scale study of distortion product otoacoustic emissions in ears with normal hearing and ears with hearing loss. Ear Hear 1997; 18: 440-455.
23. NIH Consensus Statement. Identification of Hearing Impairment in Infancy and Young Children. Bethesda, MD: NIH, 1993; 11:1-24.
24. Joint Committee on Infant Hearing. Joint Committee on Infant Hearing 1994 Position Statement. Pediatrics 1995; 95:152-156.
25. Yoshinaga-Itano C, Sedey AL, Coulter DK, et al. Language of early- and later-identified children with hearing loss. Pediatrics 1998; 102(5):1161-1171.

26. Dahle A. Longitudinal study of hearing in congenital CMV. Presented at the Annual Convention, American Academy of Audiology, 1996.

27. Pass RF, Stagno S, Myers G, et al. Outcome of symptomatic congenital cytomegalivirus infection: Results of long-term longitudinal follow-up. Pediatrics 1980; 66:758–762.

28. Walton JP, Hendricks-Munoz K. Profile and stability of sensorineural hearing loss in persistent pulmonary hypertension of the newborn. J Speech Hear Res 1991; 34:1362–1370.

29. Mullen CH, Nulton C, Neault MW, et al. Late onset of hearing loss following ECMO treatment. Presented at the American Academy of Audiology, Annual Convention, 1995.

30. Kretschmar CS, Warren MP, Lavally BL, et al. Ototoxicity of preradiation cisplatin for children with central nervous system tumors. J Clin Oncol 1990; 8(7): 1191–1198.

31. Sataloff RT, Rosen DC. Effects of cranial irradiation on hearing acuity: A review of the literature. Am J Otol 1994; 15(6):772–780.

11 The Dizzy Child

Udayan K. Shah and William P. Potsic

A visit to a playground confirms children's awareness of the dizzy sensation. The plethora of spinning, whirling, and turning games testifies to the ability of even the youngest child to enjoy dizziness in play. When his perception of this spinning is pathologic and unpleasant, he may complain of imbalance or be considered unsteady by his parents or caretakers.

Management of the dizzy child requires attention to the subtle presentations of vestibulopathy and an awareness of specific disorders that can cause dizziness in younger patients (Table 11-1). In this chapter, we discuss expedient diagnosis and successful management of these children through detailing patient evaluation, outlining general management principles, and applying an understanding of these principles to selected vestibular disorders of children. We also offer a protocol for the evaluation and management of the dizzy child to guide clinical decision making (Practice Pathway 11-1).

EVALUATION OF THE DIZZY CHILD

Dizziness is the illusion of motion. The sensation of motion is termed *vertigo*. These terms often are interchanged by practitioners and patients; for the purposes of referral and management, we consider them to be equivalent here.

A complete, precise history and a physical examination often reveal the source of a child's vestibulopathy. A pre-exam questionnaire may help the family organize their thoughts and concerns and may expedite data collection for treatment and study purposes. For some patients, a videotape of one of their dizzy episodes helps the family and the examiner speak a common language.

A young child's vertigo may be made evident by periodic "frightenings," clutching caretakers, clumsiness, or bouts of nausea or vomiting.[1] Older children may be able to describe the salient characteristics of their dizzy episodes such as inciting factors, duration, and frequency, as well as accompanying auditory, visual, neurologic, or constitutional symptoms. Delayed motor function, loss of postural control, difficulty ambulating in the dark, abnormal movements or behavior, loss of consciousness, and the presence of nystagmus may also prompt a vestibular evaluation.[2,3]

AT A GLANCE...

Signs of Dizziness in Children

- "Frightenings"
- Clutching caretakers
- Clumsiness
- Periodic episodes of nausea or vomiting
- Delayed motor function
- Loss of postural control
- Difficulty with ambulating in the dark
- Abnormal movements or behavior

The relevance of recent falls, changes in medications and trauma from diving, sports, or altercations must be assessed. Children and parents should be questioned about prescription drug use (especially of diuretics, hypoglycemics, and sedatives) and the abuse of illegal drugs, primarily alcohol. An inquiry into the mother's infectious and toxic history during gestation also may be helpful. Children with exposure to the TORCH infections (i.e., toxoplasmosis,

Pediatric Otolaryngology, Edited by R.F. Wetmore, H.R. Muntz, and T.J. McGill. Thieme Medical Publishers, Inc., New York © 2000.

Practice Pathway 11–1   RECOMMENDATIONS FOR THE EVALUATION AND MANAGEMENT OF THE DIZZY CHILD

```
                    NORMAL OTOSCOPY
              ┌───────────────┴───────────────┐
          Normal                          Hearing
          hearing                          loss
            │               ┌──────────────┼──────────────────────┐
        Medical         Normal           Poor              History of
        treatment    discrimination   discrimination   Trauma or meningitis
            │          ┌────┴────┐     ┌────┼─────┐         ┌────┴────┐
        Persistent   Diet      Lab    ABR  MRI  Genetic    ABR       CT
        symptoms  Medications  test             testing
            │                                      │                  │
          MRI                                   Surgery          Medications
            │                                                        │
        Vestibular                                                Surgery
          tests
```

Abbreviations: MRI, Magnetic Resonance Imaging; ABR, Auditory Brainstem Response; CT, Computed Tomography

rubella, cytomegalovirus, and herpes) or the human immunodeficiency virus (HIV) are at greater risk for the development of vestibular disorders, as are children who have survived neonatal sepsis or who have been treated with ototoxic medications.[2] Children with hearing loss, syndromic children, and those with craniofacial anomalies are at greater risk for vestibular dysfunction. In one small study children who presented with postmeningitic deafness before the age of 2 years were shown to have greater vestibular deficits upon testing than children with "hereditary, idiopathic" hearing loss.[4] The functional results of these postmeningitis children, who were asymptomatic at the time of the study, remains unknown.[5]

Prior otologic, ocular, craniofacial, central nervous system (CNS), or spinal surgery may impair a child's vestibular system transiently or permanently.

Family history should be reviewed for hearing loss, vertigo, migraine, and seizure disorders.[2] Motivation for malingering may be revealed by understanding the impact that the dizzy episodes have on the child's actions and status within the family and school settings. Attention should be given to any resultant secondary gain.

SPECIAL CONSIDERATION:

Children who are exposed to the TORCH infections, HIV, neonatal sepsis, and ototoxic medications are at a greater risk for the development of vestibular disorders, as are children with hearing loss, syndromic children, and children with craniofacial anomalies.

TABLE 11–1: Differential Diagnosis of the Dizzy Child

Autoimmune	Cogan's syndrome
Congenital	Cerebellar hypoplasia or agenesis
	Large vestibular aqueduct
	Perilymphatic fistula
	Syndromic
Functional	Aminoglycosides
Iatrogenic	Anticonvulsants
	Chemotherapeutic drugs
	Loop diuretics
	Quinine
	Thalidomide
Infectious	Labyrinthitis—Bacterial
	Labyrinthitis—Viral
	Meningitis
	TORCH*
	Syphilis
	Vestibular neuronitis
Neoplastic	Cholesteatoma
	Posterior fossa tumor
	Vestibular schwannoma
Vascular	Benign positional vertigo of childhood
	Migraine
Traumatic	Cerumen impaction
	Labyrinthine concussion
	Perilymphatic fistula
	Temporal bone fracture
	Tympanic membrane perforation
Toxic	Alcohol abuse
	Illicit drug abuse
Unknown	Benign paroxysmal positional vertigo
	Meniere's disease
	Multiple sclerosis
	Paroxysmal torticollis of infancy

* Toxoplasmosis, rubella, cytomegalovirus, and herpes.

Physical Examination

Efficient diagnosis is achieved by concentrating on the likely causes of childhood dizziness and by utilizing tests that are readily applicable in the initial office encounter. The sequence of tests should proceed from the least uncomfortable to the one that is most likely, on the basis of the child's history, to cause nausea or vomiting. Patent external auditory canals (EAC) and middle-ear status should be confirmed during the general otolaryngologic exam prior to embarking upon the focused vestibular exam. Patients with EAC atresia have a higher incidence of labyrinthine anomalies.[6,7]

The multisystem nature of vestibulopathy requires a broad examination with survey of labyrinthine, visual, and proprioceptive influences. Measurement of sitting and standing blood pressure and pulse, auscultation for cardiac murmers and carotid bruits, and examination of the skin for neurofibromas and "café au lait" spots are recommended.[2]

Notation of obvious dysmorphic features and development delay should be made. Complete cranial nerve examination may identify clinically-silent deficits. Olfactory testing, although not routine, may be attempted using standardized batteries.[8] Flexible fiberoptic nasopharyngolaryngoscopy in children who tolerate the exam provides useful information regarding palatal and laryngeal function as well as an assessment of the nasopharynx and the eustachian tube (ET) orifices. Videotape or photographic documentation of abnormalities is useful for follow-up, referral, and educational purposes.

> **SPECIAL CONSIDERATION:**
> Tests should proceed from the least uncomfortable to the one that is most likely, based on the child's history, to cause nausea or vomiting.

Nystagmus

Determination of underlying nystagmus, palsies, and visual field defects should be made.[2] Frenzel lenses (10-diopter[2] or 20-diopter semiopaque lenses) aid in the detection of nystagmus by removing the ability to suppress nystagmus through visual fixation.

The direction of the nystagmus is named by its fast, or corrective, component. The degree of nystagmus is defined by the position of the eye when the nystagmus is noted. *First degree nystagmus* is present only when the nystagmus occurs in the direction of gaze. *Second degree nystagmus* occurs in neutral gaze. *Third degree nystagmus* occurs in the opposite direction from gaze.

The most common cause of early-childhood nystagmus is *sensory defect nystagmus,* and it requires consultation with an ophthalmologist. *Spontaneous nystagmus* due to ocular problems is pendular, with equivalent excursions in either direction. Although children with poor visual acuity may exhibit first degree nystagmus, congenital metabolic diseases such as Chédiak-Higashi syndrome may also be responsible.[10]

Vestibular nystagmus is either rotatory, horizontal, or a combination thereof. Nystagmus due to vestibular disease is accompanied by dizziness and is rhythmic, demonstrating a slow phase followed by a compensatory fast phase.

Central nystagmus may beat in any direction and may change directions.[11] *Upbeating nystagmus* is associated with lower brainstem and anterior vermis lesions and intoxication. *Downbeating nystagmus* is seen classically in lesions at the craniocervical junction, such as with the Arnold-Chiari malformation. *Rotatory nystagmus* is due to lesions at the vestibular nuclei on the floor of the fourth ventricle. *Convergent nystagmus* due to anterior midbrain lesions, *"see-saw" nystagmus* from optic chiasm lesions, and *dissociated nystagmus* from plaques of multiple sclerosis along the MLF (median longitudinal fasciculus) all may be seen in children.[9,12]

Nystagmus may be elicited by changes in head position, as seen in the Dix-Hallpike maneuver. Such provocatory maneuvers are best performed as close to the end of the examination as possible. Pressure changes may also induce nystagmus. Pneumatic otoscopy using either the Siegel speculum or the hand-held otoscope is mandatory for the examination of the dizzy child. Ocular deviation and vertigo with the maintenance of negative pressure against an intact tympanic membrane (TM) without evidence of middle-ear disease is termed *Hennebert's sign.* Hennebert's sign initially was described in syphilis, and may be seen with labyrinthine hydrops of any etiology and with a perilymphatic fistula (PLF).[13,14] In the presence of a TM perforation, the finding of nystagmus and vertigo due to meatal pressure or the maintenance of positive insufflation is referred to as the *fistula sign* and suggests labyrinthine erosion.[2]

SPECIAL CONSIDERATION:

Ocular deviation and vertigo with the maintenance of negative pressure against an intact TM, without evidence of middle-ear disease, is termed *Hennebert's sign,* and may be seen with labyrinthine hydrops of any etiology and in PLF.

SPECIAL CONSIDERATION:

In the presence of a TM perforation, the finding of nystagmus and vertigo due to meatal pressure or the maintenance of positive insufflation is referred to as the fistula sign. This suggests labyrinthine erosion.

Electronystagmography (ENG) permits an evaluation of the relative contribution of each labyrinth to maintaining equilibrium. Motor and CNS contributions to equilibrium can be tested by examining fine and gross motor function and proprioception. Fine motor deficits can suggest specific cerebellar sites of pathology. Cerebellar hemispheric damage is displayed by failure to perform the "finger-to-nose" test (*dysmetria*), by past-pointing, or by an inability to rapidly pronate and supinate the hand (*dysdiadochokinesis*). Midline cerebellar disease is seen by trunkal ataxia and a wide-based gait.[9] Therefore, all patients should be observed as they ambulate. More subtle deficits may be elicited with the *Romberg test* (standing with eyes closed, feet together, and arms crossed or to the side) and *Unterbergers test* which requires stepping in place and like Hennebert's sign was described initially in syphilis[9]) and its modifications. Eviatar found that a normal child can stand for 7 to 10 seconds with his eyes closed, arms crossed, and one foot crossed over the other.[2] Fukuda's modification to Unterberger's test involves stepping in place over a marked cross on the floor for 1 minute. Swaying more than 45 degrees from the midline indicates ipsilateral vestibular dysfunction. Moving forwards or backwards more than 20 inches suggests bilateral vestibular involvement.[2]

Gross motor abilities may be demonstrated when the child walks in tandem gait and heel-toe, skips, or ambulates blindfolded. The child with an acute unilateral labyrinthine deficit may veer to the affected side when ambulating without visual input. Additional information may be provided by assessing pyramidal tract function via deep tendon reflexes and by muscle tone and strength.[2]

The relative contributions of the visual, vestibular, and proprioceptive systems may be distinguished qualitatively by the *"poor man's platform test."* Selective application of an opaque face shield to a child standing on the floor and then on a thick unstable cushion simulates the conditions of quantitative, dynamic, platform posturography. Alternatively, the child's stance and gait may be observed in a darkened room. As with all vestibular tests, the child's caretakers should be available readily to cajole and comfort her through the sometimes uncomfortable and frightening examination.

The immature neuromuscular control of the neonate requires different tests to determine vestibular health.[2,15] For the first 2 weeks of a term newborn's life, rotation of the child held vertically with the head flexed at 30 degrees results in eyes lagging behind the direction of head rotation (i.e., "doll's eyes"). Nystagmus, with the fast component towards the direction of rotation, develops through maturation. Rapid downward acceleration in the newborn results in head extension, arm abduction, and fanning of the hand. Righting responses may be identified as early as 6 months of age. By the fourth year, children are sufficiently developed neurologically and socially to permit formal vestibular examination and testing.

SPECIAL CONSIDERATION:

Because of immature neuromuscular control, neonates require different tests than older children to determine vestibular health; however, by 4 years of age children are sufficiently developed neurologically and socially to permit formal vestibular testing.

Audiometric Testing

All dizzy children require age-appropriate audiometric testing so that asymptomatic hearing losses may be detected and a baseline may be established. Pure tone audiometry (PTA) with tympanometry suffice in most cases.

Auditory brainstem response (ABR) testing is necessary when the hearing level cannot be ascertained otherwise or when subtle deficits in eighth nerve function are sought. In addition, ABR testing helps to distinguish peripheral from central vestibulopathies. In Meniere's disease (MD) the ABR will have a normal latency, whereas in acoustic neuromas or in granulomatous diseases interwave latencies will be increased.[16] Electrocochleography (ECoG) may show an increase in the ratio of the summating potential (SP) to the action potential (AP) in MD and other causes of endolymphatic hydrops. Otoacoustic emmisions (OAEs) may provide evidence of outer hair-cell function.

Vestibular Testing

Vestibular testing in children is performed selectively (see Practice Pathway 11-1). Common means of testing are through ENG battery, rotation testing, and platform posturography. ENG measures the ocular response to vestibular stimuli. Temple and periorbital electrodes detect the change in the electric fields that is generated by movement of the corneoretinal potentials with eye motion. These changes are recorded as vertical and horizontal movements. Rotary nystagmus does not alter the magnetic field of the corneoretinal potential and is therefore not registered in a standard ENG. Both horizontal and vertical nystagmus may be studied, although usually just left and right beating nystagmus are recorded clinically. On the horizontal measurements, an upward deflection on the tracing indicates ocular movement to the right, whereas an upward deflection on the vertical tracing indicates upward motion. The slope of the line indicates the speed of movement, with faster movement leaving a steeper slope (see Practice Pathway 11-1). Exercises to stimulate the labyrinths comprise the ENG battery.

The *Dix-Hallpike manuever* is performed to elicit benign paryoxysmal positional vertigo (BPPV). BPPV is characterized by a rotatory nystagmus that presents with latency and fatigues with repeated stimulation of the posterior semicircular canal. Because ENG does not measure the torsional component, both horizontal and vertical leads must be used to measure the degree of rotatory nystagmus. The horizontal tracing's fast phase will be away from the undermost (i.e., pathologic) ear. The fast phase of the vertical component will point upwards.

Gaze testing detects the degree of spontaneous nystagmus during fixation and movement of the eyes from 30 degrees to each side and vertically. CNS and unilateral peripheral vestibular disease are identified with this test. *Positional ENG* also measures spontaneous nystagmus as a marker of unilateral peripheral vestibular disease or CNS disease, but is performed with and without fixation, while the patient is sitting and supine, and with each ear "down." The failure of fixation suppression indicates CNS disease.

Caloric ENG testing is performed in a supine position with the head elevated 30 degrees above the horizontal plane so that the lateral semicircular canal is vertical. Cold and warm aural irrigation is used to calculate directional preponderance. A calculated difference of >30% between sides indicates a unilateral peripheral lesion. Bilateral lesions cannot be objectively studied with caloric ENG testing due to a lack of calibrated data.

The ability to follow a randomly-jumping target along a horizontal line depends on intact central and peripheral vestibular control. The resultant eye motion is termed the *saccadic response*, and it is quantified during ENG by measuring the accuracy, latency, and peak velocity of the patient's saccades. *Pursuit tracking* uses a sinusoidally-moving, to-and-fro point through slow and fast frequencies to evaluate central pathways. Ocular gain relates the velocity of horizontal eye motion to target velocity. Optokinetic nystagmus (OKN) is measured during pursuit testing.

Rotation testing provides the most sensitive test for acute unilateral and bilateral peripheral lesions. The most commonly applied rotation test is the *slow-harmonic test*, in which a light-proof, sound-dampened booth houses a chair that oscillates in the horizontal plane at frequencies ranging from 0.01 cycles/second to 0.64 cycles/second-Hz. ENG measures the phase difference between head and eye motion and the symmetry difference between right and left horizontal semicircular canals. The slow-harmonic test is superior to the cold caloric test because rotation testing stimulates the labyrinth through a wider frequency range, whereas the cold caloric test has a low-frequency thermal stimulus.[17]

The relative importance of the visual, vestibular, and proprioceptive systems is tested by *dynamic platform posturography*. In this test, two platform conditions (fixed and sway-referenced) are combined with three visual conditions (fixed, eyes closed, and sway-referenced), and the six resultant conditions allow quantification of the functional deficit and formulation of a vestibular rehabilitation strategy.

Laboratory Evaluation and Referrals

Testing of chemistries and serologies is recommended in selected cases (see Practice Pathway 11-1). Children with CNS findings or evidence of systemic disease are managed in conjunction with the appropriate specialists.

Imaging

Radiographic imaging is useful for suspected anatomic defects and for mass lesions that can dizziness. Computed tomography (CT) scanning of the temporal bone for the dizzy patient is performed ideally in the axial and coronal planes at 1 mm to 1.5 mm intervals. Three-dimensional CT (3D CT) scanning allows more detailed examination of the inner ear.[18] Contrast enhancement is not necessary. Specific disorders that require a CT scan are PLF and craniofacial syndromes. CT also may identify defects in the bony labyrinth and cholesteatoma formation in the dizzy child with chronic otitis media (OM).

Magnetic resonance imaging (MRI) with gadolinium-diethylene-triamine-penta-acetic acid (gadolinium-DTPA) enhancement is useful for children with CNS findings. Multiple sclerosis, vestibular nerve schwannomas, other tumors, and granulomatous disorders may be identified better by MRI with gadolinium than by CT scanning.[16,19,20] MRI with contrast can detect lesions as small as 2mm within the internal auditory canal (IAC).[21] Three-dimensional MRI (3D MRI) allows better delineation of membranous labyrinthine abnormalities. Functional MRI scanning and positron emmission tomography (PET) scanning are experimental and may offer insight into the metabolic aberrations found in vestibulopathies.

GENERAL MANAGEMENT OF THE DIZZY CHILD

Bed rest is recommended initially. Supportive care is provided for acute symptoms, and counseling as well as traditional and "on-line" support groups may be helpful. Pharmacologic control of vertigo is often initiated before referral to the pediatric otolaryngologist. The agents are classified by function (Table 11-2). Treatment may be offered on the initial visit before a precise diagnosis is formulated. Vestibular suppression is best used in short courses, as CNS compensation is delayed with prolonged use. Vestibular suppressants must be discontinued before quantitative vestibular testing. Meclizine and diazepam are the most helpful in children. An antiemetic, such as trimethobenzamide hydrochloride (e.g., Tigan®), provides further immediate relief. Salt restriction and fluid limits are recommended for hydropic symptoms.

Disabling vertigo refractory to maximal pharmacologic and rehabilitative care may require reduction of vestibular input by decompression of the endolymphatic sac, labyrinthectomy, or vestibular ablation. Chemical labyrinthectomy should be of-

TABLE 11–2: Drug Therapy for the Dizzy Child

Drug	Class	Action	Route	Dose	Side Effects	Warnings
diazepam (Valium)	benzodiazepine	sedative	po/im/iv	po: 0.12–0.8 mg/kg/dose im/iv: 0.04–0.2 mg/kg/dose	hypotension, respiratory depression, paradoxical excitement, dependence	cardio-respiratory monitoring at higher doses
prochlorperazine (Compazine)	phenothiazine	antiemetic	po/im	po: 0.4 mg/kg/3–4 divided doses im: 0.05–0.15 mg/kg/dose	hypotension, extrapyramidal symptoms, hyperpigmentation, urinary retention, agranulocytosis	injection has sulfites, marrow suppression, contraindicated in liver/cardiac disease or narrow-angle glaucoma
meclizine (Antivert)	antihistamine	vestibular suppressant	po	25–100 mg daily, divided per clinical response	drowsiness, dry mouth, blurred vision	not recommended for children <12 years old
clonazepam (Klonopin)	benzodiazepine	sedative	po	0.01–0.03 mg/kg/dose	hypotension, respiratory depression	contraindicated in liver disease, narrow-angle glaucoma
droperidol (Inapsine)	neuroleptic	sedative	im/iv	2.5–5.0 mg/kg/dose, q 3–4 hrs	hypotension, respiratory depression, laryngospasm	careful with electrolyte disturbance, liver or kidney disease, cardiac disease
trimethobenzamide (Tigan)		antiemetic	pr	<13 kg: 100 mg 3–4 times/day 13.6 kg–45 kg: 100–200 mg/3; 4 times/day >45 kg: 200 mg pp 3–4 times/day	hypotension, blood dyscrasias, hepatotoxicity, blurred vision, other anticholinergic or antipyramidal effects	contraindicated in patients with benzocaine allergy, injection contraindicated in children, suppository contraindicated in premature infants and neonates

Abbreviations: po, oral; im, intramuscular; iv, intravenous;
Data from Jew R, ed. *Department of Pharmacy Services. Pharmacy Handbook and Formulary 1997–1999 (The Children's Hospital of Philadelphia)*, pp. 100, 112, 266, 313. Hudson, OH: Lexi-Comp, 1998, and *Physician's Desk Reference, 52nd ed.* Montvale, NJ: Medical Economics Company, Inc, 1998, pp. 2161, 2411, 2475, 2536, 2806, 2880.

fered prior to surgical ablation. A myringotomy tube facilitates application of transtympanic gentamycin.[22] Surgical procedures to control dizziness are rarely necessary in children and usually are performed for chronic OM complicated by labyrinthine erosion or for PLF.

SPECIAL CONSIDERATION:
Surgical procedures to control dizziness in children are rarely necessary and usually are performed for chronic OM complicated by labyrinthine erosion or for PLF.

SPECIFIC DISORDERS

External Ear

Dizziness from EAC occlusion may result when debris pushes against the TM or when a pressure seal is formed by a lateral plug of cerumen or a foreign body. Removal of the offending agent is curative.[1]

Middle Ear

OM, both acute and chronic, accounts for most dizziness in children. Myringotomy with tube insertion is needed when OM otitis is refractory to drug therapy and for severe ET dysfunction. Dynamic platform posturography has demonstrated higher sway velocities and has suggested an increased dependence on visual cues for children with OM.[23] After the placement of myringotomy tubes, these children swayed less and had fewer falls.[24] Early operative treatment of OM that causes dizziness may be necessary in children with comorbidities, such as the hemophiliac whose imbalance may result in trauma and a life-threatening hemorrhage.

Chronic OM with cholesteatoma formation may lead to erosion of the bone overlying the labyrinth (usually the lateral semicircular canal) in approximately 10% of patients with cholesteatomas. Exposure of the membranous labyrinth to middle-ear contents and atmospheric-pressure changes leads to dizziness. With a TM perforation, cold exposure to either water or air can precipitate severe vertigo. Children with TM perforations must be cautioned against swimming unsupervised at depth and should avoid scuba diving.[25]

Inner Ear

Developmental disorders

Anatomic anomalies for the inner ear occur in 1/2000 live births. In descending order of frequency, the cochlea, IAC, vestibular aqueduct, and the semicircular canals may be malformed.[6]

A *large vestibular aqueduct (LVA)* most commonly presents with a progressive or fluctuating high-frequency sensorineural hearing loss (SNHL) with a down-sloping curve.[26] Some children also have vestibular symptoms. Developmental arrest during the fifth fetal week is postulated to result in LVA.[27] Precipitating events causing hearing loss and vertigo include head trauma or pressure changes due to straining, coughing, or lifting.[26] A genetic predisposition has been suggested by reports of familial cases.[28]

LVA is defined by a midaqueductal width >1.5 mm or a meatal width >2.0 mm on high-resolution CT scan. MRI with gadolinium shows a widened sac on T2-weighted images. Levenson et al found that isolated LVA was identified by CT in 0.64% of children who underwent CT scanning for all reasons.[26] Bilateral LVA is more common than unilateral LVA. Other otic capsule anomalies associated with LVA involve the lateral semicircular canal and cochlea.[26,27]

Management of the hearing loss requires attention to the possibility of progression and bilaterality. Vestibular therapy rarely is needed in children. Middle-ear exploration to improve or stabilize hearing loss due to LVA is controversial.[27]

Intrauterine toxins including thalidomide and alcohol have been linked to congenital labyrinthine malformations. Thalidomide, in particular, was associated with semicircular canal aplasia.[6] Viral effects on the cochlea and labyrinth have been reported in congenital rubella, mumps, and syphilis infection.

Craniofacial syndromes may cause dizziness due to anatomic or immunologic problems. Pars superior malformations and enlarged cochlear and vestibular aqueducts are associated with craniofacial syndromes (Table 11–3) Anatomic anomalies of the labyrinth are demonstrated in the CHARGE association. Children with the *CHARGE* anomaly have some combination of ocular *C*oloboma, congenital *H*eart anomalies, choanal *A*tresia, *R*etarded growth or CNS development, *G*enital hypoplasia, and *E*ar anomalies. A higher incidence of labyrinthine malformations and membranous deformities have been detected in these children. The possibility of vestibular deficits in these children highlights the importance of comprehensive otorhinolaryngologic and audiologic care in order to optimize their social and educational development.[29,30]

Autoimmune disorders are exemplified by Cogan's syndrome. Ocular inflammation (typically interstitual keratitis) CNS findings, and vasculitis characterize this disorder. Vestibulopathy presents as ataxia and commonly progresses to complete vestibular dysfunction with oscillopsia. Immunosuppres-

TABLE 11–3:   Syndromic Dizziness

Chromosome 13q deletion
Apert's
Branchio-oto-renal
Chromosome B minus
Cogan's
Crouzon's
DiGeorge's
Duane's
Goldenhar's
Klippel-Feil
Marfan's
Mobius'
Treacher Collins
Trisomy 13
Trisomy 18
Trisomy 21 (Down's)
Turner's XO
Vogt-Koyanagi-Harada
Waardenburg's

sion is accomplished with corticosteroids and cyclo-phosphamide.[13]

Traumatic disorders

Perilymphatic fistula (PLF) is a leak of perilymph from the membranous labyrinth. PLF may be sponta-neous (SPLF) or traumatic (TPLF) in etiology. *TPLF* occurs when a sudden jolt or pressure change (from trauma, straining, coughing, sneezing, or baro-trauma) allows increased intracranial pressure to be transmitted from the subarachnoid space. *SPLF* oc-curs without clear antecedent cause. The resulting fluid leak occurs through the round window or oval window membranes, annular ligament, or microfis-sures,[31] and leads immediately to severe vertigo and a SNHL that progresses or fluctuates over time (Fig. 11–1). Tinnitus may be present. Recurrent meningi-tis may result due to communication between the subarachnoid space and the middle-ear cleft. The child may report the Tullio phenomenon, which is vertigo induced by a loud sound.[2] The fistula test by pneumatic otoscopy may be positive. ECoG sup-ports the diagnosis of PLF when the ratio of the SP:AP is greater than 30%.[31]

Most children with PLF who have been studied have normal bony anatomy on CT. Rarely, CT identi-fies bony labyrinthine dysplasias or abnormally-

wide cochlear or vestibular aqueducts. A widened cochlear aqueduct allows a higher pressure to be transmitted through the subarachnoid fluid, placing greater tension against the oval-window membrane. Because such children with anatomic "pressure heads" are the minority of patients with PLF, CT scanning is prognostic rather than diagnostic and is useful to inform the family of an anatomic predispo-sition to further hearing loss with head trauma.

The goal of treatment is to stabilize hearing and lessen the severity of vertigo, while reducing the risk of otitic meningitis. Treatment begins with pre-scription of antiemetics and vestibular suppressants for symptomatic relief. Surgery is offered with the understanding that such surgery may improve or prevent the degradation of hearing only temporar-ily. The risks of surgical exploration are balanced against the severity of the hearing loss and imbal-ance. Exploration of the middle ear to patch the fistula is offered in both traumatic and spontaneous cases. Middle-ear endoscopy has advocated over ex-ploratory tympanotomy as a more precise means of making the diagnosis because the pooling of fluids that is seen during exploratory tympanotomy is avoided.[32,33] Valsalva's maneuver may reveal the site of fluid leak during middle-ear exploration. In-traoperative ECoG has been demonstrated to con-firm a PLF.[34] Intravenous fluorescein injection does

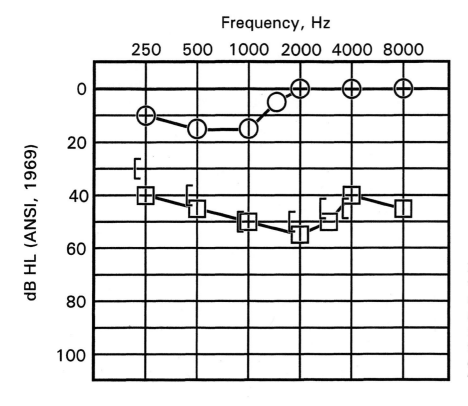

Figure 11–1: Audiogram in child with traumatic PLF. Audiogram shows left moderate SNHL with speech reception threshold (SRT) of 50 deciBels (dB HL) and discrimina-tion score with NU-6 (MLV) list of 68% at 85 dB HL presentation level. Tympanometry was normal.

not reliably indicate the presence of PLF.[35] A beta-2 transferrin level of middle-ear fluid sampled intraoperatively is diagnostic of PLF, but the difficulty of obtaining a sample that is uncontaminated by blood or serous fluid precludes routine testing. A tissue patch is applied during middle-ear exploration regardless of an obvious fistula because there is minimal morbidity to patching once the tympanotomy has been performed. After the promontory mucosa is freshened, fascia trimmed to size is placed around the round and oval windows to facilitate adhesion of the graft material. Fascia is superior to fat, which has been noted to resorb earlier and leave less of a tissue seal. Autologous tissue adhesive (fibrin glue) is useful in achieving an inflammatory reaction that promotes closure of the PLF. Preoperative preparation of blood products is required.

Whether or not exploration with patching is undertaken, serial audiograms are important to document progression of hearing loss because of the fluctuating nature of SNHL in PLF.

Head injuries in children result in as many objective lesions as in adults but fewer subjective vestibular complaints.[36] Labyrinthine concussion occurs in less than 2% of children with head injuries. Trauma to the otolithic membranes causes immediate vertigo and a mild SNHL for some. Positional nystagmus lasts until compensation occurs. The vertigo may last up to 1 year following the insult. In a series of 199 children between 2 and 16 years of age, 46% of those examined displayed spontaneous or positional nystagmus immediately after injury and 20% continued to display nystagmus 6 to 12 months later. Persistent nystagmus was seen in 18% of these children at 2 to 8 years follow-up. Central ENG findings were present in 43% of all children immediately postinjury, in 24% 6 to 12 months later, and in 12% at 2 to 8 years follow-up.[36] Labyrinthine concussion is responsive to vestibular rehabilitation.[3]

SPECIAL CONSIDERATION:

Head injuries in children result in as many objective lesions as in adults but in fewer subjective vestibular complaints.

The more deformable pediatric skull, particularly in neonates and infants, distributes the forces of impact over a greater surface area, thereby reducing the likelihood of a temporal bone fracture. In 71 patients with temporal bone fractures reviewed by Mitchell and Stone, only one child (1.4%) was reported to have vertigo.[37] Transverse temporal-bone fractures result in a higher incidence of labyrinthine damage than longitudinal fractures. Vestibular compensation accounts for the gradual disappearance of spontaneous nystagmus. The presence of high-frequency hearing loss does not correlate with the development of posttraumatic vestibulopathy.[36]

Whiplash injuries may cause vestibular membrane damage without hearing loss. Positional nystagmus is demonstrated by ENG testing. Objective documentation of vestibular abnormalities is recommended due to the possibility of litigation associated with this and all traumatic vestibulopathies. Spontaneous resolution is expected. Vestibular suppressants, muscle relaxants, a soft-collar for the neck, and vestibular rehabilitation are useful.

Infectious disorders

Infectious labyrinthitis is the most common cause of vertigo in children.[3,38] Viral causes predominate. Measles or mumps are blamed for *primary viral labyrinthitis;* rubeola, herpes, and cytomegalovirus cause *secondary viral labyrinthitis.* Serous labyrinthitis from middle-ear inflammation may also cause vertigo.[1,38]

Bacterial labyrinthitis is characterized by severe vertigo, SNHL, and severe discomfort with autonomic symptoms.[2] Spontaneous nystagmus will beat towards the normal ear, and caloric ENG will be hyporesponsive immediately after the acute episode.[1] Vestibular suppression and antibiotics are indicated.

Disorders due to ototoxic medications

Various medications may cause dizziness as a side effect or by affecting the labyrinth directly. Aminoglycosides are most often responsible for direct toxicity to the cristae and maculae of the semicircular canals, utricle, and saccule.[39] Loop diuretics (ethacrynic acid), quinine, and chemotherapeutic drugs (cisplatin[40]) also may damage the labyrinth. Anticonvulsants (carbamazepine, phenytoin), vasoactive agents, and illicit drugs may be responsible for vestibulopathy.

Idiopathic disorders

Attention to the inner ear as a focus of balance disorders began with Prosper Meniere's description of vertigo, tinnitus, low-frequency SNHL, and aural fullness. A typical attack of *Meniere's disease* (MD) lasts minutes to hours. Hydropic symptoms may be worsened in states of fluid retention, such as pregnancy and menses. Rarely, patients may report the Tullio phenomenon, in which patients with endolymphatic hydrops experience vertigo with loud noises. MD occurs less commonly in children than in adults. Variants of MD, which include cochlear MD (CMD), vestibular MD (VMD), Tumarkin's drop attacks, and Lermoyez's syndrome (which is an acute onset of hearing loss and tinnitus that is relieved by a vertiginous attack), may occur in children and adolescents.

The disease may progress by involving the contralateral side or by an exacerbation of cochlear and/or vestibular symptoms. The disease may also "burn out" leaving the patient without hearing or peripheral vestibular control. The natural history of MD in children is not described well. For adults, the development of contralateral MD occurs in 32% of all patients with the disease and is more likely the longer the duration. Nearly half of the patients who have the disease for longer than 20 years will develop bilateral symptoms. Pure VMD may be a different disease from classic MD because only 10 to 20% of all patients with VMD will go on to develop cochlear symptoms. In contrast, 80% of patients with CMD go on to develop classic MD. The natural history of MD is that of slow resolution: 71% of patients will no longer have attacks after 8 years. In general, patients with chronic MD display hearing levels at 50dB, with calorics reduced by 50%.[13]

AT A GLANCE...

Diseases Associated with Endolymphatic Hydrops

- Meniere's disease
- Endolymphatic duct or sac lesions
- Lymphoma
- Leukemia
- Syphilis
- Otitic labyrinthitis

Histopathologic temporal bone studies have shown *endolymphatic hydrops* (ELH) in patients with MD. ELH is thought to arise from inadequate absorption of endolymph or from outflow obstruction of the endolymphatic duct due to perisaccular ischemia and fibrosis,[13] inflammation, atresia or stenosis of the duct, or mass lesions.[39] Lymphoma, leukemia, syphilis,[41] and labyrinthitis secondary to OM also may cause ELH and must be considered. Viral inflammation of the endolymphatic system also may be responsible.[13]

In most cases of ELH, diagnosis depends more on description of the attacks than physical examination or formal testing. A positive Hennebert's sign, confirming saccular distension, may be present. ENG calorics, ECoG, and a glycerol test may be used to confirm the diagnosis.[13] ECoG may be used in cases of purely VMD to identify the disease so that appropriate therapy may begin.

SPECIAL CONSIDERATION:

In most cases of EHL, diagnosis depends more on description of the attacks than physical examination or formal testing.

Acute management of MD is with sedatives, suppressants, and antiemetics. Long-term pharmacologic control of MD may be possible by salt and caffeine restriction and by oral diuretics. Successful treatment with corticosteroids and plasma electrophoresis lends support to the immunologic mechanism for ELH.[13] Treatment with intratympanic steroids is experimental.[42] Chemical or surgical ablation is risky given the possibility of developing contralateral MD and the potential for complete bilateral peripheral vestibular loss. The danger of an MD episode occurring underwater must be stressed to the family—disorientation may lead to aspiration and drowing.[43] Hearing should be checked annually.

BPPV is characterized by disabling vertigo without hearing loss or tinnitus that lasts hours to days, and is accompanied by nausea. BPPV is due to cupulolithiasis of the posterior semicircular canal, and may appear after age 11. The classic nystagmus of BPPV is rotatory and geotropic, has latency, is short-lived, and fatigues with repetition. The term *geotropic* means that the direction of the rotatory nystagmus points towards the affected labyrinth when that ear is down or closest to the ground with the head tilted. Vertigo accompanies the nystagmus. The direction of the nystagmus reverses when the head is brought to the upright position. The Dix-Hallpike maneuver may be used to test the function of each labyrinth. Classically, the rotatory geotropic nystagmus of BPPV presents with latency and fatigues with repetition. The Dix-Hallpike maneuver should be performed when the history suggests BPPV. ENG is not useful in diagnosis as the rotatory component of nystagmus registers only as horizontal nystagmus on standard ENG tracings.

Initial treatment with vestibular suppression may not be as useful as expected given the severity and brevity of the vertigo and nausea. Maneuvers designed to return the offending otoliths to nonpathologic positions are popular with patients. These "particle repositioning" or "liberatory" maneuvers are effective in many cases, whether performed by the patient as described by Brandt[44] or by the physician.

The rare pediatric presentation of BPPV must be distinguished from *benign positional vertigo (BPV) of childhood* which is a disorder thought to be due to transient ischemia of the central vestibular system.[3] As such, BPV of childhood may be related to migraine not only in etiology but also in concomitant symptoms such as cyclic vomiting, abdominal pain, visual changes (scotomata and photophobia), and motion intolerance. Sudden attacks of vertigo lasting seconds to minutes begin between 1 to 4 years of age.[2] Vertigo may be precipitated by sudden changes in head position.[1] Neither hearing loss nor tinnitus are present. Paroxysmal torticollis of infancy may precede the development of BPV of childhood. BPV of childhood resolves spontaneously; migraine headache, however, is common as these children become adults. Suppressants and vestibular rehabilitation may be offered. Antimigraine treatment for BPV of childhood has been successful.[45]

Paroxysmal torticollis of infancy presents in the first year of life as periodic head tilting and truncal posturing, ataxia, vomiting, pallor, and behavioral changes.[3] The episodes last for minutes to days and are self-limited. These attacks have been considered to be a form of labyrinthitis, MD, or BPPV. Children who exhibit torticollis usually are tilting their heads to "splint" tender cervical muscles or ligaments due to infection. Rarely, vestibular and ocular torticollis is thought to arise from prolonged flexing of the head intended to diminish vertiginous visual or vestibular input.[1,46] Management of both forms is supportive. A soft collar is used to prevent muscular contracture when children maintain the abnormal head position for prolonged periods of time. Orthopedic or neurosurgical consultation may be helpful.

Vestibular nerve disorders

Vestibular neuronitis[3] is common in children and is usually viral like labyrinthitis. Adolescents most frequently experience the characteristic 1 to 2 day periodic attacks of vertigo, nausea, and vomiting.[2] Fifteen percent of children with vestibular neuronitis eventually develop BPPV.[13] Hearing is normal and the attacks gradually lessen in severity until they subside over a week's time.[1,2] ENG shows a positional nystagmus with a unilaterally hypoactive peripheral response and/or a unilateral caloric weakness. This disorder is managed with vestibular suppressants.

Tumors of the vestibular nerve cause vertigo by compression or ischemia of the nerve. Slow-growing tumors are unlikely to present with dizziness since CNS compensation will have time to take place. Associated hearing loss or tinnitus and seventh cranial nerve palsy may be present with even small eighth cranial nerve tumors. Children usually do not report hearing loss—the deficit is revealed by audiometry.[47] Larger tumors result in trigeminal signs and symptoms. Cerebral herniation is possible for tumors >3 cm in diameter.

Most tumors are vestibular schwannomas, more commonly referred to as *acoustic neuromas* (AN). Less than 20 cases of AN in children are reported in the world literature; the youngest is 6 years of age.[47] Physical examination may be abnormal only in larger tumors when cranial nerves other than the eight nerve are affected. Audiometric testing will show an SNHL with poor discrimination scores. Ipsilateral acoustic reflexes will be absent. ABR testing will show abnormal waveform or prolonged latencies on the side of the tumor. ENG may identify a unilateral reduced vestibular response. MRI with gadolinium is the most sensitive single modality for diagnosis,[48] particularly for intracanalicular tumors.[49] Surgical resection is required to cure these slow-growing neoplasms. The preservation of the cochlear nerve is of even greater importance in children with AN because the development of neurofibromatosis type II (NF II) with bilateral AN cannot always be predicted at the time of initial surgery.[47] Stereotactic radiotherapy via the "gamma knife" has been successful in controlling tumor growth in adults with AN. Patients best suited to gamma-knife irradiation are those who refuse surgical removal or those unfit for surgery.[50] MRI with gadolinium is ordered annually following tumor excision to allow for early detection of contralateral eight nerve tumors and to detect recurrence.[51]

Children with bilateral schwannomas of the eight nerves have NF II, which is also referred to as *von Recklinghausen's disease type 2.*[38] This disease is autosomal dominant and is due to a mutation of the tumor suppression gene, schwannomin, at chromosomal locus 22q12. A genetic basis for the development of unilateral AN has been suggested.[52] Progressive hearing loss with vertigo are characteristic. Other cranial nerves may be affected. Children with NF are also at higher risk for developing meningiomas.[39] Treatment generally requires surgical removal of the tumors.

Central nervous system disorders

CNS diseases frequently cause vertigo in children.[38]

Posterior fossa tumors present with hearing loss and vertigo, and in advanced cases, with brainstem deficits. These tumors include those at the cerebellopontine angle, most commonly schwannomas and meningiomas, and intrinsic tumors, medulloblastomas, astrocytomas, and gliomas.[3]

Multiple sclerosis (MS) which is a CNS disease caused by multifocal inflammatory myelin destruction, may present as early as 10 years of age, although it is usually first diagnosed after the age of 20.[39] This disease is characterized by deposition of hypercellular astrocytic plaques and atrophy in the cerebral cortex, cerebellum, and spinal cord.[53] The etiology is unclear. MS may initially simulate acute peripheral vestibular disease.[38] Hearing loss is present in 10% of patients in the later stages of the disease.

A family history of migraine headaches should be sought in children with episodic vertigo without hearing loss. *Migraine* is a vascular disorder that occurs in up to 5% of children and is associated with BPPV of childhood and paroxysmal torticollis of infancy.[3,54] Balance and headache symptoms are not necessarily concurrent or sequential. Ischemia within the occipital lobe and brainstem distribution of the basilar artery lead to *basilar artery migraine.*[3] Perioral parasthenias, vertigo, and visual

loss accompany tinnitus and drop attacks. Headaches often follow vertiginous episodes. More subtle presentations include periods of vestibular symptoms before the development of headache, and these may lead to an initial diagnosis of VMD or vestibular neuronitis. Whereas pharmacologic treatment is necessary in cases of migraine-associated vestibulopathy, dietary changes and vestibular rehabilitation may provide relief for some patients.[55] Drug therapy includes the use of vestibular suppressants and ergotamine acutely for α-adrenergic blockade. Long-term control may be possible using propranolol for β-adrenergic blockade, nifedipine for calcium-channel blockade, tricyclic antidepressants (e.g., amitryptyline), antihistamines (cyproheptadine), methysergide maleate, and the antihypertensive clonidine. Anticonvulsants may offer symptomatic relief for children with electroencephalogram (EEG) abnormalities. Dietary modifications to eliminate identifiable triggers usually requires avoidance of alcohol, tyramine containing foods (e.g., aged cheeses), sodium nitrite, monosodium glutamate (MSG), and chocolate.[54]

Vertiginous seizures present with a change in consciousness during the dizzy episode. This disorder is a form of sensory epilepsy with a temporal lobe focus. As such, the ENG is normal, while EEG abnormalities are diagnostic. Management is with anticonvulsants.

Dizziness also may result from *meningitis* that usually is due to bacterial infection; less often, it may be due to spirochetal infection[1] [i.e., *Borellia burgdorferi* (Lyme disease), *T. pallidum* (syphilis)], and rarely it may be due to granulomatous inflammation.[16] High-dose corticosteroid regimens have been shown to reduce the incidence of long-term neurologic sequelae in bacterial meningitis.[56] Their use is not routine, however.

Syphilis results from vertical (congenital) or horizontal (via mucosal or sexual contact) infection by the spirochete *T. pallidum.* Acquired syphilis in children requires evaluation for sexual abuse. Congenital transmission may occur transplacentally or by mucosal contact with active lesions along the birth canal. Early congenital syphilis presents with low-birth weight, hepatomegaly, rhinitis ("snuffles"), coryza, a maculopapular rash, and osseous, hematologic, and pulmonary abnormalities. Late congenital syphilis occurs in up to 40% of untreated infants. Bilateral vestibulocochlear deficits, interstitial keratitis, classic skull abnormalities (e.g., frontal bossing, short maxilla, saddle nose deformity, hard palate damage, and notched central incisors, or Hutchinson's incisors), and dermatologic and joint findings are seen.

Syphilitic hearing loss and dizziness result from obliterative endarteritis and gummatous destruction of the endolymphatic duct. Bony and fibrous occlusion of the semicircular canals from diffuse periosteitis also leads to imbalance. Serum venereal disease research lab (VDRL) and rapid plasma reagin (RPR) tests are diagnostic. The fluorescent treponemal antibody absorption test (FTA-ABS) is the most

sensitive diagnostic test. Treatment of early otosyphilis is with penicillin with or without corticosteroids. Late otosyphilis should be treated with corticosteroids and penicillin.[57,58]

Systemic disorders

Systemic causes for imbalance are often identified by concommitant findings. Thyroid dysfunction, diabetes mellitus, hyperlipidemias,[59] ethanol abuse, anemia, congenital heart disease and arrythmias, adrenal insufficiency, HIV infection,[60] and iatrogenic causes (e.g., medications and spinal anesthesia[61]) may all cause dizziness.[3]

Functional dizziness may correlate with school avoidance.[1] Secondary gain must be evaluated in children who are "disabled" by dizziness.

FUTURE DIRECTIONS

Continued advances in development neurobiology, genetics, and applied physics promise to broaden understanding and improve management of pediatric vestibulopathy. As vestibular hair-cell regeneration is better understood,[62,63] the appreciation of the role of neurotrophic factors in the developing cochlea[64] allows for the possibility of targeted therapy to prevent vestibular loss during embryogenesis or toxic events. Now, genetic screening exists for some of the disorders associated with imbalance in children. Interventions based upon gene therapy may be possible one day. Radiographic advances, through better labyrinthine detail using 3-D MRI and CT scanning[28] and improved assessment of CNS activity using PET scanning, help to narrow the differential diagnosis more rapidly. Improved clarity and strength of optical fibers allow smaller and brighter transtympanic endoscopes to offer less traumatic examinations, which is useful in cases of PLF. Vestibular surgery benefits from novel fiberoptic and endoscopic materials and techniques. Laser[65] and ultrasound[66] treatments require more detailed analyses of results and improved instrumentation before broader application. Increasingly-comprehensive analyses of children with craniofacial syndromes allow a better understanding of the incidence and role of vestibular disease in these complex patients.

CONCLUSION

Systematic review and an understanding of the vagaries of dizziness in children require practice and

AT A GLANCE. . .

Inner Ear Disorders

Development
large vestibular aqueduct
intrauterine toxins
craniofacial syndromes
autoimmune disorders

Traumatic
perilymphatic fistula
head injuries
labyrinthine concussion
temporal bone fracture
whiplash injuries

Infectious
infectious labyrinthitis
serous labyrinthitis
bacterial labyrinthitis

Ototoxic Medications

Idiopathic
Meniere's disease
endolymphatic hydrops
benign paroxysmal positional vertigo
benign positional vertigo
paroxysmal torticollis of infancy

Vestibular Nerve
vestibular neuronitis
acoustic neuromas
neurofibromatosis type II

Central Nervous System
posterior fossa tumors
multiple sclerosis
migraine
basilar artery migraine
vertiginous seizures
meningitis
syphilis

Systemic

patience. An appreciation of the nuances of the vestibular examination in children and of the common causes of pediatric vestibulopathy allows efficient diagnosis and treatment.

REFERENCES

1. Potsic WP, Handler SD, Wetmore RF, et al. *Primary Care Pediatric Otolaryngology, 2nd ed.* Andover, NJ: J. Michael Ryan Publishing, 1995, pp. 20-23.
2. Eviatar L. Dizziness in children. Otolaryngol Clin North Am 1994; 27:557-571.
3. Wazen JJ, Keller JL. Vestibular disorders in children. Paper presented at: Annual Meeting of the American Academy of Otolaryngology—Head & Neck Surgery. San Francisco, CA, September 1997.
4. Selz PA, Girardi M, Konrad HR, et al. Vestibular deficits in deaf children. Otolaryngol Head Neck Surg 1996; 115:70-77.
5. Anson BJ, Davies J, Duckert LG. Embryology of the Ear. In: Paparella MM, ed. *Year Book of Otolaryngology—Head & Neck Surgery.* St. Louis: Mosby, 1997, pp. 5-21.
6. Bhatt NI, Niparko JK. Imaging quiz case 2 (Vestibular dysgenesis with semicircular canal aplasia). Arch Otol Head Neck Surg 1997; 123:1011-1014.
7. Coleman B. Congenital atresia: Aspects of surgical care. Acta Otorhinolaryngol 1971; 25:925-935.
8. Doty RL, Shaman P, Kimmelman CP, et al. University of Pennsylvania Smell Identification Test: A rapid quantitative olfactory function test for the clinic. Laryngoscope 1984; 94:176-178.
9. Gibson WPR. Vestibular diagnostic tests. In: Alberti PW, Ruben RJ, eds. *Otologic Medicine and Surgery.* New York: Churchill Livingstone, 1988, pp. 487-505.
10. Johnson WG, Rapin I. Progressive genetic metabolic diseases. In: Rudolph AM, Hoffman JIE, Rudolph CD, eds. *Rudolph's Pediatrics.* Stamford, CT: Appleton & Lange, 1996, pp. 2019-2025.
11. Pickard B. Methods of examination of the ear. In: Ballantine J, Groves J, eds. *Scott-Brown's Diseases of the Ear, Nose and Throat, 3rd ed.* Philadelphia: Lippincott, 1971, pp. 1-34.
12. Apt L, Miller KM. The eye. In: Rudolph AM, Hoffman JIE, Rudolph CD, eds. *Rudolph's Pediatrics.* Stamford, CT: Appleton & Lange, 1996, pp. 2115-2116.
13. Schessel DA, Nedzelski JA. Meniere's disease and other peripheral vestibular disorders. In: Cummings CW, ed. *Otolaryngology-Head and Neck Surgery.* St. Louis: Mosby Year Book, 1993, pp. 3152-3176.
14. Morrison AW, Booth JB. Systemic disease and otology. In: Alberti PW, Ruben RJ, eds. *Otologic Medicine and Surgery.* New York: Churchill-Livingstone, 1988, pp. 855-884.
15. Eviatar L, Eviatar A. Electronystagmography and vestibular testing in children. In: Alberti PW, Ruben RI, eds. *Otologic Medicine and Surgery.* New York: Churchill Livingstone, 1988, pp. 507-521.
16. Shah UK, White JA, Gooey JE, et al. Otolaryngologic manifestations of sarcoidosis: Presentation and diagnosis. Laryngoscope 1997; 107:67-75.
17. Bojrab DI, Stockwell CW. Electronystagmography and rotation tests. In: Jackler RK, Brackmann DE, eds. *Textbook of Neurotology.* St Louis: Mosby Year Book 1994, pp. 219-228.
18. Isono M, Murata K, Aiba K, et al. Minute findings of inner ear anomalies by three-dimensional CT scanning. Intl Jrnl Pediatr Otorhinolaryngol 1997; 42: 41-53.
19. Gilman S. Imaging the brain. First of two parts. New Engl J Med 1998; 338:812-820.
20. Gilman S. Imaging the brain. Second of two parts. New Engl J Med 1998; 338:889-896.
21. Zeitouni A, Zagzag D, Cohen NL. Meningioma of the internal auditory canal. Ann Otol Rhinol Laryngol 1997; 106:657-661.
22. Monsell EM, Cass SP, Rybak LP. Chemical labyrinthectomy: Methods and results. In: Brackman DE, Shelton C, Arriaga MA, eds. *Otologic Surgery.* Philadelphia: Saunders, 1994, pp. 509-518.
23. Casselbrant ML, Redfern MS, Furman JM, et al. Visual-induced postural sway in children with and without otitis media. Ann Otol Rhinol Laryngol 1998; 107: 401-405.
24. Casselbrant ML, Furman JM, Rubenstein E, et al. Effect of otitis media on the vestibular system in children. Ann Otol Rhinol Laryngol 1995; 104:620-624.
25. Reuter SH. Underwater medicine: Otolaryngologic considerations of the skin and scuba diver. In: Paparella MM, Shumrick DA, Gluckman JL, et al. eds. *Otolaryngology.* Philadelphia: Saunders, 1991, pp. 3231-3257.
26. Levenson MJ, Parisier SC, Jacobs M, et al. The large vestibular aqueduct syndrome in children. Arch Otolaryngol Head Neck Surg 1989; 115:54-58.
27. Zalzal GH, Tomaski SW, Vezina TM, et al. Enlarged vestibular aqueduct and sensorineural hearing loss in childhood. Arch Otolaryngol Head Neck Surg 1995; 121:23-28.
28. Abe S, Usami S, Shinkawa H. Three familial cases of hearing loss associated with enlargement of the vestibular aqueduct. Ann Otol Rhinol Laryngol 1997; 106:1063-1069.
29. Admiraal RJ, Huygen PL. Vestibular areflexia as a cause of delayed motor skill development in children with the CHARGE association. Intl Jrnl Pediatr Otorhinolaryngol 1997; 39:205-222.
30. Shah UK, LA Ohlms, MW Neault, et al. Otologic management in children with the CHARGE association. Intl Jrnl Pediatr Otorhinolaryngol 1998; 44:139-147.
31. Arriaga MA, Chen DA. Surgical treatment of uncompensated vestibular disease. Otolaryngol Clinics North Am 30; 5:759-776.
32. Poe DS, Bottrill ID. Comparison of endoscopic and

surgical explorations for perilymphatic fistulas. Am J Otology 1994; 15:735-738.

33. Poe DS, Rebeiz EE, Pankratov MM. Evaluation of perilymphatic fistulas by middle ear endoscopy. Am J Otology 1992; 13:529-33.

34. Aso S, Gibson WP. Perilymphatic fistula with no visible leak of fluid into the middle ear: A new method of intraoperative diagnosis using electrocochleography. Am J Otology 1994; 15:96-100.

35. Poe DS, Gadre AK, Rebeiz EE, et al. Intravenous fluorescein for detection of perilymphatic fistulas. Am J Otology 1993; 14:51-55.

36. Vartainen E, Karjalainen S, Karja J. Vestibular disorders following head injury in children. Intl J Pediatr Otorhinolaryngol 1985; 9:135-141.

37. Mitchell DP, Stone P. Temporal bone fractures in children. Canad J Otolaryngol 1973; 2:156-162.

38. D'agostino R, Tarantino V, Melagrana A, et al. Otoneurologic evaluation of child vertigo. Intl J Pediatr Otorhinolaryngol 1997; 40:133-139.

39. Michaels L. Pathology of the inner ear. In: Alberti PW, Ruben RJ, eds. *Otologic Medicine and Surgery.* New York: Churchill-Livingstone, 1988, pp. 651-711.

40. Kitsigianis GA, O'Leary DP, Davis LL. Active head-movement analysis of cisplatin-induced vestibulotoxicity. Otolaryngol Head Neck Surg 1988; 98:82-87.

41. Darmstadt GL, Harris JP. Luetic hearing loss: Clinical presentation, diagnosis and treatment. Am J Otolaryngol 1989; 10:410-421.

42. Arriaga MA, Chen DA. Hearing results of intratympanic steroids in endolymphatic hydrops (ELH). Eastern Section Meeting of the American Otologic, Rhinologic and Laryngologic Society. New York, January 31, 1998.

43. Reuter SH. Underwater medicine: Otolaryngologic considerations of the skin and scuba diver. In: Paparella MM, Shumrick DA, Gluckman JL, et al, eds. *Otolaryngology.* Philadelphia: Saunders, 1991, pp. 3231-3257.

44. Brandt T, Daroff R. Physical therapy for benign paroxysmal positional vertigo. Arch Otolaryngol Head Neck Surg 1980; 106:484-485.

45. Telischi FF, Rodgers GK, Balkany TJ. Dizziness in childhood. In: Jackler RK, DE Brackmann, eds. *Textbook of Neurotology.* St. Louis: Mosby, 1994, pp. 555-566.

46. Tom LWC, Rossiter JL, Sutton LN, et al. Torticollis in children. Otolaryngol Head Neck Surg 1991; 105: 1-5.

47. Chen TC, Maceri DR, Giannotta SL, et al. Unilateral acoustic neuromas in childhood without evidence of neurofibromatosis: Case report and review of the literature. Am J Otology 1992; 13:318-22.

48. Zappia JJ, O'Connor CA, Wiet RJ, et al. Rethinking the use of auditory brainstem response in acoustic neuroma screening. Laryngoscope 1997; 107: 1388-1392.

49. Jeng CM, Huang JS, Lee WY, et al. Magnetic resonance imaging of acoustic schwannomas. Jrnl Formosan Med Assn 1995; 94:487-493.

50. Kamerer DB, Lunsford LD, Moller M. Gamma knife: An alternative treatment for acoustic neuronomas. Ann Otol Rhinol Laryngol 1988; 97:631-635.

51. Smith M, Castillo M, Campbell J, et al. Baseline and follow-up MRI of the internal auditory canal after suboccipital resection of acoustic schwannoma: Appearances and clinical correlations. Neuroradiology 1995; 37:317-320.

52. Bikhazi NB, Slattery WH III, Lalwani AK, et al. Familial occurrence of unilateral vestibular schwannoma. Laryngoscope 1997; 107:1176-1180.

53. Trapp BD, Peterson J, Ransohoff RM, et al. Axonal transection in the lesions of multiple sclerosis. New Engl J Med 1998; 338:278-285.

54. Harker LA, Rassekh CH. Episodic vertigo in basilar artery migraine. Otolaryngol Head Neck Surg 1987; 96:239-250.

55. Johnson GD. Medical management of migraine-related dizziness and vertigo. Otolaryngol Head Neck Surg 1987; 96:239-250.

56. Lebel MH, Freij BJ, Syrogiannopoulos GA, et al. Dexamethasone therapy for bacterial meningitis. Results of two double-blind, placebo-controlled trials. New Engl J Med 1988; 319:964-971.

57. Starling SP. Syphilis in infants and young children. Pediatr Ann. 1994; 23:334-340.

58. Darmstadt GL, Harris JP. Luetic hearing loss: Clinical presentation, diagnosis and treatment. Am J Otolaryngol 1989; 10:410-421.

59. Lehrer JF, Poole DC, Seaman M, et al. Identification and treatment of metabolic abnormalities in patients with vertigo. Arch Int Med 1986; 146:1497-1500.

60. Kohan D, Rothstein SG, Cohen NL. Otologic disease in patients with acquired immunodeficiency syndrome. Ann Otol Rhinol Laryngol 1988; 97:636-640.

61. Wemama J-P, Delecroix M, Nyarwaya J-B, et al. Permanent unilateral vestibulocochlear dysfunction after spinal anesthesia. Anesth Analg 1996; 82: 406-408.

62. Lambert PR. Inner ear hair cell regeneration in a mammal: Identification of a triggering factor. Laryngoscope 1994; 104:701-718.

63. Rubel EW, Dew LA, Roberson DW. Mammalian vestibular hair cell regeneration. Science 267:701-7.

64. Echteler SM. Developmental segregation in the afferent innervation to mammalian auditory hair cells. Proc Nat Acad Sci 89:6324-6327.

65. Anthony PF. Laser applications in inner ear surgery. Otolaryngol Clin North Am 1996; 29:1031-1047.

66. Hillerdal M, Friberg U, Svedberg A, et al. Ultrasound treatment of Meniere's disease. Otolaryngol Clin North Am 1994; 24:337-346.

12 Introduction to Pediatric Otology

William P. Potsic

Every pediatric otolaryngologist is a pediatric otologist, and every general otolaryngologist must be knowledgeable about pediatric otologic disorders as well as auditory development. Ear disease is one of the most common conditions of childhood and one of the most common reasons that patients and pediatricians seek the consultation of an otolaryngologist. Inflammatory conditions of the middle ear are the most frequently seen, but a full range of otologic conditions occur in children that require the knowledge and skill necessary to carry out diagnosis and treatment. Also, a child may present a challenge to the otolaryngologist because the condition for referral is rarely in its early stages. A primary care provider may have treated the patient for weeks, months, or years prior to the consultation. The efficient diagnosis and treatment of chronic otologic disease in children is especially important because of the developmental, intellectual, and psychosocial impact on the performance of a child. The hearing loss that accompanies many otologic diseases can impact learning, behavior, and communication throughout an entire lifetime. In today's communication-based society and service-dominated work force, poor communication skills, learning difficulty, and behavior disorders can have a devastating effect on productivity. The otolaryngologist is in a unique position to facilitate a beneficial outcome for the child, parents, and educators.

Very often, children are apprehensive about seeing the "ear doctor" because of their past experiences with multiple examinations that may have been unpleasant. They may have been examined only during an acute infection when they were experiencing pain. They may have had pain when wax was removed from the ear with a curette or by the awkward insertion of a speculum. Parents often warn the physician that their child is difficult to examine or that he usually is restrained for ear examinations. The challenge presented to the otolaryngologist is to perform the task of the otologic examination with skill and provide comfort for the child.

SPECIAL CONSIDERATION:

Otologic conditions evaluated by pediatric otolaryngologists are usually chronic, and have been treated or followed for weeks, months, or years by other physicians prior to referral.

OTOLOGIC EXAMINATION OF THE CHILD

History

As in all examinations, a careful history may reveal the child's present chief complaint, signs, and symptoms as well as provide a clear understanding of the transition from the acute episode to the current persistent condition. This history-taking phase of the evaluation is an excellent opportunity to observe the general condition of the child both physically and behaviorally. It also provides a time for the child to develop a social rapport with the examiner. Friendly recognition of the child and her age-appropriate concerns conveys a caring attitude. Small children are often reassured by a gentle but deliberate touch of the shoulder or head. It is important to include the child in the interview process and not

Pediatric Otolaryngology, Edited by R.F. Wetmore, H.R. Muntz, and T.J. McGill. Thieme Medical Publishers, Inc., New York © 2000.

just speak to the parent. Failure to interact with the patient will not go unnoticed by the child or family.

Physical Examination

The physical examination of the child should include a complete evaluation of the head and neck; however, the ears should be examined first to reassure the child that the examination will be carried out with patience, skill, and comfort. Children of all ages can be examined fully dressed, and those who do not prefer to be seated alone can be evaluated sitting on a parent's lap. Lying a child down on a table may elicit memories of shots or other unpleasant experiences. Sitting sideways allows the child to rest his head against his parent's chest for stability as well as assurance. Shifting to the opposite side provides the same stability for examining the other ear. In some cases, parents may need to hold the child's arms or legs gently to decrease motion. Rarely, a very frightened child may need to be placed on an examining table for more firm restraint, including the use of a restraint board. Regardless of the position of the examination, all procedures should be explained in simple, direct language. Mild to moderate discomfort often is well tolerated if a child is informed and not deceived. Also, children of all ages should be allowed to express their emotions honestly. If they cry, it is an expression of fear or pain and is not a personal statement about the character of the examiner.

The otologic examination should begin with inspection of the facial appearance and head. The presence of craniofacial anomalies are an immediate indicator that otologic problems may be present. The shape of the pinna as well as the skin of the scalp, face, and neck around the ear should be noted. The external meatus also should be examined with the naked eye after opening the ear canal by pulling the pinna in a posterosuperior direction and the tragus forward by placing traction on the skin in front of the ear with the opposite hand (Fig. 12-1). Using this technique, dermatologic disorders that effect the skin around the ear and of the external canal as well as cerumen or foreign bodies in the lateral portion of the ear canal may become readily apparent.

The otoscopic examination of the ear canal, tympanic membrane (TM), and middle ear is the foundation of otologic diagnosis and treatment. A brightly-illuminated pneumatic otoscope with the largest speculum that will comfortably fit in the external meatus should be used. All too often, a small otoscope is selected with the intention of providing

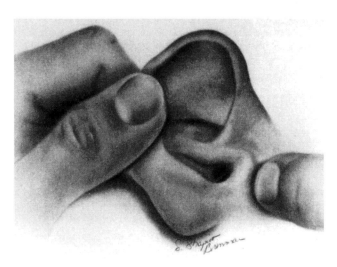

Figure 12-1: The external meatus may be opened by pulling the tragus and auricle in opposite directions.

comfort in an apparently small ear, but it limits vision and causes pain by scraping the ear canal. Abrasions may even cause bleeding, which further comprises vision and the quality of the examination. Neonates have collapsible ear canals and the otoscope may need to be introduced while applying positive pressure through the pneumatic otoscope. Halogen light provides the best light source. This type of light is available in wall-mounted and portable systems; there is currently very little difference in the intensity of the illumination from these systems. Portable units provide greater mobility, but wall units avoid the need for charging or battery changes. The otoscope should be held firmly and the heel of the hand or the fifth finger of the same hand should be rested against the child's head. In this way, if the child suddenly moves, the whole hand and otoscope move with the patient preventing the speculum from injuring the ear canal.

If cerumen is present in the ear canal but is not obstructing the view of any part of the TM, it does not need to be removed. If it does need to be removed cerumen is removed most effectively and gently with an ear curette under direct, magnified vision using illumination from a headlight. Use of the headlight also frees both hands to manipulate the ear and remove the wax. The recent, commercially-available Lumiview™ Voroscope (Fig. 12-2) is ideal for this purpose. It allows both hands to be used for manipulation and provides enhanced visualization of the ear canal, magnification, headlight illumination, and portability through battery power. Frequently, it eliminates the need for an operating microscope, even for very difficult wax im-

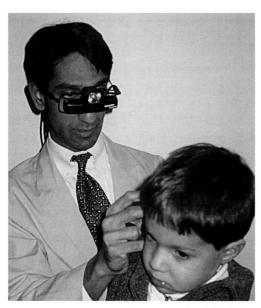

Figure 12–2: The Lumiview™ is a commercially available headlight that provides excellent illumination and magnification for examination of the external ear canal.

pactions. An otoscope with an operating head also can be used to remove wax, but it is less satisfactory.

On the rare occasion when the wax is so dry and hard that it cannot be removed comfortably by a curette, irrigation with body-temperature water may evacuate the canal. Even more infrequently, the wax may need to be softened by applying five drops of peroxide twice daily for 5 days followed by 7 days of antibiotic-containing ear drops. After soaking the wax in this way, it is usually either completely dissolved or very soft and easy to remove by irrigation or suction. However, children with atresia or stenosis of the ear canal may require examination using general anesthesia and otomicroscopy to remove impacted cerumen.

Examination of the TM includes evaluation of the medial extent of the external canal and the lateral most portion of the middle ear. The condition of the TM is, in and of itself, important. However, in the absence of disease of the ear canal, the TM reflects the effects of both acute and chronic middle-ear diseases. The appearance of thickness, tympanosclerosis, or atelectasis also may be a lagging indicator of previous middle-ear disease. The assessment of the eardrum should include a judgment on its vascularity, mobility, integrity (i.e., perforation), and position. This can be done accurately with a pneumatic otoscope. The examination should not stop at the surface of the TM. Because it is usually a translucent structure, the contents of the middle ear (e.g., ossicles, fluid and masses, etc) should be assessed also.

The position of the TM usually is found to be normal, bulging, or retracted. A bulging TM indicates acute infection. Retraction is, most often, a sign of eustachian tube (ET) dysfunction. In most early cases of TM retraction, the TM is retracted diffusely and there are no discrete pockets. As retraction progresses, pockets that, when very deep, appear to be perforations of the TM may be formed. These retraction pockets progress to form adhesions and skin-lined cysts, known as *cholesteatomas.* Early retraction pockets can be everted temporarily by applying negative pressure with the pneumatic otoscope, but this maneuver may cause considerable discomfort.

Most otolaryngologists have the capability of performing otomicroscopy in the office. This is particularly helpful when there is a need for greater magnification in order to make a judgement based on subtle findings only. Even though the Lumiview™ may be sufficient, otomicroscopy is superior for office otologic procedures such as foreign-body removal and tympanocentesis. If the microscope is connected to a video unit, it also may be of educational value to the patient and family.

Hearing Assessment

Accurate auditory assessment is possible in any child at any age. Early identification of hearing loss is possible and essential to the effective rehabilitation of children. An audiologist who is experienced in testing children must have available all of the modalities for testing in order to be able to assess hearing in all patients. A child of any age can be evaluated accurately using a combination of behavioral, mechanical, and electrophysiologic techniques.

> ### SPECIAL CONSIDERATION:
> Accurate auditory assessment is possible for any child at any age using behavioral, mechanical, and electrophysiologic techniques.

Radiographic Assessment

Plain radiography has limited application in the evaluation of the pediatric patient's ear. However, it remains useful in the evaluation of the postoperative position of a cochlear implant. Computed tomography (CT) and magnetic resonance imaging (MRI) are the most revealing, radiographic examinations used to evaluate hearing loss. CT is the most useful study for the temporal bone; MRI is most useful for the brainstem and cranial nerves. For the ear, CT is better because of its clear and accurate demonstration of the small bony structures and of the course of the facial nerve. It is also essential in the definition of congenital anomalies, fractures, and destructive lesions (e.g., cholesteatomas). CT also demonstrates soft-tissue density in the middle ear and mastoid, and is helpful in the evaluation of the internal meatus, cerebello-pontine angle masses, and early intracranial complications of inflammatory ear disease. MRI is particularly useful in identifying tumors of the eighth nerve and cerebello-pontine angle lesions. Magnetic resonance arteriography (MRA) and magnetic resonance venography (MRV) are used to help define vascular anomalies and intracranial complications such as otitic hydrocephalus and lateral sinus thrombosis.

AT A GLANCE . . .

Otologic Examination of the Child

History: provides an understanding of the child's present complaint; allows examiner to observe the child and develop rapport with her and her parents; the examiner must include the child in the interview

Physical Exam: complete evaluation of the head and neck with evaluation of the ears first; inform the child about the exam and do not deceive him; craniofacial anomalies, the shape of the pinna, and the condition of the skin around the ear should be noted; the external meatus should be examined; an otoscopic examination of the ear canal, TM, and middle ear should be done using a pneumatic otoscope; if cerumen obstructs the view of the TM, it should be removed

Hearing Assessment: an audiologist should evaluate a child using all of the available modalities for testing; a combination of behavioral, mechanical, and electrophysiologic techniques should be used

Radiographic Assessment: plain radiography is useful to evaluate the postoperative position of a cochlear implant; CT and MRI are the most revealing in the evaluation of hearing loss; MRA and MRV are useful in the definition of vascular anomalies and intracranial complications

---

OTALGIA

Otalgia, or earache, is a sensation that is interpreted by the patient to be pain in, on, or around the ear. Pain varies in its characteristics of quality, intensity, and duration. Children may be particularly difficult historians because of their variability in pain tolerance and ability to communicate. A prelingual child may be irritable, wake intermittently throughout the night, and rub his/her ear or (more often) both ears. Children with well-developed speech usually are able to describe the characteristics and location of the pain very well. An important part of the evaluation of pain is to make a judgement as to the appearance of the child's facial expression compared to the described intensity of the pain. Parents are very experienced in detecting and assessing a pained facial expression. In contrast, a child may complain of or exhibit behavior consistent with pain (such as pulling on an ear) but appear bright, happy, and inquisitive.

Ear pain may be generated by a condition of the ear itself or may be from a source that is remote from the ear (i.e., nonotogenic). The source of *otogenic pain* is diagnosed easily by inspection of the ear and ear canal using an otoscope. *Nonotogenic ear pain* is usually referred pain from the head and neck region through cervical nerves. It also may be caused by neuralgias of the cervical nerves (e.g., trigeminal neuralgia) that supply the region of the ear or may be of psychogenic origin. Table 12–1 lists the possible causes of otalgia.

Otogenic Ear Pain

Inflammatory diseases of the ear are the most common causes of ear pain in all age groups. By far, acute suppurative otitis media (ASOM) and external otitis (EO) cause the majority of otogenic pain that is constant, boring, and intense. The pain of ASOM intensifies when associated with acute mastoiditis, especially with cellulitis in the periauricular area. The pain of EO is exacerbated by movement of the ear canal, such as when chewing, pulling the ear, or pressing the tragus. *Bullous myringitis* is an infection of the TM with bulla formation on the surface of the TM that is particular painful and intense. The diagnosis of these conditions is made easily by otoscopy.

Viral infections of the middle ear are rarely painful and are usually present during an acute viral respira-

TABLE 12–1: Causes of Otalgia

Otogenic
  Acute suppurative otitis media
  Bullous myringitis
  External otitis
  Foreign body in external canal with or without infection
  Viral otitis
    Respiratory tract infection
    Herpes zoster oticus
  Chronic otitis media/cholesteatoma
  Trauma
    Barotrauma
    Lacerations
    Seroma/hematoma
  Tumors with or without infection
Nonotogenic
  Oral cavity and Pharynx
    Dental
      Erupting teeth
      Orthodontia
      Impacted molars
    Aphthous ulcers
    Pharyngitis
      Bacterial or viral infection
      Peritonsillar abscess
      Post operative tonsillectomy and adenoidectomy
    Pharyngeal tumors
    Hypopharyngeal and laryngeal lesions
  Head and neck
    Rhinosinusitis
    Lymphadenitis
    Parotitis and TMJ
    Cervical spine trauma
    Neuralgia
  Psychogenic
  Other rare conditions
    Bell's palsy
    Migraine

tory tract infection (RTI). *Viral otitis* may be associated with fluid in the middle ear and mild inflammation of the TM, but it rarely causes pain. In contrast, *Herpes zoster oticus* causes severe, excruciating pain, and is associated with vesicular eruptions on the auricle. Pharyngeal vesicles, facial paralysis, and TM necrosis may occur on the same side.

Foreign bodies and tumors of the ear canal may cause pain, but more often the pain is the result of an associated bacterial infection. Both of these conditions may be deceptive. The diagnosis of a foreign body or tumor occasionally is delayed for several weeks by treatment for a stubborn ear infection that does not respond to medical therapy. Foreign bodies are common and tumors are rare; however, both benign and malignant tumors do occur in the middle ear and ear canal of children. Rhabdomyosarcoma is a particularly destructive tumor.

Trauma to the ear usually causes acute pain that is of very short duration. Trauma to the auricle may cause a seroma or hematoma. Sharp or blunt objects poked into the ear canal may lacerate the canal skin and the TM. The pain is extreme but resolves quickly. Much more common is the pain children experience from barotrauma. Small children usually have ET dysfunction during colds. Young children who take airplane trips frequently are exposed to pressure changes that may exacerbate ET dysfunction and cause ear pain of less than an hour duration. Otoscopy of these ears in the first few days after landing may reveal small hematomas of the TM as well as hemotympanum. Because these children are rarely examined, these findings may go unnoticed and usually resolve spontaneously.

Chronic otitis media (COM) (i.e., perforation of the TM) with or without cholesteatoma rarely is associated with pain unless there is concurrent acute mastoid osteomyelitis. This is most likely due to the fact that the purulence, when present, easily drains out of the middle ear through the TM perforation.

Nonotogenic Ear Pain

Nonotogenic ear pain is frustrating for the patient, family, and physician. It is particularly difficult when the parents are convinced that their child has ear pain and they are told the ear appears normal. It is not sufficient to say that it is not from the ear. Although the parents may be relieved to know that it is not another ear infection, the source of the pain must be identified. Referred pain to the ear is usually mild to moderate in intensity, intermittent, and relieved easily by the use of nonsteroidal antiinflammatory drugs (NSAIDs). Six cranial nerves may refer pain to the ear.

As with otogenic causes of ear pain, the most common source of referred pain to the ear is an inflammatory condition in the distribution of the fifth, seventh, ninth, and tenth cranial nerves and in cervical nerves 1 (C1) and 2 (C2). These cranial nerves supply the nasosinus area, oral cavity and teeth, oropharynx, hypopharynx, larynx, and upper esophagus. Surrounding structures such as the temporomandibular joint, salivary glands, cervical nodes, and neck masses also may refer pain to the ear through their mutual innervation. Cervical spine injuries, arthritis, and disc disease may refer pain to the ear through C1 and C2. Neuralgia of any of these nerves may cause atypical pain in the presence of a normal otologic and head and neck examination.

Dental pain is common during teething, orthodontic work, and with impacted molars. Pain of dental origin is the most common cause of referred ear pain at any age.[1] Other common causes are pharyngitis, oral ulcers, rhinosinusitis, and surgery such as adenotonsillectomy. Often tonsillectomy and adenoidectomy (T&A) patients expect a sore throat but do not expect the associated referred ear pain. Rarely, ear pain may be a prodome of an impending condition, such as migraine headache or Bell's palsy.

SPECIAL CONSIDERATION:

Referred ear pain is common in children and is most often of dental origin (teething, orthodontia, and impacted molars).

When the otologic examination is normal and the complete head and neck examination reveals no likely source of referred pain, the pain may be psychogenic. Psychogenic pain is usually mild, intermittent, and refractory to pain medications, including narcotic analgesics. Pain of psychogenic origin is most common in children with depression, but anxiety disorders also may present this way. This condition is distinctly separate from the child who is malingering and complains of pain to avoid certain activities such as school. A professional usually is needed to sort out the symptoms of the psychiatric disorder that may be the cause of the pain and that may affect a child's ability to function.

In addition to the routine head and neck examination, the search for the cause of otalgia may require nasal endoscopy, nasopharyngoscopy, laryngoscopy, and esophagoscopy. A dental evaluation is essential also. Other studies may include standard radiographs with dental views. However, if radiographs of the head and neck are needed, the preferred study is a CT that includes the skull, temporal bone, and neck. Practice Pathway 12–1 summarizes the evaluation of otalgia.

OTORRHEA

Infectious Causes of Otorrhea

Otorrhea is drainage from the ear. It occurs frequently in children and is usually associated with infection of the ear canal or middle ear. The discharge can be copious and most often has a foul smell. In the presence of infection, small blood vessels frequently rupture, so a bloody tinge or frank blood in the discharge is common and usually of little long-term significance. Otorrhea itself is painless, but the underlying infection may be painful. The location and quality of the pain may help the otolaryngologist to pinpoint the source of the drainage. After several hours of drainage, the material becomes colonized with multiple strains of bacteria, so treating the bacterial infection is an important part of management of all otorrhea. In some cases, otorrhea may not be caused by infection. An example of this is a cerebrospinal fluid (CSF) leak; however, this condition usually is obvious because it occurs following severe head trauma or mastoid surgery.

External otitis

External otitis (EO) occurs more frequently during the summer months when children are swimming almost daily. Another group of children that are predisposed to EO are patients who have dermatologic conditions effecting the ear canal and immunosuppressed patients. The infection may be bacterial or fungal and typically is associated with foul drainage and pain. The infection responds to debridement (suctioning) of the ear canal and the installation of antimicrobial ototopical eardrops. Occasionally, oral antibiotics also are required.

Malignant EO is rare in the pediatric age group and usually occurs in children with compromised immune defenses.[2] These infections may be very destructive, causing tissue necrosis, osteomyelitis of the temporal bone, and cranial nerve involvement. Treatment must be aggressive using intravenous antibiotics and topical antimicrobials; it also may require surgery.

Acute suppurative otitis media

The otorrhea that occurs with *acute suppurative otitis media* (ASOM) presents suddenly with the simultaneous relief of pain a few hours into the infection. The drainage is usually copious, mucopurulent, and blood-tinged, and occurs because of necrosis and perforation of the TM; it can be compared to the spontaneous drainage of an abscess. The inflammation of the middle ear stimulates the production of large amounts of fluid that does not

Practice Pathway 12–1 EVALUATION OF OTALGIA

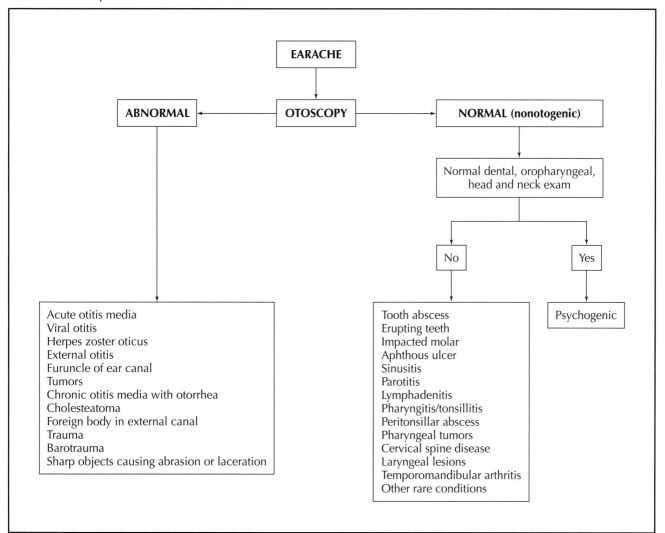

resolve until the acute infection subsides. Otorrhea also may occur through a pressure-equalization tube (PET) during acute infection of the middle ear. This most often follows an acute respiratory infection or water contamination of the middle ear.

After the ear canal is cleansed either by suctioning the drainage or removing it with a cotton swab, a small pinhole perforation that is surrounded by a rim of granulation tissue can be seen. Typically, the perforations that occur with ASOM are small and heal spontaneously after treatment of the acute OM with standard antimicrobial therapy. Infrequently, necrosis may result in a large perforation of the TM. The drainage is welcomed as a relief from the pain to the child, but to the parent it signifies that the infection is more severe than they usually experience and therefore more complicated. Parents often are very concerned about permanent hearing loss

that might occur as a result of a TM perforation. However, this is a rare occurrence.

Chronic otitis media

Chronic otitis media (COM) is defined as a persistent perforation or apparent perforation (e.g., cholesteatoma) of the TM. Chronic perforations usually result from severe, necrotizing infection. Also, PET placement or the neck of a deep retraction pocket may cause a perforation. If active infection of the middle ear is not present also, the ear is dry and no otorrhea occurs. If an infection is present in a child with COM, otorrhea occurs. The drainage is usually copious, mucopurulent, foul smelling, and often blood-tinged. The otorrhea occurs in the absence of pain. The drainage may increase or start shortly after water contamination of the ears, during an acute respiratory infection, or spontaneously with no apparent inciting event.

Specific mention of the otorrhea that occurs following PET placement is appropriate because it is seen very frequently. Many children have PETs, and the vast majority of them have dry ears. However, otorrhea may develop during a number of situations. The most frequent is when there is mucopurulent drainage through the tube during an acute respiratory infection when mucus production is copious in the nose, sinuses, and middle ear. Water contamination also is a source of infection, and it causes otorrhea through a functioning tube. This cause of otorrhea is seen more often in the summer when children are swimming frequently.

An uncommon cause of otorrhea through a PET is reflux of secretions or feedings through a patent ET in a patient with velopharyngeal insufficiency. This otorrhea occurs during feeding and is seen most often in young patients with cleft palates that have not been repaired. Although culture of this fluid often grows microbial organisms, it does not represent a chronic infection and requires only clearing of the ear canal with a cotton swab after feeding. This type of otorrhea is of little significance and stops after the palate is repaired. Similarly, otorrhea also may be associated with gastroesophageal reflux (GER). Acid inflames the ET and middle-ear mucosa causing copious otorrhea.

Bloody otorrhea also may signify the presence of granulation tissue in the middle ear. Granulation tissue is an indicator of chronic inflammation and a foreign-body reaction. Granulation polyps often form around a PET or in association with a cholesteatoma.

The management of otorrhea from COM is the same for perforation with infection, cholesteatoma, or if a PET is in place. The drainage must be evacuated from the ear canal in order to visualize the middle ear and make an accurate diagnosis. Cleaning the ear canal also clears a pathway for the application of ototopical antibiotic medications. The ototopical antibiotic and corticosteroid solutions used should be effective against *Staphylococcus aureus* and *Pseudomonas aeruginosa*. The potential ototoxicity of these preparations remains controversial; there are *no good, controlled, prospective studies* to validate the concern that these preparations are ototoxic when applied to the infected middle ear of a child.[3] The recent development of the quinalone topical preparations that are effective against *Pseudomonas aeruginosa* and *Staphylococcus aureus*

circumvents this issue of ototoxicity.[4] Oral antibiotics effective against beta-lactamase producing organisms in addition to the ototopical medications usually clear the infection and resolve the granulation tissue. When the drainage does not respond to this standard therapy, a culture of the secretions is essential to identify the resistant organisms and determine specific antibiotic sensitives. Fungal cultures may reveal a predominance of *Candida albicans* or *aspergillus.* The antifungal agent, clotrimazole, can be applied topically as a drop to eliminate the fungal component of the infection. Rarely, intravenous antibiotic therapy and daily cleansing of the ear by suctioning is required to resolve the infection.

When otorrhea does not respond in a timely fashion to treatment or recurs shortly after stopping therapy, a search should be initiated for unusual causes of drainage. In the past, one of these unusual causes was tuberculosis. In recent years, tuberculosis has made a resurgence in all populations in the United States and is no longer just seen in immigrants and immunosuppressed patients. Ears infected with tuberculosis often have multiple perforations of the TM and do not respond to conventional therapy. Bacterial cultures for the acid-fast organism and biopsy of granulation tissue will yield the diagnosis. Treatment is with antibiotic therapy, although some strains of mycobacteria tuberculosis have become increasingly resistant to treatment.

SPECIAL CONSIDERATION:

Otorrhea that is refractory to treatment or recurrent suggests the need to search for unusual causes (e.g., cholesteatoma and immunodeficiency)

Other causes of persistent purulent otorrhea that do not respond to standard therapy may be retained foreign bodies, tumors in the middle ear and external canal, and even more rarely, a vascular malformation such as a hemangioma involving the TM or the ear canal. These mass lesions do not produce the drainage but obstruct the ear canal causing secondary infection. A first-branchial-cleft sinus tract, although rare, may connect to the ear canal and if infected, produce purulent drainage. Just as cultures are required to define the offending organism in persistent cases, a high-resolution CT is indicated to examine the middle ear and temporal bone when the clinical presentation is unusual or the otorrhea persists.

Noninfectious Causes of Otorrhea

Clear drainage through perforated eardrum may indicate a CSF leak or, rarely, a perilymphatic fistula (PLF) CSF leaks through a defect in the TM usually follow head traumas that fracture the temporal bone and lacerate the TM. This CSF otorrhea usually stops spontaneously due to healing of the fracture and the dural defect; however, CSF drainage may continue through the ET after the TM heals. Small leaks of this type may go unnoticed unless the patient develops meningitis. CSF leaks and otorrhea also may follow surgery in which the dura has been violated by a surgeon or a disease process.

Similarly, PLFs rarely drain through the eardrum, unless a perforation has occurred due to a penetrat-

ing injury that causes the fistula. More likely, a child without a penetrating injury, has a PET placed for what appears to be persistent serous fluid in the middle ear but is actually perilymph. Constant clear otorrhea will result in this case. A CT scan will usually demonstrate a Mondini malformation of the labyrinth, and drainage occurs through an absent footplate or a large fistula in the center of the footplate.

The pediatric otologist frequently encounters otorrhea. The source of the drainage must be identified and the infection treated effectively. When the drainage persists or recurs frequently, a search must be carried out to identify unusual resistant organisms and unusual causes of otorrhea. High-resolution CT is most helpful in these cases. If an underlying cause is identified, it must be treated or the effort to stop the drainage is futile (Practice Pathway 12-2).

TINNITUS IN CHILDREN

Tinnitus is a persistent or intermittent noise that is perceived by the patient as being heard in the ear. Tinnitus is a symptom that is rarely volunteered by children but that is frequently obtained by a careful history. The ability of a child to describe the characteristics of the sound she hears is dependent upon the child's verbal ability and experience. The prevalence of tinnitus in children is unknown, but it is suspected that a large number of children either have it intermittently or have had it and never complained. A child may not be able to relate to the pitch and quality of the sound, but he often is able to tell the examiner that it sounds like a whistle, phone ringing, clicking sound, or paper being crumpled. Older children are better able to be very specific about the character of their tinnitus.

Tinnitus may be either *objective* (i.e., able to be heard by the examiner using auscultation) or *subjective* (i.e., unable to be heard by the examiner). The majority of children who complain of hearing noises in the ear have normal hearing or a conductive hearing loss (CHL). Few children with sensorineural hearing loss (SNHL) complain of tinnitus, in contrast to adults who frequently complain of bothersome tinnitus.

Objective tinnitus in children is usually pulsatile and of vascular origin. Similarly, vascular lesions may not produce a sound that can be heard by the examiner, but the sound is still perceived by the

---

AT A GLANCE . . .

Causes of Otorrhea

Infectious:

External Otitis: occurs more frequently during the summer when children swim more often; may be bacterial or fungal in origin; responds to suctioning of the ear canal and antimicrobial ototopical eardrops

Acute Suppurative Otitis Media: presents suddenly; drainage is copious, mucopurulent, and blood-tinged, and occurs because of necrosis and perforation of the TM; ear canal is cleansed by suctioning, and perforations usually heal spontaneously after treatment with standard antimicrobial therapy

Chronic Otitis Media: a persistent perforation or apparent perforation of the TM that results from severe, necrotizing infection retraction; drainage is usually copious, mucopurulent, foul smelling, and blood-tinged; drainage is suctioned out of ear canal and ototopical antibiotic medications and corticosteroids are used to resolve infection

Noninfectious: CSF leak following head trauma; PLF

Practice Pathway 12–2   TREATMENT OF OTORRHEA

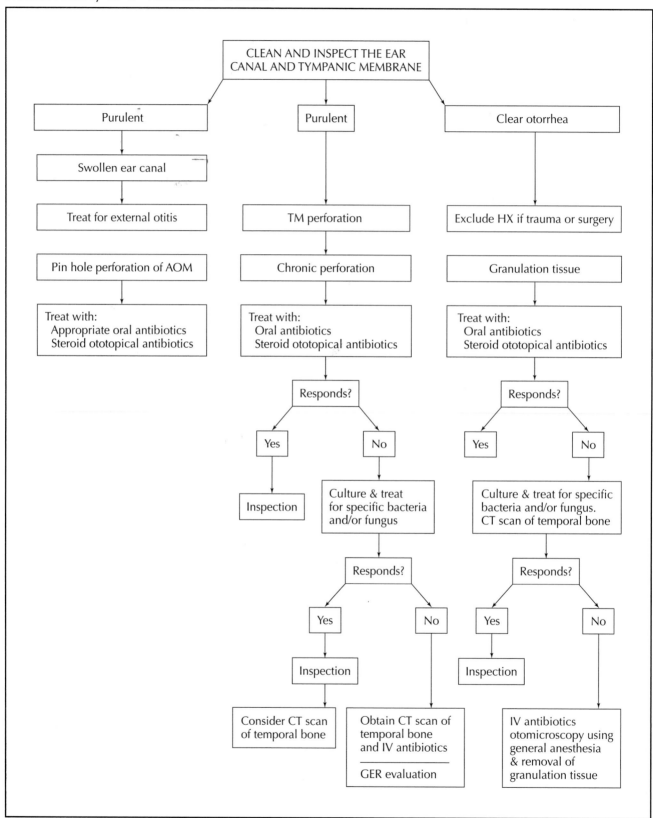

Abbreviations: AOM, acute otitis media; TM, tympanic membrane; HX, history; GER, gastroesophageal reflux.

patient. In children, the most common cause of *pulsatile tinnitus* is turbulent blood flow through normal vessels and vascular anomalies, such as an aberrant carotid artery in the middle ear that produces a bruit heard by the patient. The sound is most prominent at night when competing noises are absent. Likewise, a very high jugular bulb in the middle ear may produce a venous hum. Sounds from neck vessels in the region of the temporal bone also may be transmitted to the ear.[5]

Rare and troublesome causes of pulsatile tinnitus are hemangiomas of the middle ear and glomus tympanicum tumors. Vascular tumors may occur at a very young age.[6] Pulsatile tinnitus that occurs with these tumors may be exacerbated during times when children have a CHL, as in the presence of serous otitis media (SOM). Pulsatile tinnitus that is synchronous with the pulse and is either constant or persistently intermittent is best evaluated by CT or with MRA and MRV.

The majority of children who complain of noises in the ear do so because of a clicking sound. This is often the normal sound that we all perceive when the ET opens and closes. This crackling sound may be first apparent to the child after a PET is extruded and the child hears the sounds of normal middle-ear function. Very rarely, the rhythmic clicking sounds of palatal muscle contraction (i.e., palatal myoclonus) and middle ear muscle contraction may be troublesome to a child.

Because the majority of noises heard in the ear by a child are more apparent during a hearing loss (e.g., with an episode of OM, they are easily manageable by treating the existing condition in the middle ear. However, if there is no explanation for the tinnitus and it persists, the examiner must be as certain as possible that a potentially life-threatening condition does not exist (such as an intracranial vascular malformation, an eighth cranial-nerve tumor, a middle-ear tumor, or a cerebello-pontine angle mass). If serious temporal bone and intracranial lesions are ruled out, both the parents and the child can be reassured that a conservative, watchful approach is indicated.

When the patient notes tinnitus and a SNHL also is identified, the same approach should be taken to identify serious causes. In most of these cases, the etiology is not identified and is classified as unknown. Parents should be reassured that tinnitus is not a separate disease. Tinnitus associated with SNHL is most likely due to a neural dissynchronization that generates either a cochlear origin or a central perception of the sound. The mechanism of cochlear or centrally-produced tinnitus is a matter of speculation.

Several drugs may produce tinnitus as a side effect. The most common of these is aspirin. Because of the risk of Reye's syndrome, few children receive aspirin today. Ototoxic antibiotics and drugs used in chemotherapy also may cause SNHL and tinnitus.

Unlike adults who seem to be very bothered by tinnitus and often are willing to go to extreme measures to relieve it, children are resilient and adaptive. Children rarely are bothered enough to consider wearing an appliance to mask the sound and usually carry out their activities at school and socially with little or no difficulty. However, it should be remembered that the full spectrum of causes of tinnitus in adults also might occur in children but have a much lower prevalence. So the complaint of tinnitus from a child should not be dismissed lightly.

Practice Pathway 12–3 summarizes the evaluation for tinnitus.

HEARING LOSS IN CHILDREN

Childhood hearing loss is a frequent occurrence. Like middle-ear fluid, it is almost universally present for a period of weeks to months during respiratory infections in the first 3 years of life. OM with effusion (OME) is one of the most common chronic conditions of childhood, and when present, it causes a hearing deficit that ranges between mild and moderate. If the presence of fluid is not associated with ASOM also, parents or caretakers may not know it. Because children may have as many as seven respiratory infections per year, they may suffer between 14 and 28 weeks of hearing deficit annually during the first 3 years of life, a time when there is rapid language, speech, and communication development.

Permanent hearing deficits may be inherited or just occur by chance. Hearing losses in children are being detected earlier, and early knowledge that a hearing loss is present makes rehabilitation and treatment more effective, enhancing communication development.

Hearing assessment has reached a level of sophistication that permits the accurate definition of hearing in any child at any age with any mental status. Using a combination of behavioral, mechanical, and electrophysiologic techniques, children may be tested and screened when they are newborns and at any later age. In fact, neonatal screening has been

Practice Pathway 12–3   EVALUATION FOR TINNITUS

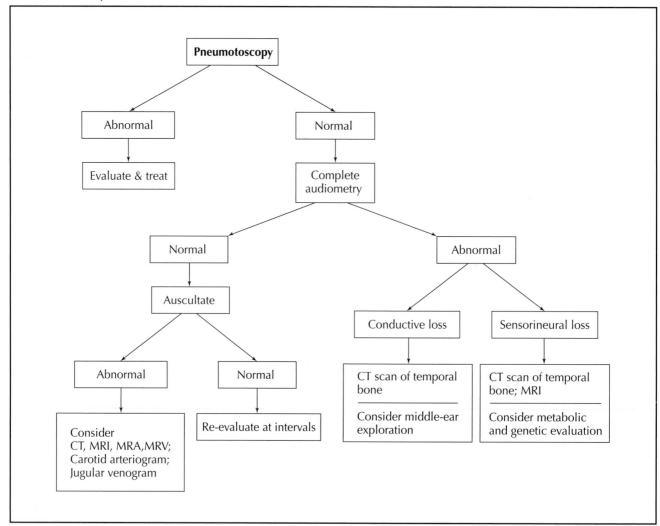

mandated in some states, and the American Academy of Pediatrics Joint Committee on Infant Hearing 1994 Position Statement recommends identification of all infants with hearing loss.[7] The sense of hearing is perceptual, and central auditory perceptual deficits may exist in spite of the fact that the peripheral auditory system is intact and functioning normally. Testing for perceptual deficits is not as well developed. Normative data must be established and standardized by age. The treatment of these central perceptual deficits is also in evolution.

Just as the diagnosis and identification of the hearing loss has advanced, the management of hearing deficits also has been evolving for children. Operative reconstructive techniques that were once reserved for adults have been refined to be just as effective for children.[8,9] Osseointegrated, bone-anchored, bone-conduction hearing aids and advances

in conventional hearing aid technology have improved the rehabilitation of hearing loss dramatically. Also, cochlear implantation is a successful mechanism for providing sound for children with no serviceable hearing. The future may bring enhancements of the current technology and embrace new frontiers such as brainstem and cortical implants.

SPECIAL CONSIDERATION:

Auditory rehabilitation has improved and is helpful for all children with hearing loss. Rehabilitation may include cochlear implantation for children with SNHL and no serviceable hearing.

Volumes of material and entire textbooks have been written on hearing loss.[10] Some of these discussions are highly academic, detailed, and exhaustive. The otolaryngologist who is seeing office patients must have a practical and useful approach to the child with hearing loss. The parents of such a child often ask questions that, although seemingly basic, have important implications to their life and the life of their child. Some of the questions parents may ask are:

1. Is a hearing loss present in one or both ears?
2. How severe is it?
3. How does it or how will it effect development of speech, language, and communication?
4. What kind of hearing loss is it (conductive or sensorineural) and is it correctable?
5. What caused it? Was it caused by something I did? Could I have prevented it?
6. Will it get worse over time? If it is in only one ear now, will it effect the other ear later?
7. What can we do to prevent further loss of hearing?
8. What can we do to maximize auditory function now to facilitate development and provide effective function both academically and socially? Some of these considerations are preferential seating in school, reconstructive surgery, hearing aids auditory-assistive devices, communication training (sign language, lip reading, and auditory verbal therapy), and cochlear implantation.

Some of these questions cannot be answered with certainty, and patients rarely require that degree of precision from their physicians. However, they can be given a good understanding of the condition, an informed but guarded prediction of the most likely possibilities, and preparation for the worst prognosis should it occur. Rehabilitation should be started immediately after the hearing loss is identified. In the event that a child loses all serviceable hearing, parents can be assured that with cochlear implantation almost all children can be helped. Exceptions include those with the most severe congenital malformations of the cochlea or an absent eighth nerve.

The three practical classifications of hearing loss are conductive, sensorineural, and mixed. *Conductive hearing loss* (CHL) is caused by an abnormality of the ear canal, TM, middle-ear space, or middle-ear ossicles. Of course, any combination of these factors may all contribute to CHL. *Sensorineural hearing loss* (SNHL) is caused by abnormalities of

the cochlea, auditory nerve or, more centrally, the auditory pathways that traverse the brainstem and end in the auditory cortex of the brain. *Mixed hearing loss* is a combination of a conductive and a sensorineural component. Hearing loss identified in childhood may be congenital, acquired, or of an unknown etiology. Although an inherited cause may be suspected, the vast majority of SNHL in children ultimately is found to be of unknown etiology.

Hearing loss may be stable, fluctuating, or progressive. The deficit may include all frequencies, but some frequencies may be affected to a greater degree than others. Audiometry that is appropriate for age and repeated at intervals defines the nature, degree, and stability of the loss.

Conductive Hearing Loss

The evaluation of a CHL requires a complete history and an otoscopic examination in addition to a thorough examination of the head and neck. CT is obtained to evaluate the structures of the temporal bone in almost all cases, except when the cause is due obviously to effusion in the middle ear. Standard radiographs rarely are helpful, and MRI may be obtained in some cases to evaluate intracranial complications of otologic diseases that are associated with a CHL.

CHL is acquired most frequently as a result of one of the most common chronic conditions of childhood—OME. Other common causes include COM and cholesteatoma with destruction of the middle-ear structures. These conditions are amenable to surgeries that ranges from myringotomy and PET placement to tympanomastoidectomy. With modern techniques and skilled hands, hearing may be returned to normal or the nearly normal range, even in the presence of some of the most destructive diseases. Acquired ossicular fixation from tympanosclerosis and otosclerosis is rarely encountered in children. *Tympanosclerosis* usually forms in the chronically-infected middle ear and is suggested when a CHL is associated with extensive tympanosclerosis of the TM. TM tympanosclerosis alone almost never causes a measurable hearing loss. *Otosclerosis* in children is seen only in patients with osteogenesis imperfecta. These children are identified easily by their history of frequent long-bone fractures and blue sclera.

Congenital CHL may be seen in conjunction with craniofacial abnormalities such as Down's syndrome or Treacher Collins syndrome. Isolated congenital malformations of the ear also may occur that are indicated only by subtle variations in the size and shape of the pinna. Severe deformity of the pinna to near absence (i.e., microtia) usually are associated with anomalies of the external ear canal and middle ear. Surgical correction of the atretic canal and the fixed ossicular chain is difficult, but in experienced hands this most often results in significant hearing improvement.

Isolated external-canal stenosis and atresia in the absence of any pinna abnormality are less common but also may have the potential for surgical correction. The surgeon must be aware that a bony plate usually replaces the TM either partially or totally and that the ossicles are malformed and fused. In all congenital malformations of the temporal bone, the facial nerve may have an abnormal course or be abnormally shaped. CT is the most useful study to determine the advisability of surgery and the likelihood of a good result.

Congenital middle-ear malformations usually are associated with abnormalities of the external ear, but isolated anomalies do occur. Isolated ossicular anomalies may vary from mild malformations that cause minimal loss of hearing to total absence of all or part of the ossicles. The ossicles also may be fused or fixed. The most common isolated middle-ear anomaly that causes a CHL is congenital fixation of the stapes. In addition, isolated middle-ear anomalies may be associated with an abnormal course of the facial nerve. Surgical reconstruction of the ossicular chain often results in substantial hearing improvement.

Sensorineural Hearing Loss

The evaluation of a child with a recently identified SNHL requires a complete medical history of the child as well as a careful family history. Although a significant amount of congenital deafness that is identified in childhood appears to be caused by genetic factors, it is extremely difficult to obtain a sufficient history to reconstruct a family pedigree.[11,12] Many parents were never evaluated as children and are unaware of a hearing loss even if they have one. Otoscopy and a complete head and neck physical examination may reveal signs of a syndrome associated with a sensorineural deficit. A CT scan is particularly helpful in identifying temporal bone abnormalities that may be associated with progressive or fluctuating hearing loss.

> ## SPECIAL CONSIDERATION:
> Although a myriad of studies can be done to evaluate SNHL, the evaluation should be targeted by clinical decision making. The CT scan of the temporal bone is very useful for detecting congenital anomalies and potentially correctable causes of hearing loss.

SNHL in children is usually congenital and of unknown etiology in spite of exhaustive efforts to identify the cause. Congenital SNHL may have been acquired during intrauterine development. The degree of loss varies and may be unilateral as well as bilateral. The parents of hearing-impaired children are usually the first to detect a hearing problem. They may just sense that something is wrong in the way the child interacts with sound and people. Mild or unilateral, congenital SNHL often goes undetected until age 3 to 5 when screening preschool hearing tests are done. Even these tests miss very mild losses that meet passing criteria for the screening test.

The majority of congenital SNHL are isolated and not associated with syndromes. Congenital SNHL usually occurs in an otherwise normal child; however, it may be associated with syndromes that effect other organ systems. Examples of these are Alport's syndrome (nephritis and SNHL), Jervell and Lange-Nielsen syndrome (arrhythmia with prolonged QT segment and SNHL), and Usher syndrome (retinitis pigmentosa and SNHL). It is important to identify these patients early so that the involved organ systems can be treated. Laboratory studies should be targeted to the suspected organ system because there is no universal battery of laboratory studies that consistently identifies the etiology of all SNHL.

SNHL also may be acquired as a result of infection. *TORCHS* studies are a group of specific immunoglobulin M antibody assays for toxoplasmosis, other agents, rubella, cytomegalovirus, herpes simplex and syphilis. This battery is useful to determine if intrauterine infection is a cause of the hearing loss. Meningitis is a common infection and often a devastating cause of SNHL. Even though the simultaneous treatment of the meningitis with antimicrobials and steroids has reduced the incidence of SNHL from meningitis, it still occurs regularly and is often associated with other neurologic sequella.[13] Because the cochlea may ossify following meningitis, making cochlear implantations difficult, children with severe SNHL due to meningitis should be considered for early implantation.

Although the laboratory evaluation of the child with SNHL should be individualized, CT of the temporal bone is particularly useful to identify potentially treatable causes of both CHL and SNHL. It also may provide some objective information to suggest that a SNHL may be progressive. The CT of the temporal bone is also essential to detect malformations of the middle ear and inner ear when evaluating children with either newly identified or sudden SNHL. Malformations of the middle ear or inner ear, such as the Mondini malformation, may be associated with a PLF that can be repaired to stabilize hearing. CT also may reveal less dramatic variations in the inner ear anatomy, such as enlarged vestibular aqueduct (EVA). Although these patients may have no hearing loss at all, EVA has been associated with progressive SNHL.[14]

Molecular biologic evaluation in nonsyndromic sensorineural autosomal recessive deafness may be helpful to identify the abnormal gene both for diagnosis and genetic counseling for the most common genetic forms of deafness.[16,17] Testing is done by deoxyribonucleic acid (DNA) sequence analysis.

A suspected hearing loss should be viewed as an opportunity to improve the long-term productivity of the child. The evaluation should be individualized. Early identification and prompt corrective action rather than watchful waiting are necessary to maximize the speech, language, cognitive, communication, and psychosocial development of the child. Maximal hearing during the early years of development appears critical for developing the neural patterns that are used throughout a lifetime. Continued vigilance by interval audiometry is required to fulfill the needs of a child that is experiencing progression of the hearing deficit.

AT A GLANCE . . .

Hearing Loss in Children

Pathogenesis: respiratory infection during the first 3 years of life, OME, COM, genetic, congenital, cholesteatoma with destruction of the middle-ear structures

Adverse Effects: delay of language, speech, cognitive, psychosocial, and communication development

Classification: *Conductive:* caused by an abnormality of the ear canal, TM, middle-ear space, or middle-ear ossicles. *Sensorineural:* caused by abnormalities of the cochlea, auditory nerve, or auditory pathways that traverse the brainstem and end in the auditory cortex of the brain. *Mixed:* a combination of conductive and sensorineural

Diagnosis: using a combination of behavioral, mechanical, and electrophysiologic techniques children may be tested accurately when they are newborns; MRI; CT

Treatment: reconstructive techniques, bone-anchored hearing aids, bone-conduction hearing aids, cochlear implants, communication training (sign language, lip reading, and auditory verbal therapy), PET.

REFERENCES

1. Nazif MM, Ruffalo RC. The interaction between dentistry and otolaryngology. Pediatr Clin North Am 1981; 28:997–1010.
2. Coser PL, Stamm AE, Lobo RC, et al. Malignant external otitis in infants. Laryngoscope 1980; 90:312.
3. Pickett BP, Shinn JB, Smith MFW. Clinical forum: Ear drop ototoxicity: Reality or myth? Am J Otol 1997; 18:782–791.
4. Barlow DW, Duckert LG, Kreig CS, et al. Ototoxicity of topical otomicrobial agents. Acta Otolaryngol (Stockh). 1994; 115:231–235.
5. Glasscock ME, Dickins JRE, Jackson CG, et al. Vascular anomalies of the middle ear. Laryngoscope 1980; 90:77–88.
6. Jacobs IN, Potsic WP. Glomus tympanicum in infancy. Arch Otolaryngol Head Neck Surg 1994; 120:203–205.
7. Joint Committee on Infant Hearing 1994, Position Statement (RE9501). American Academy of Pediatrics. 1995; 55(1):152–156.
8. Potsic WP, Winawer MR, Marsh RR. Tympanoplasty for the anterior-superior perforation in children. Am J Otol 1996; 17:115–118.
9. Kessler A, Potsic WP, Marsh RR. Type I tympanoplasty in children. Arch Otolaryngol Head Neck Surg 1994; 120:487–490.
10. Kessler A, Potsic WP, Marsh RR. Total and partial ossicular replacement prostheses in children. Otolaryngol Head Neck Surg 1994; 110:302–303.
11. Roland PS, Marple BF, Meyerhoff WL. *Hearing Loss.* New York: Thieme, 1997, pp. 1–316.

12. Gorlin R, Toriello H, Cohen M. *Hereditary Hearing Loss and Its Syndromes.* Oxford: Oxford University Press, 1995, pp. 9-21.

13. Nance WE, Sweeney A. Genetic factors in deafness of early life in sensorineural hearing loss in children: Early detection and intervention. Otolaryngol Clin North Am 1975; 8(1):19-48.

14. Lebel MH, Freij BJ, Syrogiannopoulos GA, et al. Dexamethasone therapy for bacterial meningitis. Results of two double-blind, placebo-controlled trials. N Engl J Med 1988; 319:964-971.

15. Jackler RK, De La Cruz A. The large vestibular aqueduct syndrome. Laryngoscope 1989; 99:1238-1243.

16. Zelante L, Gasparini P, Estivill X, et al. Connexin-26 mutations associated with the most common form of nonsyndromic neusosensory autosomal recessive deafness (DFNB1) in Mediterraneans. Hum Mol Genet 1997; 9:1605-1607.

17. Estivill X, Fortina P, Surrey S, et al. Connexin-26 mutations in sporadic and inherited sensorineural deafness. Lancet 1998; 351:394-398.

13 Congenital Malformations of the Ear

Edward J. Krowiak and Kenneth M. Grundfast

The incidence of congenital malformations of the ear ranges from 1/10,000[1] to 1/15,000.[2] Therefore, it is important to be familiar with the variety of ear malformations, as a multidisciplinary approach to treatment is needed in many cases. This chapter deals with malformations of the auricle, external ear canal, and middle ear up to the stapes footplate. Although congenital ear anomalies can be complex and difficult to manage, a thorough knowledge of the embryology of the ear and a familiarity with current recommendations for management of these anomalies can help the otolaryngologist achieve results that are predictable and consistent. The overall goals for otolaryngologists and other health professionals to achieve a cosmetically acceptable external ear and to create a functional pathway for sound from the external ear to the cochlea while preserving facial nerve and labyrinth function.

EMBRYOLOGY

Understanding the normal embryologic development of the ear aids in the understanding of the many possible combinations of malformations. The external ear begins developing first and then the middle and inner ear follow. Although each develops independently, determining the time of arrest of differentiation in any one segment of the ear enables prediction of expected associated anomalies of the other parts of the ear based on the time of embryologic interruption. A summary of embryologic landmarks is shown in Figure 13-1.

Pediatric Otolaryngology, Edited by R.F. Wetmore, H.R. Muntz, and T.J. McGill. Thieme Medical Publishers, Inc., New York © 2000.

Auricle

The *auricle* is formed at approximately 4 weeks gestation from the six paired hillocks of His in the mesenchymal tissue of the first and second branchial arches. The first to third hillocks form the *anterior auricle* (the tragus and crus helicis) and the fourth through sixth hillocks form the *posterior auricle* (the lobule, helix, and antihelix) by 12 weeks.[3] The conchal bowl originates from the first branchial groove. All of these elements form around the developing meatus of the external ear canal. The relationship of auricular development to that of the remainder of the ear is shown in Figure 13-1. Absence (*anotia*) or deformity (*microtia*) of the auricle therefore can be traced to approximately 7 to 8 weeks gestational age, and less severe deformities indicate that interruption of development occured closer to the end of 12 weeks. The normal size of the auricle at birth is 66% of the length and 76% of the width of the adult ear.[4]

> ### SPECIAL CONSIDERATION:
> Determining the gestational age of onset of any ear anomaly allows the otologist to predict other probable abnormalities and to plan their management.

External Auditory Canal

At approximately 8 weeks gestation, ectoderm from the first branchial cleft migrates medially to meet the mesoderm of the first groove (i.e., the developing tympanic ring). Medial to the tympanic ring is the endoderm of the first branchial pouch, which is the origin of the middle ear cavity (i.e., tympanic

Auricle and External Auditory Ear Canal	Weeks of Development	Middle Ear and Facial Nerve
	0	
	2	Membranous labyrinth development begins. Facial nerve forms.
6 Hillocks of His organize. (Early Auricle)	4	
	6	Stapedial ring forms around stapedial artery. Malleus/incus development begins. Fallopian canal development begins. Lamina Stapedialis (primitive oval window) forms.
Epithelium of 1st branchial cleft grows toward tympanic ring. (Early EAC)	8	
	10	Horizontal facial nerve above oval window. Vertical segment anterolateral to middle ear. Stapes crura bow; I-S joint forms.
Auricle is fully formed.	12	
Tympanic ring ossifies.	14	
	16	All definite facial nerve communications are formed.
	18	Incus then malleus ossification begin.
	20	Stapes ossification begins.
External canal epithelial core hollows.	22	
	24	
	26	Fallopian canal ossifies.
External canal core canalizes.	28	Mastoid pneumatization begins.
	30	
	32	
	34	

Figure 13–1:   Timeline of auricular and middle ear embryology. Abbreviations: EAC, external auditory canal; I-S, incudostapedial joint.

cavity). The *tympanic ring* begins ossification at 12 weeks and at this time also forms the bony portion of the external auditory canal (EAC). The *epithelial core* hollows at 24 weeks and begins canalization at 28 weeks.[5] Normal canalization leaves a patent EAC and a three-layered tympanic membrane, which has epithelium of the first cleft laterally, a middle fibrous layer from the mesoderm of the first groove, and endoderm from the first pouch medially lining the middle ear space. A lack of epithelial ingrowth (rare) or failure of canalization will lead to *atresia* of the EAC; thus, placing the aberrant development that causes this anomaly at 28 weeks gestation. Partial canalization results in *canal stenosis,* defined as a canal diameter of 4 mm or less, and occurs between 28 and 30 weeks. Both lack of epithelial ingrowth and incomplete canalization may be associated with maldevelopment of the tympanic ring, resulting in a bony atretic plate instead of a tympanic membrane (TM). This is due presumably to the lack of induction of differentiation of the tympanic mesenchyme secondary to failure of canalization, and is seen in almost all cases of *aural atresia.*

Middle Ear and Ossicles

The first branchial pouch grows outward from the rudimentary tympanic ring between the 4th and 6th weeks and remains filled with mesenchymal tissue until resorption and ossicular development replace this tissue.[5] The eustachian tube and mastoid development also begin at this time from the first pouch, with mastoid pneumatization taking place at 7 months gestation. The *malleus* and *incus* begin developing at 5 weeks, and are formed from Meckel's cartilage of the first arch (the neck and head of the malleus and the short process and body of the incus) and Reichert's cartilage of the second arch (the manubrium of the malleus, the long crus of the incus, and the stapes crura and base).[6] The *incudumalleolar joint* forms at 7 weeks, while middle ear mucosa develops and separates the rudimentary ossicles from their attachment to the surrounding tympanic cavity. The failure of this step results in a fused malleus-incus mass that is commonly found attached to the bony plate in patients with aural atresia. Ossification of the ossicles begins with the incus at 15 weeks and is followed closely by the malleus at 16 weeks. Ossification of the incus and malleus are complete by 24 weeks.

Ossicular development begins with the stapes at

$4\frac{1}{2}$ weeks gestation. The *stapes* is the most common congenitally-deformed ossicle due to its lengthy time of development. At 5 weeks the stapedial ring forms around the stapedial artery. Stapes development also involves the otic capsule, which begins formation at 6 weeks from precartilage surrounding the developing membranous labyrinth (from otic placode ectoderm).[5] Labyrinthine development is unrelated to the remainder of the ear and its branchial arch origins, but a depression plate (lamina stapedialis) forms on the otic capsule at 7 to 9 weeks and aids in the induction of development of the stapes footplate. Any interruption of this communication, as occurs with a dehiscent and low-hanging facial nerve, can produce a deformity or absence of the oval window.[7,8] By the 16th week, the stapes base is distinguishable from the lamina stapedialis, which continues to form the vestibular portion of the footplate and the annular ligament. Stapes crura become bowed at 12 weeks and ossification takes place between 18 and 26 weeks.[9] Anomalies of the stapes superstructure or footplate, which are not uncommon, can be traced to this 12-week point of embryologic differentiation.

Facial Nerve

Knowledge of malformations of the facial nerve is crucial, not only for avoiding injury during repair of congenital atresia, but also to be able to predict abnormalities of other middle ear structures as they relate to this nerve. For a comprehensive review of facial nerve embryology and practical applications, see Sataloff[10] and Gulya.[5]

Facial nerve development begins at 3 weeks with the appearance of the *facioacoustic primordium,* which is the nerve of the second branchial arch. At 4 to 5 weeks, the facial nerve and sprouting chorda tympani divide the mesenchymal blastema of the second arch into the stapes, the interhyale (the stapedius muscle precursor), and the laterohyale (the posterior middle ear wall precursor). Four mesenchymal lamina form at the distal end of the nerve at 6 weeks, and eventually form the intrinsic facial muscles. Five branches of the nerve appear at 7 weeks near the parotid bud. By 16 weeks all definitive communications of the facial nerve have been established. At 8 weeks, a sulcus develops on the posterior otic capsule, representing the primitive Fallopian canal, with the final, bony covering coming from the laterohyale proximally and Reichert's cartilage distally. Ossification of this canal is completed by 26 weeks. Histologic evidence of dehiscence of the canal can be demonstrated in 25[10] to 55%[11] of post-mortem human temporal bones. The dehiscence is usually near the oval window, but is not considered pathologically significant unless displacement of the nerve itself accompanies the dehiscence.

Most important to the otologist in repairing congenital aural atresia is the course of the facial nerve, which may be aberrant. At 10 weeks of development, the vertical (mastoid) segment of the nerve is anterior and lateral to the middle ear and (EAC), while the horizontal (tympanic) segment is adjacent to the otic capsule. Abnormalities of the horizontal segment of the facial nerve usually involve a more acute angle (60 degrees vs. the normal 120 degrees) at the second genu, placing the nerve anterolaterally in the middle ear cavity passing between the oval and round windows.[6] The vertical segment exhibits the most variability, and usually this variability correlates directly with the severity of microtia and atresia. Variations range from a facial nerve encased in the inferoposterior portion of atretic bony plate when making an endaural incision, to one immediately beneath the rudimentary tragus, or exiting the mastoid through the glenoid fossa. This is due to the fact that as the temporal bone develops, it separates the mastoid from the temporomandibular joint (TMJ) in an anterior to posterior direction. Normally, this forces the vertical portion of the facial nerve to grow inferiorly toward the stylomastoid foramen.[12] Without temporal bone development and mastoid pneumatization, the nerve turns abruptly anteriorly at the second genu, resulting in the range of variations mentioned above. Preoperative high-resolution computed tomography (HRCT) can aid in predicting an abnormal course of the nerve, but additional information regarding the time of developmental arrest has proved to be equally important.[10]

A variety of studies have investigated the incidence of inner ear abnormalities associated with microtia and atresia. Naunton and Valvassori[13] reported a 10% incidence of inner ear abnormalities in atresia patients based on audiometric or polytomographic findings. More recent studies generally place the incidence between 10 and 47%[14,15] of atresia patients who have documented abnormalities of the labyrinth or cochlea by HRCT.

AT A GLANCE. . .

Embryology of The Ear

Auricle: formed at approximately 4 weeks gestation from the hillocks of His in the mesenchymal tissue of the first and second branchial arches; development is complete at 12 weeks; absence or deformity can be traced to 7–8 weeks gestation; the earlier the interruption of development during the 12-week period, the more severe the deformities will be.

External Auditory Canal: at approximately 8 weeks gestation, ectoderm from the first branchial cleft meets the developing tympanic ring; at 12 weeks, the tympanic ring begins ossification, forming the bony part of the external auditory canal (EAC); canalization begins at 28 weeks; normal canalization produces a three-layered tympanic membrane, and abnormalities of the EAC are associated with this membrane's maldevelopment; failure of canalization leads to atresia, placing this abnormality at 28 weeks gestation; canal stenosis, or partial canalization, occurs between 28–30 weeks.

Middle Ear and Ossicles: the malleus and incus begin to develop at 5 weeks, and are formed from Meckel's cartilage of the first arch and Reichert's cartilage of the second arch; failure of the middle ear mucosa to develop and separate the rudimentary ossicles from the tympanic cavity results in a fused malleus-incus mass; ossification of the ossicles begins with the incus at 15 weeks, is followed by the malleus at 16 weeks, and is complete by 24 weeks; ossicular development begins at 4½ weeks with the stapes; the stapes footplate begins to develop at 7–9 weeks, and any interruption of this results in a deformed or absent oval window; stapes crura become bowed at 12 weeks and ossification takes place between 18 and 24 weeks; anomalies of the stapes superstructure or footplate can be traced to a 12-week point of embryologic differentiation.

Facial Nerve: development begins at 3 weeks, and knowledge of this nerve's possible malformations are essential to the prediction of other abnormalities of middle ear structures that are related to the nerve; abnormalities of the horizontal segment of the facial nerve usually involve an acute angle (60 degrees as opposed to the normal 120) at the second genu, which places the nerve in the middle ear cavity between the oval and round windows; the vertical segment exhibits a lot of variability that correlates with the severity of microtia and atresia.

PATIENT EVALUATION

When aural atresia is noted in a newborn, as usually indicated by the presence of microtia, several issues must be addressed. A summary of the necessary tests and interventions, both medical and surgical, is shown in Practice Pathway 13–1. Evaluation of the patient with aural atresia should include assessment by an otolaryngologist, input from plastic surgeons about possible auricular reconstruction, evaluation by audiologists for fitting of appropriate amplification devices, and genetic counseling from physicians to inform the parents of the presence or absence of a syndrome. Depending on communication skills achieved with bone-conduction hearing aids (BCHA), the child with bilateral atresia may need special education from an early age to maximize speech and language development in order to ease the transition into mainstream schooling at age 5. Radiologic assessment and consideration of surgery can usually be deferred until age 6, although some experts advocate beginning this process as early as 4 years.[16] Evaluation of unilateral atresia patients is similar, but generally no amplification or special education is necessary if the contralateral ear has normal hearing. The decision about whether to operate on unilateral atresia depends on the severity of the anatomic deformity, the hearing level of the opposite ear, the parental desire for repair, and the ability of the child to participate in postoperative care. The details of this workup and management are discussed later in the chapter.

With few exceptions (e.g., Treacher-Collins and Goldenhar's syndromes), the degree of microtia and presence or absence of aural atresia reflects the development of the middle ear and its contents. Rarely, atresia will present with a normal pinna. Isolated middle ear anomalies do occur with some frequency as well. Patients without external ear malformations who have ear canal, middle ear, or cochlear abnormalities may experience delay in diagnosis of hearing impairment. Delayed speech development may result if abnormalities that are not apparent on routine physical exam go undetected for the first year or two of life.

AURICULAR ANOMALIES

Abnormal development of the auricle generally occurs due to arrest at 4 to 12 weeks gestation. Tan[17] divides these anomalies into *malformations,* which occur early in development (e.g., microtia, anotia, cryptotia) and *deformations,* which, most likely, occur late in development and are related to external compression (i.e., lop, cup, and prominent ears). Multiple theories attempt to explain the etiology of malformations, including thalidomide and retinoid exposure in utero. These compounds as well as stapedial artery rupture have been shown in studies to lead to microtia.[18]

Microtia has a predilection for males (2:1), the right ear in unilateral cases (55–65%), and an incidence of bilaterality (approximately 10%). A family history of microtia is found in 15 to 17% of patients, and 38 to 42% are part of a syndromic condition.[1,4,19] More than two-thirds of severe microtias or anotias are associated with aural atresia, but minor deformities often present with a normal external canal, which should not diminish suspicion of possible middle ear and facial nerve anomalies.

Classification

Several classification schemes have been used for microtia, including those of Meurman[20] and of Marx[21] which are shown in Table 13–1. We prefer to use descriptors for microtia that range from a minimally deformed auricle to a peanut-shaped skin and cartilage remnant. Because there is a correlation between the morphology of the pinna and the developmental status of the middle ear, our descriptors eliminate the use of Roman numerals or other classification styles that are somewhat difficult to use in a clinical setting. Much of the literature focuses on the Marx classification, which is the basis of Jahrsdoerfer's[22] atresia scoring system (see Table 13–3). These are useful classifications, but the concept of a continuum of anomalies that may result from the interruption of embryologic development at any point must be kept in mind.

Management

Deformations of the ear can be managed by a variety of surgical techniques described in the otolaryngology and plastic surgery literature. Nonoperative measures proposed by Tan[17] and others have produced normal or near normal pinna in over 90% of cases. Splinting with a wire that is surrounded by a suction catheter within the helical folds and taping the ears back for periods of 5 to 20 weeks have produced excellent results without surgery. Early

Practice Pathway 13–1   CONGENITAL EAR MALFORMATION

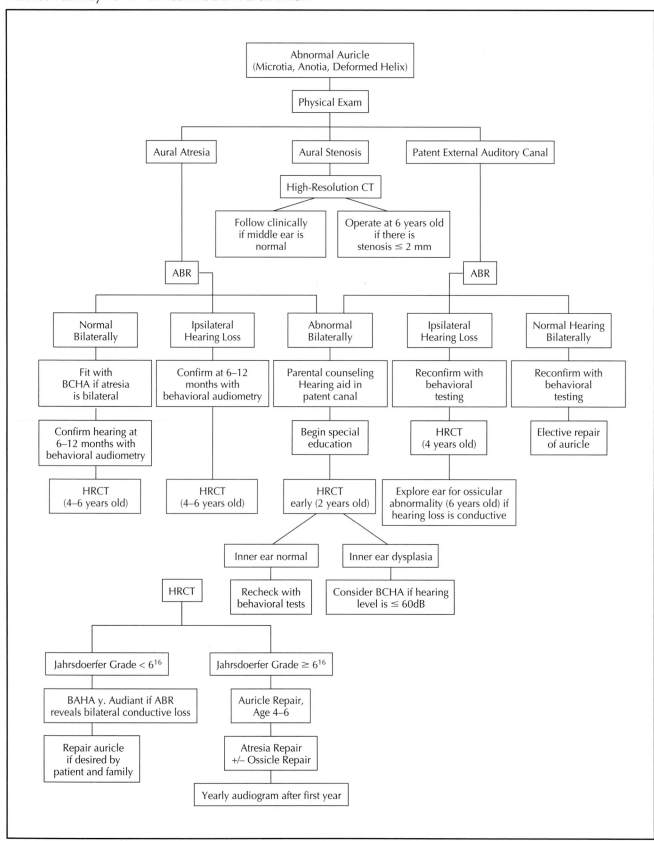

Abbreviations: HRCT, high-resolution computed tomography; ABR, auditory brainstem response BCHA, bone-conduction hearing aid; BAHA, bone-anchored hearing aid.

TABLE 13–1:   Classification Systems for Microtia

Meurman[20]	Grade I	Obviously small, malformed auricle with most of the characteristic components; atresia of the audutory meatus.
	Grade II	Vertical remnants of cartilage and skin with a smaller anterior hook; complete atresia of the canal.
	Grade III	Auricle is almost absent, except for a misplaced lobule and remnants of small skin and cartilage.
Marx[19]	Grade I	Mild deformity with an auricle that is smaller than normal, but each part is clearly distinguished.
	Grade II	The external ear is one-half to two-thirds of the normal size, but has partially retained its structure.
	Grade III	The auricle is severely malformed and usually has the shape of a peanut.

intervention is the key, as a steady decline in neonatal estrogen levels over the first 6 weeks of life decreases cartilage compliance; 100% of patients in Tan's study who were treated after 3 months of age had poor results with molding therapy.

Microtia repair has advanced greatly due to the work of several prominent surgeons who have painstakingly perfected the technique and artistry of auricular reconstruction.[4] Once the initial audiologic studies have been completed, any bone-anchored hearing aids (BAHA) must be placed well away from the auricular remnant in order to leave undisturbed tissue planes for reconstruction. Auricular reconstruction is started at 4 to 5 years of age to allow the child to enter school without a visible deformity and its attendant effects. Delay until this age is necessary to allow growth of adequate amounts of rib cartilage for harvest and for the contralateral normal ear (in unilateral cases) to achieve approximately 90% of its adult size, thus making it useful as a template for reconstruction. Brent,[4] in his series of 546 consecutive congenital microtia repairs outlined a sequence of steps to produce optimal outcome; each step, except 1 and 2, is separated by 2 to 4 month intervals. They are: (1) rib cartilage harvest and construction of framework (cartilage harvested from contralateral thorax); (2) creation of cutaneous pocket with placement of framework. Subcutaneous, silicon drains and helical-fold, petro-

latum-gauze packing ensure coaptation of skin to cartilage; (3) atresia repair or canalplasty as needed; (4) lobule transposition; (5) auricle detachment with placement of postauricular skin grafts; and (6) construction of tragus and conchal excavation. Over an average follow-up of 5.3 years, 41.6% of patients' reconstructed auricles grew in sequence with the opposite normal ear. Only four patients over this time reported 'decreased definition' of the auricle, and 40 traumatic injuries to reconstructed auricles were repaired and healed without incident.

Even though Brent and others are able to surgically create an auricle that is cosmetically acceptable, good results with auricular reconstruction are difficult to achieve. This being the case, alternative methods to surgery have been proposed, with the most success reported by Granstrom.[1] At a tertiary referral center, 101 operations for microtia were performed, including 47 surgical repairs and 73 placements of an epithesis (i.e., prosthetic ear) with bone-anchored titanium posts. 19% of Meurman grade II patients had satisfactory outcome with surgery versus 100% with epithesis placement. For grade III patients, surgical correction produced 14% satisfaction, and 100% acceptance of epithesis placements, which remained in use for over 12 years of follow-up. These numbers are skewed by the referral pattern and large number of surgical failures among the study population, but the epithesis should be considered a viable alternative to reconstructive surgery in selected cases.

ANOMALIES OF THE EXTERNAL AUDITORY CANAL

Aural Atresia

The EAC fails to form when canalization of the epithelial plug that originates from the first branchial cleft at approximately 26 to 28 weeks gestation does not occur. A multitude of factors including intrauterine toxic exposure and infection, low birth weight, and intrauterine trauma have been cited as causes of this malformation.[23] As yet, there is no experimental model that proves any of these are responsible for the arrest of embryologic development of the external canal.

TABLE 13–2: Classification for Congenital Aural Atresia

Altmann[24]	Type I	Small external canal, hypoplastic temporal bone, and tympanic membrane; normal or contracted middle ear; ossicles normal or malformed.
	Type II	Absent external canal with atretic plate; small middle ear; malleus and incus fixed and malformed.
	Type III	Absent external canal; contracted or absent middle ear with or without ossicles.
De La Cruz[6]	Minor	Normal pneumatization of mastoid; normal oval window; reasonable facial nerve—oval window relationship; normal inner ear.
	Major	Poor pneumatization; absent or abnormal oval window; abnormal course of horizontal facial nerve; inner ear abnormalities.
Ombredanne[25]	Minor	External canal normal or small; middle ear usually normal, but ossicles may be deformed and/or fixed; may have Grade I microtia (see Table 13-1).
	Major	Absent external canal and tympanic membrane; facial nerve dehiscence and displacement are common; grade II or III microtia (see Table 13-1).

Classification

Several excellent classification systems exist for aural atresia, and these are based mainly on the status of the ear canal, tympanic membrane development, middle ear cavity size, and ossicular development. Most often used are those of Altmann[23] and De La Cruz,[6] which are shown in Table 13-2, as well as that of Ombredanne.[25] As with the description of microtia, these systems are excellent for academic discussion and investigation, but are sometimes difficult to apply clinically. Again, when evaluating patients, the concept of a continuum of possible malformations must be kept in mind. Physical exam findings for the EAC should be specified as normal, stenotic, blind end, or atretic. Full evaluation of the severity of atresia cannot be made without the use of HRCT to investigate middle ear and ossicular status. Isolated atresia is not usually genetically inherited, and the syndromic association is approximately equal to that for microtia (11–47%).[26] Although atresia may occur without microtia, the opposite is rarely true.

> **SPECIAL CONSIDERATION:**
>
> Two thirds of microtia patients have associated atresia of the EAC, but isolated atresia is not rare. Minor auricle abnormalities carry a reduced but significant risk of associated aural atresia and middle ear malformations.

Evaluation

Given the close association of aural atresia with microtia, the workup for both, as outlined in Practice Pathway 13-1 will be discussed together. Initial evaluation, after physical exam of the auricle (or remnant) and external canal, involves *auditory brainstem response* (ABR) evaluation within the first few days of life. Air and bone conduction ABR thresholds are required to identify the degree of conductive hearing loss as well as to measure cochlear reserve. Although ABR is not a hearing test per se, it is the best method to evaluate auditory function in the atretic infant. In cases of bilateral atresia, ABR can distinguish individual cochlear nerve function based on a specific Wave I for each ear.[27] Limitations of ABR, which is used primarily up until the age of 6 months, are that it measures electrical activity of the eighth nerve and is not necessarily an adequate assessment of hearing level. Behavioral audiologic evaluation should be done as soon as the child is able to complete the *visual reinforcement audiometry task* (around 6 months of age). Although accurate audiologic assessment of the young child can be time consuming and difficult, the goals are to obtain pure tone and speech thresholds via both air and bone conduction as well as speech discrimination scores in older children. In patients with bilateral atresia, where masked bone conduction thresholds cannot be obtained due to a "masking dilemma," the *sensorineural acuity level* (SAL) test is used to define individual ear bone conduction thresholds. Children as young as 2½ years of age can be evaluated using the SAL, which predicts the degree of conductive component for the patient's hearing loss. Full audiologic assessment of unilateral atresia patients is necessary in all age groups due to the 10 to 25% incidence of occult conductive and sensorineural hearing loss in the normal appearing ear.[28] The average range of conductive loss for aural atresia is 45 to 60 dB. Any findings of hearing loss greater than 70 dB indicates a sensorineural component. Infants with bilateral atresia and normal cochlear function should be fit with BCHA as soon as the diagnosis of bilateral conductive hearing loss is made. For unilateral cases with normal hearing in the contralateral ear, no amplification is necessary. Parents of children with bilateral atresia need to be advised about the potential for speech and language delay, and referral for special education should be considered at the time of hearing aid fitting.

HRCT of the temporal bones in axial and coronal planes is obtained for all patients prior to the time of repair, which can be as early as 4 years of age provided that the child exhibits adequate growth for the harvesting of any needed cartilage and the ability to cooperate for postoperative care. The minimum age for repair in cases of bilateral atresia is 4 years, but often repair is delayed electively for several years in unilateral cases.[23] Important features to note in the axial and coronal CT are: (1) pneumatization of the mastoid; (2) the course of the facial nerve; the horizontal portion and its relation to the oval window and its vertical segment; (3) the presence or absence of the stapes footplate and oval window; and (4) the status of the cochlea and labyrinth. Other features to note on CT are the thickness and form of the atretic plate, the existence of cholesteatoma (reported in 8.5–14% of atretic ears[6]), the size of the middle ear cavity, and the status of the ossicles. Three-dimensional CT can be helpful in analyzing an atretic ear prior to surgery, but the limited availability of this technique and the difficulty in interpreting findings limit its use. Most pitfalls in routine two-dimensional CT interpretation involve delineation of the facial nerve course, which may vary widely. Mistaking the marrow of the styloid process for the vertical portion of the nerve has been reported.[9] Abnormalities of the vestibule or horizontal canal may be consistent with the propensity to develop perilymphatic fistula or stapes gusher intraoperatively.[27]

Grading systems and patient selection

After a thorough evaluation as outlined above, only 50% of atresia/microtia patients are surgical candidates.[29] Surgical candidates among syndromic patients, mainly Treacher-Collins and Goldenhar, are even lower, at 25%.[16,23] The absolute requirements for surgery are audiometric evidence of inner ear function and the presence of a middle ear space. Other findings, such as absence of the oval window

and absence of ossicles are relative contraindications to surgery. In contradistinction to surgery of chronic ear disease, the better ear, based on audiologic and radiographic criteria, is operated first in cases of bilateral aural atresia.

Predicting which patients were likely to have satisfactory hearing results with atresia repair was based mainly on personal experience until a grading system was proposed by Jahrsdoerfer in 1992,[16] and subsequently validated by several investigators.[22,30] The grading system gives points for anatomically normal structures such as the oval and round windows, facial nerve, and ossicles. A maximum score is 10 points. Two points are given for the presence of the stapes, though some authors dispute this heavier weighting because of the ability to place drum to footplate prostheses successfully with current techniques.[9] This grading system is shown in Table 13-3. Jahrsdoerfer was able to achieve postoperative thresholds of <20dB in 80% of patients with scores of 8 or higher. A direct correlation between increasing microtia severity and decreasing atresia scores was also shown in 200 consecutive cases.[22] Using the Marx classification of microtia (see Table 13-1) grade I average atresia score was 8.5, grade II score was 7.2, and grade III score was 5.9. This correlation allows us to predict accurately, based on appearance of the auricle and CT results,

TABLE 13–3:   Grading System of Candidacy for Congenital Atresia Surgery

Parameter	Points
Stapes present	2
Oval window present	1
Middle ear space	1
Facial nerve	1
Malleus/Incus complex	1
Mastoid pneumatized	1
Incus-Stapes connection	1
Round window	1
Appearance external ear	1
Total Available Points	10

Rating N = 10	Type of Candidate
10	Excellent
9	Very Good
8	Good
7	Fair
6	Marginal
5 or less	Poor

From reference 16, with permission.

which patients will benefit from surgical intervention and which are candidates for permanent bone anchored hearing aids (BAHA). Patients with atresia scores of 6 or less are generally poor candidates for repair and should be treated nonsurgically. Syndromic patients rarely grade above 6, which is consistent with the poor outcomes of atresia repair frequently reported in these patients.[1,31]

Repair of atresia

Coordination of the auricular reconstruction with that of the EAC and middle ear is crucial. As previously stated, staged repair of atresia (with assumed microtia for this discussion) may begin by age 4 in bilateral cases and age 6 and above for unilateral repair. Jahrsdoerfer advocates operating on all viable candidates, regardless of laterality, due to the obvious benefits of binaural hearing on speech and language development as well as on social interaction.[16,32] Others take a more conservative approach to unilateral atresia and wait until adulthood for the patients to grant fully informed consent.[19,29] Whether unilateral or bilateral, the presence of cholesteatoma on CT or a clinical facial paralysis are absolute indications for immediate surgical intervention.

Repair of the auricle proceeds in stages 1 and 2 (as outlined in the section on Management of Auricular Anomalies, i.e., cartilage harvest, framework construction, and placement in subcutaneous pocket) with adequate healing time between stages to allow for maximal vascularization and to optimize outcome once the auricle is rotated and detached posteriorly. Atresia repair is one of the most technically challenging of all otologic procedures. In addition to careful patient selection, experience, meticulous technique, and close follow-up over several years are the most important factors leading to a successful outcome.[31]

Several approaches to atresia repair are described below; the anterior approach is the most commonly used worldwide.[19,23,27] The *posterior, or transmastoid approach,* which we review briefly, is a combination of anterior and posterior procedures and is occasionally needed for difficult cases. General principals that apply to any type of atresia repair are: (1) the mandatory use of a facial nerve monitor; (2) retroplaced, postauricular incision to avoid disturbing the cartilage that has been placed for auricular reconstruction; (3) full elevation of the auricle flap to the TMJ, with exploration for an aberrant facial nerve; and (4) generous harvesting of temporalis fascia for tympanoplasty.

Anterior Approach. This overview of the anterior approach for atresia repair is taken mainly from De La Cruz,[9] and the reader is directed to this and other references for a more detailed account of the procedure.[27,32] After raising the auricular flap, drilling of the canal begins at the level of the linea temporalis, just posterior to the glenoid fossa. Occasionally, a depression will be present in the area of the atretic canal. By linking the predicted time of developmental arrest to the likely position of the facial nerve, and coupling this with CT findings, injury to the nerve can be avoided. With hypoplasia of the temporal bone in atresia, the entire middle ear cavity may be anteriorly and inferiorly displaced, placing the underdeveloped facial nerve in the region of the new external canal.[10] Further details of facial nerve anomalies associated with atresia will be discussed separately (see Congenital Facial Nerve Anomalies). Using the glenoid fossa anteriorly, middle fossa dura superiorly, and any existing mastoid air cells posteriorly as guides, a canal 1.5 times normal size (14 mm) is drilled to the level of the atretic plate. A diamond burr is used to thin the plate, and the remainder of the procedure is completed with picks and a carbon dioxide (CO_2) laser to avoid acoustic trauma from drilling, which may be transmitted to the ossicular mass. The facial nerve is usually located medial to the atretic plate infero-posteriorly, therefore entry into the middle ear space should be into the epitympanum superiorly.

A malleus-incus ossicular mass is consistently found attached to the atretic plate by the neck of the rudimentary malleus and to the wall of the tympanic cavity posteriorly and superiorly by fibrous bands. Use of the CO_2 laser to lyse these adhesions is associated with a lower incidence of postoperative sensorineural hearing loss (SNHL).[26] Several authors recommend retaining the malleus-incus ossicular mass, as long as it can be mobilized and is in continuity with the remaining ossicular chain, because it produces hearing results superior to those achieved with partial ossicular replacement prostheses (PORPs) or total ossicular replacement prostheses (TORPs).[26,29] In reviewing the results of repair in 16 major atresias, Lambert[30] found that 82% of patients with the malleus-incus ossicular mass left intact had <30dB postoperative SRT (speech reception threshold), versus a 25% incidence of similar results among patients reconstructed with prostheses.

Stapes abnormalities associated with atresia are common and usually involve the crura. A normal and mobile stapes footplate is the rule in these patients (94%), with an absent footplate found in 3 to 6% of cases.[26] Given these findings, if the malleus-incus ossicular mass is mobilized and communicates with the stapes, then no further intervention in the middle ear is necessary if presence of an oval window and footplate are confirmed by CT or intraoperatively. Absence of the stapes footplate is commonly attributed to an aberrant facial nerve that prevents interaction of the stapes mesenchyme with the lamina stapedialis of the otic capsule at 5 to 6 weeks gestation.[7,33] Early attempts to restore hearing in these patients with lateral semicircular canal fenestration had mixed results,[34] and current methods of vestibule fenestration with wire prosthesis placement show promising results.[35] Some authors show a decrement in hearing over time, even though hearing had improved initially.[7]

After a 6×6 cm split-thickness skin graft is harvested from the lower abdomen, the harvested temporalis fascia graft is trimmed to 20×15 mm and laid in place. Usually, this is placed lateral to the ossicular mass, but also may be used lateral to a TORP or PORP or as a type 3 tympanoplasty in direct communication with the stapes superstructure. De La Cruz et al use 3×6 mm tabs that are cut anteriorly and superiorly on the graft which are tucked into the epi- and protympanum to prevent graft lateralization. Lateralization, which is a major complication of this procedure that occurs in 22 to 23% of cases.[6] Others have suggested the drilling of a neosulcus at the tympanic ring with placement of a Silastic button laterally to the graft to prevent this complication.[27]

The next step of atresia repair involves "pie-crusting" the skin graft and creating a sawtooth medial edge, prior to its use as the lining of the newly created canal. The canal is packed with Gelfoam™ (Kalamazoo, Michigan) and a Merocel™ (Mystic, Connecticut) wick to prevent lateral slipping of the skin graft. Finally, a meatoplasty that is approximately 15 mm in diameter is created at the appropriate area, anterior to the reconstructed auricle, and the canal skin graft edges are sutured to the free skin edge of the meatus. These meatal sutures are removed in 7 days, and packing is removed and replaced with antibiotic-soaked Gelfoam 14 days postoperatively. This second packing is removed at 3 weeks, and antibiotic drops are continued for 8 to 12 weeks. Audiograms should be obtained at 8

weeks after surgery, at 6 months postoperatively, and then yearly.

Posterior Approach. An alternative technique, which is now rarely used, is the posterior or transmastoid approach. As with the anterior approach, elevation of the auricle and the initial drilling posterior to the TMJ are performed, but instead of using the glenoid fossa and middle fossa dura as anterosuperior guides, posterior landmarks are used. The sinodural angle, which is between the sigmoid sinus and tegmen, is located by drilling posteriorly through the mastoid air cells. The sinodural angle is followed medially into the mastoid antrum with identification of the lateral semicircular canal, facial ridge, malleus-incus complex, and atresia plate as landmarks. Entry to the middle ear follows, as in the anterior approach, and the newly created external canal is in direct communication with the mastoidectomy cavity. Bone dust pate is placed into the mastoid air cells.

In cases of poorly aerated mastoids and thick atretic plates, a combination of the above procedures is used. Initially, a transmastoid approach is used to identify the lateral canal and malleus-incus ossicular mass. Using these to gauge depth and anterior-posterior orientation, a separate hole is then drilled to create what remains as the EAC, as in the anterior approach. This method maximizes the use of anatomic landmarks, which otherwise may not be found, thereby minimizing the risk to crucial structures such as the facial nerve.

Complications of atresia repair

Lateralization of the tympanoplasty graft is the most common complication, occurring in 12 to 28% of cases.[26] Use of the above mentioned strategies can reduce the risk of this event. Stenosis of the canal or meatal opening of the auricle occurs in 7.5 to 12% of patients.[6] Creating a meatoplasty of at least 15 mm in anticipation of postoperative narrowing can reduce this number. SNHL is seen in 2 to 5% of operated patients,[9] and only rare cases of dead ears are reported.[33] Finally, permanent facial nerve injury is a complication of 1% of repairs, even with the use of adequate facial nerve monitoring.[6,9]

Results of atresia repair

De La Cruz reported a large series of atresia repairs with 87 surgeries in 302-ears[6]; 73% of patients had a residual hearing deficit of ≤30 dB at a 6-month follow-up. Chandrasekhar et al updated this report with 92 additional cases, achieving closure of the air-bone gap to ≤30 dB in 60% of primary surgeries and 54% of revisions,[26] 20% of these patients showed a 10 dB or greater loss of this hearing improvement over the 2.6-year-average follow-up.[26] Jahrsdoerfer achieved postoperative SRT of ≤25 dB in 73% of 90 patients with atresia scores of 6 or greater.[16] Given these results with large numbers of patients, the standard mark for a successful atresia repair is a patent EAC with a hearing level of 25 dB or less and closure of the air-bone gap. Using the atresia scoring system and the approach outlined, these results reflect the standard of care for congenital aural atresia patients.

SPECIAL CONSIDERATION:

Standard goals for atresia repair are a patent EAC, a hearing level of 25 dB or less, closure of the air-bone gap, and a cosmetically acceptable auricle.

Alternatives

For patients who do not meet the selection criteria of an atresia score of ≥6 (usually those who have syndromic conditions) alternative treatment using BAHA and BCHA has proven effective. Granstrom recommended BAHA for all patients with atresia scores <6, and found 100% subjective satisfaction and speech thresholds <30 dB in 39 patients. A recent study comparing the Audiant (Xomed) and BAHA HC200 (Noble Biocare, Göteborg, Sweden) bone-conducting implants showed no significant difference in the hearing gain offered by these devices,[36] and neither was effective at improving any sensorineural component of hearing loss in study patients. Cressman[23] published the following criteria for the placement of transcutaneous BCHA (1) bone conduction average <25 dB; (2) air conduction in the speech frequencies of >40 dB; (3) speech discrimination scores ≥80%; (4) age greater than 3 years; and (5) inability to wear conventional hearing aids. Use of these guidelines will provide maximal improvement in the quality of life for these patients without the risks associated with surgery, which is unlikely to be successful.

Congenital Aural Stenosis

Aural stenosis is defined as an EAC size of ≤4 mm with an hourglass type configuration. Patients with Down's syndrome or Cornelia de Langes syndrome are excluded from this criteria as hypoplasia of the external ear causes the typical uniformly narrowed and tapered ear canals. *Congenital stenosis* results from incomplete canalization of the canal epithelial plug at 28 to 30 weeks gestation, whereas the failure of canalization occurs earlier and leads to atresia. Because this is a late event in fetal development, the facial nerve is usually in the normal adult location throughout its course, making risk of injury during repair small.[10] Approximately 50% of stenotic ears have an associated hypoplastic tympanic membrane (TM), and middle ear anomalies occur with a frequency approaching that of atretic ears. An ossicular mass anchored to an underdeveloped TM is the usual finding.

Cole[37] reported a 12:1 ratio of atresia to stenosis in 600 patients. Others put the ratio at 7:1.[16] Cole found a 48% incidence of cholesteatoma among all patients; this increased to 59% if the stenosis was <2 mm and reached 90% in patients over 12 years old with a 2 mm stenosis. No cholesteatoma was found in patients under 3 years of age, and 20% of all patients had aural atresia of the contralateral ear. Presence of cholesteatoma or facial paralysis are absolute indications for surgery in this group. Otherwise, elective canalplasty should be performed between 6 and 12 years of age. All patients with stenosis of 2 mm should undergo surgery near the age of 6 to avoid cholesteatoma formation. Cholesteatoma develops medial to the stenosis in the bony EAC due to the inability of the ear to clear squamous debris.

CONGENITAL OSSICULAR MALFORMATIONS

Although ossicle and middle ear anomalies are commonly associated with aural atresia and microtia, their incidence independent of these conditions is much less than the 1:10,000 births reported for these major malformations. When isolated, ossicular deformities are generally classified with the minor deformities. Except for cases of an absent malleus or middle ear, they all appear the same on otoscopic exam and present with lifelong moderate to severe hearing loss, which may be unilateral (60–75%)[8] or bilateral, isolated or syndromic. As mentioned previously, anomalies of the stapes occur more than those of the incus, and anomalies of both of these auricles occur more than those of the malleus; the less time needed for embryologic development, the less chance there is of an anomaly occurring. Of those cases not associated with a major ear malformation, only 1/3 involve a single ossicle.[38]

The decision about whether to operate on these patients is a difficult one. An SRT <30 dB is an absolute contraindication, as a significant hearing improvement is unlikely. Audiologic testing reveals a fixed, nonprogressive conductive loss that varies in severity with the complexity of the deformity. Syndromic patients, who make up 25% of the minor anomaly population,[34] are poor candidates due to the higher incidence of inoperable inner ear anomalies. Children with Treacher Collins, Pierre Robin, or Goldenhar syndrome also have airway compromise that may complicate administration of a general anesthetic. No ear with active infection should be explored.

Radiographic investigation using axial and coronal 1 mm HRCT cuts of the temporal bones is the standard preoperative study to assess ossicular morphology and the status of the inner ear. With this technique, details such as the shape of each crus of the stapes can be seen. These findings have been shown to correlate very well with operative findings.[38,39] Stapes agenesis, crural deformity, an ab-sent or deformed incus, and incudostapedial joint separation can be diagnosed by CT, and all are amenable to surgical correction.

Classification

The list of possible middle ear and ossicle abnormalities is long, and several classification schemes have been published (Table 13-4). Using these reports as well as that of Cousins,[38] which involving over 250 cases, the most frequent anomaly is a fixed stapes footplate (ankylosis), followed by combined incus-stapes deformities, malleus-incus fusion, and malleus head fixation. Weber[40] has further subdivided abnormalities of the stapes crura base on 80 middle ear explorations for perilymphatic fistula. Type I stapes has no anterior crus and a normal posterior crus (37%), type II has a monopod or central crus (40%), and type III has a displaced anterior crus in the center of the footplate (23%). Absence of the oval window deserves special mention because of its impact on the possibility of improving hearing surgically. Twenty-four cases were reported as of 1994, and most were found to have a dehiscent facial nerve overhanging a depressed area on the otic capsule where the footplate ordinarily would be located.[41] These patients are poor surgical candidates. Round window anomalies are reported but involve effacement of the membrane or blunting of the niche and not agenesis.

TABLE 13–4:   Classification Systems for Congenital Ossicular Malformations

Teunissen[34]	Class 1	Congenital stapes ankylosis	30%
(% of 144 cases)	Class 2	Stapes ankylosis with ossicular anomaly	38%
	Class 3	Ossicular anomaly with mobile footplate	
		Ossicular discontinuity	8%
		Epitympanic fixation	14%
	Class 4	Aplasia/dysplasia of round or oval window	
		Aplasia	7%
		Dysplasia with overhanging facial nerve	2%
De La Cruz[41]	Combined	Incudomalleolar fusion	
		Fusion of all ossicles	
		Agenesis of all ossicles	
	Malleus	Head fixation	
		Absence or hypoplasia	
	Incus	Short process fixation	
		Absence or hypoplasia	
		Fibrous incudostapedial joint	
		Fusion or absence of incudostapedial joint	
	Stapes	Footplate fixation	
		Crural deformity	
		Hyperplasia	
		Stapes tendon ossification	
		Absent oval window	
		Osteogenesis imperfecta	

Surgical Intervention

Excellent hearing results can be obtained in cases of congenital ossicular malformation with careful patient selection based on audiograms and HRCT. Teunissen, performing standard stapedectomy on class 1 and 2 patients (see Table 13–4) as well as ossicular reconstruction when appropriate, closed the air-bone gap to <10 dB in 40% of cases and to <20 dB in 73% of cases.[34] Cousins' series of 68 explorations and repair for congenital conductive hearing loss produced a postoperative SRT of ≤40 dB in 47% of patients.[38] Herman,[8] in 12 cases, had an average decrease in air-bone gap of 6 dB with attempted repair. No dead ears were reported and only one case of decreased hearing was reported in these series. No reports comparing use of prostheses versus autogenous material for reconstruction or comparing use of PORP versus TORP have been published.

Agenesis of the oval window is a difficult problem to manage because of the possibility of complete hearing loss when entering the vestibule, and the usual presence of a dehiscent facial nerve in the operative field. Sterkers and Sterkers[25] reported closure of the air-bone gap to <10 dB in six cases followed over 1 to 18 years with oval window absence corrected with vestibule fenestration and wire prosthesis placement. Ossicles were mobilized as necessary, and no cases of SNHL were found postoperatively. Lambert,[7] using the same procedure in seven cases of agenesis, achieved >20dB decrease in air-bone gap in all patients, but three required revision surgery and all lost the improvement within 2 to 5 years after the surgery. No dead ears were found in either series. It must be underscored that these results were achieved only by the most experienced otologists, and surgery of this type should not be attempted without significant prior experience operating on congenital ear malformations.

CONGENITAL FACIAL NERVE ANOMALIES

The possible locations of the extratemporal portion of the facial nerve are predictable based on clues provided by associated malformations, as outlined in the section on Embryology of The Facial Nerve. Malformations of the horizontal or tympanic segment of the nerve are the most frequent, with simple dehiscence of the Fallopian canal over the area of the oval window so common (up to 55%)[19] as to consider it a normal variation. An abnormal course of this dehiscent nerve is considered pathologic and occurs in 24 to 30% of cases of atresia as diagnosed on exploration or by HRCT.[39,42] In these cases, the nerve usually pursues a medial to lateral course in the middle ear, increasing the chance of injury during middle ear exploration or atresia repair. Isolated cases of bifurcated and trifurcated facial nerves in the middle ear cavity have been reported.

Management

Jahrsdoerfer[42] proposed four criteria that should be met when considering the transposition of an anomalous facial nerve covering the oval window. He said that patients should have: (1) bilateral atresia; (2) HRCT evidence of a stapes and oval window; (3) no large vessels on the facial nerve; and (4) facial nerve integrity monitoring throughout the surgery. Even following these guidelines, his experience with six cases requiring transposition showed poor hearing results, although no permanent facial nerve injury occurred. More recently, Huang[43] reported three cases presenting as long-standing unilateral hearing loss. One patient had complete closure of a 42 dB air-bone gap, but the second case showed no improvement and the last was abandoned due to a contracted tympanic ring and stapes crura resting on the anomalous nerve. In cases with an inaccessible footplate, both authors recommend fitting of a BAHA.

CONGENITAL VASCULAR ANOMALIES OF THE MIDDLE EAR

Although vascular malformations of the ear are rare, familiarity with their presentation can prevent disastrous surgical complications. Patients with a dehiscent jugular bulb or aberrant carotid artery often present with pulsatile tinnitus, and otoscopic exam reveals a bluish mass medial to the tympanic membrane. Glasscock,[44] in a report of nine such anomalies, found all cases to occur in the right ear and 78% of patients were female. The significance of these findings is unclear.

Cadaveric studies of temporal bones reveal a 6% incidence of jugular bulbs located in the middle ear above the level of the annulus, a majority of which are dehiscent[45] Impingement on the malleus or incus, or covering of the round window by a dehiscent bulb can produce conductive hearing loss. Similarly, an aberrant internal carotid artery can produce conductive loss. Absence of the normal 0.5 mm carotid plate leading to this entity occurs in <1% of temporal bones. Finally, a persistent stapedial artery is found in 1:10,000 middle ears. This anomalous vessel courses through the obturator foramen of the stapes and appears on HRCT as an enlarged Fallopian canal and absent foramen spinosum.[39] Diagnosis of these anomalies is made with

HRCT, magnetic resonance imaging, and four-vessel angiogram. Recent improvement in magnetic resonance-angiography shows this to be a promising tool for the future, possibly as a single study for diagnosis. Associations, such as high jugular bulb in Crouzon's disease and Noonan's syndrome and an aberrant carotid in velocardiofacial syndrome, can also aid in keeping a high suspicion for these lesions.

No real possibility for repair exists with these anomalies, although some authors recommend placement of a fascia 'shield' over a dehiscent jugular bulb if encountered on exploration. Due to the lack of dural covering or a thick adventitia, the jugular bulb is highly susceptible to injury. A common occasion for such injury is during routine myringotomy. The profuse bleeding can be controlled with Surgical™ and Gelfoam™ packing, but avoidance of such complications is obviously preferred.

SYNDROMES WITH ASSOCIATED EAR MALFORMATIONS

Several syndromes mentioned throughout this text relate to specific anomalies. An examination of each syndrome and all of the otologic manifestations aids in familiarity with inherited malformations and allows prediction of certain anomalies (i.e., dehiscent jugular bulb) and avoidance of surgical complications or failure.[46]

AT A GLANCE...

Management of Ear Malformations

Auricle: *Nonsurgical:* wire splinting, taping back the ears for 5–20 weeks, epithesis (prosthetic ears). *Surgical:* auricular reconstruction using rib cartilage when the child is 4–6 years old

External Auditory Canal: *Aural Atresia:* surgery should be coordinated with auricular reconstruction; approaches to repair are anterior, which is the most popular, and posterior or transmastoid; special consideration must be given to the location of the facial nerve to avoid damage. *Aural Stenosis:* elective canalplasty for stenosis is performed between 6–12 years of age; if cholesteatoma or facial paralysis are present, exploration must be performed immediately; risk of injury to the facial nerve is small

Ossicles: patients should be selected for surgery on the basis of audiograms and HRCT; stapes agenesis, crural deformity, an absent or deformed incus, and incudostapedial joint separation are amenable to surgical correction; contraindications include an SRT <30 dB, active ear infection, and syndromes with associated ear malformations

Facial Nerve: transposition of the facial nerve in order to perform stapedectomy may be attempted if patients have bilateral atresia, HRCT evidence of a stapes and oval window, no large vessels on the facial nerve, and facial nerve integrity monitoring throughout surgery; if the patient has an inaccessible footplate, hearing aids are recommended

Middle Ear: vascular malformations of the ear are rare and no real possibility for repair exists; a fascia 'shield' placed over a dehiscent jugular bulb is recommended by some authors

---

SPECIAL CONSIDERATION:

Overall, only 25% of syndromic patients with aural atresia are candidates for surgical correction, whereas 50% of nonsyndromic patients meet the criteria for atresia repair.

Goldenhar Syndrome

Goldenhar syndrome, or hemifacial microsomia, is comprised of a spectrum of malformations involving aural, oral, and mandibular development with an incidence of 1:20,000–25,000 births. Most cases are sporadic and exhibit a 3:2 predilection for the right ear and males. Isolated microtia is considered a microform of the Goldenhar spectrum. 65% of patients have some degree of microtia, with 10 to 33% occurring bilaterally. Other ear manifestations are preauricular tags or sinuses in 40% and EACs ranging from narrow to atretic. The inner ear is usually normal on HRCT, and most hearing loss is conductive in nature. This conductive loss may be amenable to surgical repair.

Treacher Collins Syndrome

Treacher Collins syndrome is an autosomal dominant malformation of first and second arch derivatives, including down-sloping palpebral fissures, coloboma of the lower eyelids, and hypoplasia of the mandible and maxilla. These findings are bilateral and symmetrical, and occur with an unknown overall incidence. Microtia is present in 60%, and 30% have atresia with associated severe middle ear abnormalities. Hearing loss is bilateral and conductive, with inner ears normal on HRCT.

Branchio-oto-renal Syndrome

Branchio-oto-renal syndrome is an autosomal dominant syndrome with an estimated incidence of 1:40,000 births. Sixty percent of patients have branchial cleft cysts, and the association between inner ear and renal pathology is thought to be due to a shared antigen between the stria vascularis and renal glomeruli. Seventy-five percent of patients have hearing loss; 50% of the mixed type, 30% purely conductive, and 20% sensorineural. Approximately 80% have preauricular pits, and 60% have anomalies of the pinna, such as lop, cup, or flat configuration, and a narrow EAC. Malformations of the ossicles have also been described.

Other Syndromes

Crouzon's syndrome (craniofacial dysostosis) is autosomal dominant and characterized by craniosynostosis, maxillary hypoplasia, shallow orbits, and proptosis. Incidence is 1:25,000 births. Mild to moderate conductive hearing loss occurs in 55% of patients, and 13% have aural atresia.

Noonan's syndrome is characterized by craniofacial abnormalities, short stature, a webbed neck, and cardiac abnormalities. Incidence is 1:2500 births,[47] and ear manifestations consists of low-set, posteriorly-rotated ears, a folded helix, and 10 to 15% incidence of SNHL. Inner ear abnormalities such as hypoplasia of the cochlea have been reported.

Fetal alcohol syndrome, estimated to occur in 1:500 births, is characterized by midface hypoplasia, mixed hearing loss, and posteriorly-rotated ears with poorly formed concha.

AT A GLANCE...

Syndromes with Associated Ear Malformations

Goldenhar Syndrome: a range of malformations that involve aural, oral, and mandibular development; exhibits a 3:2 predilection for the right ear and males; inner ear normal on HRCT; conductive hearing loss

Treacher Collins Syndrome: malformation that includes down-sloping palpebral fissures, coloboma of the lower eyelids, and hypoplasia of the mandible and maxilla; inner ear normal on HRCT; bilateral, conductive hearing loss

Branchio-oto-renal Syndrome: association between inner ear and renal pathology may be due to an antigen that is shared between the stria vascularis and renal glomeruli; 75% of patients have hearing loss that is either mixed, conductive, or sensorineural; malformations of the pinna, EAC, and ossicles may occur

Crouzon Syndrome: characterized by craniosynostosis, maxillary hypoplasia, shallow orbits, and proptosis; mild to moderate conductive hearing loss

Noonan Syndrome: characterized by craniofacial abnormalities, short stature, webbed neck, and cardiac abnormalities; 15% have SNHL

Fetal Alcohol Syndrome: characterized by midface hypoplasia, mixed hearing loss, and posteriorly-rotated ears with poorly formed concha

CHARGE Association: characterized by coloboma, heart defects, atresia choanae, retarded growth, genital hypoplasia, and ear anomalies; mixed progressive hearing loss and deformities of the inner ear are common

---

CHARGE association (C, coloboma; H, heart defects; A, atresia choanae; R, retarded growth; G, genital hypoplasia; and E, ear anomalies/deafness) has been reported over 150 times in the literature with an unknown overall prevalence. Between 40 and

60% of patients have low-set, short, asymmetrical, cup or lop shaped ears. Mixed progressive hearing loss characterized by a wedge-shaped audiogram is common, as are deformities of the inner ear, specifically of the Mondini variety.

SUMMARY

Diagnosis and appropriate treatment of congenital anomalies of the ear is a difficult but manageable task. Considerable experience with aural atresia patients is needed to perfect the surgical techniques needed to achieve the best hearing and cosmetic results. A rational approach has been outlined to help guide all practitioners when treating patients with these developmental abnormalities.

REFERENCES

1. Granstrom G, Bergstrom K, Tjellstrom A. The bone anchored hearing aid and bone anchored epithesis for congenital ear malformations. Otolaryngol Head Neck Surg 1993; 109:46-53.
2. Farrior JP. Surgical management of congenital conductive deafness. South Med J 1987; 80:450.
3. Sando I, Ikeda M. Temporal bone histopathologic findings in oculoauriculovertebral dysplasia: Goldenhar's syndrome. Ann Otol Rhinol Laryngol 1986; 95:396-400.
4. Brent B. Auricular repair with autogenous rib cartilage grafts: Two decades of experience with 600 cases. Plast Reconstr Surg 1992; 90(3):355-374.
5. Gulya AJ, Schuknecht HF. *Anatomy of the Temporal Bone with Surgical Implications, 2nd ed.* New York: Parthenon, 1993, p. 240-270.
6. De La Cruz A, Linthicum FH, Luxford WM. Congenital atresia of the external auditory canal. Laryngoscope 1985; 95:421-427.
7. Lambert PR. Congenital absence of the oval window. Laryngoscope 1990; 100:37-40.
8. Herman HK, Kimmelman CP. Congenital anomalies limited to the middle ear. Otolaryngol Head Neck Surg 1992; 106:285-287.
9. De La Cruz A, Chandrasekhar SS. Congenital malformations of the temporal bone. In: Brackman DE, Shelton C, Arriaga MA, eds. *Otologic Surgery.* Philadelphia: Saunders, 1994, p. 69-84.
10. Sataloff RT. Embryology of the facial nerve and its clinical applications. Laryngoscope 1990; 100:969-984.
11. Baxter A. Dehiscence of the fallopian canal. J Laryngol Otol 1971; 85:587-594.
12. Crabtree JA. Congenital atresia: Case selection, complications, and prevention. Otolaryngol Clin North Am 1982; 15(4):755-762.
13. Naunton RF, Valvassori GE. Inner ear anomalies: Their association with atresia. Laryngoscope 1968; 78:1041.
14. Swartz JD, Faerber EN. Congenital malformations of the external and middle ear: HRCT findings of surgical import. Am J Radiol 1985; 144:501-506.
15. Hasso AN, Broadwell RA. Congenital anomalies. In: Som PM, Bergeron RT, eds. *Head and Neck Imaging.* St. Louis: Mosby, 1991, p. 960-966.
16. Jahrsdoerfer RA, Yeakley JW, et al. Grading system for the selection of patients with congenital aural atresia. Am J Otol 1992; 13(1):6-12.
17. Tan ST, Abramson DL, MacDonald DM, Mulliken JB. Molding therapy for infants with deformational auricular anomalies. Ann Plast Surg 1997; 38:263-268.
18. Eavey RD. Microtia and significant auricular malformation. Arch Otolaryngol Head Neck Surg 1995; 121:57-62.
19. Schuknecht HF. Congenital aural atresia. Laryngoscope 1989; 99:908.
20. Meurman Y. Congenital microtia and meatal atresia. Arch Otolaryngol 1957; 66:443-463.
21. Marx H. Die missblidungen des ohres. Handb Spez Pathol Anat Histol 1926; 12:620-625.
22. Kountakis SE, Helidonis E, Jahrsdoerfer RA. Microtia grade as an indicator of middle ear development in aural atresia. Arch Otolaryngol Head Neck Surg 1995; 121:885-886.
23. Cressman WR, Pensak ML. Surgical aspects of congenital aural atresia. Otolaryngol Clin North Am 1994; 27(3):621-633.
24. Altmann F. Congenital atresia of the ear in man and animals. Ann Otol Rhinol Laryngol 1955; 64:824-858.
25. Ombredanne H. Chirurgie des aplasies mineures. Ses resultats dans les grandes surdites congenidates par malformations ossiculaires. Ann Otolaryngol Chir Cervicodac 1964; 81:201-222.
26. Chandrasekhar SS, De La Cruz A, Garrido E. Surgery of congenital aural atresia. Am J Otol 1995; 16(6):713-717.
27. Lambert PR, Dodson EE. Congenital malformations of the external auditory canal. Otolaryngol Clin North Am 1996; 29(4):741-759.
28. Jahrsdoerfer RA. Congenital atresia of the ear. Laryngoscope 1978; 88(Suppl 13):1-48.
29. Bauer GP, Wiet RJ, Zappia JJ. Congenital aural atresia. Laryngoscope 1994; 104:1219-1224.
30. Lambert PR. Major congenital ear malformations: Surgical management and results. Ann Otol Rhinol Laryngol 1988; 97:641-648.

31. Cole RR, Jahrsdoerfer RA. Congenital aural atresia. Clin Plast Surg 1990; 17(2):367–371.

32. Jahrsdoerfer RA, Hall JW. Congenital malformations of the ear. Am J Otol 1986; 7(4):267–269.

33. Reiber ME, Schwaber MK. Congenital absence of stapes and facial nerve dehiscence. Otolaryngol Head Neck Surg 1997; 116:278.

34. Teunissen EB, Cremers WRJ. Classification of congenital middle ear anomalies: Report on 144 ears. Ann Otol Rhinol Laryngol 1993; 102:606–612.

35. Sterkers JM, Sterkers O. Surgical management of congenital absence of the oval window with malposition of the facial nerve. Adv Oto Rhino Laryngol 1988; 40:33–37.

36. Hough DA, Matthews P, Hough JVD. Bone-conduction implants for amplification: Comparison of results. Ear Nose Throat J 1997; 76(12):857–865.

37. Cole RR, Jahrsdoerfer RA. The risk of cholesteatoma in congenital aural stenosis. Laryngoscope 1990; 100:576–578.

38. Cousins VC, Milton CM. Congenital ossicular abnormalities: A review of 68 cases. Am J Otol 1988; 9(1): 76–80.

39. Fisher NA, Curtin HD. Radiology of congenital hearing loss. Otolaryngol Clin North Am 1994; 27(3): 511–531.

40. Weber PC, Perez BA, Bluestone CD. Congenital perilymphatic fistula and associated middle ear abnormalities. Laryngoscope 1993; 103:160–164.

41. De La Cruz A, Doyle KJ. Ossiculoplasty in congenital hearing loss. Otolaryngol Clin North Am 1994; 27(4): 799–811.

42. Jahrsdoerfer RA. Transposition of the facial nerve in congenital aural atresia. Am J Otol 1995; 16(3): 290–294.

43. Huang TS. Anomalously coursing facial nerves above and below the oval window: Three case reports. Otolaryngol Head Neck Surg 1997; 116:438–441.

44. Glasscock ME, Dickins JRE, Jackson CG, Wiet RJ. Vascular anomalies of the middle ear. Laryngoscope 1980; 90:77–88.

45. Overton SB, Ritter FN. A high placed jugular bulb in the middle ear: A clinical and temporal bone study. Laryngoscope 1973; 83:1986–1991.

46. Gorlin RJ, Cohen MM, Levin LS. Branchial arch and oro-acral disorders. In *Gorlin RJ, Cohen MM, Levin LS, eds. Syndromes of the Head and Neck.* New York: Oxford, 1990, p. 641–691.

47. Naficy S, Shepard NT, Telian SA. Multiple temporal bone anomalies associated with Noonan's syndrome. Otolaryngol Head Neck Surg 1997; 116:265–267.

14 Diseases of the External Ear

Ralph F. Wetmore

As the entrance and transmission of sound waves to the tympanic membrane (TM), the auricle, and the external auditory canal (EAC) play a crucial role in the hearing mechanism. The high incidence of otitis media (OM) in children mandates frequent otologic examinations in which the TM should be visualized through a patent EAC. Conditions that affect the patency of the EAC may alter hearing acuity and the ability to inspect the hearing apparatus, which is normally visible for inspection. Many times, simple removal of cerumen or debris from the canal will provide patency; however, other more serious conditions may impair the canal's function and, in the case of malignant external otitis, may even threaten the life of the patient. The pediatric practitioner needs to have a thorough knowledge of the diseases of the external ear that affect children.

NORMAL ANATOMY AND FUNCTION

The *pinna* of the ear is a skin-covered cartilaginous structure on the side of the head that is an extension of the EAC. The deepest part of the concavity, which forms the meatus of the EAC, is the *concha.* Other major cartilaginous structures of the pinna include the *antihelix* (superiorly), the *tragus* (anteriorly), and the *antitragus* (inferiorly). The skin that covers the auricle is tightly adherent to the underlying perichondrium on the lateral surface of the pinna, but is much more loosely attached medially. Most of the fat in the pinna is concentrated in the *lobule.* Sebaceous glands are found throughout the entire pinna, but are concentrated in the concha.[1]

The EAC is divided into two regions, a lateral cartilaginous portion and a medial bony portion. The *cartilaginous canal* is an S-shaped structure that extends from the concha to the tympanic ring. The cartilaginous portion of the canal makes up approximately 40% of its 2.5 cm total length. The cartilaginous canal is directed slightly upward and backward, and its shape as well as the presence of cerumen help to prevent water and foreign objects from entering the canal. In the anterior portion of the cartilaginous canal are *fissures of Santorini* that make the canal more pliable. They also provide a route for the spread of infection from the canal into the adjacent parotid and surrounding tissues. Hair follicles are numerous in the skin of the cartilaginous canal and serve to entrap foreign objects.

The *bony canal* makes up the remainder of the canal length and is directed slightly downward and anterior. The *isthmus,* which is the most narrow portion of the canal, is just medial to the cartilaginous-bony junction. Just lateral to the tympanic membrane is the *inferior tympanic sulcus,* a pocket in which debris and cerumen accumulate. There are a few small hairs and glands within the skin of the bony canal.

The sensory innervation of the EAC is complex and includes contributions from the fifth, seventh, ninth, and tenth cranial nerves. Placing an instrument in the EAC may cause nausea or coughing due to stimulation of the vagus nerve through its auricular branch (Arnold's nerve).

SPECIAL CONSIDERATION:

Instrumentation of the EAC may cause nausea or coughing due to stimulation of the vagus nerve through its auricular branch.

The skin of the entire EAC consists of *keratinizing stratified squamous epithelium,* the only keratinizing epithelium that lacks eccrine sweat glands. The skin of the cartilaginous canal is thicker and contains rete pegs, dermis, and dermal papillae. This

Pediatric Otolaryngology, Edited by R.F. Wetmore, H.R. Muntz, and T.J. McGill. Thieme Medical Publishers, Inc., New York © 2000.

skin also contains hair follicles and both sebaceous and cerumen glands. The skin of the bony canal is thinner, and lacks dermal papillae and rete pegs. A lack of subcutaneous tissue in the bony canal allows the tight attachment of the skin to the underlying periosteum. This tight attachment of the skin of the bony canal wall permits it to be easily traumatized.

SPECIAL CONSIDERATION:

The tight attachment of the skin of the bony canal wall permits it to be easily traumatized.

The normal bacterial flora of the EAC is a combination of aerobic (80%) and anaerobic (20%) organisms. Aerobic bacteria include *Staphylococcus epidermidis,* alpha-hemolytic streptococci, diphtheroids, and *Pseudomonas aeruginosa.*[2] *Propionibacterium acnes* and a variety of *Peptococcus* species make up the anaerobic flora. Bacterial and fungal infections of the EAC occur when the natural defenses break down and produce a loss of cerumen, injury to the skin of the canal, or an alteration of the normal bacterial flora.

The auditory function of the EAC is to produce a broad-banded 15 to 20 dB gain between 2000 and 5000 Hz.[3] The nonauditory function of the canal is the maintenance of a patent canal. Hairs within the cartilaginous canal prevent foreign bodies from entering the canal but may also trap cerumen and debris. Cerumen is composed of lipids that are hydrophobic, and its major function is to waterproof the canal.[4] Migration of the skin of the EAC also helps to keep the canal free of debris. The pattern of migration is from the tympanic membrane laterally and radially away from the umbo.[5]

CERUMEN IMPACTION

Cerumen is a mixture of secretions from the sebaceous glands that are found superficially in the dermis and the ceruminous or apocrine sweat glands that are located deeper. The sebaceous glands secrete sebum, an oily material, whereas cerumen glands secrete a white, milky fluid. Desquamated keratin debris is also included in the mixture. Racial

differences exist in the lipid, immunoglobulin, and lysozyme composition of cerumen. Caucasian and African-Americans produce cerumen with higher levels of lipid (wet cerumen), whereas Asians produce cerumen with higher protein levels (dry cerumen). The evolutionary advantage of wet or dry cerumen is unclear.[6]

The purpose of cerumen is to form a protective layer that protects the canal against injury. Lipids within cerumen also protect the canal from maceration due to water exposure. While the pH of cerumen is higher in males than females, the overall acidic nature of cerumen helps to inhibit the growth of bacteria and fungi.[1,7] A 3% suspension of cerumen has been shown to have a 99% in vitro bactericidal activity against both *Escherichia coli* and *Serratia marcescens,* and 30–80% activity against *Pseudomonas aeruginosa.*[8]

Cerumen may be removed safely and easily in children by several methods. Using one type of light source or another (headlight, otoscope, or microscope), cerumen may be debrided with either a suction or curette. Irrigating the EAC of a child in whom the tympanic membrane is known to be intact may remove cerumen; however, compliance in young children and the risk of perforation remain potential problems. Several commercial preparations (Debrox™, Cerumenex™) exist that soften and assist in the removal of cerumen.[9] Cerumenex™ works more quickly than Debrox™ but may cause topical allergic reactions.

EXTERNAL OTITIS

External otitis (EO) may present as either an acute or chronic illness. The sudden onset of pain and swelling of the EAC help to distinguish the acute from the chronic form of infection, which typically presents with itching and scaling. Acute infection typically requires systemic antibiotics in addition to ototopical therapy, whereas chronic infections often may be treated with meticulous cleansing and ototopical therapy. Practice Pathway 14–1 shows the diagnosis and management of EO.

Acute External Otitis

Acute EO is an infection of the EAC that results either from an alteration of the normal host defenses or trauma to the soft tissue of the canal with subse-

Practice Pathway 14–1   DIAGNOSIS AND MANAGEMENT OF EXTERNAL OTITIS

```
                              ┌─────────────────┐
                              │  External Otitis │
                              └─────────────────┘
                              ╱                 ╲
                    ┌──────────┐            ┌──────────┐
                    │  Acute   │            │ Chronic  │
                    └──────────┘            └──────────┘
                   ╱          ╲            ╱          ╲
         ┌──────────┐    ┌──────────┐  ┌──────────┐  ┌──────────┐
         │ Pain     │    │Predisposing│ │ Keratin  │  │ Pruritis │
         │ Swelling │    │ factors    │ │ debris   │  │ Scaling  │
         │ Erythema │    └──────────┘  └──────────┘  │ Erythema │
         └──────────┘         │             │        └──────────┘
              │               │             │          ╱        ╲
   ┌──────────────┐     ┌──────────┐  ┌──────────┐ ┌──────────┐ ┌──────────┐
   │ Analgesics   │     │   MBO    │  │Keratosis │ │ Atopic,  │ │Otomycosis│
   │ Oral         │     └──────────┘  │obturans  │ │ contact &│ └──────────┘
   │ antibiotics  │          │        └──────────┘ │seborrheic│      │
   │ Ototopical   │     ┌──────────┐       │       │dermatitis│ ┌──────────┐
   │ agents       │     │ CT       │  ┌──────────┐ └──────────┘ │Antifungal│
   │ Cleansing    │     │ MRI      │  │Cleansing │      │       │ drops    │
   └──────────────┘     │ Nuclear  │  │Steroid   │ ┌──────────┐ └──────────┘
          │             │ scans    │  │drops     │ │ Steroid  │
   ┌──────────────┐     └──────────┘  └──────────┘ │ drops    │
   │ Culture &    │          │                     └──────────┘
   │ IV antibiotics│    ┌──────────┐
   └──────────────┘     │IV        │
                        │antibiotics│
                        │Debridement│
                        └──────────┘
```

quent inflammation and infection. Factors that alter the normal host defenses and contribute to the development of EO are listed in Table 14-1.[1,10,11] In the early stages of EO, heat, humidity, maceration, or other factors may act to remove cerumen or change the pH of the canal. These changes may cause itching that then elicits digital manipulation or instrumentation of the canal that traumatizes the skin, thus allowing bacteria to enter the surrounding soft tissue. An increase in infection and inflammation may cause canal edema or complete obstruction of the canal in severe cases. Common bacterial pathogens that cause EO include *Pseudomonas aeruginosa*, *Staphylococcus aureus*, *Escherichia coli*, and *Proteus* species.[12]

In addition to pruritus, early symptoms of EO include pain and tenderness on palpation or manipula-

TABLE 14–1: Factors Contributing to Acute External Otitis

High humidity
Water exposure
Maceration of canal skin
High environmental temperature
Local trauma
Perspiration
Allergy
Stress
Removal of normal skin lipids
Absence of cerumen
Alkaline pH of canal

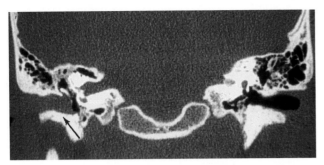

Figure 14–1: CT of the temporal bone in a child with acute external otitis. Note the complete soft-tissue obstruction of the EAC on the affected side (arrow).

tion of the tragus or EAC. Ear pain may quickly progress from mild to severe. Ear fullness and a conductive hearing loss may develop if canal swelling progresses to complete obstruction.

Physical examination of the external meatus frequently reveals erythema, swelling, and crusting. Otoscopic examination demonstrates erythema, swelling of the canal that may progress to frank obstruction, and scant discharge (Fig. 14–1). Frequently, there is an odor characteristic of *Pseudomonas* infection. In severe cases, infection may spread anteriorly through the fissures of Santorini into the parotid region and also involve postauricular and periparotid lymph nodes.

Treatment of acute EO begins with careful cleansing of the EAC with either a swab or suction. In young children this may be difficult because of poor patient compliance. In uncomplicated EO, a culture of secretions is usually unnecessary. Table 14–2 lists a variety of topical drops that may be used in the management of EO. Antiseptic and antibiotic otic preparations help to sterilize the canal. If antibiotic otic preparations are not tolerated because of pain, ophthalmic antibiotic preparations can be tried. Drops containing corticosteroids help to reduce

TABLE 14–2:   Ototopical Preparations

Antiseptics: acetic acid, boric acid, salicylic acid, ichthammol, phenol, aluminum acetate, gentian violet, thymol, Merthiolate™, Cresylate™ and alcohol, hydrogen peroxide

Antibiotics: colistin, polymyxin B, neomycin, chloramphenicol, gentamicin, tobramycin, ciprofloxacin

Corticosteroids: VoSol HC™

Antifungals: Domeboro™, Cresylate™, Sultzberger's powder, clotrimazole, amphotericin B, oxytetracycline-polymyxin

Data from references 9, 15, and 30.

canal edema, whereas anti-fungal agents may be useful if fungal elements are identified within the canal.

With severe bouts of EO, the canal may be so swollen and painful that suctioning may not be possible. Placement of a wick made of sponge or gauze provides a pathway for drops to be delivered to the EAC wall skin for 48–72 hours. Use of oral broad-spectrum antibiotics is also indicated in severe cases. To relieve pain, analgesics including narcotics may be necessary.

Episodes of EO may be recurrent, especially during the summer months. Preventing trauma to the canal and avoiding conditions that contribute to the development of EO are key to preventing recurrent infection. Use of alcohol or acetic acid drops sterilizes and restores the acidic pH of the canal, and is shown to prevent recurrent infection.[13,14]

SPECIAL CONSIDERATION

The use of alcohol or acetic acid drops sterilizes and restores the acidic pH of the canal, and is shown to prevent recurrent external otitis.

AT A GLANCE. . .

Signs and Symptoms of Acute External Otitis

- Otalgia
- Tenderness on palpation or manipulation
- Ear fullness
- Conductive hearing loss
- Erythema of meatus and canal
- Swelling and obstruction of canal
- Crusting and discharge
- Odor

Chronic External Otitis

Bacterial infection

Chronic bacterial infection of the EAC is unusual in the pediatric population. Affected patients typically complain of itching, mild discomfort, and crusting and flaking of the skin of the canal wall. Signs include evidence of mucopurulent drainage and maceration of skin. Treatment consists of frequent cleaning and the use of agents that restore the pH of the canal and the normal production of cerumen. Topical drops that dry and acidify the canal may be helpful.

Chronic dermatitis

Eczematous conditions that affect the EAC include a variety of dermatologic abnormalities such as atopic, contact, and seborrheic dermatitis and psoriasis. The usual symptom is itching, and examination of the EAC reveals erythema, edema, flaking, and crusting. Treatment includes local cleansing and the use of corticosteroid and drying agents.

Metal sensitivity is the most common form of chronic dermatitis involving the ear. Nickel is the most common offending metal, and may be released from stainless steel and other alloys, even after gold and silver plating. Women are more affected than men with approximately 10% of women being sensitized to nickel. Ear piercing is an important cause of primary sensitization to nickel.

Fungal infection (otomycosis)

Fungal infection of the EAC occurs in children who are exposed to warm, moist climates or who have a history of chronic use of antibiotic ear drops. Both of these conditions alter the cerumen and normal bacterial flora of the EAC. Symptoms of otomycotic infection include pruritus and otorrhea. Depending upon the offending fungal organism, there may be black, gray, green, yellow, or white debris in the canal. Frequently, hyphae may be identified. Common organisms include *Aspergillus* and *Candida* species. Phycomycetes, *Rhizopus, Actinomyses,* and *Penicillium* are other fungal organisms responsible for fungal EO.[13] A fungal culture may be helpful to confirm the diagnosis.

As with other types of EO, treatment begins with suctioning debris from the canal. Topical antifungal preparations such as clotrimazole (Lotrimin™), amphotericin B, oxytetracycline-polymyxin, and nystatin are usually very effective.[15] Use of drops that acidify the canal such as 2 percent acetic acid (Domeboro™), 3 percent boric acid, and 25 percent M-cresyl acetate (Cresylate™) or Sulzberger's powder

(boric acid and iodine) are also helpful in the treatment of fungal infection.[9]

Furunculosis

Formation of a *furuncle,* which is an inflammatory skin lesion that results from the infection of an obstructed apocrine or sebaceous gland, is seen commonly in the EAC due to the increased number of these glands in the canal skin. *Staphylococcus aureus* is the typical pathogen, although other organisms have been identified. The usual symptoms of a furuncle include localized pain and itching. If the furuncle is large, the canal may become obstructed, giving a sense of fullness and a conductive hearing loss. Examination of the canal is remarkable for localized erythema and swelling at the site of the abscess (Fig. 14-2). Typically, furunculosis responds to oral and topical antibiotics. Local heat may be helpful in resolving the infection, and oral analge-

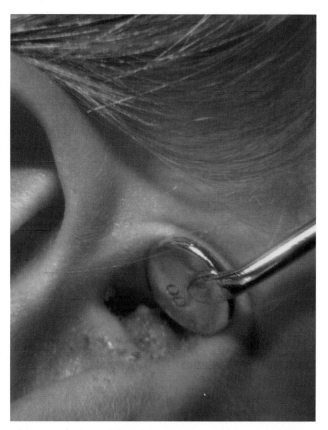

Figure 14–2: A dental mirror is used to expand the external auditory meatus, demonstrating a furuncle of the EAC. Most furuncles may be treated with oral antibiotics and warm soaks; surgical drainage may be necessary in selected cases.

sics may be necessary in some cases. In cases that fail to respond to antibiotic therapy, incision and drainage may be necessary.

Management of External Otitis

Prevention of external otitis

Prevention is key to the recurrence of both acute and chronic EO. Use of ear plugs or swim molds during recreational water activities may eliminate contamination of the canal by bacteria and maceration of the skin of the canal wall. Following exposure to water, the ear canal may be carefully dried with a blow dryer. A few drops of alcohol, which is a drying agent, may be instilled into the canal to reduce the chances of maceration also. Use of topical drops, such as acetic acid, that acidify the canal may prevent bacterial contamination.[9]

Use of ototoxic agents

Use of potentially ototoxic topical agents in the management of EO and chronic suppurative OM remains controversial. Ototoxic agents are thought to reach the cochlea by two routes: (1) direct penetration through a TM perforation into the mesotympanum and then into the cochlea via the round or oval windows; or (2) absorption into the local blood supply through the skin of the EAC. The theoretical effects of these topically applied ototoxic agents on the labyrinth are sensorineural hearing loss (SNHL) tinnitus, and/or vertigo.

Roland reviewed the English-written literature and found only four cases of SNHL that could possibly be attributed to use of topical ototoxic agents, and suggested an incidence of 1 to 10,000 or less.[16] In a survey of otolaryngologists, Lundy reported that only 3.4 percent believed that they had witnessed irreversible labyrinthine damage due to topical ototoxic agents.[17] Dispersed throughout the otolaryngologic literature are multiple reports of ototoxicity due to the application of topical agents in animals, most commonly chinchillas and guinea pigs. Several important anatomic differences exist between humans and these animals, and they are: (1) the round window niche is recessed in humans; (2) the round window is six times thicker in humans compared to either chinchillas or guinea pigs; and (3) a mucosal membrane spans the round window niche in humans and prevents most liquids from reaching the membrane.[13,16] Agents that are potentially ototoxic are listed in Table 14-3.[18,19]

TABLE 14–3: Experimental Ototoxic Agents

Solvents: propylene glycol
Antiseptics: alcohol, chlorhexidene acetate, benzalkonium chloride, iodochlorhydroxyquinolone, Cresylate™
Antifungals: Cresylate™, VoSol™, acetic acid
Antibiotics: polymyxin B, neomycin, gentamicin, tobramycin, chloramphenicol, colistin

Data from references 18 and 19.

KERATOSIS OBTURANS

Keratosis obturans results from the accumulation of large plugs of desquamated keratin in the ear canal, and differs from EAC cholesteatoma in which there is invasion of squamous tissue into a localized area of periostitis in the canal wall.[20] There appears to be no clear association between these two conditions.[20] Keratosis obturans presents with hearing loss and acute severe pain, tends to be found in a younger age group, and is usually bilateral. There also appears to be a definite relationship between keratosis obturans and both bronchiectasis and sinusitis.[21]

Examination of the child with keratosis obturans is remarkable for a plug of keratin that, when removed, reveals a thickened but otherwise normal TM.[20] In the patient with keratosis obturans, there is generalized widening of the bony EAC. With EAC cholesteatoma, the TM also may be intact; however, there is usually drainage and localized erosion of the canal lateral to the annulus. The treatment of keratosis obturans includes the mechanical removal of the epidermal plug and periodic cleansing of the canal. Granulation tissue may be managed by removal, cauterization, or the use of topical steroid drops.

AT A GLANCE...

Treatment of Keratosis Obturans

- Mechanical removal of epidermal plug
- Periodic cleansing of canal
- Management of granulation by removal, cauterization, or topical steroid drops

MALIGNANT EXTERNAL OTITIS

Malignant external otitis (MEO) begins as an infection of the EAC that spreads to the surrounding subcutaneous tissues, and that eventually may progress to osteomyelitis of the skull base. While MEO is well recognized in the adult population, it also may be seen in children.[22] The infection usually develops at the bone-cartilage junction and may spread in any direction. The most common direction of spread is anteriorly through the fissures of Santorini to involve the region between the EAC and the parotid gland. Facial paralysis as an associated complication of MEO is more common in children than adults because of the underdevelopment of the mastoid process and because the facial nerve is closer to the bone-cartilage junction in children.[23,24] Facial paralysis may be permanent in some cases.[24] Children at risk for MEO include otherwise healthy diabetics and children with an immune dysfunction, for example children suffering with a malignancy, malnutrition, or an immunodeficiency.

SPECIAL CONSIDERATION:

Facial paralysis, as a complication of malignant external otitis, is more common in children than adults because of the underdevelopment of the mastoid process and because the facial nerve is closer to the bone-cartilage junction in children.

Pseudomonas aeruginosa is the major pathogenic organism. The three factors that enhance its pathogenesis are: (1) its polysaccharide coating; (2) an exotoxin that causes a reversible neurotoxicity; and (3) the presence of enzymes that promote destruction of tissue.[25] *Proteus mirabilis* has also been seen as a causal agent in some cases.[26]

The initial presentation of MEO includes the acute onset of otalgia that may be severe and unrelenting, followed by aural drainage and swelling and erythema of the preauricular region and pinna. In children, MEO appears to progress much more rapidly than in adults. The TM is frequently necrotic, and as noted previously, facial paralysis is more common in involved pediatric patients.[23] In contrast to adults, MEO in children does not involve other cranial nerves usually.[23] Recurrent disease is also unusual in children.[23] In children, the infection may cause stenosis of the EAC due to chondritis. Occasionally, infection may spread to the mesotympanum causing ossicular disruption.[22] In infants, MEO may result in sepsis, but the high mortality rate of 20% seen in adults is not reported in children.[23,27]

The diagnosis of MEO is suggested by the documentation of a *Pseudomonas* infection that fails to resolve, especially when associated with the acute onset of a facial paralysis. In infants and young children, MEO may be difficult to distinguish from a facial paralysis that is a complication of acute OM. The identification of *Pseudomonas* as a causative organism of infection favors the diagnosis of MEO. A striking rise in the erythrocyte sedimentation rate (ESR) is also highly suspicious of MEO.[23] Computed tomography (CT) of the temporal bone is the diagnostic procedure of choice in adults, but is not as definitive in children.[23] A gallium-67 scan, in which gallium-67 citrate is taken up by granulocytes, becomes positive early in the course of the disease, but gives poor definition of the extent of the infection.[28] A positive technetium-99 bone scan is diagnostic for acute osteolytic osteomyelitis, but like the gallium scan, it demonstrates inferior detail.[28] Magnetic resonance imaging (MRI) provides an exami-

---

AT A GLANCE. . .

Malignant External Otitis

Pathogenesis: begins as an infection of the EAC and spreads to the surrounding tissue; Pseudomonas aeruginosa is the major pathogenic organism

Adverse Effects: may progress to osteomyelitis of the skull base, facial paralysis, stenosis of the EAC due to chondritis, ossicular disruption, sepsis

Symptoms and Signs: acute onset of otalgia, aural draining, swelling and erythema of the preauricular region and pinna

Diagnosis: documentation of a Pseudomonas infection; rise in ESR; CT; MRI; nuclear scans

Treatment: combination of intravenous anti-Pseudomonas antibiotics (aminoglycoside and either piperacillin or azlocillin); debridement of infected tissue

nation of the soft tissue of the base of skull that is superior to that seen with the nuclear scans.[28]

The treatment of choice for MEO includes a combination of intravenous (IV) anti-Pseudomonas antibiotics, such as an aminoglycoside and either piperacillin or azlocillin. Because of the low-recurrence rate in children, a 2–3 week course of treatment is usually sufficient. Debridement of infected tissue is very important. Hyperbaric oxygen has been used as an adjuvant in adults to prevent the need for extensive debridement; however, efficacy in children remains unclear.[25]

KELOID FORMATION

Keloid formation is usually the result of trauma to the affected region in otherwise predisposed individuals. The ear lobule is a common site of keloid formation because of trauma or chronic inflammation related to earrings. The keloid extends medially from the core of the earring hole and may become quite large (Fig. 14–3). Keloids are painless but may cause itching due to chronic inflammation. Treatment includes surgical excision and then intralesional injection with corticosteroids (triamcinolone acetonide).

PERICHONDRITIS

Perichondritis results from infection and inflammation of the pinna that frequently follows trauma to that region. Blood and/or serum collects in the potential space between the cartilage and perichondrium and infection of this fluid results in perichondritis and chondritis. The usual pathogens include *Pseudomonas* species and mixed flora. Affected children complain of pain and fever, and examination of the involved portion of the ear reveals erythema, swelling, and fluctuance (Fig. 14–4 and 14–5).

Early or mild cases of perichondritis may be treated with oral antibiotics that provide gram-positive coverage. Progression of infection necessitates aspiration of pus and a change in antibiotic therapy

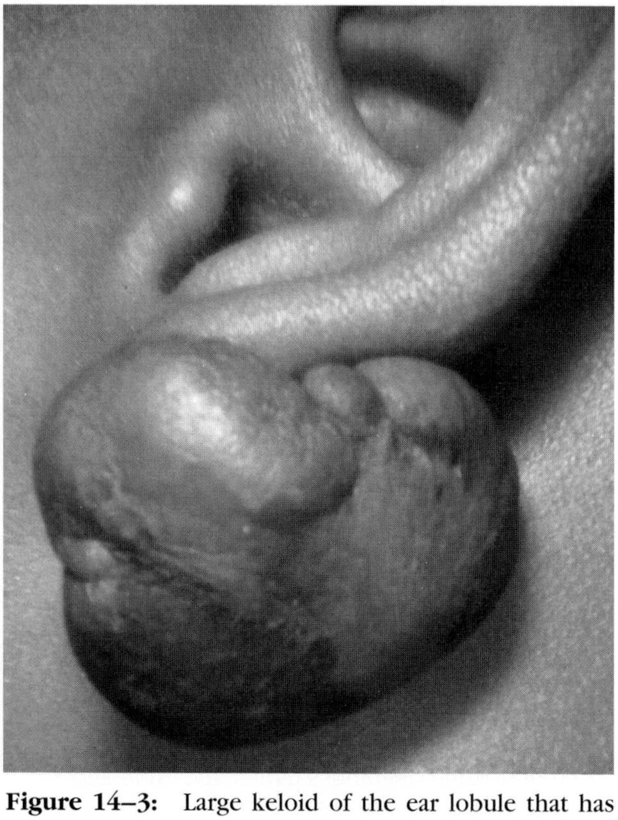

Figure 14–3: Large keloid of the ear lobule that has resulted from ear piercing. Treatment included surgical excision and corticosteroid injection of the surgical site.

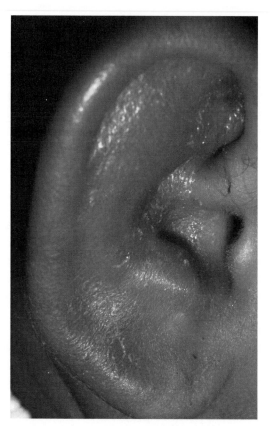

Figure 14–4: Example of perichondritis of the pinna following an episode of ear piercing. This child was treated successfully with intravenous antibiotics.

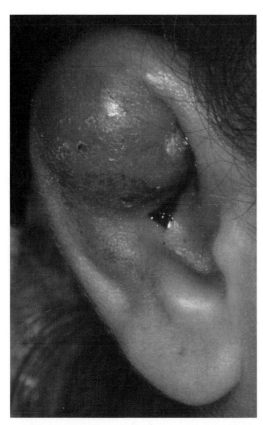

Figure 14–5: Perichondritis may progress to frank abscess formation as seen in this child who required surgical drainage in addition to intravenous antibiotics.

to include gram-negative coverage, specifically against *Pseudomonas.* If frank chondritis develops, incisions should be made in the cartilage in order to provide adequate drainage. Consideration should also be given to irrigating the involved tissue with anti-Pseudomonas antibiotics. If this method of treatment is unsuccessful, debridement of involved cartilage and overlying skin should be performed.[1]

RELAPSING POLYCHONDRITIS

Relapsing polychondritis is an uncommon progressive inflammatory disorder that may affect children, but more commonly it affects adults. Destruction of cartilage due to inflammatory infiltrates is often followed by granulation and then fibrosis and calcification. Erythema and swelling of the cartilaginous portions of the ear are associated with arthralgias involving one or several joints.[1] Tenderness of the nasal septum may progress to complete destruction of the cartilaginous septum, and ultimately to a

nasal-saddle deformity in some cases. The development of dyspnea, cough, and hoarseness may signal involvement of the laryngeal and tracheal cartilages. A conductive hearing loss may result from obstruction of the external meatus secondary to destruction of EAC cartilage.

The differential diagnosis of relapsing polychondritis in children includes rheumatoid arthritis, lymphoma, or infectious perichondritis. A weak, positive rheumatoid factor and antinuclear antibody tests may be seen with relapsing polychondritis; however, the diagnosis may depend upon biopsy of involved cartilage.[29] The usual treatment of relapsing polychondritis is with systemic corticosteroids, such as prednisone. In resistant cases, dapsone, cyclophosphamide, or azathioprine may be tried.[29]

REFERENCES

1. Senturia BH, Marcus MD, Lucente FE. *Diseases of the External Ear: An Otologic-Dermatologic Manual.* New York: Grune & Stratton, 1980, p. 5, 96, 129.
2. Brook I. Microbiological studies of the bacterial flora of the external auditory canal in children. Acta Otolaryngol 1981; 91:285–287.
3. Shaw EAG. The external ear. In: Keidel WD, Neff WD, eds. *Handbook of Sensory Physiology.* Berlin: Springer, 1974, p. 455.
4. Kelly KE, Mohs DC. The external auditory canal. Otolaryngol Clin North Am 1996; 29:725–739.
5. Alberti PW. Epithelial migration on the tympanic membrane. J Laryngol Otol 1964; 78:808.
6. Hyslop NE. Ear wax and host defense. N Engl J Med 1971; 284:1099–1100.
7. Fabricant ND, Perlstein MA. pH of the cutaneous surface of the external auditory canal. Arch Otolaryngol 1949; 49:201.
8. Chai TJ, Chai TC. Bacterial activity of cerumen. Antimicrob Agents Chemother 1980; 18:638–641.
9. Fairbanks DNF. Otic topical agents. Otolaryngol Head Neck Surg 1980; 88:327–331.
10. Linstrom CJ, Lucente FE. External otitis. In: English GM, ed. *Otolaryngology.* Vol I Philadelphia: Lippincott, 1990, p. 1–15.
11. Hughes GB, Levine SC. Disorders of the external ear. In: Hughes GB, ed. *Textbook of Clinical Otology.* New York: Thieme-Stratton, 1985, p. 271–281.
12. Ludman H. *Mawson's Diseases of the Ear, 5th ed.* Chicago: Year Book, 1989.
13. Bojrab DI, Bruderly T, Abdulrazzak Y. Otitis externa. Otolaryngol Clin North Am 1996; 29:761–782.
14. Brook I, Coolbaugh JC: Changes in the bacterial flora

of the external ear canal from the wearing of occlusive equipment. Laryngoscope 1984; 94:963–965.

15. Lopez L, Evens RP. Drug therapy of aspergillus otitis externa. Otolaryngol Head Neck Surg 1980; 88: 649–651.

16. Roland PS. Clinical ototoxicity of topical antibiotic drops. Otolaryngol Head Neck Surg 1994; 110: 598–602.

17. Lundy LB, Graham MD. Ototoxicity and ototopical medications: A survey of otolaryngologists. Presented at the Ninth Shambaugh-Shea Weekend of Otology, Chicago, Illinois, March 6–8, 1992.

18. Rohn GN, Meyerhoff WL, Wright CG. Ototoxicity of topical agents. Otolaryngol Clin North Am 1993; 26: 747–758.

19. Marsh RR, Tom LWC. Ototoxicity of antimycotics. Otolaryngol Head Neck Surg 1989; 100:134–136.

20. Piepergerdes JC, Kramer BM, Behnke EE. Keratosis obturans and external auditory canal cholesteatoma. Laryngoscope 1980; 90:383–391.

21. Morrison AW. Keratosis obturans. J Laryngol Otol 1956; 70:317.

22. Joachims HZ. Malignant external otitis in children. Arch Otolaryngol 1976; 102:236–237.

23. Rubin J, Yu VL, Stool SE. Malignant external otitis in children. J Pediatr 1988; 113:965–970.

24. Horn KL, Gherini S. Malignant external otitis of childhood. Am J Otol 1981; 2:402–404.

25. Davis JC, Gates GA, Lerner C, et al. Adjuvant hyperbaric oxygen in malignant external otitis. Arch Otolaryngol Head Neck Surg 1992; 118:89–93.

26. Coser PL, Stamm AEC, Lobo RC, et al. Malignant external otitis in infants. Laryngoscope 1980; 90: 312–316.

27. Nir D, Nir T, Danino J, et al. Clinical records: Malignant external otitis in an infant. J Laryngol Otol 1990; 104:488.

28. Gherini SG, Brackmann DE, Bradley WG. Magnetic resonance imaging and computerized tomography in malignant external otitis. Laryngoscope 1986; 96: 542–548.

29. Gilliland BC. Relapsing polychondritis and miscellaneous arthritides. In: Fanci AS, Braunwald E, Isselbacher KJ, et al, eds. *Harrison's Principles of Internal Medicine, 14th ed.* New York: McGraw-Hill, 1998, pp. 1951–1953.

30. Hirsch BE. Infections of the external ear. Am J Otolaryngol 1992; 13:145–155.

15 Diagnosis and Management of Acute Otitis Media and Otitis Media with Effusion

Margaret A. Kenna

Otitis media (OM) is the most common reason, outside of upper respiratory tract infections (URI), for young children to visit a primary care provider (PCP). Prior to the introduction of antimicrobials, OM also was responsible for significant morbidity and mortality. In a study by Rosenwasser and Adelman that looked at mortality at the Los Angeles County Hospital in the 5 years (1928–1933) preceding the introduction of sulfonamides, 1:40 deaths resulted from intracranial complications of OM.[1] Similarly, Courville noted that the death rate from OM between 1944 to 1953 was 10% of the rate between 1929 to 1933.[2] Currently, even with the widespread use of systemic antimicrobials to treat OM, morbidity and, in some parts of the world, mortality still occur.[3]

Although antimicrobials have been a "saving grace" for OM, the frequent use of these same antimicrobials is being questioned now due to the increased emergence of resistant bacterial organisms.[4] Other ongoing controversies include whether persistent middle-ear effusion has a significant impact on speech and language, and if so, whether surgical or medical therapy is the most appropriate course.

DEFINITION AND CLASSIFICATION

Otitis media means inflammation of the middle ear, without reference to etiology or pathogenesis. The other areas of the temporal bone that are contiguous to the middle ear, including the mastoid, perilabyrinthine air cells, and petrous apex, may become inflamed as well. OM can be classified further into many variants, including acute OM without effusion, acute OM with effusion, chronic OM with effusion, chronic suppurative OM with and without cholesteatoma, and atelectasis of the tympanic membrane (TM), middle ear, and mastoid. Atelectasis may or may not be associated with a prior clinical history of OM. Adhesive OM and atelectasis often are used interchangeably, although they are distinct clinical entities.[5] *OM with effusion* (OME) also is referred to as serous, mucoid, or secretory otitis; glue ear; or chronic OM. Ears with dry TM perforations also may be designated chronic OM. Although *chronic suppurative OM* (CSOM) currently refers to a nonintact TM with middle-ear otorrhea, in the older literature it also occasionally indicated an intact TM with chronic middle ear changes.

> ### SPECIAL CONSIDERATION:
> Otitis media means inflammation of the middle ear, without reference to etiology or pathogenesis.

In this chapter, *acute OME* is associated with the rapid onset of one or more of the following symptoms: otalgia, fever, otorrhea, recent onset of anorexia, irritability, vomiting, or diarrhea. These symptoms should be accompanied by otoscopic findings of a TM that is opaque, often bulging, and

Pediatric Otolaryngology, Edited by R.F. Wetmore, H.R. Muntz, and T.J. McGill. Thieme Medical Publishers, Inc., New York © 2000.

limited in mobility on pneumatic otoscopy. Erythema may or may not be present. Very early acute OM, or *myringitis,* may not have obvious middle-ear effusion, but rather just a fiery-red and sometimes thickened TM. This finding should be distinguished from the hyperemia of a normal TM in a crying child. *OME* indicates middle-ear effusion of any duration; *chronic OME* signifies middle-ear effusion that persists for 3 months or longer following a diagnosis of acute OM, or at least 3 documented months of asymptomatic OME. Actually, "asymptomatic" may be somewhat of a misnomer, as these children usually do have hearing loss in the affected ear that often is evident to a parent, teacher, or to the patient themselves. These patients also may have difficulty with balance and have tinnitus, which are symptoms that are difficult to elicit from a very young child. *CSOM* refers to middle ear-otorrhea coming through a nonintact TM with either a pressure-equalization tube (PET) (i.e., tympanostomy tube) and/or a perforation. Although there are no definite criteria for when acute otorrhea becomes chronic, 6 to 12 weeks of continuous drainage is used as a general guide. *Effusion* simply refers to the presence of fluid in the middle-ear–mastoid region, and it can be suppurative, serous, mucoid, or a combination thereof. *Atelectasis* of the middle-ear–mastoid refers to collapse of the TM. This collapse may be passive and present without an obvious history of OM, or it may be due to apparent negative middle-ear pressure with eustachian tube (ET) dysfunction. *Adhesive OM,* which is often confused with atelectasis, is actually a complication of OM. It occurs as a result of chronic inflammation of the middle ear and mastoid, resulting in proliferation of fibrous tissue. This process can limit ossicular motion, cause adhesion of a severely-atelectatic TM to the middle ear, and result in a conductive hearing loss (CHL). Finally, *retraction pockets* represent an atelectatic area of the TM, and *otorrhea* is defined as drainage of fluid from the middle ear into the external auditory canal (EAC).

SPECIAL CONSIDERATION:

Otitis media with effusion indicates middle-ear effusion of any duration. Chronic OME signifies a middle-ear effusion that persists for 3 months or longer.

AT A GLANCE . . .

Classification of Otitis Media

- Acute otitis media without effusion
- Acute otitis media with effusion
- Chronic otitis media with effusion
- Chronic suppurative otitis media with or without cholesteatoma
- Atelectasis of tympanic membrane, middle ear, and mastoid

EPIDEMIOLOGY

There are indications that the incidence and prevalence of OM is increasing.[5] Some of the factors contributing to the increased diagnosis of OM include increased awareness of the disease, improved otoscopic equipment, ready availability of tympanometers in schools and PCP's offices, and the need for working parents to keep their children healthy so that they can attend day care and the parents can continue to work. Day care attendance itself seems to be a factor in the increased occurrence of OM, due at least in part to increased exposure to multiple respiratory pathogens from the other children.[5]

SPECIAL CONSIDERATION:

Two-thirds of all children have had at least one episode of OM by 3 years of age.

The peak age-specific attack rate occurs between the ages of 6 and 18 months; and if a child has not had OM before the age of 3 years, he is statistically unlikely to develop severe or recurrent middle-ear disease. In the Boston study, the occurrence of both recurrent acute OM and OME peaked between the ages of 6 months and 13 months of age[6]; similar results have been found in other studies.[5] In a Pittsburgh study, 2% of children had experienced at least one episode of acute OM by age 2 months; by age 12 months, 34% of children had developed acute OM; and by age 24 months, 59% had developed acute OM.[7] With regard to asymptomatic middle-ear fluid, 10% had at least one episode by age 2 months; by age 12 months, 78% had at least one episode of middle-ear fluid; and finally, by age 24 months, 92% of children had been diagnosed with at least one episode of middle-ear fluid.[7] Additionally, after a single episode of acute OM, the fluid may persist for months. In the Boston study, 70% of children still had fluid at 2 weeks, 40% at 4 weeks, 20% at 2 months, and 10% at 3 months. Studies from many other centers support these observations.[6]

SPECIAL CONSIDERATION:

After an episode of acute 10% of children will still have middle-ear effusion 3 months later.

Many factors influence the incidence of OM (Fig. 15-1). Children with a first incidence of acute OM before 6 months of age or with OME before 2 months of age are statistically at an increased risk for further OM compared to children whose ear disease started later. Statistically, Native American Alaskan, and Canadian Inuit children and children who live in developing areas or crowded conditions have more middle-ear disease than other children. Until recently, there was some evidence that African-American children had less ear disease than Caucasian children, but two recent studies from Pittsburgh suggest that this is not the case and that, in fact, prevalence rates are very similar in these two populations.[8,9] Children whose biologic parents and siblings have or have had significant OM are more likely

to have an increased number of episodes and an increased duration of OM as well. Children in large day care centers are more likely to have OM than children in family day care; and those in family day care are, in turn, more likely to have OM than those in home care. Also, children exposed to "second-hand smoke" are more likely to have OM than those who are not. In some studies, breastfeeding is associated with a decreased incidence of OM.[9]

SPECIAL CONSIDERATION:

Epidemiologic factors associated with an increase incidence of OM include large group day care, a parent or sibling with OM, male sex, and second-hand smoke.

Because of underlying medical or anatomic conditions, children who are more prone to OM than others include those with cleft palate, other midface anomalies, and Down's syndrome. These children have a much higher incidence of chronic ear problems, especially chronic middle-ear effusion, than other children.[10] This is thought to be due at least in part to anatomic and physiologic abnormalities that lead to ET dysfunction. Children with altered immune systems, including hypogammaglobulinemia and human immunodeficiency virus (HIV), and children with ciliary dysfunction are much more likely to have OM and sinusitis. Finally, there has been some suggestion that gastroesophageal re-

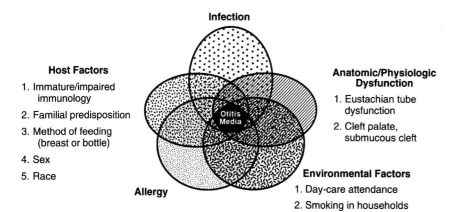

Host Factors

1. Immature/impaired immunology
2. Familial predisposition
3. Method of feeding (breast or bottle)
4. Sex
5. Race

Infection

Anatomic/Physiologic Dysfunction

1. Eustachian tube dysfunction
2. Cleft palate, submucous cleft

Allergy

Environmental Factors

1. Day-care attendance
2. Smoking in households

Figure 15–1: Factors that influence the incidence of OM.

flux (GER) especially with reflux into the nasopharynx, may cause or exacerbate OM and sinusitis.

PATHOPHYSIOLOGY

Abnormal function of the ET is the most important factor in the pathogenesis of OM. In infants and small children, the ET is shorter, more horizontal, and functionally more immature compared to the adult ET. When a child sustains an URI, there may be edema and congestion of the respiratory mucosa, including that of the middle ear, with narrowing of the ET isthmus; this results in negative pressure in the middle ear relative to the nasopharynx. When the tube opens, viruses and bacteria from the nasopharynx are aspirated into the middle ear, causing inflammation.

Many other confounding variables affecting ET function include patulous or functionally- or anatomically-obstructed tubes and abnormalities of the respiratory mucosa, including allergy, immunodeficiency, and ciliary dysfunction. Allergy has long been implicated in the etiology of OM, but the exact mechanism remains elusive. Possibilities include inflammatory swelling of the middle-ear, mastoid, and ET mucosa; allergic nasal obstruction; or middle-ear mucosa reacting as a "shock organ." As large numbers of highly-allergic children do not have significant OM and many children with significant OM do not have documented allergy, the relationship clearly is not a simple one.

AT A GLANCE . . .

Mechanism of Allergy in Otitis Media

- Inflammatory swelling of the middle ear and eustachian tube mucosa
- Allergic nasal obstruction
- Middle ear mucosa acting as "shock organ"

Although relatively small in number, children with congenital or acquired (including drug-induced) immunocompromise require special consideration because often they are more susceptible to infections in general (including OM) and are more likely to have unusual organisms. Congenital immune abnormalities include B-cell deficiencies [e.g., hypogammaglobulinemia and immunoglobulin A (IgA) deficiency]; T-cell deficiencies (e.g., DiGeorge's syndrome); combined T- and B-cell deficiencies, including ataxia telangiectasia; phagocyte defects, including Chédiak-Higashi syndrome; and others, including complement deficiencies. Acquired abnormalities include those secondary to neoplasms; inflammatory processes such as acute or chronic infections (e.g., HIV disease) and rheumatoid arthritis; and metabolic abnormalities such as diabetes. Drugs causing immune deficiencies include steroids, chemotherapeutic agents, and anti-rejection agents used in transplant patients. Although these severe forms of immune deficiency are uncommon in children, many of the otherwise normal OM-prone children may have "immature" immune systems, as documented by a poor response to polysaccharide antigen vaccines [e.g., *Hemophilus influenzae* B (HIB) tetanus, and the pneumococcal vaccine]

Physiologic or anatomic abnormalities of the palate and associated musculature, especially the tensor veli palatini, may cause or worsen ET dysfunction. For example, many craniofacial abnormalities (e.g., cleft palate, mid-face anomalies such as Crouzon's or Apert's syndrome, and Down's syndrome) are associated with abnormal skull base and/or palate anomalies with resultant ET dysfunction.

AT A GLANCE . . .

Congenital Immune Abnormalities

- B-cell deficiencies
- T-cell deficiencies
- Combined B- and T-cell deficiencies
- Phagocyte defects
- Others (complement deficiency)

MICROBIOLOGY

The most-commonly identified aerobic pathogens that are associated with acute OM are *Streptococcus pneumoniae* (30–50%), nontypable *Hemophilus influenzae* (20–30%), *Moraxella catarrhalis* (10–20%), and group A beta hemolytic streptococci

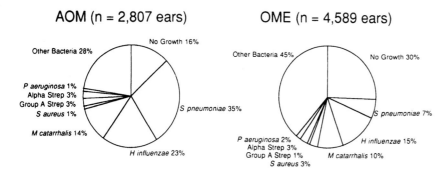

Figure 15–2: Incidence of bacterial pathogens in acute OM and OME.

(1–5%).[11] Other bacteria such as *Staphylococcus aureus* and gram-negative enteric organisms, including *Escherichia coli, Klebsiella* species, and *Pseudomonas aeruginosa,* are isolated infrequently in a small%age of patients. In neonates and young infants, *Streptococcus pneumoniae* and *Hemophilus Influenzae* are still the most-commonly isolated pathogens; however, *Staphylococcus aureus,* group B streptococci, gram-negative enteric pathogens, and other organisms associated with local and systemic infection are found up to 20% of the time. Infants and children in intensive care settings, especially if the stay is prolonged, and immunocompromised children also may have unusual organisms recovered from their middle-ear fluid. Other bacterial organisms that have been isolated occasionally from middle-ear fluid include *Mycoplasma pneumoniae, Chlamydia trachomatis,* and *Mycobacterium tuberculosis.*[5] Most recently, a new bacteria, *Alloiococcus otitidis,* has been isolated under very careful culture conditions from chronic middle-ear fluid.[12] Unusual organisms continue to be reported as isolated cases (Fig. 15–2).

Although anaerobic bacteria have been isolated in several studies of both acute and chronic OM, the consensus is that their role is a minor one. *Peptostreptococcus, Fusobacterium* species, and *Bacteroides* species are the most-commonly isolated. In CSOM, however, anaerobes are found often, and sometimes in more abundance than aerobic organisms. Despite this finding, the management of these organisms, even when isolated in large numbers, remains unclear.

Over the past 10 to 15 years, an increasing number of beta-lactamase producing bacteria have been isolated from the middle ear.[11] These include up to 40% of the *Hemophilus Influenzae,* 80 to 100% of the *Moraxella catarrhalis,* and many *Staphylococcus aureus* and anaerobes (Fig. 15–3). Fortunately,

Streptococcus pneumoniae does not make beta-lactamase yet. On the other hand, a significant%age of the *Streptococcus pneumoniae* have become resistant to penicillin and other antimicrobials; the exact%age varies with the geographic area and the population studied.[13] The mechanisms for beta-lactamase and penicillin resistance are different, so different strategies in terms of antimicrobial usage are needed for treatment. Possible clinical factors in the development of bacterial resistance include multiple and prolonged exposures to antimicrobials (including prophylaxis) not taking the entire prescribed course of antimicrobial, and inappropriate administration of medications.

AT A GLANCE . . .

Viruses Implicated in Otitis Media

- Respiratory syncytial virus (RSV)
- Rhinovirus
- Influenza viruses
- Adenovirus
- Enteroviruses
- Parainfluenza viruses
- Cytomegalovirus (CMV)
- Herpes simplex (HSV)
- Measles
- Epstein-Barr virus

Recently, viruses have gained increased attention as causative or copathogenic organisms, along with bacteria, in OM. Viruses that have been isolated directly from middle-ear fluids include respiratory syn-

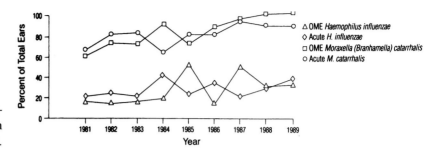

Figure 15–3: Incidence of beta-lactamase producing bacteria isolates from middle ears for both acute OM and OME.

cytial virus (RSV), rhinovirus, influenza virus, adenovirus, enteroviruses, and parainfluenza viruses.[14] Cytomegalovirus (CMV) and herpes simplex virus (HSV) also have been isolated, although in a smaller number of cases. OM also is known to accompany viral exanthems, including measles and Epstein-Barr virus.[5]

COMPLICATIONS

The complications of OM can be divided into intratemporal and intracranial. The *intratemporal complications* include hearing loss [which can be either conductive (common) or sensorineural (uncommon)] perforation of the TM, CSOM, cholesteatoma, retraction pockets, adhesive OM, tympanosclerosis, ossicular discontinuity and fixation, mastoiditis, petrositis, labyrinthitis, facial paralysis, and cholesterol granuloma. CHL is extremely common, occurring in most cases of acute or chronic OME and perforated TM. Fortunately, sensorineural hearing loss (SNHL) is very uncommon, but can occur in the setting of very long-standing CSOM or secondary to some of the other suppurative complications, including acute mastoiditis, labyrinthitis, and meningitis. Perforation of the TM may occur spontaneously due to acute OM or may result when a PET falls out and the resulting perforation fails to heal. Tympanosclerosis, adhesive otitis, ossicular discontinuity, cholesteatoma, and cholesterol granuloma usually occur secondary to chronic OM; tympanosclerosis and cholesteatoma also are known complications of PETs. Fortunately, labyrinthitis, severe mastoiditis, meningitis, petrositis, and facial paralysis are seen very infrequently; however, they can have significant morbidity if they go unrecognized.

Controversy continues as to what degree and duration of CHL affects speech, language, and short- and long-term cognitive development in children with OM.[15] Because CHL is one of the complications

of OM that guides both the medical and surgical management of the disease, much research has centered on the significance of this hearing loss. Clinical studies of this problem are especially difficult to compare because the outcomes (i.e., short- and long-term speech, language, and cognitive ability) can be evaluated using so many different methods. Additionally, the study populations often are not comparable; there is a wide range of subjects, varying from mainly Caucasian middle-class children to severely-disadvantaged minority children. Recently, some studies have focused on the long-term effects of chronic effusion and CHL on hearing and central auditory processing. Because these types of more sophisticated evaluations can be performed routinely only on children over the age of 5 years, it is difficult to know what effects hearing loss has on younger children.[5]

SPECIAL CONSIDERATION:

Prolonged middle-ear effusion associated with hearing loss may interfere with speech and language development.

Despite the variance in study design and results, there is enough significant data for both the American Academy of Pediatrics (Committee on Early Childhood, Adoption, and Dependent Care) and the Agency for Health Care Policy and Research to think that there is growing evidence for a correlation between middle-ear fluid with hearing impairment and delays in speech, language, and cognitive development. If the effusion has persisted for 3 months or longer, hearing should be assessed and communication skills evaluated. Each clinician must then decide on a course that is best for each child's current situation, remaining cognizant that too long a period of watchful waiting could be detrimental to the child.[16-20]

AT A GLANCE . . .

Intratemporal Complications of Otitis Media

- Conductive or sensorineural hearing loss
- Tympanic membrane perforation
- Chronic suppurative otitis media
- Cholesteatoma
- Retraction pockets
- Adhesive otitis media
- Tympanosclerosis
- Ossicular discontinuity and fixation
- Mastoiditis
- Petrositis
- Labyrinthitis
- Facial paralysis
- Cholesterol granuloma

DIAGNOSIS

History

The two mainstays in the diagnosis of OM are history and physical examination. The most common symptoms of acute OME are sudden onset of otalgia, otorrhea, fever, irritability, and lethargy, followed less commonly by anorexia, nausea, vomiting, diarrhea, and headache. Fever is present in up to 66% of children with acute OM, but fevers over 40°C are uncommon and may represent bacteremia or other complications. Older children also may complain of hearing loss, tinnitus, and vertigo; small children may be unable to make these complaints, but they appear off-balance or not to be hearing.[21]

Children with relatively-asymptomatic OME may complain of, or seem to have, hearing loss. Some children with subacute OME may not have the sudden onset of symptoms but may complain of intermittent otalgia, imbalance, and hearing loss. Children with acute OM and some children with chronic OME may awaken frequently and complain of pain more at night-time and during naps because the ET

is less functional when the child is lying down. In some children, the diagnosis of OME is made only incidently on routine examination or if hearing loss is suspected. Children with draining ears, especially if chronic, may have little or no pain and sleep well, but may still complain of hearing loss and have occasional low-grade fevers. Children with TM perforations are usually asymptomatic except for hearing loss or if they get water in their ears, in which case they may complain of significant discomfort. Finally, children with atelectasis of the TM are also usually asymptomatic, although many of these children have hearing loss as well.

Physical Examination

The normal TM is gray and translucent (like waxed paper) with normal mobility on pneumatic otoscopy. Middle-ear landmarks that may be seen through an intact TM include the short process of the malleus, the incudostapedial joint, and occasionally, the chorda tympani nerve. The manubrium of the malleus is the most frequently seen landmark. In acute OM, the TM is opaque, thickened, erythematous, and often bulging, and it has very limited mobility. The middle-ear landmarks may be obscured completely. Uncommonly, bullae may be seen on the TM when the disease is very acute and can be present either with or without effusion. Acutely-perforated TMs are usually erythematous and thickened, and otorrhea that is purulent, serous, or mucoid can be seen in the EAC.

In OME, the TM may be opaque but is less likely to be erythematous. Air-fluid levels or bubbles may be seen, indicating at least intermittent aeration of the middle ear. If the TM is opaque, there is usually limited mobility with obscured landmarks. If there are bubbles or an air-fluid level, the TM motion may be fairly normal, and the malleus may be seen. The TM may be in a relatively-normal position or may be retracted, but is usually not bulging. The color of the TM reflects the middle-ear contents and may be opaque and white, gray, or amber; less commonly, the TM may appear almost dark blue, a sign of either a "glue ear" or hemorrhage into the fluid. Although many older texts emphasize the presence of the "light reflex" on the TM, this reflex may be absent in entirely normal ears and present in ears with middle-ear effusion. Therefore, a light reflex is not helpful in making a diagnosis of OM.

With a TM perforation, the hole can be of any size and location within the membrane. Rarely, there may be multiple perforations, and it is common to see tympanosclerosis within the remaining TM. If the perforation is large, the ossicles may be visualized. In an atelectatic ear, the TM is often thinned-out, transparent, and draped over the promontory and the ossicles. It may move when negative pressure is applied with the pneumatic otoscope. In a TM with a significant amount of tympanosclerosis, the uninvolved portion of the membrane can be very atelectatic and retracted. Retraction pockets often occupy the site of an old PET or are found in the posterior-superior aspect of the TM in patients with ongoing ET dysfunction.

Although middle-ear effusion often is described as serous (i.e., thin and watery), mucoid/secretory (i.e., thick and viscous), purulent (i.e., pus-like), or clear [which rarely may represent a cerebrospinal fluid (CSF) leak rather than inflammation], the description of the type of fluid is made most accurately if otorrhea develops or fluid is obtained at the time of myringotomy. Treatment decisions should not be made on the basis of what type of fluid the physician thinks is in the middle ear alone. For example, serous fluid is not always sterile and may represent acute OM, for which antibiotics would be indicated often.

Hearing Evaluation

The most common complication of OM is CHL, which may result from middle-ear effusion, ET dysfunction, or pathology resulting from inflammation. Every child with recurrent OM and/or ongoing ET dysfunction should have his hearing evaluated. This hearing assessment is really two-fold and involves: (1) an audiometric evaluation to test the peripheral hearing; and (2) impedance audiometry to evaluate the stiffness of the TM and middle-ear system. The audiometric technique that is used to test a child varies with her age and maturity. In infants under the age of 6 months, *auditory brainstem response* (ABR) testing gives the most accurate thresholds and may be able to sort out a CHL from a SNHL. ABR testing also may be of great value in children who are unable to participate in behavioral testing due to age or level of disability. In young children in whom asymmetric hearing loss is suspected but not confirmed by behavioral testing, ear-specific information can be obtained with ABR. Although *otoacoustic emissions* (OAE) often are used for screening hearing in the newborn nursery, this is not a good technique to clarify the hearing status

of a child with OM, as one of the main causes of OAE failure is middle-ear fluid.

> ## SPECIAL CONSIDERATION:
> Every child with recurrent OM and/or ongoing ET dysfunction should have their hearing evaluated.

Because most children do not develop very frequent or persistent OM until 6 months of age or older, behavioral testing is the standard technique to evaluate hearing in a child with a history of OM. *Behavioral observation audiometry* (BOA) is used for infants from age 6 months to 1 year and provides an estimation of hearing, especially for the better-hearing ear. *Visual reinforcement audiometry* (VRA) is used for toddlers age 1 to 2 years and also gives results for the better-hearing ear. Although BOA and VRA can document hearing loss, they do not differentiate between CHL and SNHL. *Play audiometry* can be used with cooperative children over the age of 2 years and can provide both ear-specific data and the air and bone conduction thresholds needed to distinguish between CHL and SNHL. *Conventional audiometry* can be employed in most cooperative children >5 years of age.

Impedance audiometry includes *tympanometry,* which is a measure of the amount of sound that is reflected by the TM and middle-ear structures as well as a graphic representation of compliance changes as the ear-canal pressure is varied from −200 to +200 mm H_2O (some machines can provide more pressure). Various tympanometric patterns are associated with normal examinations, middle-ear fluid, retracted TMs, TM perforations, patent PETs, and stiff TM–middle ear systems (as in otosclerosis). Any tympanometric pattern always should be correlated with the findings on pneumatic otoscopy and other audiometric data. Two other aspects of impedance audiometry are the middle-ear muscle reflex (i.e., *acoustic reflex*) and equivalent ear-canal volume. These studies, especially the acoustic reflex, are often used by experienced audiologists to determine the level of hearing loss and middle-ear dysfunction further.[5]

Acoustic reflectometry uses a hand-held instrument that is placed next to the opening of the child's EAC and provides an 80-dB sound source that varies from 2000 to 4500 Hz in a 100-msec period. The instrument then measures the total level of reflected and transmitted sound. Some physicians find this device useful in screening for middle-ear fluid. Acoustic reflectometry is becoming more widely used by both physicians and parents, and the newer instrumentation may provide increased diagnostic accuracy and information.[22]

Other techniques that are used or that have been used in the evaluation of ET dysfunction include sonotubometry, manometry, and tympanometry using various pressure-changing maneuvers. These studies are available in research settings and are not used routinely in the evaluation of the child with OM.[5]

AT A GLANCE . . .

Methods of Hearing Assessment

Audiometry
  Behavioral observation audiometry (BOA)
  Visual reinforcement audiometry (VRA)
  Play audiometry
  Conventional audiometry
Impedance Audiometry
  Tympanometry
  Acoustic reflex
  Equivalent ear canal volume
Acoustic Reflectometry
Auditory Brainstem Response (ABR)
Otoacoustic emissions (OAE)

TREATMENT AND MANAGEMENT

Rationale

The reasons for which to treat OM are: (1) to avoid complications; (2) to treat symptomatic disease effectively; and (3) to "wait out" the URI season, buying time until the child's ET function and immune system have matured. Management options should be matched to the patient's pattern of OM, whether that is recurrent acute OM that clears in between episodes, recurrent acute OM with persistent fluid in between acute episodes, or chronic middle-ear fluid with few acute symptoms. In many cases, med-

ical therapy works well in the first example and sometimes in the second, but it is often ineffective in the third.

Acute OM has a spontaneous resolution rate of about 60 to 80%.[23] Possible reasons for this include drainage of middle-ear contents down the ET or through a perforated TM, natural resolution secondary to the body's local or systemic immune system, or acute OM that occurred as a result of viruses or some noninfectious process. Not infrequently, the diagnosis may be in error, especially in a crying child with "red" ear drums. Therefore, some physicians think that no initial antimicrobial therapy is indicated for acute OM and that agents to control the symptoms of pain and fever should be given and the child watched closely instead.[24] If after a few days the child is not significantly improved, then antimicrobial therapy can be initiated. However, several studies suggest that the resolution rate is higher and the complication rate lower if antimicrobials are given from the beginning.[5] Some studies that have evaluated middle-ear fluid several days into an acute infection have found that *Streptococcus pneumoniae* is often the cause of persistent OM. Because *Streptococcus pneumoniae* also is associated with a large number of the complications secondary to OM, nontreatment in the acute stage is at least worrisome. Based on all these factors, routine nontreatment of symptomatic acute OM is not advocated.

SPECIAL CONSIDERATION:

Acute OM has a spontaneous resolution rate of about 60 to 80%; however, several studies suggest that the resolution rate is higher and the complication rate lower if antimicrobials are given from the onset of infection.

The routine treatment of asymptomatic middle-ear fluid is at least as controversial. The child with asymptomatic middle-ear fluid typically is diagnosed during a viral URI and the fluid is noted incidentally on physical examination. The TM is often dull, but not red or bulging, its mobility is limited, and fluid or bubbles are noted. Although the parents may have noted decreased hearing, the child may have no other symptoms. In these children, watchful waiting may be entirely appropriate. The keys to management in these cases are whether the child is truly asymptomatic (i.e., no fever or pain, sleeping well at night, and not off-balance) and whether he has reliable caretakers who will make sure that he returns for follow-up and/or who will report if he develops symptoms consistent with acute OM. Of note, this type of middle-ear fluid is not necessarily sterile: bacterial organisms have been documented in 30 to 70% of cases by conventional culture techniques and in 77% by the polymerase chain reaction (PCR).[25] Over 3 months of documented middle-ear fluid is a cause for concern and treatment should be considered strongly.

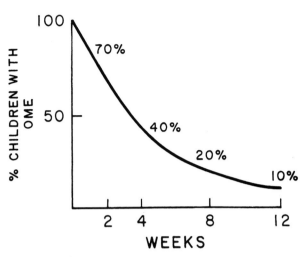

Figure 15–4: Duration of OME following an episode of acute OM.

SPECIAL CONSIDERATION:

In children with OME, bacterial organisms have been documented in 30 to 70% by conventional culture techniques and in 77% by polymerase chain reaction.

Medical Therapy

The mainstay of OM management is medical therapy using antimicrobials. The choice of drug is based on the presumed pathogen, the age of the patient (e.g., in children under the age of 2 months, sulfa should not be used routinely), the duration of disease, the other antimicrobials that have been used recently for OM, and the presence of any drug allergies. In the otherwise normal patient who probably has one of the three major bacterial organisms as a cause for his OM, amoxicillin still remains the antimicrobial of choice for the treatment of a first episode (or in frequent episodes) of acute OM. It is inexpensive, the side effects are few and well known, and compliance is usually not a problem. If the child has a prompt response to therapy with resolution of otalgia, fever and irritability and the parents think that the child is clinically well, then follow-up with the PCP can take place in 2 to 4 weeks.[26] The physician doing the follow-up must remember that, in many cases, there will be persistent middle-ear fluid after the antimicrobial is completed (Fig. 15-4). In many studies, including those in the United States and Scandinavia, there was persistent fluid after an episode of acute OM in 40% of patients at 4 weeks, in 20% at 8 weeks, and in 10% at 3 months.[5,6] Additionally, the younger the patient, the more likely the fluid is to persist. Many practitioners are inclined to prescribe further antimicrobial therapy at this point if they still see middle-ear fluid; however, in the truly asymptomatic patient it is also quite reasonable just to continue observation to see if the fluid resolves on its own. Another course of antimicrobials should be considered only if the patient develops recurrent symptoms or the fluid does not resolve spontaneously within 2 to 3 months.

In the patient who does not show significant improvement in the signs and symptoms of acute disease within 2 to 3 days, there are basically three options (Practice Pathway 15-1). The first is to continue the current regimen, perhaps at a higher dosage, for a few more days to see if there is symptomatic improvement. The second option is to change to another antimicrobial that provides either better or more selective coverage of the suspected bacterial organism(s), including consideration of those bacteria that are beta-lactamase producing or penicillin-resistant. Because it often is not possible to accomplish both goals with one antimicrobial, the clinician should be familiar with the bacterial resistance patterns in his community and base empiric therapy on that information.

The third option is used if the patient with acute OM is "toxic" with high fever, severe lethargy, and other significant symptoms. In this situation, acute

Practice Pathway 15–1 MANAGEMENT OF ACUTE OTITIS MEDIA

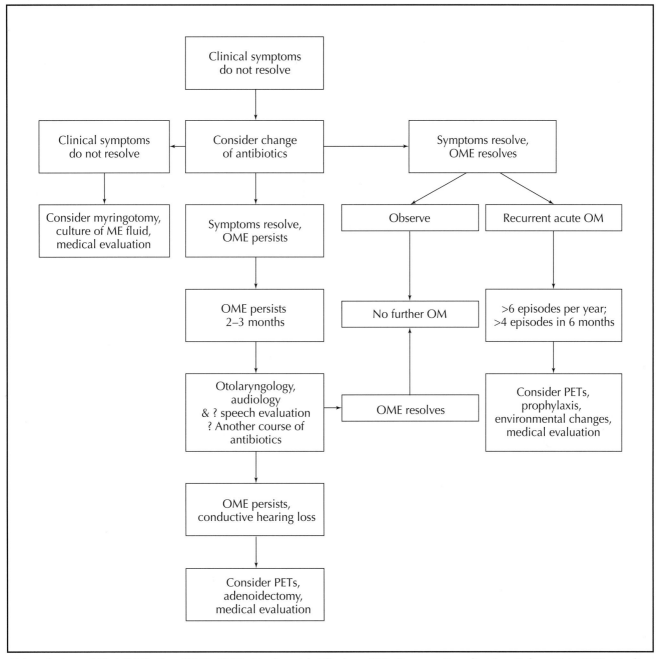

Abbreviations: ME, Middle Ear; OME, Otitis Media with Effusion; PET, Pressure Equalization Tube; OM, Otitis Media.

tympanocentesis or myringotomy with culture of the middle-ear contents may be indicated. Empiric systemic antimicrobial therapy still should be started after cultures are obtained, but may need to be changed based on the susceptibility patterns of the isolated organism. Tympanocentesis also may be indicated if an unusual organism is suspected, such as in a very young or an immunocompromised child, prior to starting antimicrobial therapy.

In the patient with only an occasional episode of acute OM that responds promptly to medical therapy, including resolution of middle-ear fluid, other treatment seldom is necessary. However, if the child has very frequent episodes of OM (i.e., more than three to four episodes in 6 months or four to six episodes in 1 year) then other management options should be considered. Until recently, long-term antimicrobial prophylaxis often was used very effectively in many children. However, with the increase in the number of resistant organisms, the enthusiasm for this mode of treatment has diminished. Amoxicillin and sulfisoxazole are the most-commonly used agents for prophylaxis. Other antibiotics can be used in allergic children. Commonly, prophylaxis is given during the winter months and often can be stopped during the summer when URIs are less common. Short-term prophylaxis in children either with or without middle-ear fluid is practical if the parents are trying to keep the child healthy over a holiday or vacation or until an upcoming surgical procedure (including PET placement.) If a child has frequent breakthrough episodes of OM while on prophylaxis, this mode of treatment is unsuccessful and other options should be considered.

In children with recurrent acute OM who have persistent fluid in between episodes, the goal of therapy is to prevent further acute symptoms and to cause resolution of fluid. Again, antimicrobial therapy is the mainstay of treatment, and the choice of antimicrobial is similar to those cases of recurrent acute OM alone. If the symptoms of recurrent acute disease are controlled with medical therapy but there is persistent middle-ear fluid for 3 months or longer, then the treatment becomes the same as for chronic middle-ear fluid.

Treatment should be considered for chronic OME that has persisted for 3 months or longer, especially if the disease is bilateral, very symptomatic, and associated with significant CHL or if SNHL is present also. As well, treatment should be considered if there are significant TM changes such as deep retraction pockets or if there is middle-ear pathology such as adhesive otitis or ossicular involvement. If the patient has been quite symptomatic, then antimicrobials and occasionally steroids may have been tried already. If not, a trial of one or two antimicrobials that are used for acute OM can be considered. However, based on multiple studies using different antimicrobials, the resolution rate is not as high as for acute OM.[5]

Multiple other medications have been tried or suggested for recurrent acute OM or chronic OME. Systemic and intranasal decongestants continue to be used frequently in children with OM despite several clinical trials demonstrating lack of efficacy in preventing or curing middle-ear disease.[5] Similarly, antihistamine–decongestant combinations frequently are prescribed for children with OM. There is no evidence that these change the clinical course or promote resolution of middle-ear fluid.[5] There is some evidence that ET dysfunction without middle-ear fluid may be helped by these agents and that

there may be improvement of nasal symptoms in children with allergic rhinitis.[5] Although these drugs, both singly and in combination, are ubiquitous on pharmacy shelves, they may have side effects and are not recommended for the treatment of OM.[5]

Systemic and topical corticosteroids have gained wide interest in the treatment of chronic middle-ear fluid. Multiple studies have been performed with varying results.[23] The studies are difficult to compare due to the lack of uniformity in the steroid type, dosage, and route of administration, as well as in the duration of effusion. Some studies included antimicrobial use and others did not; many studies were not controlled for the presence or absence of allergy. The potential side effects of corticosteroids, especially those used systemically, combined with their uncertain efficacy make routine use of them to treat chronic OME difficult to recommend.[23]

Other nonsurgical strategies that have been suggested for the management of chronic OME include mucolytics, allergy management, ET inflation, and most recently, the use of xylitol chewing gum. As previously noted, in some patients it is likely that there is a relationship between OM and allergy; however, OM as the only manifestation of allergy is unusual. If the patient has definite signs and symptoms of allergy other than those of OM, then pursuit of allergy diagnosis and management may be warranted.[27] Daily use of the Valsalva's maneuver or weekly politzerization may help to resolve effusion secondary to barotrauma or from infrequent acute serous OM; however, there is very little evidence to support their use in patients with long-standing middle-ear effusion due to chronic ET dysfunction. A few studies have attempted to evaluate autoinflation using devices that provide "feedback" to the patient (i.e., the device provides some indication of how much air is being delivered by either inflation of a balloon or a ball rising in a chamber). These studies have failed to show long-term improvement, however, in middle-ear effusion.[28,29] Limiting factors include a cooperative patient (at least 3 years of age) and differing durations and documentation methods for the middle-ear fluid. Finally, a 1996 study in the *British Medical Journal* evaluated the use of xylitol chewing gum to prevent acute OM in 5-year-old children in day care. The authors found a slight decrease in the OM rate in the children chewing xylitol gum (12.1%) versus those chewing sucrose gum (20.8%).[30] Although this is an intriguing idea, the safety of xylitol in children of any age, the older age of the children, and the very slight difference in the OM rate certainly warrant further study before this treatment can be recommended.

AT A GLANCE . . .

Medical Treatment of Otitis Media

- Antibiotics
- Corticosteroids (systemic and topical)
- Decongestants
- Antihistamine–decongestant combinations
- Mucolytics
- Allergy management
- Eustachian tube inflation
- Xylitol chewing gum

Prevention

Many strategies have been suggested for the prevention of recurrent acute OM. These include antimicrobial prophylaxis, allergic immunotherapy, tonsillectomy and/or adenoidectomy, vaccination, the administration of immunoglobulins, and elimination of environmental contributors. Antimicrobial prophylaxis has been shown to be effective in preventing new episodes of acute OM. Most studies have utilized amoxicillin–ampicillin and sulfisoxazole, although other antimicrobials have been cited also.[5] In general, younger children benefited more than older children, and the effect on the duration of middle-ear effusion was found to be insignificant. Prophylaxis should be considered in children who have had three to four or more episodes of recurrent acute OM in 6 months or four to six episodes in 1 year. Additionally, children with recurrent acute OM who are being considered for PET placement and who have not had a trial of prophylaxis are possible candidates. Children who had their first episode of acute OM during the first 6 months of life and who have siblings with severe and recurrent OM ("otitis-prone") also may be good candidates for prophylaxis. If the child on prophylaxis experiences prolonged asymptomatic middle-ear fluid, then treatment of this fluid should be considered as should other cases of chronic OME.[5]

SPECIAL CONSIDERATION:

Antibiotic prophylaxis should be considered in children who have had four or more episodes of OM in 6 months or six or more in 1 year.

Allergy management may be helpful if specific allergens can be identified. However, allergy identification and possible modification of the environment should not be done at random but in concert with an allergist or PCP, especially if major dietary changes (e.g., eliminating all milk products) are contemplated. If definite allergies that may be contributing to OM are identified; specific additional treatment of the OM, either medical or surgical, still may be needed because allergy management is often a long-term process that may take months to years to be effective. Likewise, if intravenous gammaglobulin is recommended for proven or suspected immunoglobulin deficiency, specific medical or surgical management of the OM may be needed while waiting for the immunoglobulin therapy to take effect or for the child's own immune system to mature.

Changes in contributing environmental factors include removing possible allergens, prolonging breastfeeding, removing the child from day care (or moving the child from a large daycare to a small homecare), and preventing exposure to second-hand cigarette smoke. Although a direct cause-and-effect relationship between second-hand cigarette smoke and OM has been difficult to document consistently there are enough other health hazards associated with cigarette smoking to make banning smoking around small children advisable. There is some anecdotal evidence that feeding an infant in an upright or semiupright position and not allowing the infant to fall asleep in a supine position with a bottle in her mouth also may help prevent OM.

Vaccines against OM provide an intriguing method of prevention. Until now, however, vaccines directed against the main offending bacterial pathogens have not been very effective. Most of the vaccine research has been aimed at *Streptococcus pneumoniae* and nontypable *Hemophilus influenzae*. Although the HIB vaccine has been extremely successful in preventing meningitis, epiglottitis, and soft-tissue infections due to *Hemophilus influen-*

zae, it has had little effect on OM, as <10% of *Hemophilus influenzae* otitis is due to the type B strain. A vaccine against both *Streptococcus pneumoniae* and *Hemophilus influenzae* organisms would be especially welcome as they both have developed extensive and complicated resistance patterns, making the correct choice of antimicrobial more challenging. To date, the 23 valent *Streptococcus pneumoniae* vaccine has not proven very immunogenic in children under the age of 6 years; however, several studies are underway using conjugate vaccines that are similar to the HIB vaccine to boost the immune response in patients of all ages.[5] Despite the shortcomings of the current pneumococcal vaccine, it still is recommended for children with impaired immune responses to polysaccharide antigens, as side effects are uncommon and the child may derive some benefit.

Now, as viruses are isolated commonly from middle-ear fluid, the question of vaccination against these viruses has been raised. A recent article reported that children aged 6 to 30 months who had received the influenza A vaccine had 32% fewer episodes of acute OM than those who did not.[31]

Surgical Therapy

There are three basic surgical procedures that are used routinely for the diagnosis and treatment of OM. The first, *tympanocentesis,* is used generally to relieve extreme otalgia and/or to obtain middle-ear fluid for culture. Tympanocentesis may be followed by myringotomy if wide drainage of the middle ear is desired. Both procedures can be performed at the bedside, in the outpatient clinic, or in the operating room. In the acutely-ill infant or small child, tympanocentesis can be performed under no or local anesthesia or with mild systemic sedation; the older child is more comfortable if local or general anesthesia is utilized. If a tube is to be inserted after the myringotomy, local or general anesthesia should be used for the whole procedure. If general anesthesia is required for the myringotomy, tube insertion should be considered at the same sitting, especially if there is a strong past history of OM or an intratemporal complication is present. If the tympanocentesis is being performed to obtain middle-ear cultures, the ear canal should be cleaned of cerumen thoroughly and then isopropyl alcohol instilled for 1 minute prior to the procedure. The ear canal also should be cultured after the alcohol is removed but before the tympanocentesis is per-

formed. Culture of both the canal and middle ear helps to sort out organisms that may be considered contaminants.

Pressure equalization tube (PET) insertion is used to treat both recurrent acute OM (with or without effusion) and chronic OME. In addition, a PET may be inserted urgently as part of the treatment of some complications of OM, such as acute mastoiditis or facial nerve paresis or paralysis. In recurrent acute OM, PET insertion may be indicated if the child has had four episodes of OM in 6 months or six episodes in 1 year. PET insertion should be strongly considered if there is no indication that the child is improving on medical therapy, if the patient has failed prophylaxis, or if recurrent acute OM is accompanied by chronic fluid. Less commonly, children with severe multiple antimicrobial allergies may need PETs as an alternative to medical therapy.

In children with chronic middle-ear fluid, PETs should be considered to restore hearing and avoid the possible complications of chronic OM. PET insertion should be considered in those children who have had bilateral middle-ear fluid for 3 months or longer or unilateral fluid for 6 months and who are refractory to medical therapy. Other factors that should be considered include the degree and laterality of hearing loss, the presence of clinical symptoms (e.g., otalgia, fever), and the presence of a TM retraction pocket or suspected ossicular erosion. PET insertion should be considered sooner if an underlying SNHL is present or if the child has significant speech, language, and/or learning delays that will be affected by any degree of hearing loss. If a possible source of fever needs to be eliminated in a medically-complex child (e.g., immunocompromised patients, transplant patients), early PET insertion also should be considered.

SPECIAL CONSIDERATION:

PET insertion should be considered in children who have had bilateral middle-ear fluid for 3 months or longer or unilateral fluid for 6 months.

In the patient with a minimal CHL and evidence of partial middle-ear aeration (i.e., air-fluid levels or bubbles), the decision to insert a PET may be more difficult, as the indications may not seem as strong. In the absence of other compounding factors, these children may be observed cautiously. If the hearing loss worsens, symptoms other than hearing loss develop, or the TM becomes very retracted with the development of retraction pockets, then insertion of a PET still will be indicated.

Adenoidectomy has long been advocated as an adjunct procedure in the management of OM, especially chronic OME. The results of studies looking at the effectiveness of adenoidectomy to prevent OME vary widely, with some showing modest to good effects and some showing no improvement at all.[5] Shortcomings and variations in design and method make these studies difficult to compare. Some differences between them include: (1) a nonstandard definition of OM, (including duration), (2) concurrent surgical procedures (usually tonsillectomy); (3) control for adenoid size; (4) varying adenoidectomy technique; (5) measurement of nasal and ET function not routinely performed; and (6) presence or absence of environmental allergy. In several prospective randomized trials involving children with chronic OME, modest but positive effects of adenoidectomy have been demonstrated with regard to recurrent chronic middle-ear fluid. In studies by Gates et al. and Paradise et al., time to recurrence of effusion, duration of effusion, and need for further myringotomy was improved in the adenoidectomy groups.[5] Based on these and many other studies, adenoidectomy can be recommended, especially in a slightly-older child who is having a second set of PETs placed for chronic middle-ear fluid. The efficacy of adenoidectomy without myringotomy (with or without PET placement) has not been studied extensively. Gates recommended adenoidectomy with myringotomy but without PET insertion at least partly due to the incidence of purulent otorrhea with PETs. When OM recurred after surgery, it recurred sooner in the group that had adenoidectomy and myringotomy without PET than in the group that had the same procedure plus PET insertion.[5]

SPECIAL CONSIDERATION:

In the management of chronic middle-ear fluid, an adenoidectomy can be considered in a slightly older child who is having a second set of PETs placed.

Fewer studies have evaluated the usefulness of adenoidectomy in the management of recurrent acute OM. Paradise et al. reviewed this problem as part of a large study involving adenoidectomy for children who already had one set of PETs placed and who were eligible for a subsequent set. The number of episodes of acute OM were slightly less in the adenoidectomy group than in the control group (28 vs 35%).[5]

With regard to tonsillectomy either with or without adenoidectomy, no study has demonstrated persistently any efficacy in the prevention of OM over adenoidectomy alone, although there is much anecdotal evidence that tonsillectomy is helpful. Currently, tonsillectomy for OM should be considered only if adenoidectomy alone has not helped. Other indications for tonsillectomy are sleep apnea or recurrent pharyngitis.

SPECIAL CONSIDERATION:

No study has demonstrated an efficacy of tonsillectomy with or without adenoidectomy compared to adenoidectomy alone for the prevention of OM.

Complications

The management of complications of OM often involves both medical and surgical therapy. Identification of the bacterial pathogen is highly desirable, and middle-ear cultures should be obtained early in the course of treatment. If possible, middle-ear cultures should be obtained prior to initiating antimicrobial therapy. Many of these children will have been started on therapy already, but cultures will help tailor antimicrobial coverage. For acute OM that is unresponsive to medical therapy, tympanocentesis and myringotomy with or without PET insertion is indicated often.

CONCLUSION

Although OM is common, the diagnosis and management are not always straightforward. Factors adding to controversies about treatment include increased appreciation of the high spontaneous resolution rate of OM, increased awareness of the role of viruses, emergence of resistant bacterial organisms, frequent introduction of new antimicrobials to the market, and the difficult to measure effects of OME on speech, language, and behavior. The medical care provider must be constantly aware of current research as well as the needs of each individual child when planning and recommending treatment for their pediatric patients.

REFERENCES

1. Rosenwasser H, Adelman N. Otitis complications. Arch Otolaryngol 1957; 65:225-234.

2. Courville CB. Intracranial complications of otitis media and mastoiditis in the antibiotic era. Laryngoscope 1955; 65:31-46.

3. Berman S. Otitis media in developing countries. Pediatrics 1995; 96:126-131.

4. Paradise JL. Managing otitis media: A time for change. Pediatrics 1995; 96:712-715.

5. Bluestone CD, Klein JO. Otitis media, atelectasis, and eustachian tube dysfunction. In: Bluestone CD, Stool SE, Kenna MA, eds. *Pediatric Otolaryngology, 3rd ed.* Philadelphia: Saunders, 1996, pp. 388-582.

6. Teele DW, Klein JO, Rosner B, the Greater Boston Otitis Media Study Group. Epidemiology of otitis media during the first seven years of life in children in greater Boston: A prospective cohort study. J Infect Dis 1989; 160:83-94.

7. Casselbrant ML, Mandel EM, Rockette HE, et al. Incidence of otitis media and bacteriology of acute otitis media during the first two years of life. In: Recent Advances in Otitis Media. Proceedings of the Fifth International Symposium. Decker Periodicals, 1993, pp. 1-3, Toronto.

8. Casselbrant ML, Mandel EM, Kurs-Lasky M, et al. Otitis media in a population of black American and white American Infants. Int J Pediatr Otorhinolaryngol 1995; 33:1-16.

9. Paradise JL, Rockette HE, Colborn DK, et al. Otitis media in 2253 Pittsburgh-area infants: Prevalence and risk factors during the first two years of life. Pediatrics 1997; 99:318-333.

10. Pappas DG, Flexer C, Shackelford L. Otological and habilitative management of children with Down syndrome. Laryngoscope 1994; 104:1065-1070.

11. Bluestone CD, Stephenson JS, Martin LM. Ten-year review of otitis media pathogens. Pediatr Infect Dis J 1992; 11(8 supplement):S7-S11.

12. Bosley GS, Whitney AM, Pruckler JM, et al. Characterization of ear fluid isolates of *Alloiococcus otitidis* from patients with recurrent otitis media. J Clin Microbiol 1995; 33:2876-2880.

13. Rodriguez WJ, Schwartz RH, Akram S, et al. *Streptococcus pneumoniae* resistant to penicillin: Incidence and potential therapeutic options. Laryngoscope 1995; 105:300-304.

14. Andrade MA, Hoberman A, Glustein J, et al. Acute otitis media in children with bronchiolitis. Pediatrics 1998; 101:617-619.

15. Roberts JE, Burchinal MR, Medley LP, et al. Otitis media, hearing sensitivity, and maternal responsiveness in relation to language during infancy. J Pediatr 1995; 126:481-489.

16. Nittrouer S. The relation between speech perception and phonemic awareness: Evidence form low-SES children and children with chronic OM. J Speech Hear Res 1996; 39:1059-1070.

17. Gravel JS, Wallace IF, Ruben RJ. Auditory consequences of early mild hearing loss associated with otitis media. Acta Otolaryngol (Stockh) 1996; 116:219-221.

18. Bluestone CD, Klein JO. Intratemporal complications and sequelae of otitis media. In: Bluestone CD, Stool SE, Kenna MA, eds. *Pediatric Otolaryngology, 3rd ed.* Philadelphia: Saunders, 1996, pp. 583-635.

19. Bluestone CD, Klein JO. Intracranial suppurative complications of otitis media and mastoiditis. In: Bluestone CD, Stool SE, Kenna MA, eds. *Pediatric Otolaryngology, 3rd ed.* Philadelphia: Saunders, 1996, pp. 636-645.

20. Stool SE, Berg AO, Berman S, et al. Otitis media with effusion in young children. Clinical practice guideline, number 12. AHCPR publication no. 94-0622. Rockville, MD: Agency for Health Care Policy and Research, Public Health Service, U.S. Department of Health and Human Services, 1994.

21. Casselbrant ML, Furman JM, Rubenstein E, et al. Effect of otitis media on the vestibular system in children. Ann Otol Rhinol Laryngol 1995; 104:620-624.

22. Barnett ED, Klein JO, Hawkins KA, et al. Comparison of spectral gradient acoustic reflectometry and other diagnostic techniques for detection of middle ear effusion in children with middle ear disease. Pediatr Infect Dis J 1998; 17:556-559.

23. Rosenfeld RM. What to expect from medical treatment of otitis media. Ped Inf Dis Journal 1995; 14:731-737.

24. Hoberman A, Paradise JL, Reynolds EA, et al. Efficacy of Auralgan® for treating ear pain in children with acute otitis media. Arch Pediatr Adolesc Med 1997; 151:675-678.

25. Post JC, Preston RA, Aul JJ, et al. Molecular analysis of bacterial pathogens in otitis media with effusion. JAMA 1995; 273:1598-1604.

26. Hathaway TJ, Katz HP, Dershewitz RA, et al. Acute otitis media: Who needs posttreatment follow-up? Pediatrics 1994; 94:143-147.

27. Bernstein JM. Role of allergy in eustachian tube blockage and otitis media with effusion: A review. Otolaryngol Head Neck Surg 1996; 114:562-568.

28. Chan KH, Cantekin EI, Karnavas WJ, et al. Autoinflation of eustachian tube in young children. Laryngoscope 1987; 97(6):668–674

29. Blanshard JD, Maw AR, Bawden R. Conservative treatment of otitis media with effusion by autoinflation of the middle ear. Clin Otolaryngol 1993; 18: 188–192.

30. Uhari M, Kontiokari T, Koskela M, et al. Xylitol chewing gum in prevention of acute otitis media: Double-blind randomised trial. BMJ 1996; 313:1180–1184.

31. Clements DA, Langdon L, Bland C, et al. Influenza A vaccine decreases the incidence of otitis media in 6–30-month-old children in day care. Arch Pediatr Adolesc Med 1995; 149:1113–1117.

16 Chronic Disorders of the Middle Ear and Mastoid

James W. Forsen

During one of his early explorations in search of the Nile's source, the renowned 19th century British adventurer, John Hanning Speke, was maddened by a beetle that had lodged itself in his ear canal. In an effort to relieve his discomfort, he plunged a stick into his ear. His respite was but momentary. The act caused not only pain, but also loss of hearing, vertigo, and later, chronic aural discharge. We can imagine that Speke suffered a perforation of the tympanic membrane (TM), ossicular disruption, and perhaps, a perilymph fistula. His otorrhea was the hallmark of chronic suppurative otitis media (OM), and it is quite possible that his impetuous act resulted in the formation of a cholesteatoma. At that time, understanding of otologic disease was in its infancy and there was little in the way of appropriate care, particularly in eastern Africa. The improvement in our medical capabilities during the past century has been astounding. Nonetheless, the otologic sufferings of John Speke are relived daily by thousands of children in our contemporary age. Proper understanding of the etiology, manifestations, and treatment of chronic middle-ear disease in children is a requisite for every otolaryngologist and is discussed in this chapter.

DEFINITIONS OF OTITIS MEDIA

Discussion of OM and its various forms is sometimes hampered by confusing nomenclature. Therefore, it is worthwhile to review some definitions. *Acute otitis media* (AOM) is characterized by the rapid onset of signs and symptoms of infection of the middle ear, frequently in the setting of an upper respiratory infection (URI). These symptoms include fever, otalgia, irritability, and mild hearing loss. Otoscopy

reveals an opaque to red TM that does not move freely with insufflation. There is usually a purulent middle-ear effusion. *Recurrent acute otitis media* (RAOM) is characterized by three or more discrete episodes of AOM in a 6 month period or four or more episodes in 1 year. *Otitis media with effusion* (OME) is characterized by fluid in the middle-ear space in the absence of signs and symptoms of acute inflammation. The effusion may be serious or mucoid but is usually not purulent. The effusion may be related to an earlier episode of AOM or may have developed spontaneously secondary to eustachian tube (ET) dysfunction. *Chronic suppurative otitis media* (CSOM) is characterized by persistent purulent drainage from the external auditory canal (EAC) due to infection within the middle ear. The purulence is expressed either through a perforation in the TM or through a patent pressure-equalization (tympanostomy) tube (PET) present within the TM. The term *chronic otitis media* has been used interchangeably to identify both persistent OME and

---

AT A GLANCE . . .

Definitions of Otitis Media

Acute Otitis Media: frequently occurs with an upper respiratory infection and is characterized by the symptoms of a middle-ear infection (e.g., fever, otalgia, irritability, and mild hearing loss). There is usually a purulent middle-ear effusion.

Recurrent Otitis Media: three or more discrete episodes of acute otitis media in a 6-month period or four or more episodes in 1 year.

Otitis Media with Effusion: fluid in the middle-ear space without signs or symptoms of acute inflammation.

Chronic Suppurative Otitis Media: persistent purulent drainage in the external auditory canal due to infection within the middle-ear space.

Pediatric Otolaryngology, Edited by R.F. Wetmore, H.R. Muntz, and T.J. McGill. Thieme Medical Publishers, Inc., New York © 2000.

CSOM. These are different disease states, and therefore, the term is confusing and is not used in this chapter.

INCIDENCE, EPIDEMIOLOGY, AND RISK FACTORS OF MIDDLE EAR DISEASE

Very few children will leave their early years without having suffered at least one episode of AOM. A number of longitudinal studies have attempted to determine incidence rates both in the United States and abroad. The Greater Boston Otitis Media Study Group followed more than 2500 children for several years and found that greater than 90% of these patients developed one or more episodes of AOM. By the age of 7 years, approximately 75% suffered three or more episodes.[1] However, the number of children who develop chronic ear disease and, most notably, CSOM is certainly much lower. There is little data available that accurately documents this incidence, but it would seem to be less than 1% of all children.

Certain racial groups are known to suffer significantly higher incidences of ear disease. In particular, Native Americans and both Alaskan and Canadian Eskimos are predisposed to severe attacks of AOM followed by spontaneous rupture of the TM and chronic suppuration. The Arctic Health Research team found that greater than 60% of Alaskan Inuit children suffered at least one episode of TM rupture with otorrhea.[2] Similar pathology is seen in the aboriginal natives of Australia and the Maori tribe in New Zealand. The pathophysiologic process seems related to inheritance of a patulous or semipatulous ET that allows for reflux of colonized nasopharyngeal secretions into the middle-ear space. Although this condition is clearly a defect in the protective function of the ET, the patulous state provides for adequate ventilation of the middle-ear system. This condition, coupled with the high incidence of TM perforation, seems to protect the afflicted individuals from the formation of cholesteatoma.[3]

The manifestations of chronic middle-ear and mastoid disease are myriad and, in general, the risk factors for them parallel the risk factors for AOM and OME. Virtually all children with a cleft palate experience OME because of ET dysfunction. The placement of a PET prior to repair of the cleft and,

sometimes even after, may be complicated by CSOM. Average time to recovery of ET function after cleft repair was found to be 6 years.[4] Many different craniofacial syndromes including Down's, Crouzon's, Apert's, Turner's, and Pierre-Robin are associated with chronic ear disease because of malformation or dysfunction of the ET. Defects within the host's immune system also may predispose to ear disease. These include acquired immune deficiency syndrome (AIDS), severe combined immunodeficiency (SCID), X-linked agammaglobulinemia, common variable immunodeficiency, transient hypogammaglobulinemia of infancy, selective immunoglobulin deficiencies, poor antibody response to antigens, and many others.[5] Deficiencies in immunoglobulin G (IgG) subclasses and, in particular, IgG 2 have been associated with OM, although the relationship is not understood fully.[6] Ciliary dyskinesia may exist in various forms, and in Kartagener's syndrome usually is considered a triad that includes situs inversus, bronchiectasis, and sinusitis. However, any disruption in normal ciliary transport of mucous, microbial organisms, and antigens may secondarily result in OM.[7]

The chronic debilitation that is attendant to craniofacial and immunodeficiency syndromes predisposes the afflicted individual to both acute and chronic ear disease. There are numerous other risk factors for AOM, RAOM, and OME, but the roles of these in the ultimate development of long-term otologic complications are less well known. However, they merit mentioning. These risk factors include attendance in daycare, male gender, siblings with a history of ear disease, absence of breastfeeding, lower socioeconomic status, allergy, and exposure to cigarette smoke.

AT A GLANCE . . .

Risk Factors for Otitis Media

- Attendance in daycare
- Male sex
- Family history of otitis media
- Bottle-fed
- Lower socioeconomic status
- Allergy
- Exposure to cigarette smoke

EUSTACHIAN TUBE DYSFUNCTION

Much of the pathology that constitutes chronic ear disease is an indirect result of underlying *eustachian tube dysfunction* (ETD). The normal functions of the ET are several fold. Primarily it acts to equilibrate pressure within the middle ear and mastoid system with the ambient pressure of the environment. This is an active process that requires opening of the tube by contraction of the tensor veli palatini muscle and it occurs during swallowing, yawning, and sneezing. In addition to pressure equalization, opening of the tube serves to drain the middle ear of secretions and effusions. At rest, the ET remains passively closed, which protects against insufflation, reflux, and aspiration of nasopharyngeal secretions into the middle ear.

The infant ET differs from that of the adult in several ways, all of which increase the likelihood of ear disease. In children, the tube is oriented at 10 degrees from horizontal, whereas in the adult it is oriented at 45 degrees. Subsequently, gravity plays a greater role in adults to prevent entrance of nasopharyngeal contents. The infant tube is shorter than that of the adult, averaging about 18 mm.[8] In addition, the child's ET seems to be more compliant, which makes it less effective in opening.[9]

In the resting state, the volume of air within the middle ear and, to a greater extent, mastoid cells acts as a sort of cushion that prevents the easy entrance of nasopharyngeal secretions. However, the ET usually remains passively closed. There is a gaseous pressure differential between air in the middle-ear system and the mucosal lining such that there is a net absorption of air by the mucosa; this subsequently creates negative pressure within the system. It is only through the intermittent active opening of the tube that pressure equalization occurs and high negative pressures are avoided. Interruption of this normal homeostasis defines ETD and predisposes to chronic ear disease.

ETD may exist either as a tube that is too open or patulous or one that is obstructed. A *patulous ET* allows reflux of nasopharyngeal contents into the middle ear with possible development of infection. A similar scenario may ensue when a TM perforation exists and the air cushion of the middle-ear system is released, allowing entrance of secretions from the nasopharynx. Conversely, ET obstruction can lead to middle-ear disease also. The obstruction may be functional or mechanical. A *functional obstruction* exists when the active opening process of the ET is absent, such as in the cleft palate patient. It also occurs when the tube is too compliant or "floppy." *Mechanical obstruction* may be intrinsic such as when inflammation of tubal mucosa prevents patency or when there is congenital stenosis of the tube. Mechanical obstruction also may be extrinsic such as when a large adenoid pad, nasopharyngeal tumor, or cholesteatoma result in blockage. In cases of ET obstruction, high negative middle-ear pressures may develop and lead to simple aspiration or insufflation of nasopharyngeal contents when a positive pressure is delivered to the nose, such as in sneezing. Thus, a patulous or obstructed ET may cause contamination of the otherwise sterile middle-ear system through the reflux, aspiration, and insufflation of nasopharyngeal secretions.[10]

Evaluation of the Eustachian Tube

There are many different clinical tests to assess the ET. Some are simple to perform, whereas others are more complex. No single test exists that completely and definitively evaluates ET function, and it is beyond the scope of this chapter to provide a comprehensive review. Several tests are, however, worth mentioning. The most elementary tests are those that are useful to document tubal patency but do not evaluate function. *Valsalva's maneuver* simply involves expiring against a closed mouth and nose so that air pressure is directed up the ET. If the ET is patent, the patient notices a "pop" as the TM moves laterally, and otoscopy allows the physician to see this bulging motion. Applying negative pressure through pneumatic otoscopy does not cause any further lateral movement of the drum, whereas positive pressure results in medial displacement. *Toynbee's test* involves swallowing while the nose is closed. This exerts positive pressure within the nasopharynx that is then followed by negative pressure. A patent ET allows the pressure changes to be transmitted into the middle-ear space with subsequent position changes of the TM, which may be detected by pneumootoscopy. *Politzer's test* differs from Valsalva's maneuver only in that the autoinsufflation is not generated from a breath, but from a rubber tube that is attached to a bulb at one end and inserted into one nostril at the other. Positive pressure is then delivered to the nasopharynx by squeezing the bulb. In compliant patients, Politzer's test and Valsalva's maneuver may not serve only as diagnostic tests, but also may be therapeutic in that positive pressure insufflated into the middle ear can relieve TM atelectasis.

The *inflation-deflation* and *forced response* tests are described by Bluestone.[10] Both of these are performed in individuals with nonintact TMs, and respective results may be interpreted to evaluate actual ET function. That is, in addition to verifying tube patency, these tests report opening and closing pressures of the ET and the ability of the ET to equilibrate applied negative and positive pressures. There is no test that can accurately evaluate ET function when the TM is intact.

Tympanometry may be performed with an intact or nonintact TM and is commonly used in the clinical setting. Results can be used only as indirect evaluations of ET function. By determining compliance of the TM and pressure within the middle ear, tympanometry can indicate whether the ET is providing adequate ventilation.

AT A GLANCE . . .

Evaluation of Eustachian Tube Function

- Valsalva's maneuver
- Toynbee's test
- Politzer's test
- Inflation-deflation test
- Forced response test
- Tympanometry

SENSORINEURAL HEARING LOSS

The effect of chronic ear disease upon hearing typically involves pathology of the conductive hearing mechanism. The consequences of prolonged ETD may result in atelectasis or perforation of the TM, cholesteatoma formation, ossicular dysfunction, and tympanosclerosis. These processes are discussed later in the chapter. There is also ample evidence that OM can cause sensorineural hearing loss (SNHL). Paparella et al. found that AOM and CSOM may cause temporary threshold shifts as well as permanent threshold shifts in bone conduction hearing.[11] The temporary shifts were thought to result from serous labyrinthitis and the permanent shifts

resulted from permanent dysfunction of the organ of Corti.[11] The exact pathophysiologic mechanism is not understood well, but probably results from spread of infection, toxins, or mediators of inflammation across the round-window membrane. The round-window membrane may be more vulnerable in the acute infectious stage as it is thinner and more permeable than the membrane encountered in chronic disease. The decay in sensorineural hearing (SNH) in patients with CSOM usually is seen at higher frequencies and may be related to the duration of the disease because older patients are usually more severely affected than children.

TYMPANOSCLEROSIS

Tympanosclerosis is a disease that may affect the TM middle ear, or mastoid. Clinically, it is identified as whitish plaques (Fig. 16–1). When the process is limited to the TM, it may be termed *myringosclerosis* and the plaques are located within the lamina propria or middle layer. Tympanosclerosis may involve the mucosa at any site within the middle-ear cavity, and the plaques are found within the basement membrane. This process also may involve the ossicles. It is estimated that 30% of all individuals with chronic ear disease manifest some degree of

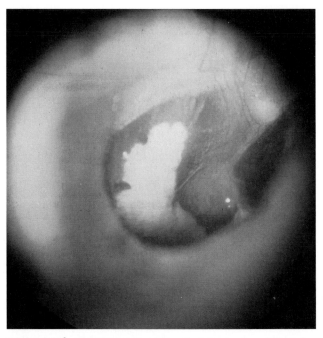

Figure 16–1: Tympanosclerotic plaque involving the posterior tympanic membrane.

tympanosclerosis.[12] The actual incidence in children remains unknown.

Tympanosclerosis is always the result of prior middle-ear inflammation, that is OM. The disease seems to be the end result of an immunologically-mediated process. Inflammation results in edema of the lamina propria with an increase in local complement and immunoglobulin components. This leads to heightened fibroblast activity and subsequent formation of collagen. Normal collagen turnover is interrupted and hyaline degeneration occurs. This is followed by deposition of calcium and phosphate ions. As noted above, any surface within the middle-ear system may ultimately become involved. An animal model using guinea pigs has been developed.[13]

The formation of tympanosclerotic plaques is a chronic process and takes months, if not years, to develop. Often a TM perforation is also present and the ear may be dry. There seems to be no direct correlation between tympanosclerosis and cholesteatoma and the two may or may not coexist. Tympanosclerosis is a separate entity from otosclerosis. When encountered in children, the plaques are usually limited to the TM. A large percentage of the surface area of the TM may be involved with little effect on hearing. However, if the entire drum is involved, giving rise to the so-called "porcelain eardrum," conductive hearing loss (CHL) results due to obvious loss of normal TM compliance. The usual finding of mild to moderate myringosclerosis requires no clinical intervention. PETs should not be placed within the plaques because the loss of local vascularity and the disturbance of the fibrous layer predisposes to the formation of a TM perforation.

SPECIAL CONSIDERATION:

PETs should not be placed within tympanosclerotic plaques because the loss of local vascularity and the disturbance of the fibrous layer predisposes to the formation of a TM perforation.

Treatment of Tympanosclerosis

The success of myringoplasty or tympanoplasty may be hindered by the presence of tympanosclerotic plaques. If the plaques are near the perforation, they

may be gently dissected from the undersurface of the drum prior to elevation of the tympanomeatal flap. This is achieved by using a right-angle hook and working through the perforation itself. Care is taken to preserve the thin outer layer of the TM.

When tympanosclerosis involves the ossicles, significant CHL may occur. The malleus head is most commonly involved and may become fixed to the epitympanum. Simple freeing of the head usually is not sufficient as refixation occurs. Definitive treatment involves removing the malleus head and incus and then using the incus to perform a stapes-to-manubrium or stapes-to-drum ossiculoplasty.

When tympanosclerosis involves the stapes and footplate, management is more complicated. Treatment involves first removing the stapes suprastructure before gently dissecting the plaque off the footplate and then performing ossiculoplasty. Use of a hearing aid, rather than surgery, is a viable option in these difficult patients.

TYMPANIC MEMBRANE PERFORATION

Perforation of the TM is one of the most common otologic pathologies to confront the pediatric otolaryngologist. Perforations are classified by their location. A *central perforation* involves any portion of the pars tensa, but does not extend to the annulus. A *marginal perforation* also involves the pars tensa with extension to or including the annulus. An *attic perforation* is actually a misnomer, and the process described is usually a deep retraction pocket of the pars flaccida, possibly with cholesteatoma present. The cause and chronicity of the perforation play significant roles in management approach. Perforations also can be subdivided into those that are *acute* and those that are *chronic*. The management of these perforations is presented in Practice Pathway 16–1.

Etiology and Treatment of Acute Perforations

The most common cause of acute TM perforation is spontaneous rupture of the drumhead during an episode of AOM. The rupture invariably occurs within the pars tensa and is due to the weakening of the drum secondary to inflammation and the high pressure exerted by the purulent middle-ear effusion. This can be seen at any age, but is most com-

Practice Pathway 16–1   MANAGEMENT OF TYMPANIC MEMBRANE PERFORATION

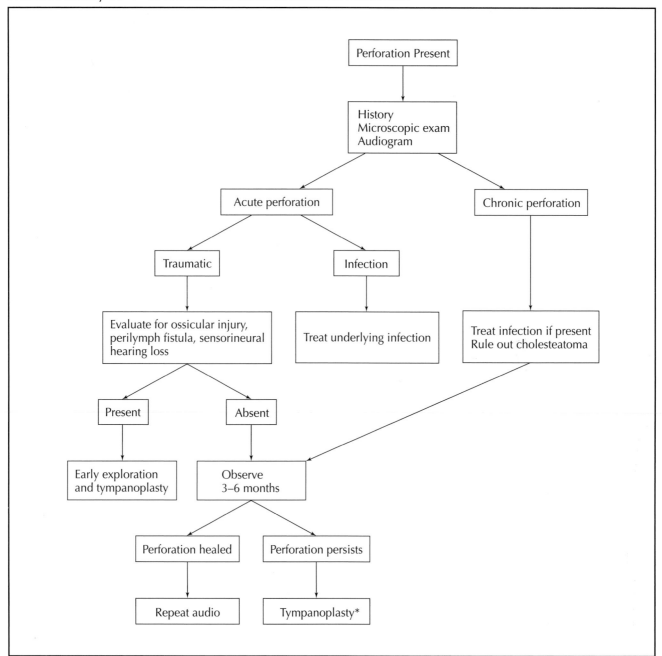

*Considerations for timing of surgery are (1) patient age; (2) bilateral hearing status; (3) eustachian tube function (observe other ear, tympanometry, consider formal eustachian tube testing); (4) past otologic history; (5) time of year.

mon in children under the age of 2 years. The classic history reported by parents is that the child initially demonstrated signs and symptoms of AOM and in particular, severe otalgia. This is followed by a rather sudden, apparent relief of pain and then the observance of otorrhea within the ear canal. Examination by the clinician is aided by the use of the operating microscope and the suctioning of the ear canal. These perforations are usually quite small and

may not be seen even with the microscope. They often are inferred simply by the presence of otorrhea. Because of their small size and the inherent treatability of the underlying etiology most of these perforations heal of their own accord within several days. Treatment involves the use of an oral antibiotic directed against the most common pathogens of AOM, *Streptococcus pneumoniae, Haemophilus influenzae,* and *Moraxella catarrhalis.* In addition, the presence of the perforation, though short-lived, allows the use of topical antibiotic drops to be instilled into the ear canal for several days.

The second most common cause of acute TM perforation is trauma. This frequently occurs after a blow to the head, such as a slap, that rapidly delivers high air pressure to the lateral surface of the drum causing implosion toward the middle-ear space. Again, the pars tensa usually is affected. Another common mechanism of injury is the presence of foreign objects in the ear canal such as sticks, bobby pins, and cotton-tipped applicators (Fig. 16–2). Because of the anatomy of the ear canal, the perforation usually is found in the posterior aspect of the TM. Other frequent causes of traumatic perforations include diving, water-skiing accidents, and temporal bone fractures. It is important for the otolaryngologist to examine these patients as soon as possible so that the extent of damage can be determined. Inner ear damage and, in particular, perilymphatic fistula should be ruled out. Ossicular disruption may be visualized or can be inferred by the degree of hearing loss. It is ideal for all of these patients to obtain an audiogram soon after the injury to determine the new hearing baseline and for medical-legal reasons. Isolated TM perforations usually result in surprisingly small deficits in conductive hearing. Within the speech frequencies (500 Hz–2000 Hz), it is estimated that a 15% perforation of the TM results in a 10 dB hearing loss, a 40% perforation causes a 20 to 25 dB loss, and a 75% perforation causes a 30 to 35 dB loss.[14] CHL > 35 dB are suspicious for ossicular injury.

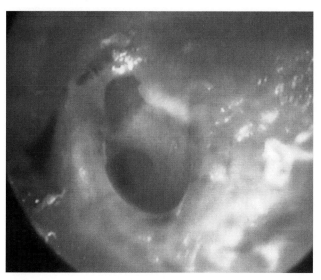

Figure 16–2: Large perforation of the tympanic membrane that was the result of injury by a foreign body.

SPECIAL CONSIDERATION:

In a child with a traumatic perforation, the presence of CHL > 35 dB should make the clinician suspicious of an ossicular injury.

Immediate management of traumatic perforations includes manual eversion of the in-folded flaps of the TM at the perforation margins. This increases the likelihood of spontaneous healing of the drum and can prevent squamous epithelial growth into the middle ear with possible cholesteatoma formation. An option is to place a small piece of micropore tape over the perforation if the child is old enough to tolerate the procedure. This helps to evert the perforation margins and acts as a scaffold for new epithelial growth.[15] If the perforation is dry, no antibiotics are necessary. If it wet, such as after a diving accident, topical antibiotic drops should be used for 3 days. At this point, watchful waiting is then the best course. Many traumatic perforations, even surprisingly large ones, close without surgical management. The patient should avoid further water contamination of the injured ear; infection of the ear decreases the likelihood of spontaneous healing and may even enlarge the perforation. The timing of surgical repair of persistent traumatic perforations is debatable, but a minimum wait of 3 months after the injury is appropriate. Longer waits are reasonable, particularly if the hole seems to be decreasing in size gradually. As we discuss below, if the patient suffers from coexistent ETD or other evidence of chronic ear disease the repair should be postponed.

Etiology and Treatment of Chronic Perforations

The most common cause of chronically-acquired TM perforations is the prior placement of PETs. This procedure is performed more than 1,000,000 times per year in the United States and published rates of permanent perforation vary widely. Certainly there are multiple factors that influence the potential for development of perforation including patient age, underlying ET function, and susceptibility to continued chronic ear disease. Regarding the PETs themselves, there seems to be a consensus that the longer a tube remains present within the drum, the higher the occurrence of permanent perforation. *Short-acting PET* are roughly defined as those that extrude within 18 months of placement. Perforation rates with these tubes range from 1 to 5%. Long-term ventilation of the middle ear is achieved with the so-called *T-tubes,* which usually remain in place 2 to 3 years or even longer. A review of several studies involving T-tubes reports a mean perforation rate of 9%.[16] Significantly higher rates can be seen if these tubes are left in place for more than 2 years. In some patients, however, use of a long-acting PET may be warranted, such as in a child with a craniofacial deformity. The higher risk of causing a perforation must be weighed against the concerns of perhaps having to place several sets of short-acting tubes. Similar questions surround the decision as to when a physician should remove a long-acting tube. If there is clinical indication of continued middle-ear disease, the tube should be left in place despite the increased risk of possibly developing a permanent perforation. This is preferable to an intact TM that subsequently may suffer persistent OME, atelectasis, retraction pocket, or cholesteatoma formation.

Patients with CSOM by definition suffer with a nonintact TM. These perforations may have originated from an initial episode of AOM and then failed to heal because the infected status of the ear was never reversed. In addition, chronic ETD and middle-ear disease can lead to the breakdown of the fibrous layer of the drum so that it becomes atrophic and prone to perforation. Also, the presence of cholesteatoma is not only a result of chronic ear disease but it also perpetuates the process, including formation and maintenance of a chronic TM perforation.

The timing of repair for a chronic perforation in a pediatric patient is still a matter of considerable controversy. All agree that the procedure should not be performed in an ear with continued purulent drainage or in one with a coexistent cholesteatoma that has not been addressed. However, even in dry ears without cholesteatoma, the presence of persistent ETD (the process most likely related to the formation of the perforation in the first place) is difficult to assess adequately.

If ET dysfunction is still present as manifested by recurrent infections and high-negative middle-ear pressure in the contralateral ear, not only is the potential for surgical repair of a perforation compromised, but it may be desirable to leave the perforation to provide ventilation. The ET matures in function around the age of 7 years,[17] and therefore

many clinicians recommend not attempting repair prior to this time. Others report high success rates in considerably younger children. It is difficult to compare success rates between authors because the respective definitions of "success" vary. The early success in closing of the perforation may later be followed by reperforation, recurrence of OME or RAOM, atelectasis of the TM, or the need for replacement of a pressure-equalization test (PET). Using stringent criteria for success, Bluestone et al. reported an overall success rate of 35% for tympanoplasty in children. They felt that preoperative measures of ET function, including pressure-equalization tests (PET) and tympanometry, were not predictive of tympanoplasty success.[18] Manning et al. found that 78% of their tympanoplasties in children resulted in an intact TM, but that only 52% ultimately obtained a healed graft *and* good middle-ear function.[19] There was a significant association between outcome and preoperative tubal function, but the prognostic value of this testing was low. They found no correlation between ultimate outcome and patient age, status of the contralateral ear, or tympanoplasty technique. Koch et al. reported a 73% success rate for tympanoplasty in children. Among several variables postulated to affect the outcome of surgery, only patient age was found to have statistical significance, and they recommended the procedure for children 8 years of age and older.[20] Shih et al. also found age to be a significant factor and that children 10 years and older had higher success rates than younger patients.[21]

SPECIAL CONSIDERATION:

There are no rigid rules defining the proper time to perform a tympanoplasty in children, primarily because a reliable and consistent method of evaluating ET function does not exist.

It is apparent that there are no rigid rules to indicate the proper time to perform a tympanoplasty in children. This is primarily because there is not a reliable and consistent method to preoperatively evaluate ET function yet. Ultimate success is based on a number of factors. However, general recommendations would be first to rule out coexisting cholesteatoma and to clear up infection of the involved ear. Continued disease in the contralateral ear and poor results on ET testing may be enough reason to delay surgery. Consideration also should be given to factors such as the duration of the perforation, whether there are bilateral perforations, and the season of the year. The older the child, the greater the likelihood of success.

When the decision has been made to perform the repair, there are numerous surgical techniques from which to choose. The terms myringoplasty and tympanoplasty are often used interchangeably. *Myringoplasty* is used to define techniques that are designed strictly to repair isolated perforations and that do not involve entering the middle-ear space. The term *tympanoplasty* actually incorporates a number of different procedures involving the TM, middle ear, and ossicles. Using the classification system designed by Wüllstein, a *Type I tympanoplasty* is similar to a myringoplasty in that the goal of the procedure is to address only a TM perforation, although the middle ear is entered by the lifting of a tympanomeatal flap.[22]

Smaller perforations including 20% or less of the cross-sectional area of the TM can be addressed with relatively simple myringoplasty techniques. First, the perforation margins are freshened by using a straight pick or applying an irritant such as trichloroacetic acid. The perforations can then be covered with a small piece of paper or filled with a wad of fat harvested from the earlobe.[23] For larger perforations, a variety of grafting materials and techniques can be used. Temporalis fascia is usually the tissue of choice because of its conducive grafting properties and the ease of harvest; tragal perichondrium, connective tissue, periosteum, and vein are also viable alternatives. Many children require a postauricular or endaural incisional approach because of narrow ear canals. Older children may allow a transcanal approach.

The two most common tympanoplasty techniques are the *underlay* and the *onlay* grafts. The first involves raising a tympanomeatal flap and then sliding the graft material beneath the TM remnant. The graft is then held in place by packing the middle ear with Gelfoam™. The underlay technique works well with moderate-sized perforations and is reasonably easy to perform. Its success rate is lower in perforations of the anterosuperior quadrant and is also compromised if continued ETD results in negative middle-ear pressure. The onlay technique involves first removing the squamous layer of the TM remnant and then applying the graft material to its lateral surface. This procedure is somewhat more difficult to perform than the underlay technique, yet it has a high rate of success in experienced hands. It works well for large perforations and anterior perforations. It also is less affected by ETD because the negative middle-ear pressure tends to "pull" the graft into proper position. Drawbacks of the onlay technique include common formation of keratin pearls in the neotympanic membrane and blunting of the anterior sulcus angle. A technique that is effective for total TM perforations is the *fasciaform myringoplasty*.[24] This surgery involves forming a new TM from a formaldehyde-fixed piece of autogenous temporalis fascia.

CHRONIC SUPPURATIVE OTITIS MEDIA

Persistent inflammation of the mucosa in the middle ear and mastoid with purulent discharge through a TM perforation or tympanoplasty tube represents CSOM. As discussed earlier, certain populations such as Native Americans, Eskimos, Maoris, and Australian aborigines are predisposed to this condition, presumably because of a patulous ET. Doyle found that Native Americans and Eskimos had anatomic differences in the bony portion of the ET as compared to caucasians.[25] A patulous ET allows reflux of nasopharyngeal bacteria into the middle ear, increasing the likelihood of AOM and possible perforation of the TM. Once a perforation is present, the protective function of the air cushion in the middle ear and mastoid is lost. This simply compounds the problem and can serve to create a cycle of continued middle-ear contamination, inflammation, and discharge. The perforation also allows bacteria within the ear canal access to the middle ear, particularly during periods of possible water contamination such as bathing or swimming. Individuals with cleft palate, other craniofacial deformities, and immune deficiencies are predisposed to this process also.

PETs are designed to treat patients with RAOM and OME (Fig. 16–3). They provide temporary ventilation for the middle ear in the hope that the ET will mature and ultimately function adequately; however, they can sometimes act to initiate or perpetuate infection. Like a TM perforation, a PET re-

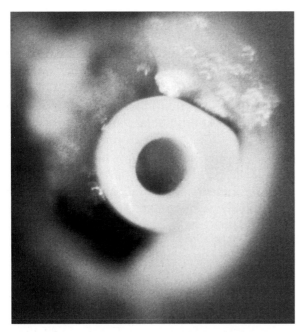

Figure 16–3: Tympanostomy tube located in the anterior-inferior portion of the tympanic membrane.

leases the air cushion of the middle-ear system and can predispose to reflux or insufflation of nasopharyngeal contents. They also pose a risk for water contamination through the ear canal. Finally, as a foreign body, a PET also may serve as a potential nidus for bacterial colonization and subsequent infection. Consequently, it is common for individuals with tubes to suffer episodes of otorrhea. Usually these are isolated occurrences and are self-limited. Mandel et al. observed acute otorrhea in 50% of children with PET.[26] Fortunately, the development of CSOM through tubes is much less frequent. McLelland reported an incidence rate of 3.6%.[27]

Etiology

The microbiology of acute suppurative OM (ASOM) differs from that of CSOM. Acute otorrhea usually is caused by the same organisms responsible for AOM, including *S. pneumoniae, H. influenzae,* and *M. catarrhalis.* These organisms are more common in children under the age of 6 years and are more frequently a problem in the winter months. *Pseudomonas aeruginosa* is an uncommon cause of acute otorrhea.[26] However, it is the most common pathogen encountered in cases of chronic suppuration. Kenna et al. found *P. aeruginosa* present in 67% of the children with CSOM[28] and Fliss et al. reported an incidence of 84%.[29] Other common agents re-

sponsible for CSOM include *Staphylococcus aureus,* diptheroids, anaerobes, and enteric gram-negative bacilli. When discussing CSOM, a distinction is often made between CSOM with cholesteatoma and CSOM without cholesteatoma. *P. aeruginosa* is often found in both disease states, but mixed infections seem to be much more prevalent in the former.[30]

History and Examination of the Patient with CSOM

Patients with CSOM often present with an extensive history of RAOM and/or OME. Frequently, they have undergone the placement of one or more sets of PETs and may have been treated with multiple courses of oral and topical antibiotics. Their primary complaints are of persistent and often malodorous discharge from the ear and hearing loss. Severe otalgia is rare and should raise suspicion for possible cholesteatoma or intratemporal complications of OM.

On examination, the clinician finds the ear canal filled with clear, purulent or perhaps bloody otorrhea and squamous debris. When suctioned away under the operating microscope, a perforation or PET is revealed. The TM remnant is thickened and may be associated with friable granulation tissue. Careful inspection should be made for possible retraction pockets, particularly in the posterosuperior quadrant and in the attic or pars flaccida region. If a retraction pocket or erosion of the scutum is noted, every effort should be made to rule out the presence of a cholesteatoma. The middle-ear mucosa is usually edematous and granular, and a polyp may extrude through the perforation. After microscopic examination, if there is still question as to the extent of disease, computed tomography (CT) scanning is warranted. This has been found to be highly sensitive to the presence of soft-tissue disease and bone erosion, and may reveal fistulae of the lateral semicircular and facial canals or exposure of the dura.[31]

Management of CSOM

Most children will present for medical care of a draining ear before the situation has become chronic. This should be approached as a complication of AOM. After the ear has been cleaned, the patient should be started on an oral antimicrobial, such as amoxicillin, which is effective against the most likely pathogens. It is also common practice to use topical antibiotic preparations such as Cortisporin®, which contains neomycin, polymyxin, and hydrocortisone. Because these drops have been associated with SNHL in animals, they should be used with caution in children.[32] The toxicity is thought to be due to permeation through the round-window membrane. There is probably little significant risk to hearing when using topical antibiotic drops in an infected ear because the generalized inflammation of the middle-ear mucosa acts to limit access to the inner ear.

If routine management of acute otorrhea is unsuccessful, the discharge should be cultured. As noted earlier, the most likely pathogen is *P. aeruginosa.* There are no currently available oral antibiotics that are active against this organism and that can be used in children. Oral ciprofloxacin has been found to be effective in adults,[33] but can disrupt bone growth in children. Ciprofloxacin also is available as a topical preparation, and it has been used successfully to treat CSOM.[34,35] There is no known contraindication to the use of topical ciprofloxacin in children. Gentamicin and tobramycin drops can also be used against *P. aeruginosa,* but potential ototoxicity should be considered.

Effective management of CSOM also entails a search for risk factors and coexisting morbidities that may complicate the clinical situation. Exposure of the ear to water contamination should be avoided. Likewise, cigarette smoke should be eliminated from the child's environment. Evaluation and treatment for possible environmental allergies and immunodeficiency are warranted. Severe gastroesophageal reflux (GER) can reach the nasopharynx and the caustic irritation may result in inflammation of the ET causing dysfunction. Affected individuals usually are managed successfully with H_2-receptor blockers and/or prokinetic agents such as cisapride. Coexisting infections, such as chronic sinusitis or adenoiditis, may perpetuate chronic ear disease and should be treated with antibiotics initially. Adenoid tissue can act as a chronic reservoir for bacteria, and adenoidectomy has been recommended as a treatment option for some patients with RAOM and OME.[36,37] The role of adenoidectomy in the treatment of CSOM has not been studied specifically, but it is reasonable to consider it as an adjuvant. The presence of a middle-ear or nasopharyngeal tumor as a cause of chronic suppuration should be ruled out. Finally, the possibility that the PET itself is acting as a foreign body and perpetuating infection

should be considered, an alternative in the treatment of CSOM is to remove the tube.

> ## SPECIAL CONSIDERATION:
> The role of adenoidectomy in the treatment of CSOM has not been studied specifically, but it remains a reasonable adjuvant.

If a patient with CSOM does not respond to oral and topical antibiotics along with management of associated risk factors, then the next recommended step is treatment with an appropriate intravenous antibiotic. The choice of antibiotic is directed by culture results and usually involves an antipseudomonas penicillin and/or an aminoglycoside. This is coupled with daily aural toilet, including debridement of granulation tissue from the TM and middle ear. Using this strategy, Kenna et al. reported that 89% of their patients initially responded with cessation of discharge within a mean duration of 10 days.[38] In a long-term follow-up of these patients, 22% of them either failed to improve or suffered recurrence of suppuration and subsequently underwent tympanomastoidectomy.[39] Leiberman et al. performed a prospective long-term study using intravenous antibiotics and aural toilet to treat CSOM.[40] All patients initially were cured with this regimen, but by 2 years post-treatment, 50% had recurrence of disease. Of those that did redevelop drainage, 80% had done so by 6 months after the initial treatment. Recurrence rate was not affected by antibiotic regimen, age of patient, duration of drainage prior to treatment, or presence of granulation tissue.

Failure of maximal medical treatment to correct CSOM mandates the use of surgery to eradicate chronic disease. The standard treatment is tympano-mastoidectomy or staged procedures with a cortical mastoidectomy followed by a tympanoplasty. The goal of the surgery is to remove granulation tissue, diseased mucosa, and chronically-infected mastoid air cells. Any patient with CSOM will also suffer chronic mastoiditis. Often the mastoid is poorly pneumatized or becomes sclerotic after prolonged osteitis. Not infrequently, a previously undiagnosed cholesteatoma will be found as the culprit of persistent discharge. In the absence of cholesteatoma, the

Practice Pathway 16–2   MANAGEMENT OF CHRONIC SUPPURATIVE OTITIS MEDIA

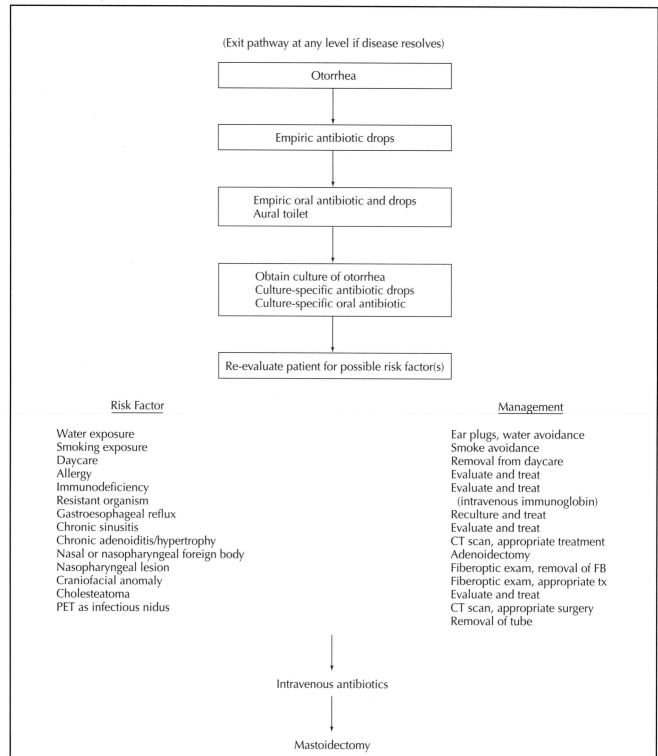

(Exit pathway at any level if disease resolves)

Otorrhea

Empiric antibiotic drops

Empiric oral antibiotic and drops
Aural toilet

Obtain culture of otorrhea
Culture-specific antibiotic drops
Culture-specific oral antibiotic

Re-evaluate patient for possible risk factor(s)

Risk Factor	Management
Water exposure	Ear plugs, water avoidance
Smoking exposure	Smoke avoidance
Daycare	Removal from daycare
Allergy	Evaluate and treat
Immunodeficiency	Evaluate and treat (intravenous immunoglobin)
Resistant organism	Reculture and treat
Gastroesophageal reflux	Evaluate and treat
Chronic sinusitis	CT scan, appropriate treatment
Chronic adenoiditis/hypertrophy	Adenoidectomy
Nasal or nasopharyngeal foreign body	Fiberoptic exam, removal of FB
Nasopharyngeal lesion	Fiberoptic exam, appropriate tx
Craniofacial anomaly	Evaluate and treat
Cholesteatoma	CT scan, appropriate surgery
PET as infectious nidus	Removal of tube

Intravenous antibiotics

Mastoidectomy

canal wall is left intact. In a large study involving adults and children with CSOM, Vartiainen achieved a 92% control rate of infection after tympanomastoidectomy.[41] Failures were most common in ears infected with *P. aeruginosa*. Persistence of disease after tympanomastoidectomy usually is due to failure to eradicate diseased air cells in the mastoid or hypotympanum.[42,43]

Other management of CSOM including lasers[44] and vaccination against *P. aeruginosa*[45] is considered experimental at this time. Practice Pathway 16-2 outlines all of the management procedures for CSOM.

CHOLESTEATOMA

The term *cholesteatoma* was coined by Müller in 1838 to describe a skin-lined cavity filled with keratinous debris.[46] This name, though the most commonly used today, is a misnomer and the lesion may also be called a *keratoma*. Cholesteatomas may be divided into two groups, those that are *congenital* and those that are *acquired*. This latter group may be further divided into *primary acquired*, which are those cholesteatomas arising from the attic or pars flaccida region of the TM without evidence of prior infection, and *secondary acquired*, which are those arising in the pars tensa region due to infection or perforation.

AT A GLANCE . . .

Classification of Cholesteatoma

- Congenital
- Acquired
  - Primary acquired
  - Secondary acquired

It is estimated that at least 5 million people in the world are affected by cholesteatoma.[47] In a metropolitan region of 300,000 in Denmark, Tos determined an annual incidence rate for cholesteatoma of 3/100,000 in children and 12.6/100,000 in adults.[48] In Iowa, Harker found an annual incidence of 6/100,000.[49] It is well known that people with cleft palates are at significant risk for cholesteatoma formation because of functional ETD; the estimated incidence is 9.2%.[50] As discussed earlier, certain groups such as Native Americans and Eskimos are unlikely to develop cholesteatoma despite chronic ear disease. Presumably this is due to the high incidence rate of TM perforations, which protect against atelectasis, retraction pockets, and subsequent cholesteatoma.

Congenital cholesteatomas are thought to originate as ectopic rests of keratinizing squamous epithelium and are located within the middle ear behind an intact TM (Fig. 16-4 and 16-5). There is no prior history of OM or TM perforation.[51] The actual incidence of congenital cholesteatoma is difficult to estimate because at the time of presentation many cholesteatomas are advanced and the site of origin is impossible to determine. In a series of 387 patients with cholesteatomas, Levenson et al. reported that 5% of the entire group and 14% of the children had lesions that fit the definition of congenital cholesteatoma.[52]

There are four proposed mechanisms for the pathogenesis of acquired cholesteatoma.[53] One suggestion is that chronic inflammation of the middle ear mucosa results in *metaplasia* of keratinizing epithelium and subsequent cholesteatoma formation. The *immigration theory* holds that squamous epithelium migrates through a defect in the TM and into the middle ear. The *basal cell hyperplasia theory* suggests that cholesteatoma forms from stimulated basal cells in the TM secondary to chronic in-

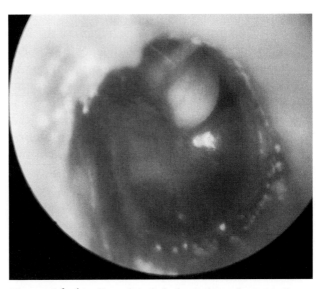

Figure 16–4: Congenital cholesteatoma just anterior to the malleus behind an intact tympanic membrane.

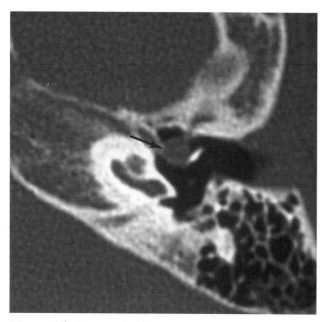

Figure 16–5: Axial CT section illustrating a congenital cholesteatoma (arrow) anterior and medial to the malleus.

flammation. Currently, the most popular theory is that ETD leads to negative pressure within the middle-ear space and that a *retraction pocket* of the TM forms. This usually occurs either within the pars flaccida or the posterosuperior quadrant of the pars tensa, as these are the most flaccid regions of the TM (Fig. 16–6).[54] As the retraction pocket deepens, the self-cleaning mechanism of the squamous epithelium is disrupted and keratin debris accumulates. The debris often becomes a nidus for bacterial infection. The TM becomes atrophic and may adhere to the ossicles or other middle-ear structures. Inflammation within the retraction pocket and of the mucosa of the middle ear ultimately leads to the entrance of the developing cholesteatoma sac into the middle ear proper. At this point, the protective integrity of the TM has been breached and a perforation may ensue. Prior to the true perforation of the TM, a retraction pocket filled with keratin debris exists as a potential cholesteatoma.[55] Wolfman and Chole demonstrated the retraction pocket theory of cholesteatoma formation in a gerbil model by cauterization of the ET.[53] These animals sequentially developed OME, TM retraction pockets, and ultimately cholesteatomas. Acquired cholesteatomas also can occur after traumatic perforation of the TM either through direct implantation of keratinizing cells into the middle ear or by allowing inward squamous migration from the margins of the perforation.

AT A GLANCE . . .

Proposed Mechanisms of Acquired Cholesteatoma

- Squamous metaplasia
- Immigration
- Basal cell hyperplasia
- Retraction pocket

A mature cholesteatoma usually exists as a sac-like structure with three components. The sac or *matrix* is formed by keratinizing squamous epithelium with an exterior fibrous stromal subepithelium. The interior of the matrix is filled with keratin debris. Cholesteatoma is often the indirect result of infection and it has the ability to perpetuate infection because of bacterial colonization within the keratin debris. Due to the chronicity of the underlying process, the most commonly cultured organism is *P. aeruginosa,* as would be expected. However, cholesteatoma also often harbors anaerobes as well as mixed infections. The greatest danger of cholesteatoma exists in its ability to destroy bone. This can occur by way of two mechanisms. The first is

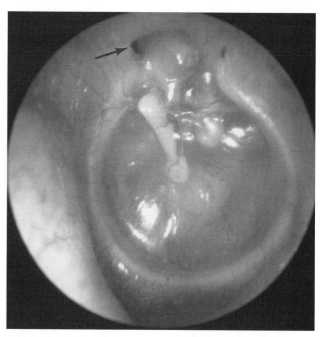

Figure 16–6: Deep attic retraction pocket (arrow) of the pars flaccida region of the tympanic membrane may develop into an attic cholesteatoma.

through infection of cortical bone known as pyogenic osteitis. The second involves production of the bone resorptive enzymes, leucine aminopeptidase and nonspecific esterase, by the subepithelial layer of the sac.[56] It is the subepithelial layer that usually is found in direct contact with either cortical or ossicular bone. The pressure exerted by the expanding cholesteatoma cyst as it fills with laminated keratin also serves to destroy bone. Keratomas can spread within the middle ear and mastoid either by gradual enlargement of the sac itself or by migrating as a sheet of epithelium. It is generally thought that cholesteatomas grow more aggressively in children than in adults. This may be related to the fact that the pediatric temporal bone is more pneumatized than the thickened, more sclerotic bone found in adults who may have experienced years of chronic ear disease. It has not been shown that the biologic activity of the cholesteatoma itself differs between children and adults. Work by Bruce Proctor detailed the development of the middle-ear spaces and helped elucidate the anatomic routes that are followed by expanding cholesteatomas as related to their respective sites of origin.[57]

SPECIAL CONSIDERATION:

It is generally thought that cholesteatomas grow more aggressively in children than in adults.

History and Examination of the Patient with Cholesteatoma

Most patients with cholesteatoma will present with a history of chronic ear disease that is manifested primarily as aural discharge. Conversely, some individuals will have a dry ear. Otalgia may or may not be a complaint, but its presence should raise the clinician's suspicion for cholesteatoma or other intratemporal or intracranial complications of OM. Hearing loss is common and may be multifactorial in origin. There is often a TM perforation or at least loss of normal compliance of the drum. Inflammation and granulation tissue within the middle ear adversely affects the sound transmission system. Ossicular erosion occurs frequently, with the long process of the incus at the greatest risk because of its

limited vascular supply. Early erosion of the incus may be masked audiologically by the cholesteatoma actually serving as a bridge between the incus and stapes, giving rise to the so-called "silent cholesteatoma" or "conductive cholesteatoma." SNHL may result from erosion into the round window or lateral semicircular canal. The latter situation may cause vertigo, particularly in the setting of labyrinthitis, or may result in unnoticed loss of vestibular function on the affected side. Facial nerve paralysis may result due to bone erosion of the fallopian canal in the middle ear or mastoid and secondary pressure effect or inflammation of the nerve sheath. Fever, headache, and vomiting may herald suppurative complications such as lateral sinus thrombosis, meningitis, otitic hydrocephalus, and brain abscess.

SPECIAL CONSIDERATION:

The long process of the incus is at greatest risk for erosion because of its limited vascular supply.

Examination under the otomicroscope allows the otolaryngologist first to culture any suppuration present and then to suction the canal clear. Squamous debris, granulation tissue, and aural polyposis are often present and usually can be cleaned to some degree. However, it should be remembered that some ears with cholesteatoma are dry and that only the presence of a retraction pocket may suggest the lesion. A pocket in the attic may be deceptively small, but it may extend deeply into the epitympanum. Crusts and debris must be cleaned diligently to determine whether the base of the pocket is visible or if there is extension into the epitympanum. A retraction pocket in the posterosuperior quadrant, if severe, will display myringoincudostapediopexy and ossicular erosion may be visible (Fig. 16-7). These retraction pockets have a tendency to be drawn into the facial recess and sinus tympani. If the intact base of the pocket cannot be visualized, then the presence of a cholesteatoma must be considered. A new development in the management of chronic ear disease is the use of angled telescopes, which can be used to evaluate retractions out of the normal field of view. They also may be passed through a TM perforation to evaluate the middle ear.

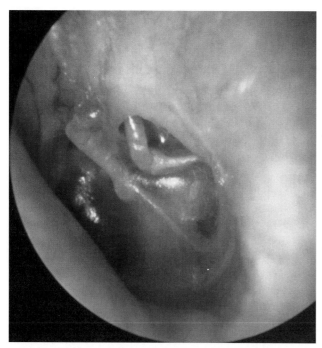

Figure 16–7: Deep retraction pocket of the posteriorsuperior quadrant of the tympanic membrane outlines the incudostapedial joint.

When present, a cholesteatoma has a characteristic pearly-white appearance; if the sac is open, the keratin debris is bright white and flaky. Small congenital cholesteatomas are diagnosed by the presence of a whitish mass behind an intact TM. Many of these originate behind the anterosuperior quadrant of the TM, just anterior to the manubrium.[58]

As with all patients suffering chronic ear disease, an audiogram with tympanogram should be obtained. CT may help in the diagnosis of cholesteatoma, although this soft-tissue mass is difficult to differentiate from granulation tissue or inspissated secretions (Fig. 16–8). The real advantage of CT is in identifying bony erosion, particularly of the scutum and ossicles. As noted earlier, the presence of labyrinthine and facial canal fistulae or dural dehiscence may be detected, which is quite helpful to know preoperatively. CT is preferable to magnetic resonance imaging (MRI) in the evaluation of chronic ear disease.[59]

Treatment of Cholesteatoma

The best treatment for cholesteatoma is prevention. When retraction of the TM is observed in a patient, ETD is clearly present and placement of a PET is

warranted. Even moderately-severe retraction pockets can sometimes be reversed by a tube, if adhesion of the drum has not occurred. Injecting sterile saline into the middle-ear space by passing a fine-gauge needle just lateral to the fibrous annulus is a technique that also will inflate and reverse a retraction pocket sometimes. When a retraction pocket will not respond to these conservative measures, more aggressive treatment is pursued usually. There is a minority school of thought that feels that if a retraction is stable, the base is clearly visible, the patient's hearing is good, and no infection is present then the situation may be followed expectantly. However, most clinicians feel that such an approach leaves too great a risk for possible ossicular erosion and/or cholesteatoma formation.

There are several surgical approaches to recalcitrant retractions that are not responding to a tube. One is an adenoidectomy in an effort to improve ET function. As an isolated procedure, this is often inadequate, although it should be considered as an adjunct. Sharp and Robinson have reported treating retraction pockets by resecting them completely and simultaneously placing a PET in the TM remnant.[60] In most cases, the TM regenerated and recurrence of atelectasis was avoided. Standard treatment of a deep retraction pocket involves a tympanoplasty procedure with either elevation or resection of the pocket. If continued ETD is anticipated, a PET may be placed or the reconstructed portion of the TM may be strengthened using tragal cartilage. This cartilage tympanoplasty technique is often successful in treating the retraction pocket, but the cartilage graft itself can mask the formation of cholesteatoma.

When the TM becomes retracted and adherent onto the ossicles and other structures of the medial wall of the middle-ear space, this is termed *adhesive otitis media*. The pathophysiologic process includes chronic negative middle-ear pressure and inflammation that results in fusion of the TM mucosa with the middle-ear mucosa. In advanced cases, there may be complete loss of the tympanic air space as the drum becomes atrophic, redundant, and retracted into the mesotympanum, hypotympanum, ET, facial recess, sinus tympani, and epitympanum. Ossicular immobility and erosion can occur with secondary hearing loss. Tympanic membrane perforation and cholesteatoma formation are possible. True adhesive OM will not respond to simple placement of a ventilation tube. This otologic com-

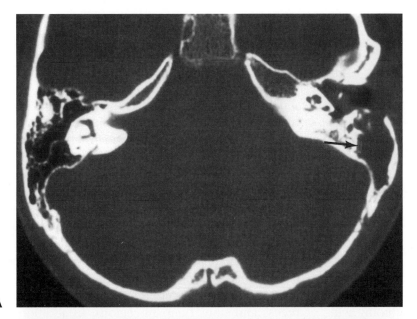

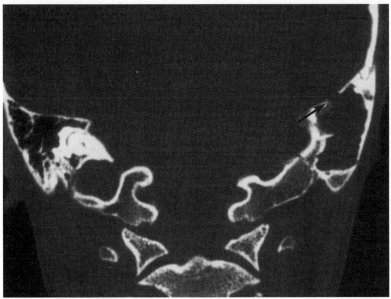

Figure 16–8: (A) CT (axial view) demonstrates a large cholesteatoma of the mastoid with bone erosion (arrow). (B) CT (coronal view) of the same patient demonstrates bone erosion of the tegmen in the region of the middle cranial fossa (arrow).

plication can be very difficult to manage surgically. The goal is to elevate all keratinizing epithelium through a tympanoplastic procedure, taking care to not create an iatrogenic cholesteatoma. The middle-ear space should be recreated and ossiculoplasty is performed if necessary. Again, cartilage support of the neotympanic membrane, along with a ventilation tube, may help prevent recurrence. Placing a small sheet of either Silastic™ or Gelfilm™ in the middle ear can also help prevent retraction of the drum onto the promontory, but the Silastic™ may extrude and will need to be removed.

When a cholesteatoma is present, the treatment is almost always surgical. Rarely, a deep retraction filled with keratin debris can be cleaned repeatedly in the office with the hope that the underlying process will reverse itself ultimately. If the retraction is adherent to bone, erosion can occur even in the absence of infection and even if the retraction is well marsupialized. Therefore, in children it is best to remove the cholesteatoma entirely. The particular surgical procedure chosen to treat a cholesteatoma is dependent on many factors including the size of the lesion, its location, the extent of damage already incurred, and the experience of the surgeon as well as his/her own biases. A complete discussion of all the various surgical techniques available is beyond the scope of this chapter, and the reader is encouraged to consult the extensive literature that exists regarding the topic. Rather, a brief overview is presented here.

SPECIAL CONSIDERATION:

True adhesive OM will not respond to simple placement of a ventilation tube.

Surgical procedures for cholesteatoma

Small congenital cholesteatomas, particularly those in the anterosuperior quadrant, are relatively easy to remove. Sometimes, a simple myringotomy will allow removal of a well-encapsulated keratin pearl. Slightly larger lesions can be excised by raising a tympanomeatal flap to gain access to the middle ear. Sometimes, it is necessary to take the TM off of the manubrium to achieve good exposure and ensure complete removal.

When the cholesteatoma is large and invades the middle ear and/or mastoid, a bigger procedure is necessary. There is great controversy regarding the appropriate approach to these lesions. On the other hand, there is consensus that pediatric cholesteatoma is aggressive and has high residual and recurrence rates. One school of thought says that the diseased ear should be exteriorized or "opened," whereas the other believes that the cholesteatoma can be removed while preserving the normal anatomy and function of the middle ear. The "open" school supports the *canal-wall-down mastoidectomy* procedure, which converts the mastoid and middle ear to a common cavity that exists as a "bowl" after the procedure is completed. This aggressive approach is thought to result in more frequent eradication of the disease because of better intraoperative exposure and because of improved postoperative surveillance with the exteriorized cavity. A single surgery is often all that is necessary. Disadvantages to this approach include poor hearing results, the need to clean debris from the mastoid bowl periodically, and a high incidence of infection with discharge. Both the *radical mastoidectomy* and the *modified radical mastoidectomy* are canal-wall-down procedures. The first involves removal of the ossicles with complete exteriorization of the middle-ear space and plugging of

the ET. The second procedure makes an attempt to preserve the transformer system by leaving the TM and ossicles intact. If it is necessary to perform TM grafting and/or ossiculoplasty, then the procedure is termed *tympanomastoidectomy*.

The "closed" school of thought supports *canal-wall-up* surgical techniques to eradicate cholesteatoma, which involves a *simple cortical mastoidectomy* to exenterate diseased mastoid air cells and allow access to the epitympanum. This procedure can be combined with a tympanoplasty if necessary. The normal anatomy of the middle ear and posterior bony ear canal is preserved, hearing results are generally better, and there is no bowl created that will require a lifetime of cleaning. However, intraoperative exposure is not quite as good as that of the canal-wall-down procedure, particularly in the facial recess and sinus tympani regions. In addition, because of the propensity for cholesteatoma to relapse or recur and because postoperative surveillance is worse it is often necessary to perform a "second-look" procedure. This second procedure involves, at the least, an exploratory tympanotomy 6 to 9 months after the initial procedure to search for the presence of recurrent or residual cholesteatoma. If discovered, necessary surgical steps are undertaken to eradicate the lesion again. This second procedure also provides the opportunity to reconstruct the ossicular system, if any ossicles were removed at the time of the first surgery.

Sheehy recommends the canal-wall-up, two-staged approach to cholesteatoma in children and reports a 36% residual disease rate.[61] Sanna et al. also prefer this technique and report a 44% incidence of residual cholesteatoma and a 9% incidence of recurrent cholesteatoma.[62] Marco-Algarra et al. report their results with both techniques and find a 37% recurrence rate with the closed approach and a 13% rate with the open approach.[63] Tos states that "no single method is superior in all cases," and that cholesteatoma surgery must be individualized to the particular pathology encountered.[64] In the face of continuing controversy, this seems to be the best advice.

Recidivistic cholesteatoma is multifactorial in origin. Rarely, does a surgeon leave behind visible cholesteatoma. However, Palva demonstrated that keratinizing epithelium may reside in normal-appearing mucosa near the matrix of the visible cholesteatoma.[65] Therefore, surgical management should treat the cholesteatoma as a type of low-grade malignancy with margins of apparently disease-free tissue removed along with the specimen itself. The initial location of the lesion also may predict the likelihood of recurrent disease. Stern found that the presence of cholesteatoma in the sinus tympani was associated with a high incidence of residual disease found during a second procedure.[66] The destructive ability of cholesteatoma also may correlate with the likelihood of recurrence, as Rosenfeld et al. reported higher rates when ossicular erosion was present at the first operation.[67]

Regardless of the surgical approach to cholesteatoma, long-term follow-up of the patient is imperative. The lesion can be aggressive, but at times its growth also can be subtle and belying. Residual disease may not declare itself for several years. Rosenfeld found that the cumulative percentage of patients who were detected with residual or recurrent disease continued for up to 6 years after initial treatment and ultimately reached 61%.[67] Therefore, even after a satisfying surgical procedure with apparently complete extirpation of the cholesteatoma, a patient cannot be safely declared "cured" for many years and should have periodic follow-up.

SPECIAL CONSIDERATION:

Regardless of the surgical approach to cholesteatoma (open or closed), long-term follow-up of the patient is imperative.

The temporal bone is anatomically and functionally complex and hence, the erosive properties of cholesteatoma can give rise to numerous complications. Labyrinthine fistula is reported to occur in approximately 5 to 10% of adult patients with cholesteatoma, but is fortunately rare in children.[64] Management of the matrix overlying the fistula is controversial, and according to Gacek, there are four factors that must be considered. These are the experience of the surgeon, the location and size of the fistula, the hearing status of each ear, and the mechanism of bony erosion of the cholesteatoma.[68] The two primary surgical decisions are whether to leave or remove the matrix and whether to perform an open or closed mastoid procedure. Some advocate complete removal of the disease at the time it is initially encountered in order to avoid further destruction.[69,70] Others recommend leaving the ma-

trix over the fistula and then removing it at a second stage when infection and inflammation have been controlled.[71] The fistulae most commonly involve the lateral semicircular canal, and to better follow the disease, most surgeons prefer a canal wall-down mastoidectomy.[70,72] Conversely, Sanna et al. recommend a canal wall-up tympanomastoidectomy.[71] Whichever procedure is chosen, the surgeon must be aware of the potential for labyrinthine fistula with every cholesteatoma in order to avoid possibly causing vertigo, compromise of vestibular function, and hearing loss. These signs and symptoms of chronic labyrinthitis also may occur in patients with CSOM without cholesteatoma. Their onset is usually more subtle than that seen in patients with acute labyrinthitis.

Facial nerve palsy is not uncommon in children during an episode of AOM. Usually, this is managed successfully by placement of a PET and use of an appropriate antibiotic. Facial paralysis is occasionally a complication of CSOM and/or cholesteatoma. In this setting, the above conservative management is inadequate and more aggressive, urgent, surgical treatment is indicated. A tympanomastoidectomy should be performed and an effort made to determine the site of nerve injury. Removal of chronic infection, granulation tissue, and cholesteatoma along with intravenous antibiotics and steroids usually results in a satisfactory return of facial nerve function.

Nonsurgical procedures for cholesteatoma

Currently, there is no accepted medical treatment of cholesteatoma. It is likely, though not certain, that the management of retraction pockets, adhesive OM, and cholesteatoma will continue to involve surgery initially. However, it would be ideal to possess a chemotherapeutic agent that could be used in a specific and nontoxic way in the middle ear and mastoid to aid in identification and/or lysis of residual keratinizing cells. This "magic bullet" has been sought and is, as of yet, elusive. The antimetabolite, 5-fluorouracil (5-FU), has been used topically to treat recurrent cholesteatoma in the mastoid defects of children after initial mastoidectomy.[73] Further epithelial growth was controlled.[74] Kiyofumi found that a combination of a liquid plant-oil soap and hydrogen peroxide was an effective solvent of keratin and surmised that this agent might help liberate tenacious cholesteatoma residua from regions difficult to access surgically.[75] Minotti et al. demonstrated that retinoic acid inhibited the unique ability of cholesteatoma epithelium to migrate in vitro, presumably by decreasing the available extracellular calcium necessary to form intercellular and substrate adhesions.[76,77] Further work on the development of a medical adjunct to the management of cholesteatoma is necessary and exciting.

OSSICULAR DYSFUNCTION

Chronic ear disease often affects the ossicles, and ossicular dysfunction can be a result of several different processes. Persistent inflammation of the middle-ear mucosa, along with the formation of granulation tissue and adhesions, may interfere with the mobility of the ossicular chain. Tympanosclerosis can lead to fixation of the ossicles. In CSOM, osteitis can cause ossicular erosion as well as destruction of other portions of the temporal bone. A retraction pocket of the posterosuperior quadrant of the TM can progress to myringoincudopexy and myringoincudostapediopexy. Initially, this may result in only mild ossicular dysfunction. If the process continues unabated, ossicular erosion may occur. Most commonly, the incus is affected, followed by the stapes. As discussed earlier, cholesteatoma can cause ossicular destruction. Also, appropriate surgical management of cholesteatoma can require removal of one or all of the ossicles.

Ossicular discontinuity or fixation is but one manifestation among a host of potential pathologies in the patient with chronic ear disease. The direct result is a degree of CHL. This can range from a mild imperceptible loss to a maximal CHL of between 50 to 60 dB. The latter scenario occurs when the ossicular chain is discontinuous behind an intact TM. On examination, otomicroscopy sometimes reveals obvious ossicular damage. Erosion of the long process of the incus can be visualized through a severe retraction pocket. Suctioning of otorrhea, granulation tissue, and keratin debris also may reveal that the ossicles have been affected. However, even if a large TM perforation is present, it is difficult to assess ossicular mobility in the awake patient.

Evaluation and Treatment of the Patient with Ossicular Dysfunction

All patients must undergo audiometric testing, which not only serves to document the current hearing baseline, but also aids in the evaluation of the pathologic process. Even large TM perforations usually result in no more than mild CHL. Hearing levels worse than 35 dB should alert the clinician to the possibility of some sort of ossicular involvement. Tympanometry also may provide information. Decreased compliance of the drum can result from a middle-ear effusion, ossicular fixation, or both. Increased compliance is associated with discontinuity. CT of the temporal bone, both in the axial and coronal planes, may show ossicular erosion, particularly in the epitympanum. These studies are not precise enough to document minor changes in the ossicular chain.

The most effective way to evaluate ossicular dysfunction is to perform an exploratory tympanotomy. This, of course, is not necessary if the middle ear has been entered already during a tympanoplasty or tympanomastoidectomy procedure. Earlier discussion in this chapter described the use of myringoplasty to repair an isolated TM perforation. The various types of tympanoplasties described by Wüllstein are indicated not only for TM defects, but also for reconstruction of the middle-ear transformer system. Wüllstein's classification reflects the degree of damage to the ossicular chain and is reviewed by Bellucci.[78] The five types of tympanoplasties are:

- Type I   Isolated repair of TM, ossicles intact
- Type II   Minor ossicular defect with TM on incus
- Type III Severe ossicular defects with TM on intact stapes
- Type IV   Stapes absent with TM on footplate
- Type V   Stapes footplate fixed with TM on a fenestration of the lateral semicircular canal

There have been numerous modifications of this classification system, and a vast number of materials have been used for ossiculoplasty. A thorough review of these techniques is not presented here. In general, management of ossicular defects in children is affected by the same concerns surrounding the treatment of TM perforations. Namely, the risk that continued ETD may compromise the repair. As discussed earlier, the timing of surgery is related to the age of the child, degree of hearing loss, unilaterality or bilaterality of disease, and the nature and severity of the underlying process. Tympanoplasty or ossiculoplasty is often a component of a second-stage surgery performed after an initial procedure to remove cholesteatoma.

Usually, it is preferable to use autologous or homologous material for ossiculoplasty in children. An eroded or cadaveric incus can be fashioned as an interposition graft between the stapes and malleus or between the stapes and the undersurface of the TM. When the stapes is absent, an incus can be fashioned to span from a mobile footplate to the malleus or TM. Treatment of a fixed footplate with stapedotomy or stapedectomy in children is controversial, and the surgeon may wish to delay this because of the risk of ETD and continued episodes of OM. Amplification of hearing using hearing aids is always an option, at least until the child is older and the likelihood of success for ossiculoplasty is greater.

A variety of synthetic prostheses are available for reconstruction of the ossicles. These are made of stable and inert materials that are designed for biocompatibility. They are generally divided into total ossicular replacement prostheses (TORP) and partial ossicular replacement prostheses (PORP). The use of synthetic prostheses is discouraged in children because of questionable long-term results and the increased incidence of extrusion. When they are used, it is recommended that tragal cartilage be placed between the prosthesis and the drum to make extrusion less likely.[79,80]

CHOLESTEROL GRANULOMA

Cholesterol granuloma is a pathologic entity of the middle ear and mastoid that results from chronic ETD and persistent OME. It has been called "idiopathic hemotympanum," but this is a misnomer because the process is not truly related to bleeding within the tympanum. Rather, chronic disease results in mucosal-gland hypertrophy and granulations with subsequent formation of a thick brown substance containing cholesterol crystals and iron. Cholesterol granuloma is not a specific lesion, but exists in varying degrees in chronically-underaerated ears. The mastoid is always involved when this process

is detected. The blue appearance of the TM seen with cholesterol granuloma is not precisely understood, but is thought to be due to light reflected back from the granuloma.[81]

There are several other middle-ear pathologies that may appear as a bluish TM on otoscopy. These include true hemotympanum, OME, a dehiscent jugular bulb, and a glomus tumor. The patient presenting with such a finding initially should be followed and treated with a course of antibiotics. Audiometry is recommended. If there is no improvement, then placement of a ventilation tube is warranted. Often the physician finds that aspiration of a middle-ear effusion will remove the blue appearance of the drum immediately. If, however, the physician finds a thick brownish material with yellow specks, then the diagnosis of cholesterol granuloma is made. The condition will not respond entirely to simple tube placement, but also requires middle-ear exploration and mastoidectomy to remove the granulation. The condition is rare in children and the prognosis for complete resolution is related to the severity of the underlying process, that is, ETD.

REFERENCES

1. Teele DW, Klein JO, Rosner B, et al. Epidemiology of otitis media during the first seven years of life in children in greater Boston: A prospective, cohort study. J Infect Dis 1989; 160:83–94.
2. Reed D, Struve S, Maynard JE. Otitis media and hearing deficiency among Eskimo children: A cohort study. Am J Public Health 1967; 57:1675.
3. Tschopp CF. Chronic otitis media and cholesteatoma in Alaskan native children. In McCabe BF, Sade J, Abramson M, eds. *Cholesteatoma: First International Conference.* Aesculapius, New York, 1977, pp. 290–292.
4. Smith TL, DiRuggiero DC, Jones KR. Recovery of eustachian tube function and hearing outcome in patients with cleft palate. Otolaryngol Head Neck Surg 1994; 111:423–429.
5. Avery ME, First LR, eds. *Pediatric Medicine 2nd ed.* Philadelphia: Williams and Wilkins, 1994, pp. 1127–1158.
6. Smith TG. IgG Subclasses. In: Barness LA, ed. *Advances in Pediatrics, Yearbook of Otolaryngology Head and Neck Surgery.* St. Louis: Mosby-Yearbook, 1992, pp. 101–118.
7. Mygind N, Petersen M. Nose, sinus and ear symptoms in 27 patients with primary ciliary dyskinesis. Eur J Respir Dis 1983; 64 (Supplement 127):96–101.

8. Sadler-Kimes D, Siegel MI, Todhunter JS. Age-related morphologic differences in the relation of the eustachian tube/middle ear system. Ann Otol Rhinol Laryngol 1989; 98:854.

9. Takahashi H, Masahiko M, Honjo I. Compliance of the eustachian tube in patients with otitis media with effusion. Am J Otolaryngol 1987; 3:154.

10. Bluestone CD, Klein JO. Intratemporal complications and sequelae of otitis media. In: Bluestone CS, Stool SE, Kenna MA, eds. *Pediatric Otolaryngology, 3rd ed.* Philadelphia: Saunders, 1996, pp. 583-635.

11. Paparella MM, Morizono T, Le CT, et al. Sensorineural hearing loss in otitis media. Ann Otol Rhinol Laryngol 1984; 93:623-629.

12. Austin DF. Reconstructive techniques for tympanosclerosis. Ann Otol Rhinol Laryngol 1988; 97:670-674.

13. Schiff M, Catanzaro A, Poliquin JF, et al. Tympanosclerosis—A theory of pathogenesis. Ann Otol Rhinol Laryngol 1980; 89:1.

14. Austin DF. Sound conduction of the diseased ear. J Laryngol Otol 1978; 92:367-393.

15. Saito H, Kazama Y, Yazawa Y. Simple maneuver for closing traumatic eardrum perforation by micropore strip tape patching. Am J Otol 1990; 11:427-430.

16. Good RL. Long-term middle ear ventilation with T-tubes: The perforation problem. Otolaryngol Head Neck Surg 1996; 115:500-501.

17. Strong MS. The eustachian tube: Basic considerations. Otolaryngol Clin North Am 1972; 5:19-27.

18. Bluestone CD, Cantekin EI, Douglas GS. Eustachian tube function related to the results of tympanoplasty in children. Laryngoscope 1979; 89:450-458.

19. Manning SC, Cantekin EI, Kenna MA, et al. Prognostic value of eustachian tube function in pediatric tympanoplasty. Laryngoscope 1987; 97:1012-1016.

20. Koch WM, Friedman EM, McGill TJI, et al. Tympanoplasty in children. Arch Otolaryngol Head Neck Surg 1990; 116:35-40.

21. Shih L, DeTar T, Crabtree JA. Myringoplasty in children. Otolaryngol Head Neck Surg 1991; 105:74-77.

22. Wüllstein H. Die tympanoplastik als gehörverbessernde operation bei otitis media chronica und ihr Resultate. Proc Fifth Internat Congress Oto-Rhino-Laryngol 1953.

23. Deddens AE, Muntz HR, Lusk RP. Adipose myringoplasty in children. Laryngoscope 1993; 103:216-219.

24. MacDonald RR, Lusk RP, Muntz HR. Fasciaform myringoplasty in children. Arch Otolaryngol Head Neck Surg 1994; 120:138-143.

25. Doyle WJ. A functiono-anatomic description of eustachian tube vector relations in four ethnic populations: An osteologic study. University of Michigan, Ann Arbor, MI, 1977. Microfilm

26. Mandel EM, Casselbrant ML, Kurs-Lasky M. Acute otorrhea: Bacteriology of a common complication of tympanostomy tubes. Ann Otol Rhinol Laryngol 1994; 103:713-718.

27. McLelland CA. Incidence of complications from use of tympanostomy tubes. Arch Otolaryngol Head Neck Surg 1980; 106:97-99.

28. Kenna MA, Bluestone CD. Microbiology of chronic suppurative otitis media in children. Pediatr Infect Dis J 1986; 5:223-225.

29. Fliss DM, Dagan R, Meidan N, et al. Aerobic bacteriology of chronic suppurative otitis media without cholesteatoma in children. Ann Otol Rhinol Laryngol 1992; 101:866-869.

30. Papastavros T, Giamarellou H, Varlejides S. Role of aerobic and anaerobic microorganisms in chronic suppurative otitis media. Laryngoscope 1986; 96:438-442.

31. O'Reilly BJ, Chevretton EB, Wylie I, et al. The value of CT scanning in chronic suppurative otitis media. J Laryngol Otol 1991; 105:990-994.

32. Meyerhoff WL, Morizono T, Wright CG, et al. Tympanostomy tubes and otic drops. Laryngoscope 1983; 93:1022-1026.

33. Esposito S, D'Errico G, Montanaro C. Topical and oral treatment of chronic otitis media with ciprofloxacin. Arch Otolaryngol Head Neck Surg 1990; 116:557-559.

34. Piccirillo JF, Parnes SM. Ciprofloxacin for the treatment of chronic ear disease. Laryngoscope 1989; 99:510-513.

35. Tutkun A, Ozagar A, Koc A, et al. Treatment of chronic ear disease. Arch Otolaryngol Head Neck Surg 1995; 121:1414-1416.

36. Paradise JL, Bluestone CD, Rogers KD, et al. Efficacy of adenoidectomy for recurrent otitis media in children previously treated with tympanostomy tube placement. JAMA 1990; 263:2066-2073.

37. Gates GA, Avery CA, Prihoda TJ, et al. Effectiveness of adenoidectomy and tympanostomy tubes in the treatment of chronic otitis media with effusion. N Engl J Med 1987; 317:1444-1451.

38. Kenna MA, Bluestone CD, Reilly JS, et al. Medical management of chronic suppurative otitis media without cholesteatoma in children. Laryngoscope 1986; 96:146-151.

39. Kenna MA, Rosane BA, Bluestone CD. Medical management of chronic suppurative otitis media without cholesteatoma in children—Update 1992. Am J Otol 1993; 14:469-473.

40. Leiberman A, Fliss DM, Dagan R. Medical treatment of chronic suppurative otitis media without cholesteatoma in children—A two-year follow-up. Int J Pediatr Otolaryngol 1992; 24:25-33.

41. Vartiainen E, Kansanen M. Tympanomastoidectomy for chronic otitis media without cholesteatoma. Otolaryngol Head Neck Surg 1992; 106:230-234.

42. Nadol JB. Causes of failure of mastoidectomy for chronic otitis media. Laryngoscope 1985; 95: 410-413.

43. Nadol JB, Krouse JH. The hypotympanum and infralabyrinthine cells in chronic otitis media. Laryngoscope 1991; 101:137-141.

44. Saeed SR, Jackler RK. Lasers in surgery for chronic ear disease. Otolaryngol Clin of N Am 1996; 29: 245-255.

45. Kent SE, Jones R. Pseudomonas vaccination in chronic ear disease. J Laryngol Otol 1988; 102: 579-581.

46. Müller J. Über den feinen bac und die formen der krankhaften gesehwulste. Berlin 1838; 1:50.

47. Sadé J. Prologue cholesteatoma and mastoid surgery. In: Sadé J, ed. *Proceedings of the Second International Conference.* Amsterdam: Kugler, 1982.

48. Tos M. Incidence, etiology and pathogenesis of cholesteatoma in children. Adv Oto-Rhino-Laryngol 1988; 40:110-117.

49. Harker LA. Cholesteatoma: An incidence study. In McCabe BF, Sadé J, Abramson M, eds. *Cholesteatoma: First International Conference.* New York: Aesculapius, 1977, pp. 308-312.

50. Harker LA, Severeid LR. Cholesteatoma in the cleft palate patient. In: Sadé J, ed. *Cholesteatoma and Mastoid Surgery.* Amsterdam: Kugler, 1977, pp. 37-40.

51. Derlacki EL, Clemis JD. Congenital cholesteatoma of the middle ear and mastoid. Ann Otol Rhinol Laryngol 1965; 74:706-727.

52. Levenson MJ, Parisier SC, Chute P, et al. A review of twenty congenital cholesteatomas of the middle ear in children. Otolaryngol Head Neck Surg 1986; 94: 560-567.

53. Wolfman DE, Chole RA. Experimental retraction pocket cholesteatoma. Ann Otol Rhinol Laryngol 1986; 95:639-644.

54. Khanna SM, Tonndorf J. Tympanic membrane vibration in cats studied by time-averaged holography. J Acous Soc Am 1972; 51:1904-1920.

55. Pfaltz CR. Retraction pocket and development of cholesteatoma in children. Adv Otorhinolaryngol 1988; 40:118-123.

56. Neely JG. Treatment of the uncomplicated aural cholesteatoma (keratoma). Self-instructional package. Am Acad Otolaryngol Head Neck Surg 1977;

57. Proctor B. The development of the middle ear spaces and their surgical significance. J Laryngol Otol 1964; 78:631-648.

58. McGill TJ, Merchant S, Healy GB, et al. Congenital cholesteatoma of the middle ear in children: A clinical and histopathological report. Laryngoscope 1991; 101:606-613.

59. Koltai PJ, Eames FA, Parness SM, et al. Comparison of computed tomography and magnetic resonance imaging in chronic otitis media with cholesteatoma. Arch Otolaryngol Head Neck Surg 1989; 115: 1231-1233.

60. Sharp JF, Robinson JM. Treatment of tympanic membrane retraction pockets by excision. J Laryngol Otol 1992; 106:882-886.

61. Sheehy JL. Cholesteatoma surgery in children. Am J Otol 1985; 6:170-172.

62. Sanna M, Zini C, Gamoletti R, et al. The surgical management of childhood cholesteatoma. J Laryngol Otol 1987; 101:1221-1226.

63. Marco-Algarra J, Gimenez F, Mallea I, et al. Cholesteatoma in children: Results in open versus closed techniques. J Laryngol Otol 1991; 105:820-824.

64. Tos M. Treatment of cholesteatoma in children. Am J Otol 1983; 4:189-197.

65. Palva T, Mäkinen J. Why does middle ear cholesteatoma recur? Arch Otolaryngol Head Neck Surg 1983; 109:513-518.

66. Stern SJ, Fazekas-May M. Cholesteatoma in the pediatric population: Prognostic indicators for surgical decision making. Laryngoscope 1992; 102:1349-1352.

67. Rosenfeld RM, Moura RL, Bluestone CD. Predictors of residual recurrent cholesteatoma in children. Arch Otolaryngol Head Neck Surg 1992; 118:384-391.

68. Gacek RR. The surgical management of labyrinthine fistula in chronic otitis media. Ann Otol Rhino Laryngol 1974; 83 (supplement 10):3-19.

69. Parisier SC, Edelstein DR, Han JC et al. Management of labyrinthine fistula caused by cholesteatoma. Otolaryngol Head Neck Surg 1991; 104:110-115.

70. Herzog JA, Smith PG, Kletzker GR, et al. Management of labyrinthine fistula secondary to cholesteatoma. Am J Otol 1996; 17:410-415.

71. Sanna M, Zini C, Gamoletti R, et al. Closed versus open technique in the management of labyrinthine fistula. Am J Otol 1988; 9:470-475.

72. Vartiainen E. What is the best method of treatment of labyrinthine fistulae caused by cholesteatoma? Clin Otolaryngol 1992; 17:258-260.

73. Smith MFW. The topical use of 5-fluorouracil in the ear in the management of cholesteatoma and excessive mucous secretion. Laryngoscope 1985; 95: 1202-1203.

74. Wright CG, Bird LL, Meyerhoff WL. Effect of 5-fluorouracil in cholesteatoma development in an animal model. Am J Otol 1991; 12:133-138.

75. Kiyofumi G, Sasaki Y. Solubilization of keratin debris in conservative treatment of middle ear cholesteatoma: An in vitro study. J Laryngol Otol 1994; 108: 113-115.

76. Minotti AM, Stiernberg CM, Cabral F. Inhibition of cholesteatoma migration in vitro with all-trans retinoic acid. Otolaryngol Head Neck Surg, 1996; 114: 768-776.

77. Minotti AM, Kountakis SE, Leighton WR, et al. Effects

of extracellular calcium on cholesteatoma migration and adhesion in vitro. Otolaryngol Head Neck Surg 1996; 115:458–463.

78. Bellucci RJ. Selection of cases and classification of tympanoplasty. Otolaryngol Clin North Am 1989; 22: 911–926.

79. East CA, Mangham CA. Composite tragal perichondrial/cartilage autografts vs. cartilage or bone paste grafts in tympanoplasty. Clin Otolaryngol 1991; 16: 540–542.

80. Jackson CG, Glasscock ME, Schwaber MK, et al. Ossicular chain reconstruction: The TORP and PORP in chronic ear disease. Laryngoscope 1983; 93: 981–988.

81. Sade J, Halevy A, Klajman A, et al. Cholesterol granuloma. Acta Otolaryngol 1980; 89:233–239.

17 Regional and Intracranial Complications of Otitis Media

Ian N. Jacobs and N. Wendell Todd

Otitis media (OM) may extend beyond the middle-ear cavity. In the preantibiotic era, intracranial complications and death were not uncommon sequelae of OM. Today, extracranial complications are more common than intracranial complications. The pathogenesis of these complications is related to bacterial virulence, host defenses including anatomic barriers, and inadequate drainage. Both intracranial and extracranial complications have become much less common since the advent of antibiotics, but grave complications may be on the rise with the emergence of bacteria that are resistant to many antibiotics. In many regions of the United States, increasing numbers of infections caused by *Streptococcus pneumoniae* have high or intermediate resistance to penicillin and other antibiotics.[1,2] For this reason, physicians may have to change their approach to common otologic infections. Clinicians should be selective in the use of oral antibiotics and should consider other therapies such as surgical drainage or vaccination. A number of authors have called for restricted use of oral antibiotics for the treatment of OM.[3-7]

Inadequate host defenses, including vulnerable anatomic barriers and congenital and acquired immunodeficiencies, contribute to complications of OM. Infections tend to spread along pathways of least resistance. Preformed channels and dehiscences are easy routes for the spread of infection. Sequestered infection in closed ear spaces with inadequate drainage (i.e., *pressurized infection*) may extend extracurricular or intracranially. The inflammatory response, specifically *edematous mucoperiosteum,* may further compromise drainage. This combination of virulent bacteria, pressurized pus, and insufficient host defenses predisposes to intracranial and extracranial complications of OM.

AT A GLANCE . . .

Factors Related to Complications of Otitis Media

- Bacterial virulence
- Host defenses
- Inadequate drainage

EVALUATION OF THE PATIENT WITH OTITIS MEDIA

Practice Pathway 17–1 outlines the steps taken in an examination.

Clinical Examination

A thorough history and physical examination are essential, and knowledge of the chronicity of middle-ear disease is important. Information concerning the development of symptoms and their time course is necessary in order to reconstruct the pathogenesis of the middle-ear process. A chronic history of otorrhea, otalgia, hearing loss, or vertigo suggest long-standing middle-ear disease. The physical examination should include an initial assessment of the child's overall condition, including the neurologic status. Constitutional signs of acute infection such as fever or lethargy should be noted. Questions to be answered are: (1) is the pinna displaced laterally? (2) is the postauricular sulcus ''filled-in'' or obliterated? and (3) is there tenderness on palpation or digital percussion of the mastoid? A good otoneu-

Pediatric Otolaryngology, Edited by R.F. Wetmore, H.R. Muntz, and T.J. McGill. Thieme Medical Publishers, Inc., New York © 2000.

Practice Pathway 17–1   CARE PATHWAY FOR INTRACRANIAL COMPLICATIONS

```
                        ┌─────────────────────────┐
                        │    History & Ear Exam    │
                        └─────────────────────────┘
                                    │
                ┌───────────────────────────────────────────┐
                │ Acute or chronic otitis media + CNS signs* │
                └───────────────────────────────────────────┘
                                    │
                    ┌─────────────────────────────────┐
                    │  CT scan of brain & temporal bone │
                    └─────────────────────────────────┘
                        │                        │
              ┌──────────────┐          ┌────────────────────────────────────────────────┐
              │    Normal     │          │                   Abnormal                       │
              └──────────────┘          └────────────────────────────────────────────────┘
```

| – Meningeal signs | + Meningeal signs | Lateral sinus thrombosis | Epidural abscess | Subdural abscess | Brain abscess |

Treat otitis media (oral antibiotics)

LP

Neurosurgical consultation, MRA

IV antibiotics, mastoidectomy

IV antibiotics, neurosurgical consultation

IV antibiotics, neurosurgical consultation

| – | + |

Treat otitis media

IV antibiotics (cefotaxime/vancomycin)

IV antibiotics
Mastoidectomy
Clot evacuation?
Internal jugular vein ligation?
Heparinization?

Burr hole? Craniotomy?

Burr hole? Craniotomy?

| AOM | COM |

BMT or Mastoidectomy

BMT

Mastoidectomy

*Central Nervous System Signs: lethargy, irritability, photophobia, stiff neck, headaches, nausea, and vomiting. Abbreviations: LP, lumbar puncture; AOM, acute otitis media; COM, chronic otitis media; BMT, bilateral myringotomids with tubes; MRA, magnetic resonance angiography.

rologic examination is crucial. The finding of facial palsy must be sought actively as youthful tissue turgor may camouflage poor motion of the muscles of expression. Any signs suggestive of increased intracranial pressure should be noted. In infants, the fontanelles should be palpated for fullness and the ocular fundi should be checked for papilledema or loss of venous pulsations.

A microscopic examination of the tympanic membrane (TM) may be quite revealing, as the TM acts as the window of the middle-ear space. The appearance of all regions of the TM should be evaluated under the microscope. Retraction pockets should be carefully examined, suctioned, and probed. Small retraction pockets may originate high in the attic and may be obscured with debris; thus, they may conceal gross cholesteatoma. Important questions to consider are whether the TM is simply inflamed or whether the inflammation is superimposed upon old scarring (e.g., myringosclerosis, fibrosis, or atrophy) and whether there is sagging of the skin of the posterosuperior bony canal from pressurized pus that has eroded through the bony canal from the mastoid antrum anteriorly and laterally.

SPECIAL CONSIDERATION:

Sagging of the posterior external-canal wall suggests bony erosion that has resulted as a complication of acute OM or cholesteatoma.

Audiologic assessment should supplement the physical examination. Even though formal audiologic examination may be inappropriate in the obtunded patient suspected of having an intracranial complication, audiometry may be helpful in the nontoxic patient with a more subtle complication. Tympanometry yields information about the eustachian tube (ET) status. Abnormal tympanograms (type B or C) indicate eustachian tube dysfunction (ETD) Pure-tone responses may indicate pathology of the sound conduction mechanism (i.e., conductive) or pathology of the cochlea or cochlear nerve (i.e., sensorineural). Elevated bone conduction thresholds are consistent with sensorineural hearing loss (SNHL). If appropriate for the patient's condition and age, vestibular testing, including electronystagomography and posturography, may suggest subtle inner ear or vestibular pathology.

Radiologic Evaluation

Beyond providing information about pneumatization and aeration of the temporal bones, plain radiographs of the mastoid are of limited value today. Plain radiographs do not adequately image the important attico-antral region, which is often the crucial site for complicating problems and not detectable by tympanoscopy. Axial and coronal noncontrast computed tomography (CT) is the study of choice for most complications of OM. Thin axial and coronal slices (1 mm) will show the fine details of the mesotympanum, attic, antrum, facial canal, hypotympanum, and cochleovestibular complex. The bony scutum and ossicles are important landmarks that are well visualized on the coronal and axial CT views (Fig. 17-1).[8] The CT study can be extended to include the brain and be done with contrast if intracranial pathology is suspected.

In addition to defining the location and extent of temporal bone pathology, the temporal bone CT should act as a "roadmap" for the surgeon. A cholesteatoma will appear as a soft-tissue mass in the mesotympanum or epitympanum; antrum bone erosion and loss of the fine detail of the scutum may be demonstrated as well (Fig. 17-2). In contrast, bone erosion and coalescence of the bony architecture of the mastoid antrum and cortex suggest acute or

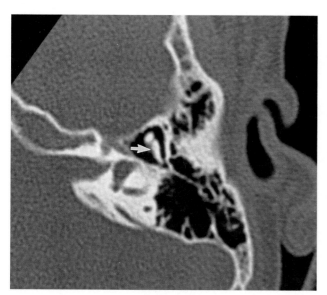
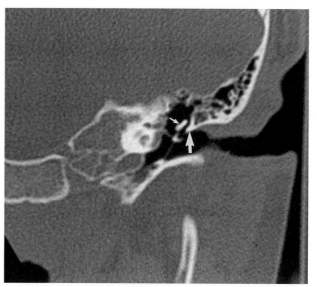

A   B

Figure 17–1: Temporal bone CT scan. (A) Axial CT of normal left ear showing incus and malleus (arrow). (B) Coronal CT scan of normal ear showing bony scutum (large arrow) and ossicles (small arrow).

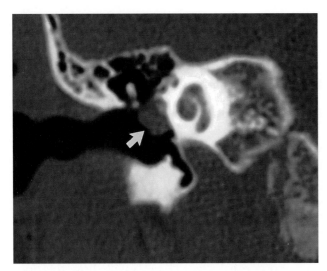

Figure 17–2: Coronal CT scan showing cholesteatoma on the promontory (arrow).

chronic otomastoiditis. Acute petrositis may be diagnosed as well on CT. Congenital anomalies such as a patent cochlear aqueduct, large vestibular aqueduct, and labyrinthine dysplasias can also be detected.[9] Magnetic resonance imaging (MRI), although not as helpful for bony detail, provides superior soft-tissue definition and with contrast, demonstrates flow within vascular structures of the head and neck. This radiologic assessment of these intracranial structures is critical for any child suspected of having an intracranial complication of OM. A more detailed discussion of radiologic temporal bone imaging can be found in Chapter 9.

EXTRACRANIAL COMPLICATIONS

Retraction Pockets/Cholesteatoma

Chronic negative pressure on the TM may lead to gradual thinning, weakening, and medialization (retraction) of portions of it. ETD is the etiologic culprit. *Retraction pockets* commonly occur in the pars flaccida region or in the posterosuperior quadrant of the pars tensa. They may evolve from a tiny dimple of desquamated epithelium that is self-cleansing to a keratin-filled sac (i.e., *frank cholesteatoma*) (Fig. 17–3).[10] However, at a given point in time, the extent of evolution may be difficult to determine on the basis of physical examination alone. The visible pocket actually may represent only the "tip of the iceberg" of the total disease.

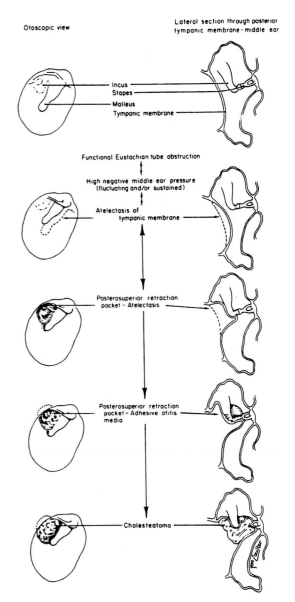

Figure 17–3: Chain of events in the pathogenesis of acquired aural cholesteatoma in the posterosuperior portion of the pars tensa or the tympanic membrane. (From reference 10, with permission.)

Diagnosis

A small dry retraction pocket may remain relatively symptom-free, and it is best detected by careful microscopic examination of the TM. It is important to examine all regions of the TM, including the pars flaccida. Pneumatic otoscopy demonstrates the normal motion of the TM and may reveal sections of it that are retracted. Probing the recesses of the retraction pocket under general anesthesia helps determine its extent. Frequently, the use of nitrous oxide may be helpful in the elevation of retraction pockets. Because a cholesteatoma sheds squamous debris, careful suctioning and cleaning of this debris are necessary to examine the full extent of the pocket and detect its site of origin.

Audiologic assessment is essential to determine the hearing level in both the diseased and contralateral ear. A conductive hearing loss (CHL) usually is found with both retraction pockets and cholesteatoma. SNHL may result from a labyrinthine fistula or labyrinthitis. The clinician should not dismiss the possibility of cholesteatoma in an ear with normal hearing and tympanometry. If a labyrinthine fistula is suspected, vestibular testing may be helpful.

If there is uncertainty about the extent of a retraction pocket then CT evaluation is necessary. The coronal view on CT shows the extent of the disease and detects bone erosion. Usually, the scutum loses its sharp definition. Soft tissue may be visualized in the attic or hypotympanum along with erosion or displacement of the ossicles.

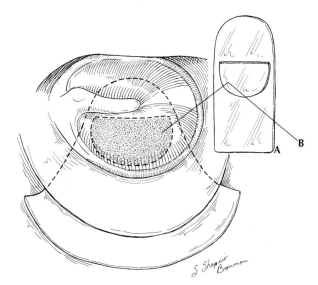

Figure 17–4: Reconstruction of a posterosuperior retraction pocket with (A) temporalis fascia and (B) tragal cartilage.

SPECIAL CONSIDERATION:

Retraction pockets of the TM need careful microscopic examinations to exclude an early cholesteatoma. CT demonstrating erosion of the scutum or evidence of soft tissue in the attic is highly suggestive of a cholesteatoma in the pars flaccida region.

Treatment

As a first step in the treatment of an early retraction pocket, the middle ear can be ventilated with a pressure-equalization tube (PET). With the administration of inhalational anesthesia, the pocket may distend, which is a good indication that the pocket is not attached to the promontory or ossicles and will reverse with middle-ear ventilation. If the retraction pocket is adhered to the promontory, it may take several months before the adhesions lyse and the TM returns to normal. Some clinicians even have described manual inflation of the ET as a means for breaking these adhesions.[11] If the retraction pocket does not normalize with middle-ear ventilation, then surgical elevation and reconstruction of the abnormal portion of the TM may be necessary. Temporalis fascia with or without tragal cartilage may

be used to graft the TM defect (Fig. 17–4).[12] A PET may be inserted to prevent recurrent retraction of the newly reconstructed TM.

Gross cholesteatoma should be excised or exteriorized completely. Depending upon the location of disease, its extent, and the experience of the surgeon, management of gross cholesteatoma may require either canal wall or intact canal-wall procedures. When the imaging study suggests that the cholesteatoma involves the epitympanum or hypotympanum and not the mastoid or sinus tympani, a mastoidotomy (e.g., transcanal atticotomy) may be performed. The mesotympanum and attic region are approached in an "inside-out" manner, which assures noninvolvement of mastoid and allows surgical access to the disease (Fig. 17–5).[13] This approach is not suitable when cholesteatoma extends into the mastoid or sinus tympani. This extent of disease requires a mastoidectomy with or without preservation of the posterior canal wall (Fig. 17–6).[14,15] When intact canal-wall procedures are employed, "second-look" middle-ear explorations are often necessary to detect and excise any recurrent or persistent disease (see Chapter 16). Cholesteatoma, uncontrollable by intact canal-wall procedures may require open-cavity procedures, such as a modified radical or radical mastoidectomy (Fig. 17–7). Creation of a mastoid cavity or bowl allows for cleaning of accumulated keratin debris or infection. Radical mastoidectomy is reserved for severe recidivistic cholesteatoma that is too extensive for a modified radical procedure.[14,15] The entire middle

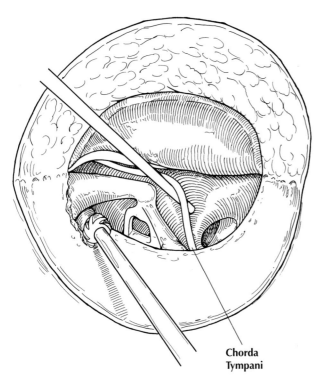

Figure 17–5: Mastoidotomy approach to cholesteatoma confined to the mesotympanum.

ear is marsupialized into the external ear canal and the ET may be blocked off. Among the disadvantages of an open-cavity mastoidectomy in a growing child is the fact that cortical bone regrowth encroaches to narrow the meatus and limit access to the bowl, requiring revision surgery (recontouring). Intraoperative electrophysiologic facial nerve monitoring may reduce the risk of facial nerve injury in selected tympanomastoid cases.[16] Such monitoring cannot substitute for either technical skill or surgi-

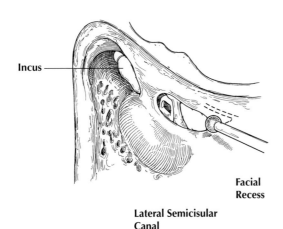

Figure 17–6: Facial recess approach to cholesteatoma in the sinus tympani and mastoid antrum.

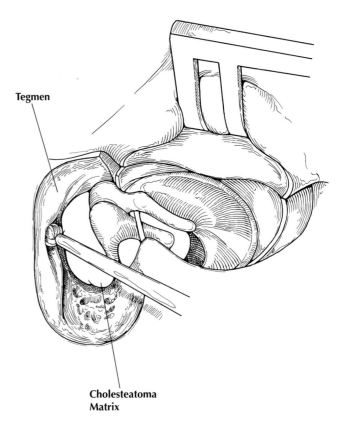

Figure 17–7: Modified radical mastoidectomy for extensive cholesteatoma of the mastoid and mesotympanum.

cal knowledge, and its use should be based on the preference of the surgeon and the complexity of the case.

Ossicular Erosion

Diagnosis and treatment

Chronic OM with or without cholesteatoma may lead to disruption of the ossicular chain either because of osteitis of the ossicles or direct invasion by cholesteatomatous debris. The lenticular process of the incus is involved most commonly because the long process of the incus has the most vulnerable blood supply. The most commonly disrupted joint is the incudostapedial joint, which is a site most frequently involved by posterosuperior retraction pockets.

A CHL, the extent of which depends on the degree of ossicular damage and the status of the TM, is frequently present. Evaluation includes a complete history and physical examination with pneumatic otoscopy. Frequently, these patients have a long standing history of chronic ear symptoms (e.g., otorrhea, hearing loss, or otalgia). Otoscopy frequently reveals a retraction pocket in the posterosuperior quadrant (Fig. 17-4). Pneumatic otoscopy may demonstrate the lack of ossicular-chain motion. CT may reveal significant erosion of the ossicles. With complete discontinuity and an intact TM, there will be a maximal CHL (average speech reception threshold = 54 dB).[17] Tympanometry in these patients may demonstrate a hypermobile ossicular unit (type AD).

Treatment depends on the degree of hearing loss, the status of the contralateral ear, current ET function, anesthetic risks, age, and wishes of the child's family. When there is mild unilateral hearing loss (SRT < 25 dB), surgery is not indicated for hearing improvement alone. Audiologic rehabilitation by successful surgery or amplification is indicated if there is moderate to severe CHL that is bilateral or if there is severe unilateral loss (SRT > 45 dB). In some children, it may be preferable to wait until ET function has normalized and active middle-ear disease has resolved before proceeding with reconstructive surgery.

Middle-ear exploration is performed with good exposure of the ossicular chain. The ossicular unit may be reconstructed utilizing a number of materials including autologous bone and cartilage as well as several synthetic materials such as hydroxyapatite or polyprolene partial ossicular replacement prostheses (PORP) or total ossicular replacement prostheses (TORP). Hearing results are generally good with both autologous and synthetic materials.[18]

Facial Nerve Paralysis

Acute facial weakness or *paralysis* can occur as a complication of both acute OM (AOM) and chronic OT. AOM is a relatively common cause of acute facial nerve paralysis in children. The presumptive mechanism is direct inflammation of the exposed or dehiscent portion of the facial nerve in the middle ear. From the surgical perspective, 60% of temporal bones have natural dehiscences along the intratympanic course (Fig. 17-8).[19] Toxins from infection may penetrate through such dehiscences and lead to infection and edema of the exposed portion of the nerve. Chronic OM with cholesteatoma also may either compress or directly invade the facial nerve and lead to acute paralysis. Facial paralysis also can occur due to osteomyelitis of the petrous portion of the temporal bone with erosion into the petrous portion of the nerve. Neoplasms such as

rhabdomyosarcoma of the temporal bone may masquerade as AOM with facial paralysis.

SPECIAL CONSIDERATION:

Acute facial weakness or paralysis can occur as a complication of both AOM and chronic OM.

Evaluation and management

Microtympanoscopy can be quite helpful in determining the etiology of facial paralysis. If AOM is diagnosed, treatment should be directed to the middle ear. CT should be considered in children with facial paralysis attributable to AOM. In cases of chronic OM with or without cholesteatoma, CT is helpful in defining the extent of disease and may suggest the site of facial nerve involvement. Electrophysiologic testing of the nerve usually is not required in cases of facial paralysis secondary to infection, cholesteatoma, or tumor, as the information obtained will not alter treatment.

Facial paralysis attributable to AOM demands wide-field myringotomy and intravenous antibiotics. Myringotomy affords decompression of the pus and a specimen for microbiologic studies (i.e., gram stain and cultures) to help direct antibiotic therapy. Some physicians prefer myringotomy with placement of a PET because of concerns of early spontaneous healing of the myringotomy. In most cases, complete recovery can be expected, although 40 percent of cases may experience persistent weakness.[20]

Facial weakness or paralysis attributable to chronic OM (with or without cholesteatoma) also demands immediate hospitalization with intravenous antibiotics and CT of the temporal bone. The surgical approach depends on the CT results. Generally, the approach is either "complete" mastoidectomy using an intact canal-wall or a canal-wall-down procedure for more extensive disease (see Chapter 16). Decompression of the involved portion of the facial nerve may be helpful as well. Usually, the area of facial involvement is in the mesotympanum or mastoid, so decompression through the mastoid and middle ear usually is adequate. Intravenous antibiotics, directed by operative cultures, help control the

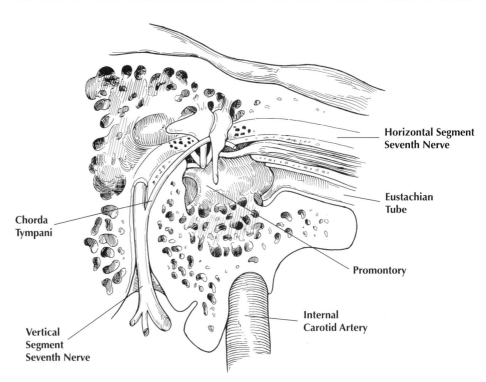

Horizontal Segment
Seventh Nerve

Eustachian
Tube

Promontory

Internal
Carotid Artery

Chorda
Tympani

Vertical
Segment
Seventh Nerve

Figure 17–8: The course of the facial nerve in the mesotympanum and mastoid. Note the regions of bony dehiscence in the middle ear.

remaining infection and should be continued until all signs of infection resolve. Facial nerve function may take several months for maximal recovery.

Acute Mastoiditis

The patient with mastoiditis may present clinically at any stage during the progression of the disease. Remember that the mastoid air-cell system is in continuity (both for ventilation and mucous clearance) with the mesotympanum via the antrum and the epitympanum. Patients with AOM routinely have some inflammation of the mastoid air-cell system. This stage of the disease typically clears in a couple of months with conservative treatment. At this stage of the disease process, radiographic studies may demonstrate clouding of the mastoid air-cell system; however, the bony architecture is largely intact.

The next stage is clinical acute mastoiditis, with pressurized pus in the mastoid antrum. This may progress to *coalescent mastoiditis* as the bony partitions between the cells dissolve. Radiographically, this manifests as open areas in the mastoid without bony septae (Fig. 17–9). The patient presents with severe retroauricular discomfort. Findings are attributable to the spread beyond the mastoid air-cell system proper. The sites of extension, which are in the pathways of least anatomic resistance, determine the clinical signs and symptoms. These clinical

findings may be masked by antimicrobial therapy or aggravated by immunodeficiencies or virulent microorganisms. Anatomically, extension occurs into six different sites:

1. **Lateral:** Extension through the mucoperiosteum into the surrounding bone and through various

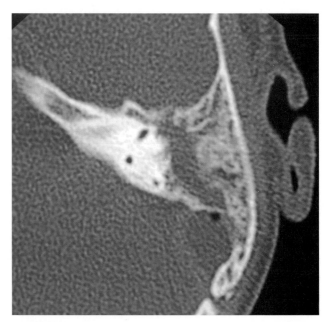

Figure 17–9: Axial CT of left ear showing coalescent mastoiditis with dissolution of the bony architecture of the mastoid.

venous channels (emissary veins) leads to inflammation of the mastoid periosteum. This periostitis is easy to recognize at this stage as severe cellulitis of the retroauricular soft tissues with lateral displacement of the pinna and blunting of the retroauricular sulcus. Later, there may be development of a subperiosteal abscess, which can rupture spontaneously and lead to a chronically draining mastoid-cutaneous fistula.

2. **Anterior:** A deceptive appearance of mastoiditis because the clinical appearance is that of external otitis confined to the posterior and slightly superior portion of the external auditory canal (EAC). The pressurized pus seems to "sag" into the ear canal.

3. **Posterior:** Spread into the sigmoid sinus or the dura mater of the posterior fossa (see section on Lateral Sinus Thrombosis).

4. **Medial:** Spread into the facial nerve, vestibular labyrinth, or petrous apex[10] (see sections on Facial Nerve Paralysis, Labyrinthitis, and Petrositis).

5. **Superior:** Spread into the dura mater of the floor of the middle cranial fossa often resulting in an epidural abscess (see section on Epidural Abscess).

6. **Inferior-Medial:** Direct extension through the mastoid tip rarely occurs, seemingly because of the tough connective tissue of the attachment of the sternocleidomastoid muscle. Instead, the infection perforates the medial aspect of the mastoid tip, then contiguously spreads down the neck to present as a deep neck or retropharyngeal abscess. This route of spread occurs if the patient has a pneumatized mastoid tip. Hence, such a Bezold's abscess is more frequent in adults and older children.

AT A GLANCE . . .

Anatomic Extension of Acute Mastoiditis

- Lateral into soft tissues of the external ear
- Anterior into the external auditory canal
- Posterior into the sigmoid sinus or posterior cranial fossa
- Medial into the labyrinth or petrous apex
- Superior into the middle cranial fossa
- Inferior-Medial into the mastoid tip

Evaluation and treatment

It is important to determine the duration of the infection. Typically, complicated cases of acute coalescent mastoiditis take several weeks to develop. Examination of the postauricular region may reveal erythema, edema, and auricular displacement in uncomplicated cases of mastoiditis with periostitis. Acute coalescent mastoiditis may result in more severe postauricular erythema and edema as well as cortical bone erosion and a postauricular fluctuance (e.g., subperiosteal abscess) or even a neck abscess (e.g., Bezold's abscess). It is important to note the overall clinical status of the child and determine whether the child is febrile or lethargic.

CT of the temporal bone is useful to evaluate the architecture of the mastoid air-cell system, if one suspects acute coalescent mastoiditis. Abnormal findings range from mild distortion and haziness of the mastoid outline to complete loss of the bony architecture (empyema) with corticol erosion (Fig. 17–9). Microscopic examination of the TM may reveal AOM or chronic OM with effusion. Diagnostic tympanocentesis may be helpful.

Treatment of uncomplicated cases of mastoiditis with periostitis (Practice Pathway 17–2) usually includes intravenous antibiotics and myringotomy with drainage. Myringotomy affords decompression of the pus and a specimen for microbial studies. Placement of a PET allows for a longer period of drainage. For the patient with minimal anterior or lateral spread of acute mastoiditis and whose clinical course is that of continued improvement in each subsequent 12 and 24 hour segment, management without a mastoidectomy is usually effective. Alternatively, for the patient with a nonimproving course or infection spread other than lateral and anterior, cortical mastoidectomy is necessary. CT is helpful in directing therapy.

During mastoid surgery for an acute complication, the surgeon has two goals. One is complete drainage of all the purulent fluid and removal of diseased bone. The other is reestablishment of attico-antral communication. Generally, a cortical mastoidectomy is performed, leaving the canal wall intact unless cholesteatoma is discovered. Diseased mastoid air-cells are removed from all areas, including the mastoid tip and perifacial (fascial recess) and zygomatic regions if involved. The tegmen and sigmoid plate are skeletonized. Cultures should be taken. Tissue specimens sent for pathologic analysis

Practice Pathway 17–2 PRACTICE PATHWAY FOR INTRATEMPORAL COMPLICATIONS

can help diagnose neoplasm or mycobacterial disease. If indicated, a PET should be placed as well. Antimicrobial therapy should be based on microbiologic data. In general, initial empirical therapy should cover for *Streptococcus pneumoniae*, Group A beta hemolytic *Streptococcus*, beta-lactamase producing *Hemophilus influenzae*, *Branhamella catarrhalis*, and *Staphylococcus aureus*. Treatment with intravenous antibiotics is continued at least until all the patient's signs and symptoms of infection have subsided and then an additional 5 to 7 days, provided that the surgeon considers that all the infection has been drained and all osteomyelitic bone debrided. Otherwise, the intravenous antibiotics should be continued longer.

SPECIAL CONSIDERATION:

The goals of mastoid surgery for an acute complication is complete drainage of pus, removal of infected bone, and restoration of the attico-antral communication.

Petrositis

Diagnosis

Petrositis is a rare complication that may develop if mastoid infection extends into the petrous portion of the temporal bone. About 30% of individuals

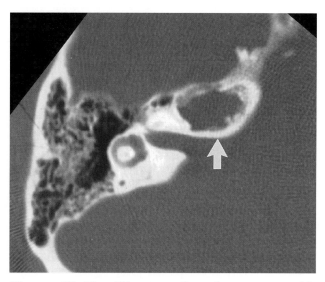

Figure 17–10: CT scan of coalescent petrositis (arrow).

have a fully pneumatized mastoid, and generally only individuals with a pneumatized petrous mastoid develop petrositis.[10,21,22] Just as AOM causes inflammation of the mastoid cells, the petrous cells may be involved also. Normally, petrous infection subsides as the middle-ear infection does. Obstructed drainage of petrous-apex-cell tracts, especially in the immunocompromised patient or in the presence of virulent microorganisms, may result in *acute coalescent petrositis.* Acute petrositis rarely occurs with AOM and usually is associated with chronic otorrhea or cholesteatoma.

Classically, petrositis leads to a triad of severe pain behind the eye (*retrobulbar*), persistent purulent otorrhea, and occasionally sixth cranial nerve (*abducens*) palsy. This triad is called *Gradenigo's syndrome.* Less often, there is facial palsy or paralysis, disequilibrium, and fever.[22] If left untreated, petrous infection may spread intracranially. Diagnosis is based on these aforementioned clinical signs and symptoms as well as CT confirmation of petrous infection (Fig. 17-10).

Treatment

Most cases of acute petrositis can be treated effectively with intravenous antibiotics and/or standard cortical mastoidectomy. Acute coalescent petrositis refractory to these measures requires aggressive surgical treatment. Shambaugh and Glasscock have described several approaches that spare the hearing.[22] The surgical approach for a particular patient is best determined by considering the location of the infection as well as hearing, vestibular, and facial functions. The simplest and most direct approach to the petrous pyramid is through the perilabyrinthine-posterior-cell tracts. After complete mastoidectomy, the three bony semicircular canals are skeletonized and the dura of the middle cranial fossa is exposed

by removing the tegmen plate (Fig. 17-11). The surgeon may follow a superior cell tract above the superior semicircular canal and posterior to the geniculate ganglion. A cell tract above the horizontal semicircular canal and behind the superior vertical canal or beneath the posterior semicircular canal can also be followed (Fig. 17-11). Small curettes, rather than cutting burrs, are safer and more useful for following these tracts.

If the posterior approach fails to eradicate the infection, a more through and complete approach would be through the anterior group of petrous apex cells just inferior and anterior to the cochlea.[22] This approach, described by Lempert and Ramadier, sacrifices a moderate degree of hearing as the surgeon first performs a radical mastoidectomy with removal of the incus, malleus, and TM.[23,24] The surgeon then explores the hypotympanum for cell tracts between the cochlear and the jugular bulb or carotid artery. If such a cell tract is not found, then the carotid artery needs to be followed to the petrous apex (Fig. 17-12). An additional approach, which preserves hearing, is through the middle cranial fossa as described by Eagleton.[25]

After the petrous apex cells are explored and exenterated, a myringotomy with placement of a PET is performed. Cultures are obtained and intravenous antibiotics are adjusted accordingly. Because it is usually impossible to remove all of the infected bone, intravenous antibiotics are essential to eradicate any remaining infection. Repeat CT scans may be necessary to rule out persistent disease.

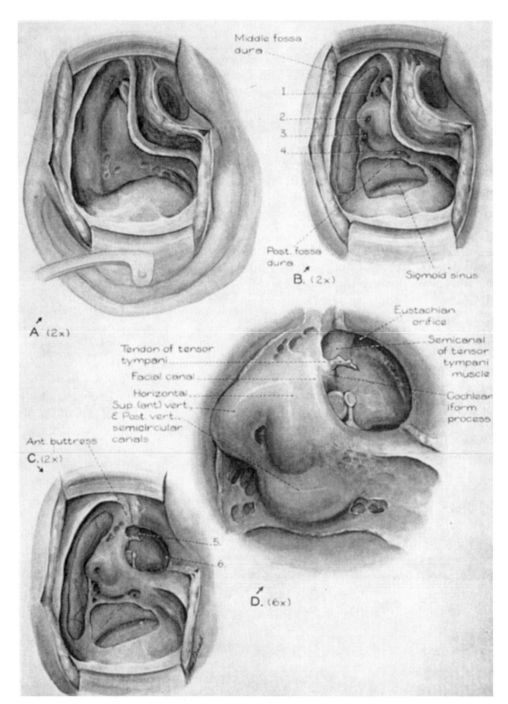

Figure 17–11:   Posterior surgical approach to petrous apex cells. (A) Initial simple mastoidectomy. (B) Exposure of dura of the middle and posterior fossae and exploration of perilabyrinthine-cell tracts. *1.* Cells between superior semicircular canal and geniculate ganglion. *2.* Arch of superior semicircular canal. *3.* Cells between superior and posterior semicircular canals. *4.* Cells beneath posterior semicircular canal. (C) Conversion to radical mastoidectomy and exploration of *5.* peritubal cells and *6.* Hypotympanic cells (D) Same, under operating microscope. (From Glasscock ME, Shambaugh GE. Aural complications of otitis media. *Surgery of the Ear, 4th ed.* Philadelphia: Saunders, 1990, p. 287, with permission.)

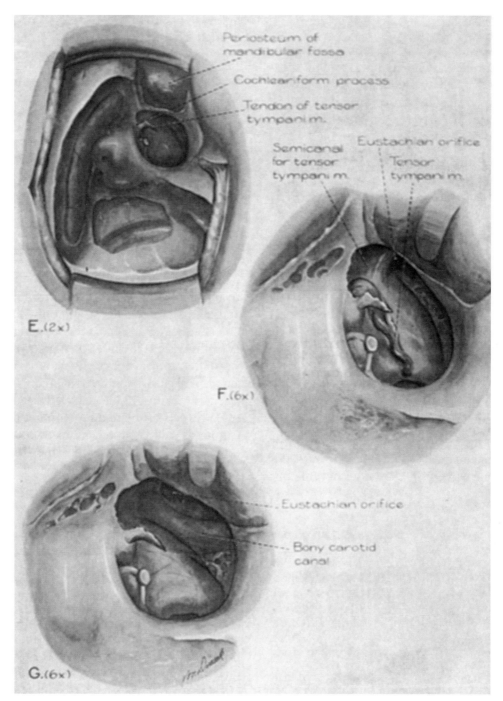

Figure 17–12:   Anterior approach to petrous apex cells. (E) Exposure of the carotid artery to the apex. (F) Exposure of the middle fossa dura to the apex. (G) Petrous cells excavated between carotid artery, middle fossa dura, geniculate ganglion, and cochlea. (From Glasscock ME, Shambaugh GE. Aural complications of otitis media. *Surgery of the Ear, 4th ed.* Philadelphia: Saunders 1990, p. 287, with permission.)

Labyrinthine Fistula

A spontaneous fistula to the labyrinth is not an uncommon occurrence in the course of cholesteatoma. This occurs as the cholesteatoma erodes through the bony capsule of the vestibule. The sac of the cholesteatoma may remain attached at the point of the fistula and minimize vestibular symptoms. Such a sac may be discovered only during mastoidectomy. In contrast, chronic noncholesteatomatous middle-ear disease is less likely to cause a labyrinthine fistula. If it does, it usually leads to fulminate suppurative labyrinthitis and severe vestibular symptoms.

Evaluation

Overt vestibular symptoms may be minimal or episodic as the fistula site may be covered by the cholesteatoma sac. Early detection may be possible only with a fistula test. This test involves the application of positive and negative pressure to the sealed TM and may be performed with the Seigel otoscope or the tympanometer. The application of positive or inward pressure may produce nystagmus with the direction of the quick component toward the affected ear. A negative fistula test does not rule out a labyrinthine fistula.

SPECIAL CONSIDERATION:

Most surgeons manage a labyrinthine fistula that results from a cholesteatoma with a canal-wall-down mastoidectomy.

Treatment

Treatment of a labyrinthine fistula involves surgical exploration of the mastoid and removal of most gross cholesteatoma; however, the matrix should be left intact in the region of the fistula. Removal of the matrix may lead to complete loss of vestibular and auditory function. For this reason, most surgeons manage the cholesteatomatous ear with labyrinthine fistula by a canal-wall-down procedure. If a fistula is exposed inadvertently, an immediate repair employing either tissue or fascia should be performed.

Serous and Suppurative Labyrinthitis

Both acute and chronic middle-ear infection may invade the labyrinth and lead to either serous or suppurative labyrinthitis. *Serous labyrinthitis* is the result of inflammation of the labyrinth only, whereas *suppurative labyrinthitis* indicates microbial invasion of the labyrinth. Serous labyrinthitis is most common and is manifested typically by vestibular symptoms. Acute infection in the middle ear cleft may spread via the annular ligament of the oval window or the membrane of the round window into the labyrinth. Labyrinthitis may occur as the result of meningitis traveling through the internal auditory meatus or, less commonly, through the cochlear aqueduct or the endolymphatic sac and duct. Presenting signs include spontaneous nystagmus toward the contralateral ear, nausea, vomiting, and ataxia. Physical examination might reveal fluid or infection in the middle-ear cleft. Neurologic exam often reveals spontaneous, constant, horizontal nystagmus as well as past pointing. Suppurative labyrinthitis, although much less common, may lead to severe consequences. This is usually heralded by worsening vestibular symptoms as well as progressive SNHL. The prognosis is poor in terms of the recovery of audiologic and vestibular function, and complete loss of vestibular and auditory function is not unusual. In addition, infection may spread in an intracranial direction, resulting in meningitis.[22]

Treatment

Treatment is directed at the underlying cause of the labyrinthitis. Treatments include myringotomy and PET placement for AOM or mastoidectomy for chronic suppurative OM. In addition, bed rest and labyrinthine-suppressant drugs afford relief of symptoms. Suppurative labyrinthitis is treated with intravenous antibiotics as well. It is important to watch for signs and symptoms of meningitis; lumbar puncture is indicated if meningeal symptoms develop. CT also should be performed if symptoms progress. If intracranial spread occurs, the labyrinth should be drained surgically to prevent further seeding to the meninges. With careful vigilance for central nervous system (CNS) complications, the overall prognosis remains excellent, but most patients do not recover labyrinthine function.[22]

AT A GLANCE . . .

Extracranial Complications of Otitis Media

Retraction Pockets/Cholesteatoma: a cyst-like mass that can evolve from a tiny dimple of desquamated epithelium to a keratin-filled sac. *Diagnosis:* microscopic examination, pneumatic otoscopy, audiologic assessment, CT. *Treatment:* ear ventilation with pressure-equalization (tympanostomy) tube (PET), surgical elevation, or reconstruction of the abnormal portion of the tympanic membrane.

Ossicular Erosion: may be caused by chronic OM with or without cholesteatoma. *Diagnosis:* complete history and physical examination with pneumatic otoscopy, CT, tympanometry. *Treatment:* audiologic rehabilitation by surgery or amplification for moderate to severe CHL; reconstruction of the ossicular unit using autologous bone and cartilage, PORP, or TORP

Facial Nerve Paralysis: can occur as a complication of AOM and chronic OM and as a result of direct inflammation of the dehiscent portion of the facial nerve in the middle ear. *Diagnosis:* microtympanoscopy, CT. *Treatment:* wide-field myringotomy with intravenous antibiotics if attributable to AOM; mastoidectomy with intravenous antibiotics if attributable to chronic OM

Acute Mastoiditis: inflammation of the mastoid antrum and cells. *Diagnosis:* CT, microscopic examination of the TM, diagnostic tympanocentesis. *Treatment:* intravenous antibiotics, myringotomy with drainage, PET, mastoidectomy

Petrositis: may develop if mastoid infection extends into the petrous portion of the temporal bone. Patient presents with severe pain behind the eye, persistent purulent otorrhea, and possibly sixth cranial nerve palsy. *Diagnosis:* based on clinical symptoms and CT. *Treatment:* intravenous antibiotics, complete mastoidectomy, myringotomy with placement of PET

Labyrinthine Fistula: occurs as the cholesteatoma erodes through the bony capsule of the vestibule. *Diagnosis:* fistula test performed with a Seigel otoscope or tympanometer. *Treatment:* exploration of the mastoid and removal of most gross cholesteatoma

Labyrinthitis: serous labyrinthitis is inflammation of the labyrinth and suppurative labyrinthitis involves microbial invasion of the labyrinth

AT A GLANCE . . . Continued

Extracranial Complications of Otitis Media

Presenting symptoms include spontaneous nystagmus toward the contralateral ear, nausea, vomiting, and ataxia. *Diagnosis:* physical and neurologic exam, CT if symptoms progress. *Treatment:* myrinotomy, PET, mastoidectomy, bed rest, labyrinthine-suppressant drugs, intravenous antibiotics

INTRACRANIAL COMPLICATIONS

Infection in the middle ear may spread to the intracranial cavity and cause a number of complications. In the preantibiotic era, AOM frequently led to intracranial problems—most commonly, purulent meningitis that was almost always fatal. From 1928 to 1933, just prior to the introduction of sulfonamides and antibiotics, 1:40 deaths at a general hospital was related to otitic intracranial complications.[26] Although the frequency of such complications decreased dramatically after the advent of antibiotics, these complications continue to occur and mortality rates for those patients who suffer intracranial complications remain high (10 to 31%).[27] Therefore, careful vigilance is essential to detect complications early in the course of the disease.

Chronic ear infection may spread intracranially by three methods: (1) direct extension through bone that has been weakened by osteomyelitis or cholesteatoma; (2) thrombophlebitis; or (3) extension along preformed pathways (e.g., oval and round windows). Infection may spread by a combination of two or three pathways. Children who are immunocompromised or infected with virulent, antibiotic-resistant microorganisms are at risk for intracranial spread. In particular, Type III *Pneumococcus* has a predilection for intracranial spread. Today, virtually all cases of otitic intracranial infections are the result of chronic ear infection. Patients with poorly pneumatized mastoids have a slightly higher incidence of CNS complications.

Diagnosis

The intracranial extension of an ear infection is fastidious in its early and treatable stages. The practi-

AT A GLANCE . . .

Methods of Intracranial Spread of Otogenic Infection

- Direct extension through bone
- Retrograde thrombophlebitis
- Extension along preformed pathways

tioner must be constantly vigilant to detect intracranial complications early. The general otologic and neurologic history and physical examination are most helpful in determining the diagnosis. Certain signs and symptoms in a child with chronic OM suggest an intracranial problem. These include severe headache, irritability, lethargy, nausea, vomiting, vertigo, and severe otalgia. Any neurologic signs, especially if focal, are important. Findings such as facial paralysis, papilledema, meningismus, seizures, or altered or fluctuating levels of consciousness suggest intracranial pathology.[28] In an infant, fontanelles may be full or distended.

Contrast-enhanced CT is usually diagnostic of most intracranial problems except meningitis where examination of the cerebrospinal fluid (CSF) is necessary; however, intracranial complications may occur with little evidence of temporal bone destruction on CT. Therefore, MRI with gadolinium may be helpful in the detection of extradural abscess formation and magnetic resonance angiography (MRA) may be helpful in the detection of sigmoid sinus thrombosis.[28] When CNS complications are being considered, appropriate neurosurgical consultation should be obtained (see Practice Pathway 17–1).

Bacterial Meningitis

Diagnosis

Otogenic meningitis continues to be the most common intracranial complication of OM. It is also the most common reason for death related to OM. In the recent literature, mortality rates as high as 30.7% have been reported for meningitis related to chronic OM.[27] The single most common microorganism is *Streptococcus.* Meningitis may occur as a result of direct spread through the dura to infect the meninges, but most commonly as the result of hematogenous spread from a distant site associated with the

ear infection. Meningitis may be localized or generalized. *Localized meningitis* is infection of the dura and pia archnoid confined to the area of the supportive focus without diffuse infection of the CSF. *Generalized meningitis* is a global infection of the entire pia archnoid with gross CSF infection.[29] Classical signs and symptoms include headache, nuchal rigidity, fever, vomiting, confusion, lethargy, and altered levels of consciousness. Kernig's sign may be positive if the leg cannot be extended beyond 135 degrees at the knee when the thigh is flexed 90 degrees at the hip. Brudzinski's sign may be positive, if passive flexion of the neck so that the chin touches the chest prompts flexion of both legs and hips.

In the initial work-up, a CT should be considered in most cases prior to lumbar puncture to exclude increased intracranial pressure that may result in brainstem herniation during the procedure. If focal neurologic signs or altered consciousness suggest an intracranial mass lesion, a brain CT should be performed. If there is uncertainty about the ear or mastoid as the source of infection, CT of the temporal bone is helpful as well. The conclusive diagnosis of meningitis is made by lumbar puncture. A tap is considered positive for bacterial meningitis if the clinician finds a grossly-cloudy fluid with more than 1000 white blood cells/mm^2 (>60% polymorphonuclear leukocytes) and a reduced glucose level. Gram stain and culture may identify the organism. In cases of localized meningitis, the CSF does not contain bacterial organisms and should be differentiated from viral meningitis. The pressure of the fluid should be noted also. A high CSF pressure may suggest *otitic hydrocephalus.* Antigen tests are available for *Haemophilus influenzae, Pneumococcus,* and *Meningococcus.* Repeat lumbar punctures are not performed routinely, but may need to be considered if meningeal signs persist.

Because OM is not an uncommon cause of meningitis, it is important to search for the source of infection in the ear. This is especially important if bacteria such as *Haemophilus influenzae* or *Streptococcus pneumoniae,* which are common to middle-ear infections, are cultured from the CSF. Obviously, a careful otologic examination is essential. The clinician must look for purulent or clear fluid in the middle-ear space; however, the ear disease may be difficult to detect on physical examination in cases involving a small cholesteatoma. A contrast-enhanced CT of the temporal bone may be necessary to identify occult ear disease, such an attic cholesteatoma or an epidural abscess. Recurrent meningitis may be caused by an abnormal communication between the middle ear or mastoid and the subarchnoid space. Such a communication may be congenital such as a perilymphatic fistula (PLF) or acquired from a temporal bone fracture. Diagnostic tests include audiometry, fistula tests, and CT cisternography; however, in cases of a PLF, the diagnosis is made after a round- or oval-window leak is found on surgical exploration of the middle ear.

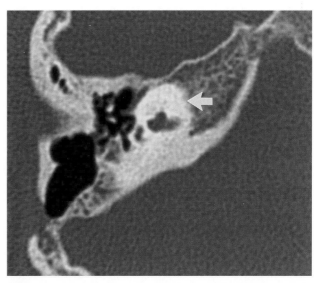

Figure 17–13: CT scan showing labyrinthitis ossificans.

SPECIAL CONSIDERATION:

Recurrent meningitis may be caused by an abnormal communication between the middle ear or mastoid and the subarachnoid space.

Treatment

The first treatment strategy is to eradicate the meningeal infection with intensive broad-spectrum antibiotics. The same bacteria that cause AOM are responsible for meningitis. Notwithstanding this fact, the care of the individual patient demands the specific identification of the microorganism. During initial "empirical therapy," vanomycin is combined with a third generation cephalosporin, such as cefotaxime, because of the potential for resistant *Streptococcus pneumoniae.* This is continued for at least 14 days.[30] Definitive culture and sensitivity should be checked and antibiotics adjusted accordingly. Infectious disease consultation should be considered.

The second treatment strategy is to eradicate the otologic source of infection. This may require surgical drainage such as myringotomy and PET placement for AOM. This would be performed as soon as the child is neurologically stable. If the child remains unstable, tympanocentesis at the bedside can be performed. If mastoiditis is diagnosed, a cortical mastoidectomy should be performed. Meningitis secondary to chronic OM with cholesteatoma is treated with the appropriate surgery to eradicate and control the cholesteatoma. In cases of recurrent meningitis, the physician must consider a middle-ear exploration for a PLF. If a history of recent trauma exists, the physician should search for a CSF leak in the mastoid or middle ear. A CT cisternogram may be followed by surgical exploration of the mastoid or middle ear.

Because the prognosis remains fair with a mortality rate of over 30% with meningitis secondary to chronic OM, early diagnosis is critical.[27] Other long-term neurologic sequelae are common, including SNHL that ranges from 6 to 37% in clinical reports.[31] This occurs as infection spreads from the meninges to the labyrinth via the internal auditory canal or the cochlear aqueduct. This may result in labyrinthitis ossificans with total loss of labyrinthine function (Fig. 17-13).

Epidural Abscess

Evaluation

An *epidural abscess* results from destruction of bone adjacent to the dura mater. The bone destruction may be attributable to chronic infection with or without cholesteatoma. Frank pus accumulates in the potential space between the dura and surrounding bone. In some cases, especially those that have been partially treated, exuberant granulation tissue forms instead of pus. Symptoms generally remain low-grade and include lateral temporal bone pain and severe otalgia. A patient with an epidural abscess may remain asymptomatic for a long time. In fact, it is not unusual to find granulation tissue in the epidural space as an incidental finding during mastoidectomy or on CT (Fig. 17-14). An Epidural abscess is dangerous because of the potential for intracranial spread.

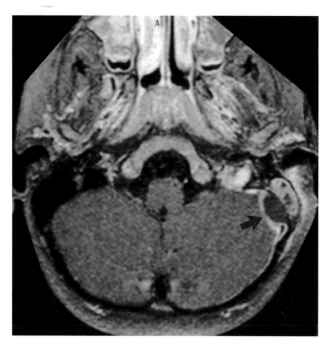

Figure 17–14:   MRI scan of epidural abscess (arrow).

Treatment

Treatment of an epidural abscess includes surgical drainage of the abscess or granulation tissue through the mastoid. If the symptoms or CT findings suggest an epidural abscess, the tegmen should be thinned to expose and explore the dura locally. Granulation should be gently removed to uncover normal dura; however, the dura should be left intact. Gross purulence should be drained. If a cholesteatoma is found, the disease should be completely exteriorized. In all cases, intravenous antibiotics should be utilized and tailored to culture results.

Subdural Empyema

Evaluation and treatment

Subdural empyema is a collection of pus in the subdural space that is the result of direct extension of infection or retrograde thrombophelebitis. It is an extremely rare but severe complication with a high mortality rate of 13 to 55%.[31] Clinically, the child with a subdural empyema presents with quite toxic symptoms and has signs of an intracranial mass effect. Symptoms include severe headaches, seizures, somnolence, obtundation, and hemiplegia. Contrast-enhanced CT or MRI scan is usually diagnostic and neurosurgical consultation is essential.

Treatment includes neurosurgical drainage either through burr holes or a craniotomy, intravenous an-

tibiotics, corticosteroids to reduce cerebral edema, anticonvulsants, and surgical debridement of the offending otogenic source. Mastoidectomy usually is performed once the patient's neurologic condition is stable, and it may be delayed several days after the neurosurgical procedure to allow for stabilization of the neurologic status. Subdural empyema may result in chronic neurologic sequelae, and mortality rates remain high.[29]

Brain Abscess

Evaluation

Brain abscess is a rare but potentially fatal complication of ear disease. The incidence of brain abscess has decreased dramatically since the advent of intravenous antibiotics, but it still occurs.[26] Brain abscess may result from direct extension of infection through the mastoid cavity or internal auditory canal or less commonly, by retrograde thrombophlebitis through preformed vascular channels. Chronic OM with cholesteatoma is thought to be the most common cause of otogenic brain abscess, but AOM also rarely may result in this complication. Initial symptoms may remain low-grade and include persistent fever, headache, nausea, vomiting, irritability, and malaise. Occasionally, convulsions may occur. The symptoms may decline during the "latent" phase, which lasts for several days or weeks. During the third stage of infection, symptoms may progress as encephalitis develops. Symptoms are related to both the mass effect and the generalized cerebral infection. An abscess in the temporal lobe may rupture into the lateral ventricle, resulting in fulminant meningitis and death. A cerebellar abscess may compress the respiratory centers leading to respiratory arrest.

Diagnosis of a brain abscess requires a high index of suspicion. Any patient with chronic OM and cholesteatoma who develops low-grade fevers, headache, and any signs of increased intracranial pressure should be followed. Localizing signs and symptoms are uncommon, but may be present. Fundoscopic exam usually reveals blurring of the disc margins or overt papilledema. Confirmation of a brain abscess is by contrast-enhanced CT or MRI. Contrast-enhanced CT may reveal a hypodense area surrounded by a dense ring ("ring sign") (Fig. 17-15). Lumbar puncture is contraindicated because of the risk of herniation.

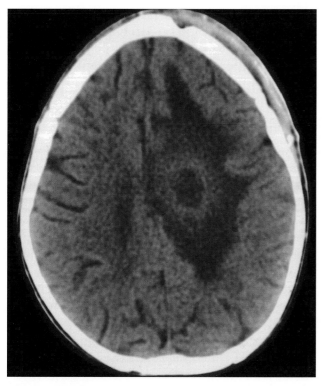

Figure 17–15: CT scan of brain showing frontal lobe abscess illustrating a classic "ring sign".

Treatment

Aggressive treatment is mandatory because of the high potential mortality. Treatment includes broad-spectrum antibiotics with good CSF penetration and anaerobic coverage, such as a third generation cephalosporin (ceftriaxone) combined with penicillin or metronidazole (Flagyl™). Intravenous corticosteroids may be given to reduce cerebral edema. Neurosurgical drainage of the abscess may be necessary. In most cases, the abscess is treated by aspiration and irrigation through a craniectomy or burr hole. The purulent fluid is sent for gram stain and culture. The abscess cavity is irrigated copiously with saline and antibiotic solution. Occasionally, open incision and drainage or possibly resection of the abscess may be necessary; however, this approach may result in a higher incidence of postoperative seizures. The ultimate approach should be determined by the neurosurgeon.

Once the patient is neurologically stable, which may take several days, "complete" intact canal mastoidectomy, modified radical mastoidectomy, or radical mastoidectomy is essential to eradicate the primary source of infection, if the CT reveals chronic otomastoiditis or cholesteatoma. In patients with a brain abscess, complete eradication of infec-

tion has priority over reconstruction of the hearing mechanism. Antibiotics with good anaerobic coverage are continued for 4 to 6 weeks. Follow-up brain CT may be necessary if neurologic symptoms persist. In general, mortality rates of 4 to 20% can be expected if the brain abscess is diagnosed early; however, patients who present with altered mental status and severe neurologic signs have an even worse prognosis.[32,33]

Otitic Hydrocephalus

Otitic hydrocephalus is a condition of increased intracranial pressure in the absence of an intracranial mass effect several weeks following an episode of AOM. It occurs most commonly in older children and adolescents. Symptoms include headache, drowsiness, nausea, and vomiting. Bilateral papilledema is common. Occasionally, ipsilateral sixth nerve palsy may occur. Other localizing neurologic signs are not present usually.[34]

Evaluation and treatment

Diagnosis of otitic hydrocephalus is confirmed by lumbar puncture that reveals increased CSF pressure with normal fluid. CT should be performed first to exclude a mass intracranial lesion. The CSF typically shows no cells, normal glucose, and normal protein. The increased pressure is due to obstruction of one or more of the venus sinuses, usually the sigmoid sinus. Treatment includes reduction of intracranial pressure with repeated lumbar punctures or lumbar drainage. Diuretics such as acetazolamide (Diamox™) may be helpful. Typically, the pressure gradually returns to normal over the course of a few weeks. As with other otogenic complications, the underlying ear disease should be treated appropriately.

Lateral Sinus Thrombosis

Evaluation

Lateral or *sigmoid sinus thrombosis* occurs from direct extension of infection into the venous sinus from the mastoid. In the preantibiotic era this was the second most common cause of death from OM after meningitis. This complication has become rare since the advent of antibiotics, but its prevalence may be on the rise again with the emergence of resistant bacteria. The most common organisms are beta hemolytic streptococci followed by *Streptococcus pneumoniae* and *Staphylococcus aureus.*[29]

The usual source of infection is coalescent mastoid infection or chronic cholesteatoma. The course of infection is through osteomyelytic bone in the dural plate. Initially, a perisinus abscess forms. This leads to an advential infection with formation of granulation tissue. Platelets, red blood cells, and fibrin adhere to this site and lead to *mural thrombus* formation. The thrombus may propagate, occlude the entire sinus, and ultimately may become embolic. Classic signs and symptoms include spiking fevers ("picket fence fevers"), headache, malaise, and signs of increased CNS pressure. Lateral sinus thrombosis should be suspected in any child with persistent OM who appears septic or spikes recurrently high fevers. Many patients may manifest generalized malaise and emaciation also. Less common signs include edema over the posterior mastoid secondary to the thrombosis of the mastoid emissary vein, known as *Griesinger's sign.* Blood cultures support the diagnosis, but negative cultures do not rule out lateral sinus thrombosis. Progressive anemia may be seen, especially after infection with beta hemolytic streptococci. The diagnosis of lateral sinus thrombosis may be suggested by MRA (Fig. 17–16), which reveals flow voids and thrombus formation within the sinus. Definitive diagnosis is made at the time of mastoidectomy when absence of blood flow is demonstrated in the sigmoid sinus. Queckenstedt's test is contraindicated because of the risk of herniation.

Treatment

Management includes broad-spectrum antibiotics (until patient-specific microbial data is available) and surgical debridement and drainage of the mastoid. A transcortical ("complete") mastoidectomy should be performed for mastoiditis without cholesteatoma. Infection related to cholesteatoma may require a canal-wall-down exteriorizing mastoidectomy. The dura overlying the sigmoid sinus and posterior fossa should be explored. The perisinus abscess should be drained and granulation tissue removed.

Treatment for the thrombosed sigmoid sinus is controversial. Intensively focused antimicrobial therapy for weeks and complete surgical debridement of the mastoid and the overlying dural plate are usually sufficient. The sigmoid sinus usually recanalizes over time. Anticoagulation is usually not required.

If the patient has signs of increased intracranial pressure attributable to the obstructed sigmoid sinus, consideration should be given to removal of the thrombus. Removal of a thrombus can be addressed by two methods. One method is with a thrombolytic agent delivered by interventional radiology. The second includes surgical exploration of the sigmoid sinus. This procedure involves aspirating the sinus with a small-gauge needle (e.g., 23 gauge) for confirmation of absent blood flow. In preparation for incision of the sinus, bone is removed several cm proximal and distal to the thrombosis so that the sinus may be compressed and packed. With attention to avoiding an air embolism, a small incision is made into the lumen of the sigmoid sinus. The clot is evacuated and, if brisk bleeding is encountered, packing with hemostatic thrombin and other agents may be performed. Once the clot is removed, the incision is closed with preplaced sutures overlaid with topical thrombin.[29]

In rare cases when there are continued signs and symptoms of sepsis and embolization, internal jugular-vein ligation may be necessary. If there is propagation of the thrombus, anticoagulation therapy may be employed. Initially, heparin is started but long-term anticoagulation therapy with coumarin

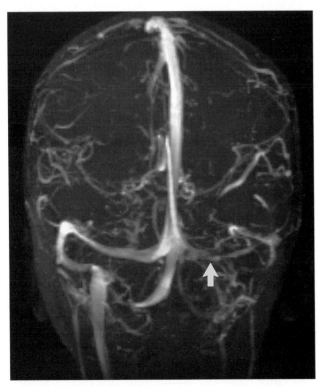

Figure 17–16:   MRA showing thrombosis of the left sigmoid sinus (arrow).

may be necessary. In most cases, infection can be controlled with intravenous antibiotics, which should be continued for an extended period of time (usually 4–6 weeks). Although the sinus usually recanalizes over time, repeat MRA studies may be necessary for confirmation. Neurosurgery consultation is essential in the management of this complication.

AT A GLANCE . . .
Intracranial Complications of Otitis Media

Bacterial Meningitis: commonly caused by *Streptococcus*. May occur as a result of direct or hematogenous spread of infection through the dura to the meninges. Patient presents with headache, nuchal rigidity, fever, vomiting, confusion, lethargy, and altered levels of consciousness. *Diagnosis:* positive Kernig's and Brudzinski's signs, CT, lumbar puncture, otologic exam, audiometry, fistula tests. *Treatment:* broad-spectrum antibiotics, myringotomy, PET, tympanocentesis, cortical mastoidectomy

Epidural Abscess: results from the destruction of bone adjacent to the dura mater. Symptoms include lateral temporal bone pain and severe otalgia. *Diagnosis:* granulation tissue found in the epidural space during mastoidectomy or on CT. *Treatment:* surgical drainage, exteriorization, intravenous antibiotics

Subdural Empyema: a collection of pus in the subdural space that is the result of extension of infection or retrograde thrombophlebitis. Symptoms include headaches, seizures, somnolence, obtundation, and hemiplegia. *Diagnosis:* contrast-enhanced CT or MRI, neurosurgical consultation. *Treatment:* neurosurgical drainage, intravenous antibiotics, corticosteroids, anticonvulsants, surgical debridement, mastoidectomy

Brain Abscess: may result from extension of ear infection through the mastoid cavity or internal auditory canal or from retrograde thrombophlebitis through preformed vascular channels. Symptoms include persistent fever, headache, nausea, vomiting, irritability, and malaise. *Diagnosis:* fundoscopic exam, contrast-enhanced CT or MRI. *Treatment:* broad-spectrum antibiotics, intravenous corticosteroids, neurosurgical drainage, mastoidectomy

AT A GLANCE . . . Continued
Intracranial Complications of Otitis Media

Otitic Hydrocephalus: increased intracranial pressure in the absence of an intracranial mass several weeks following an episode of AOM. Symptoms include headache, drowsiness, nausea, and vomiting. *Diagnosis:* lumbar puncture, CT *Treatment:* lumbar puncture and drainage, diuretics

Lateral Sinus Thrombosis: occurs from extension of infection into the venous sinus from the mastoid. Symptoms include spiking fevers, headache, malaise, and increased CNS pressure. *Diagnosis:* blood cultures, MRA. *Treatment:* broad-spectrum antibiotics, surgical debridement and drainage of the mastoid, mastoidectomy, removal of the thrombus, jugular-vein ligation, anticoagulation therapy

REFERENCES

1. Tomascz A. Multiple-antibiotic resistant pathogenic bacteria. N Engl J Med 1994; 330:1247–1251.
2. Breiman RF, Butler JC, Tenover FC, et al. Emergence of drug-resistant pneumococcal infections in the United States. JAMA 1994; 271:1831–1835.
3. Lieberman JM. Bacterial resistance in the 90's. Contemp Pediatr 1994; 11:72–99.
4. Bernstein JM. Otitis media with effusion: To treat or not to treat? J Respir Dis 1995; 16:88–99.
5. Paradise JL. Managing otitis media: A time for change. Pediatrics 1995; 96:712–715.
6. Cunningham AS. Antibiotics for otitis media, restraint, not routine. Contemp Pediatr 1994; 11:17–30.
7. Murray BE. Can antibiotic resistance be controlled? N Engl J Med 1994; 330:1229–1230.
8. Chakeres DW, Oehler M, Schmalbrock P, et al. Temporal bone imaging. In: Som P, Curtin H, eds. *Head and Neck Imaging.* St. Louis: Mosby, 1996, pp. 1319–1350.
9. Hasso AN, Casselman JW, Broadwell RA. Temporal bone anomalies. In: Som P, Curtin H, eds. *Head and Neck Imaging.* St. Louis: Mosby, 1996, pp. 1351–1390.
10. Bluestone CD, Klein JO. Intratemporal complications and sequelae of otitis media. In: Bluestone CD, Stool SE, Kenna MA, eds. *Pediatric Otolaryngology, 3rd ed.* Philadelphia: Saunders, 1996, pp. 583–635.
11. Weider D. Tympanoplasty in children. In: Hotaling AJ, Stankiewicz JA, eds. *Pediatric Otolaryngology*

for the General Otolaryngologist. New York: Igaku-Shoin, 1996, pp. 250–262.

12. Buckingham RA. Fascia and perichondrium atrophy in tympanoplasty and recurrent middle ear atelectasis. Ann Otol Rhinol Laryngol 1992; 101:755–758.

13. Glasscock ME, Shambaugh GE. The open cavity mastoid operation. In: Glasscock ME, Shambaugh GE, eds. *Surgery of the Ear, 4th ed.* Philadelphia: Saunders, 1990, pp. 228–247.

14. Potsic WP, Cotton RT, Handler SD, eds. *Surgical Pediatric Otolaryngology.* New York: Thieme, 1997.

15. Glasscock ME, Shambaugh GE. The simple mastoid operation. In: Glasscock ME, Shambaugh GE, eds. *Surgery of the Ear, 4th ed.* Philadelphia: Saunders, 1990, pp. 216–227.

16. Olds MJ, Rowan PT, Isaacson JE, et al. Facial nerve monitoring among graduates of the Ear Research Foundation. Am J Otol 1997; 18:507–511.

17. Austin DF. Acoustic mechanisms in middle ear sound transfer. Otolaryngol Clin North Am 1994; 27:641–654.

18. Wehrs RE. Incus interposition and ossiculoplasty with hydroxyapatite prosthesis. Otolaryngol Clin North Am 1994; 27:677–688.

19. Todd NW, Heindel NH, Per-Lee JH. Bony anatomy of the epitympanic. J Otorhinolaryngol 1994; 56:146–153.

20. Shapiro AM, Schaitken BM, May M. Facial paralysis in children. In: Bluestone CD, Stool SE, Kenna MA, eds. *Pediatric Otolaryngology, 3rd ed.* Philadelphia: Saunders, 1996; pp. 312–332.

21. Lindsay JR. Suppuration in the petrous pyramid. Ann Otol Rhinol Laryngol 1938; 47:3.

22. Glasscock ME, Shambaugh GE. Aural complications of otitis media. In: Glasscock ME, Shambaugh GE, eds. *Surgery of the Ear, 4th ed.* Philadelphia: Saunders, 1990, pp. 276–294.

23. Ramadier JA. L'ostéite proturde du rocher. Paris, 1933.

24. Lempert J. Complete apicectomy (mastoidotympano-apicectomy), a new technique for complete apical exenteration of apical carotid portion of petrous pyramid. Arch Otolaryngol 1937; 25:144–177.

25. Eagelton WP. Unlocking of petrous pyramid for localized bulbar meningitis secondary to suppuration of petrous apex. Arch Otolaryngol 1931; 13:386.

26. Courville CB. Intracranial complications of otitis media and mastoiditis in the antibiotic era. Laryngoscope 1955; 65:31–46

27. Gower D, McGuirt FW. Intracranial complications of acute and chronic infectious ear disease: A problem still with us. Laryngoscope 1983; 93:1028–1033.

28. Saah D, Elidan J, Gomori M. Intracranial complications of otitis media. Ann Otol Rhinol Laryngol 1997; 106:873–874.

29. Glasscock ME, Shambaugh GE. Intracranial complications of otitis media. In: Glasscock ME, Shambaugh GE, eds. *Surgery of the Ear, 4th ed.* Philadelphia: Saunders, 1990; pp. 248–275.

30. Brodie HA, Thompson TC, Vassilian L, et al. Induction of labyrinthitis ossificans after pneumococcal meningitis: An animal model. Otolaryngol Head Neck Surg 1998; 118:15–21.

31. Smith HP, Hendrick EB. Subdural empyema and epidural abscess in children. J Neurosurg 1983; 58:392–397.

32. Kaplan K. Brain abscess. Med Clin North Am 1985; 69:345–360.

33. Seydoux CH, Francioli P. Bacterial brain abscesses: Factors influencing mortality and sequelae. Clin Infect Dis 1992; 15:394–401.

34. Isaacman DJ. Otitic hydrocephalus: An uncommon complication of a common condition. Ann Emerg Med 1989; 18:684–687.

Diseases of the Cochlea and Labyrinth

Patrick E. Brookhouser

The Health and Human Services (HHS) document, "Healthy People 2000: National Health Promotion and Disease Prevention Objectives,"[4] established an objective of reducing the average age of identification of infants with significant hearing loss from 24 to 30 months to no more than 12 months.[1] Infants whose hearing losses are identified and who receive intervention before 6 months of age demonstrate a significant advantage in communicative skill development over time when compared to infants with comparable cognitive potential whose losses are identified later. Persistent, congenital, or early onset hearing loss in the moderate to profound range (41–100 dB), if undetected, can impede acquisition of literacy skills, school achievement, and social/emotional development.[2-5] Unilateral sensorineural hearing loss (SNHL) in the moderate to profound range correlates with poor academic performance, increased likelihood of repeating a grade, and school behavior problems.[6,7]

> ## SPECIAL CONSIDERATION:
>
> Infants whose hearing losses are identified and who receive intervention before 6 months of age demonstrate a significant advantage in communicative skill development compared to infants whose losses are identified later.

In developed countries, 1.0 to 2.0/1000 school age children exhibit a bilateral SNHL of 50 dB or worse, including 0.5 to 1.0/1000 whose bilateral losses exceed 75 dB.[8] In a British study, hearing loss affected 1/174 neonatal intensive care unit (NICU) babies versus 1/1278 non-NICU infants.[9] Lesser degrees of persistent hearing loss (i.e., "hard of hearing" vs. deaf) are 5 to 10 times more common than severe to profound losses.[1,10] Unilateral SNHL of 45 dB or worse among U.S. school-age children has a prevalence of about 3/1000,[11] and 13/1000 have unilateral SNHL worse than 26 dB. Most unilateral losses are detected later in life than bilateral losses (mean age in one study 8.78 years).[6]

The 1993 National Institutes of Health (NIH) consensus statement on early identification of hearing impairment in infants and young children recommends in-hospital hearing screening for all infants who are admitted to neonatal intensive care units (ICU) and screening of all other infants within the first 3 months of life.[11] Failure of rescreening warrants a comprehensive audiologic evaluation. Failure rates requiring referral can be kept in the 3% range in carefully-monitored universal screening programs.

The 1994 position statement of the Joint Committee on Infant Hearing endorses the goal of universal detection of infants with hearing loss as early as possible.[12] The position statement includes risk indicators that are associated with delayed-onset SNHL and/or conductive hearing loss (CHL) to identify infants who should be provided with periodic hearing monitoring. These indicators include: a family history of early-onset SNHL, prenatal infection (e.g., cytomegalovirus, rubella, syphilis, toxoplasmosis), neurofibromatosis type II and neurodegenerative disorders, and persistent pulmonary hypertension in the newborn period.

EVALUATION OF THE YOUNG HEARING-IMPAIRED CHILD

A child with educationally-significant hearing loss should be evaluated by a mutidisciplinary team of

Pediatric Otolaryngology, Edited by R.F. Wetmore, H.R. Muntz, and T.J. McGill. Thieme Medical Publishers, Inc., New York © 2000.

specialists that includes an otolaryngologist with pediatric experience, a pediatric audiologic team experienced with behavioral and electrophysiologic testing, a pediatrician/dysmorphologist knowledgeable of hearing loss syndromes, a genetic counselor, a pediatric ophthalmologist skilled in electroretinography, a psychologist, an educator with expertise in early intervention in children with hearing loss, and a speech/language pathologist (Practice Pathway 18-1). Consultation in pediatric neurology

and neuroradiology should be accessible as needed.

A detailed prenatal, birth, and postnatal history for the child and a complete family history should address hearing loss, speech/language disorders, ear, nose, and throat disorders; and craniofacial deformities, together with syndromic components such as kidney disorders, sudden death of a family member at a young age, thyroid disease, intracranial tumors, progressive blindness, and "café-au-lait

Practice Pathway 18-1   EVALUATION OF SENSORINEURAL HEARING LOSS

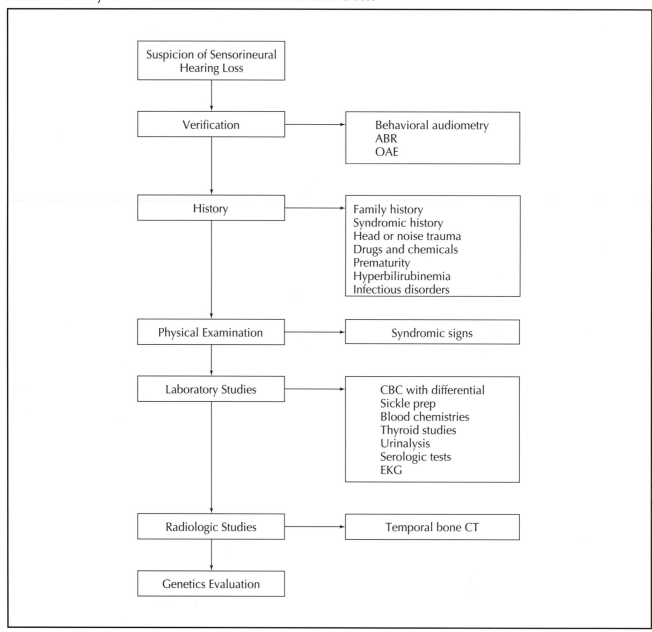

Abbreviations: ABR, Auditory Brainstem Response; OAE, Otoacoustic Emissions; CBC, Complete Blood Count; EKG, Electrocardiogram; CT, Computed Tomography.

spots.'' Any history of marital consanguinity should be noted in the family history.

AT A GLANCE . . .

Team Evaluation of the Young
Hearing-Impaired Child

- Audiologist
- Otolaryngologist
- Pediatrician/Dysmorphologist
- Genetics counselor
- Ophthalmologist
- Psychologist
- Education specialist
- Speech and language pathologist

The targeted physical examination, preferably done by a geneticist/dysmorphologist, should concentrate on subtle findings that are characteristic of hearing loss syndromes, such as preauricular or branchial pits, heterochromia irides, blue sclerae, dystopia canthorum, facial asymmetry, and café-au-lait spots. The integrity of the child's visual system should be confirmed ophthalmologically and electroretinography undertaken as indicated. Any child with early onset SNHL of uncertain etiology should have an electrocardiogram to rule out a potentially fatal cardiac conduction defect.

A reasonable array of basic laboratory studies might include complete blood count (CBC) with differential and sickle cell prep if indicated, basic blood studies, chemistries (lipids, blood sugar, creatinine, blood urea nitrogen (BUN) and thyroid studies), and urinalysis. Evidence of hematuria should prompt additional renal studies (e.g., ultrasound). Serologic tests for congenital syphilis and toxoplasmosis, which are potentially treatable conditions, may be indicated. Maternal rubella vaccination status should be confirmed by history, particularly among recent immigrants to the United States. Definitive laboratory confirmation of congenital cytomegalovirus (CMV) infection must be accomplished during the first 3 weeks or so of life because after that perinatally or postnatally acquired infection, which entails minimal risk of hearing loss, can give rise to positive antibody titers. The etiologic role, if any, of autoimmune inner ear disease in progressive

SNHL in children is unclear and a definitive diagnostic battery for youngsters has not been validated.

AT A GLANCE . . .

Laboratory Evaluation of Hearing Loss

- CBC with differential
- Sickle cell prep (if indicated)
- Chemistries
  lipids
  glucose
  creatinine
  BUN
  thyroid function studies
- Urinalysis
- Serology
  syphilis
  toxoplasmosis
  CMV

The pediatric audiologic evaluation should address the type of hearing loss (i.e., CHL, SNHL, or mixed), the degree of loss (i.e., mild, moderate, severe, profound, and anacusic), the audiometric configuration and symmetry of the impairment, and finally, with serial assessment, the stability or progression of the loss. Vestibular dysfunction can accompany hearing loss in children; this dysfunction may be attributable to genetic factors, as well as such nongenetic etiologies as bacterial meningitis and ototoxic drugs and chemicals. Pediatric vestibular evaluation requires significant modification of standard adult techniques, but computer rotational testing has facilitated serial followup of atrisk children, such as those receiving potentially ototoxic medications. Symptoms and signs of underlying vestibular dysfunction in infants and toddlers might include delayed gross motor skill development (e.g., sitting unsupported, walking, or standing on one foot). Progressive and fluctuating SNHL, with or without vertigo, should prompt a renewed search for potentially treatable conditions such as perilymphatic fistula (PLF) and congenital infections.

Variation of serial auditory thresholds in children may not reflect a permanent change in auditory sensitivity. A temporary threshold shift can follow hazardous sound exposure (including overamplification with hearing aids). Improvement in a child's ability to "tune in" more attentively to very soft sounds can yield improved thresholds. If the same audiologists evaluate a particular child's hearing over time, any variation due to methodological errors would be consistent. Fluctuation or deterioration of thresholds (in the absence of middle-ear dysfunction) at the four middle test frequencies (500, 1000, 2000, and 4000 Hz) by 15 dB or more should prompt careful reevaluation of the child.

Among 229 children with SNHL who demonstrated threshold variation over time (normal middle-ear function), the probability of contralateral threshold fluctuation if one ear fluctuated was 0.91, whereas the probability of contralateral progressive threshold deterioration if one ear progressed was 0.67.[13]

Among 65 children (110 episodes) who sustained 20 dB or greater deterioration of the three frequency average (TFA = 500, 1000, and 2000 Hz) thresholds, an improvement of 10 dB or more in the TFA, without treatment, was subsequently documented in 50% of these cases. The TFA remained stable in 45% and a 10 dB or greater decline occurred in only 4% during 6 months of follow-up (Fig. 18–1).

Genetic and nongenetic factors can lead to fluctuating and progressive childhood SNHL. Associated syndromic features can include anhidrosis, ataxia, branchial fistulas, optic atrophy, piebald trait, and preauricular pits. Acoustic neuromata associated with neurofibromatosis, particularly NF-II type, can present in younger patients. Structural inner ear anomalies, specifically Mondini aplasia and enlarged vestibular aqueduct, can be identified on temporal bone (TB) computed tomography (CT), and are associated strongly with fluctuating and progressive SNHL. This hearing loss often is exacerbated by minimal head trauma. The differential diagnosis also should include drugs and chemicals, noise trauma, ear/head trauma, mumps and congenital infections (rubella, CMV, toxoplasmosis, and syphilis), bacterial meningitis, hyperlipidemia, thyroid dysfunction, diabetes, hypercoagulability state, sickle cell disease, leukemia, autoimmune inner ear disease, and PLF.

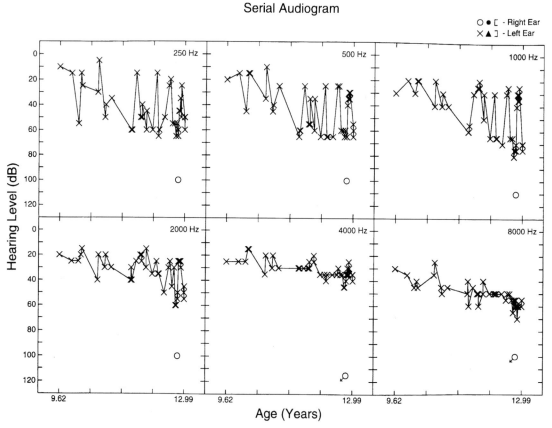

Figure 18–1: Example of a patient with fluctuating hearing loss over a period of 3+ years.

The prevalence of PLF in children with fluctuating and progressive SNHL is a matter of debate. A sensitive and specific diagnostic technique for preoperative confirmation of a PLF is not available yet, leading to surgical exploration is suspicious cases. A positive fistula test can be helpful, but a negative result can be inconclusive in many instances. TB imaging studies can identify middle-ear abnormalities known to be associated with PLF.

Following a comprehensive evaluation, the etiology of childhood SNHL may prove inconclusive in about 30 to 40% of cases, complicating family counseling about the risk of hearing loss in future offspring and the likelihood of further deterioration of their child's hearing.

GENETIC HEARING LOSS

Genetic hearing loss may be of congenital or delayed (postnatal) onset; conductive, sensorineural, or mixed type; mild to profound in degree; stable, fluctuating, and/or progressive; unilateral or bilateral and symmetrical or asymmetrical in severity and configuration; syndromic (involving identifiable characteristics in other systems) or nonsyndromic (involving only hearing loss). Over 400 different genetic syndromes, some exceedingly rare, that include hearing loss as a component have been identified. Traditionally, hearing loss syndromes have been classified according to involvement of other organ systems such as craniofacial/cervical, skeletal, integumentary, ocular, neurological, renal, metabolic, and other. Nonsyndromic hearing disorders (i.e., hearing loss only) have been characterized according to audiologic characteristics, age of onset, presence or absence of progression, and mode of inheritance. Identification of genes that are responsible for both syndromic and nonsyndromic disorders allows greater precision in classifying losses on the basis of actual genes and related gene products involved.

Various authors have estimated the distribution of dominant versus recessive versus sex-linked inheritance patterns among populations of children with genetic losses, both syndromic and nonsyndromic. There is general agreement that recessive inheritance is definitely most common and that nonsyndromic losses outnumber syndromic. Most authors attribute 75 to 80% of genetic deafness to autosomal recessive genes and 18 to 20% to autosomal dominant genes, with the remainder classified as X-linked or chromosomal disorders. Only recently has the role of mutations in the mitochondrial genome in the etiology of hearing loss been appreciated. Although as many as 200 genes may be involved in nonsyndromic hearing loss, it is becoming increasingly clear that a much smaller number of genes account for a substantial proportion of these losses, raising the possibility of clinically-useful genetic screening and diagnostic procedures in the near future.

Basic Genetic Principles

Single gene disorders

Human genes, which comprise molecular codes for inherited factors, are arranged linearly on 23 pairs of chromosomes, including 22 pairs of autosomes and one pair of sex chromosomes. The genotype for a specific trait may consist of two identical alleles (*homozygous*) or two different alleles (*heterozygous*). An autosomal allele that is dominant can be phenotypically expressed in both the homozygous and heterozygous state, whereas an autosomal recessive allele must be present homozygously to be expressed. An X-linked (i.e., sex chromosome-linked) recessive gene is expressed in the *hemizygous state* in the male because the Y chromosome does not carry a complementary allele. Dominant traits typically are transmitted from one generation to the next, with a 50% chance of an affected heterozygote transmitting the gene to each child. The children of parents who are heterozygotic (carriers) for a recessive gene experience a 25% recurrence risk. A heterozygous female may carry an X-linked recessive trait without expressing it, but her male offspring have a 50% chance of inheriting the gene that, in the absence of a second X chromosome, would be expressed. The female carrier's female offspring run a 50% risk of carrying the trait, whereas the sons of an affected male with a sex-linked trait will not be affected. All of the affected male's daughter will inherit his X chromosome carrying the defective gene.

Due to lack of penetrance, not all individuals who are heterozygous for a dominant gene manifest the disorder. Variable expressivity may cause different family members to show differing manifestations of the gene. Phenotypic expression may be influenced by environmental factors and gene-gene interaction cases.

Chromosomal disorders

Extra or absent chromosomal material may yield varied congenital anomalies and developmental delays.

Among *trisomies* (three copies of an entire chromosome being present) are *Trisomy 21* (Down's syndrome), which is more common and less severe than either *Trisomy 13* (Patau syndrome) or *Trisomy 18* (Edward syndrome). Trisomies of other autosomal chromosomes are generally lethal unless there is also a normal cell line (*mosaicism*). In contrast, the effects of extra sex chromosomes are much milder than autosomal trisomies. In other disorders, segments of one or more chromosomes may be deleted or duplicated, resulting in phenotypes that are dependent upon the quantity and origin of the involved chromosomal material.

In genetic disorders, accurate delineation of the phenotype, including a search for subtle elements of hearing loss syndromes, is essential.

Genetic Linkage Analysis and Gene Identification

Linkage analysis is a means of finding the location of a gene on a chromosome. Two genetic loci that are in close enough proximity on the same chromosome to be transmitted together more often than expected by chance are described as being linked. The location of a specific gene that is responsible for a disorder can be sought by determining if the disease is linked with one or more of markers with a known location in the genome. The absence of linkage between a disorder and a marker excludes the gene from that portion of the genome.

If a particular trait demonstrates linkage in some families but not in others, *genetic heterogeneity* is established. Through linkage analysis, genes causing different clinical subtypes of genetic syndromes have been localized. For example, Usher syndrome types 1 and 2 are distinguished on the basis of audiologic and vestibular characteristics, whereas Waardenburg syndrome types I and II differ by the presence or absence of dystopia canthorum, respectively. Other subtypes of Usher and Waardenburg syndromes that involve additional genes presently cannot be differentiated clinically. Nonsyndromic hearing loss also demonstrates a high degree of heterogeneity, with at least 18 dominant and 20 recessive genes localized. Inbred or isolated study populations reduce heterogeneity for recessive traits, whereas studies of large kindreds are helpful in reducing heterogeneity for dominant conditions.

After a gene has been localized to a specific chromosomal region, physical mapping techniques can isolate deoxyribonucleic acid (DNA) from the critical region to compare with sequences for known genes (*candidate genes*) from the region under study. Homologous genes from lower animals (e.g., mice) also can be considered as possible candidates for a human disorder. The gene is identified positively when mutations are present in that gene in all affected individuals and no mutations are detected in those who are unaffected. The precise mutation that disrupts the function of a particular gene may vary from family to family.

Inner Ear Structural Malformations

The cochlea reaches full growth (2.75 turns) by the end of the eighth week of gestation, and hearing loss may be associated with agenesis or dysgenesis of inner ear components. About 20% of children with congenital SNHL have evidence on high-resolution CT of subtle or severe abnormalities of the inner ear (approximately 65% bilateral, 35% unilateral). Jackler et al's classification system correlates the type of deformity observed with the timing of developmental insult.[14]

SPECIAL CONSIDERATION:

About 20% of children with congenital SHNL have evidence on CT of subtle to severe abnormalities of the middle ear.

Historically, inner ear malformations typically have been classified on the basis of histopathologic study into six different groups.

Michel aplasia

In *Michel aplasia,* the structures of the inner ear fail to develop with near complete agenesis of the petrous portion of the TB, probably resulting from an insult prior to the third gestational week. The external and middle ear usually remain unaffected, and the ear is anacusic. The deformity is evident on TB imaging studies, but can be confused with labyrinthitis ossificans. Neither conventional amplification nor cochlear implantation is useful in these patients, but brainstem implantation at the level of the cochlear nucleus may become feasible in the future. Mouse studies indicate that a number of dif-

ferent genes can produce Michel aplasia. Autosomal dominant inheritance has been observed, but recessive inheritance also is likely.

Mondini aplasia

In *Mondini aplasia,* only the basal cochlear coil can be identified clearly. The upper coils assume a cloacal form without an interscalar septum and the endolymphatic aqueduct typically is enlarged. A developmental arrest at approximately the sixth week of gestation is the most likely antecedent event in these cases. Mondini Aplasia is not necessarily bilateral, and both dominant and recessive, syndromic and nonsyndromic forms have been described, including occurrence with Pendred, Waardenburg, Branchio-oto-renal (BOR), Treacher Collins, and Wildervanck Syndromes. Mondini aplasia also has been associated with nongenetic etiologies, such as congenital CMV infection. Early rehabilitative intervention with conventional amplification is recommended to take advantage of residual neurosensory structures. The hearing loss may progress in some affected youngsters.

Scheibe aplasia

The bony labyrinth is normally differentiated in *Scheibe aplasia* as is the superior membranous labyrinth including the utricle and semicircular canals (SCCs). In contrast, the organ of Corti is poorly differentiated, the tectorial membrane malformed, and the scala media reduced in size by collapse of Reissner's membrane. The most common form of inner ear aplasia, Scheibe aplasia can be inherited as an autosomal recessive nonsyndromic trait and has been observed in TBs from patients with both recessive syndromes (e.g., Jervell and Lange-Nielsen, Refsum, and Usher) and dominant syndromes (e.g., Waardenburg). In some cases, conventional amplification may be beneficial.

Alexander aplasia

Alexander aplasia of the cochlear duct affects the organ of Corti and ganglion cells at the level of the basal coil and is generally associated with a high-frequency hearing loss that may benefit from amplification.

Enlarged vestibular aqueduct

An *enlarged vestibular aqueduct* (EVA), identified by TB imaging, may be associated with early-onset

SNHL that can be fluctuating or progressive. The deformity is typically bilateral and may be accompanied by vertigo or incoordination in affected children. Other cochlear and SCC deformities may be associated with EVA. Surgical intervention, including endolymphatic shunt, has not proven efficacious in these children. Some family studies suggest dominant inheritance, but recessive inheritance also is possible in sporadic cases. The deformity also has been identified in patients with Pendred's syndrome.

Semicircular canal malformations

The *semicircular canals* (SCCs) begin to form during the sixth gestational week. The superior SCC (SSCC) is the first to form and the lateral SCC (LSCC) develops last. In studies by Jackler et al., SSCC deformities were invariably accompanied by LSCC anomalies, whereas LSCC abnormalities often occurred in isolation.[14] Deformities of the LSCC are the most commonly identified inner ear malformation on radiographic imaging studies.

AT A GLANCE . . .

Inner Ear Malformations

- Michel Aplasia
- Mondoni Aplasia
- Scheibe Aplasia
- Alexander Aplasia
- Enlarged Vestibular Aqueduct
- Semicircular Canal Malformations

Autosomal Dominant Disorders

Variable expressivity, which is characteristic of dominant genes, often leads to different phenotypic characteristics in various affected members of the same family. As a result of decreased penetrance of some dominant genes, an obligate gene carrier may not have any detectable phenotypic expression (Table 18–1).

Waardenburg Syndrome

Waardenburg syndrome features include unilateral or bilateral SNHL, pigmentary anomalies (e.g., white forelock, heterochromia irides, premature graying, and vitiligo), and craniofacial features such as dystopia canthorum, broad nasal root, and synophrys. White forelock is expressed in only 20 to 30% of cases and age of initial appearance varies. Two different types of Waardenburg syndrome can be distinguished by the presence (WSI) or absence (WSII) of dystopia canthorum. Twenty percent of individuals with WSI and 50% of those with WSII demonstrate a hearing loss. Objective measures of the distances between landmarks such as the inner canthi, the pupils, and outer canthi are helpful in substantiating dystopia canthorum.

Substantially, all WSI is caused by mutations of the PAX3 gene that is located on chromosome 2q37.[27] The murine homolog of this gene produces a condition in mice called "splotch," which includes pigmentary and ocular abnormalities in the heterozygote and deafness in the homozygote. About 20% of WSII cases are attributable to a mutation of the MITF gene (microphthalmia transcription factor) on chromosome 3p.[28] Analysis of the specific mutations within the PAX3 in various families has correlated the array of phenotypic traits expressed with the class of mutation that is present. Forty-two known mutations were grouped in five categories ranging from amino acid substitution in the paired domain to deletion of the entire gene. The odds of having eye pigment abnormality, skin pigmentation, and white forelock was from 2 to 8 times greater among affecteds who had homeodomain deletions and Pro-Ser-Tjr-rich region than among those who had an amino acid substitution in the gene's homeodomain. Gene products resulting from different types of mutations within the same gene appear to lead to the expression of different components of the phenotype.

Stickler syndrome

The traits associated with *Stickler syndrome* include a small jaw, often accompanied by a cleft palate (Pierre Robin sequence); severe myopia, which may lead to retinal detachment or cataracts; hypermobility and joint enlargement with early adult onset arthritis; and spondyloepiphyseal dysplasia in some cases. Significant SNHL or mixed hearing loss, often progressive, is found in approximately 15% of affected individuals, with lesser degrees of hearing loss being present in up to 80% of cases. Variable expressivity can make diagnosis challenging, and various mutations of the type II collagen gene

TABLE 18–1:   Identified Genes Causing Hearing Impairment in Humans

Disorder (MIM#)*	Inheritance	Linkage	Gene	Reference
Alport syndrome	AR	xq22	COL4A5	Barker et al., 1990[15]
Alport syndrome	AR	2q36–q37	COL4A3, COL4A4	Mochizuki, 1994[3]
Branchio-Oto-Renal syndrome (BOR)	AD	8q13.3	EYA1	Abdelhak et al., 1997[16]
Jervell & Lange-Nielsen (JLNS1)	AR	11p15.5	KVLQT1	Neyroud et al., 1997[17]
Jervell & Lange-Nielsen (JLNS2)	AR	21q22.1–q22.2	KCNE1	Tyson et al., 1997;[18] Schulze-Bahr et al., 1997[19]
Norrie Disease	XL	Xp11.3	Norrin	Berger et al., 1992;[20] Chen et al., 1992[21]
Pendred syndrome	AR	7q21–34	PDS	Everett et al., 1997[22]
Stickler syndrome (STL1)	AD	12q13.11–q13.2	COL2A1	Williams et al., 1996[23]
Stickler syndrome (STL2)	AD	6p21.3	COL11A2	Vikkula et al., 1995[24]
Stickler syndrome (STL3)	AD	1p21	COL11A1	Richards et al., 1996[25]
Treacher Collins syndrome	AD	5q32–q33.1	TCOF1	Treacher Collins Syndrome Collaborative Group, 1996[26]
Waardenburg syndrome type I (WSI)	AD	2q35	PAX3	Tassabehji et al., 1992[27]
Waardenburg syndrome type II (WSII)	AD	3p14.1–p12.3	MITF	Tassabehji et al., 1992[28]
Waardenburg syndrome type III	AD	2q35	PAX3	Hoth et al., 1993[29]
Waardenburg syndrome type IV	AD	13q22	EDNRB	Attie et al., 1995[30]
Waardenburg syndrome type IV	AD	20q13.2–q13.3	EDN3	Edery et al., 1996[31]
Waardenburg syndrome type IV	AD	22q13	SOX10	Pingault et al., 1998[32]
Usher Syndrome				
USH1A	AR	14q32	Unknown	Kaplan et al., 1992[33]
USH1B	AR	11q13.5	MYO7A	Weil et al., 1995[34]
USH1C	AR	11p15.1	Unknown	Smith et al., 1992[35]
USH1D	AR	10q	Unknown	Wayne et al., 1996[36]
USH1E	AR	21q	Unknown	Chaib et al., 1997[37]
USH1F	AR	10	Unknown	Wayne et al., 1996[36]
USH2A	AR	1q41	USH2A	Kimberling et al., 1990;[38] Eudy et al., 1998[39]
USH2B	AR	5q14.3–q21.3	Unknown	Pieke-Dahl et al., 1998[40]
USH3	AR	3q21–q225	Unknown	Sankila et al., 1995[41]

Adapted from Van Camp G Smith RJH. Hereditary Hearing Loss Homepage. World Wide Web
*Mendelian Inheritance in Man.

(COL2A1) on chromosome 12 have been found in some individuals.[42] Kneist syndrome and congenital spondyloepiphyseal dysplasia which also include progressive SNHL, are associated with other mutations of the same COL2A1 gene.

Branchio-oto-renal (BOR)

Branchio-oto-renal (BOR) or *Melnick-Fraser Syndrome* includes ear pits (rarely tags) and cervical fistulae together with renal involvement that ranges in severity from agenesis and renal failure to minor asymptomatic dysplasia that is detectable by ultrasound or intravenous pyelography. Hearing loss in BOR patients may be sensorineural, conductive, or mixed, and Mondini aplasia is present in some individuals. The gene, identified on chromosome 8q, is the human homolog of the developmental Drosophila gene eyes absent.[16]

Treacher Collins syndrome

Abnormalities comprising *Treacher Collins syndrome* (mandibulofacial dysostosis) may be microtia, aural meatal atresia, and in about 30% of cases, conductive hearing impairment that may be accompanied by SNHL and vestibular dysfunction. Typical facial findings include malar hypoplasia, downward slanting palpebral fissures, coloboma of the lower eyelids, and a hypoplastic mandible. Bilateral symmetrical facies and eyelid coloboma serve to distinguish Treacher Collins syndrome from the similar, but unilateral, findings observed in Goldenhar's syndrome and other oculoauricular vertebral syndromes. Although ossicular malformation often is present in these disorders, otologic reconstructive surgery in these youngsters can be challenging even in the hands of experienced surgeons. Diminished middle-ear volume and an extremely-aberrant location of the facial nerve may preclude surgical intervention in some cases. Treacher Collins syndrome is transmitted as an autosomal dominant pattern with high penetrance that may result from a new mutation in about 60% of cases, whereas the oculo-auriculo-vertebral (OAV) spectrum is sporadic and probably multifactorial. The TCOF1 gene for Treacher Collins syndrome on chromosome 5q codes for a protein named treacle, which appears to function in early craniofacial development.[26,43] Variable expression within families suggests that other genes can modify expression of the treacle protein.

Neurofibromatosis

"Café-au-lait spots" (i.e., light brown, variable-sized pigmented spots) and multiple fibromas are the cardinal traits of neurofibromatosis, which genetically is heterogeneous with two distinct forms. *Classic neurofibromatosis (von Recklinghausen disease or NFI)* occurs in 1:3000 persons and is characterized by a large number of café-au-lait spots and cutaneous neurofibromas together with plexiform neuromas, pseudoarthrosis (e.g., tibia), Lisch nodules (hamartomas) of the iris, and optic gliomas. Mental retardation, blindness, or hearing loss resulting from central nervous system (CNS) lesions is relatively uncommon. True acoustic neuromas that are nearly always unilateral occur in only 5% of cases. Longitudinal audiologic follow-up is crucial in children with this disorder.

Central neurofibromatosis (NFII), a genetically distinct disorder, involves bilateral acoustic neuromas (vestibular schwannomas) that tend to be slow-growing until young adulthood when tinnitus and vestibular dysfunction become the presenting features. Café-au-lait spots and cutaneous neurofibromas are fewer in number than with NFI. Both NFI and NFII are inherited as autosomal dominants with high penetrance but variable expressivity. A nerve growth factor gene on chromosome 17 is responsible for NFI,[44] whereas NFII is attributable to a mutation of a tumor suppressor gene on chromosome number 22.[45]

AT A GLANCE . . .

Autosomal Dominant Disorders

Waardenburg Syndrome: unilateral or bilateral SNHL, pigmentary anomalies (white forelock, heterochromia irides, etc.), craniofacial features (dystopia canthorum, broad nasal root, synophrys)

Stickler Syndrome: SNHL or mixed hearing loss, Pierre Robin sequence, severe myopia, hypermobility and joint enlargement, spondyloepiphyseal dysplasia

Branchio-Oto-Renal (BOR): SNHL, CHL, or mixed hearing loss; ear pits; renal abnormalities

Treacher Collins Syndrome: SNHL and CHL, microtia and aural atresia, malar and mandibular hypoplasia, downward slanting palpebral fissures, coloboma of the lower eyelids

Neurofibromatosis: *NFI* (classic neurofibromatosis): café-au-lait spots, cutaneous neurofibromas, pseudoarthrosis, Lisch nodules of iris, optic gliomas, and rarely, mental retardation, blindness, or hearing loss. *NFII* (central neurofibromatosis): bilateral acoustic neuromas, café-au-lait spots, cutaneous neurofibromas

---

Otosclerosis

In some cases, *otosclerosis* is inherited as an autosomal dominant trait with decreased penetrance, estimated at 25 to 40%, with a possible hormonal influence suggested by a preponderance of affected males. Measles virus particles identified within the bony overgrowth suggest a possible interaction with the viral genome. One gene causing otosclerosis has been localized to chromosome 15.[45a]

Nonsyndromic Autosomal Dominant Hearing Loss

Konigsmark and Gorlin distinguished several types of nonsyndromic, autosomal dominant hearing loss.[46]

Dominant progressive hearing loss

Dominant progressive hearing losses (DPHL) are nonsyndromic and noncongenital SNHLs that have varying ages of onset and rates of progression. Idiopathic as regards etiology, DPHL differ from otosclerosis by the absence of ossicular and otic capsule involvement and from presbycusis by the earlier age of onset. Although certain varieties of DPHL inexorably progress in degree to severe and profound hearing losses, initial frequency involvement may be quite different among families. Konigsmark and Gorlin described early onset, high-frequency, mid-frequency, and low-frequency dominant progressive losses.[46] Advances in gene identification are having an important impact in our understanding of DPHL and should lead to identification of subclasses grouped according to the involved gene. Thus far, at least 19 genes causing DPHL have been localized. Two DPHL genes have been identified, both on 5q. DFNA1 is due to a mutation in a gene that is homologous to the Drosophila gene diaphanous and is thought to be related to actin polymerization. DFNA15 is due to mutations of POU4F3, a transcription factor. How these genes cause hearing loss is still unknown (Table 18-2).

Recessive Disorders

Approximately 80% of childhood genetic deafness is inherited in an autosomal recessive pattern, with about 50% of cases involving recognizable syndromes. Identification of recessively-inherited syndromes is not obscured generally by decreased penetrance and variable expressivity as with dominant conditions. Identification of recessive hearing loss syndromes requires a diligent search for the other syndromic components.

Usher syndrome

Usher syndrome, characterized by SNHL and progressive retinitis pigmentosa, has an estimated frequency of 3/100,000 in Scandinavia and 4.4/100,000 in the United States. Three clinically distinct subtypes have been described that differ with regard to severity or progression of the hearing loss and the extent of vestibular system involvement. Usher *type 1* (USH1) patients manifest congenital bilateral profound hearing loss and absent vestibular function,[33] whereas *type 2* (USH2) patients sustain moderate, usually downward sloping, SNHL and normal vestibular function.[38] Most *type 3* (USH3) patients, who demonstrate progressive hearing loss and variable vestibular dysfunction, have Norwegian ancestry.[27] USH2 is the most common type, accounting for 50% or more of cases in some reported series.[26] Genetic heterogeneity has been documented within as well as between these subtypes (see Table 18-1). Gene localization studies have identified at least six

TABLE 18–2: Genes Causing Nonsyndromic Hereditary Hearing Loss: Dominant

Locus Name	Type of Loss	Location	Gene	Reference
DFNA1	Progressive	5q31	HDIA1	Leon et al., 1992;[47] Lynch et al., 1997[48]
DFNA2	Progressive	1p34	GJB3 kCNQ4	Coucke et al., 1994[49]
DFNA3	Congenital	13q12	GJB2	Chaib et al., 1994;[50] Denoyelle,[51] 1998
DFNA4	Progressive	19q13	unknown	Chen et al., 1995[52]
DFNA5	Progressive	7p15	DFNA5	van Camp et al., 1995[53]
DFNA6	Progressive	4p16.3	Unknown	Lesperance et al., 1995[54]
DFNA7	Progressive	1q21-q23	Unknown	Fagerheim et al., 1996[55]
DFNA8	Congenital	11q22-24	TECTA	Krischhofer et al., 1998;[56] Verhoeven et al., 1998[57]
DFNA9	Progressive	14q12-q13	COCH	Manolis et al., 1996[58]
DFNA10	Progressive	6q22-q23	Unknown	O'Neill et al., 1996[59]
DFNA11	Progressive	11q12.3-q21	MYO7A	Tamagawa et al., 1996;[60] Liu et al., 1997[61]
DFNA12	Progressive	11q22-q24	TECTA	Verhoeven et al., 1997;[62] Verhoeven et al., 1998[63]
DFNA13	Unavailable	6p21	Unknown	Brown et al., 1997[64]
DFNA14	Unavailable	4p16	Unknown	Van Camp et al., 1997[65]
DFNA15	Unavailable	5q31	POU4F3	Vahava et al., 1998[66]
DFNA16	Unavailable	2q24	Unknown	Fukushima et al., 1998[67]
DFNA17	Unavailable	22q	Unknown	Lalwani et al., 1998[68]
DFNA18	Unavailable	3q22	Unknown	Boenschet et al., 1998[69]
DFNA19	Unavailable	10 pericentromeric	Unknown	Green et al., 1998[70]

Adapted from Van Camp G, Smith RJH. Hereditary Hearing Loss Homepage. World Wide Web URL:http://dnalab-www.uia.ac.be/dnalab/hhh/. Retrieved November, 1998.

different genes for type 1 and at least two for type 2. Only type 3 appears to be attributable to a single gene. Usher syndrome *type 1B* (USH1B) results from mutations in a gene that codes for the unconventional myosin VIIA, which appears to have a role in trafficking vessicles in photoreceptors and hair cells in the cochlea. The USH2A gene on the long arm of chromosome 1q41 encodes a protein that has laminin epidermal growth factor and fibronectin type III motifs. These motifs are generally found in proteins that are components of the basal lamina and extracellular matrix and in cell adhesion molecules.

An ophthalmologic evaluation, critical in the diagnostic work-up of suspected Usher syndrome patients, should include electroretinographic (ERG) studies that have been reported as subnormal in 2- to 3-year-old patients utilizing periorbital electrode placement. If Usher syndrome is diagnosed early, it can influence rehabilitative and educational program plans that make allowances for a gradual decrease in visual acuity as the child ages.

Pendred syndrome

In *Pendred syndrome,* early onset, often progressive, SNHL is associated with abnormal iodine metabolism, producing a euthyroid goiter. There is a high likelihood of a Mondini aplasia or enlarged vestibular aqueduct in Pendred patients. The perchlorate discharge test demonstrating an abnormal organification of nonorganic iodine yields the highest level of diagnostic certainty (a few false positives), although it involves some exposure to radioactive material and should be utilized only in selected cases. The therapy of choice is exogenous thyroid hormone, whereas surgical extirpation of the gland has proven ineffective and is not recommended.

Recessive inheritance is demonstrable clearly in a large number of Pendred families, but several reported pedigrees in which hearing loss and/or thyroid problems occur in other generations raise the possibility of dominant inheritance with variable expression. A gene for Pendred syndrome has been identified on chromosome 7q in a number of families with clear autosomal recessive inheritance.[22] This gene produces a protein called pendrin, which appears to be a sulfate transporter. Additional studies will clarify questions regarding possible heterogeneity and whether expression may occur in some heterozygotes.

Jervell and Lange-Nielsen syndrome

Jervell and Lange-Nielsen syndrome patients have a recessively-inherited congenital SNHL in conjunction with a cardiac conduction defect that can lead to syncopal episodes and even sudden death. The hearing loss is usually severe and an electrocardiogram reveals large T-waves and prolongation of the Q–T interval, which can manifest itself in bouts of syncope as early as the first 2 to 3 years of life. Beta-adrenergic blocking agents are efficacious in managing the cardiac component of the syndrome, reiterating the need to obtain an electrocardiogram on children with early-onset hearing loss of uncertain etiology. Mutations of a potassium channel gene. KVLQT1 on chromosome 11p, have been implicated in some but not all forms of Jervell and Lange-Nielsen syndrome.[17] The dominantly-inherited long Q–T syndrome (*Romano-Ward syndrome*) is attributable to other mutations in the same gene. Heterozygous carriers for Jervell and Lange-Nielsen show a prolonged Q–T interval that can remain asymptomatic.

AT A GLANCE . . .

Recessive Disorders

Usher Syndrome: SNHL, progressive retinitis pigmentosa
Pendred Syndrome: SNHL, euthyroid goiter
Jervell and Lange-Nielsen Syndrome: SNHL, cardiac conduction defect

---

Recessive Nonsyndromic Hearing Loss

Based on clinical studies, Konigsmark and Gorlin's classification of nonsyndromic recessive SNHL comprised three subtypes: congenital severe-to-profound; congenital moderate; and early-onset, with typical onset at age 1.5 years progressing to profound loss by age 6 years.[46] Gene linkage studies have identified at least 20 loci for recessive nonsyndromic hearing loss (Table 18–3).

SPECIAL CONSIDERATION:

Gene linkage studies have identified at least 20 loci for recessive nonsyndromic hearing loss.

TABLE 18–3:   Genes Causing Nonsyndromic Hereditary Hearing Loss: Recessive

Locus Name	Type of Loss	Location	Gene	Reference
DFNB1	Congenital	13q12	GJB2	Guilford et al., 1994;[71] Kelsell et al., 1997[72]
DFNB2	Congenital	11q13.5	MYO7A	Guilford et al., 1994;[73] Liu et al., 1997;[74] Weil et al., 1997[75]
DFNB3	Congenital	17p11.2	MYO15	Friedman et al., 1995;[76] Wang et al., 1998[77]
DFNB4	Congenital	7q31	PDS	Baldwin et al., 1995;[78] Li et al., 1998[79]
DFNB5	Congenital	14q12	Unknown	Fukushima et al., 1995[80]
DFNB6	Congenital	3p14–p21	Unknown	Fukushima et al., 1995[81]
DFNB7	Not available	9q13–q21	Unknown	Jain et al., 1995[82]
DFNB8	Not available	21q22	Unknown	Veske et al., 1996[83]
DFNB9	Congenital	2p22–p23	OTOF	Chaib et al., 1996[84]
DFNB10	Congenital	21q22.3	Unknown	Bonne-Tamir et al., 1996[85]
DFNB11	Not available	9q13–q21	Unknown	Scott et al., 1996[86]
DFNB12	Congenital	10q21–22	Unknown	Chaib et al., 1996[87]
DFNB13	Unknown	7q34–36	Unknown	Mustapha et al., 1998[88]
DFNB15	Not available	3q21–q25 19p13	Unknown	Chen et al., 1997[89]
DFNB16	Not available	15q21–q22	Unknown	Campbell et al., 1997[90]
DFNB17	Not available	7q31	Unknown	Greinwald et al., 1998[91]
DFNB18	Not available	11p14–15.1	Unknown	Jain et al., 1998[92]
DFNB19	Not available	18p11	Unknown	Green et al., 1998[93]

Adapted from Van Camp GI, Smith RJH. Hereditary Hearing Loss Homepage. World Wide Web URL:http://dnalab-www.uia.ac.be/dnalab/hhh/. Retrieved November, 1998.

The gene DFNB1 on chromosome 13q11–12 codes for connexin 26 (CX26), and mutations in this gene may account for as much as half of nonsyndromic recessive hearing loss[20] A class of membrane proteins, *connexins,* form gap-junction channels with similar connexins in other cells to allow the exchange of electrolytes, second messengers, and metabolites. About 13 different connexins have been identified in mammals, and many are distributed widely. CX26 is downregulated in tumor tissue and significantly upregulated in synchronized cells. Cochlear histopathology in animals have identified CX26 in two cell groups, including such nonsensory cells as interdental spiral limbus cells, inner sulcus cells, and organ of Corti supporting cells, as well as connective-tissue cells such as spiral limbus and spiral ligament fibrocytes, basal and intermediate stria vascularis cells, and mesenchymal cells that line the scala vestibuli. The most common CX26 mutation identified in families with DFNB1 is called 30delG, which represents a G deletion at a point that appears to be a hot spot for mutation (Fig. 18–2). The homozygous frequency for the mutation is estimated at about 1/10,000 which would suggest that this particular mutation may be responsible for about 20% of hereditary childhood hearing loss.

Sex-Linked Disorders

Sex-linked inheritance of hearing loss may account for as much as 6% of nonsyndromic profound losses in males (Table 18–4).

Norrie syndrome

The sex-linked disorder *Norrie syndrome* includes congenital or rapidly-progressive blindness, pseudoglioma development, opacification, and ocular degeneration resulting in eventual microphthalmia. Progressive SNHL, with onset in the second or third decade, is found in about one-third of Norrie patients. The Norrie syndrome gene has been localized to Xp11.4, and a number of families demonstrate variable deletions of chromosomal material in this region.[99]

Oto-palato-digital syndrome

Hypertelorism (increased interocular distance), flat midface, small nose, and cleft palate are all components of *Oto-palato-digital syndrome.* Affected individuals have short stature with broad fingers and toes that are variable in length. The space between the first and second toe is also excessively wide.

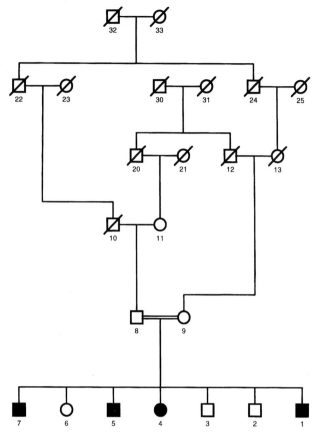

Figure 18–2: Gene for connexin 26—recessive nonsyndromic hearing loss. Pedigree demonstrates consanguinity.

An ossicular malformation, potentially amenable to surgical correction, accounts for the associated conductive component of the hearing loss. Some mild manifestations of this disorder have been documented in female carriers of the gene, which has been to localized to Xq28.[100]

Wildervanck syndrome

Wildervanck syndrome encompasses the *Klippel-Feil malformation* (i.e., fused cervical vertebrae),

SNHL or mixed hearing loss attributable to a bony inner ear malformation, and sixth cranial nerve paralysis resulting in retraction of the eye on lateral gaze (i.e., *Duane retraction syndrome*). The disorder affects females almost exclusively, suggesting the possibility of X-linked dominant inheritance or polygenic inheritance that is lethal in males. About one-third of individuals with isolated Klippel-Fell sequence also have hearing loss, whereas fewer than 10% of those with Duane retraction syndrome also suffer hearing loss.

Alport syndrome

Alport syndrome involves progressive SNHL and renal disease of varying severity. The hearing loss may not be detected until adolescence, whereas the nephritis, which can manifest itself as hematuria in infancy (e.g. ''red diaper''), is typically asymptomatic for several years prior to onset of renal insufficiency. The renal involvement in males tends to be severe, and prior to the advent of renal dialysis and transplantation often caused death from uremia before age 30 years. Although most cases of Alport syndrome are due to an X-linked mutation of a type 4 collagen gene (COL4A5), the disorder is genetically heterogeneous. Mutation of an autosomal type 4 collagen gene leads to a recessively-inherited form of Alport syndrome, but the disorder is still more severe in affected males.

Nonsyndromic X-Linked Hearing Loss

It is known that the X chromosome contains at least six genetic loci for nonsyndromic hearing loss. Patients who have X-linked stapes fixation with a perilymphatic gusher present with a progressive mixed hearing loss and apparent stapes fixation. Attempts at stapedotomy carry a high risk of perilymphatic gusher, resulting in significant attendant SNHL. Sen-

TABLE 18–4:   Genes Causing Nonsyndromic Hereditary Hearing Loss: X-Linked

Locus Name	Type of Loss	Location	Gene	Reference
DFN1	Progressive	Xq22	DDP	Tranebjaerg et al., 1995[94]
DFN2	Congenital	Xq22	Unknown	Tyson et al., 1996[95]
DFN3	Progressive Mixed (Gusher)	Xq21.1	POU3F4	de Kok et al., 1995[96]
DFN4	Congenital	Xp21.2	Unknown	Lalwani et al., 1994[97]
DFN6	Progressive	Xp22	Unknown	del Castillo et al., 1996[98]

Adapted from Van Camp G, Smith RJH. Hereditary Hearing Loss Homepage. World Wide Web URL:http://dnalab-www.uia.ac.be/dnalab/hhh/. Retrieved November, 1998.

syndrome (oculo-auriculo-vertebral dysplasia) appears to be transmitted in an autosomal dominant pattern, but this may represent fortuitous clustering of cases.

tinel preoperative findings include an enlarged internal auditory canal (IAC) with thinning or absence of bone at the base of the cochlea. The gene for this disorder has been identified as the POU3F4 gene at Xq21, which is located in close proximity to a choroideremia gene. Deletion of both genes yields the contiguous gene syndrome of choroideremia, hearing loss, and mental retardation. Stapes surgery should be undertaken with caution in any male child or adolescent, particularly one with an X-linked family history or with choroideremia.

Multifactorial Genetic Disorders

Examples of disorders that are attributable to an array of genetic factors that interact with environmental influences include clefting (i.e., cleft lip/palate) syndromes that involve CHL and the microtia/hemifacial microsomia/Goldenhar Spectrum that encompasses preauricular tags/pits, vertebral anomalies such as hypoplastic or hemivertebrae in the cervical region, epibulbar dermoids, and coloboma of the upper lid. In some families, *Goldenhar*

Autosomal Chromosomal Syndromes

Autosomal chromosomal syndromes often involve general developmental delays. In Down's syndrome (Trisomy 21), middle ear and mastoid disease is typical but residual SNHL also may be present. Infants with the more severe Trisomy 13 often succumb as neonates, but significant SNHL may occur in survivors.

Turner's syndrome, resulting from monosomy for all or part of one X chromosome, often is detected during evaluation of a girl for delayed puberty. Typical findings include gonadal dysgenesis, short stature, webbed neck, and/or shield chest. SNHL or mixed hearing loss, which often progresses in adulthood, may be the initial presentation in prepubertal girls.

Mitochondrial Inheritance

Mitochondria, small intracytoplasmic organelles, contain pieces of nonnuclear DNA in ring form. A typical mitochondrion may contain two to ten copies of the mitochondrial genome (about 16 kilobases), comprising genes for messenger, ribosomal, and transfer RNAs that are necessary for mitochondrial protein synthesis. Interacting with proteins encoded by nuclear DNA, mitochondrial proteins facilitate energy production through adenosine triphosphate (ATP) synthesis and oxidative phosphorylation. Mitochondrial gene mutations produce a disproportionate effect on tissues, such as muscle that requires high levels of energy production. Mutations are more common in mitochondrial DNA as compared with nuclear DNA, whereas mitochondrial DNA repair mechanisms are less effective. Of the hundreds of mitochondria in each cell, only a fraction may contain a specific mutation, a condition known as *heteroplasmy,* and different proportions of mutated mitochondria may be present in different tissues. Mitochondrial disorders are likely to involve progressive neuromuscular degeneration with ataxia, ophthalmoplegia, and progressive hearing loss. Ragged red fibers identified histopathologically on muscle biopsy are a classic finding in mitochondrial disorders with muscle involvement. Known mitochondrial disorders include Kearns-Sayre, MELAS (mitochondrial encephalopathy, lactic acidosis, and stroke), MERRF (myoclonic epilepsy with ragged red fibers), and Lebers Hereditary Optic Neuropathy. Mitochondrial DNA mutations that produce isolated progressive hearing loss also have been discovered.

Matrilineal inheritance that affects male and female offspring equally is characteristic of mitochondrial disorders because sperm transmit few if any mitochondria and nearly the entire contribution originates from the egg. All of the offspring of a mother who is homoplasmic for a mitochondrial mutation will be affected. A mitochondrial deletion has been found responsible for a disorder involving diabetes, progressive hearing loss, and stroke. Nonsyndromic hearing loss in a few families has been attributed to the combined action of a mitochondrial mutation along with a recessive mutation in a nuclear gene. One example involves nucleotide #1555 in a large Arabic kindred. This identical mutation, as well as several other mitochondrial mutations, leads to enhanced sensitivity to the ototoxic effects of aminoglycosides such as streptomycin. Milder hearing loss often is observed in family members having these mutations but who are not exposed yet to aminoglycosides. Maternal relatives of individuals who sustain hearing loss following standard therapeutic doses of aminoglycosides should be screened for these mutations.

Evaluation and Genetic Counseling

Before starting genetic counseling, it is important to search for the etiology of the hearing loss. If no evidence of nongenetic etiology exists, a genetic disorder must be suspected. A detailed family history, including construction of a pedigree chart to include third-degree relatives, should be coupled with queries regarding the hearing status of other family members and the occurrence of subtle syndromic manifestations such as ear pits in the family. Previous family audiologic data is useful in identifying a familial progressive hearing loss. Consanguinity should be ruled out, particularly among geographically and culturally isolated populations where multiple intermarriages among families are more common.

A careful prenatal, perinatal, and postnatal medical history should precede a thorough physical examination by a clinical geneticist/dysmorphologist who is cognizant of subtle syndromic features. Further evaluation including TB imaging, laboratory tests, electroretinograms, electrocardiograms, and perchlorate discharge studies may be indicated in selected cases.

Pedigrees from families with inherited hearing impairment may contain marriages between deaf individuals with hearing losses of uncertain etiology. Family tradition may attribute each person's loss to a different nongenetic etiology, such as noise exposure, head trauma, or childhood infections. All reported losses should be plotted on the pedigree and excluded as noninformative only after careful analysis.

Counselors should be aware that many deaf adults are proud of their cultural heritage and unique language (American Sign Language), and they may not regard having a deaf child as particularly burdensome. Boughman et al. have developed specific signs for communicating genetic terminology, and it is essential that an interpreter be available.[101]

Recurrence risks for autosomal dominant disorders depend upon the gene's usual pattern of penetrance. If full penetrance is expected, offspring of an affected individual have a 50% chance of inheriting the disorder, whereas children of unaffected parents are not at risk. If the gene demonstrates decreased penetrance, offspring of an affected parent inherit the gene 50% of the time but may not exhibit the full phenotype. If the gene is nonpenetrant in some cases, a carrier capable of transmission to the next generation may appear unaffected.

Approximately 25% of children born of two heterozygous carriers of an autosomal recessive gene will exhibit deafness, and 50% of offspring will be carriers. The recurrence risk for offspring of a person with recessively-inherited deafness relates to the genetic status of his/her mate. Recurrence risk for heterozygotic carriers of a recessive gene depends upon the frequency of the specific gene in the general population.

Sons of a mother who carries an X-linked recessive disorder gene stand a 50% chance of being affected, whereas daughters have a 50% risk of being carriers. An affected male passes the gene (i.e., X chromosome) to all his daughters but to none of his sons. Recurrence risk for both multifactorial disorders and chromosomal disorders, when both parents have normal karyotypes, can be quite low. The risk for transmission of a mitochondrial disorder is determined by whether the mother is homoplasmic or heteroplasmic, and if other genetic or nongenetic factors are requisite for expression. Offspring of a male with a mitochondrial disorder are not at risk. Empiric risk tables developed by Bieber and Nance take into account various possibilities, including the number of affected and unaffected children in the family.[102] The range of recurrence risk for future offspring, cited for a family with an only child who has an unexplained hearing impairment, is 10 to 16%. Each subsequent normal hearing offspring decreases the empiric recurrence risk, whereas the converse is true if additional children with hearing loss are born.

Historically, reports derived from pupil records at schools for the deaf have attributed about 50% of childhood SNHL to genetic etiologies. About 20 to 25% of cases generally are assigned to identifiable nongenetic causes operative during the prenatal, perinatal, and/or postnatal periods, with the remaining 25 to 30% being of uncertain etiology. Singleton cases of nonsyndromic hearing loss are undoubtedly represented in this latter group.

Introduction of effective vaccines against once prevalent nongenetic SNHL etiologies, including rubella, measles, mumps, and *Hemophilus influenzae* B (HIB) meningitis, has led to their near disappearance in developed countries having mandatory immunization programs. Conjugate vaccines, against *Neisseria meningitidis,* Escherichia coli, nontypable *Hemophilus influenzae,* and pneumococcal

disease, are presently in clinical trials. A conjugate vaccine strategy also is being pursued for CMV infections because of fears regarding the carcinogenic potential of the currently available Towne vaccine. A safe and effective CMV vaccine administered to sexually-active adolescent girls and younger mothers whose young children attend day care centers (known reservoirs of CMV infection) could reduce the incidence of congenital CMV infections significantly. Prenatal diagnosis of intrauterine infections such as toxoplasmosis, utilizing polymerase chain reaction (PCR) technology, facilitates prompt and aggressive prenatal treatment of newly-infected expectant mothers together with their infants in utero. This strategy, coupled with postnatal therapy for congenitally-infected infants, shows promise of ameliorating such sequelae as SNHL. As the prevalence of nongenetic SNHL etiologies is reduced, genetic SNHL assumes greater importance among future cohorts of affected children.

INFECTIOUS ETIOLOGIES

Viruses may access the inner ear from the bloodstream, middle ear, or cerebrospinal fluid (CSF). An inflammatory response generally occurs in the cochlea within 48 hours, and as inflammatory cells disappear from the cochlear duct, the remaining matrix may undergo obliterative calcification. Prenatal rubella, mumps, rubeola, or CMV produce histopathologic changes that are compatible with an endolymphatic labyrinthitis affecting the cochlear duct, saccule, and utricle, suggesting spread via the vessels within the stria vascularis. Direct spread to the perilymphatic spaces along meningeal and neural structures can occur during measles, mumps, or CMV meningoencephalitis leading to eventual fibrosis.

Congenital and Early-Onset Infections

Accurate diagnosis of congenital infections is facilitated by serological testing on maternal and infant sera that is collected concurrently. Transplacentally-transmitted maternal immunoglobulin G (IgG) antibodies gradually decline over the first 6 months of life so that an infant's titer, which is four or more times greater than the mother's, is highly suggestive of active infection. Detection of neonatal immunoglobulin M (IgM) antibodies, which are not transferred transplacentally, aids in diagnosing congenital toxoplasmosis, rubella, and CMV infection.

Cytomegalovirus infection

Approximately 30,000 to 40,000 infants who are born annually in the United States are congenitally infected with CMV herpes group virus. The virus may be transmitted transplacentally during maternal viremia (i.e., from mother to child) or perinatally and postnatally through prolonged (i.e., months) viral shedding in secretions such as breast milk, saliva, urine, semen, and cervical/vaginal fluids. In utero infection of the fetus may occur during both primary maternal infection and following reactivation of latent virus in immune women, although primary infection is nine times more likely to produce significant sequelae in the newborn. Approximately 1 to 4% of susceptible women will experience primary CMV infection during pregnancy, yielding a fetal infection rate of 40%. Reinfection with one of several antigenically-distinct CMV strains also is possible. CMV has a demonstrated affinity for VIII cranial nerve neurons and ependymal cells lining the ventricles of the brain.

Epidemiologically, the overall U.S. infection rate is about 2% per year, but a significantly-increased risk occurs among women being treated in sexually transmitted disease (STD) clinics (35%). As well, child care center employees who are exposed to infants and young children experience an annual seroconversion rate of 11%. Youngsters who acquire CMV during out-of-home care can transmit the virus to their pregnant mothers. Nearly 40% of seronegative mothers who had young children (under 3 years) who were excreting CMV experienced seroconversion during 12 months of observation. Whereas about 1% of live born children have manifest congenital CMV infection, an additional 4 to 10% acquire the infection perinatally and postnatally from virus in cervical secretions, virus in breast milk, and blood transfusions. Among seronegative infants exposed to breast milk from a seropositive mother for more than 1 month, the seroconversion rate is about 40 to 60%.

In order to confirm true congenital CMV infection, the virus must be isolated from the neonate's secretions (e.g., urine or saliva) during the first 2 to 3 weeks of life, following which perinatally-or postnatally-infected infants also may begin shedding virus. Symptoms and signs are observed in only 10 to 15% of congenitally infected infants. Of those,

90% manifest typical cytomegalic inclusion disease (CID) involving the CNS and reticuloendothelial systems with an eventual mortality rate approaching 30%. Common presenting findings include hepatosplenomegaly, petechiae, jaundice, microcephaly, intrauterine growth retardation, and prematurity. By 2 years of age, nearly all CID infants will experience severe mental and perceptual deficits, including severe to profound sensorineural hearing impairment and such ocular abnormalities as chorioretinitis and optic atrophy in 25 to 30% of cases.

Among the 90% of congenitally-infected CMV infants who are asymptomatic at birth, SNHL that ranges from mild to profound is a common sequela that eventually affects 10 to 15% of asymptomatic infants. This SNHL often develops or progresses after the first year of life and is bilateral in about 50% of cases and variable in severity (50–100 dB).[103] A greater risk for delayed-onset CMV hearing loss in asymptomatic infants has been correlated with periventricular radiolucencies or calcifications on neonatal CT and significantly-elevated maternal titers of envelope glycoprotein gB antibodies throughout the pregnancy.

> ### SPECIAL CONSIDERATION:
> Of the 90% of infants who are infected congenitally with CMV and are asymptomatic at birth, 10 to 15% will develop SNHL ranging from mild to profound.

The attenuated live-virus Towne vaccine against CMV has demonstrated capability to induce antibodies in some populations, but it has not found widespread acceptance because of its possible carcinogenic potential. Recent vaccine development efforts have employed noninfectious viral subunits, specifically a portion of the viral envelope consisting of a glycoprotein gB.

Histopathologic study of TBs from victims of CID reveal characteristic inclusion bodies in the superficial cells of the stria vascularis, Reissner's membrane, the limbus spiralis, saccule, utricle, and SCCs. The organ of Corti, cristae, and/or ganglion cells do not have inclusion bodies, but endolymphatic hydrops are observed in at least a portion of each cochlear duct.

Congenital toxoplasmosis

Felines are the natural host for the protozoan parasite *Toxoplasma gondi,* which typically is spread to humans through food contaminated with oocysts from cat feces or consumption of tissue cysts in undercooked meat products. Excreted oocysts sporulate at about 1 to 5 days to the infectious sporozoite form that, after human ingestion, penetrates the intestinal mucosa and spreads throughout the body. This spread may include the placenta that then serves as a route for fetal infection.

In contrast with CMV, only primary maternal infection during pregnancy leads to congenital toxoplasmosis in the fetus at a rate that varies from 15% in the first trimester to 30% during the second trimester and 60% during the third trimester. Although transmission to the fetus is most likely from maternal infection in close proximity to delivery, the severity of fetal involvement is greatest with earlier infection. Weighing both factors, it has been estimated that the greatest risk of severe congenital toxoplasmosis is associated with primary maternal infection during weeks 10 to 24 of pregnancy. About 75% of infants with congenital toxoplasmosis are asymptomatic at birth, another 15% have only ocular lesions, and the remainder are affected severely often manifesting the classic triad of chorioretinitis, hydrocephalus, and intracranial calcifications. A neurologically-dominant type of involvement is more common than a disseminated variety that affects multiple organ systems leading to chorioretinitis, microphthalmia, cataracts, hydrocephalus, generalized intracranial calcifications, microcephaly, thrombocytopenia, hepatosplenomegaly, and jaundice. Untreated infants with subclinical infection are at risk for later chorioretinitis with decreasing visual acuity (up to 85% by age 20), progressive CNS involvement with decreased intellectual function, deafness, and precocious puberty. Studies such as the New England Newborn Screening Program revealed that 90% of babies with congenital toxoplasmosis were judged on the basis of standard physical examination to be clinically normal at discharge from the newborn nursery.[104] In contrast, targeted diagnostic studies of these same infants (e.g., cranial CT, CSF examination, and ophthalmologic examination including retinoscopy) de-

tected evidence of the disorder in 40% of these infants.

> ### SPECIAL CONSIDERATION:
> The greatest risk of severe congenital toxoplasmosis is associated with primary maternal infection during weeks 10 to 24 of pregnancy.

The recommended treatment protocol for acute toxoplasmosis in an expectant mother includes a combination of pyrimethamine plus a sulfonamide of the sulfapyrimidine type (sulfadoxine or sulfadiazine) to minimize transmission to the fetus and the sequelae if fetal infection occurs. In France, prenatal treatment of infected mothers yielded a 0.6% fetal infection rate during preconceptual or early first trimester maternal infection, a 3.7% infection rate for maternal infection during the sixth to the sixteenth week of gestation, and a 20% rate if the infection occurred during the sixteenth through twenty-fifth week.[105-108] Treatment for up to 1 year with alternating courses of pyrimethamine and sulfonamide (sulfadiazine) coupled with folinic acid to prevent pyrimethamine complications is recommended for infants born of mothers with confirmed prenatal toxoplasmosis. If intensive treatment of congenitally-infected infants is instituted at birth, the risk of subsequent chorioretinitis is reduced from 60 to 10%. No SNHL was documented during the initial followup of 57 congenitally-infected infants who were treated in a Chicago-based study.[109] TB histopathology in infants with toxoplasmosis-related SNHL revealed calcified scars, predominantly in the stria vascularis, that were comparable to those observed in the CNS.

Recommendations for prevention of maternal prenatal toxoplasmosis include careful personal hygiene, cleaning of fruits and vegetables before ingestion, thorough cooking of meat products, and avoidance of exposure to cat litter boxes. A recently-developed antitoxoplasma vaccine for administration to feline carriers may help diminish the risk of human exposure.

Syphilis

The risk for transplacental transmission of *Treponema pallidum* to the developing fetus, which can occur at any stage of maternal disease, is highest during primary syphilis (70–100%) and lowest (30%) in the late stage of the disease. Maternal illicit drug use (e.g., cocaine addiction) significantly increases the likelihood of congenital syphilis in their infants.

Among pregnant women with untreated syphilis, the likelihood of delivering a normal full term newborn is about 20%. Fetal death occurs in about 25% of cases and an additional 10 to 20% who are born alive die during the perinatal period. Approximately 33% of infants with congenital syphilis manifest some findings at birth. Maternal infection during the first trimester is most apt to produce serious sequelae at birth including low birth weight with hepatosplenomegaly and mucocutaneous involvement such as rhinitis ("snuffles") and a diffuse, maculopapular, desquamating skin rash that typically involves the palms and soles of the feet. More commonly, the classical stigmata of congenital syphilis such as SNHL, interstitial keratitis, Hutchinson's teeth (notched incisors), mulberry molars, Clutton joints (bilateral painless knee effusions), nasal septal perforation, and saddle deformity emerge over the first several years of life. Other common manifestations include frontal bossing of the skull, as well as osteochondritis and periostitis of the long bones, leading to "saber shin" deformity. Radiographic findings including serrated metaphyseal ends, thickened periosteum, and metaphyseal defects of long bones such as the upper medial tibia may be the only presenting sign in up to 20% of early onset congenital syphilis. Offspring of mothers whose syphilis was treated by an apparently-adequate regimen also should be treated unless a four fold decrease in nontreponemal maternal antibody following treatment was documented.

Prevalence estimates of SNHL among congenital syphilis patients range from 3 to 38%. Thirty-eight percent of cases present prior to age 10 years, 51% between 25 and 35 years of age, and 12% become apparent later in life. Longitudinal audiologic follow-up of congenital syphilitic babies is necessary because few will present with SNHL during the neonatal period. The hearing loss may present as a sudden, bilateral, profound loss with a flat audiogram configuration and little or no vertigo. Speech discrimination scores are typically worse than would be predicted by the pure tone loss. Loudness recruitment can be severe, and caloric responses are usually weak to absent. It may be possible to elicit a positive labyrinthine fistula test (Hennebert's sign)

and a history of dysequilibrium in response to loud sounds (Tullio's phenomenon).

Sensitivity rate of the fluorescent treponema antibody absorption test (FTA-ABS) is high during all stages of syphilis, and the specificity rate (few false positives) has approached 98% in large studies. A positive FTA-ABS is often confirmed by the more costly microhemagluttination assay for *Treponema Pallidum* (MHA-TP) and the tremponema pallidum inhibition test. Whereas both antitreponemal IgM and IgG antibodies are present during active infection, only IgG antibodies should persist following efficacious successful treatment. Definitive diagnosis of congenital syphilis during the neonatal period can be challenging, so offspring of seropositive mothers should be followed carefully. Serial lumbar punctures with CSF examination at 6 month intervals should be done for infants with neurologic involvement.

The preferred treatment of nonpenicillin allergic infants and children with otosyphilis is high-dose parenteral penicillin. It is important to comply with current Centers for Disease Control (CDC) recommendations for treatment and follow-up in cases of congenital syphilis. Administered as an adjunct to antibiotics, systematically-administered corticosteroids (generally oral prednisone) have proven effective in stabilizing or improving hearing in approximately 50% of patients with syphilitic deafness, but the risks and benefits of extended steroid therapy in pediatric patients must be weighed carefully.

Among TB histopathologic findings in cases of congenital otosyphilis are obliterative endarteritis, mononuclear cell infiltrates, osteitis of the otic capsule, and varying degrees of tissue necrosis. Round cell infiltration of the labyrinthine structures and VIII cranial nerve can be observed in cases of early congenital syphilis, which alternatively may present as a meningolabyrinthitis. Atrophy of the organ of Corti may be accompanied by involvement of the stria vascularis, spiral ganglion, and VIII cranial nerve. Gummatous changes involving the ossicles can add a conductive component to coexisting SNHL.

Rubella

Transplacental transmission of the rubella virus, an enveloped ribonucleic acid (RNA) togavirus, to a developing fetus occurs during viremia 5 to 7 days following initial exposure of the expectant mother. The observations of Gregg[110] as well as Swan et al.[111] linked prenatal maternal rubella with the triad of congenital deafness, congenital cataracts, and heart defects. The 1964 to 1965 rubella epidemic in the United States resulted in about 11,800 cases of congenital rubella hearing loss. Almost 90% of infants who contract congenital rubella during the first trimester will manifest some sequelae. Congenital rubella infection may affect as many as 50% of infants whose mothers experience the infection during gestational weeks 11 to 20, but only 25 to 50% of these manifest sequelae, primarily hearing loss. Significant sequelae rarely occur following maternal infections after the 20th week of gestation. Studies of infants with laboratory-confirmed congenital rubella led to the description of an expanded congenital rubella syndrome, comprising cataracts/congenital glaucoma, congenital hearing disease (i.e., patent ductus arteriosus or peripheral pulmonary artery stenosis), hearing loss, and pigmentary retinopathy. Other findings may include purpura, jaundice, microcephaly, splenomegaly, mental retardation, meningoencephalitis, or radiologic evidence of long bone lucencies. The most pervasive disability is SNHL that may represent the sole finding in infants infected after the fourth month of gestation. In large series, hearing loss generally ranges in severity with some asymmetry in degree and configuration. The most typical audiogram shows the greatest loss in the middle frequencies between 500 and 2000 Hz. Longitudinal follow-up has confirmed a progressive decrease of auditory acuity in 25% of cases.

Histopathologic study of TBs of patients with laboratory-confirmed congenital rubella revealed Scheibe-type cochleosaccular changes with the utricle, SCCs, and spiral ganglion remaining relatively unaffected. Partial Reissner's membrane collapse with adherence to the stria vascularis and organ of Corti was noted, and the tectorial membrane was rolled in the internal sulcus in some sections. The organ of Corti was relatively unaffected, but the stria vascularis demonstrated cystic dilatation at the junction of Reissner's membrane and the spiral ligament.

Accurate clinical diagnosis of acute rubella must be founded upon a positive viral culture, the presence of rubella-specific IgM antibody, or a significant rise in IgG antibody in paired acute (within 7–10 days of onset) and convalescent sera (preferably 2–3 weeks later).

Following the isolation of the rubella virus in 1962, efforts were directed toward the development of an effective and safe vaccine that was li-

censed initially in 1969 and superseded in 1979 by a safer and more immunogenic strain. The incidence of rubella in the United States fell from 57,686 cases (58/100,000 population) in 1969 to fewer than 1000 cases (<0.5 cases/100,000 population) in 1983.

Neonatal sepsis

In 1990, 50% of approximately 15,000 reported cases of Group B streptococcal disease (GBS) in the United States involved neonates, and about 80% of neonatal GBS infections that occur during the first week of life begin on the first day of life. The most common disabilities affecting GBS survivors include hearing loss, vision problems, and developmental delay. Meningitis is a common occurrence in neonatal sepsis patients and auditory brainstem response (ABR) testing should be carried out on all survivors.

Prevention of neonatal GBS is best accomplished by obtaining maternal vaginal and rectal cultures within 5 weeks (typically 35–37 weeks gestation) of expected delivery, coupled with the administration of intrapartum antibiotics to all culture-positive mothers and all mothers who deliver preterm.

Herpes simplex encephalitis

Of the two herpes simplex virus (HSV) serotypes, HSV-I and HSV-II, the latter is implicated in most recurrent genital herpes cases. Primary maternal genital herpes infection near the time of delivery increases the risk of neonatal infection (30–50%), whereas the risk of transmission is low for women who have a history of recurrent herpes at term or whose primary infection occurred during the first half of pregnancy (3%). Delivery by C-Section may be recommended to minimize the risk of neonatal infection in high-risk cases.

Although uncommon, 20 to 30% of herpes simplex encephalitis (HSE) occurs in the pediatric age group. Neonatal infections are most likely attributable to intrapartum or postpartum exposure, with only 5% arising from intrauterine transmission. One-fourth to one-third of the neonates with disseminated HSV infection also experience meningoencephalitis, presenting with abnormal CSF findings in more than 90% of cases. Focal meningoencephalitis may be evident on electroencephalographic and imaging studies [CT, magnetic resonance imaging (MRI)]. Brain biopsy, positive in 33 to 55% of HSV patients, is the only definitive diagnostic study. Typically HSV occurs during the second or third postpartum week with about half being related to a history of maternal or paternal infection. Therapeutic recommendations include systemic acyclovir 30–60 mg/kg/day for 10 to 21 days.

AT A GLANCE . . .

Congenital and Early-Onset Infectious Hearing Loss

- Cytomegalovirus (CMV)
- Toxoplasmosis
- Syphilis
- Rubella
- Neonatal sepsis (Group B Streptococcus)
- Herpes simplex encephalitis

Late-Onset Infections

Measles and mumps

The mumps RNA paramyxovirus initially replicates in the nasopharynx and regional nodes leading to a 3- to 5-day period of viremia between day 12 and 25 that disseminates the infection to tissues such as the salivary glands and meninges. Approximately 5/10,000 mumps patients will sustain a SNHL that tends to be sudden in onset and 80% unilateral with associated tinnitus, vertigo, nausea, and vomiting in many cases.

Isolation of the mumps virus can be accomplished during the initial 5 days of illness from saliva, urine, and CSF specimens. Administration of the Jeryl-Lynn strain of live attenuated mumps virus vaccine, initially licensed in late 1967, led to a decline from an estimated 212,000 cases in 1964 to about 3000 (1.3/100,000 population) annually in the United States by 1983.

Measles, a single-strand RNA paramyxovirus, was isolated in 1954 and has a single antigenic type. Initial replication in the respiratory epithelium nasopharynx is followed by a primary viremia 2 to 3 days following exposure and a second viremia 5 to 7 days after initial infection, spreading the virus to other organs. A positive enzyme-linked immune sorbent assay (ELISA) test documenting elevated IgM antibody for measles, which is drawn early in the infection, establishes the diagnosis. One or more measles complications occur in nearly 30% of reported cases, with acute encephalitis being reported in about 0.1% of cases. Measles encephalitis has a fatal outcome in about 15% of cases and fully 25% of survivors sustain neurologic sequelae, including SNHL. Widespread use of the measles vaccine as part of the measles/mumps/rubella (MMR) series administered to infants has brought about a 98% decline in reported cases except for a resurgence in 1989 to 1991 that was attributable to since-remedied deficiencies in the immunization program.

If hearing loss associated with measles or mumps occurs in the absence of meningoencephalitis, the virus apparently accesses the inner ear via the stria vascularis during the viremia phase. Histologically, inflammatory changes are followed by degeneration and scarring of the stria vascularis, the organ of Corti, the tectorial membrane, and peripheral cochlear neurons, proceeding from the cochlear base to the apex. Collapse of Reissner's membrane has been described. The perilymphatic system, vestibular end organs, and content of the IAC generally remain.

TB findings in mumps or measles meningoencephalitis cases are compatible with those observed with meningogenic bacterial labyrinthitis such as severe degeneration of neural elements in the modiolus and lesser involvement of neural structures in the cochlear duct. Infant TBs, reflecting the acute stage of meningoencephalitis, reveal lymphocytic infiltration along nerves and vessels in the IAC but no involvement of the stria vascularis. TBs from survivors of the acute disease process revealed patterns of intralabyrinthine fibrosis and osteogenesis in perilymphatic spaces.

Bacterial meningitis and vaccine development

Escherichia coli and group B hemolytic streptococci are responsible for most neonatal meningitis but, historically, HIB, *Neisseria meningitidis,* and *Streptococcus pneumoniae* have been responsible for about 80% of bacterial meningitis cases throughout the world. The introduction of effective antibiotics markedly reduced the mortality of childhood meningitis from more than 90% to 2 to 3% for patients older than 1 month of age, but did little to ameliorate sequelae such as SNHL. The development of safe and effective vaccines for the most common meningitis pathogens holds the greatest promise of reducing the incidence of postmeningitic SNHL.

In the past, about 60% of invasive HIB disease has occurred prior to 12 months of age, with most children acquiring natural immunity to HIB by age 5 to 6 years through asymptomatic exposure. A vaccine with enhanced immunogenicity in infancy was developed by Robbins et al. who utilized covalent linkage of the bacterial capsular polysaccharide (CP) to a protein carrier (i.e., conjugation), transforming the CP from a T lymphocyte-independent to a T cell-dependent antigen.[111a] The resultant HIB conjugate vaccine has been in use since 1990 and is approved for initial dose at 2 months of age. It has helped reduce the incidence of HIB disease by 98% in the United States. Prior to the development of the HIB vaccine, this organism constituted the predominant etiology (i.e., 70%) of bacterial meningitis in infants and children under 5 years of age, with a case fatality rate of about 5%. An additional 15 to 30% of survivors sustained neurologic sequelae, including SNHL.

Before introduction of the HIB vaccine, approximately 20% of all meningitis cases were attributable to *Neisseria meningitidis,* with a case mortality rate across all age groups of around 10%. Among the 12 meningococcal serotypes, type B (50%) and C (20%) are implicated in most meningococcal meningitis in the United States. A polyvalent protein conjugate vaccine that elicits antibodies against both Group A and C meningococcus and *Escherichia coli* K1 is currently undergoing clinical trials. In the case of Group B meningococcus, noncapsular antigens are being utilized for vaccine development.

Approximately 13% of bacterial meningitis cases in the United States have been caused by *Streptococcus pneumoniae,* with children under 2 years of age having the greatest susceptibility. The overall mortality rate for pneumococcal meningitis can be as high as 25%. Of the 84 known pneumococcal serotypes, types 4, 6, 14, 18, 19, and 23 are implicated most often in childhood infections. Pneumococcal polysaccharide has been linked with tetanus toxoid in a conjugate vaccine that demonstrates enhanced immunogenicity in children ages 2 to 5 years. Unfortunately, each serotype must be conjugated individually, which limits the number of serotypes that can be contained in a single vaccine.

In a 1995 study of bacterial meningitis in the United States, group B streptococcus was still found to be the most common pathogen in the neonatal period: 76% of bacterial meningitis among infants aged 1 to 23 months was attributable to *Streptococcus pneumoniae* (45%) and *Neisseria meningitidis*

(31%).[112] The most common pathogen among those in the 2- to 18-year age bracket was *Neisseria meningitidis,* which accounted for 59% of cases. Notably, the median age of patients with meningitis rose from 15 months in 1986 to 25 years in 1995, with only 31% of cases involving children under age 5 years.

Postmeningitic hearing loss Postmeningitic SNHL, affecting 15 to 20% of survivors, has its onset early in the course of the disease. The majority of losses result in permanent, bilateral, severe to profound SNHL. A longitudinal study by Richardson et al. in England, who performed serial hearing evaluations of children with meningitis from the time of hospital admission, revealed that all study children who demonstrated a SNHL at any time during the study had abnormal otoacoustic emissions (OAE) at the time of first evaluation.[113] A subgroup (i.e., 10%) of children with abnormal OAEs and normal tympanograms at initial evaluation demonstrated normal hearing within 5 days of diagnosis, confirming the occurrence of rapidly-reversible SNHL early in the course of meningitis in about 10% of cases. A meningitic child who exhibits a normal ABR after the first few days of inpatient antibiotic therapy is highly unlikely to develop later SNHL. Fluctuating losses have been observed in some children for as long as 1 year following the meningitis, and late progression of postmeningitic SNHL after years of stability can occur.

> **SPECIAL CONSIDERATION:**
> Sensorineural hearing loss following meningitis affects 15 to 20% of survivors.

Bacteria and bacterial toxins can access the inner ear via the cochlear aqueduct or IAC, leading to perineuritis or neuritis of the cochleovestibular nerve and/or suppurative labyrinthitis. Serous or toxic labyrinthitis, thrombophlebitis or embolization of labyrinthine vessels, and hypoxia/anoxia of the eighth cranial nerve and central auditory pathways have been postulated as additional pathophysiologic mechanisms that result in postmeningitic SNHL.[114]

Both direct bacterial action on nervous tissue

and/or the inflammatory response elicited by bacterial breakdown products after antibiotic treatment is initiated may be important causes of postmeningitic sequelae. Dexamethasone inhibits the inflammatory response triggered by both interleukin-1 beta and tumor necrosis factor (TNF) from astroglia. Corticosteroids are known to inhibit the activity of phospholipase with consequent decrease in prostaglandin E, thromboxane, and leukotriene formation. Although corticosteroids (e.g., dexamethasone) initially showed promise in decreasing the indices of meningeal inflammation at 24 hours and ameliorating neurologic sequelae, the effectiveness of this regimen has not been demonstrated conclusively. The most encouraging benefits of corticosteroid administration as an adjunct to antibiotic treatment were observed with HIB meningitis, which is rapidly declining in importance. A Finnish study compared the efficacy of oral glycerol (an osmotic diuretic) with dexamethasone in preventing neurologic and auditory sequelae in meningitis. Only 7% of glycerol-treated patients suffered sequelae as compared with 19% of those receiving dexamethasone.[114a]

TB histopathologic changes following acute bacterial meningitis revealed suppurative labyrinthitis in 49% of specimens, cochlear involvement (most often only perilymphatic spaces) in all cases, and vestibular labyrinth changes (principally LSCC) only 50% of the time. The remaining TBs revealed eosinophilic staining in the absence of inflammatory cells. This finding represents a probable pathologic correlate of serous labyrinthitis that was found principally in the vestibular labyrinth, including the superior (100%) and posterior (86%) SCCs. Cochlear involvement was present in only 40% of these specimens. Sensory and neural structures were preserved in most specimens with suppurative and serous-type changes raising hope for possible preventive intervention. Severe degeneration of spiral ganglion cells in 12% of TBs confirmed that this group of patients would be unlikely to benefit from cochlear implantation.

AT A GLANCE . . .

Late-Onset Infectious Hearing Loss

- Mumps
- Measles
- Bacterial meningitis

OTOTOXIC DRUGS AND CHEMICALS

The serum half-life of parenterally-administered aminoglycosides in patients with normal renal function is about 2 hours, whereas urinary concentrations may reach 100 times serum concentrations in the presence of renal impairment. Even in renal patients, however, inner ear concentrations do not rise above serum levels. Brownell[115] determined that high concentrations of gentamicin per se will not damage outer hair cells unless the drug is enzymatically pretreated, yielding a cytotoxic gentamicin metabolite ("gentatoxin"), which was isolated by Schacht.[116] Strategies to prevent or ameliorate the ototoxic effects of gentamicin initially centered on glutathione (GSH), an antioxidant, to retard free radical formation. An alternative approach exploits gentamicin's role as a chelator. This approach promotes the production of free radicals in the presence of iron salts by utilizing competitive, less toxic chelators (e.g., deferoxamine) that do not impede gentamicin's antimicrobial properties. Histopathologic damage from aminoglycoside ototoxicity observed in TB sections includes injury to the stria vascularis, suprastrial spiral ligament, pericapillary tissues in the spiral prominence, the outer sulcus, and Reissner's membrane. Outer hair cells sustain the earliest damage that proceeds from the basilar turn toward the cochlear apex, but inner hair cells are typically spared. Type I vestibular hair cells of the crista ampullaris generally incur greater damage by streptomycin, kanamycin, and gentamicin than type II cells, and supporting cells are spared largely.

The specific toxicity of aminoglycosides varies. Neomycin is the most ototoxic over-all. Streptomycin, gentamicin, and tobramycin are primarily vestibulotoxic, and kanamycin and amikacin are principally cochleotoxic. Coexistent factors thought to enhance the risk of ototoxicity include preexisting hearing loss, concurrent noise exposure, age, duration of therapy, previous aminoglycoside use, impaired nutritional status, and concomitant use of other ototoxic drugs such as loop diuretics (e.g., ethacrynic acid and furosemide). Administration of an aminoglycoside prior to a loop diuretic increases the ototoxic risk than the reverse order of administration. Transplacental passage of aminoglycosides to the fetus has been confirmed, but the degree of risk to hearing and balance function has been a matter of debate.

Families with point mutations, 1555 A-G in the mitochondrial 12S riboxomal RNA, show exquisite sensitivity to ototoxic effects of aminoglycosides administered even at ostensibly "safe" dosage levels. Prescreening for this mutation before initiating aminoglycoside therapy will no doubt become a standard of care in the not too distant future.

The loop diuretics, such as ethacrynic acid and furosemide, can have ototoxic effects when administered in isolation (0.7% incidence with ethacrynic acid; 6.4% with furosemide), but ototoxicity is enhanced significantly when these drugs are administered concurrently with standard doses of aminoglycosides. Ototoxicity studies with animals have documented post-treatment changes in the stria vascularis and significant hair cell loss. It has been postulated that furosemide and ethacrynic acid have distinct mechanisms of action on the cochlea.

Bilateral SNHL, typically associated with tinnitus and vertigo, has been reported by adults with coexisting renal and/or hepatic failure who received erythromycin doses of 2 gm per day. A toxic effect on the stria vascularis has been suggested as the pathphysiologic mechanism.

Reversible hearing loss and tinnitus are a well-documented side effect of high therapeutic doses of salicylates (levels exceeding 20 mg/dL). Salicyclates are known to promote a reduction in the levels of transaminases and cochlear adenosine triphosphate, as well as cochlear blood flow.

Vancomycin blood levels, exceeding 45 mg/L in adults, are likely to be nephrotoxic and ototoxic. Increased half-life of the drug in premature neonates places them at highest risk for vancomycin ototoxicity. Emerging resistant bacterial strains, necessitating more widespread clinical use of vancomycin, may increase the number of children at risk for vancomycin ototoxicity.

Side effects of cisplatin (cis-diamminedichloroplatinum) include myelosupression, neurotoxicity, and nephrotoxicity, but ototoxicity effectively imposes dosage limits in clinical practice. Cisplatin-related hearing loss initially affects the 10,000 to 18,000 Hz range with progressive involvement of frequencies below 8000 Hz with continued exposure. Drug-mediated blockade of outer hair cell transduction channels, with a concurrent decrease in adenylate cyclase, has been suggested as pathphysiologic mechanisms by which this drug exerts it ototoxic effects. Initial outer hair cell loss in the basal turn of the cochlea may progress to gradual involvement of inner hair cells proceeding toward the cochlear apex. Strial atrophy and Reissner's membrane collapse also have been observed.

The risk of cisplatin ototoxicity varies across audiometric frequencies. Dreschler and colleagues determined that dosage levels exceeding 3 to 4 mg/kg pose a definite risk of ototoxicity.[117] High-frequency hearing loss (40 dB or greater at 1000 Hz and above) has been confirmed in about 50% of all children treated with a standard therapeutic dose (60–100 mg/m2 per course). Permanent bilateral high-frequency SNHL was documented in 88% of children receiving cisplatin doses over 450 mg/m2. There is a direct relation between the degree of cochlear damage and cumulative cisplatin doses exceeding 279 mg/m2, whereas an inverse relationship exists with the age of the child. A synergy between noise exposure (85 dB sound pressure level or greater) and cisplatin ototoxicity has been noted in animal studies.

Ingestion of quinine in therapeutic doses by expectant mothers has been associated with severe to profound hearing impairment in their infants. Chloroquine taken during pregnancy has been linked to both retinopathy and hearing loss in infants. The pathophysiologic mechanism appears to be vasculitis and ischemia in the inner ear, leading to degenerative changes of the stria vascularis, organ of Corti, and neuronal elements.

Retinoid (e.g., isotretinoin) administration during pregnancy can lead to spontaneous abortion or severe malformations including CNS, cardiovascular, and respiratory anomalies; cleft lip; cleft palate; and external ear defects, which may include canal agenesis.

AT A GLANCE . . .
Ototoxic Drugs and Chemicals

- Aminoglycosides
- Loop diuretics
- Erythromycin
- Salicylates
- Vancomycin
- Cisplatin
- Quinine/chloroquine
- Retinoid

ANOXIA/HYPOXIA

Perinatal *anoxia/hypoxia* is statistically correlated with subsequent SNHL in the child. Postanoxic changes in the brainstem reticular formation and cochlear nuclei include reductions in cell numbers and volume in direct proportion to the duration and severity of oxygen deprivation. Persistent fetal circulation, with associated chronic hypoxemia, carries a 20% incidence of SNHL, 75% of which is in the moderate to severe range and 25% of which is profound.

HYPERBILIRUBINEMIA

When bilirubin crosses the blood-brain barrier and is deposited in a neonate's basal ganglia (i.e., kernicterus), particularly the ventrocochlear nucleus, neurologic sequelae including SNHL can result. Elevated bilirubin levels in neonates may result from inadequate bilirubin conjugation, impaired albumin binding, or increased unconjugated bilirubin production. Reversible ABR changes (absence of the wave IV-V complex), which have been documented in about 33% of neonates with bilirubin levels in the 15 to 25 mg/dL range, are compatible with transient encephalopathy. About half the infants with kernicterus will die, and survivors may suffer from cerebral palsy, mental retardation, and hearing loss. Exhaled carbon monoxide levels, which help identify infants with hemolysis-related hyperbilirubinemia, can predict which infants would benefit from aggressive preventive intervention. Hemeoxygenase inhibitors (e.g., tinmesoporphyrin Sn-mesoporphyrin) bind hemeoxygenase more aggressively than heme itself, thus impeding access of heme to its natural binding site and reducing heme degradation and bilirubin production.

PREMATURITY AND FULL-TERM LOW BIRTH WEIGHT

Outcome studies of premature infants reveal a 20-fold increase in risk for severe hearing loss compared with full-term, normal birth weight infants. Significant SNHL is found in approximately 2% of all infants with birth weight of 3 pounds or less.

EAR AND HEAD TRAUMA

Trauma to the middle and inner ear, including explosive and penetrating injury as well as blunt skull trauma which can lead to TB fracture, can result in transient or permanent hearing loss. Although mild to moderate CHL is the most common finding, intralabyrinthine injury can produce a SNHL, most often affecting the high frequencies initially. A PLF may present with fluctuating or progressive SNHL, often associated with imbalance or in a smaller percentage of cases true vertigo. Of children admitted to the hospital following head injury, 7% are found to have temporal bone fractures and 13% of these children experience SNHL.

NOISE-INDUCED HEARING LOSS

Exposure to sounds of sufficient loudness and duration can result in temporary or permanent hearing loss. Potentially harmful noise sources at home, on the farm, and in recreational environments can place children and adolescents at risk for noise related hearing loss.

U.S. Department of Labor regulations establish the boundary between acceptable and damaging noise in the workplace for 8 hours of continuous exposure at 85 dB(A). Ear damage resulting from hazardous noise exposure is classified as either acoustic trauma or noise-induced hearing loss (NIHL). Acoustic trauma, which is immediate and severe and results in permanent hearing loss, may occur from exposure to intense sounds [>140 dB(A)] of short duration (e.g., gunfire, explosion). A temporary threshold shift (TTS) can result from moderate periods of exposure to less intense, but potentially damaging sounds. Continued exposure at hazardous levels produces a permanent NIHL that typically begins in the 3000 to 6000 Hz range and produces a characteristic "notch" audiometric configuration. Outer hair cells are most vulnerable to noise damage, and extensive hair cell damage eventually may be reflected in the loss of auditory nerve fibers and alterations in auditory areas of the CNS. Histopathologic correlates of TTS include swelling of hair cells and afferent nerve fiber terminals that resolves during a rest period away from loud sounds.

Short duration impulse noises, such as discharge

of a firearm, produce very high sound intensity up to 132 to 170 dB(A) during the initial acoustic pulse. Sound levels emanating from toy weapons measured at a distance of 50 cm showed mean peak values from 143 to 153 dB(A), and firecrackers produced peak levels measured at 3 meters of 125 to 156 dB. Personal cassette players (PCP) can generate sound levels in excess of 110 to 115 dB(A) at a child's ear. Studies of PCP use in the midelementary school age group revealed that 80% of the youngsters own PCPs and 5 to 10% listen at potentially hazardous volume levels for extended periods.

REFERENCES

1. U.S. Department of Health and Human Services, Public Health Service. Healthy people 2000: National health promotion and disease prevention objectives. Washington, D.C.: U.S. Government Printing Office, 1990.

2. Bess FH, Paradise JL. Universal screening for infant hearing impairment: Not simple, not risk-free, not necessarily beneficial, and not presently justified. Pediatrics 1994; 93(2):330-334.

3. Mochizuki T, Lemmink HH, Mariyama M, et al. Identification of mutations in the alpha 3(IV) and alpha 4(IV) collagen genes in autosomal recessive Alport syndrome. Nat Genet 1994; 8(1):77-81.

4. Weisel A. Early intervention programs for hearing impaired children—evaluation of outcomes. Early Child Dev Care 1990; 41:77-87.

5. Greenberg MT. Family stress and child competence: The effects of early intervention: Am Am Deaf 1983; 128(3):407-417.

6. Bess FH, Klee T, Culbertson JL. Identification, assessment and management of children with unilateral sensorineural hearing loss. Ear Hear 1986; 7:43-51.

7. Brookhouser PE, Worthington DW, Kelly WJ. Unilateral hearing loss in children. Laryngoscope 1991; 101(12):1264-1272.

8. Brookhouser PE. Incidence and Prevalence. Presented at National Institutes of Health Consensus Development Conference on Early Identification of Hearing Impairment in Infants and Young Children. Bethesda, Maryland, March 1-3, 1993.

9. Davis A, Wood S. The epidemiology of childhood hearing impairment: Factors relevant to planning of services. Br J Audiol 1992; 26:77-90.

10. White KR, Maxon AB. Universal screening for infant hearing impairment: Simple, beneficial, and presently justified. Int J Ped Otorhinolaryngol 1995; 32:201-211.

11. National Institutes of Health. Early Identification of Hearing Impairment in Infants and Young Children. Consensus Development Conference on Ear identification of Hearing Impairment in Infants and Young Children, 1993.

12. Joint Committee on Infant Hearing. 1994 Position Statement. ASHA 1994; 36:38-41.

13. Brookhouser PE, Worthington DW, Kelly WJ. Fluctuating and/or progressive sensorineural hearing loss in children. Laryngoscope 1994; 104(8):958-964.

14. Jackler RK, Luxford WM, House WF. Congenital malformations of the inner ear: A Classification based on embryogenesis. Laryngoscope 1987; 97(40):2-14.

15. Barker DF, Hostikka SL, Zhous J, et al. Identification of mutations in the COL4A5 collagen gene in Alport syndrome. Science 1990; 248(4960):1224-1227.

16. Abdelhak S, Kalatzis V, Heilig R, et al. A human homologue of the Drosphilia eyes absent gene underlies Branchio-Oto-Renal (BOR) syndrome and identifies a novel gene family. Nat Genet 1997; 12(2):157-164.

17. Neyroud N, Tesson F, Denjoy I, et al. A novel mutation in the potassium channel gene KVLQT1 causes the Jervell and Lange-Nielsen cardioauditory syndrome. Nat Genet 1997; 12(2):186-189.

18. Tyson J, Tranebjaerg L, Bellman S, et al. IsK and KVLQT1: Mutation in either of the two subunits of the slow component of the delayed rectifier potassium channel can cause Jervell and Lange-Nielsen syndrome. Hum Mol Genet 1997; 6(12):2179-2185.

19. Schulze-Bahr E, Wang Q, Wedekinds H, et al. KCNE1 mutations cause Jervell and Lange-Nielsen syndrome. Nat Genet 1997; 17(3):267-268.

20. Berger W, Meindl A, van de Pol TJ, et al. Isolation of a candidate gene for Norrie disease by positional cloning. Nat Genet 1992; 1(3):199-203.

21. Chen ZY, Hendriks RW, Jobling MA, et al. Isolation and characterization of a candidate gene for Norrie disease. Nat Genet 1992; 1(3):204-208.

22. Everett LA, Glasser B, Beck JC, et al. Pendred syndrome is caused by mutations in a putative sulphate transporter gene (PDS). Nat Genet 1997; 17(4):411-422.

23. Williams CJ, Ganguly A, Considine E, et al. A-2àG transition at the 3' acceptor splice site of IVS17 characterizes the COL2A1 gene mutation in the original Stickler syndrome kindred. Am J Med Genet 1996; 68(3):461-467.

24. Vikkula M, Mariman EC, Lui VC, et al. Autosomal dominant and recessive osteochondrodysplasias associated with the COL11A2 locus. Cell 1995; 80(3):431-437.

25. Richards AJ, Yates JR, Williams R, et al. A family

with Stickler syndrome type 2 has a mutation in the COL11A1 gene resulting in the substitution of glycine 97 by valine in alpha 1(XI) collagen. Hum Mol Genet 1996; 5(9):1339–1343.

26. The Treacher Collins Syndrome Collaborative Group. Positional cloning of a gene involved in the pathogenesis of Treacher Collins syndrome. Nat Genet 1996; 12(2):130–136.

27. Tassabehji M, Read AP, Newton VE, et al. Waardenburg's syndrome patients have mutations in the human homologue of the PAX-3 paired box gene. Nature 1992; 355(6361):635–636.

28. Tassabehji M, Newton VE, Read AP. Waardenburg syndrome type 2 caused by mutations in the human microphthalmia (MITF) gene. Nat Genet 1994; 8(3): 251–255.

29. Hoth CF, Milunsky A, Lipsky N, et al. Mutations in the paired domain of the human PAX3 gene cause Lkein-Waardenburg syndrome (WS-III) as well as Waardenburg syndrome type I (WS-I). Am J Hum Genet 1993; 52(3):455–462.

30. Attie T, Till M, Pelet A, et al. Mutation of the endothelin-receptor B gene in Waardenburg-Hirschsprung disease. Hum Mol Genet 1995; 4(12): 2407–2409.

31. Edery P, Attie T, Amiel J, et al. Mutation of the endothelin-3 gene in the Waardenburg-Hirschsprung disease (Shah-Waardenburg syndrome). Nat Genet 1996; 12(4):442–444.

32. Pingault V, Bondurand N, Kuhlbrodt K, et al. SOX10 mutations in patients with Waardenburg-Hirschsprung disease. Nat Genet 1998; 12(2):171–173.

33. Kaplan J, Gerber S, Bonneau D, et al. A genet for Usher syndrome type I (USH1A) maps to chromosome 14q. Genomics 1992; 14(4):979–987.

34. Weil D, Banchard S, Kaplan J, et al. Defective myosin VIIA gene responsible for Usher syndrome type 1B. Nature 1995; 374(6517):60–61.

35. Smith RJ, Coppage KB, Ankerstjerne JK, et al. Localization of the gene for branchiootorenal syndrome to chromosome 8q. Genomics 1992; 14(4): 841–844.

36. Wayne S, Der Kaloustain VM, Schloss M, et al. Localizationo fo the Usher syndrome type ID gene (USH1D) to chromosome 10. Hum Mol Genet 1996; 5(10):1689–1692.

37. Chaib H, Kaplan J, Gerber S, et al. A newly identified locus for Usher syndrome type I, USH1E, maps to chromosome 21q21. Hum Mol Genet 1997; 6(1): 27–31.

38. Kimberling WJ, Weston MD, Moller C, et al. Localization of Usher syndrome type II to chromosome 1q. Genomics 1990; 7(2):245–249.

39. Eudy JD, Weston MD, Yao S, et al. Mutation of a gene encoding a protein with extracellular matrix motifs in Usher syndrome type IIA. Science 1998; 280(5370):1753–1757.

40. Pieke-Dahl S, Kelly PM, Astuto LM. Localization of USH2B to 5q14.3–q21.3. (Abst. 88) Presented at the Molecular Biology of Hearing and Deafness Conference. Bethesda, October 10, 1998.

41. Sankila EM, Pakarinen L, Kaariainen H, et al. Assignment of an Usher syndrome type III (USH3) gene to chromosome 3q. Hum Mol Genet 1995; 4(1): 93–98.

42. Brunner HG, van Beersum SE, Warman ML, et al. Stickler syndrome gene is linked to chromosome 6 near the COL11A2 gene. Hum Mol Genet 1994; 3(9):1561–1564.

43. Edwards SJ, Gladwin AJ, Dixon MJ. The mutational spectrum in Treacher Collins syndrome reveals a predominance of mutations that create a premature-termination codon. Am J Hum Genet 1997; 60(3):515–524.

44. Shen MH, Harper PS, Upadhyaya M. Molecular genetics of neurofibromatosis type 1 (NF1). J Med Gent 1996; 33(1):2–17.

45. Rouleau CA, Merel P, Lutchman M, et al. Alteration in a new gene encoding a putative membrane-organizing protein causes neuro-fibromatosis type 2. Nature 1993; 363(6429):495–496.

45a. Tomek MS, Brown MR, Mani SR, Ramesh A, Srisailapathy CR, Couke P, Zbar RI, Bell AM, McGuirt WT, Fukushima K, Willems PJ, Van Camp G, Smith RJ. Localization of a gene for otosclerosis to chromosome 15q25–q26. Hum Mol Genet 1998; 7(2): 285–290.

46. Konigsmark BW, Gorlin RJ, (eds). Genetic Hearing Loss with No Associated Abnormalities. *Genetic and Metabolic Deafness.* Saunders, Philadelphia: 1976, pp. 7–48.

47. Leon PE, Raventos H, Lynch E, et al. The gene for an inhereited form of deafness maps to chromosome 5q31. Proc Nat Acad Sci USA 1992; 89(11): 5181–5184.

48. Lynch ED, Lee MK, Morrow JE, et al. Nonsyndromic deafness DFNA1 associated with mutation of a human homolog of the Drosophilia gene diaphanous. Science 1997; 278(5341):1315–1318.

49. Coucke P, Van Camp G, Djoyodiharjo B. Linkage of autosomal dominant hearing loss to the short arm of chromosome 1 in two families. N Engl J Med 1994; 18:331(7):425–431.

50. Chaib H, Lina-Grande G, Guilford P, et al. A gene responsible for a dominant form of neurosensory non-syndromic deafness maps to the NSRD1 recessive deafness gene interval. Hum Mol Genet 1994; 3(12):2219–2222.

51. Denoyelle F. et al. Connexin 26 gene linked to a dominant deafness. Nature 1998; 28:393(6683): 319–320.

52. Chen AH, Ni L, Kukushima K, et al. Linkage of

a gene for dominant non-syndromic deafness to chromosome 19. Hum Mol Genet 1995; 4(6): 1073–1076.

53. van Camp G, Coucke P, Balemans W, et al. Localization of a gene for non-syndromic hearing loss (DFNA5) to chromosome 7p15. Hum Mol Genet 1995; 4(11):2159–2163.

54. Lesperance MM, Hall JW, Bess FH, et al. A gene for autosomal dominant nonsyndromic hereditary hearing impairment map to 4p16.3 Hum Mol Genet 1995; 4:1967–1972.

55. Fagerheim T, Nilssen O, Raeymaekers P, et al. Identification of a new locus for autosomal dominant non-syndromic hearing impairment (DFNA7) in a large Norwegian family. Hum Mol Genet 1996; 5(1): 1187–1191.

56. Kirschhofer K, Kenyon JB, Hoover DM, et al. Autosomal-dominant, prelingual, nonprogressive sensorineural hearing loss: Localization of the gene (DFNA8) to chromosome 11q by linkage in an Austrian family. Cytogenet Cell Genet 1998; 82(1–2): 126–130.

57. Verhoeven K, Van Laer L, Kirschhofer K, et al. Mutations in the human alpha-tectorin gene cause autosomal dominant non-syndromic hearing impairment. Nat Genet 1998; 19(1):60–62.

58. Manolis EN, Nadol JB, Eavey RD, et al. A gene for non-syndromic autosomal dominant progressive postlingual sensorineural deafness maps to chromosome 14q12-13. Hum Mol Genet 1996; 5(7): 1047–1050.

59. O'Neill ME, Marietta J, Nishimura D, et al. A gene for autosomal dominant late-onset progressive non-syndromic hearing loss maps to chromosome 6-DFNA10. Hum Mol Genet 1996; 5(6):853–856.

60. Tamagawa Y, Kitamura K, Ishida T, et al. A gene for a dominant form of non-syndromic sensorineural deafness (DFNA11) maps within the region containing the DFNB2 recessive deafness gene. Hum Mol Genet 1996; 5(6):849–852.

61. Liu XZ, Walsh J, Tamagawa Y, et al. Autosomal dominant non-syndromic deafness caused by a mutation in the myosin VIIA gene. Nat Gen 1997; 17(3): 268–269.

62. Verhoeven K, Van Camp G, Govaerts PJ, et al. A gene for autosomal dominant nonsyndromic hearing loss (DFNA12) maps to chromosome 11q22-24. Am J Hum Genet 1997; 60(5):1168–1173.

63. Verhoeven K, Van Laer L, Kirschhofer K, et al. Mutations in the human alpha-tectorin gene cause autosomal dominant on-syndromic hearing impairment. Nat Genet 1998; 19(1):60–62.

64. Brown MR, Tomek MS, Van Laer L, et al. A novel locus for autosomal dominant nonsyndromic hearing loss, DFNA13, maps to chromosome 6p. Am J Hum Genet 1997; Oct;61(4):924–927.

65. Van Camp G, Willems PJ, Smith RJ. Nonsyndromic hearing impairment: Unparalleled heterogeneity. Am J Hum Genet 1997; 60(4):758–764.

66. Vahava O, Morell R, Lyunch ED, et al. Mutation in transcription factor POU4F3 associated with inherited progressive hearing loss in humans. Science 1998; 279(5358):1950–1954.

67. Fukushima K, Ueki Y, Nishizaki K. Autosomal; dominant non-syndromic deafness locus (DFNA 16) maps to chromosome 2q24. (Abst. 103) Presented at The Molecular Biology of Hearing and Deafness Conference, Bethesda, Maryland, October 10, 1998.

68. Lalwani AK, Wilcox ER, Castelein CM. DFNA17, new locus for nonsyndromic hearing loss maps to chromosome 22. (Abst. 104) Presented at The Molecular Biology of Hearing and Deafness Conference, Bethesda, Maryland, October 10, 1998.

69. Boensch D, Scheer P, Storch P, Neuman C, Deufel T, Lamprecht-Dinnesen A. Mapping of a further type of autosomal dominant, non-syndromic hearing impairment (DFNA18) to chromosome 3122. Presented at the American Society of Human Genetics Meeting, 1998, Bethesda, MD.

70. Green, et al. Molecular Biology of Hearing and Deafness. Bethesda, MD, October 8–11, 1998.

71. Guilford P, Ben Arab S, Blanchard S, et al. A non-syndrome form of neurosensory, recessive deafness maps to the pericentromeric region of chromosome 13 q. Nat Gent 1994; 6(1):24–28.

72. Kelsell DP, Dunlop J, Stevens HP, et al. Connexin 26 mutations in hereditary non-syndromic sensorineural deafness. Nature 1997; 387(6628):80–83.

73. Guilford P, Ayadi H, Blanchard S, et al. A human gene responsible for neurosensory, non-syndromic recessive deafness is a candidate homologue of the mouse sh-1 gene. Hum Molec Genet 1994; 3: 989–993.

74. Liu XZ, Walsh J, Mburu P, et al. Mutations in the myosin VIIA gene cause non-syndromic recessive deafness. Nat Gent 1997; 16(2):188–190.

75. Weil D, Kussel P, Blanchard S, et al. The autosomal recessive isolated deafness, DFNB2, and the dUsher 1B syndrome are allelic defects of the myosin-VIIA gene. Nat Genet 1997; 16(2):191–193.

76. Friedman TB, Liang Y, Weber JL, et al. A gene for congenital, recessive deafness DFNB3 maps to the pericentromeric region of chromosome 17. Nat Genet 1995; 9(1):86–91.

77. Wang A, Liang Y, Fridell RA, et al. Association of unconventional myosin MY015 mutations with human nonsyndromic deafness DFNB3. Science 1998; 280(5368):1447–1451.

78. Baldwin CT, Weiss S, Farrer LA, et al. Linkage of congenital recessive deafness (DFNB4) to chromosome 7q31 and evidence for genetic heterogeneity

in the Middle Eastern Bruze population. Hum Mol Genet 1995; 4(9):1637–1642.

79. Li XC, Everett LA, Lalwani AK, et al. A mutation in PDS causes non-syndromic recessive deafness. Nat Genet 1998; 18(3):215–217.

80. Fukushima K, Ramesh A, Srisailapathy CR, et al. Consanguineous nuclear families used to identify a new locus for recessive non-syndromic hearing loss on 14q. Hum Mol Genet 1995; 4(9):1643–1648.

81. Fukushima K, Ramesh A, Srisailapathy CR, et al. An autosomal recessive nonsyndromic form of sensorineural hearing loss maps to 3p-DFNB6. Genome Res 1995; 5(3):305–308.

82. Jain PK, Fukushima K, Deshmukh D, et al. A human recessive neurosensory nonsyndromic hearing impairment locus is a potential homologue of the murine deafness (dn) locus. Hum Mol Genet 1995; 4: 2391–2394.

83. Veske A, Oehlmann R, Younus F, et al. Autosomal recessive non-syndromic deafness locus (DFNB8) maps on chromosome 21q22 in large consanguineous kindred from Pakistan. Hum Mol Genet 1996; 5:165–168.

84. Chaib H, Place C, Salem N, et al. A gene responsible for a sensorineural nonsyndromic recessive deafness maps to chromosome 2p22-23. Hum Mol Genet 1996; 5(1):155–158.

85. Bonne-Tamir B, DeStefano AL, Briggs CE, et al. Linkage of congenital recessive deafness (gene DFNB10) to chromosome 21q22.3. Am J Hum Genet 1996; 58(6):1254–1259.

86. Scott DA, Carmi R, Elbedour K, et al. An autosomal recessive nonsyndromic-hearing loss locus identified by DNA pooling using two inbred Bedouin kindreds. Am J Hum Genet 1996; 59(2):385–391.

87. Chaib H, Place C, Salem N, et al. Mapping of DFNB12, a gene for a non-syndromal autosomal recessive deafness, to chromosome 10q21–22. Hum Mol Genet 1996; 5(7):1061–1064.

88. Mustapha M, Chardenoux S, Nleder A, et al. A sensorineural progressive autosomal recessive form of isolated deafness, DFNB13, maps to chromosome 7q34-q36. Eur J Hum Genet 1998; 6(3): 245–250.

89. Chen A, Wayne S, Bell A, et al. New gene for autosomal recessive non-syndromic hearing loss maps to either chromosome 3q or 19p. Am J Med Genet 1997; 71(4):467–471.

90. Campbell DA, McHale DP, Brown KA, et al. A new locus for non-syndromal, autosomal recessive, sensorineural hearing loss (DFNB16) maps to human chromosome 15q21-q22. J Med Genet 1997 Dec; 34(12)1015–1017.

91. Greinwald JH, Wayne S, Chen AH, et al. Localization of novel gene for nonsyndromic hearing loss (DFNB17 to chromosome region 7q3) Am J Med Genet 1998; 78(2):107–113.

92. Jain PK, Lalwani AK, Li XC, Singleton TL, Smith TN, Chen A, Deshmukh D, Verma IC, Smith RJ, Wilcox ER. A gene for recessive nonsyndromic sensorineural deafness (DFNB18) maps to the chromosomal region 11p14–p15.1 containing the Usher syndrome type 1C gene. Genomics 1998; 50(2): 290–292.

93. Green, et al. Molecular Biology of Hearing and Deafness. Bethesda, MD, October 8–11, 1998.

94. Tranebjaerg L, Schwartz C, Eriksen H, et al. A new X-linked recessive deafness syndrome with blindness, dystonia, fractures and mental deficiency is linked to xq22. J Med Genet 1995; 32(4):257–263.

95. Tyson J, Bellman S, Newton V, et al. Mapping of DFN2 to Xq22. Hum Mol Genet 1996; 5(12): 2055–2060.

96. De Kok YJ, van der Maarel SM, Bitner-Glindzicz M, et al. Association between X-linked mixed deafness and mutations in the POU domain gene POU domain gene POU3F4. Science 1995; 267(5198): 685–688.

97. Lalwani AK, Brister R, Fex J, et al. A new nonsyndromic X-linked sensorineural hearing loss linked to Xp21.2. The Association for Research in Otolaryngology. (ARO) 1994; (Abstract):402.

98. del Castillo I, Villamar M, Sarduy M, et al. A novel locus for non-syndromic sensorineural deafness (DFN6) maps to chromosome Xp22. Hum Mol Genet 1996; 5(9):1383–1387.

99. Kelley PM, Harris DJ, Comer BC, et al. Novel mutations in the connexin 26 gene (GJB2) that cause autosomal recessive (DFNB1) hearing loss. Am J Hum Genet 1998; 62:792–799.

100. Biancalana V, LeMarec B, Odent S, et al. Oto-palato-digital syndrome type I: Further evidence for assignment of the locus to Xq28. Hum Genet 1991; 88(2): 228–230.

101. Boughman JA, Shaver KA. Responsibilities in genetic counseling for the deaf. Am J Hum Genet 1983; 35(6):1317–1319.

102. Bieber FR, Nance WE. Hereditary hearing loss. In: Jackson LG, Schimke RN eds. *Clinical Genetics: A Sourcebook for Physicians.* New York: John Wiley & Sons, 1979, pp. 443–461.

103. Stagno S, Pass RF, Dworsky ME, et al. Congenital cytomegalovirus infection: The relative importance of primary and recurrent maternal infection. N Engl J Med 1982; 306(16):945–949.

104. Lynfield R, Eaton RB. Teratogen update: Congenital toxoplasmosis. Teratology 1995; 52:176–180.

105. Desmonts G, Couvreur J. Congenital toxoplasmosis: A prospective study of 378 pregnancies. N Engl J Med 1974; 290:1110–1116.

106. Daffos F, Forestier F, Capella-Pavlovsky M, et al. Prenatal management of 746 pregnancies at risk for congenital toxoplasmosis. N Engl J Med 1988; 318(5):271–275.

107. Decoster A, Darcy F, Caron A. IgA antibodies against P30 as markers of congenital and acute toxoplasmosis. Lancet 1988; 2:1104–1106.

108. Stepick-Biek P, Thulliez P, Araujo FG, et al. IgA antibodies for diagnosis of acute congenital and acquired toxoplasmosis. J Infect Dis 1990; 162(1):270–273.

109. Roizen N, Swisher CN, Stein MA, et al. Neurologic and developmental outcome in treated congenital toxoplasmosis. Pediatrics 1995; 95(1):11–20.

110. Gregg NM. Congenital cataract following German measles in the mother. Ophthal Cos Aust 1941; 3:35–46.

111. Swan C, Tostevin AL, Moore B, et al. Congenital defects in infants following infectious diseases during pregnancy with special reference to relationship between German measles and cataracts, deafmutism, heart disease and microcephaly and to period of pregnancy in which occurrence of rubella is followed by congenital abnormalities. Med J Aust 1943; 2:201–210.

111a.Robbins JB, Schneerson R, Anderson P, Smith DH. Prevention of systemic infections, especially meningitis, caused by Haemophilus influenzae type b. Impact on public health and implications for other polysaccharide-based vaccines. JAMA, 276(14):1181–1185, 1996.

112. Schuchat A, Robinson K, Wenger JD, et al. Bacterial meningitis in the United States in 1995. Active surveillance team. N Engl J Med 1997; 337(14):970–976.

113. Richardson MP, Reid A, Tarlow MJ, et al. Hearing loss during bacterial meningitis. Arch Dis Child 1997; 76(2):134–138.

114. Nadol JB Jr. Medical progress—Hearing loss, review article. N Eng J Med 1993; 1092–1102.

114a.Kilpi T, Peltola H, Jauhiainen T, Kallio MJ. Oral glycerol and intravenous dexamethasone in preventing neurologic and audiologic sequelae of childhood bacterial meningitis. The Finnish Study Group. Pediatr Infect Dis J 1995; 14(4):270–278.

115. Brownell WE, Bader CR, Bertrand D, et al. Evoked mechanical responses of isolated cochlear outer hair cells. Science 1996; 227:194–196.

116. Schacht, J. Molecular mechanisms of drug-induced hearing loss. Hear Res 1986; 48:297–304.

117. Dreschler WA, Hulst RJAM, Tange RA. The role of high-frequency audiometry in early detection of ototoxicity. Audiology 1985; 24:387–395.

19 Pediatric Cochlear Implantation

Audie L. Woolley and Rodney P. Lusk

Cochlear implants are now firmly established as effective options in the enablement and rehabilitation of select children with profound hearing impairment. Since the Federal Drug Administration (FDA) approved the Nucleus 22 channel-cochlear implant for children ages 2 to 17 in June 1990, approximately 4000 children have received cochlear implants worldwide,[1] and approximately 600 children have received the Clarion cochlear implant. The key to successful implantation lies in the appropriate selection of candidates, skillful surgery, and experienced rehabilitation. This involves a multidiscipline approach that encompasses pediatric audiology, speech and language evaluation, expert radiographic evaluation, and a thorough medical examination prior to selecting each candidate.

DEVICE DESCRIPTION

All cochlear implants have two major components:[2] the internal or implanted component and the external component, which is worn on the body. The *internal component* consists of one or more electrodes that are implanted into the cochlea. An internal receiver is imbedded into the temporal bone above and behind the auricle.

The *external components* consist of a microphone, an external transmitter, and a signal processor. The *signal processor* is responsible for transporting the sound stimulus that is received by the microphone and preparing it for transmission to the external transmitter and then to the internal receiver.

The incoming sound is analyzed by the signal processor and computed into fundamental acoustical information that represents key elements of human speech. The analysis results in coding for the appropriate electrode, current amplitude, and stimulus rate. The processed signal is sent transdermally via radio frequency transmission to the internal receiver. The message is decoded so that separate bipolar pairs of electrodes are activated to stimulate segments of the auditory nerve.[2]

CANDIDATE SELECTION

Practice Pathway 19–1 outlines the evaluation procedures for the standard cochlear implant candidate.

The selection criteria for cochlear implantation in children are as follows.[3]

- 2 years of age or older
- Profound bilateral sensorineural hearing loss (SNHL)
- No appreciable benefit from hearing aids
- No medical contraindications
- High motivation and appropriate expectations
- Enrollment in a program that emphasizes development of auditory skills

PREOPERATIVE EVALUATION

Practice Pathway 19–2 summarizes the medical and psychologic evaluations prior to cochlear implantation, as well as the contraindications to implantation.

Audiologic and Speech Evaluation

Once a child is referred for cochlear implant candidacy determination, a multidisciplinary evaluation should begin. The cochlear implant team should include a surgeon, an audiologist, a speech-language pathologist, and teachers for the deaf; each of these

Pediatric Otolaryngology, Edited by R.F. Wetmore, H.R. Muntz, and T.J. McGill. Thieme Medical Publishers, Inc., New York © 2000.

Practice Pathway 19–1   STANDARD COCHLEAR IMPLANT
CANDIDATE EVALUATION

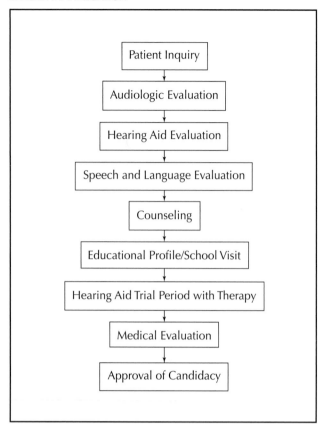

specialists plays a crucial role in the preimplant evaluation. The preimplant evaluation begins with the audiologic assessment. Unaided and aided hearing thresholds are obtained with the use of conventional amplification. The potential implant candidate must have bilateral, profound SNHL with a pure tone and an unaided threshold in the better hearing ear equal to or greater than 95 dB. In children less than 6 years of age, auditory brain stem testing is performed frequently to confirm the hearing loss.

SPECIAL CONSIDERATION:

The potential implant candidate must have bilateral, profound SNHL with a pure tone and an unaided threshold in the better hearing ear ≥95 dB.

Once the hearing loss is confirmed, a trial amplification is carried out to assess the child's benefit

from hearing aids. Discrimination testing is performed with the hearing aid that provides the best warble-tone threshold. Over a 6 month period of time, the child's aided performance on the discrimination tests is compared with the results of children using cochlear implants. Children who demonstrate no response to warble tones in the sound field with the appropriate hearing aids or whose responses suggest only vibrotactile responses rather than auditory sensations become implant candidates and need medical assessment.

Once the hearing loss is identified, a thorough medical evaluation is performed. Medical assessment includes a careful review of the otologic history, a physical examination, and radiographic evaluation of the cochlea. Every effort is made to establish the etiology of the deafness. With few exceptions, experience with cochlear implants demonstrates that auditory neural elements that can be stimulated seem to be present, regardless if the cause of deafness is congenital or acquired.[4] Prior to implantation, particular attention is paid to the status of the tympanic membrane (TM) and middle ear. An otologically-stable condition should be present prior to implantation. The TM should be intact, and there should be no evidence of infection. If the child is otitis prone and has recurrent otitis media (OM), the condition should be treated appropriately. Conventional antibiotic therapy usually accomplishes this. If medical management fails, then myringotomy tubes are inserted until the middle ear becomes infection free. We prefer to remove the myringotomy tube from the ear that is to be implanted approximately 4 to 6 weeks prior to implantation. This allows time for the TM to heal. The incidence of acute OM actually drops 35 to 60% in the implanted ear after surgery.[5] When a middle ear effusion occurs in an ear in which a cochlear implant device was placed previously, no treatment is required as long as the effusion remains uninfected.

Radiographic Assessment

High-resolution, thin-section, computer tomography (CT) scanning of the cochlea and temporal bone is performed during the preoperative evaluation. CT is vital in helping the surgeon assess the feasibility of implantation in a particular candidate. It assists in the decision of which ear to implant, and allows the surgeon to ensure that the inner ear morphology is normal, including patency of the cochlea. A checklist created by the Children's Hos-

Practice Pathway 19–2   EVALUATION PROCEDURES FOR COCHLEAR IMPLANTATION

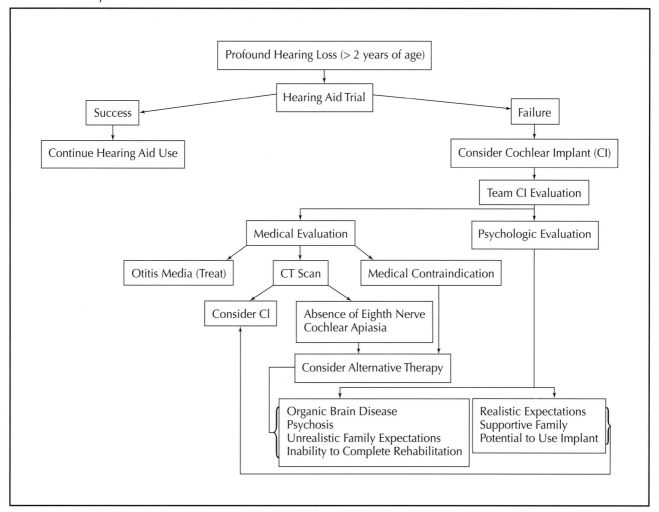

pital of Alabama, will aid the surgeon and radiologist in identifying potential risks and complications as shown in Table 19-1.[6] Congenital cochlear abnormalities do not necessarily preclude implantation, but need to be identified preoperatively in order to assist in the surgical planning. Likewise, although cochlear ossification does not exclude the patient from implantation, it may influence the type and length of the electrode array and the surgical approach used; as well, it may help to predict the overall postimplanted performance.

Absolute contraindications to implantation include cochlear aplasia or absence of the auditory nerve.[7] In any case where the internal auditory canal (IAC) is less than 2 mm in size, magnetic resonance imaging (MRI) should be performed to confirm the presence of the cochlear nerve (Fig. 19-1).[7] Likewise, if soft tissue obliteration of the cochlea is suspected secondary to meningitis, MRI should be ob-

tained because soft tissue obliteration usually will not be seen on CT.

SPECIAL CONSIDERATION:

Congenital cochlear abnormalities and cochlear ossification do not necessarily preclude implantation, but need to be considered in surgical planning. Absolute contraindications to implantation include cochlear aplasia or absence of the auditory nerve.

Psychologic and Social Considerations

The parents and family members should become an integral part of the implant team. The parents need

TABLE 19–1:   Cochlear Implant Radiographic Evaluation

I. Mastoid Aeration (Circle one)	Grade	I	II	III
II. Middle Ear Abnormalities (Circle one)				
Yes		No		
Explain _____				
III. Cochlear Anatomy (Circle one)				
	LEFT	RIGHT		
Normal	_____	_____		
Incomplete partition	_____	_____		
Hypoplasia	_____	_____		
Common cavity	_____	_____		
Aplasia	_____	_____		
IV. Cochlear Ossification (Circle one)	Yes	No		
	LEFT	RIGHT		
Site of Ossification	_____	_____		
Round Window Niche	_____	_____		
Basal Turn (mm from niche)	_____	_____		
Mid-Turn (mm from niche)	_____	_____		
Apical Turn (mm from niche)	_____	_____		
V. Vestibular Aqueduct (Circle)				
LEFT Normal	Enlarged	RIGHT: Normal	Enlarged	
VI. Internal Auditory Canal				
LEFT: Normal	<1.5 mm	RIGHT: Normal	<1.5 mm	
SHAPE: Symmetric		Symmetric		
Asymmetric _____		Asymmetric _____		
_____		_____		

From reference 6, with permission.

to understand that a tremendous amount of the postoperative rehabilitation is carried out at home. Parents must be willing to spend extra time with their child, carrying out implant-oriented exercises during their daily interactions. The educational setting

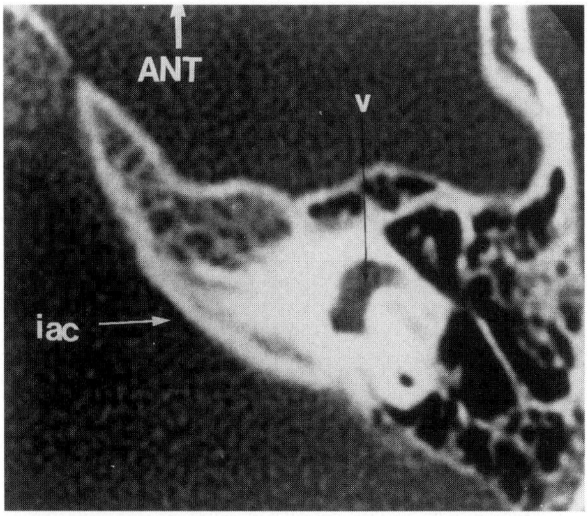

Figure 19–1:   Axial CT of the temporal bone at the level of the IAC. Note complete absence of the IAC. The arrow points to the location where the IAC should be, and V indicates the vestibule. This particular patient had intact facial nerve function, but no eighth nerve function. (Photo courtesy of William Gibson, MD.)

into which the child is enrolled must cooperate in placing special emphasis on auditory training.

At the current time, psychologic and social considerations for a successful candidate include:[2,8]

- No evidence of severe organic brain damage
- No evidence of psychosis
- No evidence of mental retardation
- No behavioral or personality traits that would make completion of the program unlikely
- No unrealistic expectations about the goals of the implant
- A pattern of parent/child interaction that indicates that the family will be able to follow the postimplant rehabilitative program effectively

COCHLEAR IMPLANTATION

Ear Selection

In choosing which ear to implant, the surgeon carefully reviews the audiologic evaluation and CT to make a selection. If no acoustical difference between the ears exists, the implant is placed in the better surgical ear as determined by CT. If both ears are identical, the implant is placed on the side with the dominant hand in order to facilitate device manipulation. If the ears are different, according to peripheral factors, the surgeon should implant the better-hearing ear provided that there is no significant hearing in it. For example, in a child with different durations of profound hearing impairment in each ear, better results usually are obtained when the ear with the shortest duration of deafness is implanted.[9] For the candidate who has bilateral profound hearing loss but who has used a hearing aid for sound awareness in one ear with little or no benefit as determined by the audiologist, we encourage placing the implant in the ear that has received the most auditory stimulation.[9] We inform the family that although we expect that particular ear to be the best for implantation, the child will likely lose whatever residual hearing is in that ear.

Surgical Procedure

In children, flap design is crucial because of the delicate tissues and small dimensions. The skin incision that is described by Dr. Richard Miyamoto has eliminated the need to develop a large post auricular flap.[3]

After induction of anesthesia, electrodes for monitoring the facial nerve are placed. The position of the internal component of the implant is determined and marked on the external skin surface with a methylene-blue, marking pen. This position may vary with the different implants. By making a template of the implant 1 to 2 cm behind the postauricular crease, the incision begins 2 cm from the edge of the implant. The inferior extent of the incision is made posterior to the mastoid tip (Fig. 19–2) to preserve the branches of the posterior auricular artery. The incision is directed posteriorly-superiorly and then superiorly without a superior-anterior limb. The flap is elevated anteriorly as a skin-muscle, periosteal flap to provide access to the mastoid process. A canal, wall-up mastoidectomy with an extended, facial recess approach is performed. Working through the facial recess, the round window niche is identified 2 mm inferior to the stapes. Occasionally, the round window niche is not well visualized through the facial recess in children. The round window niche may be obscured by an overlying facial nerve in the vertical segment, a prominent pyramidaleminence or, in some cases, by ossification. It is very important for the surgeon to realize the relationship of the round window to the stapes and oval window because this prevents the surgeon from being misdirected by prominent hypotym-

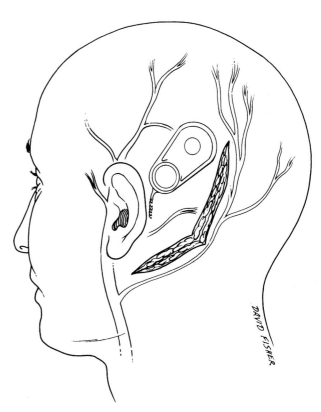

Figure 19–2: Skin incision for cochlear implantation in children.

panic air cells. Entry into the cochlea is carried out with a small fenestration placed anteriorly and slightly inferiorly to the annulus of the round window membrane. A 1.5 mm diamond burr is used to drill down to the white endosteum and then a 1 mm diamond burr is used to create an opening in the bone that is approximately 1.2 to 1.5 mm in diameter. The bone is then removed and its edges smoothed with a large McGee cochlear rasp (Storz, St. Louis, MO). This approach bypasses the hook area of the scala tympani, allowing direct insertion of the active electrode array.

SPECIAL CONSIDERATION:

It is very important for the surgeon to realize the relationship of the round window to the stapes and oval window because this prevents the surgeon from being misdirected by prominent hypotympanic air cells.

Returning to the mastoid cortex, the site of the template is outlined on the skull. A circular-shaped well is drilled through the cortex and down to the inner table of the skull. In children, it is important to create as deep a well as possible so that the implant is adequately recessed. In very young children, the inner table of the skull is removed, and the implant is placed directly on the dura. The surgeon should attempt to preserve the inner table of the skull, thinning it down so that the bone is able to be "egg-shelled" over the dura.

SPECIAL CONSIDERATION:

In creating a well for the implant in children, it is important to make it as deep as possible so that it will be recessed adequately.

The electrode and as many retaining rings as possible are inserted into the scala tympani through the cochleostomy. Next, the cochleostomy is packed and sealed with fascia, preventing electrode migration and perilymphatic fluid leakage. Then, the implant is placed into the circular well, which has been created in the cortex of the skull, and secured with 2.0 prolene sutures that are placed through the preserved mastoid cortex. Finally, the skin is closed in two layers using absorbable sutures. A drain is not used routinely.

Surgery usually takes 1.5 to 2.5 hours, and the patients are discharged on the day following surgery. The first postoperative visit is at 1 week to check the wound. Approximately 4 to 6 weeks later, after flap edema has resolved, the fitting and the mapping of the signal processor begins.

Special Surgical Situations

Cochlear Ossification

Ossification of the labyrinth and the scala tympani especially is a common complication of bacterial meningitis. It may also be seen in other common causes of profound deafness.[10] In an earlier report of cochlear implants in children who were deafened by meningitis, 20 out of 25 (80%) were noted to have some degree of ossification.[11] Ossification of the cochlea makes electrode insertion quite diffi-

cult. The degree and location of the cochlear ossification defines the surgical approach that should be taken. If successful implantation is carried out, the hearing outcomes in patients with partially ossified cochleae appear to be quite similar to those patients with nonossified cochlea. Good hearing results have also been obtained with a variety of surgical procedures for totally ossified cochleae.[11-14]

If obstruction is limited to the inferior segment of the cochlea (i.e., the category of cochlear ossification most frequently seen following meningitis), the obstruction may be removed or a tunnel may be created through the obstruction to reach an open window within the cochlea.[12] This technique is successful if the obstruction is limited to 8 to 10 mm, measured from the round window membrane. In those cases, the new bone formation will be recognized as being less dense and a lighter color. Following this bone anteriorly leads into a patent scala tympani, if the obstructed inferior segment is short. Complete electrode insertion is possible if the obstruction is limited to the inferior segment, and results in these cases are equivalent to implanted patients with patent cochleae.[12]

If obstruction extends apically into the ascending segment, the scala vestibuli can be opened by widening the cochleostomy 1 to 2 mm superiorly. Steenerson et al have reported successful electrode insertion in the scala vestibuli of patients with obstruction of the scala tympani.[13] It is thought that meningogenic osteoneogenesis occurs through the cochlear aqueduct, which opens into the scala tympani. In some cases, ossification may be limited to the scala tympani, sparing the scala vestibuli.[10]

If the scala vestibuli is also obstructed, the only way to achieve a complete electrode insertion in the cochlea is to drill an open trough around the modiolus, as described by Gantz et al.[12,15] This technique is performed by beginning with a radical mastoidectomy. The skin and mucosa are removed from the middle ear, including the TM, malleus, and incus. Drilling begins by sketching the location of the carotid artery in the middle ear so that it can be identified and avoided. Then, an inferior tunnel that is approximately 8 to 10 mm is created at the usual site of the cochleostomy. Next, a second trough, which is approximately 6 to 8 mm, is created anteriorly from the oval window, and then the two troughs are connected by carefully drilling around the modiolus. Great care must be taken not to drill into the modiolus. Once the trough has been drilled around the modiolus, the electrode is curled into it and held in place by fascia and tissue glue. Although experience with this surgery is limited, the results with patients implanted by Gantz's procedure have been encouraging.

Although CT is quite helpful in identifying osteoneogenesis within the cochlea, it can be misleading also. Jackler et al. reported that a normal, preoperative CT does not exclude the possibility of compromised cochlear patency.[16] In their series, a 48% false-negative rate existed because of subtle degrees of osseous or fibrous obliteration of the cochlea that were beyond the resolution of CT.[16] In any child with postmeningitic deafness, the cochlear-implant surgeon must be prepared to encounter some degree of ossification, even when CT is normal. MRI scans may be helpful in identifying soft-tissue obstruction within the cochlea.

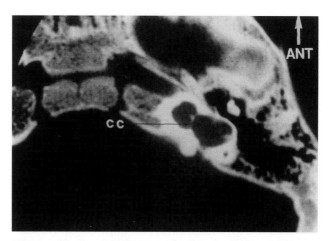

Figure 19–3: Axial cut at the level of the cochlea reveals a large, common, cavity deformity of the cochlea; a dysplastic lateral semicircular canal; and enlargement of the vestibular aqueduct. The large, white arrow points to the anterior and CC points to the common, cavity deformity.

SPECIAL CONSIDERATION:

In any child with postmeningitic deafness, the surgeon must be prepared to encounter some degree of ossification, even when the CT is normal.

Congenital inner ear malformations

There are well-documented risks in performing cochlear implantation in a patient with inner ear malformations. In cochlear malformations, the cribiform area between the modiolus and IAC is often very thin and may actually be absent (Fig. 19–3).[17,18] In the ear with an enlarged vestibular aqueduct, the endolymphatic sac and duct are known to be grossly dilated, allowing communication with the cerebrospinal fluid (CSF) and increasing the risk of CSF leak during the cochleostomy.[19] Malpositions of the facial nerve are also more common in patients with congenital inner ear malformations.

A gusher is managed by allowing the CSF reservoir to drain off. Once the CSF leak slows, the electrode may be inserted into the cochlea, followed by packing around the cochleostomy with fascia and muscle. Although this usually seals the leak, occasionally a lumbar drain may be used to reduce the CSF reservoir until a satisfactory seal has occurred.

AT A GLANCE . . .

Risks of Cochlear Implantation in Children with Congenital Cochlear Malformations

- Cribiform area may be thin or absent
- CSF leak
- Malpositions of facial nerve
- CSF gusher

Revision Surgery

Unfortunately, revision surgery still occurs because of device failure or infection. Revision is possible because significant degeneration of the remaining viable neural tissue due to mechanical trauma does not appear to occur.[20] The implant can usually be reimplanted in the same ear. It is not difficult to remove and reinsert a cochlear implant electrode into the scala tympani. Two difficulties that may be encountered are an exposed facial nerve from previous surgery and extensive fibrosis filling the scala tympani. It may be difficult to obtain a full insertion in revision cases because of fibrosis. This soft tissue can be removed through the cochleostomy.

Implants potentially may fail because of manufacturing defects or use-related trauma. Ninety five percent of the Nucleus 22 implants are still functioning after 9 years. Current implants include self-test circuitry that allows objective device monitoring. Re-implantation of the same ear is usually possible, and so far, individual auditory performances after reimplantation have equaled or exceeded that seen with the original implant.

Complications

Fortunately, complications with cochlear implantation done by experienced surgeons have been infrequent. In a recent review of complications,[21] the most frequently encountered problems were those associated with the incision and flap. Using the incision described above in the pediatric population, we have not had any flap breakdown in over 135 children implanted. Facial nerve injury can be avoided by careful dissection of the facial recess. The facial nerve should be left encased in bone when working through the facial recess toward the mesotympanum, and care must be taken so that the shaft of the burr does not rotate against the nerve.

Force must not be used when inserting the long Nucleus 22 channel electrode. Excessive force may lead to damage of intracochlear tissue with loss of the stimulative neuronal population and kinking of the electrode.[22] Routine anterior and posterior skull films should be obtained in the operating room prior to extubation to document electrode position and lack of electrocompression when using this particular implant (Fig. 19–4). In children with congenital deafness, there is a greater risk that the facial nerve may follow an aberrant course within the temporal bone. The preoperative CT should be helpful in predicting this anomaly.

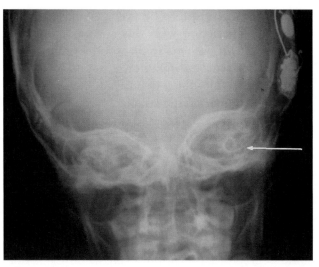

Figure 19–4: Anterior and posterior skull film confirming position of a Nucleus 22 channel-cochlear implant coiled into the cochlear (arrow). Note lack of electrode compression.

SPECIAL CONSIDERATION:

Excessive force when inserting the electrode may lead to damage of intracochlear tissue with loss of the stimulative neuronal population and kinking of the electrode.

REHABILITATION

A key portion of the rehabilitation process is carried out prior to implantation. Four to 6 weeks before surgery, the child is introduced to the equipment

by loaning a dummy speech processor, transmitter, and microphone to the family for use at home. Approximately 4 to 6 weeks after surgery, the child is seen for the initial mapping and tune-up session, which is scheduled over a 2 day period. During this session, the child is fit with the external equipment, and the parents and child are given instructions in the maintenance of the unit. Thresholds and comfort level are obtained for each of the active electrodes. The *threshold* is defined as the minimum amount of current that is required for the child to indicate that a sound is perceived.[23] At least two audiologists are necessary to properly set the threshold and comfort level in young children. Educators for the deaf and speech therapists proficient in sign language can assist in communicating with children who are not oral communicators.

Every child is unique with respect to mapping. The parents' active participation during the sessions helps them realize the benefits and limitations of the implant and gives them practice in working with the child. Depending upon the device and a child's age and needs, the rehabilitation process may require daily sessions for 1 to 2 weeks until the map is set. The time commitment on the part of the parents must be understood before the child undergoes implantation.

Speech therapists and educators for the deaf are vital liaisons to the school system. These individuals assist in the transition of the child from the rehabilitation program to the educational setting and help parents make educational decisions for their child. They also bring expertise regarding classroom placement and communication issues for each child. It is clear that the educational programs for children with cochlear implants must include auditory and speech instruction using auditory information provided by the implant.

RESULTS

Several factors, including age at the time of deafness, age at the time of implantation, duration of deafness, status of the remaining nerve fibers, educational setting, type of implant, and length of time with the implant, all play a role in the success of the implant. The definition of success, however, varies from patient to patient and family to family.

Children with congenital deafness and children with prelingually-acquired-meningitic deafness achieve similar auditory performance, if the cochlear implant is received before the age of 6. In general, the etiology of hearing loss does not appear to affect auditory performance in either children or adults, as long as the cochlear nerve is intact.[24]

Children with a memory of previous auditory experience and a short period of deafness have a distinctive advantage over children who are prelingually hearing impaired; however, the difference between children with postlingual and prelingual or perilingual onset of deafness lessens with time. Postlingual deaf subjects showed dramatic improvement on all perceptual tests after only 6 months of implant use because of the advantage of previous hearing.[25] Prelingual hearing impaired children show large improvements in speech perception skills, but over a longer, protracted course.[25] Perceptual performance increases on average with each succeeding year after implantation. The results from Miyamoto et al. suggest that the most important factor contributing to individual differences among implant users is the amount of experience that the users have with the device.[26]

In a report by Miyamoto et al., the speech perception skills of 50 prelingually hearing-impaired children who underwent cochlear implantation and were followed for more than 5 years were graded and compared to those of age-appropriate children who used hearing aids.[27] The hearing aid users were grouped into gold, silver, and bronze groups based on pure tone averages (PTA). The gold hearing aid

users were children with a mean PTA of 90 to 100 dB HL; the silver group had a mean PTA of 101 to 110 dB HL; and the bronze group had a mean PTA of 110 dB HL. Two years following implantation, the speech perception performance of the implanted children surpassed that of the silver hearing aid users, and by 3½ years, the mean scores of the implant users were 20 to 40% higher than the silver hearing aid users and were similar to the gold hearing aid users. Likewise, the speech intelligibility of the children with cochlear implants improved from 0 to 40% after 3½ years and exceeded those of the silver hearing aid users. This advantage has continued to increase over time.

In children with prelingual hearing loss who received implants, Gantz et al reported that 4 years following implantation 80% of children achieved open-set, sound-only, word understanding. Speech perception skills continue to develop and do not reach a plateau.[25] Some of the prelingual hearing-impaired children actually achieved higher scores than some of the postlingually deaf children. Of significance, no subject demonstrated a deterioration in performance over the observation period.

In their evaluation of prelingual hearing-impaired children who were implanted before the age of 3 years and then followed for 2 to 5 years, Waltzman et al found significant improvement in the perception of all aspects of the speech signal.[28] Mean, postoperative, sound-field threshold improved from 36 to 39 dB HL at the first postoperative year to 15 to 25 dB HL at 5 years postoperatively in some children. All of the children demonstrated open-set speech recognition, used oral language as their primary means of communication, and attended regular schools.

Age at the time of implantation is important. It is likely, that the auditory and central nervous system have a critical period for learning, and these systems must be stimulated before a certain age in order to achieve speech perception.[25] The age at which auditory information provided by cochlear implants becomes less useful to deaf individuals is unknown. Speech production results, in a limited number of children with prelingual hearing loss, suggest that children with early-onset deafness (prior to 4 years of age) demonstrate more improvement of speech production skills than those who receive an implant after 10 years of age.[29] However, results have shown that prelingually deaf children up to 13 years of age can obtain substantial speech perception from multichannel implants.[25] Because older children on the whole tend to perform more poorly, they should be assessed in a much more intensive manner to ensure proper selection of the appropriate candidate.

AT A GLANCE...

Results of Cochlear Implantation

- In general, if the cochlear nerve is intact, the etiology of hearing loss does not appear to affect auditory performance.

- Age at the time of implantation is especially important because the auditory system and CNS may have a critical period for learning.

- Children who are prelingually deaf take longer to show improvement with cochlear implants than children who are postlingually deaf, but their performance improves each year. Experience is the biggest contributing factor to success with cochlear implants.

- Children who are postlingually deaf have an initial advantage over children who are prelingually deaf, and they show dramatic improvement after only 6 months of implant use.

CONCLUSION

Currently, children at least 2 years of age and older with profound deafness are candidates for implantation. Auditory performance with cochlear implants varies among individuals, but data indicate that performance is better in children who have shorter durations of deafness, who have acquired speech and language before hearing loss, and who have received implants before the age of 6 (if prelingual) Auditory performance does not appear to be affected by the etiology of the hearing loss. Access to optimal education and rehabilitation services is vitally important for children to maximize the benefits available from cochlear implantation. Cochlear implants continue to improve and the current generation of intracochlear, multichannel implants with spectrally-based speech processors provides a substantial improvement over the devices of the previous generation. Advances that have been made in improving speech perception in cochlear implant users should continue to improve with changes in electrode design and signal processing strategies.

REFERENCES

1. Parisier S, Chute P, Popp A. Cochlear implant mechanical failures. Am J Otol 1996; 17:730–734.
2. Kveton J, Balkany T. American academy of otolaryngology—head and neck surgery subcommittee on cochlear implants: Status of cochlear implantation in children. J Pediatr 1991; 118:1–7.
3. Miyamoto RT. Cochlear implants in children. In: Bluestone C, Stool S, Kenna M, eds. *Pediatric Otolaryngology. 3rd ed.* Philadelphia: Saunders, 1996, pp. 671–675.
4. Hinojosa R, Marion M. Histopathology of profound sensorineural deafness. Ann NY Acad Sci 1983; 405: 459–484.
5. House W, Luxford W, Courtney B. Otitis media in children following cochlear implantation. Ear Hear 1985; 6:24S–26S.
6. Woolley A, Oser A, Lusk R, Bahadori R. Preoperative temporal bone computed tomography scan and its use in evaluating the pediatric cochlear implant candidate. Laryngoscope 1997; 107:1100–1106.
7. Shelton C, Luxford W, Tonokawa L, Lo W, House W. The narrow internal auditory canal in children: A contraindication to cochlear implants. Arch Otolaryngol Head Neck Surg 1989; 100:227–231.
8. Hartrampf R, Lesinski A, Allum D, Dahm M, Lenarz T. Reasons for rejected candidacy for cochlear implantation in children. Adv Otolaryngol 1995; 50: 14–18.
9. Luxford W. Surgery for cochlear implantation. In: Brackmann D, Shelton C, Arriaga M, eds. *Otologic Surgery.* Philadelphia: Saunders, 1994, pp. 426–436.
10. Green J Jr, Marion M, Hinojosa R. Labyrinthitis ossificans: Histopathologic considerations for cochlear implantation. Otolaryngol Head Neck Surg 1991; 104:320–326.
11. Eisenberg L, Luxford W, Becker T, House W. Electrical stimulation of the auditory system in children deafened by meningitis. Otolaryngol Head Neck Surg 1984; 92:700–705.
12. Balkany T, Gantz B, Steenerson R, Cohen N. Systematic approach to electrode insertion in the ossified cochlea. Otolaryngol Head Neck Surg 1996; 114: 4–11.
13. Steenerson R, Gary L, Wynens M. Scala vestibuli cochlear implantation for labyrinthine ossification. Am J Otol 1990; 11:360–363.
14. Telian S, Zimmerman-Phillips MS, Kileny P. Successful revision of failed cochlear implants in severe labyrinthitis ossificans. Am J Otol 1997; 17:53–60.

15. Gantz B, McCabe B, Tyler R. Use of multichannel cochlear implants in obstructed and obliterated cochleae. Otolaryngol Head Neck Surg 1997; 98:72-81.

16. Jackler R, Luxford W, Schindler R, McKerrow W. Cochlear patency problems in cochlear implantation. Laryngoscope 1987; 97:801-805.

17. Monsell EM, Jackler RK, Motta G, Linthicum FH. Congenital malformations of the inner ear. Laryngoscope 1987; 97:18-24.

18. Schuknecht H. Mondini dysplasia: A clinical and pathological study. Ann Otol Rhinol Laryngol 1980; 89:3-23.

19. Hirsch BE, Weissman JL, Curtin HD, Kamerer DB. Magnetic resonance imaging of the large vestibular aqueduct. Arch Otolaryngol Head Neck Surg 1992; 118:1124-1127.

20. Jackler R, Leake P, McKerrow W. Cochlear implant revision: Effects of reimplantation on the cochlea. Annals of Otology, Rhinology, & Laryngology 1989; 98:813-820.

21. Cohen N, Hoffman R, Stroschein M. Medical or surgical complications related to the Nucleus multichannel cochlear implant. Ann Otol Rhinol Laryngol 1988; 97:8-13.

22. Cohen N. Cochlear implant soft surgery: Fact or fantasy? Otolaryngol Head Neck Surg 1997; 117:214-216.

23. Parisier S, Chute P, Nevins M. Pediatric cochlear implants: Surgical and rehabilitative issues. *Highlights of Instructional Courses,* num 7. St. Louis: Mosby Yearbook, 1994, pp. 145-154.

24. NIH Consensus Development Panel on Cochlear Implants in Adults and Children. Cochlear implants in adults and children. JAMA 1995; 274:1955-1960.

25. Gantz B, Tyler R, Woodworth G, Tye Murray N, Fryauf-Bertschy H. Results of multichannel cochlear implants in congenital and acquired prelingual deafness in children: Five year follow-up. Am J Otol 1994; 15:1-7.

26. Miyamoto RT, Osberger MJ, Todd SL, et al. Variables affecting implant performance in children. Laryngoscope 1994; 104:1120-1124.

27. Miyamoto RT, Kirk K, Robbins A, Todd S, Riley A. Speech perception and speech production skills of children with multichannel cochlear implants. Acta Otolaryngol 1996; 116:240-243.

28. Waltzman S, Cohen N, Gomolin R, Shapiro W, Ozdamar S, Hoffman R. Long-term results of early cochlear implantation in congenitally and prelingually deafened children. Am J Otol 1994; 15:9-13.

29. Staller S, Beiter A, Brimacombe J, Mecklenburg D, Amdt P. Pediatric performance with the Nucleus 22 channel-cochlear implant system. Am J Otol 1991; 12:126-136.

20 Traumatic Injury to the Ear and Temporal Bone

Ronald W. Deskin

The otolaryngologist is commonly called upon to evaluate and manage children who have suffered trauma to the ear. Some of these injuries may be relatively minor, involving small specific areas of the ear (such as the pinna), or may be a component of a major injury that requires evaluation and management from a multidisciplinary group. Protocols and practice pathways provide the most direct approach to management and improve the possibilities of a more successful outcome.

First, consideration should be given to the general principles of trauma management (Table 20-1). Injuries to the head and neck require initial evaluation of airway status, circulation, and the cervical spine. Careful evaluation of these should be carried out prior to any ear assessment. A general neurologic evaluation is also mandatory. In adolescents and teenagers, the concomitant use of drugs and alcohol must also be taken into consideration during this initial assessment. Radiographic and more specialized examinations may be necessary to detect leakage of cerebral spinal fluid (CSF) and presence of cranial nerve deficits. The initial otolaryngologic exam should be as complete and detailed as the patient's condition allows.

OTOLOGIC EVALUATION

The most frequent symptoms of temporal bone involvement resulting from head trauma are: (1) unconsciousness; (2) bleeding from the ear; (3) loss of hearing; (4) vertigo; (5) facial paralysis; (6) CSF otorrhea; and (7) tinnitus.[1]

Unconsciousness is usually of short duration, but may last longer depending on the extent of the head injury. Unconsciousness has been reported in 50-100 percent of head-trauma patients that suffer an otologic injury.[1]

Bleeding from the ear canal is usually not profuse and is of short duration, unless a major vessel such as the carotid artery or jugular vein is involved. In severe cases, blood may follow the path of least resistance through the eustachian tube and appear in either the mouth or the nose. Bleeding from the ear may be secondary to external auditory canal (EAC) laceration, temporomandibular joint (TMJ) injury with canal laceration, tympanic membrane (TM) perforation, or temporal bone fracture.

Complaints of hearing loss may arise from obstruction of the EAC with blood or displaced skin and cartilage, TM perforation, ossicular discontinuity, or labyrinthine damage that results from either concussion injury or temporal bone fracture. Tinnitus may accompany traumatic hearing loss.

Vertigo occurs in a small percentage of patients. It is usually the result of concussion injury or a temporal bone fracture that involves the vestibular labyrinth. Facial nerve paralysis typically results from a temporal bone fracture and the prognosis is worse if documented immediately after the injury.

The initial evaluation of a child with trauma to the ear should include a thorough examination of the head and neck for associated injuries. Because ear trauma may be the result of physical abuse (Fig. 20-1), the examiner should carefully search for other signs of abuse to the head and neck as well as to other areas of the body. Inspection of the external ear should include the identification of lacerations or hematomas of the pinna. Ecchymosis over the mastoid tip (i.e., Battle's sign) is suggestive of a temporal bone fracture. After inspecting the external ear for injury, the EAC should be examined with an otoscope or, preferably, an operating microscope and cleaned using an aseptic technique. Lacerations of the EAC or perforations of the TM should

Pediatric Otolaryngology, Edited by R.F. Wetmore, H.R. Muntz, and T.J. McGill. Thieme Medical Publishers, Inc., New York © 2000.

1. Airway
2. Breathing
3. Circulation
4. Neurologic evaluation
5. Search for other injuries
6. Radiographic and more specialized examinations

be noted. The examiner should always be alert to the presence of a foreign body or a displaced ossicle within the canal. Careful pneumatic otoscopy may be necessary to confirm the presence of a perforation or a positive fistula test.

> ## SPECIAL CONSIDERATION:
>
> Because ear trauma may be the result of physical abuse, the examiner should search carefully for other signs of abuse both to the head and neck and to other areas of the body.

The evaluation of hearing in a child who has suffered head trauma may be difficult. Bedside assessment of hearing acuity using tuning forks may be erroneous due to the presence of blood or debris

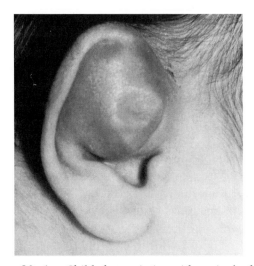

Figure 20–1:   Child abuse victim with auricular hematoma. (From Gilmer, PA. Trauma of the auricle. In: Bailey BJ, ed. *Head and Neck Surgery—Otolaryngology.* Philadelphia: Lippincott, 1993, p. 1557 with permission.)

within the canal. Tuning-fork testing is often not reliable in young children. As soon as the child is medically able, formal audiologic testing should be performed. In the unconscious or uncooperative child, auditory brainstem response (ABR) testing may give an indication of hearing acuity.

Computed tomography (CT) is essential in the evaluation of a child with temporal bone trauma, and should include thin sections to evaluate for small fractures, ossicular displacement, or facial nerve injury. Magnetic resonance imaging (MRI) is of less value in the assessment of the temporal bone, but is an important part of the overall neurologic evaluation.

Vestibular testing may be necessary in patients who complain of persistent vertigo or dizziness. A complete electronystagmography (ENG) examination, including positional and caloric testing, should be performed in children with these complaints. Electrical stimulation testing of the facial nerve should help to predict recovery from a facial nerve paralysis. Electromyographic (ENG) studies may also be helpful in facial nerve paralysis patients, and should be performed approximately 7–10 days following the injury.[2]

> ## AT A GLANCE. . .
> Otologic Evaluation
>
> **Initial Evaluation:** exam of head and neck for injuries; cleaning of ear canal with aseptic technique
>
> **Audiologic Exam:** tuning forks, conventional audiology, ABR
>
> **Radiologic Exam:** CT for bone evaluation and possibly MRI for soft tissue detail
>
> **Vestibular Exam:** fistula test, positional testing, calorics, ENG
>
> **Facial Nerve Exam:** acoustic reflex, threshold testing, EMG

INJURY TO THE EAR AND TEMPORAL BONE

Injury to the External Ear

Because it projects from the head, the external ear is in a precarious location and is prone to shearing-type injuries. *Ecchymosis* of the pinna may occur from the rupture of blood vessels in the plane between the anterior perichondrium and the auricular cartilage. This type of injury usually occurs on the lateral surface and rarely on the medial surface because the lateral surface has a cushion of subcutaneous fat that allows the skin to slide over the cartilage. The presence of a medial hematoma usually indicates a complete fracture of the cartilage. Partial absorption of the devascularized cartilage may result in the formation of dense, fibrous tissue, which becomes the "cauliflower ear" deformity (Table 20–2).

The treatment of ecchymosis, when it occurs alone, includes cold compresses for 24 hours. The formation of a seroma or hematoma may be treated with needle aspiration as long as the clot has not become organized. Perichondrium should be reapproximated to cartilage by placing saline-soaked cotton over the area and covering with a mastoid dressing. The mastoid dressing is removed and the area reevaluated in 24 hours. If fluid has reaccumulated, either the procedure should be repeated or an incision and drainage should be performed. Incision and drainage is indicated if aspiration is unsuccessful, if the child presents 72 hours after trauma, or if the treatment requires general anesthesia. Incision and drainage is carried out either in the skin crease of the anterior surface or through the cartilage from the posterior aspect. A drain is left in place for 48 hours. The anterior surface is packed with cotton that has been soaked in mineral oil in order to maintain the ear shape and a mastoid dressing is applied for 24 hours.

Abrasions and lacerations of the external ear are common in children (Practice Pathway 20–1). Contaminated wounds are best managed by examination under general anesthesia, which permits thorough cleaning and debridement. When there is no large tissue defect, skin edges should be undermined and trimmed before closure. The cartilage and perichondrium are closed with white, nonabsorbable sutures. The subcutaneous tissue is closed

TABLE 20–2: Complications of Auricular Trauma

Diagnosis	Complications
Hematoma	Cauliflower ear
Frostbite	Tissue necrosis
Burn	Chondritis
Keloid	Recurrence, subcutaneous atrophy after steroid injection

From reference 3, with permission.

with absorbable sutures, and the skin edges are approximated with fine, 7–0, monofilament suture. Dressings are usually unnecessary. The wound should be cleaned twice daily and antibiotic ointment applied. Broad-spectrum oral antibiotics should be given to reduce the chance of infection. The 7-0 sutures are usually removed under magnification in 4 to 5 days.

The external ear has an abundant blood supply from the posterior and deep auricular arteries and from the superficial temporal arteries. The entire ear may survive, even when it is left hanging only by EAC skin or a portion of the ear lobe. If the ear has a shattered appearance, be work should be done from "known to unknown" areas. Reassembling the helical rim will often cause other parts of the pinna to realign in a satisfactory fashion. The ear has remarkable powers of secondary epithelialization, which may be complete in 7 to 10 days following an abrasive injury.

SPECIAL CONSIDERATION:

The entire external ear may survive even when it is left hanging only by the EAC skin or a portion of the ear lobe; the ear has remarkable powers of epithelialization, which may be complete in 7–10 days.

If a partial-thickness avulsion occurs and perichondrium is exposed, a split-thickness skin graft can be obtained from the postauricular area. If the perichondrium is also missing, treatment should include a wedge resection, with primary closure for small peripheral injuries, or a local flap using preauricular or postauricular skin. Open treatment with frequent dressing changes may be carried out until granulation occurs and then a split-thickness skin graft applied. Of note is that excision of cartilage and skin grafting usually results in poor cosmesis.

In a full-thickness avulsion, if the ear segment is not available for reattachment, one of the following methods may be employed:

(1) Open treatment and delayed reconstruction is performed in an ear that is badly chewed from human or animal bites. Treatment is with debridement, antibiotic compresses, and systemic antibiotics.

Practice Pathway 20–1   AURICULAR TRAUMA OR EXPOSURE

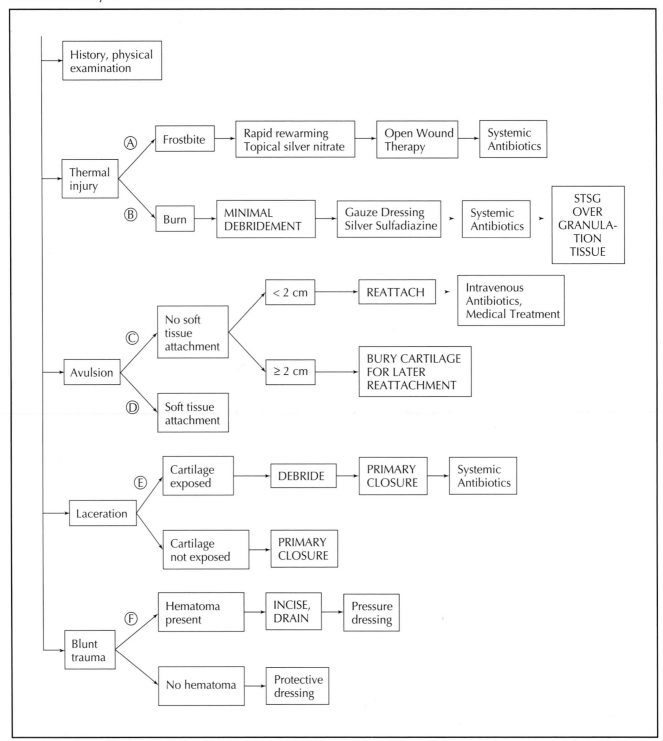

Abbreviations: STSG, split thickness skin graft. From Thomas JR. Auricular trauma. In: Holt CR, Mattox DE, Gates GA (eds) *Decision Making in Otolaryngology*. Philadelphia: B. C. Decker, 1984; pp. 158–159, with permission.

(2) Simple skin closure is used only in a severely-injured patient with poor prognosis. The ear is reconstructed later if the patient survives.

(3) Wedge excision with a radial, triangular resection is used for defects up to 2 cm along the helical rim.

(4) Postauricular attachment (mastoid flap) is used for broad, shallow defects. Rib or concha cartilage may be added in this technique to provide helical form.

(5) *Cephaloauricular flap* is a one-step modification of the mastoid flap. A *chondrocutaneous flap* is an advancement flap used for full defects that involve 3 cm or less of the helical rim (Fig. 20-2).

If the avulsed portion is available for reattachment, the following techniques may be useful:

(1) The composite-free graft is replaced within 4 hours of the injury. The best success is in segments < 2 cm in size.

(2) The *pocket principle* is useful when the severed ear part is > 2 cm and in good condition and the postauricular skin is undamaged. The following steps are involved: first, the amputated portion is dermabraded and attached to the ear stump; next, subcutaneous pocket is developed through a postauricular incision; then, the ear is inserted in the pocket and removed 10 to 14 days later. This technique should not be employed for human bite injuries.

(3) If the postauricular skin has been damaged, the ear may be covered with a large, scalp flap that is rotated over the dermabraded postauricular area and left for 3 weeks. Then, the flap is rotated back to the donor site and a split-thickness skin graft is used to cover the postauricular area.

These reconstructive techniques should only be carried out by a head and neck surgeon with extensive facial-plastic experience.

Burns and frostbite to the pinna involve cellular damage and small vessel injury. A first-degree burn includes erythema of the skin; a second-degree burn produces bulla formation; a third-degree burn involves full-thickness skin loss: and a fourth-degree burn involves complete auricular tissue loss. These burns may be complicated by perichondritis or chondritis. Usually, these complications occur 3 to 4 weeks after the burn and may be seen even in an apparently healed ear. Typically, children with perichondritis and chrondritis complain of severe pain. Physical examination initially reveals erythema and edema and then a loss of auricular contours. In severe cases, abscess formation occurs. These complications are almost always the result of *Pseudomonas* infection.

First-degree auricular burns are treated by cold compresses and analgesics. Second-degree and third-degree burns are treated with general burn principles. Hyperbaric oxygen may be employed in select cases. Prophylaxis against perichondritis may be improved by injecting the auricle with gentamicin and dressing the area in moist compresses of 0.5% silver nitrate. Bullae should not be broken. Clean granulation tissue may be grafted with an un-

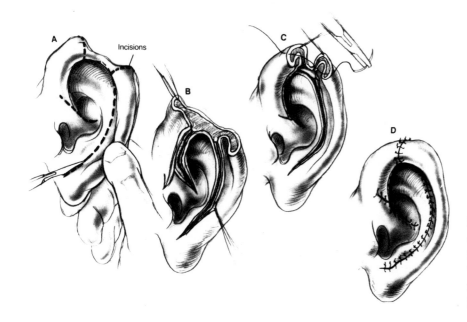

Figure 20-2: Creation of chondrocutaneous flap to close helical rim defect. (Redrawn from Antia NH, Buch VI. Chondrocutaneous advancement flap for the marginal defect of the ear. Plast Reconstr Surg 1967; 39:475.)

meshed split-thickness skin graft. A fourth-degree burn is treated with excision of necrotic tissue with primary closure and delayed reconstruction.

Frostbite is treated by rewarming the ear rapidly with saline pledgets at 38° to 42°C. These pledgets should be applied gently, and excessive manipulation should be avoided. The ear should then be treated as a burn. It may take days to weeks for demarcation of the involved tissue to occur. Mummified tissue requires debridement and grafting.

Perichondritis is initially managed with intravenous (IV) antibiotics. If this is unsuccessful, incision and drainage under general anesthesia may be necessary. Fenestrated angiocaths may be used for irrigation with antibiotic solution that contains gentamicin (80 mg in 1 L of normal saline) or another antibiotic that is determined from culture sensitivity. Irrigation is carried out several times a day for 7 days. When chondritis and chondronecrosis have occurred, some authors recommend total excision of involved cartilage with preservation of the soft tissue should be considered.

Injury to the External Auditory Canal

Lacerations of the pinna may extend into the EAC. A longitudinal wound may require closure with sutures. With small lacerations, packing the edges together with antibiotic-soaked Gelfoam™ may be all that is required. On the other hand, circumferential or multiple lacerations in the outer cartilaginous segment may have a tendency to heal with stenosis. Stenting with iodoform gauze may be helpful as well as placement of a soft-hearing-aid mold.[4] Lacerations of the ear canal from mandibular displacements usually do not require treatment, unless there is extensive narrowing of the bony canal. A permanent step-off deformity may be noted in the ear canal after a temporal bone fracture, but most do not usually require treatment.

Injuries to the skin of the canal wall may occur in a variety of ways. The child may sustain a self-induced injury caused by placing a foreign body in the canal. The parent may try to clean the canal with a cotton swab or other similar object and injure the canal. A health professional may injure the canal attempting to remove cerumen during an otologic examination. The skin of the cartilaginous canal is less likely to be injured than that covering the bony canal because it is thicker and less adherent to the underlying tissue. A hematoma is the usual EAC injury and the skin will usually regenerate over this area. If there is concern that a canal stenosis will result, stenting with gauze packing may be preventive.

Injury to the Tympanic Membrane

Traumatic perforations of the TM can be classified according to their etiology and include: compression injuries, blast injuries, penetrating injuries, and lightning injuries.[4,5]

Compression injuries occur when a sudden burst of air pressure is applied to the EAC, such as with an open-hand slap to the head. With a water-skiing accident, or by the direct hit with a ball on the external meatus during sporting events. Water injuries frequently lead to immediate contamination and purulent otorrhea within 48 hours. Most compression injuries involve the pars tensa, and may range from a pin-point perforation to a total loss of the pars tensa. Cholesteatoma may result from transplantation of squamous epithelium in a small percentage of patients. Systemic antibiotics are given if water contamination has occurred with the injury, and topical antibiotic drops may be necessary if the drainage is persistent. Ossicular damage is uncommon, and most perforations will heal spontaneously within 3 months. If there is inversion of the TM flap, many authors advocate patching of the TM immediately with eversion of the flaps over a bed of Gelfoam™ and an external paper patch to splint the TM.[5] Persistent conductive hearing loss with a healed TM is an indication for exploratory tympanotomy. Children with severe vertigo, visible injury to the ossicles or round window or with a suspected perilymph fistula should undergo immediate exploration. Blast injuries produce an injury similar to a compression injury. Rupture of the round or oval window may occur with blast injury but rarely is the ossicular chain involved.

AT A GLANCE. . .

Treatment of Tympanic Membrane Injury

Injury	Treatment
Inverted TM edges	Evert edges and patch
Water contamination	Systemic antibiotics, otic drops and culture if continues to drain
Persistent perforation after 3 months	Tympanoplasty
Ossicular damage	Reconstruction

Direct penetration of the TM by a sharp object is a frequent occurrence. Most injuries involve the posterior half of the TM and are frequently stellate-shaped with torn edges rolled beneath the residual TM. Frequently, more than 50% of the TM may be affected. Small perforations will generally heal spontaneously. Larger perforations may be treated by the same method used to fix inverted edges. Ninety percent of these perforations heal spontaneously within 3 months, if there are no inverted edges.[6] Persistent perforations after 3 months should be repaired surgically. As with compression injuries, those patients with severe vertigo, visible injury to the ossicles, or a suspected perilymph fistula should be considered for early exploration.

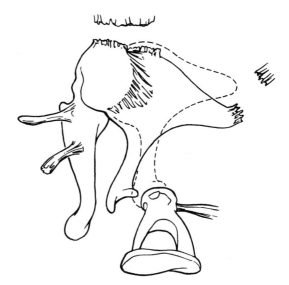

Figure 20–3: Dislocation of the incus with a separation of the incudostapedial joint is the most common type of ossicular injury. (From Bluestone C, Stool S, Kenna M, eds. *Pediatric Otolaryngology,* 3rd ed. Philadelphia: Saunders, 1996, p. 701, with permission.)

SPECIAL CONSIDERATION:

Most perforations of the TM will heal spontaneously within 3 months, if there are no inverted edges.

Lightning injuries may damage the EAC, TM, ossicles, cochlea, vestibular labyrinth, and facial nerve.[7] TM injuries due to lightning are usually resistant to repair secondary to the effect of the burn on the soft tissue of the ear canal. Because these burn injuries affect the vascularization of the canal and TM, definitive repair should be avoided for several months.

Ossicular Damage

In addition to TM injury, the ossicular chain also may be disrupted by penetrating wounds, accidents during cleaning of the ear, or removal of foreign bodies.[1,2] Closed head injuries may also involve ossicular chain damage.[4]

Incudostapedial (I-S) joint separation is the most common ossicular mishap (Figs. 20–3 and 20–4). This injury is thought to result from an interplay of numerous forces, including vibratory and concussive forces that separate the joint, inertial forces that occur during deceleration injury, the action of the stapedius and tensor tympani muscles causing stress on the joint, torsion from fracture or concussive deformation of the mesotympanum, and twisting of the I-S joint. The I-S joint acts as a univer-

sal joint, and with severe disruption, the joint may be separated. Dislocation of the incus may occur in a high percentage of cases and causes more trauma than simple I-S separation (Fig. 20–5). In severe cases, the incus may be displaced completely from the middle ear.

Fracture and displacement of the stapes occurs less frequently, and involves fracture of the annular ligament and bone surrounding the oval window with avulsion of the entire stapes or the crural arch and displacement of the stapes superstructure. The weakest anatomical point is at the junction of the arch and the footplate.

Fracture and displacement of the malleus occurs less commonly, and is usually associated with major injury to the remainder of the ossicular chain (Fig. 20–6). Rarely, the malleus head may be avulsed into the mesotympanum.

SPECIAL CONSIDERATION:

I-S joint separation is the most common ossicular injury; incus dislocation causes more trauma than I-S separation; fracture and displacement of the stapes and malleus occur less frequently.

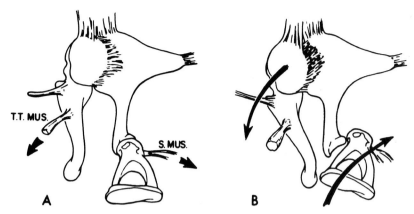

Figure 20–4:   A traumatic blow to the head causes an abrupt contraction of the middle-ear muscles. (A) The stapedius muscle (S. MUS.) rotates the stapes laterally and posteriorly out of the oval window (arrow). The tensor tympani muscle (T.T. MUS.) pulls the malleus handle medially toward the promontory (arrow). (B) The simultaneous reflex contraction of these two muscles creates a tension that pulls the malleus in an opposite direction from the stapes (arrows), and this may be a factor in producing a dislocation of the incus. (From Bluestone C, Stool S, Kenna M, eds. *Pediatric Otolaryngology,* 3rd ed. Philadelphia: Saunders, 1996, p. 702, with permission.)

A secondary repair of an ossicular-chain injury is usually recommended, so that inflammation of the TM and EAC caused from the primary injury is allowed to resolve. Repair of I-S joint separation involves restoration of the ossicular chain by interposing a displaced ossicle between the malleus and stapes superstructure or footplate. An alternative re-

pair utilizes an ossicular-chain prosthesis between the TM and the head of the stapes or stapes footplate.[8,9] A bone graft that is harvested from the posterior canal wall may also be used to repair an I-S joint separation. Damage to either the incus or malleus may be repaired either by reposition of the ossicle or use of an ossicular prosthesis. Treatment of

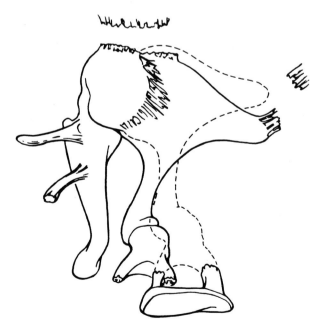

Figure 20–5:   Dislocation of the incus: fracture of the stapes crura. (From Bluestone C, Stool S, Kenna M, eds. *Pediatric Otolaryngology,* 3rd ed. Philadelphia: Saunders, 1996, p. 701, with permission.)

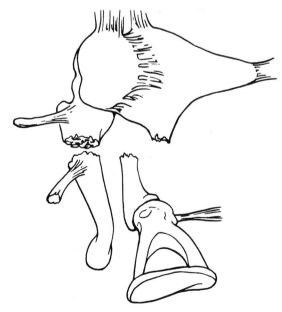

Figure 20–6:   A fracture of the malleus is generally accompanied by other ossicular injuries. (From Bluestone C, Stool S, Kenna M, eds. *Pediatric Otolaryngology,* 3rd ed. Philadelphia: Saunders, 1996, p. 702, with permission.)

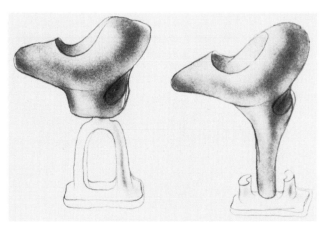

Figure 20–7: The two principal types of prostheses used to repair defects of the ossicular chain between 1964 and 1987. (A) Notched incus with short process. (B) Notched incus with long process. (From reference 7, with permission.)

a stapedial arch fracture includes either repositioning of a sculpted incus from the footplate to the malleus or use of an ossicular prosthesis (Figs. 20-7 and 20-8.

In children who have suffered an ossicular injury, it is also important to evaluate for a cochlear injury because concussive forces may be transmitted through the ossicular chain into the cochlea. When a child exhibits symptoms of ossicular damage, as well as symptoms of cochlear damage, an exploratory tympanostomy should be performed as soon as the child's medical condition permits. A search should be made for an ossicular fracture with fistula formation through either the stapes footplate or round window membrane. The oval window is the most vulnerable site of such a fistula because of the inward displacement of the ossicles. In this case, the fragments of the stapes footplate must be removed and a facial or perichondrial graft used to seal the defect.

Penetrating wounds to the middle ear may also injure the facial nerve in its tympanic segment. As with a labyrinthine injury, a facial nerve injury mandates exploration of the middle ear as soon as the child's condition permits. Decompression or grafting of the nerve may be necessary.

Temporal Bone Fracture

The head may be injured in various ways. Some objects traveling at high speed, such as a bullet, have great penetration power, but very little compression or concussion power. On the other hand, a moving head may come into contact with a large blunt object, a moving blunt object may come into contact with a stationary head, or a head may be compressed between two blunt objects. These blunt, compression forces are the most common cause of head trauma. In children with head trauma, a 3:1 male predominance has been noted, and most patients are under 12 years of age. The most common etiology is a fall, followed by motor vehicle and bicycle accidents.[10]

The temporal bone is frequently involved in cranial-cerebral injury.[2,4,11] Because the cochlear and vestibular mechanisms, as well as the facial nerve, are housed in the skull, these injuries can have serious sequelae. In studies that review pediatric head injuries, 6 to 14% result in a basilar skull fracture.[9]

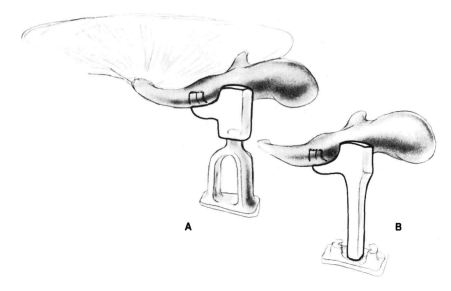

A   **B**

Figure 20–8: Prostheses of hydroxyapatite have been available since 1986. (A) The incus prosthesis, which replaces the notched incus with short process. (B) The incus-stapes prosthesis, which substitutes for the notched incus with long process. (From reference 7, with permission.)

Practice Pathway 20–2 SUSPECTED TEMPORAL BONE INJURY

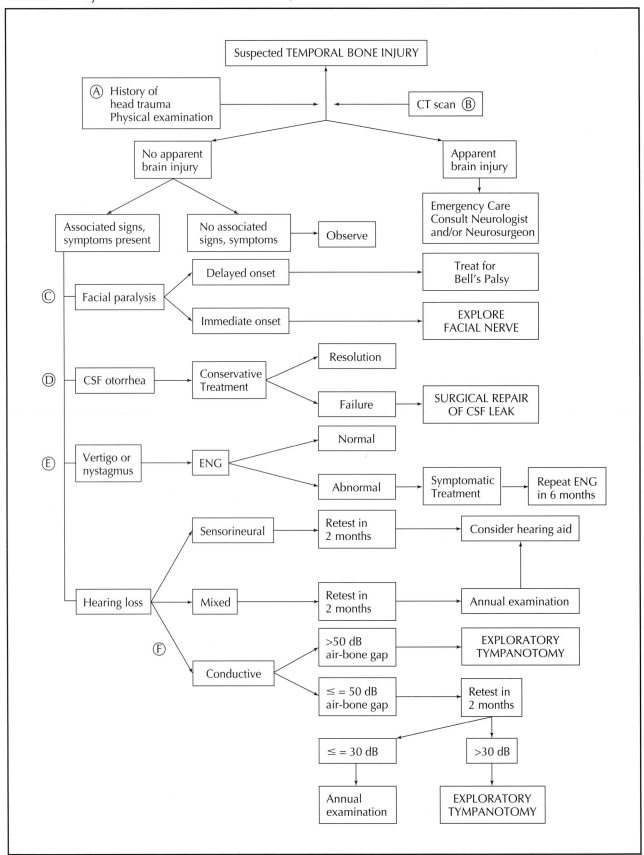

From Olson JB. Temporal Bone Injury. In: Holt CR, Mattox DE, Gates GA (eds) *Decision Making in Otolaryngology.* Philadelphia: B. C. Decker, 1984; pp. 158–159, with permission.

The temporal bone has been shown to be involved in more than 20% of basilar skull fractures.[9] Practice Pathway 20-2 outlines the symptoms and management of temporal bone injuries.

> ## SPECIAL CONSIDERATION:
> Because the cochlear and vestibular mechanisms, as well as the facial nerve, are housed in the skull, cranial-cerebral injuries can have serious sequelae.

Temporal bone fractures may be divided into longitudinal or transverse fractures (Table 20-3), depending upon the direction of the fracture line in relation to the long axis of the temporal bone. Temporal or parietal blows cause tearing forces in the anterior-posterior direction with resultant longitudinal fractures of the temporal bone. Occipital and frontal blows cause transverse fractures. Many fracture lines are variations or combinations of transverse and longitudinal fractures. CT remains the radiographic procedure of choice in diagnosis (Fig. 20-9). One millimeter CT sections through the temporal bone may provide additional information as to ossicular disruption, facial canal involvement, or otic capsule damage.

The *longitudinal fracture* is an extra-labyrinthine fracture, and accounts for 80% of temporal bone

fractures. Thirty to forty percent are bilateral. Longitudinal fractures run parallel to the internal auditory canal (IAC) and disrupt the bony annulus. TM, and ossicles, but typically spare the otic capsule, the auditory nerve, and the intracanalicular segment of the facial nerve. Bleeding tends to occur through the TM perforation, and any hearing loss is usually conductive. CSF leaks are uncommon. Facial nerve paralysis occurs in less than 20% of longitudinal fractures and is usually delayed due to compression by edema rather than transection of the nerve. The labyrinth is not fractured, but concussion forces may cause hemorrhage into the inner ear. Middle ear damage is the result of a torn TM with ossicular-chain fracture and disruption. Longitudinal fracture will cause a conductive hearing loss in 80 percent of cases with a contralateral, sensorineural hearing loss (SNHL) in as many as 50% of cases.[9,10,12]

Twenty percent of temporal bone fractures are transverse or mixed. Much more force is required to create these fractures, and a child is usually more significantly injured, often with life-threatening consequences. *Transverse fractures* may disrupt the otic capsule, the IAC, and the seventh and eighth cranial nerves, resulting in severe SNHL and vestibular abnormalities. The TM may remain intact, such that hemotympanum occurs rather then otorrhea. CSF leak is more common in transverse fractures. Fifty percent of transverse fractures have facial nerve involvement, and most of these are immediate in onset. Early recognition of a facial paralysis is crucial because early exploration and decompres-

TABLE 20-3: Classification of Temporal Bone Fractures

	Longitudinal Fractures	Transverse Fractures
% of temporal bone fractures	80%	20%
Point of impact	Temporoparietal area	Frontal or occipital area
Force of impact	Moderate to severe	Severe
Loss of consciousness	Not always present	Present
Associated Otologic Findings		
Ear canal bleeding	Frequent	Infrequent
Tympanic membrane perforation	Frequent	Infrequent
Hemotympanum	Common	Less Common
Hearing loss	Variable: conductive, mixed, and sensorineural	Profound sensorineural loss
Vertigo	Variable frequency and severity	Frequent; severe
Facial nerve		
Injury	Variable severity	Severe
Frequency	25%	50%
Paralysis	May be incomplete; onset may be delayed	Immediate onset; complete paralysis

From Bluestone C, Stool S, Kenna M, eds. *Pediatric Otolaryngology 3rd ed.* Philadelphia: Saunders, 1996, p. 697, with permission.

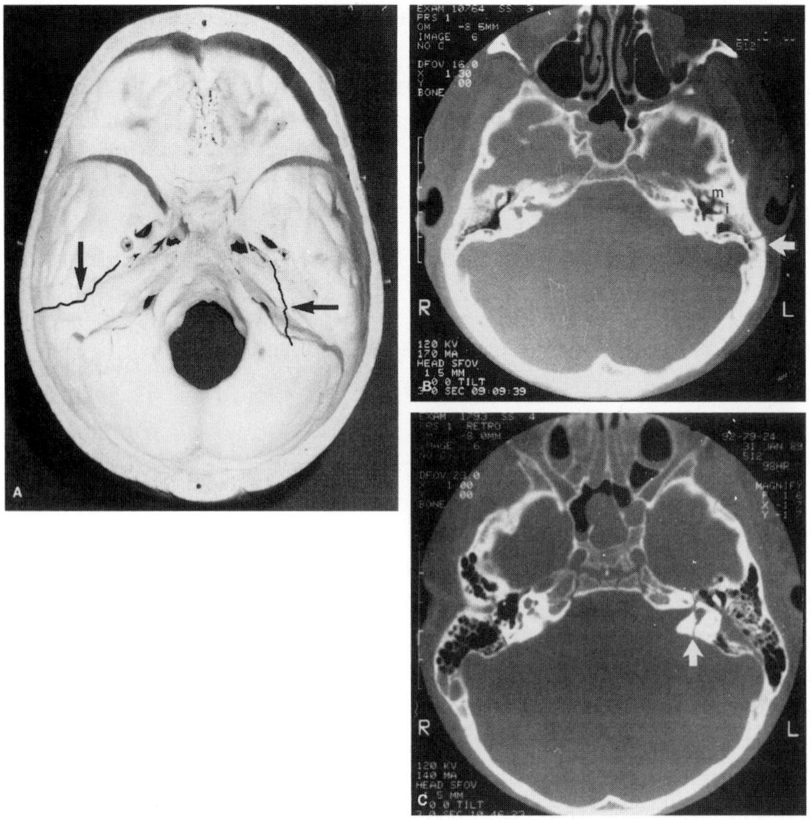

Figure 20–9: (A) Arrows point to a characteristic longitudinal fracture in the left temporal bone and a transverse fracture on the right. (B) Longitudinal fracture (arrow) of the temporal bone with ossicular disruption. m, malleus; i, incus; (C) Transverse fracture (arrow) of the temporal bone extends through the otic capsule. (From reference 2, with permission.)

sion, if the fracture line has disrupted the facial canal, may allow return of nerve function. Naturally, early exploration of a facial nerve injury can only be performed if the child's medical condition permits.

Transverse fractures may cause complete cochlear and vestibular disruption. Labyrinthine concussion without fracture causes a shock wave or pressure and hemorrhage into the perilymphatic and endolymphatic spaces with resultant fibrous and bony formation. Pressure waves transmitted into the inner ear may also cause violent disruption of the delicate cochlear membranes. Since contralateral injury is common, a transverse fracture may cause complete deafness in the ear on the involved side and SNHL in the contralateral ear.

Blunt trauma to the head may result in a labyrinthine concussion because of a shock wave to the contents of the otic capsule. Vestibular disturbances are usually of a delayed onset and normally self-limiting. High-frequency SNHL may occur from direct concussion to the cochlea. Fluctuating SNHL, particularly if associated with vertigo, is suggestive of a perilymph fistula. Injuries may be bilateral even though the trauma occurred on one side of the head. The most common vestibular dysfunction is *positional vertigo,* and this is thought to be due to cupu-

lolithiasis with free floating otoconia. Treatment includes avoiding sudden positional changes and the occasional need for vestibular suppressants. *Posttraumatic endolymphatic hydrops* is thought to occur from hemorrhage into the membranous labyrinth. Over time, this injury may cause distension of the endolymphatic system, producing episodic vertigo similar to that of Meniere's disease.

Rarely, a newborn infant may have peripheral facial paralysis due to a temporal bone fracture during labor and delivery. Unless a transverse fracture has occurred with transection of the facial nerve, spontaneous recovery usually occurs, and facial nerve decompression is rarely indicated.

OTHER CAUSES OF TRAUMATIC EAR INJURY

Barotrauma

Airplane travel and scuba diving are activities that may expose children and adolescents to rapid changes in pressure. The use of hyperbaric oxygen as part of various medical treatments may also result in *barotrauma*. The principle of Boyle's law states that, at a constant temperature, the volume of a gas varies inversely with the pressure. As atmospheric pressure increases, the volume decreases. This may result in pain, hearing loss, TM rupture, and vestibular injury. Middle ear barotrauma occurs, for instance, during the descent of an airplane, when a relative negative pressure develops in the middle ear. The activity of swallowing causes the eustachian tube lumen to open, equalizing the pressure between the middle ear and atmosphere. These same events occur during scuba diving. If the eustachian tube fails to open, negative pressure in the middle ear causes the TM to retract, resulting in a transudation of serous fluid from the middle ear mucosa. If pressure changes are severe and sudden, bleeding into the mesotympanum may occur or the TM may rupture. Flying or diving during an upper respiratory tract illness may precipitate these events.[4] The effects of barotrauma can be decreased by using topical or systemic nasal decongestants and encouraging children to swallow during periods of pressure change. An infant may take a bottle or an older child may chew gum. Persistent middle ear fluid or blood following this event may eventually require myringotomy and/or ventilation tube insertion.

Labyrinthine barotrauma is less frequent than middle ear barotrauma, but may result in permanent SNHL and persistent vestibular symptoms. The primary treatment is bed rest with head elevation. If a fistula is suspected or symptoms worse, exploratory tympanostomy for a possible fistula may be necessary.

Acoustic Trauma

Exposure of a child's ear to loud sounds that are a result of explosions, such as firecrackers or gunfire, may produce an immediate SNHL. Massive sound waves produced by such explosive events may be transmitted through the TM and ossicular chain to the basilar membrane, causing hair-cell damage. Chronic exposure to loud sound from motorcycles, snowmobiles, power tools, or music amplified by headphones or at concerts also has been shown to result in SNHL.[4,13] Hearing loss from chronic noise exposure is the result of metabolic changes within the cochlea. Depending upon the intensity of the noise and the length of exposure, the resultant hearing loss may be temporary or permanent.

Noise-induced hearing loss can be prevented by the use of ear protectors that reduce the exposure to the traumatic noises. A cotton ball is ineffective. Ear plugs and specially designed ear muffs that attenuate sound are the most effective preventive measures. In addition, preventing children from exposure to loud tools and firecrackers as well as controlling the intensity of amplified music will decrease the risk of this type of injury.

SUMMARY

In summary, trauma to the ear in children is common and may range from minimal soft tissue injury with spontaneous healing to severe ossicular chain damage with conductive hearing loss, permanent sensorineural hearing loss, vestibular symptoms and severe intracranial deficits. Most penetrating injuries can be managed early as these are usually isolated injuries. Other severe otologic injuries occur with trauma to other systems, and the timing and extent of management is dictated by the extent of the other injuries. Evaluation and management protocols and pathways support a complete approach with a better chance of satisfactory functional and cosmetic outcomes.

REFERENCES

1. Hough, JVD. Otologic trauma. In: Paparella M, Shumrick D, eds. *Otolaryngology 2nd ed.* Philadelphia, Saunders, 1980, p. 1656.
2. Kamerer, DB. Middle ear and temporal bone trauma. In: Bailey BJ, ed. *Head and Neck Surgery—Otolaryngology.* Philadelphia: Lippincott, 1993, p. 1623.
3. Gilmer, PA. Trauma of the auricle. In: Bailey BJ, ed. *Head and Neck Surgery—Otolaryngology.* Philadelphia: Lippincott, 1993, p. 1557.
4. Parisher, SC, McGuirt, WF Jr. Injuries of the ear and temporal bone. In: Bluestone C, Stool S, Kenna M, eds. *Pediatric Otolaryngology.* Philadelphia, Saunders, 1996, p. 687.
5. Donaldson, JD. Otologic trauma. In: Healy GB, ed. *Common Problems in Pediatric Otolaryngology.* Chicago, Yearbook Medical Publishers. 1990, p. 131.
6. Kinney SE. Trauma to the middle ear and temporal bone. In: Cummings CW, Fredrickson JR, Harker LA, et al. *Otolarygology Head and Neck Surgery,* 3rd Ed. St. Louis: Mosby, 1998, p. 3082.
7. Bergstrom L, Neblett L, Sando I, et al. The lightning-damaged ear. Arch Otolaryngol 1974; 100:117–121.

8. Wehrs, RE. Reconstruction of the tympanic membrane and ossicular chain. In: Bailey BJ, ed. *Head and Neck Surgery—Otolaryngology* Philadelphia: Lippincott, 1993, p. 1666.

9. Hough, JVD, Stuart, WD. Middle ear injuries in skull trauma. Laryngoscope. 1968; 78:899–937.

10. McGuirt, WF Jr. Stool, SE. Temporal bone fractures in children. Clin Pediatr. 1992; 31:12–18.

11. Friedman, EM, Deskin, RW. Pediatric otolaryngology. In: Morris PJ, Malt RA, eds. *Oxford Textbook of Surgery.* New York: Oxford, 1994, p. 2105.

12. Williams. WT, Ghorayeb, BY. Pediatric temporal bone fractures. Laryngoscope 1992; 102:600–603.

13. Dobie, RA. Noise-induced hearing loss. In: Bailey BJ, ed. *Head and Neck Surgery—Otolaryngology.* Philadelphia: Lippincott, 1993, p. 1782.

21 Neoplasms of the Ear and Temporal Bone

Michael J. Cunningham

Benign and malignant neoplasms of the ear and temporal bone constitute a very small percentage of pediatric head and neck tumors. In a review of 241 children with head and neck malignancies, the temporal bone was the primary site only in 1.5% of cases.[1] Although few in absolute number, a wide variety of neoplastic and paraneoplastic lesions may involve the ear and temporal bone in the pediatric age group (Table 21–1). The embryologic development of the temporal bone and aural structures may explain the occurrence of certain pathologies. Whereas the petrous portion of the temporal bone is of endochondral origin and is completely formed at birth, the squamous, tympanic, and mastoid portions are of membranous origin and continue to develop postnatally. These active growth centers predispose to the development of mesenchymal neoplasms, which predominate in this region.

SPECIAL CONSIDERATION:

The active growth centers of the squamous, tympanic, and mastoid portions of the temporal bone predispose to the development of mesenchymal neoplasms, which predominate in this region.

CONGENITAL MALFORMATIONS AND PARANEOPLASTIC PROCESSES

Langerhans' Cell Histiocytosis

The term *histiocytosis X* was proposed by Lichtenstein in 1953 to describe a group of disorders

that had an idiopathic proliferation of histiocytes, which produced either local or systemic manifestations, in common.[2] Modern pathologic techniques have revealed that histiocytosis X disorders uniquely involve a histiocyte called the *Langerhans' cell,* hence the more appropriate term *Langerhans' cell histiocytosis* (LCH).[3-5] Whether LCH represents a proliferation of abnormal Langerhans' cells or a pathologic accumulation of normal Langerhans' histiocytes remains unclear.[6] The disorder is not malignant in the classic pathologic sense, as the lesional cells are not shown to be monoclonal, do not have cytogenetic alterations, and do not demonstrate atypia (Fig. 21–1).

Manifestations of LCH

The clinical manifestations of LCH are protean. Patients may present with histiocytic infiltration of a variety of organ systems, including bone, skin, lymph nodes, paranasal sinuses, liver, spleen, lung, bone marrow, and central nervous system (CNS). Three classic, clinical syndromes—eosinophilic granuloma, Hand-Schüller-Christian syndrome, and Letterer-Siwe disease—have been described.[7]

AT A GLANCE . . .

Classic Syndromes of Langerhans' Cell Histiocytosis

- Eosinophilic granuloma
- Hand-Schüller-Christian syndrome
- Letterer-Siwe disease

Eosinophilic granuloma generally implies osseous disease alone. One bony site typically is af-

Pediatric Otolaryngology, Edited by R.F. Wetmore, H.R. Muntz, and T.J. McGill. Thieme Medical Publishers, Inc., New York © 2000.

TABLE 21–1:   Lesions of The Middle Ear, Mastoid, and Temporal Bone

Anatomic Variations	Paraneoplastic Lesions	Benign Neoplasms	Malignant Neoplasms	Congenital Malformations
Aberrant or aneurysmal carotid artery High jugular bulb	Choristoma Fibromatosis Fibrous dysplasia Hamartoma Langerhans' cell histiocytosis Teratoma	Adenoma Carcinoid Chondroblastoma Chondromyxoid fibroma Giant cell bone tumor Granular cell tumor Hemangiopericytoma Leiomyoma Lipoma Meningioma Neurofibroma Ossifying fibroma Osteoblastoma Osteoma Paraganglioma Plasmacytoma Schwannoma	Adenocarcinoma Adenoid cystic carcinoma Chondrosarcoma Ewing's sarcoma Fibrosarcoma Hemangiosarcoma Leukemia Liposarcoma Lymphoma Melanoma Metastases (breast, lung, kidney) Mucoepidermoid carcinoma Neuroblastoma (metastatic) Rhabdomyosarcoma Squamous cell carcinoma	Aneurysmal bone cyst Cholesterol cyst Congenital epidermoid cyst Encephalocele Hemangioma Meningocele Vascular malformation

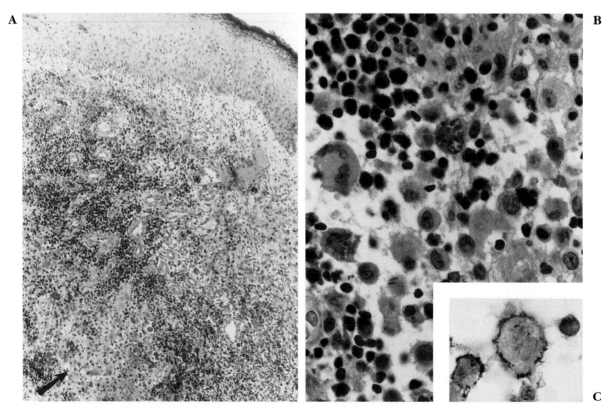

Figure 21–1:   Langerhans' cell histiocytosis. (A) Clusters of characteristic histiocytes (arrow) may be obscured by the darkly stained eosinophils (H & E, × 97). (B) The Langerhans' histiocyte is the sine qua non of the diagnosis; the eosinophils may be variable in their presence (H & E, × 290). (C) Inset shows peanut agglutinin decorating the surface of the Langerhans' cell with a circumferential striking pattern (peroxidase diaminobenzidine, × 550).

fected, although multifocal osseous involvement does occur. The most frequent site is the skull. Additional sites of involvement include the long bones of the extremities, the pelvis, ribs, mandible, maxilla, and vertebrae. Localized bone pain, often with an accompanying soft-tissue mass, is the frequent presentation. Although eosinophilic granuloma can occur at any age, approximately 50% of patients are diagnosed before the age of 5 years and 75% before the age of 20 years.[8] The clinical course is typically benign with an excellent prognosis.

Letterer-Siwe disease, in contrast, is a disseminated histiocytosis that characteristically presents in children below the age of 3 years. Multiorgan involvement is the rule, and clinical features at presentation may include fever, rash, lymphadenopathy, hepatosplenomegaly, dyspnea, and blood dyscrasias. Historically, the disease course is one of progressive, frequently rapid deterioration with a high-mortality rate.

Hand-Schüller-Christian syndrome is also a systemic histiocytosis with a clinical severity between that of localized eosinophilic granuloma and disseminated Letterer-Siwe disease. Children between the ages of 1 and 5 years are afflicted typically, although the disease can present in young adulthood. The syndrome is characterized chiefly by multifocal osseous lesions associated with limited extraskeletal involvement of skin, lymph nodes, and viscera. The classic triad of osteolytic skull lesions, exophthalmos secondary to orbital bone involvement, and diabetes insipidus secondary to posterior pituitary and/or hypothalamic disease is actually present in less than 25% of cases.[9,10] The clinical course of Hand-Schüller-Christian syndrome is characteristically chronic with significant associated morbidity.

The three classic syndromes evolved as a clinically useful way to subclassify LCH. The clinical heterogeneity of this disease, however, makes it difficult to categorize many individual cases. Within the Letterer-Siwe and Hand-Schüller-Christian categories, some children demonstrate a more favorable or more fulminant course than others.

These observations led to the identification of specific clinical prognostic factors applicable to every patient with LCH. The younger the age of the child at diagnosis, the worse the prognosis; children younger than 2 years of age, and especially those below 6 months, do particularly poorly.[11] Likewise, the greater the extent of the disease at presentation, as defined by the number of organ systems involved, the worse the prognosis.[12] Organ failure, rather than organ involvement per se, appears to be of the greatest prognostic significance, especially when there is clinical evidence of liver, lung, or bone marrow dysfunction.[13] Several staging systems for LCH have been developed based on these prognostic indices.[13-15] Health professionals advocate the use of a standardized classification system so that study populations at different institutions can be compared more precisely and treatment regimens can be assessed more effectively.

SPECIAL CONSIDERATION:

With Langerhans' cell histiocytosis, the younger the age of the child at diagnosis, the worse the prognosis. Likewise, the greater the extent of the disease at the time of diagnosis, the worse the prognosis.

The frequency with which otologic manifestations are reported in patients with LCH varies between 11 to 61% (Table 21-2).[16-24] This wide range is attributed to the observation that ear and temporal bone involvement is more likely to occur in children with multisystemic disease; studies limited to children with multisystemic LCH are expected to include a higher percentage of children with otologic involvement. The diligence with which otologic findings are sought influences their reported incidence also; the systemic manifestations of LCH

TABLE 21–2: Incidence of Otologic Manifestations in Langerhans' Cell Histiocytosis

Study	Overall Incidence (%)	Incidence as Presenting Manifestation (%)
Tos (1966)[16]	61	25
McCaffrey & McDonald (1979)[17]	15	5
Schloss et al (1981)[18]	40	—
Smith & Evans (1984)[19]	21	—
Anonsen & Donaldson (1987)[20]	38	20
Cunningham et al (1989)[21]	29	10
DiNardo & Wetmore (1989)[22]	11	—
Alessi & Maceri (1992)[23]	28	9
Irving et al (1994)[24]	19	—

can be so dramatic that ear and temporal bone involvement may be overlooked.

Otologic signs and symptoms can be the sole presenting manifestations of LCH (see Table 21–2). The otologic findings in these children often are attributed initially to acute or chronic infectious ear disease. Bilateral ear involvement, documented in up to 30% of patients with LCH, should increase suspicion of a possible uncommon diagnosis.[25] Failure of response to routine therapy should prompt investigation for a noninfectious cause.

Children with otologic LCH usually present with otorrhea and/or postauricular swelling; otalgia is reported infrequently. Physical examination often reveals nonsuppurative external or middle-ear granulation tissue. Aural polyp formation is common, and erosion of mastoid disease through the osseous canal wall into the posteromedial ear canal is reported. Primary eczematous involvement of the skin of the auricle and external ear canal can occur also.[26]

Conductive hearing loss (CHL) commonly is present secondary to soft-tissue infiltration and ear-canal obstruction. Tympanic-membrane (TM) perforation may occur in the presence of secondary infection. The histiocytic mass may erode the ossicles. The otic capsule appears less susceptible to erosion; however, bony labyrinth destruction with secondary sensorineural hearing loss (SNHL) and vertigo has been described.[27,28] Such histiocytic infiltration of inner-ear structures may be facilitated by previous middle-ear surgery.[29]

Facial-nerve paralysis is notably rare.[30] LCH does not invade neural tissue, but appears to interrupt the blood supply to the facial nerve by destruction of its surrounding osseous canal. The involvement of other cranial nerves, in addition to the seventh and eighth nerves, suggests extension of the disease to the base of skull or CNS.[31]

Diagnosis of LCH

The typical, radiologic, osseous findings in LCH of the temporal bone are nonsclerotic, radiolucent defects with a punched-out appearance.[32] Early lesions may demonstrate an accompanying periosteal reaction. Computed tomography (CT) best delineates the extent of temporal bone involvement (Fig. 21–2).[33] The sharply-marginated, lytic lesions are seen readily on bone-window algorithms, and erosion of the small structures of the ossicular chain and otic capsule is potentially demonstrable. Intravenous contrast enhancement allows delineation of the soft-tissue margins of the histiocytic mass relative to the extratemporal tissues and CNS. Magnetic resonance imaging (MRI) provides additional valuable information in this latter regard.[34]

The diagnosis of temporal-bone LCH is established ultimately by biopsy of the most accessible

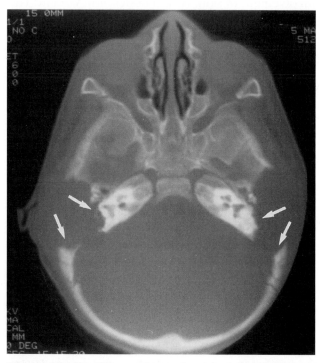

Figure 21–2: CT scan (bone algorithm) demonstrating sharply-marginated, bone erosion (arrows) characteristic of Langerhans' cell histiocytes.

AT A GLANCE . . .

Symptoms and Signs of Otologic Langerhans' Cell Histiocytosis

- Otorrhea
- Postauricular swelling
- Conductive hearing loss
- Eczematous involvement of skin of auricle and canal
- Granulation or polyp in external canal
- Perforation of tympanic membrane
- Erosion of mastoid disease through the posterior canal wall

area of involvement by either a transcanal or trans-mastoid approach. Definitive histopathologic techniques, such as immunohistochemistry and electron microscopy, require only small amounts of tissue for diagnosis. Care must be taken to avoid superficial biopsy specimens that yield solely nondiagnostic granulation tissue. The osseous destruction that is typical of LCH can obliterate anatomic landmarks and place the facial nerve at risk for injury during biopsy. Careful review of the preoperative, temporal-bone CT can help avoid such complication. In certain cases, a transmastoid biopsy actually may pose less risk to vital ear structures.

In biopsy-confirmed cases, a laboratory evaluation subsequently is necessary to assess for systemic disease. Complete blood count (CBC), liver function enzymes, chest roentgenogram, and skeletal survey constitute the recommended workup; in addition, bone-marrow aspirate or biopsy, liver–spleen scan, and lumbar puncture are necessary in selected patients.

Therapy for LCH

Therapeutic options for unifocal, temporal-bone LCH include intralesional steroid injections,[35] limited surgical resection,[36] radiation therapy,[37] or a combination of these. Recalcitrant otitis externa responds well to topical nitrogen mustard.[38] LCH lesions that are limited to the mastoid cortex can be treated by surgical curettage. Extensive tympanomastoidectomy procedures generally are avoided due to the increased surgical risk that is related to disease destruction of anatomic landmarks. Large LCH lesions with both middle ear and mastoid involvement, small lesions arising within the petrotympanic portions of the temporal bone, and recurrent or residual temporal-bone disease warrant radiation therapy. Radiation therapy, alone or in combination with surgical curettage, is used in many centers to treat all symptomatic, temporal-bone lesions regardless of size.[39] Typically, otorrhea, postauricular swelling, and CHL either clear or improve considerably after radiation therapy; only SNHL secondary to otic-capsule disruption appears irreversible. A treatment course of 600 to 1000 cGy (centigray) in 200 cGy daily fractions is recommended. Such dosages appear clinically therapeutic, while still being low enough to avoid complications. Cure rates for unifocal, osseous LCH are greater than 90%, regardless of the therapy chosen. The prognosis is so good that there is some argu-

ment for allowing asymptomatic, unifocal, osseous lesions that are localized to the mastoid cortex to heal spontaneously without treatment.[40]

> **SPECIAL CONSIDERATION:**
> Radiation therapy, alone or in combination with surgical curettage, is used in many centers to treat all symptomatic, temporal-bone lesions.

When the temporal bone is one of multiple sites involved in multifocal, osseous LCH without visceral (extraskeletal) involvement, either radiation therapy or chemotherapy may be utilized. Often, chemotherapy is used in young children due to their increased likelihood for developing disseminated disease and because of the long-term, sequelae concerns of radiation therapy.[41]

The more common scenario is temporal bone involvement in the presence of multisystemic LCH. When otologic symptoms are severe or hearing is significantly compromised, local treatment should proceed as outlined. Concurrent systemic therapy is also administered. This is typically chemotherapy, although immunologic manipulations, such as injection of thymic hormone preparations, or biologic-response modifiers, such as alpha-interferon, have also been used.[42-44] Chemotherapeutic agents reported to be effective in treating LCH include corticosteroids, methotrexate, 6-mercaptopurine, etoposide, vincristine, chlorambucil, and cyclophosphamide. Current practice is to initiate therapy with the least toxic agent(s) possible.[41] A vinca alkaloid or an antimetabolite, with or without high-dose corticosteroids, is a common initial choice. If there is obvious progression of disease after a 4 to 6 week trial, a change to a different drug or to a combination of drugs is indicated. Failure of response to one chemotherapeutic agent does not preclude a response to others. It is hoped that the clinical staging systems that were discussed previously will prove to be a useful guide for therapy, ensuring that patients with poor prognostic features receive adequate treatment and avoiding the hazards of drug toxicity in prognostically favorable cases.

A response to initial therapy, even in unifocal,

osseous LCH, does not ensure cure. Long-term follow-up of these children is necessary. Monthly or bimonthly otologic examinations are suggested over the first year. In the absence of clinical symptoms, a follow-up CT scan in children with temporal-bone disease is recommended 12 to 18 months after completing treatment. Skeletal surveys are far more sensitive than radioisotope scans in detecting recurrent, asymptomatic, osseous disease.[45] Residual hearing loss and radiotherapy-induced otitis are potential long-term otologic problems. Hypopituitarism, hepatic insufficiency, pulmonary failure, and neuropsychiatric disabilities are potential risks of both chronic, indolent LCH and toxic therapies.[46] Children who successfully undergo treatment of multisystemic LCH warrant yearly examinations into young adulthood, not only because of the chance of LCH recurrence but also because of the risk of a second, therapy-related malignancy.[47]

Choristoma

Choristoma and the analogous terms *heterotopia, ectopia,* or *aberrant rest* all refer to a developmental anomaly in which mature tissues with a normal architectural arrangement occur in an abnormal location; in other words, the lesion is not local or indigenous to the area in which it is found.[48] Choristomas present clinically in benign neoplasm-like fashion.

Salivary choristomas are the most common choristomas of the middle ear.[49] They have been reported in association with facial-nerve or ossicular abnormalities and in patients with developmental anomalies of the external ear and face, thus supporting a congenital origin.[50,51] There is a left-ear preponderance, and bilateral lesions have been described. Children as young as 5 years have been diagnosed. The lesions grow slowly, if at all, and typically produce no morbidity other than progressive hearing compromise. Otomicroscopic examination may reveal a middle-ear mass. Audiologic evaluation often will document CHL. Surgical excision is both diagnostic and therapeutic, although there is a risk of additional hearing loss as well as facial-nerve paresis/paralysis due to the presence of associated anatomic anomalies. Operative examination typically reveals a firm, lobulated mass. Well-formed serous and mucinous acini in a random or lobular formation characterize the histologic appearance. The possibility of a salivary neoplasm arising from chori-

stomatous middle-ear tissue is remote; only one mixed tumor has been reported.[50]

Middle-ear choristomas that consist of heterotopic neural tissue (glioma),[52] fatty tissue (lipoma),[53] and dental elements (odontoma)[54] have been reported in children also. All these lesions present in a fashion similar to that described for salivary choristomas.

Hamartoma

A *hamartoma* is a developmental anomaly that is comprised exclusively of tissues that are indigenous to the site in which it arises; a disorganized, nonencapsulated, architectural pattern is characteristic.[48,55] Perhaps the most common hamartoma of the middle ear is the *extracanalicular osteoma*. Extracanalicular osteomas can occur anywhere in the temporal bone, but the mastoid and squamous portions are involved most commonly. Osteomas of the middle ear are comparatively rare.[56] Slowly-progressive CHL due to impingement on the ossicular chain or TM is the characteristic presentation. Audiologic evaluation confirms a CHL. CT documents a bony mass within the middle-ear cavity. A familial tendency or the occurrence of bilateral lesions suggest a congenital etiology.[57]

Teratoma

Teratomas are rare lesions that usually, but not always, contain tissues that arise from all three germ-cell layers (i.e., the ectoderm, mesoderm, and endoderm) in various degrees of maturity.[48] Teratomas occur in 1:4000 births, and approximately 10% of cases originate within the head and neck, particularly in the cervical region and the nasopharynx.[58] Teratomas are detected frequently either prenatally or immediately at birth. Although the presence of immature fetal tissue sometimes is regarded as a sign of malignant potential, infantile teratomas of the head and neck are clinically benign lesions with an excellent prognosis, despite their typical incorporation of such immature elements.[59]

The *hairy polyp* is a subset of benign teratoma that is distinguished by its clinical and histopathologic features. It is a solid lesion that characteristically arises within the nasopharynx. It consists primarily of fibroadipose tissue, vascular tissue, foci of smooth and striated muscle, bone or cartilage, and glandular tissue. It is bigeminal (i.e., ectodermal and mesodermal) in origin and specifically lacks endodermal derivatives. Aural–nasopharyngeal hairy polyps with contiguous involvement of the middle ear, eustachian tube, and nasopharynx in a dumb-bell-shape fashion have been described.[60] Additionally, some children with aural–nasopharyngeal hairy polyps have auricular malformations, suggesting that such lesions may represent heterotrophic accessory auricles without the growth potential of a true teratoma.[61]

Cystic Lesions of the Petrous Apex

Lesions arising within the petrous apex portion of the temporal bone deserve separate mention due to the insidious fashion in which they present. Potential manifestations of an expanding lesion in the petrous apex include: CHL due to middle-ear effusion secondary to eustachian-tube obstruction; headache from petrous-bone erosion and secondary meningeal irritation; diplopia related to secondary involvement of the third and sixth cranial nerves; facial hyperesthesia caused by compression of the fifth cranial nerve; or vertiginous symptoms attributed to changes in labyrinthine vascular circulation.[62] The complex anatomic composition of the petrous apex potentially gives rise to lesions of epithelial, bone-marrowy, osseous, cartilaginous, neural, or vascular etiology. Such lesions may be divided into solid or cystic categories (a useful differentiation based principally on the imaging techniques used to assess this region). In the pediatric population, two cystic lesions—congenital epidermoid cyst and cholesterol cyst—are predominant, although isolated reports of other lesions do exist.[63]

Congenital or acquired cholesteatoma arising within the middle-ear–mastoid air-cell system is a common pediatric problem. *Congenital epidermoid cysts* of the petrous apex occur much less frequently and, due to the anatomic isolation of the apical temporal-bone segment, typically do not reach a size large enough to cause symptoms until adolescence or young adulthood.[64] Like primary middle-ear cholesteatoma, such epidermoid cysts are believed to arise from embryonic epithelial remnants.

Cholesterol cysts are clinically granulomatous lesions that histologically contain cholesterol crystals. The factors necessary for the development of a cholesterol cyst are hemorrhage, interference with clearance of drainage, and absence of air exchange or ventilation.[65,66] A petrous-apex cholesterol cyst is suspected to be the end result of complete obstruction of an air-cell tract within the petrous apex; the contralateral petrous apex in such patients usually is well pneumatized, suggesting that the involved side was pneumatized similarly early in development.

CT demonstrates both congenital epidermoid cysts and cholesterol cysts to be sharply-marginated, expansile lesions of the petrous apex that cause remodeling and possible erosion of bone.[67,68] The lesions are avascular, do not enhance with contrast, and are isodense either with brain tissue (congenital epidermoid cysts) or cerebrospinal fluid (CSF) (cholesterol cyst). MRI differentiates between these lesions (Table 21–3). Cholesterol cysts uniquely demonstrate high-signal intensity on both T1- and T2-weighted images, which is attributed to their cholesterol crystals and hemorrhagic by-products; cholesteatomas, in contrast, demonstrate low-to medium-signal intensity on T1-weighted images and high-signal intensity on T2-weighted images.

AT A GLANCE . . .

Manifestations of Expansile Lesion
of Petrous Apex

- Conductive hearing loss (otitis media with effusion)
- Headache (petrous-bone erosion/meningeal irritation)
- Diplopia (involvement of third and sixth cranial nerves)
- Facial hyperesthesia (involvement of fifth cranial nerve)
- Vertigo (changes in labyrinthine blood supply)

SPECIAL CONSIDERATION:

MRI differentiates between a congenital epidermoid cyst and a cholesterol cyst of the petrous apex.

Surgical intervention is recommended for cystic lesions of the petrous apex that: (1) manifest obvious bone erosion with exposed dura; (2) are asso-

TABLE 21–3: Roentgenographic Features Distinguishing Cystic Petrous Apex Lesions

	Cholesteatoma	Cholesterol Cyst
Computed Tomography		
Margins	Sharply, marginated, expansile lesion with remodeling and possible erosion of bone	Sharply-marginated, expansile lesion with remodeling but rarely erosion of bone
Density	Isodense to brain	Isodense to cerebrospinal fluid
Contrast enhancement	None	None
Magnetic Resonance Imaging		
T1-weighted signal intensity	Low to medium	High
T2-weighted signal intensity	High	High
Gadolinium enhancement	None	None

Adapted from references 67 and 68.

ciated with persistent or recurrent cranial-nerve deficits; or (3) are documented in a patient with persistent or recurrent headaches.[62] The justification for surgery in such cases is the prevention of disabling or lethal complications. Specific surgical management is dictated by lesion type, size, and extension. Cholesterol cysts are best managed by marsupialization, decompression, and establishment of normal pneumatization; total removal is not necessary. In contrast, complete extirpation of congenital epidermoid cysts is attempted if possible; in some cases only permanent exteriorization will be possible. The infra-labyrinthine approach is the procedure of choice in most institutions, when hearing preservation is a desired therapeutic goal.

Infantile Myofibromatosis

Representative of the aggressive fibromatoses, *infantile or congenital myofibromatosis* (IM) is a rare, benign, proliferative process that occurs almost exclusively in infants and young children.[69] The term *desmoid tumor* is applied more commonly to somewhat similar fibroblastic proliferations occurring in older children and adults. Typically, the temporal bone is one of several multicentric IM sites, although rare cases of solitary temporal-bone involvement are reported.[70] The characteristic presentation of IM is focal, painless swelling. This lesion is important because of its histopathologic similarity to the soft-tissue sarcomas; electron microscopy examination often is necessary to differentiate this lesion from fibrosarcoma and rhabdomyosarcoma (RMS). Once the diagnosis is established, therapeutic intervention by means of surgical resection is recommended if the lesion causes functional compromise or significant cosmetic dis-

figuration. Although total removal may be curative, a relatively high rate of local recurrence is reported. Radiation therapy or chemotherapy is considered only for symptomatic lesions that are situated where surgical extirpation is not possible.[41]

Fibrous Dysplasia

Fibrous dysplasia (FD) is a benign, slowly-progressive, fibro-osseous disorder of unknown etiology that most often appears initially in the first or second decade of life. The pathologic process consists of the resorption of normal, cancellous bone and its replacement by immature, woven bone. The clinical manifestations of FD depend on the site of the lesion and subsequent alterations in the form, size, stability, and function of the involved bone.

Three subtypes of FD are described classically.[71] A *monostotic form* that involves one osseous site is the most common subtype, accounting for 70% of cases. A *polyostotic form* that involves multiple osseous sites is the next most common. The least common form is a polyostotic subtype with associated extraskeletal abnormalities, such as abnormal pigmentation of the skin and mucous membranes, endocrinopathies, and disturbances of growth and sexual maturation; this combination of findings is also known as the *McCune-Albright syndrome.*

The incidence of craniofacial involvement varies with the subtype of FD; it is approximately 10% in the monostotic form, 50% in the polyostotic form, and almost universal in patients with polyostotic FD with extraskeletal involvement.[72] FD of the craniofacial skeleton demonstrates a predilection for the frontal and sphenoid bones. Comparatively, temporal-bone involvement is much less frequent, but interestingly is more common in patients with monostotic disease.[73] Two common clinical manifestations of temporal-bone FD are bony occlusion of the external auditory canal (EAC) with secondary CHL and progressive mastoid expansion with post-auricular swelling and pinna displacement. Less frequent findings include: secondary cholesteatoma formation behind an obstructed EAC; dysplastic involvement of the ossicles and/or otic capsule causing CHL and/or SNHL; and monocranial or polycranial neuropathies secondary to progressive bony expansion with fifth, sixth, or seventh cranial nerve entrapment.

The initial radiographic evaluation of any expansile, temporal-bone process is best performed by CT. Characteristic findings of FD include expansile growth, thinning of the surrounding cortical bone, and displacement rather than destruction of adjacent structures. The otic capsule is spared usually and may appear to "float" within the lesion.

The differential diagnosis of such a lytic temporal-bone lesion in a child includes congenital epidermoid cyst cholesteatoma, cholesterol granuloma, LCH, ossifying fibroma, giant cell bone tumor, aneurysmal bone cyst, osseous hemangioma, meningioma, and metastatic neuroblastoma. Although the clinical, radiologic, and in some cases, biochemical findings help distinguish these possibilities, diagnostic confirmation requires an histologic examination of bone. The typical histopathologic features of FD include irregular trabeculae of woven bone that are loosely embedded in vascular, connective-tissue stroma. The woven pattern, rather than the lamellar osseous pattern, differentiates FD from similar bony disorders.

AT A GLANCE . . .

Differential Diagnosis of Lytic Temporal Bone Lesion

- Congenital epidermoid cyst cholesteatoma
- Cholesterol granuloma
- Langerhans' cell histiocytosis
- Ossifying fibroma
- Giant cell bone tumor
- Aneurysmal bone cyst
- Osseous hemangioma
- Meningioma
- Metastatic neuroblastoma

Conservative management is recommended.[74] Surgery should be performed when function is threatened or when deformity becomes substantial. For cosmetic purposes, simple recontouring of the expanded bone back to its normal dimensions is usually effective. Stenosis of the internal auditory meatus or fallopian canal may be associated with impairment of cranial nerve function, and in selected cases, may warrant surgical decompression. Progressive narrowing of the EAC with secondary cholesteatoma formation or significant CHL is the most common indication for surgical intervention. Canal reconstruction in patients with FD is difficult because restenosis is common; repeated procedures may be required until disease activity ceases.

Sarcomatous malignant degeneration of FD lesions may occur. Clinical manifestations in such patients include local pain, rapid swelling, or sudden elevation of alkaline-phosphate levels. Notably, over 50% of FD patients with documented subsequent malignancy have received prior radiotherapy.[75] In patients who have been irradiated, the incidence of sarcoma is increased 400 times above the spontaneous rate, whereas the overall risk of malignant change is estimated to be approximately 1:200 cases, if FD is left untreated.[76] Therefore, radiation therapy is contraindicated in the treatment of this disease.

BENIGN NEOPLASMS

Adenomatous Tumors

Primary nonsalivary *adenomatous tumors* of the middle ear are diagnosed in adulthood typically, but have been reported in patients as young as 14 years.[77] The vast majority of these lesions are benign adenomas with an indolent biologic course. Adenomatous tumors of the middle ear can display a carcinoid appearance with histopathologic documentation of neurosecretory granules and serologic detection of a variety of peptide hormones.[78] The typical presentation is progressively decreasing, unilateral hearing loss in association with a sense of aural fullness, tinnitus, or other otologic symptoms. Occasionally, the tumor may be visualized behind or against the TM on otomicroscopic examination. Intraoperatively, adenomas are firm to rubbery, nonvascular masses that may fill the middle-ear space with possible mastoid extension. Regardless of size, most of these tumors prove to be tightly adherent to the middle-ear mucosal surface, and show a similar adherence to the ossicles and TM when these structures are involved. Osseous destruction is not a feature of these lesions and, if present, signifies the possibility of carcinoma.[79] The vast majority of middle-ear–mastoid adenomatous tumors are able to be completely resected and seldom recur.

Paragangliomas

Paragangliomas of the ear and temporal bone arise from the jugulotympanic paraganglia, which, like other extra-adrenal paraganglia, are derivatives of the neural crest neuroectoderm. The exact role of the jugulotympanic paraganglia is not known completely; it is proposed that their granule-containing chief cells function to control afferent or efferent excitation in the autonomic nervous system.

Jugulotympanic paragangliomas are classified based on their site of origin. Those that arise within the middle ear from the region of Jacobson's nerve and the promontory plexus are termed *tympanic paragangliomas* or *glomus tympanicum*. Paragangliomas that arise from the jugular-bulb region are termed *glomus jugulare.*

Paragangliomas usually present in middle age with a peak incidence in the fourth decade of life; they are rare in children.[80] Approximately a dozen pediatric cases have been reported in the literature, with the youngest child being 6 months of age.[81-84] Although paragangliomas are more common in women than men, a hereditary form in which the sexes are equally affected exists.

Diagnosis of paragangliomas

The most common clinical characteristics are unilateral pulsatile tinnitus and a sense of aural fullness due to CHL. Associated bleeding, otalgia, SNHL, vertiginous symptoms, or cranial nerve palsies signify more advanced lesions. Otoscopic examination often reveals a red or purplish mass behind the TM. More detailed otomicroscopic examination may allow distinction between a promontory mass (glomus tympanicum) or a hypotympanic mass (glomus jugulare); a presumptive diagnosis of the latter is made if the mass extends inferior to the fibrous annulus. In those cases in which the paraganglioma impinges on the TM, the application of positive pressure on pneumatic otoscopy will blanch the TM and cease associated pulsations, a finding known as *Brown's sign.*

Various anatomic anomalies can be confused clinically with paragangliomas, including aberrant internal carotid artery, internal carotid artery aneurysm, high jugular bulb, and persistent stapedial artery. Particularly in the pediatric population, paragangliomas have been mistaken to be hemorrhagic middle-ear effusions until failure of response to standard otitis media management prompts additional workup.

Typically, tympanometry documents increased impedance and, in classic cases, pulse synchronous undulations. Audiometry often will reveal conductive hearing compromise; SNHL is seen only in rare cases of labyrinthine invasion. Radiologic evaluation provides more specific diagnostic information. Contrast-enhanced CT will reveal a diffusely-enhancing lesion. A glomus tympanicum usually does not show bony destruction. A glomus jugulare will often have associated demineralization or osseous erosion. MRI with gadolinium enhancement defines both lesion vascularity and soft tissue more precisely, especially intracranial extension. Either study can be used to confirm the potential existence of additional head and neck paragangliomas; this is of particular importance in children in whom paragangliomas are suspected to be of congenital origin and therefore more likely to be multifocal.[85] Arteriography is recommended in the evaluation of larger lesions to demarcate the major contributing arterial and venous circulation as a prelude to embolization.

SPECIAL CONSIDERATION:

With a paraganglioma of the temporal bone, tympanometry may demonstrate pulse synchronous undulations.

Additional symptoms such as profuse sweating, periods of hyperactivity or nervousness, tachycardia, palpations, or hypertension suggest the possibility of a catecholamine-secreting paraganglioma. There is some evidence to suggest that paragangliomas in children may be more likely to secrete such vasoactive substances.[86] Since catecholamine production is intermittent, a 24-hour urine collection that assesses vanillylmandelic acid and metanephrine levels is more useful than sporadic serum screening. Patients documented to have catechol-

TABLE 21–4:   Jackson-Glasscock Classification of Jugulo-Tympanic Paraganglioma

	Glomus Tympanicum	Glomus Jugulare
Type I	Small tumor limited to promontory	Small tumor involving jugular bulb, middle ear, and mastoid
Type II	Tumor completely filling middle-ear space	Tumor extending under internal auditory canal; may have intracranial extension
Type III	Tumor filling middle-ear space and extending into mastoid	Tumor extending into petrous apex; may have intracranial extension
Type IV	Tumor filling middle ear, extending into mastoid or through TM to fill EAC	Tumor extending beyond petrous apex into clivus or infratemporal fossa; may have intracranial extension

From reference 87, with permission.

amine-secreting tumors require preoperative therapy with both alpha-blocking and beta-blocking agents.

Therapy for paragangliomas

The definitive treatment of jugulotympanic paraganglioma is surgical resection. The operative approach utilized is determined by the size and location of the tumor as summarized by the Jackson-Glasscock staging system (Table 21–4).[87] Small, circumscribed glomus tympanicum tumors of the mesotympanum can be removed via a transcanal tympanomeatal flap approach. A postauricular transcanal hypotympanotomy is recommended for middle-ear glomus tumors with hypotympanum extension. Larger, middle-ear–mastoid tumors necessitate a canal wall down mastoidectomy approach for wider-field exposure. Paragangliomas extending outside the confines of the temporal bone require a combination of tympanomastoidectomy and skull base techniques. Preoperative arteriography with embolization is recommended in such cases, and there is a significant risk for postoperative neurologic deficits.

Radiation therapy is sometimes chosen as a less invasive means of treating paragangliomas in elderly patients; in children it is reserved for lesions that cannot be resected with intracranial extension. There have been too few cases to determine appropriate radiation dosing; typically prognosis has been poor in such cases.[88]

MALIGNANT NEOPLASMS

Rhabdomyosarcoma

RMS is the most common soft-tissue malignancy in the pediatric age group and the most common neo-plasm of the ear and temporal bone in children. Approximately 35 to 40% of pediatric RMS, arise within the head and neck, and the orbit, nasopharynx, middle ear-mastoid region, and the sinonasal cavities are the most common sites in descending order of frequency.[89] Approximately 70% of children with RMS present before the age of 12 years, and more than 40% are younger than 5 years. There is no apparent sex predilection. RMS is, however, four times more common in Caucasian children than in any other racial group.[90]

AT A GLANCE . . .

Most Common Sites of Rhabdomyosarcoma of the Head and Neck (in descending order)

1. Orbit
2. Nasopharynx
3. Middle-ear–mastoid region
4. Sinonasal cavities

The tissue of origin of RMS is striated skeletal muscle.[91] The normal development of skeletal muscle begins with the *rhabdomyoblast,* which is a primitive round cell, then proceeds to a spindle cell form and finally to mature multinucleated muscle fibers. This progression is recapitulated in RMS in a highly-disorganized manner. Four histopathologic subtypes of RMS have been described: *pleomorphic, embryonal, alveolar,* and *botryoid.* Often there is a mixture of subtypes in any individual case; however, there is always one predominant pattern. Embryonal RMS is the most common subtype found in the middle ear-mastoid region in children.

The presentation of aural RMS is often insidious. Typical initial symptoms and signs such as serosanguinous otorrhea and nonsuppurative granulation tissue often mistakenly are diagnosed as otitis media or otitis externa.[92] Refractoriness to standard medical therapy eventually prompts further workup. Findings at the time of definitive diagnosis include a mass in the region of the ear or a polyp in the EAC in over 50% of patients.[93] Approximately 20% of patients with aural RMS have neurologic findings by the time the proper diagnosis is determined, with the facial nerve being involved most commonly.[94] Multiple cranial nerve palsies suggest extension of disease to the base of skull or the CNS.[95,96] This is particularly common when RMS initially arises within the petrous portion of the temporal bone; such children often manifest minimal ear pathology until late in the course of their disease with headache, abducens nerve palsy, trigeminal nerve dysfunction, and Horner's syndrome being the more characteristic findings.[97]

The natural history of RMS of the ear and temporal bone is that of a highly-aggressive, locally-destructive, invasive lesion with a significant propensity for distant hematogenous metastases; regional lymph node metastatic disease is comparatively rare.[98] Potential routes of local RMS extension from the middle ear–mastoid region include: invasion and destruction of the fallopian canal with secondary infiltration of the facial nerve; extension via the internal auditory canal to the leptomeninges and CNS; direct middle cranial fossa extension from the mastoid; inferior base of skull extension along the vascular sheaths of the jugular vein and carotid artery; and bidirectional extension along the eustachian tube to and from the nasopharynx.[99] Approximately 20% of children who have RMS of the middle-ear–mastoid present with distant hematogenous metastases at the time of diagnosis with the lung, bone, and bone marrow being the most common sites.[100]

Diagnosis of rhabdomyosarcoma

Clinical suspicion of middle-ear–mastoid RMS should prompt a thorough neuro-otolaryngologic evaluation by both physical and radiographic means. A combination of CT and MRI is recommended to best determine lesion size, extent, and anatomic site(s) of involvement (Figs. 21–3, 21–4, and 21–5). These roentgenographic studies, together with lumbar puncture for cytologic examination of CSF, are essential for detection of intracranial, base of skull, and meningeal extension.

The diagnosis of RMS is established ultimately by biopsy. Adequate tissue sampling is crucial as superficial biopsies may reveal only inflammatory granulation tissue. A tympanomastoidectomy approach may prove necessary to obtain diagnostic specimens. Once the histopathologic diagnosis is confirmed, a thorough metastatic evaluation must be

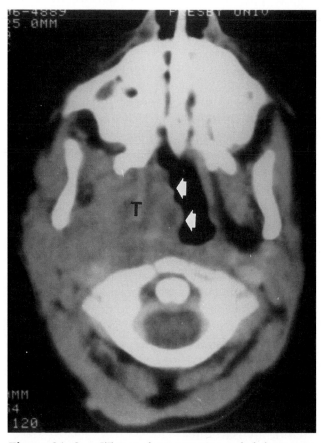

Figure 21–3: CT scan demonstrating a rhabdomyosarcoma of the oropharynx (arrows) and parapharyngeal space (T).

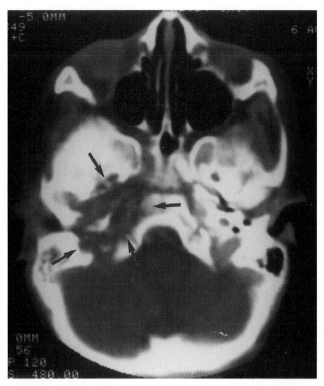

Figure 21–4: Same contiguous tumor as Figure 21-3 causing extensive destruction of the petrous portion of the temporal bone (arrows).

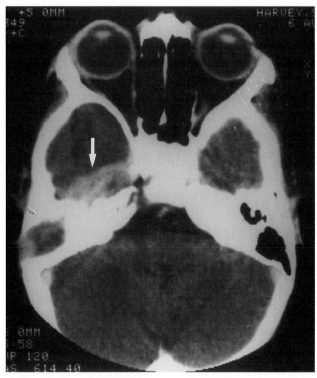

Figure 21–5: Intracranial temporal-bone extension (arrow) of the same tumor as Figure 21-3.

performed including CBC, chest radiograph, bone scan, liver-spleen scan, and possible bone-marrow aspirate in addition to the lumbar puncture previously mentioned.

Therapy for rhabdomyosarcoma

The treatment of children with RMS is determined by the primary site of involvement and the clinicopathologic stage of disease as established by the Intergroup Rhabdomyosarcoma Studies (IRS). The unique IRS staging system is based on the extent of disease (i.e., local, regional, or systemic) and whether excision of the local/regional disease can be accomplished (Table 21-5).[101] This staging system is problematic because surgical definitions of the ability to resect the disease vary among institutions.[102]

The IRS have established the superiority of multimodality therapy—surgery, radiotherapy, and chemotherapy—over single modality therapy in treating this disease.[103] The exact protocol chosen varies principally with disease stage. Tumor excision is indicated when removal of the primary tumor imposes no major functional disability and when excision of the primary tumor will permit either the elimination of postoperative irradiation or a significant reduction in radiation dose. Because the parameningeal location of many middle-ear–mastoid RMSs is not amenable to complete resection, radiation therapy typically is required. Almost all children with RMS receive some form of systemic

TABLE 21–5: Intergroup Rhabdomyosarcoma Study (IRS) Clinical Grouping Staging System

Stage	Definition
Group I	A. Localized disease confined to muscle or organ of origin, completely resected
	B. Localized disease with contiguous involvement or infiltration outside the muscle or organ of origin, completely resected
Group II	A. Localized disease (lymph nodes negative), grossly resected with microscopic residual
	B. Regional disease (lymph nodes positive), completely resected
	C. Regional disease (lymph nodes positive), grossly resected with microscopic residual
Group III	A. Local or regional gross residual disease after biopsy
	B. Local or regional gross residual disease after ≥50% resection of primary tumor
Group IV	Distant metastatic disease present at diagnosis

From reference 101, with permission.

chemotherapy because microscopic metastases are presumed present even when metastatic work up is negative.

Prior to the IRS, the overall 5-year survival for RMS of the head and neck, all sites considered, ranged from 8 to 20% with an average survival time of 7 to 12 months for children with middle-ear–mastoid RNS.[104] Survival rates have improved progressively since. The final report of the IRS-I study documented a 5-year, relapse-free survival rate of 46% for patients with primary paramengingeal (i.e., middle-ear–mastoid, sinonasal, nasopharyngeal, and infra-temporal fossa) disease.[105] Two groups of these children did particularly poorly: those with distant metastases (Group IV) and those with evidence of either base of skull or CNS extension from their parameningeal primary sites (Group III). Survival in these groups remained less than 12 months. In IRS-II, an effort was made to protect the CNS in such high-risk patients by the addition of prophylactic cranial irradiation and intrathecal chemotherapy.[106] This approach has proven efficacious in patients with Group III disease with improved 5-year, relapse-free survival rates of 67 to 79%.[107-109] The present IRS-IV protocol addresses the control of disease in patients with distant metastases by employing trials of new pairs of chemotherapeutic agents prior to the introduction of standard chemotherapy and radiotherapy.[104,110] IRS-IV also assesses the value of hyperfractionated radiation compared with conventional radiation for selected patients with residual tumor after surgery. This modification is the result of concerns regarding the effects of radiotherapy on facial growth as well as the later appearance of presumed radiation-induced second neoplasms. Such concerns have also revitalized debate about the potential role of initial ablative surgery, particularly given recent advances in skull base surgery and reconstructive microsurgical techniques.[111]

The most meaningful prognostic variable is response to treatment, as children who fail to achieve complete response do not survive.[112,113] Individuals who are free of recurrence 2 years after treatment are probably cured, but long-term follow-up is necessary because of an increased risk of second therapy-related neoplasms.[114]

Other Soft Tissue Sarcomas

There are rare, reported cases of temporal bone involvement by other sarcomatous neoplasms such as fibrosarcoma, malignant fibrous histiocytoma, lipo-

sarcoma, mesenchymal chondrosarcoma, and extraskeletal Ewing's sarcoma.[115,116] In some instances, the eustachian tube or temporalis muscle is the site of origin; in other cases the primary tumor appears to arise within the middle-ear–mastoid region. These various lesions typically present as firm, progressively-enlarging masses in the periauricular–temporal bone region. Radiographic evaluation typically demonstrates extensive areas of lytic osseous destruction reflective of their aggressive nature.

The management of extraskeletal Ewing's sarcoma employs a combination of surgery, radiotherapy, and multidrug chemotherapy similar to that utilized in patients with RMS.[117,118] The treatment of the other sarcomatous neoplasms is generally as complete as possible surgical excision without the loss of vital structures; unfortunately, there is little proven response of these various lesions to adjuvant therapy.[119] Local recurrence and hematogenous metastases are common. Prognosis is generally poor.

Endodermal Sinus (Yolk Sac) Tumors

Endodermal sinus (yolk sac) tumors are rare malignancies that contain cysts resembling yolk-sac vesicles and neoplastic germ cells that differentiate into extraembryonic structures.[120] Temporal bone involvement has been reported.[121] The serum alpha-fetoprotein level is elevated in most children with endodermal sinus tumors; this antigen can serve as a useful tumor marker for supporting the diagnosis and monitoring therapy.

Leukemia

Acute lymphocytic or *lymphoblastic leukemia* is the predominant malignancy of childhood. Involvement of the ear and temporal bone occurs in approximately 20% of leukemic patients, with a reported range of 16 to 35%.[122] Rarely, aural manifestations can be the initial leukemia presentation. Leukemic infiltration of ear and temporal-bone structures may result in hemorrhagic mucosal ulceration of the external auditory meatus and middle ear, thickening of the TM and middle-ear mucosa, and both seventh and eighth cranial nerve deficits.[123] Temporal-bone manifestations including facial-nerve palsy, hearing loss, and vertigo do improve with successful medical treatment of the underlying leukemia.[124] Surgical management is restricted typically to obtaining tissue for diagnosis and controlling associated infection.

Lymphoma

Primary lymphoma of the ear and temporal bone is rare.[125-127] Involvement of the middle ear and mastoid is seen more typically in children with disseminated lymphoma, particularly non-Hodgkin's. The signs and symptoms of temporal-bone lymphoma are similar to those described with leukemic temporal-bone involvement, and are also reversed by appropriate and timely systemic lymphoma treatment.

Other Lesions

The malignant neoplasms that commonly involve the middle-ear–mastoid region in adults, such as squamous cell carcinoma, malignant melanoma, and tumors of salivary gland origin such as adenocarcinoma, adenoid cystic carcinoma, and mucoepidermoid carcinoma, are extremely rare in children and will not be discussed in this chapter.

SUMMARY

The presenting signs and symptoms of many of the neoplastic and paraneoplastic lesions of the ear and

Practice Pathway 21–1   CHILD WITH CHRONIC OTITIS MEDIA UNRESPONSIVE TO MEDICAL MANAGEMENT

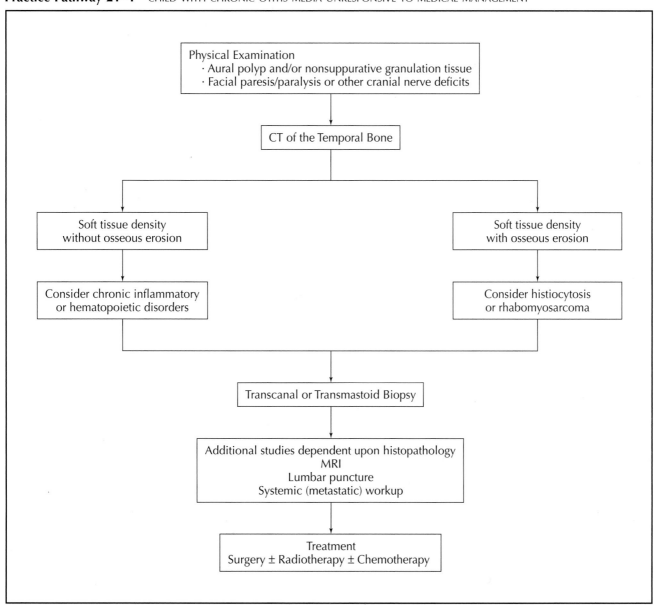

Practice Pathway 21–2   CHILD COMPLAINING OF HEARING LOSS WITH OTOSCOPIC DOCUMENTATION OF A MIDDLE EAR MASS

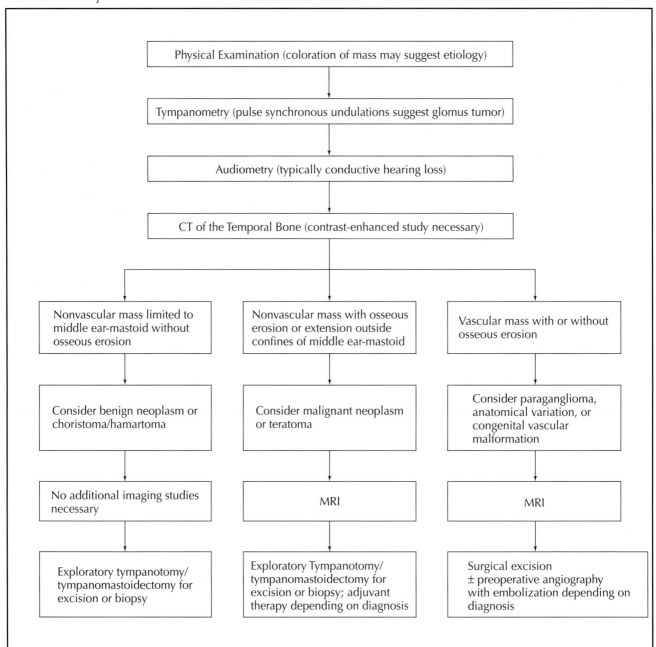

temporal bone in children initially mimic those of common inflammatory otologic disorders. Unfortunately, delays in diagnosis are common. Failure of response to standard medical management or the associated presence of an aural polyp, periauricular mass, or facial paralysis should all increase suspicion of a worrisome underlying etiology (see Practice Pathways 21-1, 21-2, and 21-3). Detailed otomicroscopic examination, proper audiologic and roentgenographic assessment, and eventual tissue

Practice Pathway 21–3   CHILD WITH A NONINFLAMMATORY POSTAURICULAR MASS

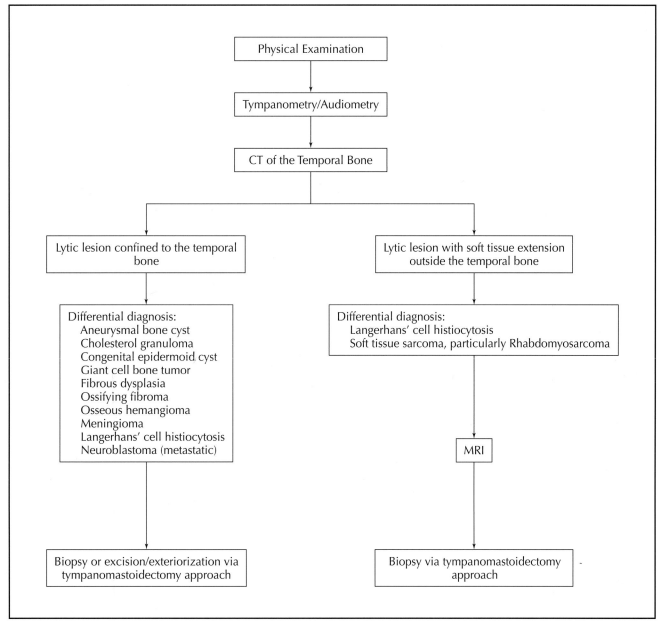

biopsy by excisional or incisional means are critical for establishing the correct diagnosis and determining proper management.

REFERENCES

1. Cunningham MJ, Myers EN, Bluestone CD. Malignant tumors of the head and neck in children: A twenty year review. Int J Pediatr Otorhinolaryngol 1987; 13:279–292.

2. Lichtenstein L. Histiocytosis X. Arch Pathol Lab Med 1953; 56:84–102.

3. Nezelof C, Bassett F, Rousseau MF. Histiocytosis X: Histogenetic arguments for a Langerhans' cell origin. Biomedicine 1973; 18:365–371.

4. Favara BE, Jaffe R. Pathology of Langerhans' cell histiocytosis. Hematol Oncol Clin North Am. 1987; 1:75–97.

5. Chu T, D'Angio GJ, Favara B, et al. Histiocytosis syndromes in children. Lancet 1987;2:41–42.

6. Jaffe R. Pathology of histiocytosis X. Perspect Pediatr Pathol. 1987; 9:4–47.

7. Devaney KO, Putzi MJ, Ferlito A, et al. Head and neck Langerhans' cell histiocytosis. Ann Otol Rhinol Laryngol 1997; 106:526-532.

8. Slater JM, Swarm OJ. Eosinophilic granuloma of bone. Med Pediatr Oncol 1980; 8:151-164.

9. Christian HA. Defects of membranous bone, exophthalmos and diabetes insipidus; An unusual case of dyspituitarism. Med Clin North Am 1919; 3:849.

10. Hand A. Defects of membranous bone, exophthalmos, and polyuria in childhood: Is it dyspituitarism? Am J Med Sci 1921; 162:509.

11. Lahey ME. Prognosis in reticuloendotheliosis in children. J Pediatr 1962; 60:664-671.

12. Lahey ME. Histiocytosis X: Comparison of three treatment regimens. J Pediatr 1975; 87:179-183.

13. Komp DM, Herson J, Starling KA, et al. A staging system for histiocytosis X: A southwest oncology group study. Cancer 1981; 47:798-800.

14. Greenberger JS, Crocker AC, Vawter G, et al. Results of treatment of 127 patients with systemic histiocytosis. Medicine 1981; 60:311-338.

15. Lavin PT, Osband ME. Evaluating the role of therapy in histiocytosis X: Clinical studies, staging and scoring. Hematol Oncol Clin North Am 1987; 1:35-47.

16. Tos M. A survey of Hand-Schüller-Christian's disease in otolaryngology. Acta Otolaryngol 1966; 62:217-228.

17. McCaffrey TV, McDonald TJ. Histiocytosis X of the ear and temporal bone: Review of 22 cases. Laryngoscope 1979; 89:1735-1742.

18. Schloss MD, Klein A, Black MJ. Histiocytosis X of the head and neck. J Otolaryngol 1981; 10:189-194.

19. Smith RJ, Evans JN. Head and neck manifestations of histiocytosis X. Laryngoscope 1984; 94:395-399.

20. Anonsen CK, Donaldson SS. Langerhans' cell histiocytosis of the head and neck. Laryngoscope 1987; 97:537-542.

21. Cunningham MJ, Curtin HD, Jaffe R, et al. Otologic manifestations of Langerhans' cell histiocytosis. Arch Otolaryngol Head Neck Surg 1989; 115:807-813.

22. DiNardo LJ, Wetmore RF. Head and neck manifestations of histiocytosis X in children. Laryngoscope 1989; 99:721-724.

23. Alessi DM, Maceri D. Histiocytosis X of the head and neck in the pediatric population. Arch Otolaryngol Head Neck Surg. 1992; 118:945-948.

24. Irving RM, Broadbent V, Jones NS. Langerhans' cell histiocytosis in childhood: Management of head and neck manifestations. Laryngoscope 1994; 104:64-70.

25. Jones RO, Pillsbury HC. Histiocytosis X of the head and neck. Laryngoscope 1984; 94:1031-1035.

26. DeMarino DP, Dutcher PO Jr, Parkins CW, et al. Histiocytosis X: Otologic presentations. Int J Pediatr Otorhinolaryngol 1985; 10:91-100.

27. Lopez-Rios G, Benitez JT. Histiocytosis: Histopathological study of the temporal bone. Ann Otol Laryngol Rhinol 1968; 77:1171-180.

28. Cohn AM, Satalof J, Lindsay JR. Histiocytosis X (Letter-Siwe disease) with involvement of the inner ear. Arch Otolaryngol Head Neck Surg 1970; 91:24-29.

29. Kimmelman CP, Nielsen E, Snow JB. Histiocytosis X of the temporal bone. Otolaryngol Head Neck Surg 1984; 92:588-590.

30. Tos M. Facial palsy in Hand-Schüller-Christian's disease. Arch Otolarngol 1969; 90:563-567.

31. Sivalingam S, Corkill G, Ellis WG, et al. Focal eosinophilic granuloma of the temporal lobe. J Neurosurg 1977; 47:941-945.

32. Hadjigeorgi C, Parpounas C, Zarmakoupis P, et al. Eosinophilic granuloma of the temporal bone: Radiological approach in the pediatric patient. Pediatr Radiol 1990; 20:546.

33. Cunningham MJ, Curtin HD, Butkiewioz BL. Histiocytosis X of the temporal bone: CT findings. J Compt Assist Tomogr 1988; 12:70-74.

34. Angeli SI, Luxford WM, Lo WM. Magnetic resonance imaging in the evaluation of Langerhans' cell histiocytosis of the temporal bone: Case report. Otolaryngol Head Neck Surg 1996; 44:120-124.

35. Cohen M, Zornoza J, Cangir A, Murray JA, et al. Direct injection of methylprednisolone in the treatment of solitary eosinophilic granuloma of bone. Radiology 1980; 136:289-293.

36. Angeli SI, Alcalde J, Hoffman HT, et al. Langerhans' cell histiocytosis of the head and neck in children. Ann Otol Rhinol Laryngol 1995; 104:173-180.

37. Cassady JR. The current role of radiation therapy in the management of histiocytosis X. Hematol Oncol Clin North Am. 1987; 1:123-129.

38. Hadfield PJ, Birchall MA, Albert DM. Otitis externa in Langerhans' cell histiocytosis: The successful use of topical nitrogen mustard. Int J Pediatr Otorhinolaryngol 1994; 30:143-149.

39. Richter MP, D'Angio GJ. The role of radiation therapy in the management of children with histiocytosis X. Am J Pediatr Hematol Oncol 1981; 3:161-163.

40. Womer RB, Raney RB, D'Angio GJ. The rate of healing of treated and untreated bone lesions in histiocytosis X. Pediatrics 1985; 76:286-288.

41. Raney RB. Chemotherapy for children with aggressive fibromatosis and Langerhans' cell histiocytosis. Clin Orthoped Related Research 1991; 262:58-63.

42. Osband ME, Lipton JM, Lavin P, et al. Histiocytosis X: Demonstration of abnormal immunity, T-cell histamine H2-receptor deficiency and successful treatment with thymic extract. N Engl J Med 1981; 304:146-153.

43. Davies EG, Levinsky RJ, Butler M, et al. Thymic hormone therapy for histiocytosis X? N Engl J Med 1983; 309:493-494.

44. Osband ME: Immunotherapy of histiocytosis X. Hematol Oncol Clin North Am. 1987; 1:131-145.

45. Siddiqui AR, Tashjian JG, Lazarus K, et al. Nuclear medicine studies in evaluation of skeletal lesions in children with histiocytosis X. Radiology 1981; 140: 787-789.

46. Komp DM, Mahdi AE, Starling KA, et al. Quality of survival in histiocytosis X: A southwest oncology group study. Med Pediatr Oncol 1980; 8:35-40.

47. Komp DM. Long-term sequelae of histiocytosis X. Am J Pediatr Hematol Oncol 1981; 3:163-168.

48. Ferlito A, Devaney KO. Developmental lesions of the head and neck: Terminology and biologic behavior. Ann Otol Rhinol Laryngol 1995; 104: 913-918.

49. Kartush JM, Graham MD. Salivary gland choristoma of the middle ear: A case report and review of the literature. Laryngoscope 1984; 94:228-230.

50. Moore PJ, Benjamin BNP, Kan AE. Salivary gland choristoma of the middle ear. Int J Pediatr Otorhinolaryngol 1984; 8:91-95.

51. Saeger KL, Gruskin P, Carberry JN. Salivary gland choristoma of the middle ear. Arch Pathol Lab Med 1982; 106:39-40.

52. Gulya AJ, Glasscock ME III, Pensak ML. Neural choristoma of the middle ear. Otolaryngol Head Neck Surg 1987; 97:52-56.

53. Selesnick SH, Edelstein DR, Parisier SC. Lipoma of the middle ear: An unusual presentation in a 4 year old child. Otolaryngol Head Neck Surg 1990; 102: 82-84.

54. Bellucci RJ, Zizmor J, Goodwin RE. Odontoma of the middle ear. Arch Otolaryngol 1975; 101: 571-573.

55. Mahataphongse VP, Conner GH. Middle ear hamartoma. Trans PA Acad Ophthalmol Otolaryngol. 1977; 30:49-51.

56. Glasscock ME III, McKennan KX, Levine SC. Osteoma of the middle ear: A case report. Otolaryngol Head Neck Surg 1987; 97:64-65.

57. Yamasoba T, Harada T, Okuno T, et al. Osteoma of the middle ear. Arch Otolaryngol Head Neck Surg 1990; 116:1214-1216.

58. Kountakis SE, Minotti AM, Mallard A, et al. Teratomas of the head and neck. Am J Otolaryngol 1994; 15:292-296.

59. Batsakis JG, El-Naggar AK, Luna MA. Teratomas of the head and neck with an emphasis on malignancy. Ann Otol Rhinol Laryngol 1995; 104:496-500.

60. Forrest AW, Carr SJ, Beckenham EJ. A middle ear teratoma causing acute airway obstruction. Int J Pediatr Otorhinolaryngol 1993; 25:183-189.

61. Heffner DK, Thompson LDR, Schall VG, et al. Pharyngeal dermoids ("hairy polyps") as accessory auricles. Ann Otol Rhinol Laryngol 1996; 105: 819-824.

62. Gacek RR. Cystic lesions of the petrous apex. In: JB Nadol Jr, HF Schuknecht, eds. Surgery of the Ear and Temporal Bone. New York: Raven Press, 1993, p. 423.

63. Goldsmith AJ, Myssiorek D, Valderrama E, et al. Unifocal Langerhans' cell histiocytosis (eosinophilic granuloma) of the petrous apex. Arch Otolaryngol Head Neck Surg 1993; 119:113-116.

64. Horn KL, Shea JJ III, Brackmann DE. Congenital cholesteatoma of the petrous pyramid. Arch Otolaryngol 1985; 111:621-622.

65. Matt BH, Myer CM III, Bellet PS. Cholesterol granuloma presenting in the ear canal. Ann Otol Rhinol Laryngol 1990; 99:672-673.

66. Kerstetter JR, Dolan KD. Middle ear cholesterol granuloma. Ann Otol Rhinol Laryngol 1991; 100: 866-868.

67. Goldofsky E, Hoffman RA, Holliday RA, et al. Cholesterol cysts of the temporal bone: Diagnosis and treatment. Ann Otol Rhinol Laryngol 1991; 100: 181-187.

68. Ferlito A, Devaney KO, Rinaldo A, et al. Ear cholesteatoma versus cholesterol granuloma. Ann Otol Rhinol Laryngol 1997; 106:79-85.

69. Chung EB, Enzinger FM. Infantile myofibromatosis. Cancer 1981; 48:1807-1818.

70. Hutchinson L, Sismanis A, Ward J, et al. Infantile myofibromatosis of the temporal bone: A case report. Am J Otol 1991; 12:64-66.

71. Nager GT, Kennedy DW, Kopstein E. Fibrous dysplasia: A review of the disease and its manifestations in the temporal bone. Ann Otol Rhinol Laryngol 1982; 91(supplement 92):1-52.

72. Kessler A, Wolf M, Ben-Shoshan J. Fibrous dysplasia of the temporal bone presenting as an osteoma of the external auditory canal. Ear Nose Throat J 1990; 69:197-199.

73. Sharp M. Monostotic fibrous dysplasia of the temporal bone. J Laryngol Otol 1970; 84:697-708.

74. Donnelly MJ, McShane DP, Burns H. Monostotic fibrous dysplasia of the temporal bone with associated lymphadenopathy. Ear Nose Throat J 1994; 73: 328-330.

75. Schwartz DT, Alpert M. The malignant transformation of fibrous dysplasia. Am J Med Sci 1964; 247: 35-54.

76. Williams DM, Thomas RS. Fibrous dysplasia. J Laryngol Otol 1975; 89:359-374.

77. Batsakis JG. Adenomatous tumors of the middle ear. Ann Otol Rhinol Laryngol 1989; 98:749-752.

78. Krouse JH, Nadol JB Jr, Goodman ML. Carcinoid tumors of the middle ear. Ann Otol Rhinol Laryngol 1990; 99:547-552.

79. Pallanch JF, Weiland LH, McDonald TJ, et al. Adeno-carcinoma and adenoma of the middle ear. Laryngoscope 1982; 92:47–54.

80. Spector JG. Paragangliomas of the temporal bone. In: Nadol JB Jr, Schuknecht HF, eds. *Surgery of the Ear and Temporal Bone*. New York: Raven Press, 1993, p. 369.

81. Jacobs IN, Potsic WP. Glomus tympanicum in infancy. Arch Otolaryngol Head Neck Surg 1994; 120: 203–205.

82. Choa DI, Colman BH. Paraganglioma of the temporal bone in infancy: A congenital lesion? 1987; 113:421–424.

83. Yaniv E, Sade J. Glomus tympanicum tumors in a child. Int J Pediatr Otorhinolaryngol 1983; 5:93–97.

84. Magliulo G, Cristofari P, Terranova G. Glomus tumor in pediatric age. Int J Pediatr Otorhinolaryngol 1996; 38:77–80.

85. Kohout E, Stout AR. The glomus tumor in children. Cancer 1961; 14:555–556.

86. Bartels LJ, Gurucharri M. Pediatric glomus tumors. Otolaryngol Head Neck Surg 1988; 99:392–395.

87. Jackson CG, Glasscock ME III, Nissen AJ, et al. Glomus tumor surgery: The approach, results, and problems. Otolaryngol Clin N Am 1982; 15: 897–916.

88. Kim J-A, Elkon D, Lim M-L, et al. Optimum dose of radiotherapy for chemodectomas of the middle ear. Inter J Rad Oncol Biol Phys 1980; 6:815–819.

89. Newton WA Jr, Soule EH, Hamoudi AB, et al. Histopathology of childhood sarcomas. Intergroup Rhabdomyosarcoma Studies I & II: Clinicopathologic correlations. J Clin Oncol 1988; 6:67–75.

90. McGill T. Rhabdomyosarcoma of the head and neck: An update. Otolaryngol Clin North Am 1989; 22:631–636.

91. Donaldson SS. Rhabdomyosarcoma: Contemporary status and future directions. Arch Surg 1989; 124: 1015–1020.

92. Schwartz RH, Movassaghi N, Marion ED. Rhabdomyosarcoma of the middle ear: A wolf in sheep's clothing. Pediatrics 1980; 65:1131–1133.

93. Prat J, Gray GF. Massive neuroaxial spread of aural rhabdomyosarcomas. Arch Otolaryngol 1977; 103: 301–303.

94. Dehner L, Chen K. Primary tumors of the external and middle ear. A clinical pathologic study of embryonal rhabdomyosarcoma. Arch Otolaryngol 1978; 104:399–403.

95. Leviton A, Davidson R, Gilles F. Neurologic manifestations of embryonal rhabdomyosarcoma of the middle ear cleft. J Pediatr 1972; 80:596–602.

96. Fleischer A, Koslow M, Rovit R. Neurological manifestations of primary rhabdomyosarcoma of the head and neck in children. J Neurosurg 1975; 43: 207–214.

97. Canalis R, Gussen R. Temporal bone findings in rhabdomyosarcoma with predominately petrous involvement. Arch Otolaryngol 1980; 106:290–293.

98. Raney RB Jr, Lawrence W, Maurer HM, et al. Rhabdomyosarcoma of the ear in childhood: A report from the Intergroup Rhabdomyosarcoma Study—I. Cancer 1983; 51:2356–2361.

99. Wiatrak BJ, Pensak ML. Rhabdomyosarcoma of the ear and temporal bone. Laryngoscope 1989; 99: 1188–1192.

100. Sutow W, Lindberg R, Gehan E, et al. Three-year relapse-free survival rates in childhood rhabdomyosarcoma of the head and neck. Cancer 1982; 49: 2217–2221.

101. Maurer HM, Moon T, Donaldson M, et al. The Intergroup Rhabdomyosarcoma Study: A preliminary report. Cancer 1977; 40:2015–2026.

102. Donaldson SS, Belli JA. A rational clinical staging system for childhood rhabdomyosarcoma. J Clin Oncol 1984; 2:135–139.

103. MacArthur CJ, McGill TJ, Healy GB. Pediatric head and neck rhabdomyosarcoma. Clin Pediatr 1992; 31:66–70.

104. Mandell LR. Ongoing progress in the treatment of childhood rhabdomyosarcoma. Oncology 1993; 7: 71–83.

105. Maurer HM, Beltangady M, Gehan EA, et al. The Intergroup Rhabdomyosarcma Study—I: A final report. Cancer 1988; 61:209–220.

106. Maurer HM. The Intergroup Rhabdomyosarcoma Study—II: Objectives and study design. J Pediatr Surg 1980; 15:371–372.

107. Raney R Jr, Tefft M, Newton W, et al. Improved prognosis with intensive treatment of children with cranial soft tissue sarcomas arising in nonorbital paramengingeal sites: A report from the Intergroup Rhabdomyosarcoma Study—II. Cancer 1987; 59: 147–155.

108. Crist WM, Gransey L, Beltangady MS, et al. Prognosis in children with rhabdomyosarcoma: A report of the Intergroup Rhabdomyosarcoma Studies I and II. J Clin Oncol 1990; 8:443–452.

109. Maurer HM, Foulkes M, Gehan EA: Intergroup Rhabdomyosarcoma Study (IRS)—II: Preliminary report. Proc Am Soc Clin Oncol 1983; 2:70.

110. Raney RB Jr, Tefft M, Maurer HM, et al. Disease patterns and survival rates in children with metastatic soft tissue sarcoma: A report from the Intergroup Rhabdomyosarcoma Study (IRS)—IV. Cancer 1988; 62:1557–1566.

111. Healy GB, Upton J, Black PM, et al. The role of surgery in rhabdomyosarcoma of the head and neck in children. Arch Otolaryngol Head Neck Surg 1991; 117:1185–1188.

112. Rodary C, Rey A, Olive D, et al. Prognostic factors in 281 children with non-metastatic rhabdomyosar-

coma (RMS) at diagnosis. Med Pediatr Oncol 1988; 16:71–77.

113. Treuner J, Suder J, Keime M, et al. The predictive value of initial cytostatic response in primary unresectable rhabdomyosarcoma in children. Acta Oncol 1989; 28:67–72.

114. Meadows AT, Silber J. Delayed consequences of therapy for childhood cancer. CA-A Cancer Journal for Clinicians 1985; 35:271–286.

115. Miser J, Pizzo P. Soft tissue sarcomas in childhood. Pediatr Clin N Am 1985; 32:779–800.

116. Chabalka J, Creagan E, Fraumeni J Jr. Epidemiology of selected sarcomas in children. J Natl Cancer Inst 1974; 53:675–679.

117. Rosen G, Caparros B, Mosende C, et al. Curability of Ewing's sarcoma and considerations for future therapeutic trials. Cancer 1978; 41:888–899.

118. Soule EH, Newton W, Jr, Moon TE, et al. Extraskeletal Ewing's sarcoma. A preliminary review of 26 cases encountered in the Intergroup Rhabdomyosarcoma Study. Cancer 1978; 42:259–264.

119. Jenkin D, Sonley M. Soft tissue sarcomas in the young: Medical treatment advances in perspective. Cancer 1980; 46:621–629.

120. Dehner LP, Mills A, Talerman A, et al. Germ cell neoplasms of the head and neck soft tissues: A pathologic spectrum of teratomatous and endodermal sinus tumors. Hum Pathol 1990; 21:309–318.

121. Stanley RJ, Scheithauer BW, Thompson EI, et al. Endodermal sinus tumor (yoke sac tumor) of the ear. Arch Otolaryngol Head Neck Surg 1987; 113:200–203.

122. Paparella MM, Berlinger NT, Oda M, et al. Otologic manifestations of leukemia. Laryngoscope 1973; 83:1510–1526.

123. Zechner G, Altman F. Histologic studies of the temporal bone in leukemia. Ann Otol Rhinol Laryngol 1969; 78:375–387.

124. Levy R, Har-el G, Segal K, Sidi J. Acute myelogenous leukemia presenting as facial nerve palsy. A case report. Int J Pediatr Otorhinolaryngol 1986; 12:49–53.

125. Tucci DL, Lambert PR, Innes DJ Jr. Primary lymphoma of the temporal bone. Arch Otolaryngol Head Neck Surg 1992; 118:83–85.

126. Welling DB, McCabe BF. American Burkitt's lymphoma of the mastoid. Laryngoscope 1987; 97:1038–1042.

127. Scott SN, Burgess RC, Weber P, Gantz BJ. Non-Hodgkin's lymphoma of the middle ear cleft. Otolaryngol Head Neck Surg 1997; 117:S203–S205.

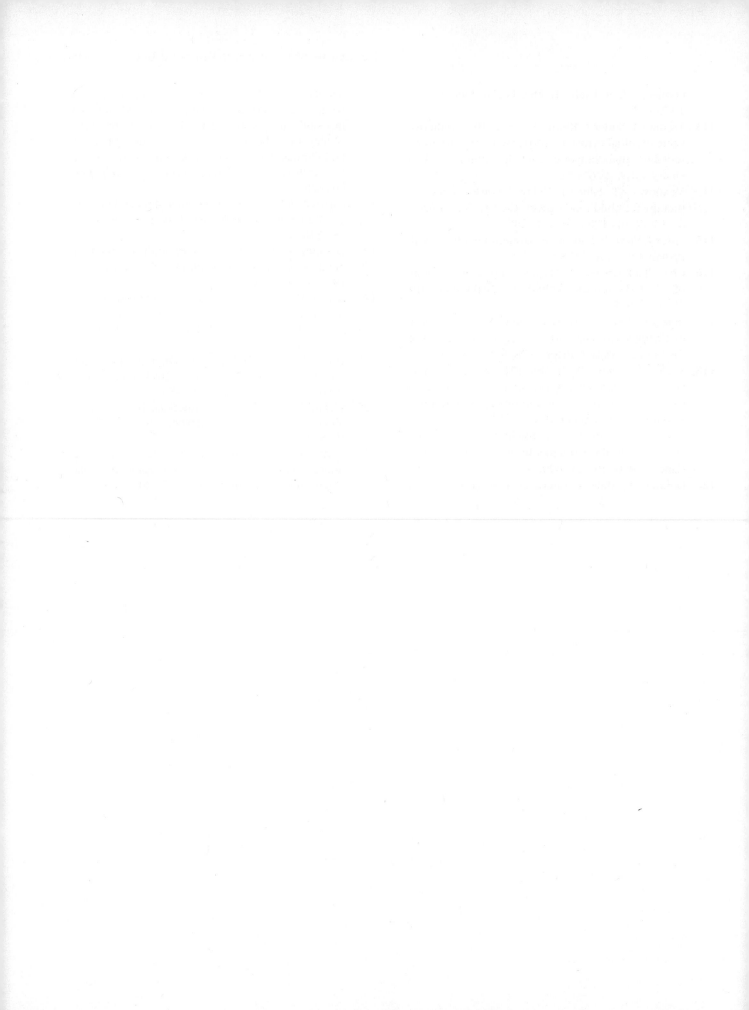

III

THE NOSE, PARANASAL SINUSES, AND ORBIT

22 Structure and Function of the Nose, Paranasal Sinuses, and Nasopharynx

Lawrence W.C. Tom

Nasal and paranasal sinus complaints are among the most common reasons children are referred to an otolaryngologist. Nasal congestion, rhinorrhea, and epistaxis are frequent symptoms of young children, whereas adolescents often are concerned with the appearance of their noses. Although most of these symptoms are caused by benign conditions that are easily treated they often produce much parental anxiety.

To manage these children properly, an understanding of the normal anatomy and physiology of the nose, nasopharynx, and paranasal sinuses is essential. With the advent and development of nasal endoscopy for both the evaluation and treatment of nasal and paranasal sinus disease, a thorough knowledge of the anatomy of this region has become increasingly important.

NASAL ANATOMY

External Nose

The *nose* is a pyramidal structure that rests on a bony pear-shaped opening in the facial skeleton, which is known as the the *pyriform aperture* (Fig. 22-1). For aesthetic purposes, the nasal pyramid can be divided into thirds, consisting of the bony pyramid, cartilaginous vault, and lobule. It is separated in the midline by the nasal septum.

The *bony pyramid* forms the superior third of the nose. It is composed of the nasal bones, which are joined medially, and the ascending (frontal) processes of the maxillae, which articulate with the nasal bones laterally. Superiorly, the nasal bones ar-

ticulate with the frontal bones, and the midline point where these bones meet is the *nasion.* The underlying nasal spine of the frontal bone provides superior support for the nasal bone, whereas the perpendicular plate of the ethmoid adds posteroinferior support. Inferiorly, the undersurface of the nasal bones is attached firmly to the upper lateral cartilages, and the *rhinion* is the point in the midline where these structures meet.

The *cartilaginous vault* consists of the upperlateral cartilages and the dorsum of the quadrangular cartilage of the nasal septum. Medially, the upper-lateral cartilages are attached firmly to the quadrangular cartilage, except at their most caudal extent where they depart from the septum and end as a free edge. The caudal margin of the upper-lateral cartilages articulates with the lower-lateral cartilages, and the upper-lateral cartilages are attached laterally to the maxilla by dense fibroareolar tissue. The cephalic portion of the cartilaginous vault is immobile and stable, whereas the caudal aspect is more mobile and flexible, permitting nostril dilatation and contraction; also, because of its flexibility the caudal aspect is able to withstand a moderate degree of trauma more easily.[1]

The *lobule* is the mobile, caudal third of the nose and includes the tip, ala, columella, and vestibule. It is composed primarily of the lower-lateral (alar) cartilages and secondarily by skin, fibroareolar tissue, and muscle. The U-shaped lower-lateral cartilages, which vary widely in shape and configuration, provide the skeletal support of the lobule and consist of medial and lateral crura. The *crura* blend together giving the lobule its rounded appearance. The *tip* is the most-anterior, soft-tissue projection of the lobule and is defined by the highest, medial, cephalic portion of the lateral crura. The *ala* is the most lateral portion of the lobule. Both medial crura articulate loosely with each other in the midline to

Pediatric Otolaryngology, Edited by R.F. Wetmore, H.R. Muntz, and T.J. McGill. Thieme Medical Publishers, Inc., New York © 2000.

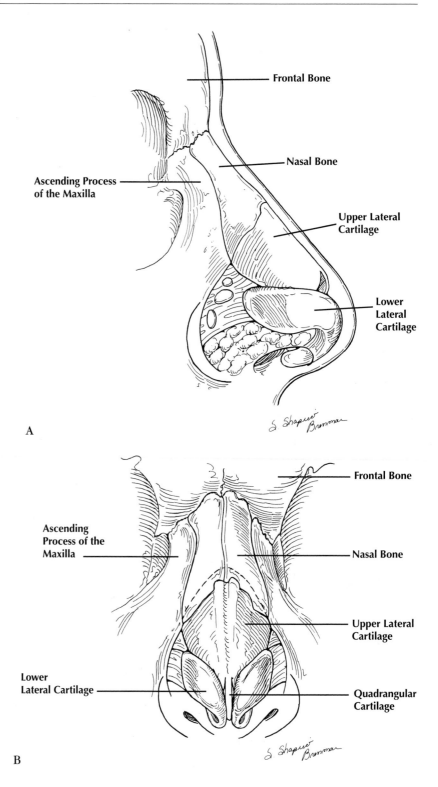

Figure 22–1: Lateral (A) and frontal (B) views of the bony and cartilaginous structures of the external nose.

form the cartilaginous skeleton of the *columella,* which is the most caudal midline structure of the nose. The *vestibule* is not a structure but rather the internal region into which the nares opens. Caudally, it is bordered by the ala and columella, and posteriorly, by the *pyriform aperture,* which leads into the nasal cavity. The anterior vestibule is lined with hair-bearing, keratinized, squamous epithe-

lium, and respiratory epithelium is found posteriorly.

Nasal Muscles

The nasal muscles play important roles in nasal physiology and animation. Fibers from different muscles tend to overlap, and functions are achieved by combinations of muscles rather than by an individual one. The *procerus* and *forehead muscles* elevate the skin of the dorsum. Compression of the nares is accomplished by *transverse nasalis* and compressor *narium minor.* The anterior and posterior *dilator nares* and *levator labii superioris alaeque* portion of the *quadratus muscle* dilate the nares. The *depressor septi* and *alar nasal* depress the nose.

Internal Nose

The internal nose consists of paired, pyramidal cavities that begin at the pyriform aperture just posterior to the nasal vestibule and end at the posterior choanae. A cross section of each cavity demonstrates a triangle with its base at the floor of the nose and its apex at the roof. The sides of the triangle are represented by the septum, medially, and nasal wall, laterally.

The roofs of the nasal cavities are formed by several bones. The nasal and frontal bones contribute to their anterior border. In their midportions, both the cribiform plate of the ethmoid bone and frontal bone form the roofs and the posterior borders are formed by the undersurface of the sphenoid bone.

An understanding of the anatomy of the midportion of the roof is necessary for any surgeon performing intranasal surgery. The cribiform plate of the ethmoid bone is the thin, horizontal plate that holds the ethmoid together and comprises the medial aspect of the nasal roof. It contains many perforations through which the olfactory filaments pass and is closely associated with the subarchnoid space. Lateral to the cribiform plate, the ethmoid

bone is open superiorly, and the frontal bone covers this open area. The lateral roof of the nasal cavity is actually formed by the thicker frontal bone and is more resistant to trauma than the medial roof. Both the course of the ethmoid roof and its relationship to the cribiform plate vary considerably, and differences may exist between both on each side.[2] To avoid injury to the thin vulnerable cribiform plate, it is essential that the surgeon recognize these individual variations through analysis of coronal sections of a patient's computed tomography (CT).

> ## SPECIAL CONSIDERATION:
>
> To avoid injury to the cribiform plate, the surgeon must be aware of the course of the ethmoid roof and its relationship to the cribiform plate.

The *hard palate* forms the floor of the nasal cavity. The anterior three-quarters is composed of the palatal process of the maxilla, and the posterior one-quarter consists of the horizontal process of the palatine bone. If these processes fail to fuse medially, a *cleft palate* develops.

The *nasal septum* divides the nose into two cavities. It is composed of bone and cartilage, and is an important support for the bony and cartilaginous vaults (Fig. 22–2). Its major components are the quadrangular cartilage, perpendicular plate of the

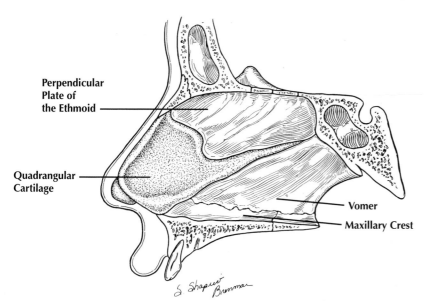

Figure 22–2: The bony and cartilaginous structures of the nasal septum.

ethmoid, and vomer. The quadrangular cartilage together with the columella and membranous septum forms the *anterior septum*. The *quadrangular cartilage* articulates inferiorly with the nasal spine and maxillary crest of the maxilla and posteriorly with the perpendicular plate of the ethmoid and vomer, both of which form the *posterior septum*. The septum is rarely straight but usually deviates from the midline in varying degrees. Significant deviations may obstruct the nasal cavity, and spurs are common inferiorly at the articulation of the quadrangular cartilage and vomer with the maxillary crest.

The lateral nasal wall is the most complex region of the nasal cavity. Safe, successful endoscopic nasal surgery requires a thorough understanding of its anatomy. The *lateral nasal wall* is formed by the nasal surface of the maxilla, the inferior turbinate, the ethmoid bone (which contains the middle, the superior, and the occasionally-present supreme turbinates) and the perpendicular plate of the palatine bone (Fig. 22–3).

The *turbinates* are prominent, ridge-like structures that extend horizontally along the lateral nasal wall and protrude into the nasal cavity. The inferior turbinate is a separate bone, whereas the middle, superior, and supreme turbinates are part of the ethmoid bone. The *middle turbinate* is an important surgical landmark (Fig. 22–4). The basal lamella is formed by the insertion of the middle turbinate and separates the anterior ethmoid air cells from the posterior cells. Its anterior attachment is 1 cm inferior to the cribiform plate, and its posterior two-thirds is attached to the lamina papraycea. The posterior end of the middle turbinate is in close proximity to the sphenopalatine foramen, through which run the sphenopalatine artery and a branch of the maxillary nerve. This foramen is a site for the administration of local anesthesia and may be a site of intraoperative bleeding.

There are several clefts that are associated with the turbinates. The *sphenoethmoid recess* lies medial to the superior or the supreme turbinate and is the location for the ostium of the sphenoid sinus. The *meatus* are spaces that are inferior to each turbinate, and each meatus is named after the turbinate that covers it. If it is present, the supreme meatus has no clinical significance. The *superior meatus* contains several openings through which the posterior ethmoid air cells drain.

The *middle meatus* is the most complex and contains several structures. Two bony prominences, the uncinate process, a thin leaflet, and the ethmoid bulla (which is the wall of the most constant and usually the largest anterior ethmoid air cell) project into the middle meatus and form the anterior and posterior borders of the hiatus semilunaris. The *hiatus semilunaris* is a passage that connects the middle meatus with the ethmoid infundibulum. The *ethmoid infundibulum* is a cleft into which the maxillary sinus ostia, anterior ethmoid air cells, and

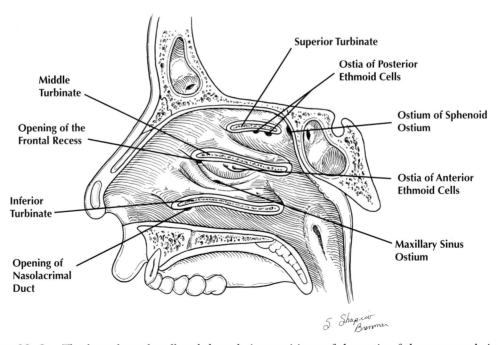

Figure 22–3:   The lateral nasal wall and the relative positions of the ostia of the paranasal sinuses.

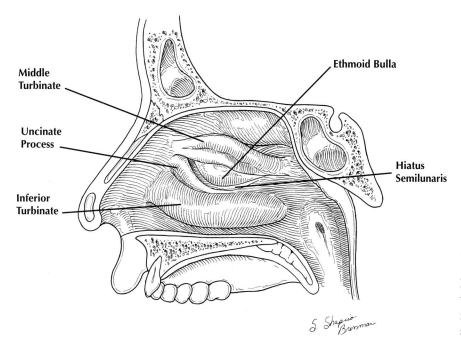

Middle
Turbinate

Uncinate
Process

Inferior
Turbinate

Ethmoid Bulla

Hiatus
Semilunaris

Figure 22–4: The lateral nasal wall with the middle turbinate partially removed to reveal important structures affecting the sinuses.

frontal recess open. This area is known as the *ostio-meatal unit,* and inflammatory processes involving any of these areas can spread easily to adjacent ones (Fig. 22–5).[3]

The *nasolacrimal duct* is the only structure that drains into the inferior meatus. Its opening is in the anterosuperior aspect of the meatus and can be injured during maxillary sinus surgery.

Blood Supply

The internal and external carotid arteries provide the blood supply to the nose. Within the orbit, the *ophthalmic artery,* which is a branch of the internal carotid artery, divides to form the anterior and posterior ethmoidal arteries, which penetrate the lamina papyracea to enter the ethmoid sinuses (Fig.

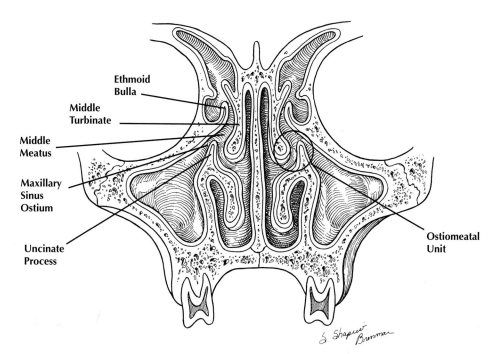

Ethmoid
Bulla

Middle
Turbinate

Middle
Meatus

Maxillary
Sinus
Ostium

Uncinate
Process

Ostiomeatal
Unit

Figure 22–5: Coronal section through the anterior ethmoid and maxillary sinuses showing the osteomeatal complex.

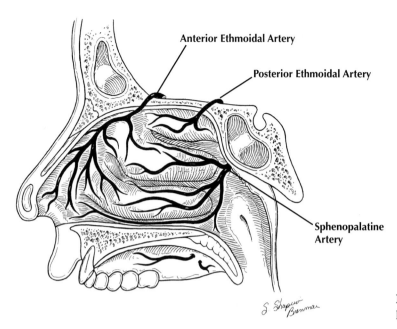

Figure 22–6: The arterial blood supply of the lateral nasal wall.

22-6). The *ethmoidal arteries* traverse the roof of the ethmoid sinuses and are usually protected within bony canals. The anterior ethmoidal artery supplies the anterior portions of the inferior and middle turbinates and the anterosuperior septum; the posterior ethmoidal artery distributes to the superior turbinate and posterosuperior septum. The bony canal covering the anterior ethmoidal artery may be dehiscent, exposing portions of the artery, and the anterior skull base is the weakest in the region of this artery. During intranasal surgery, caution must be taken when working in the vicinity of this artery to prevent injury and penetration of the anterior cranial fossa.[2]

The internal maxillary and facial arteries, which are branches of the external carotid system, also supply blood to the nose. The *internal maxillary artery* courses through the pterygopalatine fossa where it gives rise to the sphenopalatine and descending palatine arteries (Fig. 22-7). The *sphenopalatine artery* enters the nose at the sphenopalatine foramen and provides blood to the posterior region of the middle and inferior turbinates and septum. The *greater palatine artery,* which is a branch of the descending palatine artery, exits the greater palatine foramen to anastomose with branches of the sphenopalatine, anterior ethmoidal, and superior labial arteries in the region of the caudal septum called either *Little's area* or *Kisselbach's plexus,* which is a common site of epistaxis. The superior labial and angular arteries, which are terminal divi-

sions of the facial artery, provide the major blood supply to the external nose.

The venous drainage of the nose accompanies the arterial supply. The ethmoid veins drain into the ophthalmic veins, which empty into the cavernous sinus. The sphenopalatine and descending palatine veins flow into the pterygoid plexus within the infratemporal fossa. The *pterygoid plexus,* which is an extensive network of veins, may drain into the cavernous and superior sagital sinuses and the jugular vein. The *facial vein* is a tributary of either the external or internal jugular vein and drains the anterior nasal cavity and external nose. Anastomoses between branches of many veins allow blood to flow from one area into distant sites. This is especially true for the facial vein, which has no valves. Retrograde flow from the external nose may, thus, empty into the cavernous sinus.

Innervation

Innervation of the nose plays a key role in nasal physiology. In addition to general sensation, the nervous system provides autonomic innervation and the special sensation of olfaction.

The *maxillary division* (V_2) of the trigeminal nerve supplies the majority of general sensory fibers. The maxillary nerve originates from the semilunar ganglion and exits the middle cranial fossa through the foramen rotundum. This nerve then crosses the roof of the pterygopalatine fossa, passes

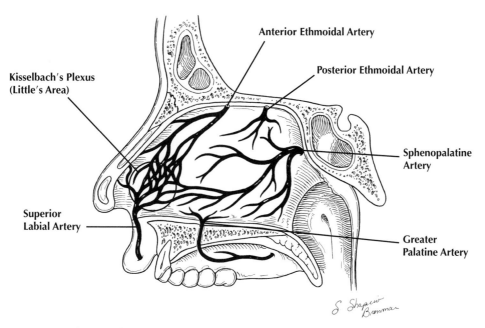

Figure 22–7:   The arterial blood supply of the nasal septum.

through the infraorbital fissure, traverses the infraorbital canal, and exits at the infraorbital foramen. Its terminal branches innervate the lateral bridge of the nose, ala, and several areas of the face. Branches of the maxillary nerve course through the pterygopalatine fossa, and some enter the nose through the sphenopalatine foramen. The posterolateral nasal and nasopalatine nerves supply the lateral nasal wall and septum, respectively. Other branches continue through the fossa and provide sensation to the teeth, gingiva, and palate.

The *ophthalmic division* (V_1) of the trigeminal nerve provides additional sensory fibers. Within the orbit, its nasociliary branch divides into the anterior and posterior ethmoidal nerves, which penetrate the lamina papyracea through their respective foramina. The posterior ethmoidal nerve supplies a small region near the superior turbinate and a corresponding area on the septum. The anterior ethmoidal nerve divides into the internal and external nasal nerves. The *internal nasal nerve* innervates the anterior lateral wall and septum, and the *external nasal nerve* passes between the upper-lateral cartilage and nasal bone to innervate the dorsum and nasal tip.

The *autonomic nervous system* (ANS) regulates the production of nasal secretions and the vascular supply to the nasal mucosa, which helps regulate the heating and humidification of inspired air. The maxillary division of the trigeminal nerve also serves as the conduit for both parasympathetic and sympathetic fibers. *Parasympathetic fibers* originate in the superior salivary nucleus, exit the brainstem, join with fibers of the facial nerve in the internal auditory canal (IAC), and traverse the geniculate ganglion. After leaving this ganglion, these fibers become the greater petrosal nerve, and in the pterygoid canal, combine with the deep petrosal nerve and carry sympathetic fibers to form the *vidian nerve.* These fibers then enter the pterygopalatine fossa, continue to the sphenopalatine ganglion to synapse with postganglionic cells, enter the sphenopalatine foramen, and travel to the mucus glands of the nasal mucosa with branches of the maxillary nerve.

Sympathetic fibers originate from the intermediolateral cell column of the spinal cord in the area of T-1, course through the first thoracic sympathetic ganglion, and synapse in the superior cervical ganglion. Postganglionic fibers accompany the internal carotid artery and exit the carotid canal as the deep petrosal nerve, which becomes part of the vidian nerve. They accompany parasympathetic fibers through the pterygoid fossa and sphenopalatine foramen and are distributed to the blood vessels of the nose with branches of the maxillary nerve.

Olfactory cells, or bipolar neuroepithelial cells, are found in the superior midportion of the nasal cavity, in the mucosa of the nasal septum, and in the superior turbinate. A superficial process known as an *olfactory hair* extends beyond its epithelial surface; a deep process joins neighboring processes to form *olfactory nerves.* Within the submucosa, there are several bundles of these nerves that pass through the formina of the cribiform plate as the *fila olfactoria* and then synapse in the olfactory bulb.

ANATOMY OF THE NASOPHARYNX

The *nasopharynx* is the rhomboid-shaped cavity that forms the superior aspect of the pharynx. Unlike the rest of the pharynx, which is surrounded by muscles, the nasopharynx is surrounded by bone and is thus always patent. It begins 1 cm behind the posterior border of the inferior turbinates, and the posterior choanae form its anterior limit. Its roof and posterior wall are continuous, and are formed by the sphenoid and occipital bones and the first two cervical vertebrae. Adenoid tissue (pharyngeal tonsil) is found along the posterosuperior surface.

The sphenoid bone forms the lateral walls of the nasopharynx. The eustachian tube orifice is located along its lateral wall. The *torus tubarius,* which is a prominent cartilaginous ridge, marks the posterior boundary of the orifice. Just behind the torus tubarius is a deep recess, known as the *fossa of Rosenmüller.*

The anterior aspect of the inferior border is formed by the soft palate, and posteriorly an orifice, the pharyngeal isthmus, opens into the oropharynx. During speech, the isthmus is closed by coordinated actions of the salpingopharyngeus, palatopharyngeus, and levator veli palatini muscles and the contraction of the sphincteric fibers of the superior constrictor muscles of the pharynx. During contraction, these sphincteric fibers may rise to form *Passavant's ridge.* The tensor veli palatini contributes to closure of the isthmus during swallowing.

ANATOMY OF THE PARANASAL SINUS

The *paranasal sinuses* are air-filled cavities within the skull. There are four pairs of sinuses: the maxillary, ethmoid, sphenoid, and frontal. Each sinus is lined with respiratory mucosa that is contiguous with that of the nasal cavity, and communicates with the nasal cavity through various ostia.

Not only are the size and proportion of the si-

nuses different in children and adults, but there are also significant differences among children of different ages. These age differences are related to the development of the skull and dentition. Since intranasal surgery is frequently performed in children of all ages, an understanding of the developmental anatomy of the paranasal sinuses is necessary for proper management of pediatric sinus disease.

Maxillary Sinus

The *maxillary sinus* is the first sinus to develop, and it originates as an air cell between the ethmoid bulla and uncinate process during the third fetal month. In the newborn, it is found as a pouch in the lateral nasal wall, but cannot be demonstrated radiologically until 4 to 5 months of age. Growth of the maxillary sinus is biphasic, with a period of rapid growth from birth to 4 years and another from 8 to 12 years. During the initial growth phase, the sinus expands to the infraorbital nerve and to the floor of the inferior turbinate to the level of attachment. By 7 years, the sinus floor has only descended to the level of the middle of the inferior meatus, and prior to age 8 fenestration of the maxillary sinus via the inferior meatus is hazardous. The tooth buds can easily be injured and the small dimensions of the sinuses increase the risk of injury.[4] During the second phase, pneumatization extends to the lateral orbital wall and the floor reaches the level of the floor of the nasal cavity. From 12 years until 22 to 24 years when development is complete, much of the growth of the sinus is related to the pneumatization of the alveolar process following eruption of the permanent teeth, when the sinus floor comes to lie below that of the nasal cavity.

The maxillary sinus, which is the largest paranasal sinus, occupies the body of the maxilla. The *maxilla* is a pyramid: its base in the lateral nasal wall and its apex points toward the zygomatic process. The anterior wall forms the facial surface of the maxilla, and the posterior wall becomes the infratemporal surface, separating the sinus from the pterygopalatine fossa. The orbital surface of the maxilla forms the roof of the maxillary sinus. The infraorbital canal, carrying the infraorbital nerve, usually projects into the sinus as a ridge traversing the roof. The sinus floor is formed by the alveolar process of the maxilla. Within the floor, bony processes (which cover the roots of the second premolar and the first and second molars) project into the sinus. In some cases, these roots may break through the bone and extend into the sinus cavity. In children, the floor lies above or at the floor of the nose; in adults it may be located between 4 to 10 mm below the floor of the nasal cavity.

The *maxillary sinus ostium* is located along the medial wall and drains into the ethmoid infundibulum. In children, its location within the middle meatus is more anterior and inferior than in adults. Accessory ostia are found in 10 to 30% of individuals and are usually posterior to the true ostium.[5] Within the maxillary sinus, mucociliary clearance is directed toward the natural ostium, not toward the accessory ostia. It is critical to identify and enlarge the true ostium when performing a middle meatal antrostomy in order to re-establish physiologic sinus drainage.[3,6]

Ethmoid Sinus

The *ethmoid sinus* or *labyrinth* are pneumatized cells within the ethmoid bone. They can be divided into two groups: the anterior cells drain into the ethmoid infundibulum and the posterior cells drain into the superior meatus.

The *anterior ethmoidal cells* first appear as sacs in the middle meatus during the third fetal month, and the *posterior ethmoidal cells* develop from the superior meatus shortly afterward. At birth, they are well developed, and three to four distinct cells can be identified. They expand rapidly during the first 4 years, and are more developed than the other sinuses. They can be demonstrated radiographically by 1 year. The ethmoidal cells are almost completely developed by 12 years.

The limits of the ethmoid sinus are not well defined because of the variability in their pneumatization. There are usually between two and eight anterior ethmoidal cells. The *ethmoid bulla* is the most constant and usually the largest anterior cell; it is found in 92% of patients.[2] The *agger nasi cells* are located anterior to the most anterosuperior insertion of the middle turbinate and occur in 80% of individuals.[5a] The *basal lamella* is the bony attachment of the middle turbinate and separates the anterior and posterior cells; the anterior cells lie anterior and inferior to it and the posterior cells lie posterior and superior. There are usually between one and eight posterior cells.

The superior, lateral, and posterior walls of the ethmoid sinus are well defined. The fovea ethmoidalis of the frontal bone forms the roof of the air cells, and the lamina papyracea is the lateral wall that sep-

arates the ethmoid sinus from the orbit. The posterior wall is formed by the thick sphenoid bone.

Air cells may extend beyond the limits of the ethmoid sinus. The *concha bullosa* represents an aerated cell within the middle turbinate. *Haller cells* are ethmoid cells that develop along the roof of the maxillary sinus near the ostium. *Onodi cells* are posterior ethmoid cells that extend lateral to and even superior to the body of the sphenoid bone. It is important to recognize the presence of Onodi cells, because the optic nerve and even the carotid artery may traverse along their lateral wall.

> ### SPECIAL CONSIDERATION:
>
> The optic nerve and carotid artery may traverse along the lateral wall of Onodi cells.

Sphenoid Sinus

The *sphenoid sinus* is a pneumatized cavity within the body of the sphenoid bone. It begins as a mucosal sac in the sphenoethmoidal recess in the fourth fetal month. At birth, it remains undeveloped and has not extended into the sphenoid bone yet. After 5 years, pneumatization of the sphenoid bone accelerates and the sinus grows rapidly. The sinus reaches the sella turcica by 7 years and develops completely between 12 and 15 years.

The extent of pneumatization varies considerably, and rarely are these sinuses symmetrical. The sides are usually separated by a bony intrasinus septum. The ostium of the sphenoid sinus lies medially along the anterior face of the sinus, approximately 10 mm above the floor, and empties into the sphenoethmoidal recess, which is located medial to the superior or supreme turbinate. During endoscopic sinus surgery, the surgeon may entered the sphenoid sinus through the natural ostium by way of the sphenoethmoidal recess or through the anterior wall of the sphenoid sinus. If the approach is through the anterior wall, a total ethmoidectomy must be performed first, and then the sphenoid sinus is entered superior and lateral to the natural ostium.

Several structures are in close proximity to the sphenoid sinus, including the hypophysis, cavernous sinus, maxillary nerve, superior orbital fissure with its cranial nerves, optic nerve, and internal carotid artery. Traversing the lateral wall of the sphenoid sinus are two bulges: a superior one that is formed by the optic nerve and an inferior one that is formed by the internal carotid artery. Depending upon the degree of sinus pneumatization, these bulges may be imperceptible or very prominent. Although the artery and nerve are usually covered by bone, in a significant percentage of patients they will be dehiscent, increasing the risk of injury to these structures during surgery.

Frontal Sinus

The *frontal sinus* develops from the anterior pneumatization of the frontal recess or infundibulum into the frontal bone. It is the last sinus to develop, and at birth cannot be differentiated from the ethmoid sinus. The so-called ''frontal cell'' grows slowly, and pneumatization of the frontal bone begins between 4 and 8 years. The frontal sinus does not become fully developed until the late teenage years. Pneumatization of the frontal bone is quite variable. Asymmetry of the sinuses is common, and although

aplasia is rare, significant hypoplasia of one or both sinuses occurs in 2 to 20% of individuals.[7]

The frontal sinus has a thick anterior wall or table that is composed of diploic bone and a thin posterior table that separates the sinus from the anterior cranial fossa. The frontal ostium is found along the posteromedial sinus floor and is contiguous with the frontal recess. Medial to the recess is the thin lamella of the cribriform plate, which is a common site for injury and potential cerebrospinal fluid (CSF) leak.[8] The frontal recess may empty directly into the middle meatus or infundibulum.

NASAL FUNCTION

The primary function of the nose is the preparation of inspired air for the lower respiratory tract. This is accomplished mainly by the nasal mucosa, which regulate airway resistance and provide for the humidification, temperature regulation, cleansing, and filtration of inspired air. In addition, specialized nasal epithelium is responsible for olfaction.

The anterior vestibule is lined with hair-bearing, keratinized, squamous epithelium, and respiratory epithelium is found posteriorly. The *nasal mucosa* is made primarily of respiratory epithelium that consists of ciliated, pseudostratified, columnar squamous epithelium with many goblet cells. Within the submucosa are numerous mucinous and seromucinous glands and a rich vascular network of venous plexus and specialized arteriovenous anastomoses. This network regulates the erectile tissue of the nose and is especially prominent in the inferior and middle turbinates. The ANS controls both mucus secretions and the vascular supply to the submucosa. Olfactory mucosa containing ciliated, olfactory epithelium is located along the superior turbinate and adjacent septum, and it makes up 1.25% of the nasal mucosa.[8] In the posterior nasal cavity, the epithelium changes to moist, nonkeratinizing, stratified squamous epithelium, which aids the conduction of inspired air.

Respiration

The major function of the nose is to provide a passage to the lower respiratory tract (LRT). Breathing may occur through the nose or mouth, but nasal breathing is preferred. The deeper, shallower respirations and greater airway resistance that are associated with nasal breathing allow for more efficient

---

AT A GLANCE. . .

Sinus Development

Maxillary Sinus: the first sinus to develop, it can be seen radiologically at 4 to 5 months of age; growth is biphasic with rapid growth from birth to 4 years and another growth period between 8 to 12 years; growth continues from 12 years until 22 to 24 years, when it is then complete.

Ethmoid Sinus: anterior ethmoidal cells first appear during the third fetal month and posterior ethmoidal cells develop shortly after; these cells are well developed at birth, grow rapidly during the first 4 years, and can be seen radiographically by 1 year; development is almost complete by 12 years.

Sphenoid Sinus: begins development in the fourth fetal month; at birth, it remains undeveloped and does not begin to grow rapidly until after 5 years; development is complete between 12 to 15 years.

Frontal Sinus: the last sinus to develop, it cannot be differentiated from the ethmoid sinus at birth; pneumatization of the frontal bone begins between 4 to 8 years; does not develop fully until the late teenage years.

alveolar ventilation. Nasal breathing results in a 10 to 20% greater oxygen uptake than does mouth breathing.[9] Pulmonary function is affected both by nasopulmonary reflexes, which regulate respiration and bronchiolar tone, and by passive nasal-airway resistance, which is essential to maintain the elasticity of the lungs.[8]

Nasal resistance may provide up to 50% of the total airway resistance, and varies depending upon these multiple factors: the orientation of the nasal ala; the size of the pyriform aperture, nasal cavity, and posterior choanae; and the velocity of air flow. The size of the nasal cavity is the most variable factor; it is altered by the vasomotor responses of the vasculature of the nasal mucosa and turbinates to hormones, activity, emotions, environment, posture, and pharmacologic agents. Vasomotor control is mediated primarily by the sympathetic system, with a lesser contribution from the parasympathetic system. A sympathetic response causes vasoconstriction with mucosal shrinkage, an increase in nasal patency, and a decrease in nasal resistance; a parasympathetic response results in vasodilatation and a subsequent increase in nasal resistance.

Three separate areas within the nasal airway regulate nasal resistance. Anteriorly, the nasal vestibule is supported by the lower lateral cartilages. During inspiration, negative pressure tends to collapse the vestibule, increasing resistance, but the action of the dilator nares muscles help to reduce this collapse. The vestibule accounts for one-third of nasal resistance.

The *nasal valve area* is a triangular region that is bordered inferiorly by the floor of the pyriform aperture, medially by the nasal septum and laterally by the caudal border of the upper lateral cartillage and the anterior edge of the inferior turbinate. The nasal valve area is the narrowest point of the nasal cavity, and the most important nasal resistor, contributing approximately two-thirds of the nasal airway resistance. Minor alterations in the vasomotor control of the septal mucosa and inferior turbinates will have a profound effect on the nasal valve and subsequently nasal resistance. Deviations of the nasal septum and scarring in this region will have similar effects.

SPECIAL CONSIDERATION:

The nasal valve is the most important nasal resistor, accounting for approximately two-thirds of nasal resistance.

The lateral nasal wall that is posterior to the pyriform aperture is a minor nasal resistor. The degree of this resistance is determined by the amount of vasodilatation of the turbinates and septum.

Although there may be short-term fluctuations, nasal resistance remains constant in individuals over longer periods of time. This nasal resistance is regulated by the *nasal cycle,* the process by which one nasal cavity opens with the production of mucus and serous secretions while the opposite cavity closes with the cessation of secretions. The nasal cycle maintains a constant nasal pressure to help provide adequate lower airway resistance and optimal heating and humidification of inspired air. The average cycle ranges from 30 minutes to 4 hours. In adults, the ANS controls the cycle. However, young children do not have a nasal cycle, and although older children may demonstrate regular changes in nasal resistance, the exact mechanism may not be the same as adults.[10]

Heating and Humidification

The nose plays a vital role in the heating and humidifying of inspired air. Optimal gas exchange within the alveoli requires warm moist air. Failure to heat and humidify inspired air also results in impaired mucociliary activity, increased viscosity of nasal secretions, decreased resistance of the pulmonary mucosa to bacteria, and breakdown in pulmonary surfactant.

Humidification and warming primarily occur adjacent to the vascular mucosa of the septum and turbinates and are controlled by the ANS. Cold dry air stimulates the parasympathetic system, causing vasodilatation of the mucosa with subsequent transudation of fluid as well as an increase in mucus secretions by goblet cells, resulting in the moisturization of the passing air. After flowing through the nose, inspired air becomes 75 to 95% saturated.[11]

Vasodilatation also results in swelling of the nasal mucosa and in an increase in mucosal temperature. As air flow crosses the septum and turbinates, heat is transferred to the inspired air. The amount of warming is dependent on the external temperature.

Filtration and Protection

The nose provides the initial defense for the respiratory system. Inspired air first passes through the vibrases, or the hairs of the nasal vestibule, which filter large particles and sweep them out of the nose.

The remainder of the protective functions is furnished by the *mucociliary system,* which consists of ciliated, pseudostratified, columnar squamous epithelium; mucus secreting goblet cells; submucosal mucinous and seromucinous glands; and the mucus blanket. The *mucus blanket* is composed of two layers: the superficial layer is thick and vesicoelastic, forming a protective sheet; the deeper layer consists of thin serous fluid. Cilia beat within the serous layer, generally posteriorly, directing the mucus into the nasopharynx. This nasal mucus blanket is renewed every 10 to 20 minutes. Drying, cold temperatures, and viral disease impede ciliary activity and may even cause its cessation. This decrease in activity increases the penetration and growth of infectious agents.

The mucociliary system removes particulate matter and bacteria from the air and supplies protection for the nasal mucosa. 70 to 80% of particles 3 to 5 mu in diameter and 60% of particles 2 mu in diameter are filtered out of the inspired air. Particles <1 mu in diameter will pass into the lungs. Debris is entrapped in the mucus blanket, especially along the anterior portions of the middle and inferior turbinates, and ciliary activity directs it posteriorly into the nasopharynx. The mucus blanket not only provides a physical barrier, but contains antibacterial and antiviral substances. Mast cells, polymorphonuclear leukocytes, eosinophils, immunoglobulins, and interferon all have been found within the mucus blanket.

Olfaction

Although humans do not rely upon the sense smell as much as other animals, olfaction still plays a vital role in everyday life. It is important for food choices, social interactions, and protection against noxious and toxic substances.

The olfactory epithelium, which is found along the superior turbinate and adjacent septum, occupies only 1.25% of the nasal mucosa.[8] This is a small, relatively-concealed area and many odors are never sensed because they do not reach the olfactory epithelium in sufficient quantities to stimulate a response. Odor detection is dependent upon the amount of stimulation within a given time. Sniffing increases the detection of odors by increasing air flow to the olfactory mucosa.

To be detected, the odorant must have a vapor pressure and be relatively lipid and water soluble so that it can be absorbed into the nasal mucosa

and diffused to the olfactory receptor cells. It is believed that when an odorant interacts with receptor cells, an action-potential is generated and sent through nerve fibers to the olfactory bulb and then to the cortex for processing. The exact mechanism for odor identification and recognition remains unknown.[12]

AT A GLANCE. . .

Nasal Function

- Respiration
- Heating and Humidification
- Filtration and Protection
- Olfaction

FUNCTION OF THE PARANASAL SINUSES

The significance of the paranasal sinuses is unknown. The only accepted role of the sinuses is to supply mucus to the nasal cavity. Several other theories regarding sinus function have been postulated, but none has been proven. These theories include the humidification and heating of inspired air, the assistance in the regulation of intranasal pressure, the decrease of the weight of the skull, and the increase in the surface area of the olfactory membrane.[13]

The sinuses develop as evaginations of the nasal cavity. Their mucosa is contiguous with that of the nasal cavity and has the same mucociliary system. Within each sinus, the cilia beat in the direction of the natural ostium, moving the mucus blanket toward the nose. Under normal conditions, the cilia are effective in clearing mucus and preventing infection. The mucociliary system may be disrupted by a variety of conditions including cold temperature, drying conditions anatomic obstruction, infections, and inflammation. Sinusitis may result when the mucociliary system is disrupted.

When mucosal surfaces come into contact, mucociliary clearance becomes impeded, resulting in impaired sinus ventilation and retained secretions. This contact provides an ideal environment for viral and/or bacterial growth and increases the likelihood of infection. Infection may lead to mucosal hyperplasia, and these areas of hyperplasia may become foci of reinfection.[13] Mucosal contact is most likely to occur in the narrow passages of the middle meatus and anterior ethmoidal complex, which is termed the *ostiomeatal unit.*[14] This is the primary location for inflammatory disease of the nose and sinuses.[15] Because the ostiomeatal unit is the location through which the anterior ethmoid, maxillary, and frontal sinuses drain, inflammation of this region may result in occlusion of these sinuses and subsequent infection. Resection of the inflammatory tissue and/or anatomic abnormalities in the ostiomeatal unit results in the restoration of normal sinus ventilation, mucociliary clearance, and the resolution of anterior ethmoid, frontal, and maxillary sinus disease. This concept forms the basis for functional, endoscopic, sinus surgery.

SPECIAL CONSIDERATION:

Contact between mucosal surfaces impedes mucociliary clearance, leading to impaired sinus ventilation, retained secretions, and infection.

REFERENCES

1. Tardy ME, Brown RJ. *Surgical Anatomy of the Nose.* New York: Raven Press, 1990, p. 55.
2. Stammberger H. *Functional Endoscopic Sinus Surgery.* Philadelphia: Decker, 1991, p. 52.
3. Kennedy DW, Zinreich SJ, Kuhn F, et al. Endoscopic middle meatal antrostomy: Theory, technique, and patency. Laryngoscope 1987; 70(Supplement 43):1.
4. Wolf G, Anderhuber W, Kuhn F. Development of the paranasal sinuses in children: Implications for paranasal sinus surgery. Ann Otol Rhinol Laryngol 1993; 102:705.
5. Van Alyea OE. *Nasal Sinuses: An Anatomic and Clinical Consideration.* Baltimore: Williams & Wilkins, 1955, p. 12.
5a. Graney DO, Rice DH: Anatomy. In Cummings CW, Frederickson JM, Harker LA, et al, eds. Otolaryngology-Head and Neck Surgery, Vol 2. St. Louis: Mosby Year Book, 1998, p. 1062.
6. May M, Sobol SM, Korzec K. The location of the maxillary os and its importance to the endoscopic sinus surgeon. Laryngoscope 1990; 100:1037.
7. Lang J. *Nasal Cavity and Paranasal Sinuses.* New York: Thieme, 1989 p. 62.
8. Jafek BW. Ultrastructure of human nasal mucosa. Laryngoscope 1983; 93:1576.
9. Barelli PA. Nasopulmonary Physiology. In: Timmons BH, Ley R, eds. *Behavioral and Psychological Approaches to Breathing Disorders.* New York: Plenum, 1994, p. 47.
10. Van Cauwenberge PB, Deleye L. Nasal cycle in children. Arch Otolaryngol 1984; 10:108.
11. Meyerhoff WL, Schaefer SD: Physiology of the Nose and Paranasal Sinuses. In Paparella MM, Shumrick DA, Gluckman JL, et al, eds. Otolaryngology, Vol 1, Philadelphia: WB Saunders, 1991, p. 322.
12. Doty RL, Snow JB. Olfaction. In: Goldman JL, ed. *The Principles and Practice of Rhinology.* New York: Wiley, 1987, p. 761.
13. Amedee RG. Sinus Anatomy and Function. In: Bailey BJ, Johnson JT, Kohut RI, et al, eds. *Head and Neck Surgery-Otolaryngology.* Philadelphia: Lippincott, 1993, p. 346.
14. Stammberger H. Endoscopic endonasal surgery—Concepts in treatment of recurring rhinosinusitis. Part I. Anatomic and pathophysiologic considerations. Otolaryngol Head Neck Surg 1985; 94:143.
15. Naumann H. Pathologische anatomie der chronischen rhinitis und sinusitis. In: *Proceedings VIII International Congress of Oto-rhino-laryngology.* Amsterdam: Excerpta Medica, 1965, p. 80.
16. Kennedy DW, Zinreich SJ, Rosenbaum AE, et al. Functional endoscopic sinus surgery: Theory and diagnostic evaluation. Arch Otolaryngol 1985; 111:576.

23 Radiology of the Paranasal Sinuses

Benjamin C.P. Lee

IMAGING TECHNIQUES

Plain radiograph, computed tomography (CT), and magnetic resonance imaging (MRI) scans are used to evaluate paranasal sinus diseases. Plain radiograph and CT scans involve ionizing radiation that is potentially hazardous, especially in sensitive regions such as the cornea of the eye. As the radiation dose is cumulative, these harmful effects can be diminished by spreading the exposures over time.[1,2] The three factors that are involved in the delivery of radiation in diagnostic examinations are: voltage in kilovolts (kV), current in milliamperes (mA), and the time of exposure in seconds. In general, the voltage used is standard (around 120 kV), but different currents and times are used to image various body parts. Radiation dose is related to the product of the current and the time known as mAs. Bony structures are evaluated adequately with low mAs, whereas soft tissue requires higher mAs techniques, especially in places where this tissue is enclosed within thick bone. The dosages of radiation for various imaging techniques are shown in Table 23-1.[3] It is believed that exposures in excess of 100 rem over a short time may result in cataracts. Although the dosage for CT is higher than plain radiographs, it should be remembered that each CT section is collimated to 2 to 3 mm, and thus the radiation exposure is limited to the region that is scanned. In contrast, the entire face and skull is radiated during each radiograph exposure. Irrespective of the differences in radiation exposure between these two techniques, it is prudent to limit the number of examinations each year.

Plain Radiography

Although the *plain radiograph* has been the mainstay in evaluation of paranasal diseases in the past, its role is now limited to screening in the emergency room and primary care facilities.[4] The primary reason for this is the difficulty in interpretation due to the overlap of structures within the direction of view. Overlap of anterior/posterior structures can be overcome partially by directing the X-ray beam at different directions in AP radiographs. Overlap of lateral structures can only be corrected partially by the use of oblique lateral views. Unlike CT scans, plain radiographs are useful only for detecting bony structures and calcium; all soft tissue shows up in various degrees of opacity, but it is not possible to determine whether these are solid, fluid, or blood.

SPECIAL CONSIDERATION:

The harmful effects of radiation doses can be diminished by spreading the exposures over time.

Because of these limitations, plain radiographs are useful only for visualizing gross bony destruction, displacements, and the presence of opacities and calcium within air-containing structures. Essentially, they play no role in the evaluation of inflammatory sinus disease and may, in fact, be confusing.[4,5]

SPECIAL CONSIDERATION:

Plain radiographs are useful only for visualizing gross bone destruction, displacements, and the presence of opacities and calcium within air-containing structures.

Pediatric Otolaryngology, Edited by R.F. Wetmore, H.R. Muntz, and T.J. McGill. Thieme Medical Publishers, Inc., New York © 2000.

TABLE 23–1: Radiation Doses for Various Imaging Techniques

Sinus radiograph (4 views)	7 mrems
Sinus CT (3mm 160mAs)	51 mrems
Head CT (5mm 300mAs)	110 mrems

Computed Tomography

CT is the gold standard in the evaluation of paranasal sinus disease.[3,4,6-8] CT may be performed using individual 2D sections or with the spiral technique. In 2D scans, *coronal sections* are constructed at right angles, and *axial sections* are constructed parallel to the orbito-meatal line with 3 mm between each section. The scans may be the same thickness or 4 to 5 mm overlapped at 3 mm. Where high resolution views are necessary for evaluation of subtle fractures or for 3D surface rendering, 2 mm contiguous cuts are performed. The radiation dose is approximately 250 mAs.[9,10] In *spiral scans,* sections are performed using a nominal thickness of 3 mm and mAs of approximately 125. Images are reconstructed with a soft-tissue algorithm. In cases where bone detail is necessary, the scans are reconstructed with a bone algorithm. Spiral and individual 2D sections each have advantages and disadvantages (Table 23-2). The spiral technique is fast. Each turn of the spiral takes one second and the entire examination may be completed in a few seconds, depending upon the number of turns used. The total examination time for 2D technique is longer as each individual scan takes 2 to 3 seconds to complete. On the other hand, any section that is degraded by patient movement may be repeated. Spiral scans are acquired continuously so there is no time for cooling of the X-ray tube; this limits the mAs that can be used and results in images that are less detailed (lower signal: noise) and have poorer gray scale in comparison to 2D images that are performed with higher mAs. In addition, because of the geometry of the spiral rotations, spiral scans are not as sharp as

TABLE 23–2: Advantages and Disadvantages of Spiral and Individual Scans

	2D	Spiral
Speed	+	+ + +
Soft-tissue-detail/gray scale	+ +	+
Spatial resolution	+ +	+
3D-surface rendering	–	+ +

individual sections of 2D scans. Three-dimensional surface reconstructions from spiral scans are smoother than those from 2D images, which have 'step-ladder' artifacts.

A *limited sinus CT* technique has been used in adults and is helpful in screening or inflammatory diseases.[11] As the paranasal sinuses are relatively large in this population, it is possible to visualize them with widely-spaced CT sections. However, the paranasal sinuses in children are smaller and it is difficult to be sure that they are adequately visualized with this technique. In children supplementary CT sections must be added to evaluate structures that are missed on the initial examination. In cases where movement of the subject has occurred, it is also likely that the scans will have to be repeated several times. Radiation exposure is not reduced and it may even be increased compared with a conventional CT examination. For this reason, the limited sinus technique should not be used in children.

> ## SPECIAL CONSIDERATION:
>
> A limited sinus technique should not be used on children because radiation exposure may be increased compared with a conventional CT exam.

CT is the method of choice for evaluating bony and most soft-tissue structures. Compared with plain radiography, structures are seen as thin sections and are not obscured by overlapping structures. CT is more sensitive to subtle changes and has a considerably greater dynamic range than plain radiography. It is thus possible to differentiate between fluid and soft tissues and to detect calcification and blood. The coronal view is most useful for viewing the ostiomeatal complex, sinus pathology, and bony lesions. Axial views are used mainly to evaluate extension of sinus disease into the orbits, cranial cavity, and the skull base. These views are complimentary and both may be necessary in the full evaluation of some diseases. Sagittal views can be reconstructed from axial or coronal scans. As a general principle, displacement and destruction of bony structures are best seen when these are at right angles to the direction of the imaging plane.

Magnetic Resonance Imaging

MRI is a technique that depends on differences in relaxation characteristics in tissues. It has no known risks compared with X-rays. It is extremely sensitive in detecting changes in soft tissues, is considerably better in differentiating fluid from solid, and is better at characterizing changes in soft tissues.[12,13] Although this technique is sensitive in evaluating marrow, it is unable to detect changes within bone and calcium, both of which appear as signal loss. Currently, the main use of MRI is in evaluating extension of sinus disease into the orbit and intracranial cavity, as well as in characterizing lesions that originate from these locations, such as encephaloceles or tumors. Although this technique is excellent in detecting fluid and soft tissues, MRI is thought to be overly sensitive in the evaluation of inflammatory changes in the paranasal sinuses. MRI has been used in evaluating temporal changes of the nasal cavity

(i.e., nasal cycling).[14] It obviously has potential application in the epidemiologic study of the natural history of sinusitis in cohorts of otherwise healthy children.

Ultrasonography and Angiography

Ultrasonography may be used to detect fluid in the frontal and maxillary sinuses. Its only advantage is that it does not involve ionizing radiation. Otherwise, it is extremely insensitive. It plays practically no role in the evaluation of paranasal sinus diseases. *Angiography* has a limited role in the evaluation of the paranasal sinuses, but is invaluable in evaluating the blood supply of vascular lesions. It is used mainly for vascular malformations and in the diagnosis and preoperative embolization of vascular tumors such as juvenile angiofibromas.

AT A GLANCE . . .

Imaging Techniques

Plain Radiograph: useful only for detecting bony structures and calcium. Soft tissue shows up but it is not possible to determine if it is solid, fluid, or blood.

Computed Tomography: structures are seen as thin sections and not obscured by overlapping structures as in plain radiographs. There is differentiation between fluid and soft tissues and detection of calcification and blood *Axial View:* used to evaluate sinus disease in the orbits, cranial cavity, and skull base. *Coronal View:* used for viewing the ostiomeatal complex, sinus pathology, and bony lesions.

Magnetic Resonance Imaging: extremely sensitive in detecting changes in soft tissues, better than other imaging techniques in differentiating fluid from solid, and better at characterizing soft tissues. It is unable to detect changes within bone and calcium.

Ultrasonography: an extremely insensitive techniques that is used to detect fluid in the frontal and maxillary sinuses.

Angiography: invaluable for evaluating the blood supply of vascular lesions. Used in the diagnosis and preoperative embolization of vascular tumors.

ANATOMY OF THE PARANASAL SINUSES

The *paranasal sinuses* include the maxillary, ethmoid, frontal, and sphenoid sinuses. The *ethmoid* and *maxillary sinuses* are usually present at birth, although the latter continue to grow until almost 12 years of age.[15] The *sphenoid* and *frontal sinuses* are not aerated until 1 to 2 years of age and 5 to 7 years of age, respectively.[16-18] The paranasal sinuses drain into the nasal cavity through a number of complex channels.[6,15,18-22]

The nasal cavity is divided by bony structures known as the *superior, middle,* and *inferior turbinates* (conchi) that arise from the roof and lateral walls of the nasal cavity. The turbinates demarcate the nasal cavity into superior, middle, and inferior meati, which are situated lateral to their respective turbinates. The *middle meatus* is the most important compartment for sinus drainage and constitutes the epicenter of the ostiomeatal unit. This compartment is demarcated medially by the middle turbinate, which is attached anteriorly to the nasolacrimal bone and posteriorly and laterally to the basal lamina and the lamina papyracea. The space between the posterolateral attachment and the ethmoid bulla (sinus lateralis) further drains the anterior ethmoid. The posterior ethmoid cells and the sphenoid sinuses eventually empty into the *superior meatus.* The nasolacrimal duct drains into the

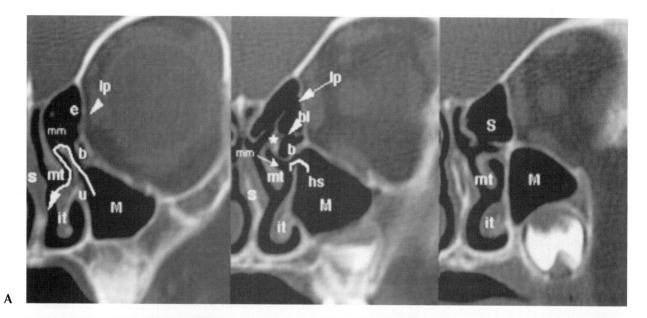

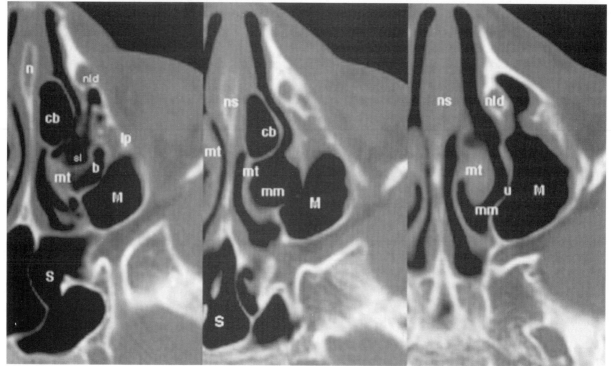

Figure 23–1: (A) Normal, Coronal CT. (Left panel) at level of ostiomeatal unit: arrow shows drainage from maxillary sinus (M) through infundibulum into the middle meatus (mm). (Middle panel) at posterior aspect of ostiomeatal unit: passage through hiatus semilunaris (hs). (Right panel) behind ostiomeatal unit. (b, ethmoid bulla; bl, basal lamina; e, ethmoid air cell; hs, hiatus semilunaris; it, inferior turbinate; lp, lamina paprycea; mm, middle meatus; mt, middle turbinate; s, nasal septum; S, sphenoid sinus; *, attachment of middle turbinate to basal lamina.) (B) Normal, Axial CT. (Left panel) superior section shows the relationship of the maxillary sinus (M) with the bulla of the ethmoid sinus (b) and nasal cavity. An incidental concha bullosa of the turbinate is noted (cb). (Middle panel) at the level of the ostiomeatal unit shows communication of the maxillary sinus (M) with the middle meatus (mm). (Right panel) inferior section shows relationship of the maxillary sinus (M) and middle turbinate (mt). (b, ethmoid bulla; bl, basal lamina; cb, concha bullosa; lp, lamina paprycea; M, maxillary sinus; mm, middle meatus; mt, middle turbinate; nld, nasal lacrimal duct; n, nasal septum; u, uncinate process.)

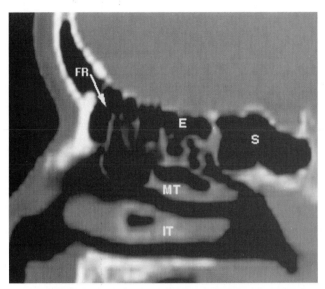

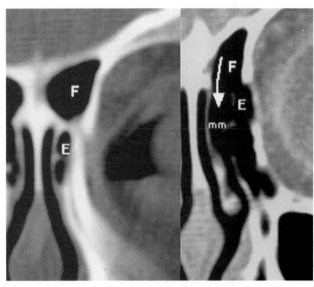

C

D

Figure 23–1 Continued: (C) Normal, Lateral CT. (Paramedian view) shows drainage of the frontal sinus via the frontal recess (FR) into the anterior ethmoid. (E, ethmoid sinus; IT, inferior turbinate; MT, middle turbinate; S, sphenoid sinus.) (D) Normal, Coronal CT. (Left panel) shows relationship of the frontal sinus (F) with the ethmoid sinus (E). (Right panel) Posteriorly the frontal sinus drains through the frontal recess (arrow) into the middle meatus (mm). (E, anterior ethmoid air cells (agger nasi cells); F, frontal sinus; mm, middle meatus.)

inferior meatus. The frontal, anterior ethmoid and maxillary sinuses drain into the middle meatus through the area known as the *ostiomeatal complex* (Fig. 23-1A and 23-1B).[3,7,16,23-25] Defective drainage in this region is thought to be responsible for the majority of sinus inflammation and infections.[3,16,24]

The frontal sinus drains into the anterior portion of the middle meatus close to the midline through the frontal recess. Inferior, anterior, and lateral to this recess are the *agger nasi cells,* which are the most anterior ethmoid air cells. These cells also drain into the middle meatus in the region of the infundibulum (Fig. 23-1C and 23-1D). The maxillary sinus is an inverted cone with an ostium at the apex that opens into the middle meatus of the nasal cavity via the infundibulum. The *infundibulum* is bounded by the uncinate process, the medial orbital wall, and the anterior ethmoid bulla. The *uncinate process* is the superior extension of the medial maxillary wall. The posterior portion of the infundibulum is known as the *hiatus semilunaris* and is bounded inferiorly by the hook-like portion of the uncinate process and superiorly and laterally by the ethmoid bulla (see Fig. 23-1A).

Anatomic Variants

There are many variations in the degree of aeration of the paranasal as well as many configurations of the septa within the frontal, ethmoid, and sphenoid sinuses; these are generally incidental findings.[22,23,26-28] Variants of the ostiomeatal complex, on the other hand, may be significant; although, there is controversy as to whether some of these anomalies predispose to the development of obstruction of the drainage passages.[29] Common variants include paradoxical middle turbinates, aeration of the turbinates (i.e., concha bullosa), extension of ethmoid bulla into the infundibulum (i.e., Haller-infraorbital cells), atelectatic deviations of the uncinate process, and deviation of the nasal septum (Fig. 23-2).

SPECIAL CONSIDERATION:

Variations in the degree of aeration of the paranasal sinuses or in the configuration of the septa are generally considered incidental, whereas variations of the ostiomeatal complex may be significant.

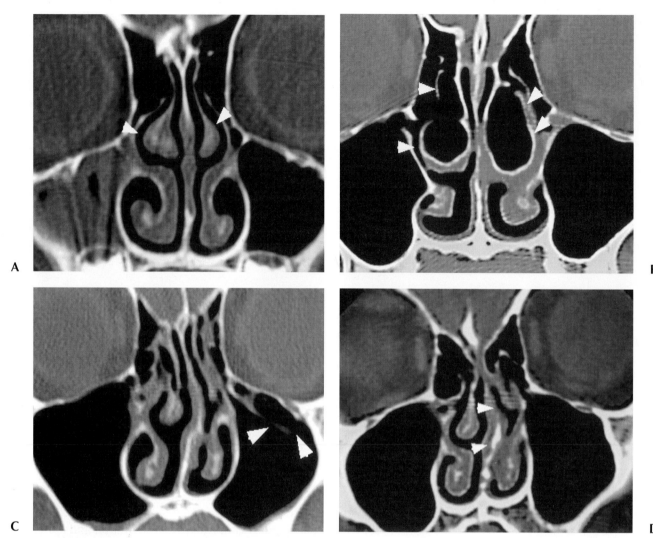

Figure 23–2:   Normal variants—Coronal CT views. (A) Paradoxical middle turbinates (arrowheads) extend laterally and narrow the middle meatus. (B) Concha bullosa (arrowheads) are aerated middle turbinates. (C) Haller cells are extension of the ethmoid air cells into the maxillary sinus (arrowhead). (D) Deviated nasal septum (arrowheads).

DISORDERS OF THE PARANASAL SINUSES

Sinusitis

Sinusitis may be bacterial, viral, fungal, or allergic in etiology. The clinical presentation and course of the symptoms determine whether the abnormality is acute or chronic; rarely is it possible to predict either the organism or the chronicity of the inflammation on imaging alone. Diagnostic imaging should be used to confirm disease, to evaluate the extent of the sinus involvement, to determine whether there is an underlying anatomic abnormality, and to assess complications of sinus disease.

SPECIAL CONSIDERATION:

Diagnostic imaging alone does not allow prediction of the cause or chronicity of inflammation, but it should be used to confirm disease, evaluate the extent of the sinus involvement, determine if there is an underlying anatomic abnormality, and assess complications of sinus dura.

Opacity within the paranasal sinuses is, in general, an indication of sinusitis, except in children under 4 years of age in whom there is a poor correlation with clinical symptoms.[29-36] Abnormalities include mucosal thickening, retention cysts, polyps, and air-fluid levels. Mucosal thickening is the most common abnormality and suggests chronicity in cases where there is associated thickening of the wall and hypoplastic development of the affected sinus (Fig. 23–3). This is to be distinguished from osteomyelitis that is demonstrated as an irregularity in addition to thickening of the wall (Fig. 23–4). Retention cysts are most common in the maxillary sinus and are radiologically synonymous with inflammatory polyps (Fig. 23–5 and Fig. 23-6). Air-fluid levels are seen with bacterial infection, and less commonly with chronic sinusitis and allergic sinus disease. Unilateral sinus disease is common with bacterial infection.

Obstruction of the infundibulum commonly leads to *maxillary sinus disease,* whereas more extensive involvement of the ostiomeatal unit may result in additional blocking of drainage from the frontal and anterior ethmoid sinuses. Anatomic variants are often observed, but there is no clear evidence to indicate that these are responsible for sinus disease directly.[29] It is important, nevertheless, to note these anomalies as they are landmarks for functional endoscopic sinus surgery (FESS).[22,23,25,37-39] A suggested scheme for surveying the paranasal sinuses involves observation of the following drainage patterns: (1) anterior drainage from the ostiomeatal

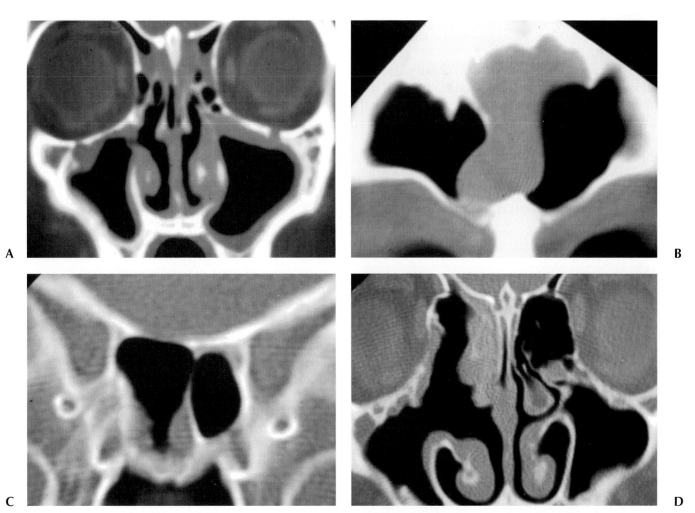

A

B

C

D

Figure 23–3: Mucosa thickening. Coronal CT shows mucosal thickening in the (A) maxillary, (B) frontal, and (C) sphenoid sinuses. Note obstruction of the ostiomeatal unit in the maxillary sinus (arrowhead). (D) Shows mucosal thickening of right ethmoid. Note the typical postoperative appearance following endoscopic sinus surgery with removal of the middle turbinate and part of the medial wall of the maxillary sinus.

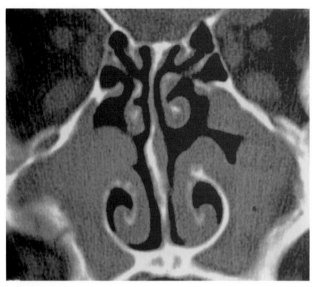

Figure 23–4: Osteomyelitis. Coronal CT demonstrates thickening and periosteal reaction of the wall of the left maxillary sinus.

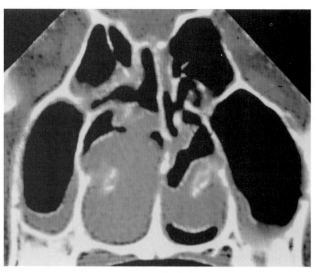

Figure 23–6: Nasal polyps. Coronal CT shows swollen turbinates causing nasal obstruction.

unit and middle meatus (maxillary sinus through the infundibulum and hiatus semilunaris and frontal sinus through the frontal recess and agger nasi cells); and (2) posterior drainage from the posterior ethmoid and sphenoid sinuses.

Severe protracted sinus infection may result in osteomyelitis and may erode the bone, extending into the orbital and intracranial cavity.[40-42] These

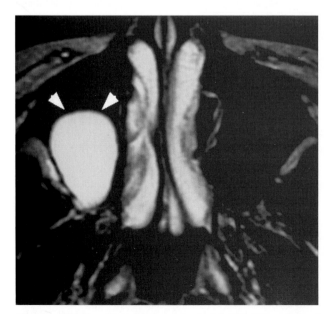

Figure 23–5: Retention cyst. Axial MR T2-weighted image shows a fluid-containing cyst in the right maxillary sinus (arrowheads).

complications are most common with ethmoid and frontal disease (Fig. 23-7). Axial views, in addition to the conventional coronal views, are essential for evaluating these complications.

A *mucocele* results from chronic obstruction of the paranasal sinuses and is most common in the frontal and ethmoid sinuses. It is less common in the maxillary and sphenoid sinuses.[43] The affected sinus is filled completely with no residual air and is always expanded. Depending on the chronicity of the lesion, the wall may be mildly sclerotic to frankly eroded. There is no evidence of infection, and the lesion presents as a expansile mass effect with displacement of adjacent structures. The density of the mucocele varies depending upon its age. Initially, it contains fluid and is of low density, but eventually it becomes desiccated and may have a somewhat higher density (Fig. 23-8). Similarly, depending upon the amount of desiccation a MRI signal may range from low on T1 and high on T2 (reflecting fluid) to an increased signal on T1 and an increased or decreased signal on T2 images (see Fig. 23-8).

Fungal infection of the paranasal sinuses does not have specific radiologic features, although some findings are suggestive of this etiology. Clinical histories suggestive of such infections include an association with diabetes, immunocompromised states, transplantation patients, and those with blood dyscrasias. The radiologic findings of acute fungal infection are nonspecific, although involvement of the cheek is reported to be a common clinical finding

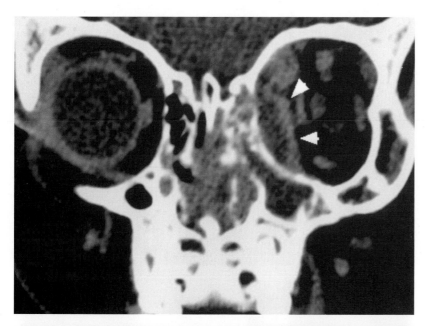

A

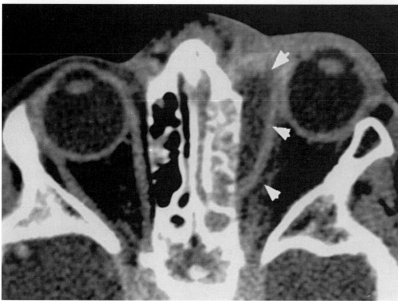

B

Figure 23–7: Orbital abscess. Contrast CT shows opacification of the ethmoid sinus and nasal cavity with extension into the orbit (arrowheads). The abscess does not enhance with contrast. (A) Coronal. (B) Axial.

due to the extension of the infection through the anterior face of the maxillary sinus.[44] Chronic infection may have CT attenuation and MRI signal changes similar to mucoceles; specifically, a slight increased density on CT, an increased signal on T1 MRI images, and a decreased signal on T2 MRI images (Fig. 23-9).[45,46] The presence of sclerosis of the sinus wall may be helpful in differentiating a fungal infection from a mucocele.[47] *Allergic sinusitis* may be associated with aspergillosis of the affected paranasal sinuses. The radiologic appearance in this condition includes mucosal thickening and polyp formation but no air-fluid levels.

SPECIAL CONSIDERATION:

Radiologic findings of acute fungal infection are nonspecific, although involvement of the cheek is reported to be a common clinical finding due to the extension of infection through the anterior face of the maxillary sinus.

Total opacification of all the paranasal sinuses is a characteristic finding in cystic fibrosis (CF).[48,49]

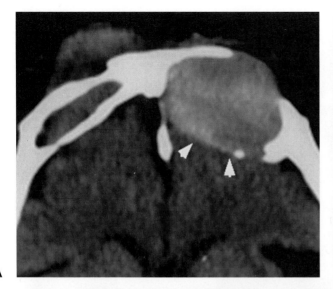

A

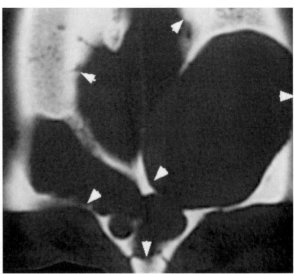

B

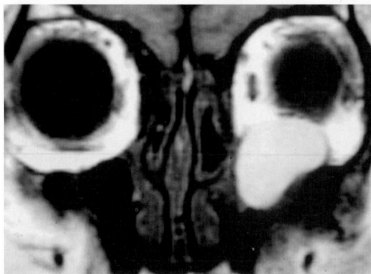

C

Figure 23–8: Mucocele. (A) Axial CT shows a mass with increased density within the left frontal sinus (arrowheads) and breakdown of the anterior wall. (B) Coronal CT (bone window) shows expansion with erosion and thinning of the margins of the sinuses (arrowheads). (C) MRI (T1-weighted image) another case shows increased signal within the mucocele.

In addition, the sinuses often are slightly expanded and the walls may be thinned. In spite of these findings, patients may not have the clinical picture of chronic sinusitis. The radiologic appearance probably is caused by the presence of thick viscous secretions and does not imply that there is active sinus infection. The presence of nasal polyps in children is highly suggestive of CF. Destructive mucoceles, especially involving the ethmoid sinuses, also are seen almost exclusively in children with CF.

SPECIAL CONSIDERATION:

The presence of nasal polyps in children is highly suggestive of CF.

Nasal Masses

Masses in the nasal cavity include congenital lesions and benign and malignant tumors.

Encephaloceles are herniations of the brain and meninges through congenital defects in the skull base. They may arise in the midline and laterally. Only midline and paramedian defects involve the nasal cavities. Midline frontal defects herniate through an enlarged foramen cecum into the superior nasal cavity; large encephaloceles may cause nasal obstruction. (Fig. 23-10). Paramedian defects may allow brain and meninges to herniate into the ethmoid sinuses. Posterior midline defects are rare and present into the sphenoid sinus and the nasopharynx. The defects are visible, have sclerotic margins, and are occasionally seen on plain radiography. It is important to ascertain whether the

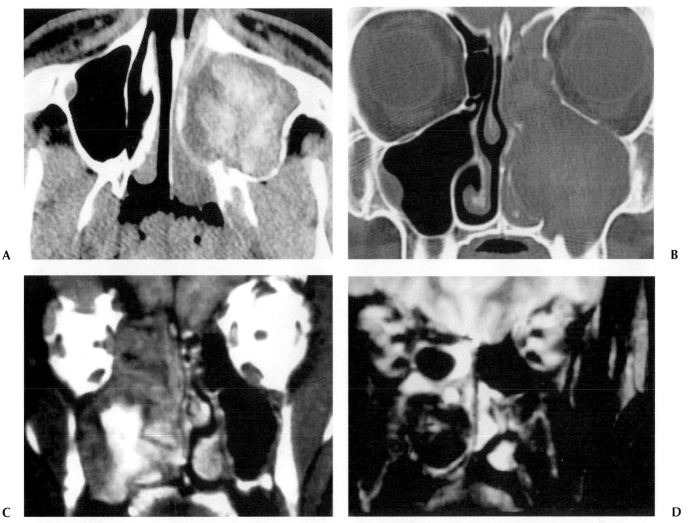

Figure 23–9: Fungal infection. (A) Axial and (B) Coronal CT shows a mass with increased density within the left maxillary sinus that is also expanded. MRI coronal (C) T1- and (D) T2-weighted images in another patient show soft-tissue mass with regions of increased signal on T1 and decreased signal on T2 images.

herniated tissue contains only cerebrospinal fluid (CSF) or also includes brain. Although it is possible to make this determination by CT, MRI is more reliable (see Fig. 23–10).

Dermoids, lipomas, and *hemangiomas* are lesions that occur in the frontonasal groove and that may extend deeply, and sometimes intracranially, through the foramen cecum. Although visible on CT, they are best evaluated by MRI in the sagittal plane (Fig. 23–11). The term nasal glioma is a misnomer, because the lesion is not a tumor but merely brain tissue and surrounding meninges that have grown through a defect in the foramen cecum. Unlike an encephalocele, this ectopic brain has lost its communication with the intracranial cavity.

A *juvenile nasopharyngeal angiofibroma* (JNA)

occurs in males and originates from the pterygopalatine fossa. It extends through the sphenopalatine foramen to involve primarily the sphenoid sinus, but may extend anteriorly into the superior orbital fissure and also into the ethmoid and maxillary sinuses. This tumor is highly vascular and must be surgically treated following angiographic embolization of its blood supply. Failure to diagnose this tumor accurately may result in fatal hemorrhage. This is one of the few lesions with a characteristic plain radiographic finding: anterior bowing of the posterior wall of the maxillary sinus or pterygoid plates. On CT, JNA presents as a soft tissue mass posterior to the maxillary sinus in the pterygopalatine fossa with displacement but no destruction of the adjacent bone. This lesion enhances with contrast

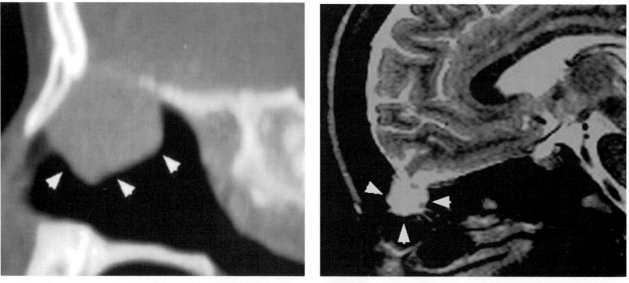

A

B

Figure 23–10:   Frontal meningoencephalocele. (A) Reformatted sagittal CT scan shows mass extending from the intracranial cavity through a bony defect into the nasal cavity (arrowheads). (B) Sagittal MRI (T2-weighted image) shows that the lesion is an meningocele because the signal intensity is similar to that of cerebrospinal fluid.

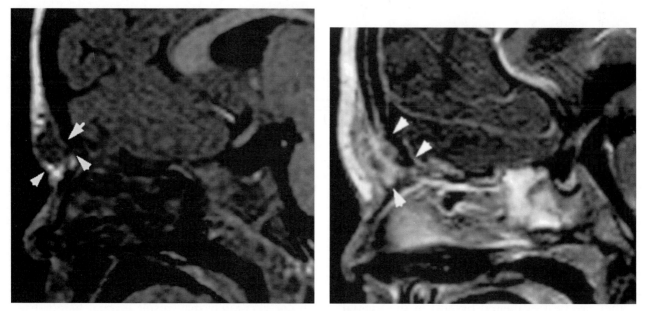

A

B

Figure 23–11:   Nasal dermoid. Sagittal MRI (T1-weighted). (A) Noncontrast image shows soft tissue in the frontonasal region (arrowheads). (B) Contrast image shows enhancement of this lesion (arrowheads) with intracranial communication.

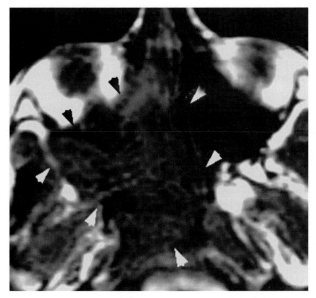

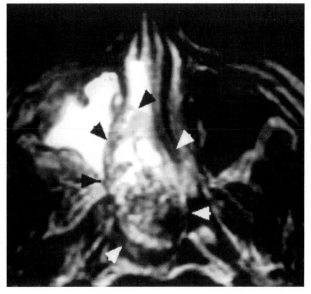

A

B

Figure 23–12: Juvenile nasopharyngeal angiofibroma. Axial MRI. (A) Noncontrast T1-weighted image shows large mass situated in the pterygopalatine fossa (arrowheads). (B) T2-weighted image shows the inhomogenous signal intensity of the tumor (arrowheads) compared with the homogenous increased signal of secondary fluid retention within the maxillary sinus and nasal cavity.

(Fig. 23–12). Although it may be confused with inflammatory sinus disease when the tumor involves the sphenoid, ethmoid, and maxillary sinuses, its site of origin belies its pathologic nature. Associated sinus disease is due to obstruction of the ostiomeatal complex.

Rhabdomyosarcoma occurs in young children and characteristically arises from the skull base, orbit, nasopharynx, or temporal bone. It is highly

destructive, but has no other distinguishing features.

Malignancies of the nasal cavity are rare in the pediatric age group and typically present during adolescence. These include osteogenic sarcoma and olfactory neuroblastoma (Fig. 23–13).

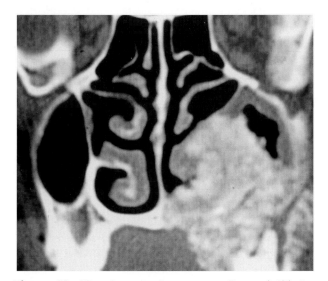

Figure 23–13: Osteogenic sarcoma. Coronal CT view shows a mass with enlargement and gross destruction of the maxillary sinus walls. The increased density of the mass is due partly to ossification.

AT A GLANCE . . .

Types of Nasal Masses

- Encephaloceles
- Dermoids
- Lipomas
- Hemangiomas
- Juvenile nasopharyngeal angiofibroma
- Rhabdomyosarcoma

REFERENCES

1. Jones DJ, Wall BF. Organ doses from medical x-ray examinations calculated using Monte Carlo tech-

niques. London: National Radiological Protection Board, 1985, R186.

2. Curry TS, Dowdey JE, Murry RC. *Christensen's Physics of Diagnostic Radiology, 4th ed.* Philadelphia: Lea & Febiger, 1990, pp. 372–391.

3. Zinreich S. Imaging of inflammatory sinus disease. Otolaryngol Clin North Am 1993; 26:535–547.

4. McAlister WH, Lusk RP, Muntz HR. Comparison of plain radiographs and coronal CT scans in infants and children with recurrent sinusitis. AJR 1989; 153: 1259–1264.

5. MacLeod B. Paranasal sinus radiography. Emerg Med Clin North Am 1991; 9:743–755.

6. Som PM. CT of the paranasal sinuses. Neuroradiology 1985; 27:189–201.

7. Pollei S, Harnsberger HR. The radiological evaluation of the sinonasal region. Postgrad Radiol 1989; 9: 242–266.

8. Kronemer KA, McAlister WH. Sinusitis and its imaging in the pediatric population. Pediatr Radiol 1997; 27:837–846.

9. Marmolya G, Wiesen EJ, Yagan R, et al. Paranasal sinuses: Low-dose CT. Radiology 1991; 181: 689–691.

10. Babbel R, Harnsberger HR, Nelson B, et al. Optimization of techniques in screening CT of the sinuses. AJR 1991; 157:1093–1098.

11. Wippold II FJ, Levitt RG, Evens RG, et al. Limited coronal CT: An alternative screening examination for sinunasal inflammatory disease. Allergy Proc 1995; 16:165–169.

12. Teresi L, Lufkin R, Hanafee W. Low cost MRI of the paranasal sinuses. Comp Med Imag Graphics 1988; 12:165–168.

13. Lloyd GAS, Lund VJ, Phelps PD, et al. Magnetic resonance imaging in the evaluation of nose and paranasal sinus diseases. Brit J Radiol 1987; 60:947–968.

14. Zinreich SJ, Kennedy DW, Kumar AJ, et al. MR imaging of normal nasal cycle: Comparison with sinus pathology. J Comp Assist Tomogr 1988; 12: 1014–1019.

15. Schatz CJ, Becker TS. Normal CT anatomy of the paranasal sinuses. Radiol Clin North Am 1984; 22: 107–118.

16. Youssem DM, Kennedy DW, Rosenberg S. Osteomeatal complex risk factors for sinusitis: CT evaluation. J Otolaryngol 1991; 20:419–424.

17. Aoki S, Dillon WP, Barkovish AJ, et al. Marrow conversion before pneumatization of the sphenoid sinus: Assessment with MR imaging. Radiology 1989; 172:373–375.

18. Simonson TM, Kao SCS. Normal childhood developmental patterns in skull bone marrow by MR imaging. Pediatr Radiol 1992; 22:556–559.

19. Dolan KD. Paranasal sinus radiology, Part 1A: Intro-

duction and the frontal sinuses. Head Neck Surg 1982; 4:301–311.

20. Dolan KD. Paranasal sinus radiology, Part 2A: Ethmoid sinuses. Head Neck Surg 1982; 4:486–496.

21. Dolan KD. Paranasal sinus radiology, Part 3A: Sphenoid sinus. Head Neck Surg 1982; 5:164–176.

22. Zinreich SJ, Benson ML, Oliverio PJ. Sinonasal Cavities. In: Som P. Curtin HD, eds. *CT Normal Anatomy, Imaging of the Osteomeatal Complex, and Functional Endoscopic Surgery Book 1.* St. Louis: Mosby, 1996, pp 97–125.

23. Lang FJ, Smoker WRK. The ostiomeatal unit and endoscopic surgery: Anatomy, variation, and imaging findings in inflammatory diseases. AJR 1992; 159: 849–857.

24. Wallace R, Salazar JE, Cowles S. The relationship between frontal sinus drainage and osteomeatal complex disease: A CT study in 217 patients. AJNR 1990; 11:183–186.

25. Zinreich SJ, Kennedy DW, Rosenbaum AE, et al. Paranasal sinuses: CT imaging requirements for endoscopic surgery. Radiology 1987; 163:769–775.

26. Bolger WE, Butzin CA, Parsons DS. Paranasal sinus bony anatomic variations and mucosal abnormalities: CT analysis for endoscopic sinus surgery. Laryngoscope 1991; 101:56–64.

27. Earwaker J. Anatomic variants in sinonasal CT. Radiographics 1993; 13:381–415.

28. Zinreich SJ, Mattox DE, Kennedy DW, et al. Concha bullosa: CT evaluation. J Comp Assist Tomogr 1988; 12:778–784.

29. Youssem DM. Imaging of sinonasal inflammatory disease. Radiology 1993; 188:303–314.

30. Towbin R, Bunbar JS. The paranasal sinuses in childhood. Radiographics 1982; 2:253–279.

31. Odita JC, Akamaguna AI, Ogisi FO, et al. Pneumatisation of the maxillary sinus in normal and symptomatic children. Pediatr Radiol 1986; 16:365–367.

32. Glasier CM, Ascher DP, Williams KD. Incidental paranasal sinus abnormalities on CT of children: Clinical correlation. AJNR 1986; 7:861–874.

33. Glasier CM, Mallory GBJ, Steele RW. Significance of opacification of the maxillary and ethmoid sinuses in infants. J Pediatr 1989; 114:45–50.

34. Diament MJ, Senac MOJ, Gilsanz V, et al. Prevalence of incidental paranasal sinuses opacification in pediatric patients: A CT study. J Comp Assist Tomogr 1987; 11:426–431.

35. Babbel RW, Harnsberger HR, Sonkens J, et al. Recurring patterns of inflammatory sinonasal disease demonstrated on screening sinus CT. AJNR 1992; 13: 903–912.

36. Lesserson JA, Kieserman SP, Finn DG. The radiographic incidence of chronic sinus disease in the pediatric population. Laryngoscope 1994; 104: 159–166.

37. Zinreich SJ, Kennedy DW, Gayler BW. Computed tomography of nasal cavity and paranasal sinuses: An evaluation of anatomy for endoscopic sinus surgery. Clear Images 1988; 2-9.

38. Lusk RP, Lazar RH, Muntz HR. The diagnosis and treatment of recurrent and chronic sinusitis. Pediatr Clin North Am 1989; 36:1411-1421.

39. Babbel RW, Harnsberger HR. A contemporary look at the imaging issues of sinusitis: Sinonasal anatomy, physiology, and CT techniques. Semin Ultrasound CT MR 1991; 12:526-540.

40. Clary RA, Cunningham MJ, Eavey RD. Orbital complications of acute sinusitis: Comparison of CT scan and surgical findings. Ann Otol Rhinol Laryngol 1992; 101:598-600.

41. Clayman GL, Adamas GL, Paugh DR, et al. Intracranial complications of paranasal sinusitis: A combined institutional review. Laryngoscope 1991; 101: 234-239.

42. Williams BJ, Harrison HC. Subperiosteal abscesses of the orbit due to sinusitis in children. Aust NZ J Ophthalmol 1991; 19:29-36.

43. Van Tassel P, Lee YY, Jing BS, de Vana CA, et al. Mucoceles of the paranasal sinuses: MR imaging with CT correlation. AJR 1989; 153:407-412.

44. Shugar JMA, Som PM, Robbins A, et al. Maxillary sinusitis as a cause of cheek swelling. Arch Otolaryngol 1982; 108:507-508.

45. Som PM, Dillon WP, Curtin HD, et al. Hypointense paranasal sinus foci: Differential diagnosis with MR imaging and relation to CT findings. Radiology 1990; 176:777-781.

46. Som PM, Dillon WP, Fullertin GD, et al. Chronically obstructed sinonasal secretions: Observations on T1 and T2 shortening. Radiology 1989; 172:515-520.

47. Zinreich SJ, Kennedy DW, Malat J, et al. Fungal sinusitis: Diagnosis with CT and MR imaging. Radiology 1988; 169:439-444.

48. Cuyler JP, Monaghan AJ. Cystic fibrosis and sinusitis. J Otolaryngol 1989; 18:173-175.

49. Hasso AN. CT of tumors and tumor-like conditions of the paranasal sinuses. Radiol Clin North Am 1984; 22:119-130.

24 Introduction to Pediatric Rhinology

Rodney P. Lusk and Harlan R. Muntz

Nasal symptomatology is a constant companion of the young child. Frequent or chronic nasal drainage is believed by some to be the routine in children. Recurrent upper respiratory infections in association with a developing immune system predispose the young child to nasal symptoms. Severe exacerbations of infection that lead to periorbital and intracranial complications are the exception but are significant enough that the physician should not disregard nasal symptoms in children. Many children present with nasal symptoms that fall between these two extremes, having troublesome symptoms and signs but not life-threatening complications.

Pediatric rhinology has been poorly studied and understood. In the past, the nasal examination of a child was only a cursory evaluation of the anterior nasal vestibule. Instrumentation that was adopted promptly for the adult is reserved for only the most stoic child in the outpatient arena. In the past, the sinuses were difficult to evaluate clinically and radiographic evaluation in the young child was always considered less than ideal.

Changes in cultural practices and medical technology have prompted the otolaryngology community to examine more closely the problem of nasal symptoms in children. With the increased popularity of day care, and hence early socialization, children are exposed at an earlier age to many organisms, both viral and bacterial. The developing immune system must learn to fight these organisms, but the result in some children is more symptomatic infections. Working parents have little time for their child to be ill. Day-care settings often refuse to admit children with rhinorrhea or fever.

The medical community has been pressured to treat nasal symptoms with antibiotics, even if the infection is not bacterial. This injudicious use of antibiotics in the general population has likely been one of the primary reasons for the development of the numerous resistant strains of bacteria. The development of the endoscopic approach to sinus surgery and the discovery of a scientific basis for the development of chronic sinus infections in adults allowed the pediatric community to consider pediatric rhinology more seriously. Although there has been significant and increasing controversy in this discipline, the eventual outcome should be an improved understanding of the nose and sinuses in children and the ability to improve the quality of life for those who suffer from nasal symptoms.

AT A GLANCE . . .

Symptoms of Rhinitis and Sinusitis

- Nasal obstruction
- Headache or facial pain
- Irritability
- Cough
- Rhinorrhea
- Symptoms suggestive of allergy or immunodeficiency

CLINICAL ASSESSMENT OF THE NOSE AND SINUSES

The clinical evaluation of a child with a nasal or sinus disorder begins with a careful history. Typically, this history is elicited from the primary caregiver, although an older child or adolescent may

Pediatric Otolaryngology, Edited by R.F. Wetmore, H.R. Muntz, and T.J. McGill. Thieme Medical Publishers, Inc., New York © 2000.

440   The Nose, Paranasal Sinuses, and Orbit

provide important details. Important symptoms include the presence, frequency, and duration of symptoms such as nasal obstruction, headache, or facial pain, irritability, and cough. Questions about the color and consistency of rhinorrhea are also important. Associated symptoms of infection in the cars, throat, or chest also may be helpful. In addition, one should carefully question the caregivers for symptoms suggestive of underlying conditions such as allergy or immunodeficiency.

Like other examinations of the head and neck in children, the evaluation of the nose and sinuses should take place in a calm and reassuring setting. Seating the child on the caregiver's lap often provides reassurance and allows the caregiver to assist in restraint if necessary. Allowing the child to see and touch instruments may also prove helpful in allaying fear.

A variety of illumination sources is available for the examiner. Although the use of a head mirror, separate light source, and nasal speculum provide adequate visualization of both nasal cavities, their use may be intimidating to a young child. Good illumination and magnification can be achieved with the hand-held otoscope. In a cooperative older child or adolescent, the nasopharynx can be visualized with a small nasopharyngeal mirror. After anesthetizing the nasal cavities with topical lidocaine and a vasoconstrictor (0.125% or 0.25% phenylephrine or oxymetazoline), a flexible nasopharyngoscope can provide excellent visualization of the nasopharynx. Likewise, insertion of a 90-degree telescope (Storz Hopkins rod system™) through the oral cavity and into the pharynx also provides an excellent view of the nasopharynx. As with other aspects of the head and neck examination in children, the use of general anesthesia may be necessary if the child is young or uncooperative.

The examination of the nose should include inspection of the external framework of the nose. The dorsum should be straight and palpation should be performed to exclude displacement or step-off deformity of the nasal bones. A pit or mass over the nasal dorsum suggests a dermoid cyst. Occasionally, a large hemangioma appears on the dorsum of the nose. Further evaluation of such masses is required to exclude obstruction of the nasal airway.

The internal examination of the nose is initiated by upwardly elevating the tip of the nose and examining the nasal vestibule for signs of infection or trauma. Assessment of the patency of the nasal cavities and evaluation of the caudal septum can be per-

formed to check for evidence of dislocation. Inspection of Little's area in the anterior nasal septum for signs of fresh hemorrhage is important in the evaluation of epistaxis. The anterior edge of the inferior turbinates and the floor of the nasal cavities are other sites of recurrent epistaxis.

Determining the patency of the nasal cavities is especially important in the neonate who is an obligate nasal breather. Because it may be difficult to pass a nasopharyngoscope through the nasal cavity of an infant, the initial assessment of nasal patency can be performed by either passing small catheters through the nose or placing a small mirror near the nares and looking for fogging.

In a cooperative older child, the nasal examination may include use of either the flexible nasopharyngoscope or a small 90-degree telescope to inspect the middle meati for signs of infection. Nasal polyps in children are suggestive of cystic fibrosis (CF). Unilateral nasal drainage usually accompanies a chronic nasal foreign body.

It is now well recognized that plain radiographs do not adequately image the paranasal sinuses of children.[1,2] A lateral neck radiograph, however, can be used to assess the size of the adenoid pad and the degree of nasopharyngeal obstruction. Because of its ability to demonstrate bone–mucosal interfaces, computed tomography (CT) is currently the state-of-the-art study for evaluating the sinuses.[1-4] Disease in each of the sinuses can be documented, as can complications such as mucoceles, pyomucoceles, allergic fungal sinusitis, and fungal sinusitis. CT should be obtained after aggressive medical management has failed and surgical intervention is contemplated. If surgery is not considered a therapeutic option by either the surgeon or the family, CT may not be indicated because the findings will not change the management. One must understand that when CT is performed and disease is documented, even if it is not major, some parents will demand surgical intervention. It is best to advise parents that evidence of disease on CT is not the sole criteria for surgery. Duration and severity of symptoms should remain the most important indicators for possible intervention.

SPECIAL CONSIDERATION:

Computed tomography is currently the state-of-the-art study for evaluating the sinuses.

Magnetic resonance imaging (MRI) is not useful in evaluating chronic sinusitis because the bony walls of the sinuses are not well imaged and the test requires more time to perform. In addition, there is some concern that the false-positive rate is very high with MRI. For example, allergic rhinitis may be identified as sinusitis on MRI.[5–7] MRI is useful for assessing a soft tissue nasal mass such as an encephalocele or angiofibroma and other soft tissue anomalies of the nasal cavity.

EVALUATION OF THE CHILD WITH NASAL OBSTRUCTION AND RHINORRHEA

The clinician must be aware of the symptoms of nasal obstruction (Practice Pathway 24-1) and rhinorrhea (Practice Pathway 24-2). Several parameters can be used to characterize the nature of these symptoms. It should be noted if the obstruction is unilateral or bilateral, complete or partial. If present from birth, the lesion is congenital rather than acquired. The age of the patient may limit the differential diagnosis. Congenital lesions that are obstructive are more likely to be due to anatomic variations or mass lesions. Older children have a higher incidence of infectious disease problems that may result in nasal symptoms.

Lesions in the Neonate and Infant

Because the neonate is more likely to have anatomic variations, the physical examination is crucial for making the diagnosis. The physician must pay attention to both the internal and external nose and related structures. Because the infant is an obligate nasal breather, bilateral anomalies of the nasal airway can present with significant respiratory distress. The degree and duration of obligate nasal breathing are variable. Nasal breathing may last for few months, but typically children are obligate nasal breathers for the first 6 months of life. Respiratory distress that results from neonatal nasal obstruction is manifested by intermittent cyanosis, apnea, and failure to thrive and may be life-threatening. Obstructive lesions may occur anywhere in the nose, from the vestibule to the nasopharynx. Therefore, complete examination of the nasal airway is essential.

Practice Pathway 24–1   NASAL OBSTRUCTION

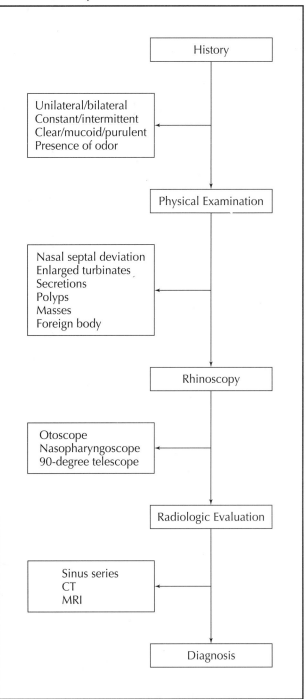

SPECIAL CONSIDERATION:

Respiratory distress that results from neonatal nasal obstruction is manifested by intermittent cyanosis, apnea, and failure to thrive and may be life-threatening.

Practice Pathway 24–2   RHINORRHEA

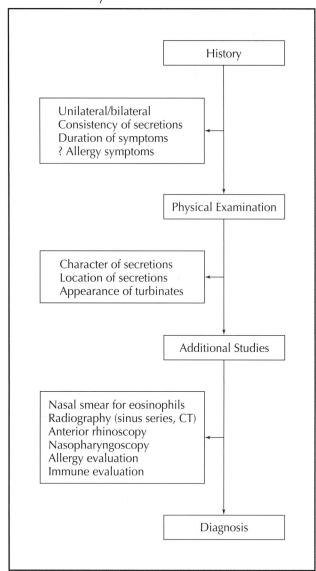

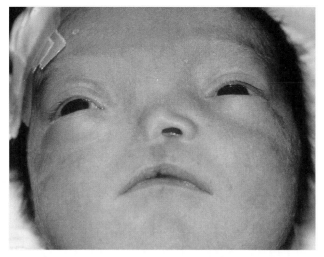

Figure 24–1:   Agenesis of the right side of the nose.

methods of measuring nasal resistance in the neo-nate or infant have not be developed. Acoustic rhi-nometry may hold some promise but it is not yet an effective diagnostic tool in the neonate.[9] The most effective means of diagnosis is direct examination with flexible endoscopy of the nasal cavity. Flexible endoscopy can be performed in even the smallest infants without sedation and should be attempted prior to obtaining a CT scan.

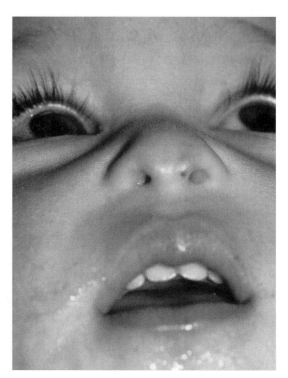

Figure 24–2:   Abnormal lower lateral cartilages in a ne-onate that resulted in airway distress.

Some congenital anomalies are associated with syndromes that are readily diagnosed and are associ-ated with nasal airway obstruction. Common exam-ples of these anomalies include Treacher Collins and Crouzon's syndromes. Agenesis or partial agenesis of the nose has been reported and, if bilateral, is associated with airway distress (Fig. 24-1).

Lesions of the nasal valve area are rare but can occur in the newborn. Abnormal lower lateral carti-lages (Fig. 24-2), severe anterior septal deviation of the septum, and bony stenosis of the nasal vault can cause significant nasal airway resistance and ob-struction. The smaller cross-sectional area of the in-fant nose results in approximately four times the nasal resistance found in adults.[8] However, practical

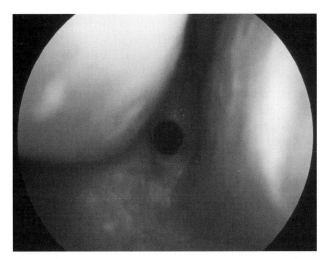

Figure 24–3: Endoscopic view of a choanal stenosis.

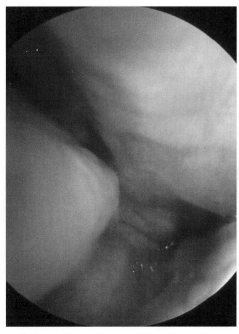

Figure 24–4: Endoscopic view of choanal atresia.

Choanal atresia and stenosis are causes of nasal obstruction and respiratory distress in the neonate (Fig. 24-3). The incidence of choanal atresia ranges from 1 in 5000 to 8000 live births.[10] Unilateral choanal atresia is more common than bilateral atresia.[11] There is a high incidence of associated anomalies, which have been characterized with the acronym CHARGE: *c*oloboma, *h*eart disease, *a*tresia, *r*etardation, *g*enital anomalies, and *e*ar anomalies.[12] The diagnosis of CHARGE is justified if four of the six anomalies are present.[13]

Bilateral choanal atresia frequently presents with severe respiratory distress during the newborn period; the neonate with bilateral choanal atresia requires intubation or immediate correction of the obstruction. The diagnosis of choanal atresia is usually excluded by passing a catheter through each nasal cavity during the neonatal examination. The diagnosis also can be confirmed with flexible nasopharyngoscopy (Fig. 24-4), but axial CT (Fig. 24-5) is required to assess the thickness and extent of bone in the atresia plate. Thin atresia plates are more likely to be membranous and are easier to correct.

Choanal stenosis, which is defined as narrowing of the choanae, may be unilateral or bilateral. In general, unilateral lesions are not associated with respiratory distress and are not diagnosed until 4 to 5 years of age. Choanal stenosis usually presents as intermittent nasal airway obstruction in the neonate and may be associated with significant feeding problems.[14] Not infrequently these children require nasogastric tube feedings. The nasogastric tube occupies one nasal cavity and the other nasal airway is frequently used as a port for suctioning, which accounts for the high number of children who present with airway distress. Placing an oral gastric tube rather than an nasogastric tube and discontinuing the nasal suctioning usually improves the airway. Judicious use of topical decongestants also helps to relieve the symptoms of nasal obstruction.

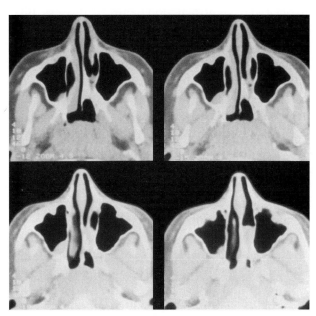

Figure 24–5: Axial CT sections demonstrating unilateral choanal atresia.

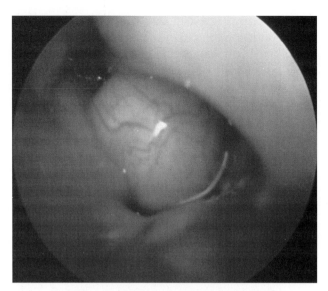

Figure 24–6: Endoscopic view of a lacrimal duct cyst in a neonate that caused airway distress.

sions that cause nasal airway obstruction. Adenoid hypertrophy in neonates is very rare. The pharyngeal bursa (Thornwaldt's bursa) in the midline of the nasopharynx may be patulous at birth but may close, becoming cystic, inflamed, and obstructive. This diagnosis is best confirmed endoscopically or with CT or MRI. Other rare lesions that may present in the nasopharynx include hamartomas, craniopharyngiomas, chordomas, and teratomas.

Fetal alcohol syndrome has been shown to be associated with anomalies of the nose including nasal hypoplasia, choanal stenosis, and a narrow nasal vault.[15] Midface hypoplasia (64%) is also a common feature of fetal alcohol syndrome.[16] Nasal trauma during delivery can cause significant deviation of the septum, septal hematoma, and nasal obstruction. It is unusual, however, for this to present as airway obstruction.

SPECIAL CONSIDERATION:

Choanal stenosis usually presents as intermittent nasal airway obstruction in the neonate and may be associated with significant feeding problems.

Rarely, tumors or cysts may present in the nasal cavity, and depending on their size, there may be associated nasal obstruction or airway distress. Bilateral nasal lacrimal duct cysts also can be a source of nasal obstruction in the neonate (Fig. 24–6). If only one side is involved, the child usually breathes adequately and does not present with airway distress. Other cysts that present as neonatal nasal obstruction include dermoid cysts, nasoalveolar (incisive canal) cysts, and dentigerous and mucous cysts of the floor of the nose. Meningocele (meninges alone), meningoencephalocele (meninges and brain), or nasal glioma (glial tissue with no connection to the brain) may present high in the nasal cavity and usually originate from the medial side of the middle turbinate. Usually these lesions are noted on careful anterior nasal rhinoscopy. Lesions that arise high in the nose require a thorough evaluation including CT and MRI to minimize the risk of cerebrol spinal fluid leaks with surgical correction.

Rarely, neonates present with nasopharyngeal le-

AT A GLANCE . . .
Obstruction in the Neonate

- Nasal Cysts
  Nasal lacrimal cysts
  Dermoid cysts
  Nasoalveolar cysts
  Dentigerous cysts
  Mucous cysts
- Nasopharyngeal Lesions
  Adenoid hypertrophy
  Thornwaldt's bursa
  Hamartomas
  Craniopharyngiomas
  Chordomas
  Teratomas

Lesions in the Child

As the child becomes older, infectious processes play a more prominent role in the causes of nasal airway obstruction and rhinorrhea. Adenoid hypertrophy is the most common anatomic lesion associated with nasal airway obstruction. Enlarged adenoid tissue may or may not be associated with recurrent adenoiditis. Longstanding nasal airway obstruction may be associated with the development of craniofacial anomalies such as the long-face syndrome or adenoid facies.

The most frequent cause of nasal disease in children is inflammation of the mucosa secondary to infections, allergy, or toxic agents. Symptoms usually are confined to the nasal cavity and/or sinuses. The child with a viral upper respiratory infection initially presents with clear rhinorrhea, which occurs secondary to a vasomotor reaction.[7-21] Rhinorrhea is thinner in acute infections and becomes thicker in chronic infections.[22-25] The most common cause of purulent nasal discharge is the development of a secondary bacterial infection that may follow a viral rhinitis. Likewise, bacterial sinusitis is also secondary to an infection that starts in the nasal cavity. Therefore, it is better to think of the disease process as rhinosinusitis, and it is very rare for an infection of the sinus to occur without an antecedent infection of the nasal cavity.

Children have immature immune systems and frequently are infected easily when exposed to viruses. Viral rhinitis is associated with acute inflammation, vascular dilatation, and an exudation of protein-rich fluid that causes nasal airway obstruction. During this acute phase a number of chemotactic agents are released that potentiate the inflammatory reaction. As a result of this acute inflammatory reaction, there is a variable amount of mucosal damage that can inhibit or completely destroy ciliary function. Disruption of mucociliary transport results in obstruction of the ostia of the sinuses, which creates an environment for acute bacterial sinusitis. Microabscesses also may form within the nasal mucosa, leading to a chronically infected state, which can affect not only the nasal mucosa, but also the mucosa of the sinuses.

Wald et al.[21] reported that the average infant experiences approximately six to eight viral upper respiratory infections each year. It is now understood that children in day care settings are exposed to a greater number of viral infections and therefore are more likely to develop purulent rhinorrhea and nasal airway obstruction. Parents, caretakers, and physicians must be cognizant that day care may play a significant factor in the health of their child. Secondary smoke exposure is being increasingly recognized as a risk factor for otitis media;[27,28] it is reasonable to suspect that it is also an equally high risk factor for sinusitis. It is believed that smoke causes a toxic inflammatory reaction of the nasal mucosa and inhibits ciliary function. Children with nasal symptoms should avoid smoking environments.

SPECIAL CONSIDERATION:

Day-care attendance and secondary smoke exposure are risk factors for both otitis media and rhinosinusitis.

Acute bacterial sinusitis may present in two forms. The more severe type is associated with a fever exceeding 39° C, purulent rhinorrhea, and facial pain. The second type presents as a prolonged upper respiratory infection that lasts more than 10 days with cough and nasal discharge.[17,22,29,30] It is thought that up to 90% of episodes of acute sinusitis resolve spontaneously, but the remainder develop into chronic infection.[26] The duration of symptoms is an important factor in differentiating between upper respiratory infections, acute sinusitis, and chronic sinusitis. An upper respiratory infection typically lasts no more than 2 weeks. Symptoms lasting 2 to 6 weeks suggest bacterial rhinosinusitis. If symptoms are persistent for greater than 3 months, the infection should be considered chronic. Unless the child with chronic sinusitis is treated with an appropriate course of antibiotics (4 to 6 weeks), the symptoms frequently return within days of discontinuing the medication.

Unilateral symptoms in any age group lead one to consider anatomic lesions first. It is very unusual to see unilateral chronic sinusitis unless it is associated with an anatomic anomaly, allergic fungal sinusitis (Fig. 24-7), inverting papilloma, or a unilateral foreign body that is causing a concomitant sinusitis (Fig. 24-8). In children, foreign bodies are a frequent cause of unilateral purulent nasal discharge and must be ruled out. A foul smelling nasal discharge is almost always associated with a foreign body. Bilateral disease is less likely to be associated with anatomic abnormalities and more likely to be associated with systemic abnormalities.

Sinusitis and otitis media are commonly associated with one another. Whenever the triad of sinusitis, otitis media, and recurrent bronchitis or pneumonia appears, an underlying systemic condition should be suspected. Immunodeficiency is a common condition that predisposes to chronic sinusitis. Shapiro et al.[31] reported that up to 33% of children with refractory sinusitis have an underlying immunodeficiency. Therefore, immunoglobulin (Ig) lev-

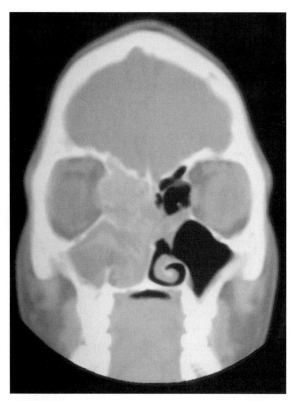

Figure 24–7: CT scan (coronal view) of a patient with complete obstruction of the right nasal cavity due to fungal sinusitis.

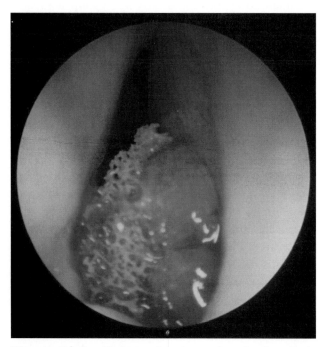

Figure 24–8: Endoscopic view of a foreign body (sponge) in the nasal cavity. Note the granulation tissue that has surrounded it.

els (IgG, IgA, IgM) should be obtained as a part of the initial evaluation of any child with chronic or recurrent sinus infection. There is a spectrum of immunodeficiencies that range from selective antibody deficiency to human immunodeficiency virus (HIV). If the symptoms persist after aggressive medical or surgical management, it is reasonable to perform IgG subclass evaluations. The most common type of immunodeficiency associated with chronic sinusitis is an IgG2 or IgG2IgG4 subclass deficiency with an associated IgA deficiency or a selective antibody deficiency.[32] IgG3 deficiency appears more frequently in adults and is rare in children. A word of caution about the interpretation of IgG subclass deficiencies is in order. Approximately 10% of normal asymptomatic children have IgG subclass deficiency, and there appear to be no good norms for comparison. In children with significant underlying immunodeficiencies, the only therapy that may be helpful is monthly Ig replacement therapy. Patients with transient immunodeficiencies have the best long-term prognosis.[33]

SPECIAL CONSIDERATION:

Immunoglobulin levels should be obtained as part of the initial evaluation of any child with chronic or recurrent sinusitis.

CF is another systemic disease that can have a major impact on the health of the nose and paranasal sinuses. In some children, the only manifestation of CF may be rhinosinusitis. Ciliary dyskinesia is another rare disorder that may present with chronic rhinosinusitis. Abnormalities of the cilia may result in altered mucociliary transport, retained secretions, and subsequent infection of the nose and sinuses. Biopsy of the nasal or tracheal mucosa and electron microscopy, which identifies structural abnormalities of the cilia, are necessary for diagnosis. Regional ciliated abnormalities have not been reported; however, transient ciliary dysfunction secondary to viral infections is common.

Allergies are unquestionably associated with nasal symptoms. The most common nasal symptoms include nasal airway obstruction, clear rhinorrhea, and an itchy nose. The exact role of allergic sinusitis in the development of chronic sinusitis remains unclear. However, it is appropriate to evaluate patients for allergic rhinitis if they have rhinorrhea and nasal airway obstruction. Children with significant sinus disease and allergic rhinitis usually do not improve significantly with immunotherapy alone. Seasonality and duration of symptoms are important factors in diagnosing allergy. Nonseasonal allergic symptoms may occur throughout the year. Seasonal allergic symptoms occur primarily during the spring and fall. Upper respiratory tract infections and sinusitis occur primarily during the winter months and infrequently during the summer months. Allergic symptoms are usually prolonged, whereas symptoms of upper respiratory tract infections and acute sinusitis are shorter in duration. Allergy should always be considered if the patient has prolonged symptoms for several months.

EVALUATION OF THE CHILD WITH HEADACHE

Frequently the child with nasal pathology will present with complaints of headache or may appear irritable (Practice Pathway 24–3). Because infants and toddlers are unable to verbalize their pain and discomfort, they may exhibit a noticeable change in attitude. There may be unexplained fussing, increased separation anxiety, outbursts of anger including hitting or biting, and frequent crying. It is thought that these behavioral symptoms are the result of discomfort or pain.

Headache is a common complaint in children with sinusitis, allergy, a nasal foreign body, and other nasal pathology. The pathogenesis of these headaches is not completely understood but is thought to have both mechanical and biochemical derivations.

Contact headaches that result from mechanical pressure have been described in the adult population. During the normal nasal cycle, the nasal mucosa typically goes through a cycle of swelling and shrinking, changing the airway resistance from side to side. This process is affected by the ambient humidification and temperature of the inspired air. At times, the mucosa may swell to the point that it almost touches the mucosa of the opposite wall of the nasal cavity. If there is a significant septal spur, concha bullosa, or abnormality of the lateral nasal wall, the opposing mucosal surfaces impact, resulting in discomfort. Treatment of these anatomic ab-

Practice Pathway 24–3   HEADACHE

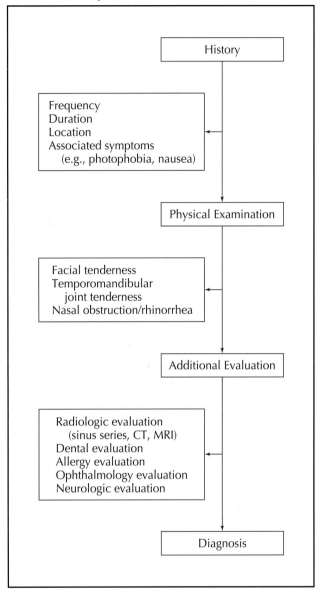

normalities through the use of either medication or surgery may result in headache relief. Contact headaches can be identified in the cooperative child. Clinical evaluation during a headache and identification of the offending contact point can be made if the headache disappears when the area is anesthetized.

The pressure contact theory does not explain all nasal related headaches. The person suffering from nasal allergies can have headaches due to nasal congestion from increased secretions. This symptom may be especially severe during episodes of flying or diving when secretions block the normal sinus ostia, resulting in barotrauma.

Neurotransmitters are now thought to be an important cause of nasal related headaches. Pain perception in the nose and sinuses seems to be related to a small unmyelinated C-nerve fiber that transmits signals of pain to the cerebral cortex. One of the C-fiber transmitters is substance P, which can be released through even minimal mucosal contact. Substance P also can be released by other irritants such as chemicals, temperature changes, and infections.[34] Unfortunately, a cycle of pain may ensue with the release of substance P, followed by edema and additional pressure, which cause further release of substance P. Other neurotransmitters and local inflammatory cell mediators may add to the development of discomfort.

Capsaicin is an extract from red peppers that has been shown to selectively destroy afferent C fibers. It has enjoyed widespread use in Europe for the treatment of sinus related headaches.[35] Capsaicin can be locally administered in increasing concentrations in a nasal spray. Because the administration of the currently used capsaicin as a spray is irritating to the nasal mucosa, it may not be well accepted by the pediatric population.

Migraine is the most common additional cause of headache in children. Often childhood migraine will present with dizziness in addition to, or instead of, pain. A family history of migraine can be a helpful clue to diagnosis. Children may present with the symptoms of classic unilateral head pain associated with photophobia and nausea, but they also may present with atypical symptoms. Because the diagnosis of migraine may be difficult to confirm, careful exclusion of severe nasal pathology or a central nervous system tumor is necessary prior to instituting treatment.

> ## SPECIAL CONSIDERATION:
> Children may have migraine headaches with associated symptoms of photophobia and nausea.

EVALUATION OF THE CHILD WITH COUGH

Cough can be a primary symptom and sign of nasal pathology. Cough is seen in association with chronic and acute sinusitis, nasal allergies, a nasal foreign body, nasal polyposis, and tumor. Unfortunately, it is a nonspecific sign that can be seen in lower airway diseases such as asthma or bronchitis as well.

It is commonly thought that the predominant cause of cough is mucous drainage. In the lower airway, the cough associated with pneumonia and bronchitis seems to result from the thick mucous irritating the airway at the carina. This reflex is protective, allowing the removal of a potential obstruction by the cough. If the reflex is lost or diminished, the ability to clear secretions is compromised and complications are likely. The cough reflex can also be stimulated by nasal mucous dropping into the hypopharynx or near the larynx. The nose and sinuses constantly produce mucous that is directed posteriorly from the sinuses and nasal cavity by the mucociliary blanket. An increase in the flow or a change in the character of nasal secretions may trigger the cough reflex.

Studies in asthmatic patients have demonstrated that cough is not predicated on mucous flow alone. A neural pathway has been postulated for a nasal-induced cough. The trigeminal nerve is thought to provide the afferent fibers for this pathway and the vagus nerve is thought to provide the efferent fibers.[36] Humoral mediators also have been implicated in the development of a cough. In the presence of nasal or sinus inflammation, there is a release of substances such as leukotrienes, prostaglandins, and histamines. The resultant inflammatory cascade releases mediators that have more distal effects and cause coughing.[37]

In the child with sinusitis, cough is frequently worse at night but may be present during the day as well.[17,18,38] A diagnosis of asthma should be considered is the child with only a night-time cough. Cough may be so severe as to lead to gagging or even vomiting.[39,40] Posttussive syncope is a rare but possible scenario.

> ## SPECIAL CONSIDERATION:
> In the child with sinusitis, cough is frequently worse at night but may be present during the day as well. If there is only night-time cough, the diagnosis of asthma should be considered.

Habitual cough or psychogenic cough are seen in some children and are often misdiagnosed or treated unsuccessfully. Habitual cough is usually nonproductive and associated with other unusual disturbing habits such as flailing of the hands. The diagnosis is usually made by excluding other pathology.

EVALUATION OF THE CHILD WITH EPISTAXIS

The nose is a highly vascular structure. The lateral wall is supplied by the anterior ethmoidal, sphenopalatine, posterior lateral nasal, ascending palatine, and greater palatine arteries. The anterior ethmoidal, posterior ethmoidal, posterior nasal septal, and nasopalatine arteries supply the septum, which comprises Kisselbach's plexus of vessels in Little's area in the anterior nasal septum. The venous drainage of the nose is by way of the anterior facial, sphenopalatine, and ethmoidal veins. The ethmoidal veins drain into the superior ophthalmic veins and subsequently into the cavernous sinus, forming a direct pathway for the spread of nasal infection intracranially.

Epistaxis may result from trauma tumor or vascular abnormality and can be exacerbated by a coagulopathy (Practice Pathway 24-4). Unlike adults, hypertension is rarely contributory in children. On the other hand, children with coagulopathies frequently suffer from epistaxis. Epistaxis as the only symptom of bleeding does not signal the need for coagulation studies; however, if it is found in combination with other episodes of bleeding or easy bruising, or if a family history of bleeding problems has been noted, an aggressive evaluation is necessary.

The most common cause of childhood epistaxis is trauma to Kisselbach's plexus in the anterior septum. Children are prone to digital trauma of this area. Dry crusted mucus from allergy or infection can lead to itching or discomfort, and injury of the septal mucosa during removal is common. The cycle of inflammation and reinjury sets the stage for recurrent epistaxis. Septal injury is possible even after minor nasal trauma, with a resultant nasal septal deviation. The increased turbulence of inspired air at this location may contribute to the crusting and subsequent risk of trauma. Physical examination usually reveals dilated, fragile vessels, with or without excoriation of the mucosa.

Practice Pathway 24–4   EPISTAXIS

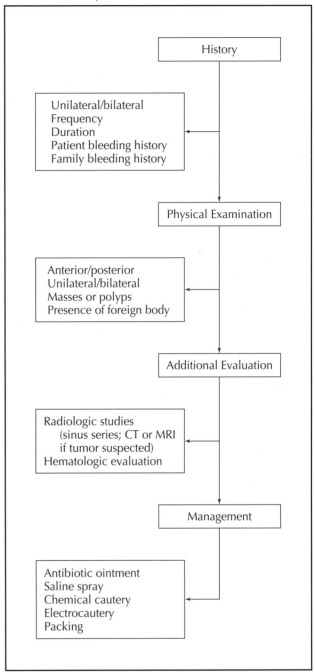

Epistaxis in children is typically self-limited. In the child with an acute bleed, it is best to control the bleeding by applying pressure over the bleeding site. Pinching the nasal alae to put pressure on the anterior septum is often sufficient. Phenylephrine (0.25%) or oxymetazaline can be used to vasoconstrict the bleeding vessels. Anterior nasal packing can be performed using ointment-coated gauze or absorbable oxycellulose packing material. Placement and removal of packing is often difficult in the child because they are unable to cooperate. The application of a topical anesthetic (i.e., 4% lidocaine) prior to packing may make the experience more tolerable for both the child and physician. Although posterior nasal packing is often necessary in the adult with epistaxis, it is rarely required in the child except in cases of major facial trauma or tumor bleeding. Oral antibiotics should be given while nasal packing is in place to reduce the risk of toxic shock syndrome and sinusitis.

SPECIAL CONSIDERATION:

If nasal packing is placed, the child should be placed on oral antibiotics to prevent the development of toxic shock syndrome or sinusitis.

In the case of recurrent epistaxis, the initial treatment should include the use of an antibiotic ointment, typically applied to Little's area, to reduce the low-grade infection and to keep the area lubricated and free of crusts during healing. Most often, this therapy is effective and the episodes are eliminated. Silver nitrate may be topically applied to the vessels in Kisselbach's plexus. The area of concern is identified and circumscribed by the caustic.

Some children are unresponsive to these conservative measures and continue to have problems with recurrent epistaxis. In these patients, electrocautery of the vessels of Kiesselbach's plexus should be considered. Individual vessels can be identified and selectively cauterized. Care must be taken to prevent extensive cautery, which may compromise the vascular supply to the cartilaginous septum with resultant perforation. Nasal electrocautery is usually performed under general anesthesia in most children, although local anesthesia may suffice in adolescents. Postoperatively, the family should be instructed to apply topical antibiotic ointment to the involved septum until healing has completed.

A limited septoplasty has been advocated for recurrent epistaxis, that is difficult to control. It has been demonstrated to be effective even in the case of Glanzmann's thrombasthenia.[41] Dermal grafts to the anterior nasal septum have been used for the chronic management of conditions such as hereditary hemorrhagic telangiectasia.[42]

If a tumor (e.g., juvenile angiofibroma) or vascular abnormality is suspected, arteriography or magnetic resonance angiography can be helpful in identifying the bleeding site, the extent of disease, and the vessels supplying the tumor. Embolization may be helpful for the acute management of bleeding as well as for decreasing the blood flow to the tumor or vascular abnormality, which allows surgical excision with reduced blood loss. Embolization is similarly useful for arteriovenous malformations and aneurysms.

REFERENCES

1. McAlister WH, Lusk RP, Muntz HR. Comparison of plain radiographs and coronal CT scans in infants and children with recurrent sinusitis. Am J Roentgenol 1989; 153:1259–1264.
2. Lazar RH, Younis RT, Parvey LS. Comparison of plain radiographs, coronal CT, and intraoperative findings in children with chronic sinusitis. Otolaryngol Head Neck Surg 1992; 107:29–34.
3. Kopp W, Stammberger H, Fotter R. Special radiologic imaging of paranasal sinuses. A prerequisite for functional endoscopic sinus surgery. Eur J Radiol 1988; 8:153–156.
4. Zinreich SJ. Imaging of chronic sinusitis in adults: X-ray, computed tomography, and magnetic resonance imaging. J Allergy Clin Immunol 1992; 90:445–451.
5. Stankiewicz JA, Newell DJ, Park AH. Complications of inflammatory diseases of the sinuses [review]. Otolaryngol Clin North Am 1993; 26:639–655.
6. Zinreich SJ. Paranasal sinus imaging. Otolaryngol Head Neck Surg 1990; 103:863–868.
7. Druce HM. Emerging techniques in the diagnosis of sinusitis. Ann Allergy 1991; 66:132–136.
8. Lacourt G, Polgar G. Interaction between nasal and pulmonary resistance in newborn infants. J Appl Physiol 1971; 30:870–873.
9. Pedersen OF, Berkowitz R, Yamagiwa M, Hilberg O. Nasal cavity dimensions in the newborn measured by acoustic reflections. Laryngoscope 1994; 104:1023–1028.
10. Theogaraj SD, Hoehn JG, Hagan KF. Practical management of congenital choanal atresia. Plast Reconstr Surg 1983; 72:634–642.
11. Skolnik EM, Kotler R, Hanna WA. Choanal atresia. Otolaryngol Clin North Am 1973; 6:783–789.
12. Pagon RA, Graham JM, Jr., Zonana J, Yong SL. Coloboma, congenital heart disease, and choanal atresia with multiple anomalies: CHARGE association. J Pediatr 1981; 99:223–227.
13. Dobrowski JM, Grundfast KM, Rosenbaum KN, Zajtchuk JT. Otorhinolaryngic manifestations of CHARGE association. Otolaryngol Head Neck Surg 1985; 93:798–803.

14. Jaffe BF. Classification and management of anomalies of the nose. Otolaryngol Clin North Am 1981; 989-1004.

15. Usowicz AG, Golabi M, Curry C. Upper airway obstruction in infants with fetal alcohol syndrome. Am J Dis Child 1986; 140:1039-1041.

16. Jones KL, Smith DW. The fetal alcohol syndrome. Teratology 1975; 12:1-10.

17. Rachelefsky GS, Goldberg M, Katz RM, et al. Sinus disease in children with respiratory allergy. J Allergy Clin Immunol 1978; 61:310-314.

18. Wald ER, Milmoe GJ, Bowen A, et al. Acute maxillary sinusitis in children. N Engl J Med 1981; 304:749-754.

19. Wald ER, Pang D, Milmoe GJ, Schramm VI, Jr. Sinusitis and its complications in the pediatric patient. Pediatr Clin North Am 1981; 28:777-796.

20. Paul D. Sinus infection and adenotonsillitis in pediatric patients. Laryngoscope 1981; 91:997-1000.

21. Jaffe BF. Chronic sinusitis in children. Comments on pathogenesis and management. Clin Pediatr 1974; 13:944-948.

22. Wald ER. Diagnosis and management of acute sinusitis. Pediatr Ann 1988; 17:629-638.

23. Wald ER, Reilly JS, Casselbrant M, et al. Treatment of acute maxillary sinusitis in childhood: A comparative study of amoxicillin and cefaclor. J Pediatr 1984; 104:297-302.

24. Bluestone CD. Otitis media and sinusitis in children. Role of Branhamella catarrhalis. Drugs 1986; 31:132-141.

25. Wald ER. Epidemiology, pathophysiology and etiology of sinusitis. Pediatr Infect Dis 1985; 4:51-54.

26. Wald ER, Guerra N, Byers C. Upper respiratory tract infections in young children: Duration of and frequency of complications. Pediatrics 1991; 87:129-133.

27. Anonymous. Environmental tobacco smoke: A hazard to children. American Academy of Pediatrics Committee on Environmental Health. Pediatrics 1997; 99:639-642.

28. Collet JP, Larson CP, Boivin JF, et al. Parental smoking and risk of otitis media in pre-school children. Canadian Journal of Public Health 1995; 86:269-273.

29. Wald ER. Special series: Management of pediatric infectious diseases in office practice. Klein JO, Marcy SM, eds. Acute sinusitis in children. Pediatr Infect Dis 1983; 2:61-68.

30. Wald ER. The diagnosis and management of sinusitis in children. Diagnostic considerations. Pediatr Infect Dis 1985; 4:61-64.

31. Shapiro GG, Virant FS, Furukawa CT, et al. Immunologic defects in patients with refractory sinusitis. Pediatrics 1991; 87:311-316.

32. Umetsu DT, Ambrosino DM, Quinti I, et al. Recurrent sinopulmonary infection and impaired antibody response to bacterial capsular polysaccharide antigen in children with selective IgG-subclass deficiency. New Engl J Med 1985; 313:1247-1251.

33. Lusk RP, Polmar SH, Muntz HR. Endoscopic ethmoidectomy and maxillary antrostomy in immunodeficient patients. Arch Otolaryngol Head Neck Surg 1991; 117:60-63.

34. Stammberger H, Wolf G. Headaches and sinus disease: The endoscopic approach. Ann Otol Rhinol Laryngol Suppl 1988; 134:3-23.

35. Lundblad L, Brodin E, Lundberg JM, Anggard A. Effects of nasal capsaicin pretreatment and cryosurgery on sneezing reflexes, neurogenic plasma extravasation, sensory and sympathetic neurons. Acta Otolaryngol (Stockh) 1985; 100:117-127.

36. Casale T. Neuromechanisms of asthma. Ann Allergy 1987; 59:391-399.

37. Bardin PG, Vanheerden BB, Joubert JR. Absence of pulmonary aspiration of sinus contents in patients with asthma and sinusitis. J Allergy Clin Immunol 1990; 86:82-88.

38. Herz G, Gfeller J. Sinusitis in paediatrics. Chemotherapy 1977; 23:50-57.

39. Rachelefsky GS. Sinusitis in children—diagnosis and management. Clin Rev Allergy 1984; 2:397-408.

40. Holinger LD. Chronic cough in infants and children. Laryngoscope 1986; 96:316-322.

41. Guarisco JL, Cheney ML, Ohene-Frempong K, et al. Limited septoplasty as treatment for recurrent epistaxis in a child with Glanzmann's thrombasthenia. Laryngoscope 1987; 97:336-338.

42. Zohar Y, Sadov R, Shvili Y, et al. Surgical management of epistaxis in hereditary hemorrhagic telangiectasia. Arch Otolaryngol Head Neck Surg 1987; 113:754-757.

25 Congenital Malformations of the Nose, Nasopharynx, and Sinuses

Robert F. Ward and Max M. April

Congenital malformations of the nose, nasopharynx, and sinuses are rare anomalies that encompass a variety of lesions. These lesions may vary from an incidental malformation to severe, life-threatening abnormalities. Although usually detected at birth, they may not be recognized until much later in life. The main concern in all of these malformations is the possibility of an intracranial communication or central nervous system (CNS) malformation as well. Congenital malformations generally fall into two categories—those with nasal obstruction and those without. Because the vast majority of newborns are obligate nasal breathers, those lesions that present with respiratory obstruction present early in the neonatal period.

The pathogenesis of congenital malformations of the nose and its related structures remains obscure because the process occurs early in embryogenesis.[1,2] During the fourth week of gestation, several swellings or prominences appear on the fetal face. The normal nasal development is initiated by the migration of neural crest cells from the dorsal neural folds. They migrate laterally around the eye and traverse the frontonasal process.[3] By the ninth week of gestation, the neural crest cells have migrated beneath the epithelium and, once positioned, undergo rapid proliferation and differentiation into a matrix of mesenchymal tissue. This tissue is transformed into muscle, cartilage, and early bone formation to form the human facial form eventually.[4] The whole nasofacial architecture is completed by the twelve week of gestation. Alterations in embryogenesis during this critical developmental period are

thought to be responsible for the development of a variety of these malformations. The more common malformations typically include choanal atresia (CA), midline nasal masses (i.e., nasal dermoids, nasal gliomas, encephaloceles), and anterior pyriform aperture stenosis. In addition, there are other malformations that are understood less well.

CHOANAL ATRESIA

Choanal atresia (CA) is a rare congenital anomaly that presents in one in 10,000 births.[5] Approximately 50% of cases are unilateral and 50% are bilateral. In the past, it was reported that the atresia plate was bony in 90% of the cases and membranous in 10% of the cases. A recent literature review demonstrated that 29% of cases are pure bony atresias and 71% are mixed bony-membranous. None are purely membranous.[6] This study was based on modern methods of evaluation, including computed tomography (CT) and nasal endoscopy (Fig. 25–1). The pathogenesis of CA remains controversial.

> ### SPECIAL CONSIDERATION:
>
> A recent literature review of choanal atresia demonstrated that 29% of cases are pure bony, 71% are mixed bony and membranous, and none is purely membranous.

Bilateral CA usually presents at birth with airway obstruction. Affected infants have episodes of respi-

Pediatric Otolaryngology, Edited by R.F. Wetmore, H.R. Muntz, and T.J. McGill. Thieme Medical Publishers, Inc., New York © 2000.

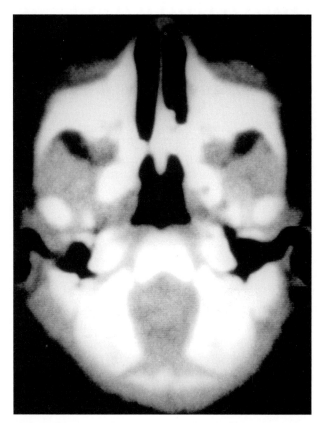

Figure 25–1: CT scan demonstrating bilateral CA. Note the prominent lateral bony overgrowth from the pterygoid plates.

ratory distress with cyanosis that is relieved with crying (*paradoxical cyanosis*). Initial treatment includes an oral airway or a McGovern nipple (i.e., a standard nipple that has an enlarged hole and that is secured with tracheotomy tape as a tie). Diagnosis is made in a stepwise fashion. First, a mirror under the nares does not fog with expiration. An 8-French soft catheter cannot be passed beyond 3.5 cm from the anterior nasal vestibule. Flexible fiberoptic exam after topical decongestion can confirm the atresia, but axial CT is necessary to assess the thickness of the atresia plate, the degree of lateral pterygoid plate and medial vomerine involvement, and to plan for surgical intervention.[7]

Up to 70% of children with CA have associated abnormalities and the CHARGE association must be considered (Table 25–1). Appropriate consultations from ophthalmology, cardiology, neurology, and nephrology should be obtained. CA in CHARGE association often involves a more severe medialization of the pterygoid plate and repair of this type of atresia may be much more difficult. For patients with this condition, a tracheotomy may be recommended

TABLE 25–1: CHARGE Association

C	Coloboma of the eye
H	Heart anomaly
A	Atresia of the choanae
R	Retardation of growth and/or development
G	Genital hypoplasia
E	Ear anomalies and/or deafness

with resultant surgical repair of the CA when the child is older.[8]

Unilateral CA often presents with unilateral rhinorrhea and persistent obstruction between the ages of 2 and 5 years. Rarely, an infant with unilateral CA may present early because of a contralateral nasal obstruction such as a deviated septum (Fig. 25–2).

Management

There has been a great variability in the methods of repair of CA. In the early literature, repair was performed transnasally with an almost blind puncture and curettage of the posterior vomer and lateral pterygoid plates. Later, the transpalatal approach was advocated, particularly for bilateral CA. Transpalatal repair may lead to a maldevelopment of the upper dental arch with a resultant crossbite.[9]

Management of CA has undergone recent

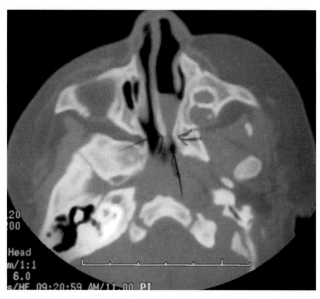

Figure 25–2: CT scan of unilateral CA. Arrows indicate the stenotic area. This patient presented with nasal obstruction caused by the CA in conjunction with a deviated nasal septum to the opposite side of the atresia.

changes. With the advance of rigid nasal endoscopes, transnasal endoscopic repair is now favored
over a transpalatal approach by many. The use of
powered instrumentation, especially with a small
drill and continuous suction irrigation, improves visualization and allows for precise removal of tissue
and bone improving the results.[10,11] This technique
includes the use of a 120° telescope through the
oral cavity with a tonsillar mouth gag in place to
determine intermittently how far to drill laterally
and superiorly. The back-biting forceps is employed
to remove the posterior portion of the vomer,
which at times is quite thick. For bilateral cases with
a thick atresia plate, stenting should be used. For
all unilateral atresias or bilateral atresias with a thin
plate, stenting may not be necessary. Suspected gastroesophageal reflux (GER) should be treated.[12]

One of the more difficult conditions faced by otolaryngologists is recurrent scarring and cicatrix formation in patients with CA and stenosis. This problem is encountered more frequently in children
with bilateral atresia and in syndromic patients. In
those cases of recurrent scarring at the surgical site,
an approach similar to one used commonly in laryngotracheal reconstruction may be employed.[13] In a
severe bilateral atresia or in a revision case, a second-look procedure is performed approximately 3
weeks after the initial surgical repair at the time of
stent removal or if no stenting was employed. During this second-look procedure any granulation tissue or granuloma formation can be removed as
would be done in a subglottic or tracheal repair.
Some have recommended against blind dilation
after stent removal because this procedure may act
to irritate and injure the healing process. Additionally, wound healing may be modulated with the use
of mitomycin-C, in order to promote epithelial
growth over fibroblastic proliferation.[14] This medication is applied topically after revision surgery.

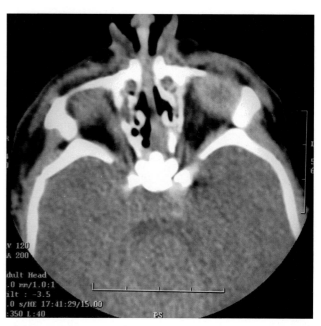

Figure 25–3:   CT showing narrowing of the anterior pyriform aperture from bony overgrowth.

similar to that seen with bilateral CA. Typically, a
newborn with CNPAS presents with nasal airway
obstruction that may lead to respiratory distress and
failure. In its milder form, it may present as feeding
difficulties with episodes of cyclical cyanosis that
are usually relieved by crying.[17] Examination of the
nasal cavities may reveal an extremely-narrowed
nasal vestibule; however, this may be difficult to
determine in an active newborn. Similar to CA, it
may be difficult to pass small nasal catheters. The
pathoneumonic sign is the inability to pass a stan-
dard-size fiberoptic, flexible nasopharyngoscope
(3.5 mm) through the nasal passage. Thin-section
CT with special attention to the pyriform region is
the imaging study of choice when CNPAS is suspected. CNPAS can occur as an isolated anomaly or
in association with other congenital anomalies.

CONGENITAL NASAL PYRIFORM APERTURE STENOSIS (CNPAS)

Premature fusion and overgrowth of the medial
nasal processes can result in a narrowing of the anterior nasal pyriform aperture (Fig. 25–3). This malformation is recently described;[15] however, there were
earlier reports of nasal obstruction due to restriction
of the bony nasal inlet, and these contained suggested surgical corrections.[16] The clinical picture is

SPECIAL CONSIDERATION:

The clinical picture of congenital nasal pyriform aperature stenosis is similar to that seen
with bilateral choanal atresia.

In a significant number of children, premature
fusion of the nasal medial processes may lead to a

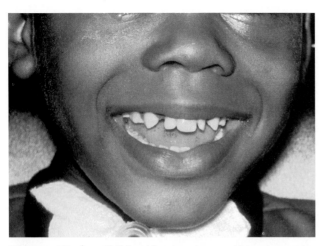

Figure 25–4: Child with anterior pyriform aperture stenosis and a megaincisor. Note that the patient still has a tracheotomy in place.

fusion of the central upper incisors leading to a single, central megaincisor (Fig. 25-4).[15-17] These patients also may have abnormalities of the pituitary-adrenal axis. In 1992, Arlis et al. suggested that CNPAS might represent a developmental field defect, such as a microform of holosprosencephaly.[18] In those patients with a coinciding finding of CNPAS and a central megaincisor on CT or the eruption of teeth, an assumption may be raised that the child may have a microform of holoprosencephaly. Chromosomal analysis, evaluation of parents and other relatives, CT to search for CNS malformations, and an assessment of the hypothalmic-pituitary-adrenal axis may be necessary in these patients.[17] In a recent report of the largest series of children with CNPAS, 12 of 20 patients (60%) had a single central incisor demonstrated by CT. These children also had morphologic abnormalities of the pituitary on magnetic resonance imaging (MRI).[17]

Management

Strategies for treatment and management of CNPAS include conservative medical therapy with the use of a McGovern nipple as well as initial gavage feedings until the infant learns to adjust to the nasal obstruction. If this fails, surgical enlargement of the nasal pyriform aperture should be performed. This surgery typically is approached via a sublabial incision in order to preserve the nasal mucosa. Nasal stenting is employed to prevent stenosis of the surrounding soft tissues. The nasal stents are left in place from 1 to 2 weeks.

CONGENITAL MIDLINE NASAL MASSES

Congenital midline nasal masses are rare anomalies that are estimated to occur in about 1:20,000 to 40,000 births.[19] The majority of these lesions fall into the category of nasal dermal sinus cysts, nasal gliomas, or encephaloceles.[19-21] *Nasal dermoids* are the most common, followed by *dermal sinus tracts* that end as a blind pouch in the deep structures of the nose. As mentioned previously, the pathogenesis of these lesions remains obscure because the developmental process occurs quite early in embryogenesis. The prenasal space theory, as described by Grunwald, outlines the embryogenic steps that occur in normal development (Fig. 25-5).[20] Early in development, a projection of dura lies in the prenasal space as a diverticulum. In the same region, the fronticulus frontalis separates the frontal bone from the nasal bones. As the embryo develops, the diverticulum regresses and the fora-

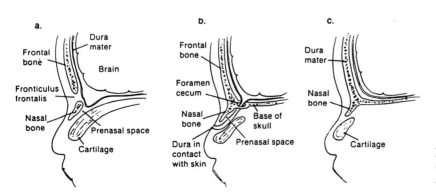

Figure 25–5: The embryogenesis of the nasofrontal area as described by Grunwald. (From ref. 20, with permission.)

men cecum develops in the region anterior to the christa galli.[19]

Faulty closure of the anterior neuropore may result in a defect in the fonticulus frontalis, foramen cecum, cribiform plate, or the sphenoid and ethmoid bones. The nasal dermal sinus cyst is theorized to result from an error in the involution of the dural diverticulum. If the dural element remains attached to the nasofrontal epidermis, a small dimple or pit presents on the external surface of the nose. This dimple is the external opening of the dermal sinus tract. If a portion of the brain tissue is isolated extracranially after fusion of the cranial bones, a *nasal glioma* develops. When a bony defect allows herniation of the dura mater and brain tissue extracranially, an *encephalocele* may develop (Fig. 25-6).

Midline nasal masses may present as an asymptomatic finding in the newborn.[19] Some lesions, such as the nasal dermal sinus cyst, may be quite subtle and therefore not recognized in the small infant. Typically, small hairs may protrude from the dermal opening and a cheesy material may be expressed from the tract (Fig. 25-7). Prior to any planned excision, it is imperative to delineate as best as possible any intracranial extension. Preoperative studies may typically require both CT and MRI of the nasofrontal and intracranial region (Figs.

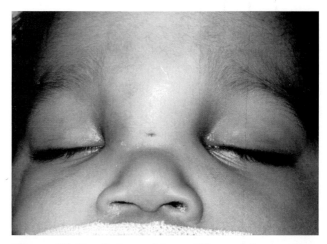

Figure 25–7: Patient with a midline nasal tract. Note the presence of small hairs at the skin site.

25-8 and 25-9). CT is necessary to delineate the bony detail, whereas MRI (sagittal view) is essential for visualizing an intracranial connection. A positive study obviously is helpful in any surgical planning; however, a negative study does not exclude completely the possibility of an intracranial connection.

Complications associated with these lesions may be severe, particularly if intracranial extension is present (Fig. 25-10). Local nasal complications include cellulitis, abscess formation, and potential

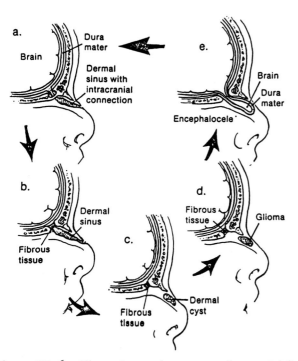

Figure 25–6: The variety and spectrum of potential disorders that involve the prenasal space and its disruption. (From ref. 20, with permission.)

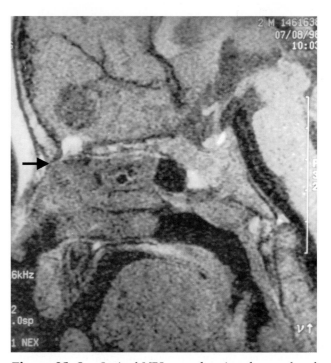

Figure 25–8: Sagittal MRI scan showing the nasal and intracranial extension of a nasal pit. The arrow points to the tract that extends intracranially.

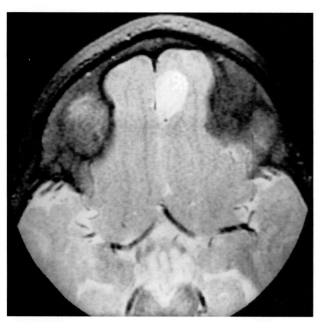

Figure 25–9: Coronal MRI of the same patient as in Figure 25-8 showing the intracranial dermoid that was present. This was removed by a combined neurosurgical and otolaryngologic approach.

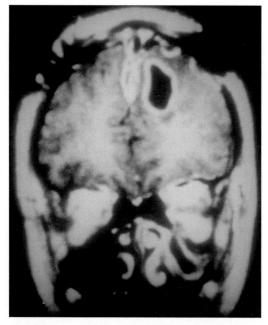

Figure 25–10: Large intracranial abscess that resulted from an infection in a nasal dermal sinus pit with an obvious intracranial connection. Prior to the development of the abscess, the intracranial connection was not visualized on CT and MRI.

cosmetic deformities. Unless treated properly, the development of a cerebrospinal fluid (CSF) leak, frontal lobe abscess formation, and recurrent meningitis are potential problems.[22]

Nasal gliomas (also known as nasal cerebral heterotopias) were first described in 1952;[20] since then, over 150 cases have been reported. Nasal gliomas may present as an intranasal mass or extranasally. It is estimated that 20% of nasal gliomas have an intracranial communication via a thin fibrous stalk. *Intranasal gliomas* typically present as a polypoid mass in the nasal cavity and are usually attached to the lateral nasal wall. They also may arise from the nasopharynx. On physical examination, *extranasal gliomas* are typically firm and noncompressible. They occur most often over the dorsum of the nose and grow slowly over time in proportion to the child's growth. These masses typically are composed of dysplastic brain tissue consisting primarily of astrocytes and gliosis, and they are reported to have no malignant potential. Because of the possibility of an intracranial connection, any nasal mass in an infant should be evaluated completely with imaging studies prior to any planned biopsy or removal.

> ## SPECIAL CONSIDERATION:
>
> Because of the possibility of intracranial connection, any nasal mass in an infant should be evaluated completely with imaging prior to any planned biopsy or removal.

Encephaloceles clinically present as soft, compressible masses with spontaneous pulsations. They may have a bluish coloring and may vary in size with crying, Valsalva's maneuver, or with positioning. The Furstenberg test (i.e., compression of the internal jugular vein that causes enlargement of an encephalocele) is usually positive. *Extranasal encephaloceles* extend through the fonticulus frontalis and may be visible at the nasofrontal angle. *Intranasal encephaloceles* extend through the cribiform plate and arise medially in the nasal cavity. Most of these lesions present as an asymptomatic mass; however, symptoms may include nasal obstruction, epistaxis, and CSF rhinorrhea. The concern of developing meningitis and/or brain abscess mandates early sur-

Practice Pathway 25–1   EXTRANASAL MASSES

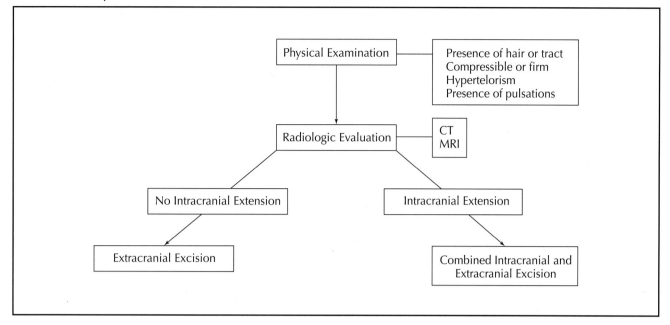

gical removal after a thorough evaluation has been performed.

Management

The management of midline nasal masses depends upon the presence of an intracranial extension (Practice Pathways 25-1 and 25-2). Most nasal der-

moids may be treated with excision of the cyst and the tract extending to the skin. Likewise, most nasal gliomas may be managed extracranially, although the physician must be prepared to close a resultant CSF leak through either an intracranial or nasal endoscopic approach. Encephaloceles frequently require a combined approach that includes a craniotomy with closure of the dural defect and then

Practice Pathway 25–2   INTRANASAL MASSES

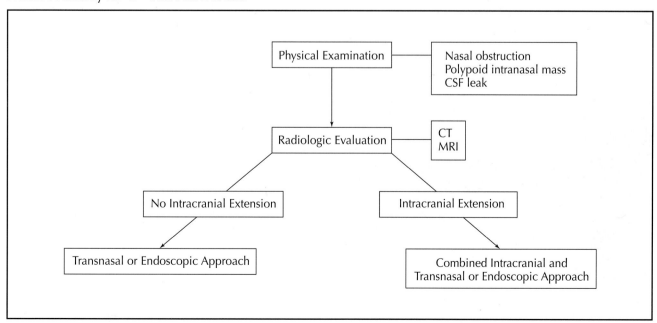

removal of the extracranial tissue through either the craniotomy incision or later via either a rhinotomy or local sagittal approach.

AT A GLANCE . . .

Congenital Midline Nasal Masses

- Nasal dermal sinus cysts
- Nasal gliomas
- Encephaloceles

CONGENITAL TERATOMAS

Teratomas are rare germ cell tumors derived from embryonic origin. A teratoma is a developmental tumor consisting of mature elements from all three germinal layers including endoderm, mesoderm, and ectoderm. Hair, skin, bone, respiratory tissue, gastrointestinal lining, cartilage, and cranial elements all have been identified within these tumors. Congenital teratomas of the head and neck comprise only 5% of all neonatal teratomas with the majority located in the sacrococcygeal region.[23] In the head and neck, teratomas are found most commonly in the cervical region, followed by the nasopharynx (Fig. 25–11). Some authors report that nearly half

of all head and neck teratomas are found in the nose or nasopharynx.[24] Typically, these lesions present as sessile or pedunculated masses in the nasopharynx, but they may extend into the oropharynx and even the oral cavity.

Respiratory distress in infants with nasopharyngeal lesions is well described and also may occur in cases of cervical teratomas if the tumor compresses the trachea. If ultrasound yields a prenatal diagnosis of an obstructing head and neck lesion, airway management may be planned prior to delivery with attempts to maintain maternal-fetal circulation.[25] Management of head and neck teratomas includes careful diagnostic evaluation, airway considerations, surgical excision, and appropriate follow-up.

After establishment of a safe airway either by intubation or tracheotomy, CT and/or MRI are necessary for preoperative assessment to aid in surgical planning and to determine the presence of intracranial extension. Surgical excision is the treatment of choice and typically results in an excellent prognosis. These tumors are often encapsulated or pseudoencapsulated with no surrounding tissue infiltration, facilitating dissection of the mass from surrounding structures. Tumor recurrence is rare. For some nasopharyngeal lesions, a transoral endoscopic removal may be possible.[26]

Despite the fact that congenital teratomas are most often benign, routine follow-up should be included in the management plan. CT and/or MRI should be considered at regular intervals for up to 2 years to insure no recurrence. Recent reports describe the use of alpha-fetal protein (AFP) in evaluating and following patients with massive tumors.[26,27] It has been recommended that serial AFP measurements should be taken for several months following surgery to ensure that there is no recurrence of tumor activity.

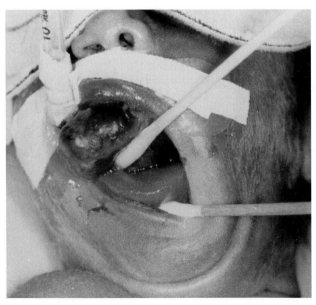

Figure 25–11:   Large nasopharyngeal teratoma with extension into the oral cavity.

FRONTONASAL DYSPLASIA

Midline facial clefting results from a failure in embryonic development of fusion of the medial nasal processes. *Frontonasal dysplasia* and *median cleft syndrome* are exceeding rare and thought to be a sporadic condition, although there has been some evidence to suggest that it may be associated with an autosomal or X-linked inheritance.[28] Affected patients may be divided into two groups. In one group

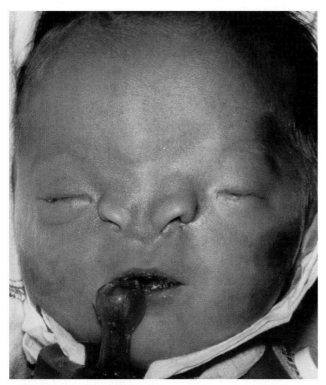

Figure 25–12: Facial clefting with severe frontonasal dysplasia.

the clefting involves the upper lip, hard palate, and occasionally the nose, and may be associated with agenesis of the corpus callosum, optic nerve dysplasia, basal encephaloceles, and other CNS abnormalities. In the other clefting group the cleft involves the nose and forehead and also may involve the lip and hard palate (Fig. 25–12). There may be associated narrowing of the anterior pyriform apertures or even complete agenesis of the nasal aperture. Additional anomalies may include frontoethmoidal and intraorbital encephaloceles, microphthalmus, anophthalmus, intracranial lipomas, and rarely, agenesis of the corpus callosum. The vast majority of these median clefts are associated with hypertelorism.[29] If there are associated intracranial midline defects such as holoprosencephaly, there may be hypotelorism rather than hypertelorism.

Pathogenetically, frontonasal dysplasia is heterogeneous and thought to represent a regional developmental defect. This may be the result of a single developmental field defect or a sequence abnormality.[30,31]

Frontonasal dysplasias and median clefts are not associated commonly with upper airway obstruction. In those cases in which there is a severe nasal deformity or if there is a large nasoethmoidal en-

cephalocele, there may be blockage of the nasal passages with accompanying respiratory distress. This airway obstruction may be treated initially in a conservative manner with the use of an oral airway (such as a McGovern nipple) until the exact nature and extent of the congenital malformation can be established. In certain cases, there may be a need for a tracheotomy to prevent neurologic compromise from repeated episodes of cyanosis and oxygen desaturation. Repair of median clefts and frontonasal dysplasias is complex and often requires the skills of a craniofacial team, consisting of a plastic and reconstructive surgeon, otolaryngologist, neurosurgeon, oral surgeon, ophthalmologist, pediatrician, psychologist, social worker, and geneticist.

DEVIATED SEPTUM

Nasal septal deviation in the neonatal period is encountered occasionally. A majority of septal deflections are likely the result of prolonged pressure due to intrauterine positioning. Neonatal septal deviation represents a type of deformation and not a true septal dislocation. Most correct spontaneously within the first few months of life. It is estimated that up to 1% of neonates have nasal septal deviation that results from birth trauma. With changes in the techniques of delivery, particularly with the decreased use of forceps, the incidence of traumatic deviations appears to be decreasing. In the uncommon situation with significant external deformity and airway compromise, a closed reduction of the septal deformity can be attempted. This procedure should be performed within a few days of life after placing a topical anesthetic agent in each nostril.

If the infant presents with severe nasal obstruction that interferes with feeding and sleeping, the associated mucosal edema overlying the deviated septum may be treated with decongestant and steroid drops.[32] This airway compromise may be particularly problematic if the infant develops an upper respiratory infection. At such times, saline drops and the use of a humidifier may be of help. With nasal growth and development, the critical airway narrowing decreases.

RARE NASAL ANOMALIES

Complete Agenesis of the Nose (Arhinia)

Complete absence of the nose or nasal cavities is a rare anomaly with only a handful of reported cases.[33] Affected infants should be expected to have respiratory distress due to their obligate nasal breathing. Reconstruction involves establishing both a patent airway and reconstruction of an external nasal skeleton. This reconstruction should be performed in stages with creation of an airway by drilling through the maxilla and lining the nasal cavities with skin grafts. The external nasal skeleton can be created with the use of tissue expanders, bone, cartilage, and regional flaps.

Proboscis Lateralis

With this anomaly, a tubular structure of skin and soft tissue forms lateral to the remaining nose, which may vary from normal to complete agenesis. Presenting symptoms and signs of respiratory distress are dependent upon the patency of the nasal airway. Preoperative evaluation includes CT, MRI, or both to identify both bony and soft-tissue abnormalities and exclude any associated CNS abnormalities. Depending upon the condition of the remaining nose, the proboscis lateralis can be excised or used to reconstruct the external nasal skeleton.

Polyrhinia (Double Nose)

This rare anomaly usually is associated with pseudohypertelorism and CA. Surgical reconstruction requires removal of the medial portions of both noses and anastomaosis of both lateral halves in addition to the CA repair.[34]

REFERENCES

1. Mazzola RF. Congenital malformations in the frontonasal area: Their pathogenesis and classification. Clin Plast Surg 1976; 3:573–610.
2. Grunwald L. Bettrage zur Kenntnis Kongenitaler Geschwulste und missbildungen an ohr und nase. Ztsch f Ohrenhik 1910; 60:270.
3. Hengerer AS, Oas RE. Congenital anomalies of the nose: Their embryology, diagnosis and management. Amer Acad Otolaryngol Manual, 1980.
4. Hengerer AS, Strome M. Choanal atresia: A new embryologic theory and its influence on surgical management. Laryngoscope 1982; 92:913–921.
5. Harris J, Robert E, Kallen B. Epidemiology of choanal atresia with specific reference to CHARGE association. Pediatrics 1997; 99:363–367.
6. Brown OE, Pownell P, Manning SC. Choanal atresia: A new anatomic classification and clinical management applications. Laryngoscope 1996; 106:97–101.
7. Crockett DM, Healy GB, McGill TJ, et al. Computed tomography in the evaluation of choanal atresia in infants and children. Laryngoscope 1987; 97: 174–183.
8. Morgan D, Bailey M, Phelps P, et al. Ear nose throat abnormalities in CHARGE association. Arch Otolaryngol Head Neck Surg 1993; 119:49–54.
9. Pirzig W. Surgery of choanal atresia in infants and children. Int J Ped Otorhinolaryngol 1986; 11: 153–170.
10. April MM, Ward RF. Choanal atresia repair: The use of powered instrumentation. Oper Tech Otolaryngol Head Neck Surg 1996; 7:248–251.
11. Josephson GD, Vickery CL, Giles WC, et al. Transnasal endoscopic repair of congenital choanal atresia. Arch Otolaryngol Head Neck Surg 1998; 124: 537–540.
12. Beste DJ, Conley SF, Brown CW. Gastroesophageal reflux complicating choanal atresia repair. Int J Pediatr Otorhinolaryngol 1994; 29:51–58.
13. Ward RF, April MM. Modifications of airway reconstruction in children. Ann Otol Rhinol Laryngol 1998; 107:365–369.
14. Ward RF, April MA. Mitomycin C in the treatment of tracheal cicatrix after tracheal reconstruction. Int J Pediatr Otorhinolaryngol 1998; 44:221–226.
15. Brown OE, Myer CM, Manning SC. Congenital nasal pyriform aperture stenosis. Laryngoscope 1989; 99: 86–91.
16. Shetty R. Nasal pyramid surgery for correction of bony inlet stenosis. J Laryngol Otol 1977; 91: 201–208.
17. Van Den Abbeele T, Triglia JM, Francois M. Congenital nasal pyriform aperture stenosis: Diagnosis and management of 20 cases. Submitted to Ann Otol Rhinol Laryngol. (in press).
18. Arlis H, Ward RF. Congenital nasal pyriform aperture stenosis: Isolated abnormality vs. developmental field defect. Arch Otolaryngol Head Neck Surg 1992; 118:989–991.
19. Hughes GB, Sharpino G, Hunt W, et al. Management of the congenital midline nasal mass. Head Neck Surg 1980; 2:222–223.
20. Sessions RB. Nasal dermal sinuses: New concepts and explanations. Laryngoscope 1982; 92 (supplement 29):1–28.
21. Badwray R. Midline congenital anomalies of the nose. J Laryngol Otol 1967; 81:419–429.
22. Grundfast KM, Mihail R, Majd M. Intraoperative detection of cerebrospinal fluid leak in surgical removal of congenital nasal masses. Laryngoscope 1986; 96: 211.
23. Azizkhan RG, Haase GM, Appelbaum H, et al. Diagnosis, management and outcome of cervicofacial terato-

mas in neonates: A Children's Cancer Group study. J Pediatr 1995; 30:312–316.

24. Heffner DK. Problems in pediatric otorhinolaryngic pathology: III. Teratoid and neural tumors of the nose, sinonasal tract and nasopharynx. Int J Pediatr Otorhinolaryngol 1983; 6:1–21.

25. Rothschild MA, Catalano P, Urken M, et al. Evaluation and management of congenital cervical teratoma. Arch Otolaryngol Head Neck Surg 1994; 120: 444–448.

26. April MM, Ward RF, Garelick JM. Diagnosis, management and follow-up of congenital head and neck teratomas. Laryngoscope 1998; 108:1398–1401.

27. Billmore DF, Grofeld JL. Teratomas in childhood: Analysis of 142 cases. J Pediatr surg 1986; 21: 548–551.

28. Fryburg JS, Persing JA, Lin KY. Frontonasal dysplasia in two successive generations. Am J Med Genet 1993; 46:712–714.

29. Nadich TP, Osborn RE, Bauer BS, et al. Embryology and congenital lesions of the midface. In: Som PM, Bergeron RT, eds. *Head and Neck Imaging.* St. Louis: Mosby, 1991, pp. 1–17.

30. Guio-Almeida ML, Richieri-Costa A, Saavedra D, et al. Frontonasal dysplasia: Analysis of 21 cases and literature review. Int J Oral Maxillofac Surg 1996; 25: 91–97.

31. Optiz JM. The developmental field concept in clinical genetics. J Pediatr 1982; 101:805–809.

32. Prescott CA. Nasal obstruction in infancy. Arch Dis Child 1995; 72:287–289.

33. Gifford GH, Swanson L, MacCollum DW. Congenital absence of the nose and anterior nasopharynx. Plast Reconstr Surg 1972; 50:5–12.

34. Hengerer AS, Yanofsky SD. Congenital malformations of the nose and paranasal sinuses. In: Bluestone CD, Stool SE, Kenna MA, eds. *Pediatric Otolaryngology.* Philadelphia: Saunders, 1996, pp. 840–842.

Acute Inflammatory and Infectious Disorders of the Nose and Paranasal Sinuses

Randall A. Clary

At what point does a "nose cold" become an illness that should be treated medically? As we enter an era in which respiratory pathogens are becoming increasingly resistant, the answer to this simple question takes on profound importance. After decades of thoughtful research, the answer is still elusive for several reasons.

First, the nose cold tends to be a self-limiting disease in which the sufferer gets better without treatment. Therefore, aggressive interventions are not warranted. Next, even if we needed to investigate "colds," the process is not straightforward. The nasal cavity is very narrow and very sensitive to noxious stimuli. Currently, we have very limited access to the paranasal cavities in awake children. In short, physicians always will question the value of submitting cold-sufferers to painful, investigative procedures because most sufferers get better without intervention.

In addition to these practical concerns, the etiology of nasal inflammation is multifactorial. For instance, in an otherwise healthy patient, an isolated bacterial infection requires an antecedent condition. Viral infections or noninfectious inflammatory processes, such as allergies, typically are responsible for disturbing the function of the nose and paranasal sinuses. As a result, poor clearance of the mucus promotes stasis and the growth of bacteria. The inability to differentiate readily allergic hypersensitivity reactions from viral infections with simple exam or lab tests continues to plague clinicians. Likewise, distinguishing between viral and bacterial infections is not a simple task. Recent data by Gwaltney suggests that even computed tomography (CT)

cannot differentiate between the two.[1] In patients with acute rhinitis, CT demonstrates sinus changes that are similar to those found in patients with chronic sinus disease. For this reason, routine use of radiologic imaging studies is not helpful in the evaluation of acute rhinitis.

SPECIAL CONSIDERATION:

Routine use of radiologic imaging studies usually is not helpful in the evaluation of acute rhinitis.

Thus, the simple question of when to treat a "nose cold" is not straightforward. Management strategies are provided, but the reader should keep in mind the limitations of diagnosis that have been discussed above. Practice Pathway 26-1 outlines the management strategies for acute rhinitis and sinusitis.

DEFINITIONS

In reviewing acute disease processes of the nose and sinuses, the reader often is struck by the confusing terminology that is the result of multiple types of organisms infecting multiple sites. For instance, *rhinosinusitis* encompasses all inflammatory processes of the nose and paranasal sinuses. *Viral rhinitis* suggests a mild infection of the nasal cavity despite radiographic evidence that the sinuses are involved. *Sinusitis* refers to a bacterial infection of

Pediatric Otolaryngology, Edited by R.F. Wetmore, H.R. Muntz, and T.J. McGill. Thieme Medical Publishers, Inc., New York © 2000.

Practice Pathway 26–1   MANAGEMENT OF ACUTE RHINITIS AND SINUSITIS

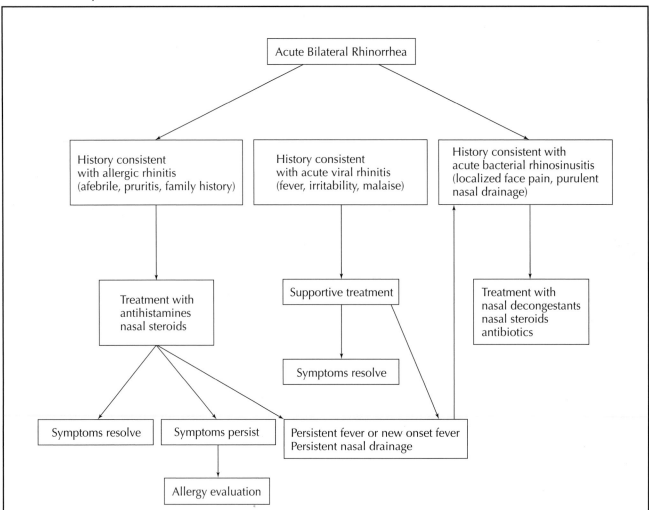

the sinuses, and yet rhinitis is usually a necessary antecedent. This chapter uses specific modifiers, such as viral and bacterial, to emphasize the origin as well as the involved location.

VIRAL RHINITIS

The overwhelming culprit of nasal symptoms in children is viral rhinitis. Several types of viruses use many different mechanisms of cellular damage to incite inflammatory changes. Damage to cilia has been associated with the influenza virus, respiratory syncytial virus, parainfluenza virus, and adenovirus.[2] Other viruses, such as rhinovirus, appear to alter mediator pathways without damage to the cellular structure.

AT A GLANCE . . .

Viral Pathogens in Acute Rhinitis

- Influenza virus
- Respiratory syncytial virus
- Parainfluenza virus
- Adenovirus
- Rhinovirus

The introduction of viral particles into the nasal cavity or nasopharynx results in a cascade of inflammatory mediators that produce the symptoms seen with viral rhinitis. Typically, the clinical picture includes general feelings of malaise, myalgia, fatigue, irritability, headache, and fever. A history of nasal symptoms without these prodromal features should make the diagnosis of viral rhinitis suspect. The nasal symptoms are typically copious, clear rhinorrhea and nasal obstruction. After the initial few days, the secretions may thicken and change color. The symptoms of a viral illness should stabilize and improve between 1 and 2 weeks. The diagnosis of bacterial involvement is considered in the section *Bacterial Rhinitis.*

AT A GLANCE . . .

Symptoms of Viral Rhinitis

- Nasal obstruction
- Copious, clear rhinorrhea
- Malaise
- Myalgia
- Fatigue
- Irritability
- Headache
- Fever

During the office examination, the child may be irritable and mouth breathing with a low-grade fever and the exhibition of bright red nasal mucosa. The mainstays of treatment for viral rhinitis continue to be prevention and supportive care. During the fall months, influenza vaccination is recommended to abbreviate illness that may be caused by many of the most likely pathogens. Once the patient is ill, use of fluids and antipyretics continues to be the mainstay of treatment. Nasal saline irrigation helps to clear abnormal secretions. There is no role for antibiotics in presumed viral illnesses.[3] The use of antiviral agents, such as amantadine, has not been encouraged in otherwise healthy children.

Topical vasoconstricting agents such as oxymetazoline (e.g., Afrin®) and phenylephrine (e.g., Neosynephrine®) improve nasal and ostial obstruction. These agents are associated with rebound congestion after prolonged use and are a common source of addiction for patients with nasal obstruction. Alternatively, similar results can be obtained with an oral agent such as pseudoephedrine. Oral agents

can trigger cardiovascular changes, problems with sleep, and loss of appetite. The use of antihistamines for viral rhinitis remains controversial. Ipratropium bromide in a nasal spray has been shown to decrease rhinorrhea that accompanys acute viral infections.[4]

SPECIAL CONSIDERATION:

After prolonged use, topical vasoconstricting agents are associated with rebound congestion and addiction in patients with nasal obstruction.

The importance of viral rhinitis in children is twofold: these illnesses are particularly common in children and the inflammatory changes that result from viral rhinitis are believed to be the most common cause of bacterial infections of the ears and sinuses. Viral rhinitis occurs more frequently in younger children because of the following: (1) their immunologic immaturity; (2) their contact with the nasal and oral secretions of other children; and (3) their frequent, close proximity with other children in this age group. Parents should be reassured that during the cold season viral rhinitis episodes may be separated by as little as 4 to 6 weeks. This difference in frequency between pediatric and adult viral illnesses is unanticipated by many first-time parents and can be a source of concern. Again, there is no role for antibacterial therapy in otherwise healthy children with a viral illness.

SPECIAL CONSIDERATION:

There is no role for antibacterial therapy in otherwise healthy children with a viral illness.

ACUTE BACTERIAL RHINITIS

The diagnosis of acute bacterial rhinitis underscores the difficulty in identifying the location and organism that is causing nasal symptoms and signs. The distinction between viral and bacterial rhinitis often is not clear because both maladies may present with mucopurulent nasal drainage, low-grade fever, and malaise. In addition, acute nasopharyngitis (i.e., adenoiditis) and acute bacterial sinusitis typically present with a similar clinical scenario. Because acute bacterial rhinitis, nasopharyngitis, and acute sinusitis are often the sequelae of an episode of viral rhinitis, it is often difficult to determine when one entity ends and another begins. Thus, objective evidence as to which location is the source of the infection is difficult to obtain, and even cultures of selected regions within the nasal cavity (e.g., the middle meatus) may not be truly representative of the organism causing the infection.

In addition to viral and allergic rhinitis, several other factors predispose to the development of a bacterial infection of the nose. Impaction of a nasal foreign body usually leads to the development of unilateral, odoriferous nasal discharge within a few days. Conditions that lead to stasis of nasal secretions such as adenoid hypertrophy, nasal polyps, or nasal septal deviation favor bacterial infection of the nasal cavities. Factors that adversely affect local nasal defenses, for example immunodeficiency or cystic fibrosis, also lead to acute and chronic nasal infections. Pathogens that cause acute bacterial rhinitis are the same organisms that infect other regions of the head and neck, such as the ears and pharynx, and include the streptococcal species *Hemophilus influenzae, Moraxella catarrhalis,* and *Staphylococcus aureus.*

AT A GLANCE . . .

Conditions Predisposing to Bacterial Rhinitis

• Viral rhinitis
• Allergic rhinitis
• Immunodeficiency
• Nasal foreign body
• Adenoid hypertrophy
• Nasal polyps
• Nasal septal deviation
• Other anatomic disorders

In addition to symptomatic relief with antipyretics and decongestants, the major decision is when

to institute antibiotic therapy. The end of an episode of viral rhinitis usually is marked by a thickening of secretions; however, this change in secretions may be difficult to distinguish from the onset of a bacterial superinfection, which is an event common to many young children. The decision to treat with antibiotics is dependent upon clinical findings that include factors such as the duration of infection, exposure to pathogens (e.g., day care), and severity of symptoms such as fever and irritability. The choice of antibiotic also is dependent upon the severity of illness and the incidence of resistant organisms in the community. Amoxicillin remains the drug of choice, but cephalosporins, amoxicillin-clavulanic acid (e.g., Augmentin®), clarithromycin, azithromycin, and erythromycin are all acceptable alternatives.

Symptoms of nasal congestion in newborn infants rarely may suggest infection with two other bacterial organisms. *Chlamydia trachomatis* may present in the newborn period with nasal symptoms of congestion and discharge, protracted cough, and the absence of fever.[5] Because this organism is difficult to culture, suspected cases of chlamydial infection should be treated with erythromycin or azithromycin.[6] Infants infected congenitally with syphilis (i.e., *Treponema pallidum*) present with symptoms that include a diffuse copper-colored maculopapular rash, bone lesions that may result in pseudoparalysis and snuffles, and a rhinitis characterized by a watery discharge. Chronic, unrecognized infection may result in destruction of the nasal septal cartilage and a saddle nose deformity. The diagnosis of syphilis should be confirmed by serologic testing, and penicillin remains the antibiotic of choice.[6]

Special Consideration:

Chlamydial infection in the newborn may present with nasal symptoms of congestion and discharge and protracted cough in the absence of fever.

ACUTE BACTERIAL SINUSITIS

As with acute bacterial rhinitis, the diagnosis of acute bacterial sinusitis continues to be subjective because of the difficulties encountered in determining the specific bacterial pathogen objectively. Nevertheless, clinicians regularly are called upon to declare an infection to be bacterial and initiate antibiotics. Wald has elucidated two characteristics of bacterial sinusitis that can be helpful in distinguishing bacterial infections from antecedent viral infections.[7] First, the persistence of an infection for 10 days without evidence of improvement is considered ample evidence to suggest that an infection has a bacterial component. Second, a high fever (39° C) with 3 days of purulent nasal drainage also is ample reason for initiating treatment.

SPECIAL CONSIDERATION:

A persistent infection that lasts more than 10 days, a high fever of 39° C, and 3 days of purulent nasal drainage is indicative of a bacterial infection.

The typical clinical presentation of childhood acute sinusitis includes cough (especially nocturnal), halitosis, headache and facial pain, fever, and irritability. Coughing typically originates from the throat and may induce vomiting of swallowed secretions. Headaches can be vague and require asking the child to use one finger to point to the area of pain. Irritability may be manifested in peculiar behaviors such as increased biting of other children during play.

AT A GLANCE . . .

Symptoms of Acute Sinusitis

- Cough
- Halitosis
- Headache/facial pain
- Fever
- Irritability

The pathogenesis of acute bacterial sinusitis in children is fundamentally the same process as with adults: the local defense mechanisms are unable to prevent the adherence and invasion of the sinus mucosa. The two main factors that promote the development of sinusitis are: (1) malfunction of the mucociliary clearance mechanism allows organisms to invade the mucosa; and (2) blockage of the sinus ostium by mucosal swelling promotes stasis.

There are environmental antagonists that predispose to the development of sinusitis. Tobacco smoke and air pollutants can decrease the motility of the cilia of the nose and sinuses. Parents should be counseled about the importance of tobacco smoke as a contributor to their child's health. Frequent exposure to viral illness, either from contact with older siblings or in daycare facilities, increases the likelihood of progression to sinusitis. Children with hypersensitivity to inhalants have mucosal inflammation that predisposes them to bacterial sinusitis. This factor is particularly important in children with asthma that is exacerbated by sinus infection.

Lastly, children with underlying immunodeficiencies or mucociliary clearance abnormalities suffer from sinusitis more frequently. Children with frequent sinusitis, middle-ear disease, and chest infections should be evaluated for structural aberrations of the cilia. In children with frequent sinusitis and chest infections, the diagnosis of cystic fibrosis (CF) should be entertained. A history of meconium ileus, failure to attain growth parameters, or nasal polyps should suggest CF. Referral to a pulmonary specialist for a sweat test and additional evaluation is appropriate.

The bacteria responsible for acute sinusitis are similar to those of other upper respiratory infections. Wald et al. demonstrated that the three most common organisms are *Streptococcus pneumoniae, Moraxella catarrhalis,* and *Hemophilus influenzae.*[8] Other streptococcal species such as *Staphylococcus aureus* and anaerobes have been isolated also. Patients with underlying immune or ciliary disorders tend to demonstrate the same profile of organisms. Children with CF frequently harbor a *Pseudomonas* species or *Staphylococcus aureus.*

Most episodes of acute bacterial sinusitis do not require radiologic confirmation. As mentioned previously, even CT that is suggestive of acute infection in the sinuses may not allow differentiation between viral and bacterial infections.[1] Plain radiographs of the sinuses still have a limited role in screening for acute sinus infection. In young children, it may be difficult to distinguish between acute and chronic

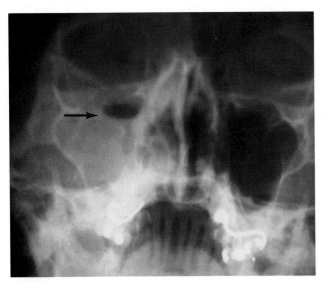

Figure 26–1: Plain sinus radiograph (Waters view) illustrates an air-fluid level (arrow) of the right maxillary sinus that is consistent with an acute infection.

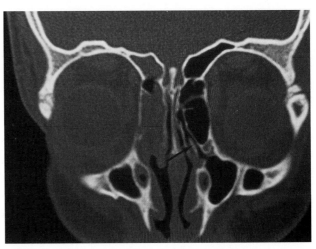

Figure 26–3: CT (coronal view) shows opacification of the right ethmoid sinus. A patent ostiomeatal complex can be visualized on the left side (arrow).

infection of the maxillary sinuses because of their small size. CT is rarely necessary for the diagnosis of acute bacterial sinusitis, unless a regional or intracranial complication is suspected (Figs. 26–1 to 26–3).

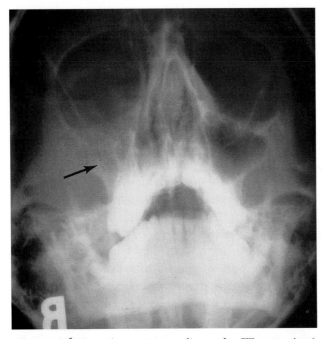

Figure 26–2: Plain sinus radiograph (Waters view) demonstrates a mucous-membrane thickening of the right maxillary sinus (arrow) that typically is seen with chronic, rather than acute, sinus infection.

The goal of treatment is two-fold: to support the clearance mechanism of the sinus and to eradicate invading organisms. Therapies directed at enhancing the clearing of the sinus include agents that reduce inflammation of the mucosa.[9] Topical vasoconstrictors (e.g., oxymetazoline) or oral decongestants reduce peripheral blood flow in the nasal mucosa. Some authors have raised the concern that alpha-adrenergic agents will decrease blood flow, and hence the delivery of antibiotics, defending white blood cells and oxygen level in the nasal mucosa. Irrigation with nasal saline can remove inspissated secretions that can block ostia. Topical, steroid, nasal sprays are recommended to reduce the inflammatory response accompanying infections.

AT A GLANCE . . .

Treatment of Acute Sinusitis

- Topical vasoconstrictors
- Oral decongestants
- Nasal saline
- Topical nasal steroids
- Antibiotics

The antibiotic treatment chosen should be based on the child's previous history and the community's bacterial-susceptibility profile.[10] In an otherwise healthy child, the use of amoxicillin as a first-line agent is still appropriate. Unfortunately, in the last decade there has been a substantial increase in antibiotic resistance. It is common to see 90% of community *Moraxella catarrhalis* and 50% of *Hemophilus influenzae* produce beta-lactamases. Children whose symptoms do not respond or who have recurrent episodes of sinusitis should be treated with antibiotics, such as third-generation cephalosporins (e.g., Vantin®) and amoxicillin-clavulanic acid combinations (e.g., Augmentin®) that have activity against beta-lactamase-producing organisms.

> ## Special Consideration:
> The antibiotic treatment chosen should be based on the child's previous history and the community's bacterial-susceptibility profile.

More recently, *Streptococcus pneumoniae* has demonstrated increasing resistance to penicillins and cephalosporins due to synthesis of penicillin-binding proteins (PBPs) with decreased affinity. Other classes of antibiotics that include the macrolides (e.g., clarithromycin, azithromycin) and sulfa-combination drugs (e.g., trimethoprim-sulfamethoxazole, sulfisoxazole-erythromycin) may be useful alternatives. If the organism is gram-positive or anaerobic, clindamycin may be a reasonable choice. Unfortunately, penicillin-resistant *Streptococcus pneumoniae* also may be acquiring resistance mechanisms for other drug classes.

With the increasing resistance of bacteria, the need to obtain culture specimens from the nose and sinuses also will increase. Aspiration of sinuses in children is difficult, and has been used selectively in children who have compromised immunity or a serious complication of sinusitis. More recently, evidence that selective aspiration of purulent secretions from the region of the middle meatus may be a reliable alternative.[11] Nasopharyngeal cultures may be sensitive but not necessarily specific in identifying the organism involved. Lastly, nonpathogenic organisms may secrete beta-lactamases that contribute to the virulence of normal pathogens.[12] These frustrating factors make the diagnosis of sinusitis a persistent challenge and a continuing area of research.

ALLERGIC RHINITIS

The most common cause of acute rhinitis in childhood is the viral upper-respiratory infection (URI). Allergic hypersensitivity to inhalants is the second most common cause. As mentioned above, both of these acute inflammatory conditions of the nose are the common antecedents to sinusitis.

Allergic rhinitis is more thoroughly discussed in Chapter 3. The nasal symptoms of allergic rhinitis include nasal airway obstruction, clear watery rhinorrhea, itching of the nose, and irritation of the throat. The child typically presents with mouth breathing, uses his hand to brush the end of his nose (the "allergic salute"), and has a cough that clears pharyngeal secretions. The child's eyes may be injected symmetrically (as opposed to unilateral, infectious conjunctivitis) with edema of the eyelids. Parents may complain of the child's peculiar pharyngeal noises, which are a response to increased pharyngeal secretions and palatal itching. These children frequently have a night-time cough that also results from pharyngeal secretions.

> ## AT A GLANCE . . .
> Symptoms of Allergic Rhinitis
>
> - Nasal airway obstruction
> - Clear watery rhinorrhea
> - Itching of the nose
> - Irritation of the throat
> - Cough
> - Throat clearing
> - Conjunctival injection

The management of allergic rhinitis in a child depends on the severity of symptoms. For the child with mild seasonal nasal symptoms, the use of either antihistamines or topical, steroid nasal sprays may be therapeutic. Children with more debilitating perennial symptoms or with accompanying reactive airway symptoms may require more intensive therapy including immunotherapy or oral/inhaled steroids. Cromolyn-sodium nasal spray helps to minimize symptoms when used prior to inhalant exposure.

NASAL VESTIBULITIS

The nasal vestibule may be colonized with organisms such as *Staphylococcus aureus* and Group A beta-hemolytic streptococcus. Impetigo, the honey-crusted erythematous skin infection from either of these organisms, may develop by inoculating the skin with contaminated fingers (Fig. 26–4). These infections can be spread between family members or schoolmates.

Cellulitis or even an abscess can develop in the nasal vestibule. The patient typically complains of a tender nasal tip. Mild erythema and induration may be seen on the involved nares and lower lateral cartilage area. Close inspection of the vestibule is essential because an abscess between the upper and lower cartilages can be subtle in appearance. The presence of tender, boggy fullness in this area suggests an abscess that needs to be incised to prevent a more serious infection (Fig. 26–5). The cellulitis should be treated with an antistaphylococcal antibiotic.

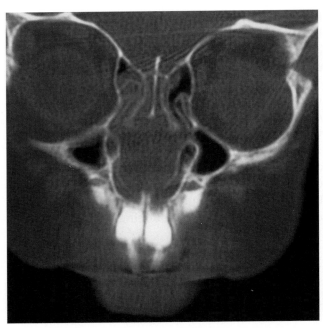

Figure 26–5: CT of the nose (coronal view) demonstrates widening of the septum due to a septal abscess.

CONCLUSION

With viral or bacterial rhinitis, chronic adenoiditis, nasal vestibulitis, and sinusitis as diagnostic possibilities, the determination of the cause of a nasal infection may be difficult. The history and physical examination help to narrow the differential diagnosis. Cultures of nasal secretions may be misleading. Medical management typically includes decongestants, antihistamines, nasal steroids, and/or antibiotics tailored to those bacteria found in the community.

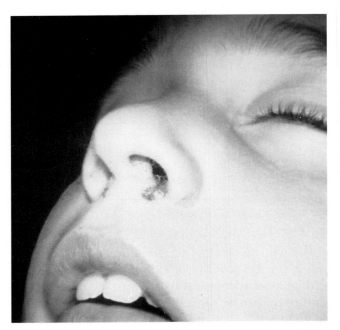

Figure 26–4: Typical appearance of nasal vestibulitis with honey-crusting and erythema.

REFERENCES

1. Gwaltney JM Jr, Phillips CD, Miller RD, et al. Computed tomographic study of the common cold. New Engl J Med 1994; 330:25–30.
2. Carson JL, Collier AM, Hu SS. Acquired ciliary defects in nasal epithelium of children with acute viral upper respiratory infections. New Engl J Med 1985; 312(8): 463–468.
3. Schwartz RH, Freij BJ, Ziai M, et al. Antimicrobial prescribing for acute purulent rhinitis in children: A survey of pediatricians and family practitioners. Pediatr Infect Dis J 1997; 16:185–190.

4. Hayden FG, Diamond L, Wood PB, et al. Effectiveness and safety of intranasal ipratropium bromide in common colds. A randomized, double-blind, placebo-controlled trial. Ann Intern Med 1996; 125:89–97.

5. Beem MO, Saxon EM. Respiratory-tract colonization and distinctive pneumonia syndrome in infants infected with *Chlamydia trachomatis*. N Engl J Med 1977; 296:306–310.

6. The choice of antibacterial drugs. Med Lett Drugs Ther 1998; 40:33–42.

7. Wald ER. Diagnosis and management of sinusitis in children. Adv Pediatr Infect Dis 1996; 12:1–20.

8. Wald ER, Reilly JS, Casselbrant M, et al. Treatment of acute maxillary sinusitis in childhood: A comparative study of amoxicillin and cefaclor. J Pediatr 1984; 104:297–302.

9. Zeigler RS. Prospects for ancillary treatment of sinusitis in the 1990s. J Allergy Clin Immunol 1992; 90:478–495.

10. Green M, Wald ER. Emerging resistance to antibiotics: Impact on respiratory infections in the outpatient setting. Ann Allergy Asthma Immunol 1996; 77:167–173.

11. Vaidya AM, Chow JM, Stankiewicz JA, et al. Correlation of middle meatus and maxillary sinus cultures in acute maxillary sinusitis. Am J Rhinol 1997; 11:139–143.

12. Brook I. Microbiology and management of sinusitis. J Otolaryngol 1996; 25:249–256.

27 Diagnosis and Management of Chronic Sinusitis

Harlan R. Muntz

Nasal drainage in childhood is a frequent finding. A developing immune system, early socialization, and a lack of attention to some aspects of hygiene place children at risk for recurrent viral infections. Often, the pathologic bacteria that are present in the nose and nasopharynx use this as an opportunity for invasion.

The natural history of chronic sinusitis in children has not been delineated clearly. The child who has repeated episodes of acute sinusitis may have enough injury to the mucosa to reduce the efficiency of mucus clearance. Additionally, other non-infectious disease processes may play key roles in the development of chronic infection.

Acute sinusitis may be characterized by its sudden onset and obvious symptoms of high fever, pain, and nasal drainage. Other symptoms may include cough, halitosis, and exacerbation of asthma. If a child has symptoms of an upper respiratory infection (URI) for longer than 10 days without improvement, the physician also should consider the diagnosis of sinusitis.[1]

If these symptoms persist beyond 1 month, the diagnosis of *subacute sinusitis* is considered.[2,3] The evaluation of the microbiology of acute and subacute sinusitis has shown organisms that are similar to those seen in acute otitis media (OM). These common pathogens include *Streptococcus pneumoniae, Moraxella catarrhalis,* and *Haemophilus influenzae.*[3,4] The treatment of acute and subacute sinusitis consists of antibiotics and comfort measures. In some difficult cases, the improvement of sinus drainage by mucosal shrinkage with a vasoconstrictor should be considered.

Chronic sinusitis is a complex disease of the nose and paranasal sinuses. The chronicity is defined as greater than 3 months, but most children present to the otolaryngologist with a longer duration.[5] The disease process of chronic sinusitis is poorly understood, especially in children. Much debate surrounds both its impact on the child and the appropriate treatment. The range of symptoms, the broad differential diagnosis, and the effect of other disease processes on the sinuses all contribute to the debate. This chapter tries to approach these problems in a way that clarifies at least some of the controversial issues while proposing a more rational approach that neither undertreats or overtreats the child.

SYMPTOMS

Unfortunately, there is no single test that objectively confirms the diagnosis of sinusitis in childhood. This leaves the clinician with the task of sorting through an often complex history and a less than perfect physical exam to arrive at a working diagnosis.

Most children with chronic sinusitis have a low-grade, indolent disease with occasional exacerbations. This is a disease that affects the child's and family's quality of life; it rarely is seen as a life-threatening disease process. Symptoms include, but are not limited to, nasal drainage, day and night-time cough, irritability, headache, nasal-airway obstruction, and facial swelling.[4-6] These symptoms may be present in a variety of diseases and conditions, and the child's history must be considered carefully in order to arrive at any conclusion.

Nasal drainage is frequently seen in normal children. The presence of nasal drainage as the only finding in a child should not point to a diagnosis of sinusitis. More commonly, nasal drainage is seen in a child with frequent viral URIs. The average child may have more than eight URIs per year, most commonly during the fall and winter months.[7] This could give the impression of chronic nasal catarrh even without true chronic sinus disease. Overt al-

Pediatric Otolaryngology, Edited by R.F. Wetmore, H.R. Muntz, and T.J. McGill. Thieme Medical Publishers, Inc., New York © 2000.

lergy also is present in as many as 20% of children. Nasal drainage may accompany allergic rhinitis and may be chronic over many seasons. Adenoid enlargement with posterior nasal obstruction may contribute to chronic drainage without sinus disease. Nasal septal deviation, nasal foreign bodies, vasomotor rhinitis, and choanal atresia all may present with nasal drainage without the diagnosis of chronic sinusitis. On the other hand, the lack of normal mucus flow or the increase of mucus volume from these conditions may predispose to chronic sinus disease.

SPECIAL CONSIDERATION:

Overt allery may be present in as many as 20% of children.

Nasal crusting can be an irritating problem. Behind the crusts, growth of bacteria can increase local inflammation and contribute to infection. *Ectodermal dysplasia* is a disease that affects the skin and mucous membranes. Often, children present with a diagnosis of chronic sinusitis due to nasal crusting when in fact they have sinusitis rarely. Treatment with long-term antibiotics does not reduce the problem. Nasal hygiene with saline washes can control crusting and reduce symptoms.

Nasal-airway obstruction can be caused by nasal mucosal edema from allergy, rhinitis medicamentous, mechanical or chemical irritation, and inflammation. Adenoid enlargement, nasal foreign body, nasal septal deviation, and inferior-turbinate hypertrophy can likewise cause obstruction.

Headaches are not a common complaint during childhood. The younger child does not voice the concern, and there is no objective measure of the presence or degree of headache. Often, the discomfort may produce irritability, crying, and moodiness, but there is no way to document its cause. Holding the head, resting the head on a cold tile floor, pulling out hair, and head banging have been seen as indicators of headache in the child who is unable to verbalize the discomfort. As the child grows older, he may be able to express the location of the discomfort and to some extent the degree of discomfort. Although headaches may result from chronic sinus infection, they also may represent vascular headaches (i.e., migraines) or be due to stress.

SPECIAL CONSIDERATION:

Although headaches may result from chronic sinus infection, they also may represent vascular headaches or be due to stress.

Cough is seen in URI, asthma, bronchitis, pneumonia, and allergy. The cough in sinusitis often is felt to be triggered by nasal drainage, but actually may be initiated by neural or humoral factors related to the mucosal inflammation and edema. Typically, the cough is worse at night, but it may not have a night-time component. A daytime cough is a more reliable indicator of chronic sinusitis.[7] If the cough is only at night, cough-variant asthma should be considered high in the differential diagnosis. If the cough is dry, unusual sounding, and nonproductive without any night-time symptoms, the clinician should consider factious or habit cough. Often the cough in chronic sinusitis causes sleep disturbance, vomiting, and shortness of breath; it also may be the presenting complaint. Holinger studied a cohort of children with chronic cough and found sinusitis to be the second, most-common cause.[8]

SPECIAL CONSIDERATION:

Daytime cough is a more reliable indicator of chronic sinusitis than night-time cough.

Halitosis often is seen in patients with chronic sinusitis. Parents may even suggest that they can predict symptoms by the smell. Dental disease, including gingivitis and severe caries, can leave an anaerobic smell in the mouth. Chronic tonsillitis with tonsilloliths also produces a foul odor.

Fever is usually of low grade.[9] High fever is often a sign of an additional intercurrent illness, frequently an acute exacerbation of sinusitis. If increased severity of symptoms is associated with a high fever, the physician should consider a change in the plan of treatment and evaluation for other contributing problems.

In the assessment of children with chronic sinus problems, it is helpful to establish a practice of detailed documentation of the symptom complex, rating severity as perceived by the parent but with as much objectivity as possible. This allows monitoring the effect of treatment and reduces the parental bias. Some parents feel that their child should never have a runny nose, whereas others are resigned to the fact that chronic nasal symptoms are a part of childhood. The clinician's job is to sift through the parental anxiety and determine if the child does have any significant disease.

AT A GLANCE . . .

Symptoms of Chronic Sinusitis

- Nasal drainage
- Nasal crusting
- Nasal-airway obstruction
- Headache
- Cough
- Halitosis
- Fever

PATHOPHYSIOLOGY

The treatment of chronic sinusitis must be based on understanding the pathophysiology of the disease process. Unfortunately, there is no good data that describes the natural history of the disease. There have been few prospective randomized trials of treatment or nontreatment. The majority of reports focus on the outcome of intervention. Our limited understanding has resulted in a proposal of reasonable management strategies for the child with chronic sinusitis.

The underlying cause of chronic sinusitis appears to be due to mucostasis.[10,11] In the normal nose and paranasal sinuses, there is a complex system of mucus production, with a precise flow of the mucociliary blanket toward the natural ostium of the sinus and a systematic flow first toward the nasopharynx and then the oropharynx.

The nose is colonized naturally with many bacterial organisms. The normal mucociliary transport keeps these bacteria from causing inflammation and disease. Mucociliary flow can be limited by increases in the viscosity and amount of mucus, injury

to the cilia,[12] and anatomic obstruction to the mucus flow.[13]

A viral URI predisposes a child to sinusitis. Many viral and bacterial illnesses injure the cilia, which may not recover.[14] Mucus is an environment perfect for the overgrowth of bacteria, especially if the oxygen tension is low.[15] The small child with a developing immune system is plagued by viral URIs. Estimates of more than eight infections per year in a reasonably healthy child demonstrate the potential for chronic infection.[7] If the majority of the viral URIs are in the fall and winter months, the child may exhibit nearly constant infection symptoms. Repeated injury to the mucosa may fail to allow complete recovery.

Repeat acute bacterial sinusitis can effect the mucosa in the same way. Edema and inflammation usually subsides as the infection resolves. Repeat infection, however, can set up a chronic pattern of inflammation that reduces the normal mucus flow. Acute infection with mucosal breakdown may lead to scar formation. The region most likely to be affected is the infundibulum, where the pathway is the narrowest.[13]

Allergic rhinosinusitis also increases the thickness of the nasal and sinus mucosa.[16] In turn, this can result in the occlusion of the ostia of the sinuses and preclude normal mucus flow. In addition, the viscosity of the mucus may be increased in allergic states, which is a factor that may affect mucociliary transport of the mucus. Allergy also may trigger the immune cascade causing an increase in inflammation and both local and humoral symptoms.

Environmental conditions also can affect the nasal and sinus mucosa. Most notable is tobacco smoke, which is a well established cause of mucosal injury and mucus thickening and which is implicated in the development of OM and sinusitis. Usually, the child's exposure is from passive smoking due to the parent or caregiver smoking. Also implicated in the development of sinusitis is the use of wood-burning heat; it is not known whether the injury is from small particulate matter or the dry air. Some children are affected by swimming in a chlorinated pool. Chlorine may be a direct irritant to the nasal mucosa. Other children seem to do better if allowed to swim year round, possibly because of nasal irrigation while swimming.

Anatomic variations also have been implicated in the development of chronic sinusitis. Children may have many of the same abnormalities that are described in the adult nose and sinuses.[13] Theoreti-

TABLE 27–1:   Bacteriology of Chronic Sinusitis

Coagulase-negative staphylococcus
Alpha-hemolytic streptococci
Staphylococcus aureus
Haemophilus influenzae
Streptococcus pneumoniae
Moraxella catarrhalis
Anaerobes

cally, these abnormalities may reduce the normal flow of mucus and contribute to mucostasis. Nasal septal deviation, concha bullosa, infraorbital cells, enlarged agar nasi cells, and paradoxical turbinates all have been implicated in the etiology of chronic sinusitis. In itself, the presence of the abnormality does not signify sinus disease, but it may be a component in the development of this multifactoral process.

Sinusitis is an inflammatory process within the sinus mucosa that can be caused by or contributed to a bacterial infection. As described earlier, the bacteriology of the acute and subacute sinusitis mirrors that of OM. The studies of the bacteria in chronic sinusitis suggest a different set of organisms. Brook's studies of the maxillary sinus show a preponderance of anaerobic organisms.[17,18] The lower, partial pressure of oxygen in the maxillary sinus (as contrasted to the ethmoid sinus) may explain this finding. The aerobic organisms that are found in his study correspond to the aerobes that are seen in the ethmoid sinuses in chronic sinusitis (Table 27–1).

The organisms seen in cultures of ethmoid tissue in chronic sinusitis suggest a less invasive infection.[19,20] The presence of coagulase-negative *Staphylococcus aureus* in many of the cultures could signify colonization, but some suggest that the overgrowth of the commensal could actually contribute to the inflammation and therefore mucostasis. Alpha-hemolytic streptococci are not considered very aggressive organisms. *Staphylococcus aureus* also is frequently seen in the nose of healthy children; however, it may be a pathogen in some cases.[19] The normal pathogens seen in acute OM and acute sinusitis are not a frequent finding in children with chronic sinusitis. It is unclear whether the low percentage of these bacteria are the result of the aggressive antibiotic management that precedes the cultures of if they only represent a different set of pathogens for chronic sinusitis.

Children with cystic fibrosis (CF) will display the normal CF pathogens in their chronic sinusitis specimens (i.e., *Pseudomonas aeruginosa* and *Staphylococcus aureus*.[21] Because the mucosa is colonized, removal of polyps alone will not eliminate the offending bacteria completely.

Some children with immunodeficiencies also present with bacteria that are dependent upon the nature of the immunodeficiency. "Lacunar defects" are noted when the child is unable to create an antibody reaction to *Streptococcus pneumoniae* or *Haemophilus influenzae*.[22] The child with an immunodeficiency frequently harbors resistant organisms because of chronic antibiotic usage due to poor humoral or cellular response to infection.

AT A GLANCE . . .

Factors Predisposing to Chronic Sinusitis

- Recurrent viral URIs
- Recurrent acute bacterial sinusitis
- Allergic rhinosinusitis
- Environmental conditions (e.g., smoke, chlorine)
- Anatomic variations
- Cystic fibrosis
- Immunodeficiencies

MANAGEMENT

Practice Pathway 27–1 outlines the management of chronic sinusitis.

Nonsurgical

As bacteria play a major role in the development of chronic sinusitis in children, it is imperative to choose correctly an antibiotic that attacks the most common organisms. Unfortunately, nasal cultures do not reflect the cultures of the sinuses accurately.[24] In the older, more cooperative child, a culture of the mucus that leaves the infundibulum may be a better representation. The difficulty of obtaining such a culture and the lack of well-documented specificity and sensitivity reduce the overall reliance on such techniques. Certainly, it is appropriate to consider this technique in searching for resistant

Practice Pathway 27–1   DIAGNOSIS AND MANAGEMENT OF CHRONIC SINUSITIS

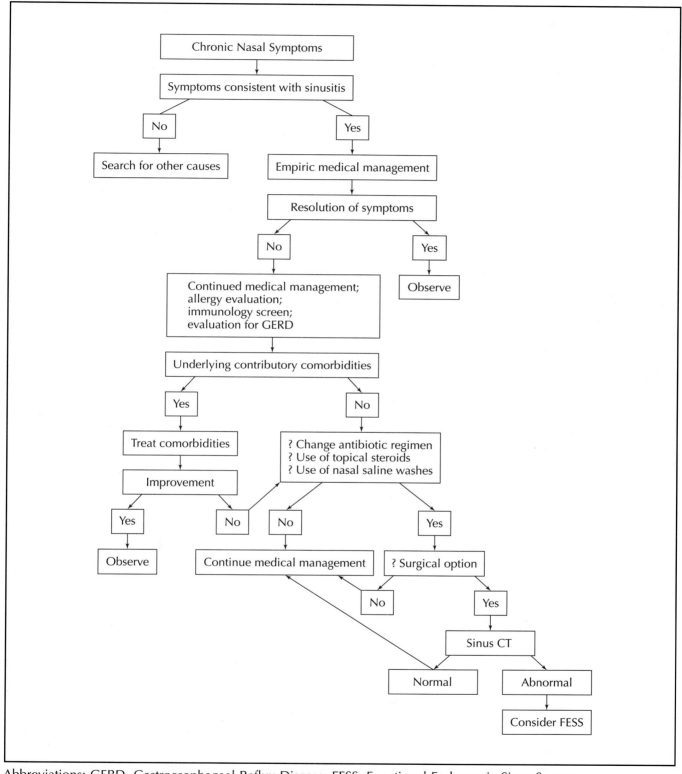

Abbreviations; GERD, Gastroesophageal Reflux Disease; FESS, Functional Endoscopic Sinus Surgery

organisms. Presence of a resistant organism in the mucus from the infundibulum directs a change in the antibiotic coverage.

In chronic sinusitis, the duration of treatment is an important consideration. In most infectious diseases, the duration of treatment depends on a combination of empiric and anecdotal data. The standard treatment of 10 days for many childhood infectious diseases is based mostly on the studies of streptococcal throat treatment. Only recently, there are studies in OM that suggest that for some antibiotics a full 10 days may not be necessary. In chronic sinusitis, there are no prospective studies on the duration of antibiotic treatment; however, it seems that short-term treatment is not sufficient to keep the infection controlled long enough to reverse the mucosal damage. It is suggested that a course of antibiotic therapy as long as 4 to 8 weeks should be tried before considering any failure of medical management.[5,6,25] In difficult-to-treat infections, the clinician should consider the use of oral medicines that also cover anaerobes.[25]

> ## SPECIAL CONSIDERATION:
> With chronic sinusitis, a course of antibiotic therapy as long as 4 to 8 weeks should be tried before considering any failure of medical management.

Topical, nasal, steroid sprays have been used with success in the management of sinusitis in children.[4,26] No prospective randomized trials have been performed in adults or children, but from a pathophysiologic point of view, these sprays should be an effective tool in treatment. Decreased edema and inflammatory response from the steroid spray should improve mucociliary clearance. Nasal steroids have been shown to be effective for the treatment of allergic rhinitis. Similarly, a nonallergic nasal and sinus mucosa edema should respond to the nasal steroids because the steroid effect is nonspecific. The reduction of mucus obstruction by mechanically improving the dimension of the pathways of flow also should reduce the risk of chronic sinusitis. In allergic rhinitis, there seems to be a reduction of mucus production as well. This reduced volume of mucus could impact positively on the

symptoms of chronic sinusitis. Interestingly, there appears to be a greater success in the treatment of children with chronic sinusitis if topical nasal steroids are used.

The thick nasal mucus that is seen in both allergic rhinitis and chronic sinusitis contributes to the development of both an increasing bacterial load and inflammation because the mucus sits in the nose and normal nasal bacteria multiply. Drying of this nasal mucus causes crusting, and within these crusts, bacteria may flourish. Mechanical debridement by nose blowing can be helpful, but few children are expert at nose blowing. Saline douche is an excellent way to remove the thick mucus from the nose mechanically. Large volume washes, if tolerated by the child, can improve the mucus clearance, reduce the chance of bacterial overgrowth, and improve the nasal airway. Parsons[27] has suggested that hypertonic-nasal-saline solutions do even better. The hypertonicity and (if made with baking soda) the increased pH act as a deterrent to bacteria growth. A concentrated effort of the parents is required to get the children to use this douche. Many children become comfortable with the process if given the opportunity. The use of a few drops of saline most probably adds nothing to the treatment as it merely stays in the nose with the mucus and contributes to bacterial overgrowth as well. Large volumes of saline are the key to the prevention of crusting. The use of a Water Pick® can be considered for the older child or patients with allergic fungal sinusitis.

> ## SPECIAL CONSIDERATION:
> Large-volume nasal washes can improve mucus clearance, reduce the chance of bacterial overgrowth, and improve the nasal airway.

Some experts have suggested the use of antibiotics in the nasal irrigant. This method has been effective in some children with CF in the postoperative period to control recolonization.[28] The routine use of this method for children with sinusitis has not been studied; however, caution should be exercised as the development of resistant organisms remains a real concern, especially if the concentration of the antibiotic that reaches the sinus is low enough to select out only the strains that have a greater resistance. In addition, some concerns have been raised about sensitization to the antibiotic.

If the child is allergic, attention should be addressed to the environmental factors causing the allergy. Allergic testing can identify some of the antigens. However, the clinician should remember that allergy testing is not always accurate in the young child who has a developing immune system and that the amount of available skin for testing is limited. It is wise to consider testing for animal danders and food allergies because elimination may be done more easily than control of dust mite or mold.

Other environmental factors include reduction or preferably elimination of exposure to tobacco smoke. Fortunately, the present social climate and general societal knowledge of the risks of tobacco smoke make it easier to encourage the parents to stop smoking or at least to eliminate the smoke from the child's environment. Smoking cessation is still very difficult to accomplish, and referral to smoking cessation programs and to the parents' or caretaker's physician for other adjuvant therapies is in order. Frank discussions with the family about smoking should be pursued.

Estimates of the frequency of childhood immunodeficiency is less than 0.5%.[29] If a child is documented to have an immunodeficiency, the medical and surgical management of the child's sinusitis is compromised without the management of the immunodeficiency.[30] Characterization of the defect may be a difficult and laborious task. Some immunodeficiencies will not be found in the routine screening evaluations. Suspicion must be high in the child with multisystem infections. Aggressive use of antibiotics along with the other listed modalities can be helpful but is not typically curative. The use of intravenous immunoglobulins has been a salvation for many children.[31] The control of sinus symptoms in these children may correspond to the immunoglobulin levels at any given time. Similarly, sinus surgery can be helpful in reducing the symptoms of chronic sinusitis, but it does not address the underlying pathology and the children often continue with sinus symptoms, albeit reduced, until the immunodeficiency resolves.

Surgical

Sinus surgery in children should be a rare occurrence. Aggressive treatment using the medical ra-

tionale as described above should control most of the chronic sinusitis in children. The younger and smaller the child, the greater the surgical risks and potential difficulties with technique. More importantly, children have a developing immune system, and improvement of the symptoms will, we hope, be seen as the child ages.

If the child demonstrates severe symptoms and has not responded to long-term aggressive medical management, the child may be considered as a candidate for surgical intervention. Given the data on recurrent URIs in childhood, the physician should be hesitant to consider surgery unless symptoms have been present for longer than 6 months. Multiple long-term courses of antibiotics should be employed because of both the lack of sensitivity of cultures and the poor sinus-tissue penetration of antibiotics. Chronic use of nasal steroids and saline sprays should be considered a necessary part of the therapy. Environmental control and treatment of gastroesophageal reflux also may help to limit symptoms.

If all of the above has been tried and the child still remains symptomatic, computed tomography (CT) of the paranasal sinuses in the coronal plane should follow a 4-week trial of antibiotic therapy. Because an URI causes mucosal thickening, the clinician should obtain CT at the conclusion of treatment when the child is at his best. CT may show areas with potentially nonreversible disease that need to be addressed surgically. Areas of anatomic deformity and narrowing can be defined. Normal areas of the sinus need no surgery, unless they are to be traversed for access to a more distal sinus.

Plain sinus radiographs are not useful in the evaluation of the child with chronic sinusitis. It is difficult to identify pathology accurately because the overlying bone and soft tissue reduces the sensitivity and specificity as compared to CT. McAllister et al. showed a lack of correlation between sinus radiography and CT in nearly 75% of the patients.[32]

Surgery should be reserved for those with abnormalities on CT after aggressive medical management. A normal CT scan confirms that medical management should control the disease process. Routine and frequent use of sinus surgery in children should be condemned.

The surgical techniques employed should focus on the preservation of as much normal tissue as possible. A functional approach allows for the opening of the sinuses through natural ostia based on the understanding of the normal flow of sinus and nasal mucus.[4,11] Impediments to the normal flow contribute to disease and the attempt to create flow other than in a predetermined route can cause disease as well.

The introduction of the endoscope to operate meticulously in the sinuses has improved the sinus care of both adults and children.[4,11,13,24,33] Special instrumentation has been developed to meet the size limitations of the child. The addition of the microdebrider also has allowed the atraumatic removal of mucosa and polyps.[34]

The removal of the uncinate process improves the drainage from the maxillary, anterior ethmoid, and frontal sinuses. Enlargement of the maxillary ostium is suggested to improve maxillary sinus drainage.[5] The creation of an accessory ostium for the maxillary sinus in that area can cause continued sinus infections and symptoms because of deviation from the normal pattern of mucus flow.

The anterior ethmoid sinuses are located anterior to the basal lamella. There are often two sets of cells—those at the bullae ethmoidalis and those above the insertion of the middle turbinate. Usually, these are opened to develop an ethmoid cavity from the lateral aspect of the middle turbinate to the lamina papyracea. If the superior cells are not diseased, they are left intact. The posterior ethmoid cells are opened through the basal lamella. The sphenoid and frontal sinuses in children should be left untouched, unless there is specific isolated disease. These sinuses frequently clear with resolution of disease in the maxillary and ethmoid sinuses. Surgical intervention in the sphenoid and frontal sinuses also carries a high risk of complications, such as visual loss or cerebrospinal fluid (CSF) leak. Scaring in the frontal recess also may contribute to long-standing frontal disease that becomes progressively harder to treat.

SPECIAL CONSIDERATION:
Surgical intervention in the sphenoid and frontal sinuses carries a high risk of complications.

Sinus surgery in childhood should be conservative. Normal tissue should be preserved if at all possible. Normal landmarks such as the middle and su-

perior turbinates should be preserved. In the rare case, a portion of the middle turbinate can be removed for access to the middle meatus. Extreme care should be taken to leave mucosal surfaces on the laminae papyracea and middle turbinate to reduce the risk of scaring. Assured identification of the maxillary ostium is essential to avoid the creation of an accessory ostium that allows recirculation of mucus in the infundibulum.

SPECIAL CONSIDERATION:
Sinus surgery in children should be conservative.

Stenting of the middle meatus after surgery has been proposed to reduce the likelihood of scar formation between the middle turbinate and the lateral nasal wall. The use of stenting, however, in both children and adults remains controversial. Because postoperative debridement is not possible in children without general anesthesia, the stent may be removed during debridement a few weeks following the initial surgery.

During the postoperative healing phase, the continued use of antibiotics and nasal steroids should be encouraged until the cavities are healed. Oral corticosteroids should be utilized if there is significant edema at the time of surgery.

Success of surgical management of chronic sinusitis, as measured by a reduction in sinus-related symptoms, has been shown in many case series.[4,5,26] Asthma exacerbations also have been reduced in frequency and severity.[35] Success, however, may be limited by comorbidities such as allergies and immunodeficiency.[30] Appropriate parental expectation is important, as children may improve but still have persistent symptoms due to recurrent URIs and nasal allergy.

Children with nasal polyposis secondary to CF present with nasal-airway obstruction, headache, reduction of pulmonary function, and in the long run, facial deformity. Because the disease process is due to abnormalities in the sinus mucosa, as mucosa regrows, the tendency for polyp formation continues. The use of similar techniques as described above allows the surgeon access to the sinuses for debulking of polyps. The microdebrider has facilitated this debulking greatly. It has been shown that the more aggressive the surgical approach, the less frequently that surgery needs to be performed.[36]

> ## SPECIAL CONSIDERATION:
> In CF patients, it has been shown that the more aggressive the surgical approach, the less frequently that surgery needs to be performed.

Allergic fungal sinusitis also presents with nasal polyposis.[37-40] Although the debridement of the polyps is the mainstay of therapy, allergic fungal sinusitis is frequently recurrent. The polypoid response to saprophytic fungi can be aggressive and require frequent surgery. Some children may respond to sinus polypectomy in combination with nasal steroids and saline douches, without resorting to more aggressive long-term oral corticosteroids.

Complications of medical management include adverse reactions to long-term antibiotic therapy and nasal steroid use. Chronic diarrhea, pseudomembranous colitis, and the development of resistant organisms are all possible reactions to antibiotic therapy. Nasal steroid use has been associated with epistaxis. Theoretical concerns about glaucoma or cataract formation have not been confirmed in children. The Federal Drug Administration has approved most nasal steroid preparations for use in children as young as age 6 years. Parents of children under 6 years should be informed of the presumed low risk and the potential benefits of nasal steroids.

In most reported pediatric-case series, there has been little documented morbidity or mortality of endoscopic sinus surgery. These case series certainly are not large enough to suggest safety unequivocally, but it does seem that in capable hands with careful attention to technique, the procedure is not exceptionally hazardous. Most series report very few complications and acceptable revision rates.[4,5,24,26]

The potential risks of sinus surgery are many. Anesthesia, bleeding, and infection are possible with any surgical procedure. Injury to the carotid artery in the sphenoid sinus is possible, although some protection may be afforded in the poorly developed sphenoid sinus because the overlying bone may be thicker. Attention should be paid to the use of potential anticoagulants perioperatively, especially the use of nonsteroidal antiinflammatory agents.

Orbital complications are also of great concern.[41] The optic nerve can be injured in the area of the sphenoid or posterior ethmoid sinuses. If the lamina is traversed, the medial rectus can be injured. The lacrimal duct may be violated in the region of the anterior fontanelle or at the lacrimal bone.[42] Epiphora, as a complication, is possible but rarely seen in children.

Intracranial complications include CSF leak and meningitis. Care must be taken, especially in the anterior superior ethmoid and frontal recess, to avoid fracturing the fovea ethmoidalis.[41,43]

Preoperative analysis and intraoperative referral to the CT does not eliminate the possibility of untoward and unexpected complications completely, but they can help the surgeon to know the danger areas and can facilitate in reducing the risk. It is appropriate to stop the surgery and repeat the scan if the surgeon is unsure as to the precise surgical location of disease. The use of systems for localizing the surgical area on CT in real time should result in a decreased incidence of complications.

> ## AT A GLANCE . . .
> Complications of Endoscopic Sinus Surgery
>
> Anesthesia
> Bleeding
> Infection
> Vascular injury
> Orbital complications
>   optic nerve injury
>   medial rectus injury
>   lacrimal duct injury
> Intracranial complications
>   CSF leak
>   meningitis

CONCLUSION

Chronic sinusitis is a real concern in the child. The symptom complex overlaps with many other disease entities. Careful attention to the diagnosis is important as a first step to proper management. Medical management usually is successful in treating this disease, but at times it must be aggressive and long-term. If medical management fails, surgery is an option, but it should be reserved for those patients with long-standing severe disease.

REFERENCES

1. Wald ER. Sinusitis in children. [Review]. N Engl J Med. 1992; 326:319-323.
2. Wald ER, Byers C, Guerra N, et al. Subacute sinusitis in children. J Pediatr 1989; 115:28-32.
3. Wald ER, Milmoe GJ, Bowen A, et al. Acute maxillary sinusitis in children. N Engl J Med 1981; 304: 749-754.
4. Lusk RP, Muntz HR. Endoscopic sinus surgery in children with chronic sinusitis: A pilot study. Laryngoscope 1990; 100:654-658.
5. Parsons DS, Phillips SE. Functional endoscopic surgery in children: A retrospective analysis of results. Laryngoscope 1993; 103:899-903.
6. Arjmand EM, Lusk RP. Management of recurrent and chronic sinusitis in children. [Review]. Am J Otolaryngol 1995; 16:367-382.
7. Wald ER. Diagnosis and management of acute sinusitis. Pediatr Ann 1988; 17:629-638.
8. Holinger LD. Chronic cough in infants and children. Laryngoscope 1986; 96:316-322.
9. Cherry JD, Dudley JP. Sinusitis. In: Cherry JD, ed. *Textbook of Pediatric Infectious Diseases.* Philadelphia: Saunders, 1981, pp. 104.
10. Messerklinger W. On the drainage of the normal frontal sinus of man. Acta Otolaryngol (Stockh) 1967; 63: 178-181.
11. Kennedy DW, Zinreich SJ, Rosenbaum AE, et al. Functional endoscopic sinus surgery. Theory and diagnostic evaluation. Arch Otolaryngol 1985; 111: 576-582.
12. Fontolliet C, Terrier G. Abnormalities of cilia and chronic sinusitis. Rhinology. 1987; 25:57-62.
13. Stammberger H. Endoscopic endonasal surgery—concepts in treatment of recurring rhinosinusitis. Part I. Anatomic and pathophysiologic considerations. Otolaryngol Head Neck Surg 1986; 94: 143-147.
14. Wilson R, Sykes DA, Currie D, et al. Beat frequency of cilia from sites of purulent infection. Thorax 1986; 41:453-458.
15. Drettner B. Pathophysiology of paranasal sinuses with clinical implications. Clin Otolaryngol 1980; 5: 272-284.
16. Shapiro GG. Role of allergy in sinusitis. Pediatr Infect Dis J 1985; 4:S55-S59.
17. Brook I. Aerobic and anaerobic bacterial flora of normal maxillary sinuses. Laryngoscope 1981; 91: 372-376.
18. Brook I, Thompson DH, Frazier EH. Microbiology and management of chronic maxillary sinusitis. Arch Otolaryngol Head Neck Surg 1994; 120:1317-1320.
19. Muntz HR, Lusk RP. Bacteriology of the ethmoid bullae in children with chronic sinusitis. Arch Otolaryngol 1991; 117:179-181.
20. Orobello PW Jr, Park RI, Belcher LJ, et al. Microbiology of chronic sinusitis in children. Arch Otolaryngol Head Neck Surg 1991; 117:980-983.
21. Shapiro ED, Milmoe GJ, Wald ER, et al. Bacteriology of the maxillary sinuses in patients with cystic fibrosis. J Infect Dis 1982; 146:589-593.
22. Umetsu DT, Ambrosino DM, Quinti I, et al. Recurrent sinopulmonary infection and impaired antibody response to bacterial capsular polysaccharide antigen in children with selective IgG-subclass deficiency. N Engl J Med 1985; 313:1247-1251.
23. Axelsson A, Brorson JE. Bacteriological findings in acute maxillary sinusitis. J Otorhinolaryngol Relat Spec 1972; 34:1-9.
24. Stankiewicz JA. Pediatric endoscopic nasal and sinus surgery. Otolaryngol Head Neck Surg 1995; 113: 204-210.
25. Brook I. Bacteriology of chronic maxillary sinusitis in adults. Ann Otol Rhinol Laryngol 1989; 98:426-428.
26. Lazar RH, Younis RT, Gross CW. Pediatric functional endonasal sinus surgery: Review of 210 cases. Head Neck 1992; 14:92-98.
27. Parsons OS. Chronic sinusitis: A medical or surgical disease? Otolaryngol Clin North Am 1996; 29:1-9.
28. Moss RB, King VV. Management of sinusitis in cystic fibrosis by endoscopic surgery and serial antimicrobial lavage. Reduction in recurrence requiring surgery. Arch Otolaryngol Head Neck Surg 1995; 121: 566-572.
29. Stiehm ER, Chin TW, Haas A, et al. Infectious complications of the primary immunodeficiencies. Clin Immunol Immunopathol 1986; 40:69-86.
30. Lusk RP, Polmar SH, Muntz HR. Endoscopic ethmoidectomy and maxillary antrostomy in immunodeficient patients. Arch Otolaryngol Head Neck Surg 1991; 117:60-63.
31. Roifman CM, Lederman HM, Lavi S, et al. Benefit of intravenous IgG replacement in hypogammaglobulinemic patients with chronic sinopulmonary disease. Am J Med 1985; 79:171-174.
32. McAlister WH, Lusk RP, Muntz HR. Comparison of plain radiographs and coronal CT scans in infants and children with recurrent sinusitis. Am J Roentgenol 1989; 153:1259-1264.
33. Stammberger H. Endoscopic endonasal surgery—concepts in treatment of recurring rhinosinusitis. Part II. Surgical technique. Otolaryngol Head Neck Surg 1986; 94:147-156.
34. Settlif RC. Minimally invasive sinus surgery: The ra-

tionale and the technique. Otolaryngol Clin North Am 1996; 29:115–129.

35. Manning SC, Wasserman RL, Silver R, et al. Results of endoscopic sinus surgery in pediatric patients with chronic sinusitis and asthma. Arch Otolaryngol Head Neck Surg 1994; 120:1142–1145.

36. Crockett DM, McGill TJ, Healy GB, et al. Nasal and paranasal sinus surgery in children with cystic fibrosis. Ann Otol Rhinol Laryngol 1987; 96:367–372.

37. Waxman JE, Spector JG, Sale SR, et al. Allergic aspergillus sinusitis: Concepts in diagnosis and treatment of a new clinical entity. Laryngoscope 1987; 97: 261–266.

38. Hartwick RW, Batsakis JG. Sinus aspergillosis and allergic fungal sinusitis. [Review]. Ann Otol Rhinol Laryngol 1991; 100:427–430.

39. Cody DT, Neel HB, Ferreiro JA, et al. Allergic fungal sinusitis: The Mayo Clinic experience. Laryngoscope 1994; 104:1074–1079.

40. Manning SC, Vuitch F, Weinberg AG, et al. Allergic aspergillosis: A newly recognized form of sinusitis in the pediatric population. Laryngoscope 1989; 99: 681–685.

41. May M, Levine HL, Mester SJ, et al. Complications of endoscopic sinus surgery: Analysis of 2108 patients—incidence and prevention. Laryngoscope 1994; 104:1080–1083.

42. Bolger WE, Parsons DS, Mair EA, et al. Lacrimal drainage system injury in functional endoscopic sinus surgery. Incidence, analysis, and prevention. Arch Otolaryngol Head Neck Surg 1992; 118:1179–1184.

43. Freije JE, Donegan JO. Intracranial complications of transnasal ethmoidectomy. Ear Nose Throat J 1991; 70:376–380.

28 Regional and Intracranial Complications of Sinusitis

Mark A. Richardson

Sinusitis, as it exists in children, must be an exceedingly common occurrence given the frequency of upper respiratory illnesses (URI) and the accompanying nasal congestion. In fact, there are objective studies that confirm that sinusitis is indeed a common accompaniment with the presence of an URI.[1] Sinusitis that requires therapy, such as antibiotics, is less common, and complications from infection must be rarer still. However, the complications from sinusitis, when it is constituted by a bacterial infection, can be exceedingly severe and when unchecked and untreated, catastrophic to the individual. The complications of sinusitis do not seem to be decreasing despite increasing and widespread use of antibiotics. A recognition of the potential complications, their signs and symptoms, and diagnosis and treatment must be within the capacity of every practitioner who treats patients with sinusitis of any etiology. The deliberate induction of immune suppression as part of the therapy for individuals with certain malignancies probably has increased the overall number of patients who require surgical management of aggressive infections. These infections, which are usually fungal, are a part of a spectrum of regional complications associated with sinusitis. Anatomic relationships, organisms involved, pathways of invasion, types of complications, and interventional steps to take and when to take them are key elements to the successful management of the complications associated with sinusitis.

> ### SPECIAL CONSIDERATION:
>
> Regional and intracranial complications of sinusitis do not appear to be decreasing despite increasing and widespread use of antibiotics.

Pediatric Otolaryngology, Edited by R.F. Wetmore, H.R. Muntz, and T.J. McGill. Thieme Medical Publishers, Inc., New York © 2000.

ORBITAL COMPLICATIONS

Orbital complications are by far the most common. They can be the result of sinusitis that involves any of the sinuses, but most commonly the ethmoid (Figs. 28-1 through 28-3). These complications are so common because of the proximity and intimate anatomic relationships between the orbital contents and all four groups of paranasal sinuses. There are a variety of anatomic factors that may lead to the spread of infection from the sinuses to the orbit, and these include:

1. The bone is generally thin, especially the lamina papyracea, and may have natural (although variable and unnamed) dehiscences that permit the spread of infection.
2. The sinuses and the orbit are supplied by a rich venous system that is valveless and also connects to the cavernous sinus.
3. There are multiple neurovascular foramina present in the orbit that are also pathways for the spread of infection.[2]

Orbital Anatomy

Orbital septum

The periosteum of the orbit is called the *periorbita.* As it reflects from the orbital rims to the eyelids and tarsal plate, it becomes the *orbital septum,* which acts as a barrier to infection. Infections located anterior to the orbital septum usually do not extend intraorbitally. So, although these infections may cause significant eyelid swelling, there is no gaze restriction, proptosis, or visual disturbance. These types of infections are called *preseptal. Postseptal infections* are those that occur within the confines of the bony orbital walls. They may create orbital cellulitis, subperiosteal abscess, orbital abscess, or cavernous sinus thrombosis.[3] Unfortunately, the distinction be-

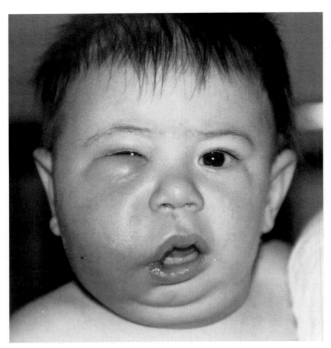

Figure 28–1: Right facial cellulitis secondary to ethmoid and maxillary sinusitis.

tween pre- and postseptal infection is not demonstrated clearly in clinical situations. Postseptal infections often cause eyelid edema, and preseptal infections may cause enough swelling to prevent the adequate evaluation of a young child to determine if significant clinical signs of orbital processes are present.

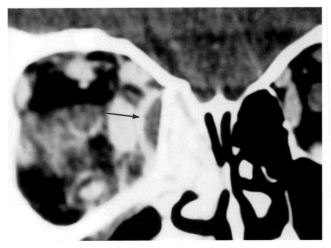

Figure 28–2: Subperiosteal abscess of the right orbit (arrow) secondary to acute sinusitis of the right ethmoid sinus.

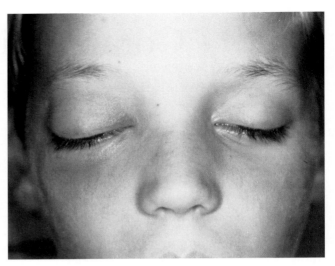

Figure 28–3: Proptosis of the right eye secondary to subperiosteal abscess of the right orbit.

Orbital Swelling

Chandler's classification system that was developed in 1970 remains largely unchanged (Practice Pathway 28-1). Fortunately, since Chandler's day, computed tomography (CT) has become available to help us guide our intervention.[4] All patients with a presumed postseptal infection should be evaluated initially in an ophthalmologic examination and placed on intravenous antibiotics to prevent further spread of inflammation. Many report that at least 80 percent of their patients may be controlled with such intervention without the need for surgery.[4]

Unfortunately, CT is not infallible when assessing the presence of abscesses either subperiosteally or intraorbitally. A worsening clinical picture of chemosis, visual disturbance, proptosis, or discomfort should trigger the potential need for surgical drainage. Pain is an important indication of disease progression and should not be discounted.

Bacteriology

The causal organisms vary somewhat by age. *Hemophilus influenzae* is reportedly the most common infection in young children, but the use of the HiB vaccine may be widening the spectrum of infection to involve *Streptococcus pneumonae* more commonly. Staphylococci, *Moraxella,* and bacteroides species also may be found. Antibiotic therapy should be directed towards these organisms. Cephtriaxone, a third generation cephalosporin with good penetration of the blood brain barrier, is a

Practice Pathway 28–1   ORBITAL SWELLING

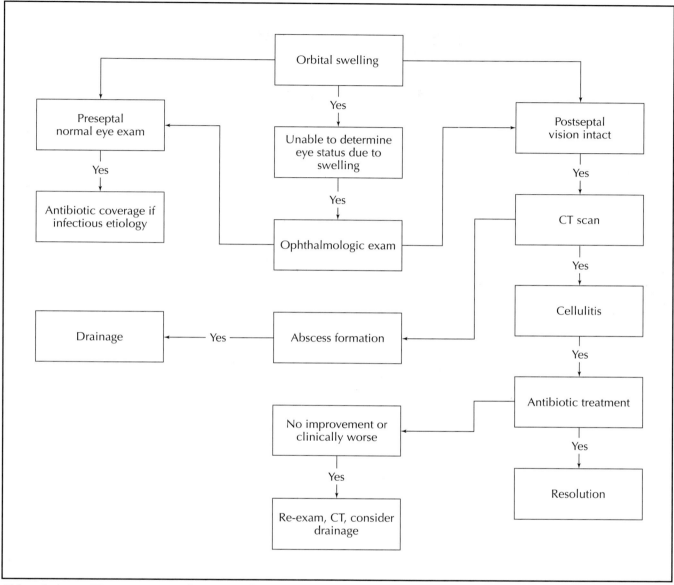

Abbreviations: CT, computerized tomography.

logical choice. The addition of clindamycin will help with anaerobic coverage.

As children age, the organisms that cause infection also change somewhat. Mixed aerobic and anaerobic infections become more common. *Klebsiella, Eikanella,* and microaerophilic streptococci all can be found in conjunction with the usual spectrum of aerobic bacteria in younger children. These pathogens may spread beyond the local area to produce septicemia or intracranial complications. Age differences may be significantly related to: (1) positive blood cultures, which are much more likely to

be positive in children under 4 years of age; and (2) complications that extend intracranially, which seem to be higher in children 9 years and older.

Treatment

After evaluating the patient and determining the nature of infection present, antibiotics are instituted. If concern exists as to the status of the eye examination or visual acuity, ophthalmologic consultation is essential to document progression of disease and the degree of visual acuity present prior to any therapeutic intervention. The ophthalmologist also may have additional suggestions for treatment of an intraorbital process. If an abscess is confirmed on CT, the safest treatment is surgical drainage. Although, in some cases, repeated examination and careful observation may be successful in management, preservation of function is the highest priority. If an abscess is not confirmed but clinical signs are deteriorating, drainage is necessary to preserve vision.[5]

The advent of endoscopic sinus surgery and its instrumentation has made the drainage of ethmoid sinusitis and orbital extensions of infection possible intranasally.[6] However, if the location of the abscess is superior or lateral, the endoscopic approach may not be possible. Additionally, the inflammation present may present problems with bleeding and edema, compounding surgical difficulty. Endoscopic management calls for a highly-experienced surgeon. The external approach for drainage is simple, time-honored, and successful.

SPECIAL CONSIDERATION:

Although a subperiosteal abscess of the orbit can be drained via an endoscopic approach, an external drainage procedure is simple, time-honored, and successful.

Orbital Apex Syndrome

The posterior ethmoid and sphenoid sinuses are situated in direct proximity to the orbital apex. Direct spread of inflammation from these areas may cause injury to the optic nerve and visual loss without periorbital edema or proptosis. Ophthalmoplegia, failing vision, and pain are the presenting symptoms that require rapid intervention to avoid blindness. Optic nerve decompression is the surgical treatment of choice. Fortunately, this is a rare complication because the bone usually is thick in this area, the periosteum is tightly adherent, and few foramina are present medially to permit rapid spread of the infection.

Cavernous Sinus Thrombosis

When infection spreads from the supraorbital or infraorbital veins, *cavernous sinus thrombosis* may

occur. This disease process is actually a phlebitis that may develop from any site that drains to this area, including (of course) most of the midface such as the nose, upper lip, and cheeks.[7] Cavernous sinus thrombosis usually begins unilaterally but evolves to bilateral extensions within a few hours. Headache, meningismus, eye pain, and decreasing vision occur. Temperature spikes from thromboembolic phenomenon are seen. Patients are profoundly ill. Proptosis, ophthalmoplegia, chemosis, and blindness along with a dismal prognosis are the norm in this significant complication. Retinoscopy may suggest venous engorgement, which is an early sign, and progressive infarction.

Evaluation beyond the physical examination and retinoscopy should consist of CT or magnetic resonance imaging (MRI), with MRI being more sensitive. Treatment, in addition to intravenous antibiotics, is similar to orbital apex syndrome and constitutes drainage of the infection and decompression of the optic nerve if vision is impaired. The use of anticoagulants is controversial.

AT A GLANCE . . .

Orbital Complications of Sinusitis

Orbital Swelling: most commonly caused by *Hemophilus influenzae* and *Streptococcus pneumonae;* mixed aerobic and anaerobic infections are more common in older children; antibiotic treatment is with cephtriaxone and clindamycin; surgical drainage is used when abscess is confirmed on CT.

Orbital Apex Syndrome: spread of inflammation from the posterior ethmoid and sphenoid sinuses may cause injury to the optic nerve and visual loss; optic nerve decompression is the surgical treatment of choice.

Cavernous Sinus Thrombosis: may occur when infection spreads from the supraorbital or infraorbital veins; proptosis, ophthalmoplegia, chemosis, and blindness may occur; diagnosis may be made with retinoscopy, CT, and MRI; treatment consists of intravenous antibiotics, drainage of the infection, and decompression of the optic nerve.

INTRACRANIAL COMPLICATIONS

The most common source of intracranial complications is the frontal sinus (Fig. 28–4), followed by

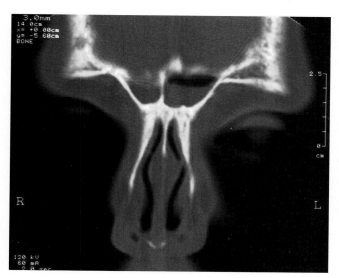

Figure 28–4: Complete opacification of the right frontal sinus and air-fluid level of the left frontal sinus consistent with acute frontal sinusitis. The patient presented with fever, headache, pain, and tenderness over the frontal region. An endoscopic drainage procedure was performed when symptoms failed to resolve with intravenous antibiotics.

the ethmoid, sphenoid, (Fig. 28–5) and maxillary sinuses. The incidence of intracranial complications from frontal sinusitis ranges from 3 to 10% among hospitalized patients.[8] Because younger patients have rudimentary frontal sinuses, intracranial complications, excluding meningitis, are more common in adolescents. The increased incidence of intracra-

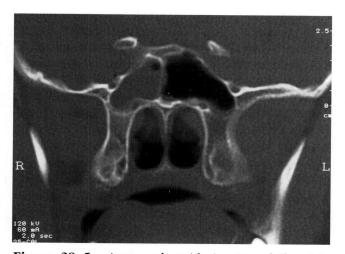

Figure 28–5: Acute sphenoid sinusitis of the right sphenoid sinus. The patient presented with fever, headache, and pain. When symptoms persisted in spite of adequate antibiotic coverage, an endoscopic drainage procedure was performed.

nial complications as a result of frontal sinusitis also may be a result of the organisms involved and the vascularity of the diploic system. The diploic veins communicate extensively with the veins of the dura and superior sagittal sinus. These veins are valveless and may permit retrograde thrombophlebitis. Osteomyelitis that is present in the bone also may permit direct extension of infection. Olfactory foramina in the roof of the ethmoid may be another pathway for spread of infection. Meningitis may occur through septicemia, which is more common in younger children. Infections may be in the form of meningitis, epidural abscess, subdural abscess or empyema, intracerebral abscess, venous sinus thrombosis, and osteomyelitis.

SPECIAL CONSIDERATION:

Because young patients have rudimentary frontal sinuses, intracranial complications of acute sinusitis, excluding meningitis, are more common in adolescents.

Epidural Abscess

Epidural abscess usually is a slowly-developing process with very subtle neurologic findings. Increased intracranial pressure may produce severe headache and vomiting. CT or MRI are best for diagnosis, but MRI has the edge in sensitivity.[9] Any bony defect suggests the development of an abscess.

Complete drainage of the sinus and abscess is the key to treatment, which may require cranialization of the frontal sinus if that is the source. If possible, the removal of granulation tissue over the dura should be accomplished without penetrating the dura.

Subdural Abscess

Subdural abscess or *subdural empyema* is defined as pus between the dura and brain. Subdural empyema is rare (10%) of all intracranial complications), more common in young men and adolescents, and associated with high morbidity and mortality. Aerobic and anaerobic streptococci along with *Staphylococcus aureus* are the most common bacteria encountered. Symptoms include headache, meningismus, fever, and changes in the level of consciousness.[10] As the infection progresses, hemipare-

Practice Pathway 28–2   INTRACEREBRAL ABSCESS

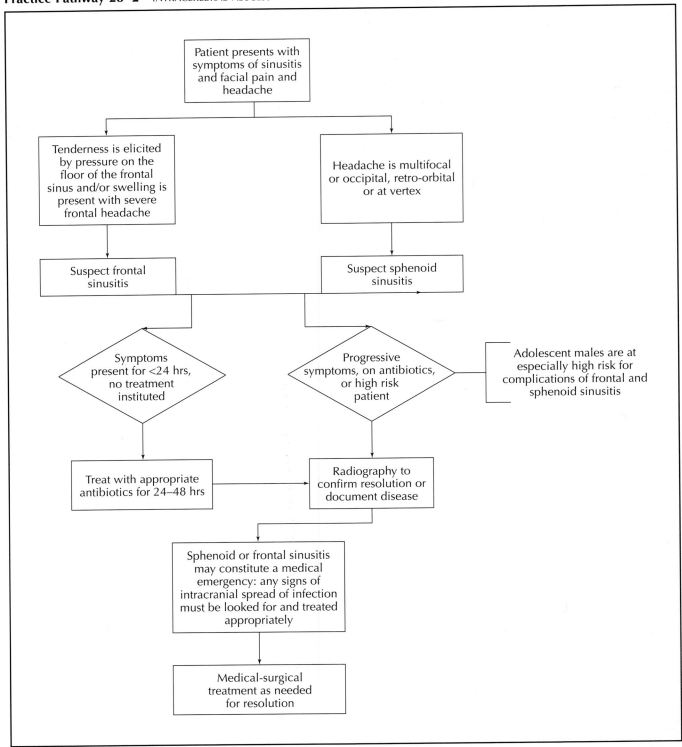

TABLE 28–1: Stages of Brain Abscess

Stage	Characteristics
I	Early cerebritis. Bacterial seeding in focal necrosis with local inflammation.
II	Late cerebritis. Pus formation leads to enlargement of necrotic center. Maximal edema is present.
III	Early abscess capsule formation.
IV	Late abscess capsule formation.

sis and seizures may occur. Lumbar puncture is not always diagnostic and, again, MRI may be the most sensitive study for diagnosis. Treatment should be directed towards draining all collections of purulent material through a craniotomy, drainage of the frontal sinus, and debridement of the affected bone if that is felt to be the source.

Intracerebral Abscess (Practice Pathway 28–2)

Brain abscesses of paranasal sinus origin develop most commonly in the frontal lobe and are secondary to infections in the frontal or ethmoid sinuses. The pathogenesis is usually through retrograde thrombophlebitis or extension of subdural empyema. The intraparenchymal infection begins as a cerebritis and progresses with liquefactive necrosis to abscess formation over a 10 to 14 day time period (Table 28–1). Headache, lethargy, fever, and agitation are hallmark symptoms.[11] When the abscess forms, an intracranial mass lesion is present with signs of increased intracranial pressure such as seizure or focal neurologic signs. Frontal lobe abscesses are notorious for producing mood changes at least initially.

MRI and CT identifies cerebritis and localized abscesses. Lumbar puncture is to be avoided because of increased intracranial pressure and the risk of brain herniation. Additionally, lumbar puncture does not provide specific information. Symptoms progress as the abscess enlarges or ruptures into the ventricles.

SPECIAL CONSIDERATION:

In a patient with a brain abscess, lumbar puncture should be avoided because of increased intracranial pressure and the risk of brain herniation.

Treatment

The most common causative organisms related to intracranial abscesses are *Staphylococcus aureus*, *Streptococcus pneumoniae*, *Hemophilus influenzae*, and beta-hemolytic streptococci. Anaerobes play a role, but due to difficulty with their recovery during culturing, their real incidence is unknown.[12]

Drainage of the abscess is the most common management, but intravenous antibiotic therapy as the sole treatment is advocated by some for small (<2 cm) lesions.[8] Recent mortality rates range between 5 to 10%. Treatment of the underlying sinus infection appropriately is also critical to resolution of any complications.

Osteomyelitis, Pott's Puffy tumor (which is a subperiosteal abscess of the frontal bone), and mucoceles also can result from frontal sinusitis and require surgical debridement and antibiotic therapy.

AT A GLANCE . . .

Intracranial Complications of Sinusitis

Epidural Abscess: a slowly-developing process with subtle neurologic findings; symptoms may consist of headache and vomiting; diagnosis is made with CT or MRI; treatment is drainage of the sinus.

Subdural Abscess: defined as pus between the dura and the brain; caused by aerobic and anaerobic streptococci and *Staphylococcus aureus*; symptoms include headache, meningismus, fever, and changes in levels of consciousness; diagnosis is made with MRI; treatment is directed towards draining all collections of purulent material through a craniotomy, drainage of the frontal sinus, and debridement of affected bone if necessary.

Intracerebral Abscess: develops most commonly in the frontal lobe secondary to infections in the frontal or ethmoid sinuses; infection begins as a cerebritis and progresses to abscess formation; usually caused by *Staphylococcus aureus*, *Streptococcus pneumoniae*, *Hemophilus influenzae*, and beta-hemolytic streptococci; symptoms include headache, lethargy, fever, and agitation; diagnosis is made with MRI or CT; treatment includes drainage of the abscess and intravenous antibiotics.

INVASIVE FUNGAL SINUSITIS (Practice Pathway 28-3)

Treatment of malignancies and HIV as well as chronic use of antibiotics have led to an increased incidence of *fungal sinusitis.* If the fungal infection becomes invasive, early diagnosis and treatment are essential for patient survival. The bone-marrow-transplant population is a good example of a group of patients at high risk for fungal disease; the mortality rate is approaching 60 to 80%, and there is an overall incidence of 1.7 to 2.6% in patients being transplanted.

Diagnosis

The most common presenting symptom is fever despite multi-drug antibiotic coverage. Facial pain, paranasal sinus congestion, and rhinorrhea are asso-

Practice Pathway 28–3   INVASIVE FUNGAL SINUSITIS

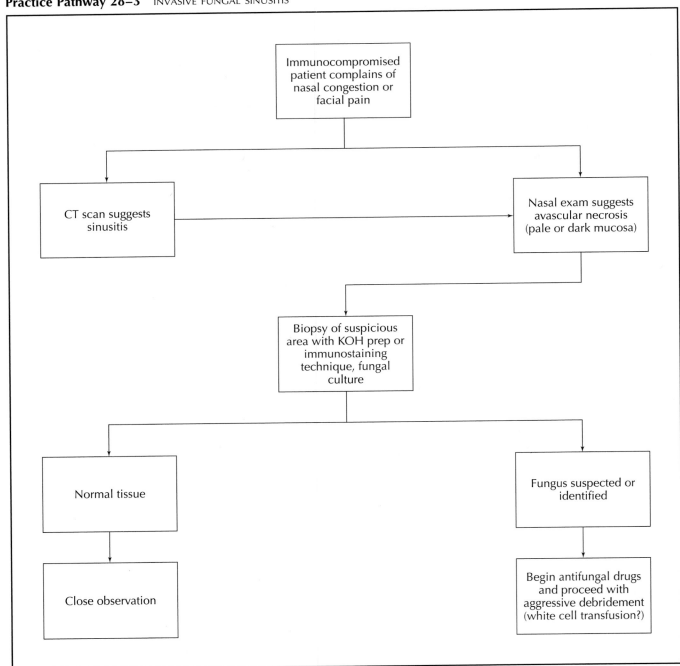

CT, computerized tomography; KOH, potassium hydroxide.

ciated symptoms. The appearance of affected mucosa varies from pale and avascular to dark with eschar formation. Biopsy of the nose results in minimal bleeding, which is an important sign used to determine the degree of resection required if the diagnosis is confirmed. Definitive diagnosis is made by histologic identification of fungal organisms within biopsy tissue.[13] Potassium hydroxide (KOH) preparations of tissue may result in rapid identification of fungal elements. Staining of the material with hemotoxolin and eosin, periodic-acid Schiff, and silver methenamine should identify the specific organism. Septate hyphae with dichotomous branching at 45 degrees (*Aspergillus*) or broad nonseptate hyphae (*Mucor*) can be seen. *Aspergillus* species are the most common fungi recovered but *Alternaria, Mucor,* and others also may be responsible for the infection.[14]

The rapid spread of infection may be related to the fungal predilection for arterial invasion. Ischemia and necrosis result from thrombosis, which allows for further spread of the fungus. The infection usually spreads from intranasal sites (septum, turbinate) to paranasal sinus or the palate.

Absolute white counts are not predictive of the outcome. In bone-marrow-transplant patients, the transplant must be successful for ultimate survival as well as recovery from neutropenia. The most important factors predicting recovery from fungal sinus infection are orbital or intracranial involvement diagnosed by imaging studies and biopsy.[15]

Treatment

Antifungal medication, primarily amphotericin B, and white-blood-cell transfusions are used as treatment. Surgical debridement of infection is also critical. Removal of necrotic, thrombosed tissue facilitates penetration of antifungal medications. Progression is common and reexcision often is necessary until the infection is controlled and the immune response has improved.

REFERENCES

1. Gwaltney JM, Phillips D, Miller RD, et al. Computed tomographic study of the common cold. N Engl J Med. 1994; 330:25-30.

2. Stammberger H. Complications of acute sinusitis. In: Hawke M, ed. *Functional Endoscopic Sinus Surgery.* Philadelphia: B.C. Decker, 1991, pp. 362-367.

3. Osguthorpe DJ, Hochman M. Inflammatory sinus diseases affecting the orbit. Otolaryngol Clin North Am 1993; 26(4):657-668.

4. Healy GB. Classics from the laryngoscope. Chander et al. The pathogenesis of orbital complications in acute sinusitis. Laryngoscope 1997; 107:441-446.

5. Pereira KD, Mitchell RB, Younis RT, et al. Medical management of medical subperiosteal abscess of the orbit in children—a 5 year experience. Int J Pediatr Otorhinolaryngol 1997; 38:247-254.

6. Wolf SR, Gode U, Hosemann W. Endonasal surgery for rhinogen intraorbital abscess: A report of six cases. Laryngoscope 1996; 106:105-110.

7. Odabasi AO, Akgul A. Case report—Cavernous sinus thrombosis: A rare complication of sinusitis. Int J Pediatr Otorhinolaryngol 1997; 39:77-83.

8. Giannoni CM, Stewart MG, Alford EL. Intracranial complications of sinusitis. Laryngoscope 1997; 107: 863-867.

9. Conlon BJ, Curran A, Timon CV. Pitfalls in determination of intracranial spread of complicated suppurative sinusitis. J Laryngol Otol 1996; 110:673-675.

10. Lerner DN, Zalzal GH, Choi SS, et al. Intracranial complications of sinusitis in childhood. Ann Otol Rhinol Laryngol 1995; 104:288-293.

11. Singh B, Van Dellen J, Ramjettan S, et al. Sinogenic intracranial complications. J Laryngol Otol 1995; 109:945-950.

12. Dolan RW, Chowdhury K. Diagnosis and treatment of intracranial complications of paranasal sinus infections. J Oral Maxillofac Surg 1995; 53:1080-1087.

13. Perez-Jaffe LA, Lanza DC, Loevner LA, et al. In situ hybridization for aspergillus and penicillium in allergic fungal sinusitis: A rapid means of speciating fungal pathogens in tissues. Laryngoscope 1997; 107: 233-240.

14. Seibert RW, Bower CM. Invasive fungal rhinosinusitis—The method of Robert W. Seibert. In: Gates GA, ed. *Current Therapy in Otolaryngology—Head and Neck Surgery.* St. Louis: Mosby, 1998, pp. 386-388.

15. Kendall KA, Senders CW. Rhinocerebral mucormycosis. In: Gershwin ME, Incaudo GA, eds. *A Comprehensive Textbook of Diagnosis and Treatment.* Totowa, NJ: Haman Press, 1996, pp. 349-355.

29 Pediatric Facial Trauma

Craig W. Senders

In the United States, trauma is the leading cause of death for children < 14 years of age, accounting for 40% of the mortality in this age group.[1] It is estimated that 15,000 children die of trauma each year.[2] In spite of this incidence, the occurrence of facial fractures is relatively low, accounting for 1.5 to 15% of trauma admissions.[3-7]

Younger children are less likely to sustain facial fractures than older children, and the majority of fractures occur in the teenage population.[8] This higher incidence in the teenage population reflects the maturation and sinus aeration of the facial skeleton as well as changes in lifestyle (Fig. 29–1). Young children live in a protected environment, whereas teenagers tend towards a riskier lifestyle (Table 29–1).[9,10] Some studies show a slight male predominance,[8,11] whereas others show an equal pattern across the genders.[12] As motor vehicle accidents account for the majority of facial fractures, one might expect gender neutrality.

During the past 15 years, rigid fixation has been the dominant method of treating facial fractures in adult patients. The use of these techniques in children remains controversial for fear of inhibiting facial growth.[2,3,5] The use of rigid fixation across suture lines has been demonstrated to inhibit skeletal growth in the animal model.[13,14] Experience in craniofacial surgery has demonstrated that plates applied to the skull of a growing child can migrate intracranially.[15] There is evidence that stripping the periosteum, which is required to apply the plates and align the fracture, also may inhibit growth independently.[16] The paradox for the treating physician is that facial fractures themselves inhibit facial growth and that the methods of reconstruction additionally inhibit craniofacial growth. Resolving this paradox is not entirely possible. This chapter presents a rational approach that should provide consistent results when treating children with facial fractures.

INITIAL MANAGEMENT

The basic tenets of trauma management apply to children. The child's airway, breathing, and circulation (i.e., the ABCs) must be assessed. For most fractures, careful positioning of the child will manage the airway. Suctioning of blood and secretions from the oral cavity is also helpful. The oral cavity must be assessed for loose foreign bodies that have a potential for aspiration.

SPECIAL CONSIDERATION:

As with any patient suffering trauma, the basic tenets of trauma management (i.e., airway, breathing, and circulation) apply to children who have sustained a facial fracture.

If careful positioning or suctioning of the oral cavity is not adequate to maintain the airway, intubation or an emergency cricothyrotomy is appropriate. Prior to manipulation of the neck, radiologic evaluation of the cervical spine should be obtained; however, cervical spine injuries are relatively infrequent in this population.[8] After the airway is established, packing the nose or nasopharynx may be necessary to prevent further blood loss.

PHYSICAL EXAMINATION

After airway, breathing, and circulation have been assessed and stabilized, a careful and orderly exami-

Pediatric Otolaryngology, Edited by R.F. Wetmore, H.R. Muntz, and T.J. McGill. Thieme Medical Publishers, Inc., New York © 2000.

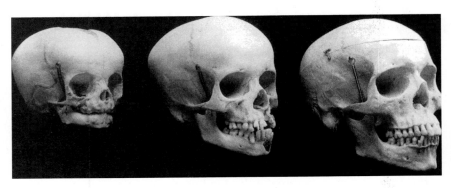

Figure 29–1: The proportion between the size of the cranium and the facial bones changes dramatically with age. (From Ferraro JW. *Fundamentals of Maxillofacial Surgery*. Columbus, OH: Springer, 1996, p. 216, with permission.)

nation should be made of the head and neck that includes an examination for injuries of the central nervous system (CNS), cervical spine, orbital contents, nose, oral cavity, and facial skeleton. The external auditory canals (EAC) should be examined carefully to exclude a temporal bone fracture associated with mandibular trauma. The presence of a hemotympanum is suggestive of a temporal bone fracture, although it may be the result of epistaxis that is common in trauma patients. Nasoseptal hematoma or significant cerebrospinal fluid (CSF) rhinorrhea can be diagnosed by anterior rhinoscopy.

SPECIAL CONSIDERATION:

The presence of a hemotympanum on otoscopic examination may suggest a temporal bone fracture, but also may be only the result of the epistaxis seen in many facial trauma patients.

The facial skeleton should be examined for edema, crepitation, hematomas, focal tenderness,

TABLE 29–1: Mechanism of Pediatric Facial Fracture by Age Category

Age Group (yr)	Traffic Accident	Falls	Sports-related and Altercations	Other
<3	1	9	0	2
3 to 5	12	8	4	1
6 to 12	32	12	9	4
13 +	23	3	15	2
Total	68	32	28	9

From reference 10, with permission.

and asymmetries. Tenderness of the zygomatic arch or trismus suggests a fracture. Evaluation of the orbital rim should include palpation for step-offs, tenderness, and asymmetry. Movement of the extraocular muscles should be evaluated carefully. In cooperative older patients, forced duction tests should be performed if there is suspicion that gaze is limited. The orbit should be evaluated carefully for proptosis or enophthalmos. Any suggestion of a visual loss or restriction of gaze always should be confirmed by ophthalmologic consultation.

Mobility of the midface can be assessed by grasping the upper incisor teeth and rocking the maxilla while the head and nasal bridge are held steady with the opposite hand. The gingivolabial sulcus should be examined carefully for ecchymosis that is suggestive of an underlying fracture. Subject changes in occlusion should be assessed also. The occlusion should be examined carefully, looking for changes that might suggest a fracture. If the child is cooperative, biting on a tongue blade can illicit pain that suggests a fracture or dental trauma. Paresthesia of any of the divisions of the trigeminal nerve also suggests a fracture.

RADIOLOGIC EVALUATION

The gold standard for evaluating the cranium and midface is computed tomography (CT).[17,18] Axial CT sections are easy to obtain and are the only CT sections that are appropriate with a suspected cervical spine injury. For complex facial fractures, both coronal and axial sections should be obtained. Three dimensional (3D) CT reconstruction should be considered for complex fractures.[19]

Although axial CT sections can be used to evaluate the mandible, plain radiographs are preferred. An orthopantograph (panorex) provides an excellent overall view of the mandible. A Towne's view specifically allows evaluation of the condyle. A lateral oblique projection is useful for evaluating the mandibular ramus, angle, and body.

Simple nasal fractures do not require radiologic evaluation, and often radiologic evaluation is misleading in these patients. In patients with a significant nasal/midfacial injury, CT is appropriate to evaluate for nasoethmoid fractures, as well as other midfacial fractures.

MANAGEMENT OF FACIAL FRACTURES

Often, facial fractures in children can be managed by a *closed technique* or a *limited open technique.* This is especially true for nasal fractures, fractures of the zygomatic arch, and fractures of the mandible. Advances in craniofacial surgery have led to the development and popularity of minimally-visible incisions that allow complete exposure of the midface and mandible.

Fractures of the Midface

The upper third of the face including the zygomatic arches and the superior, lateral, and medial orbital rims can be exposed through a coronal incision. The lower orbital rim and orbital floor can be exposed through an extended transconjunctival incision or a subcilliary incision. The face of the maxilla, nasomaxillary, and zygomaxillary buttresses can be exposed via an upper gingivolabial sulcus incision. The gingivolabial sulcus incision can be combined with the coronal incision to approach nasoethmoid fractures. Bilateral gingivolabial sulcus incisions can be extended into a midfacial degloving incision for additional exposure. In cases where exposure is difficult or a coronal incision is not required for other fractures, some nasoethmoid fractures are still best approached with an (modified Lynch) external ethmoidectomy. Typically, the resultant scar from an external ethmoidectomy is aesthetically acceptable.

Coronal incision

The *coronal incision* is camouflaged in the hairline. Beginning 1 to 2 cms above the level of the tragus in the preauricular crease, it continues across the cranium to the opposite ear. The scalp flap is ele-

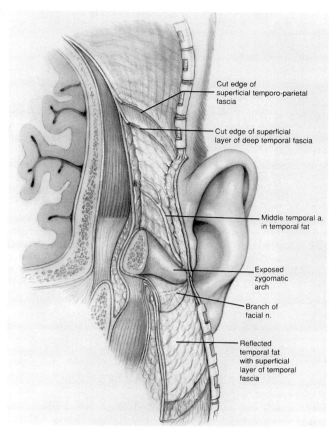

Figure 29–2: The coronal flap is elevated in the subgaleal plane until 2 cm above the superior orbital rim when it is elevated in the subperiosteal plane. (From Kellman RM, Marentette LJ. *Atlas of Craniomaxillofacial Fixation.* New York: Raven Press, 1995, p. 100, with permission.)

vated superficially to the periosteum of the calvarium and the temporalis fascia (subgaleal plain). The flap is then pulled forward with a plain of dissection being above the periosteum and the temporalis fascia (Fig. 29-2).

The temporalis fascia is incised sharply inferior to the level of the temporal line and parallel to the zygomatic arch (Fig. 29-3). Inferior to the temporal line, the temporalis fascia splits to form the superficial and deep layers that envelope the superficial temporal fat pad (Fig. 29-4). The elevation continues inferiorly just deep to the superficial temporalis fascia. This technique protects the frontal branch of the facial nerve, which passes very closely to the periosteum of the zygomatic arch.[2,20]

The periosteum is incised sharply over the cranium, approximately 2 cm above the superior orbital rims (Fig. 29-2). The supraorbital nerve must be freed from its foramen with an osteotome or drill.

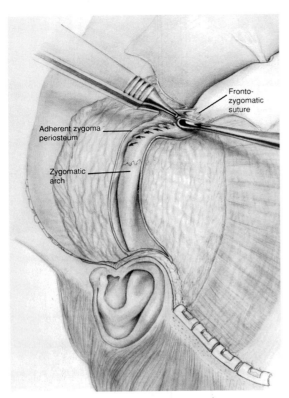

Figure 29–3: The superficial layer of the temporalis fascia is incised just inferior to the temporal line. (From Kellman RM, Marentette LJ. *Atlas of Craniomaxillofacial Fixation.* New York: Raven Press, 1995, p. 101, with permission.)

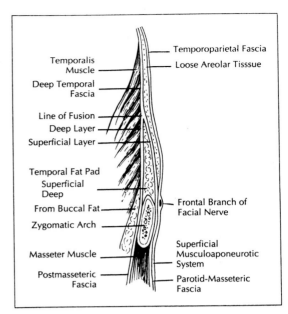

Figure 29–4: As the temporal branch of the facial nerve crosses over the zygoma, it is intimately involved with the temporal parietal fascia. By approaching the zygoma deep to the superficial layer of the temporalis fascia, the nerve is protected. (From Frodel JL, Marentette LJ. The coronal approach. Anatomic and technical consideration and morbidity. Arch Otolaryngol Head Neck Surg 1993; 119:203, with permission.)

In this plane, the entire superior orbit, including the medial wall, roof, and lateral wall, can be exposed (Fig. 29-5). With detachment of the lateral canthal ligament, the lateral portion of the inferior orbital rim can be exposed. Upon closure, the lateral canthal ligament should be reattached. The medial canthal ligaments are reachable using this technique.

The lacrimal sac and duct limit exposure of the inferior orbital rim medially. To approach the inferior orbital rim, either a transconjunctival[12,21,22] or the subciliary[23] incision may be used (Fig. 29-6). The transconjunctival incision has gained popularity because it is hidden completely over its infraorbital course. Additionally, there is less lid edema following this incision. The conjunctiva is incised inferior to the lower border of the tarsus (Fig. 29-7).[12] The dissection is begun anterior to the orbital septum. At the orbital rim, the periosteum is incised, exposing the orbital rim and floor. For all but the simplest of fractures, improved access can be obtained by combining this approach with a lateral canthotomy. At the completion of the case, the

conjunctiva can be closed with a buried, running 6-0 chromic suture. The lateral canthal ligament must be restored with a long-lasting absorbable or permanent suture.

Frontozygomatic suture approach

The *frontozygomatic suture* can be approached directly through a lateral brow incision. Alternatively, it can be approached through an extended lateral canthotomy incision when the inferior orbital rim is exposed.

External ethmoidectomy

An *external ethmoidectomy incision* is far from hidden, but in most patients it is barely visible over time. If inadequate exposure is obtained through the coronal incision or the gingivolabial incision, the surgeon should not hesitate to add this incision in order to achieve an appropriate esthetic and functional result. This approach is most helpful in the child with a difficult nasoethmoid fracture. The incision is started midway between the punctum of the

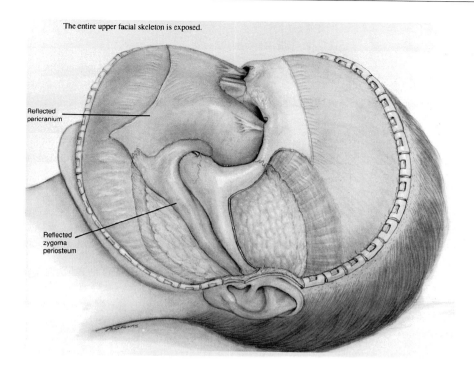

The entire upper facial skeleton is exposed.

Reflected pericranium

Reflected zygoma periosteum

Figure 29–5: By staying in the subperiosteal plane and detaching the lateral canthal ligament, the lateral orbital wall as well as the lateral portion of the inferior orbital wall can be approached through the coronal incision. (From Kellman RM, Marentette LJ. *Atlas of Craniomaxillofacial Fixation.* New York: Raven Press, 1995, p. 107, with permission.)

eye and the dorsum of the nose, and should extend in a gentle curve. Superiorly, it should blend into the interior portion of the brow, and inferiorly it should flow toward the nasal facial crease. For approaches to the nasoethmoid area, the incision generally should be 3 cm in length. The incision should be made at a right angle to the skin through the periosteum of the nasal bone.

Gingival incision

The *gingivolabial sulcus incision* is used to approach the face of the maxilla, and more importantly, the nasomaxillary and zygomaticomaxillary buttresses (Fig. 29-8). The nasoethmoid region can be exposed through this approach as well. The incision is begun 2 to 3 mm on the labial side of the gingivolabial sulcus. Leaving this small cuff of mucosa aids in placing sutures during closure. The dissection is then continued to bone, and the soft tissue is elevated subperiosteally off the face of the maxilla. The infraorbital nerve should be identified and preserved. To give full exposure to the zygomaticomaxillary buttress, the masseter muscle may need to be elevated.

Degloving approach

A *degloving approach* to the nasal ethmoid region can be accomplished by joining bilateral gingivolab-

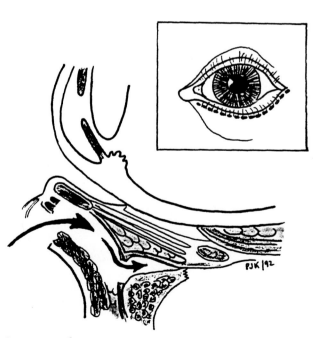

Figure 29–6: The subcillary incision is made 2 mm inferior to the lash border. The obicularis oculi muscle and skin flap is elevated leaving the periorbita intact. At the orbital rim, the periosteum is incised and the plane is continued subperiosteally. (From reference 12, with permission.)

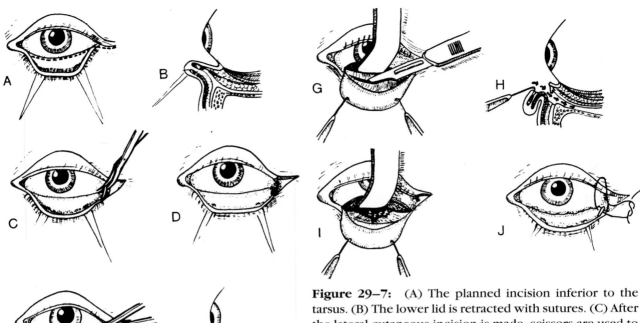

KOLTAI/92

Figure 29–7: (A) The planned incision inferior to the tarsus. (B) The lower lid is retracted with sutures. (C) After the lateral cutaneous incision is made, scissors are used to divide the lower lateral canthal tendon. (D) After division of the lateral canthal tendon. (E) Using scissors or a knife an incision is made in the conjectiva inferior to the tarsus. (F) The incision should be carried just inferior to the tarsus external to the periorbita. (G) The exposed periosteum is cut sharply. (H) The dissection is subperiosteal. (I) Exposure of the orbital floor. (J) The conjectival incision is closed with a buried, running 6-0 chromic suture. The inferior lateral canthal tendon is reattached to its stump or its superior lateral canthal tendon with a permanent or slowly-resorbing suture. (From reference 12, with permission.)

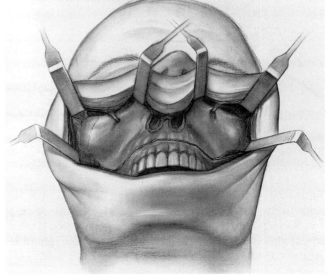

Figure 29–8: The gingivolabial incision is elevated in a subperiosteal plane. The infraorbital nerve is identified and protected. When necessary, this incision may be connected across the midline to give complete exposure of the inferior maxilla and pyriform apertures. When appropriate, this can be extended into a degloving incision. (From Kellman RM, Marentette LJ. *Atlas of Craniomaxillofacial Fixation.* New York: Raven Press, 1995, p. 113, with permission.)

ial incisions. This incision connects to a circumferential nasovestibular incision that includes a transfixion incision medially and an intercartilaginous incision superiorly. The nasal skin is elevated from the upper lateral cartilages, and the elevation is continued in the subperiosteal plane over the nasal bones. This approach gives complete exposure to the midface and nasal ethmoid region. The circumferential nasovestibular incision places a risk for postoperative nasal stenosis, particularly in young patients. For this reason, its use should be limited to the adolescent.

> ## SPECIAL CONSIDERATION:
> In young patients, the circumferential nasovestibular incision places the patient at risk for postoperative nasal stenosis, and so its use should be limited to the adolescent.

Fractures of the Mandible

With the retractors that are available today, the open reduction of a mandible fracture should be managed through an intraoral approach.[24,25] Again, the gingivolabial sulcus incision is utilized to approach the fracture. The incision is made 2 to 3 mm towards the labial side from the gingivolabial sulcus. The incision should be made at a right angle to the bone, and the periosteum should be elevated. The inferior alveolar nerve is identified and preserved. This nerve can be damaged easily if care is not taken. For exposure posterior to the inferior alveolar nerve, visualization should be accomplished intraorally also.

Drilling and screw placement is performed directly through the cheek. After exposing the fracture intraorally, a small superficial skin incision parallel to the relaxed skin tension lines is made at the site of the fracture. Blunt dissection protects the facial nerve and connects the skin incision to the intraoral exposure. Sleeves are then placed through this opening to protect the overlying soft tissue from instrumentation.

Management of fractures of the mandible (Prac-

tice Pathway 29–1) in children differs from that of adults because the child's mandible is still growing and heals rapidly, there are differences in dentition and the plasticity of pediatric dentition, and there is the propensity of the child's bone to remodel. In patients < 13 years of age, intermaxillary fixation with arch bars is much more difficult to achieve because of the presence of deciduous or mixed dentition. Placement of rigid fixation is difficult because of concern for tooth roots or tooth buds.

The tenet of immobilization applies to pediatric patients, but is much more forgiving than in the adult. In the patient with mixed dentition, applying intermaxillary fixation can be both a challenge and a cause of frustration. Even with the use of a cap splint, arch bars, circummandibular wires, and pyriform aperture suspension, complete immobilization is not always obtained for longer than a few weeks. Nevertheless, despite the problems with immobilization, it is exceedingly rare that a nonunion would result. Patients who are older than 13 years of age can be treated in the same manner as adults.

> ## SPECIAL CONSIDERATION:
> In the management of mandibular fractures, the tenet of immobilization applies to pediatric patients but is much more forgiving than in the adult.

Fractures of the Condyle

Most fractures of the condyle in the mixed or deciduous dentition can be treated conservatively with a soft diet. In patients with unilateral or bilateral fractures of the condyle with normal occlusion, moderate to normal range of motion, and no evidence of an open bite deformity, a soft diet and exercises are all that is appropriate. Range of motion exercises prevent trismus and ankylosis. If there is an anterior open bite deformity, then the patient should be treated with 2 to 3 weeks of intermaxillary fixation followed by the use of elastics. In pediatric patients with marked displacement of the condylar head, long-term follow-up radiographs demonstrate complete remodeling of the condyle.[26,27]

Practice Pathway 29–1 MANDIBULAR FRACTURE

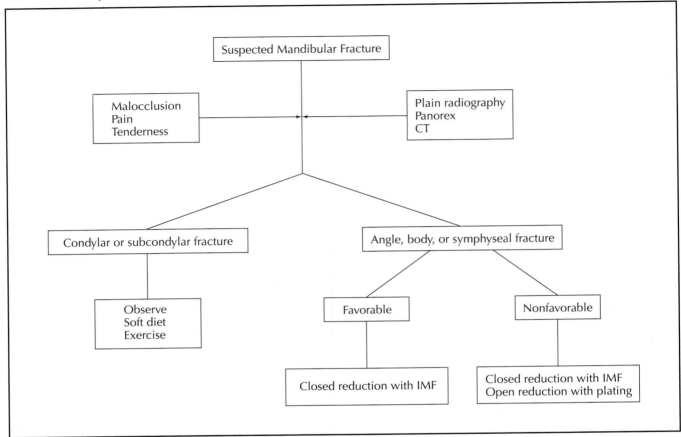

Abbreviation: IMF, Intermaxillary Fixation.

Fractures of the Mandibular Arch

Many mandibular fractures in the pediatric age group are greenstick. Fractures that are nondisplaced or minimally displaced (favorable) can be treated by a soft diet and observation. A Barton's bandage can be used to provide comfort (Fig. 29–9). In one study involving 220 fractures in 157 patients, the majority were managed without open reduction.[9] In another study, 30% were managed without surgery, and 30% were managed with intermaxillary fixation alone.[10]

> ### SPECIAL CONSIDERATION:
>
> Because many mandibular arch fractures in children are greenstick, most of these nondisplaced or minimally-displaced fractures can be treated with a soft diet and observation.

In fractures with significant displacement or malocclusion, intermaxillary fixation with arch bars and cap splints is appropriate. In a young child with mixed or absent dentition, occlusion can be restored in the operating room using an acrylic splint that is held in place with submandibular wires.

In the young child with comminuted fractures, use of monocordical miniplates along the inferior mandible can avoid damaging tooth roots. Stabilization of the fracture is optimized when use of miniplates is combined with intermaxillary fixation. Compression plates can be used in the older child. In some cases, placing plates along the inferior border of the mandible may require an external incision.

Dental Alveolar Fractures

Avulsed teeth

An attempt should be made to reimplant all teeth whether deciduous or permanent unless the root is

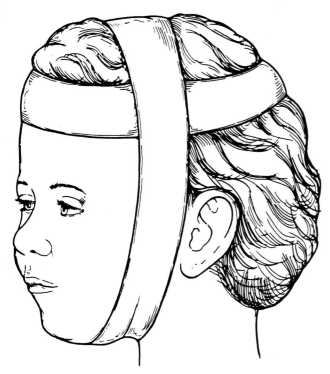

Figure 29–9: A Barton's bandage may be all that is required in young patients with nondisplaced mandibular fractures. (From Potsic WP, Cotton RT, Handler SD, eds. *Surgical Pediatric Otolaryngology.* New York: Thieme, 1997, p. 574, with permission.)

reabsorbed significantly (which indicates pending eruption of the permanent tooth). Not reimplanting a deciduous tooth results in less dental alveolar height. More importantly, it may be difficult to distinguish between a permanent and a deciduous tooth during a period of mixed dentition. Therefore, reimplantation always is recommended within the first 1 to 2 hours following the injury. If the parents cannot be convinced to attempt reimplantation on their own, they should store the tooth in milk or a moist gauze. After reimplantation, the tooth should be stabilized to nearby teeth using wire or an acrylic cap. The child's dentist should be involved in the long-term management of the reimplanted tooth.

Alveolar ridge fracture

An alveolar ridge fracture typically involves one or more teeth and the surrounding alveolar ridge bone. Often there are associated avulsed teeth. The fracture should be repositioned and avulsed teeth should be reimplanted, using wire or an acrylic cap to stabilize loose fragments to surrounding teeth.

Any associated gingival lacerations should be repaired. A soft diet is appropriate for six weeks. Dental consultation for long-term care is appropriate.

Zygomatic Complex Fractures

Surgical correction of zygomatic complex fractures is appropriate when there is significant bony displacement or extraocular muscle entrapment (Practice Pathway 29–2). Suspicion of this fracture is best assessed with a careful physical examination and with CT. Physical examination may be limited by edema that may take several days to resolve.

The surgical exposure is best accomplished through either a transconjunctival or subciliary incision (Figs. 29–6 and 29–7).[12] The incision can be extended laterally or combined with a brow incision to expose the frontozygomatic suture. In fractures that are displaced significantly, the zygomaticomaxillary buttress should be exposed through a gingivolabial incision. In comminuted fractures that involve the body and the arch, a hemicoronal approach is necessary.

Most fractures can be repaired with two point rigid fixation at the frontozygomatic suture (miniplate) and along the intraorbital rim (microplate) after realigning the bony fragments. In more complex fractures, the zygomaticomaxillary buttress requires an additional plate. If there is significant prolapse of orbital contents into the maxillary sinus, the floor can be reconstructed using a calvarial bone graft or slowly-absorbing mesh. Septal cartilage should not be used in a growing face.

Fractures of the Superior Orbital Rim

This type of fracture is unusual in the pediatric age group due to nonaeration of the frontal sinus. Cases in which the superobital rim is involved usually have a significant frontal bone fracture. If there is significant displacement of the frontal bone fragments, correction may require the assistance of a neurosurgeon. If a craniotomy is necessary, the superior orbital rim can be repaired through that approach, otherwise a brow incision provides adequate exposure.

The older pediatric patient with a large frontal sinus is treated in a manner similar to the adult. Nondisplaced anterior frontal sinus wall fractures do not require intervention. Fractures of the posterior sinus wall, especially centrally, should be addressed surgically to prevent mucocele formation.[28,29] An osteoplastic flap with fat obliteration is

Practice Pathway 29–2 ZYGOMATIC COMPLEX FRACTURE

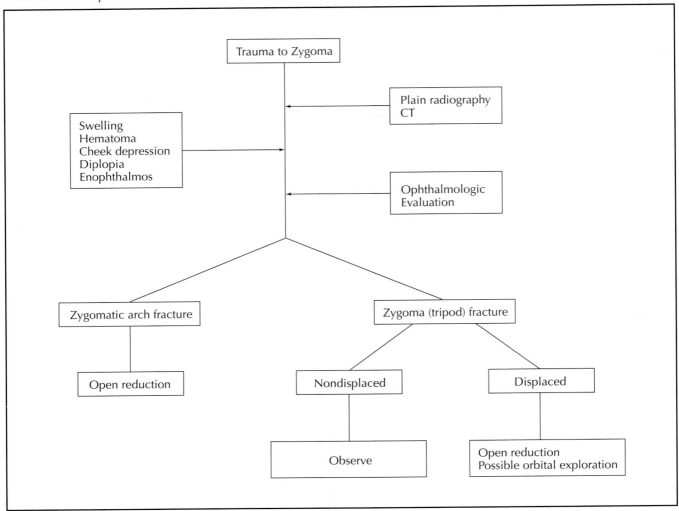

the easiest and most practical approach. In patients with severe intercranial injuries that require a neurosurgical procedure, cranialization is appropriate. In both of these techniques, all mucosa from the frontal sinus needs to be removed by curettage and drilling. The nasofrontal duct should be occluded with fascia. Practice Pathway 29-3 outlines the management of frontal sinus fractures.

Nasoethmoid Complex

CT is the most valuable tool in assessing nasoethmoid fractures (Practice Pathway 29-4). Both axial and coronal cuts are beneficial, although the axial cuts give a better assessment of retrodisplacement of the nasoethmoid complex. The physical examination may provide only minimal information due to severe edema in this region. An intercanthal distance > the length of the palpebral fissure suggests a nasoethmoid injury.

Nasoethmoid complex fractures are best treated with open reduction and rigid fixation through a bicoronal incision, nasal degloving, or an external ethmoidectomy. Nasal degloving should be avoided in the young child. In cases with retrodisplacement, the bicoronal approach is recommended. The goals of treatment are reduction of the retrodisplacement of the nose and restoration of the normal medial

Practice Pathway 29–3   FRONTAL SINUS FRACTURE

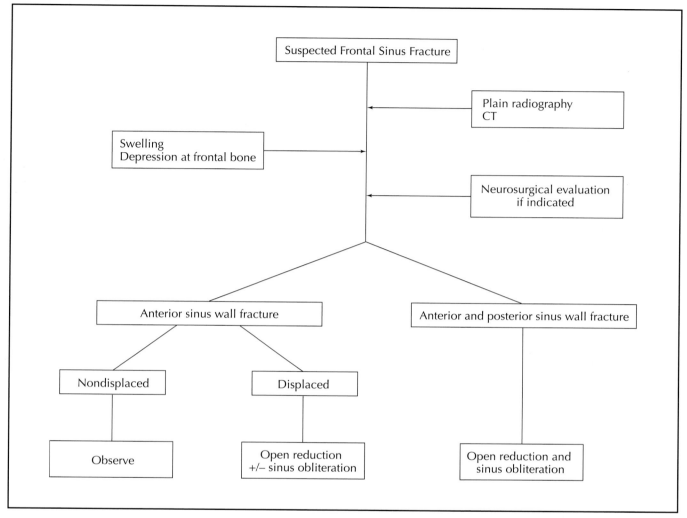

canthal distance. Using distraction forceps, the anterior position of the nasoethmoid complex is displaced anteriorly and secured. A cantilever calvarial bone graft may be used to restore dorsal height primarily or secondarily. The tip of the cantilever graft should be placed deep to the cephalic border of the lower lateral cartilages. To prevent resorption, the cantilever graft should be fixed rigidly to the frontal bone.

The medial canthal tendon typically is attached to a large bony fragment that can be reconstructed using microplates. If the tendon has been completely detached, a transnasal canthopexy can be performed. Stainless steel wire (28 or 30 gauge) may be passed from one canthal tendon to the other for stabilization. This wire is tightened in an effort to overcorrect the deformity, because there may be chronic separation.

Fractures of the Maxilla

Classification

Maxillary fractures in children can be classified using the Le Fort classification system. A *Le Fort I fracture* separates the palate from the maxilla. This horizontally-oriented fracture passes through the pterygoid plate, maxillary sinus, and the floor of the nose. A *Le Fort II fracture* separates the midface (palate and nose subunit) from the cranium with a fracture that extends through the pterygoid plates, lateral and anterior maxillary wall, inferior orbital rim, medial orbital wall nasofrontal suture, and bony septum. A *Le Fort III fracture* separates the entire face from the cranium extending through the pterygoid plates, lateral orbital wall, frontozygomatic suture, medial orbital wall, nasofrontal suture, and bony septum. The Le Fort classification system is

Practice Pathway 29–4   NASOETHMOID COMPLEX

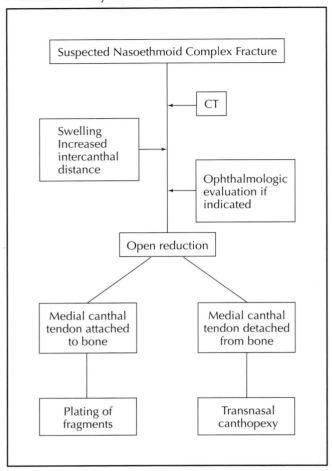

(Practice Pathway 29–5). For fractures with significant displacement, open reduction and rigid fixation through a gingivolabial incision is appropriate. If there are associated mandibular fractures, intermaxillary fixation is also appropriate.

For patients with Le Fort II or III fractures, the airway may be at risk and a tracheotomy appropriate. Le Fort II fractures can be approached through a gingivolabial incision and a transconjunctival or subcillary incision. Stabilization can be provided by intermaxillary fixation. If there is significant displacement, a bicoronal approach should be used to secure the nasofrontal suture rigidly. Le Fort III fractures or comminuted Le Fort II fractures can be approached through bicoronal, transconjunctival, or subcillary and gingivolabial incisions. All are necessary to achieve an appropriate esthetic and functional result. Consistent results can be obtained by establishing dental occlusion first, followed by reduction of the zygomatic complex and midfacial components.

Practice Pathway 29–5   MIDFACIAL FRACTURE

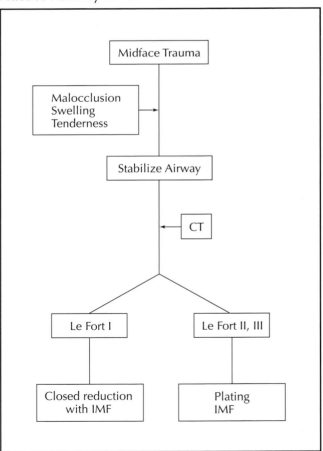

quite simplistic and does not take into account the degree of comminution, which has the highest correlation with ultimate results.

AT A GLANCE . . .

Classification of Fractures of the Maxilla

Le Fort I: separates the palate from the maxilla.

Le Fort II: separates the midface from the cranium.

Le Fort III: separates the entire face from the cranium.

Treatment

In Le Fort I fractures that are minimally displaced, intermaxillary fixation alone may be appropriate

Abbreviations: IMF, Intermaxillary Fixation.

Removal of plates

It is controversial as to whether plates should be removed in a pediatric patient. Experimental evidence has shown that rigid fixation across suture lines inhibits facial growth.[13-15] Additionally, plates placed during craniofacial surgery on a child with a growing brain have later been found intracranially.[30] Experience at the University of California Davis, shows that plates in the pediatric patient can be overgrown completely by bone, presumably through appositional growth. Periosteal stripping also inhibits facial growth.[31] Removing the plates requires a second anesthetic and may require multiple approaches in a complex midfacial fracture. Additionally, a repeat transconjunctival or subciliary approach to the inferior orbital rim may result in an ectropion.

Nasal Bone Fractures

In young children, the profile of the nose is less prominent than that of adolescents and adults, and the nose consists mostly of cartilage that is elastic and able to withstand blows to the face that would otherwise fracture other bony structures. For this reason, although nasal injuries are common in young children, nasal bone fractures are not. As the child matures and the nose projects more from the maxilla, fractures of the nasal bones become more frequent.

If the child is seen immediately following the nasal injury, the assessment for a fracture may be easy. On the other hand, if the evaluation occurs several hours later, swelling may make it difficult to determine the severity of the nasal injury. In either case, examination of a child or an adolescent with a nasal injury should always include the evaluation of surrounding bony structures (especially the orbit) for evidence of other injuries. The nasal dorsum should be examined for deviation of the nasal bones or septal cartilage. Likewise, the nasal bones should be palpated for either a step-off or instability. Examination of the nasal cavities with either an otoscope or a nasal speculum should include evaluation of the septum for either a hematoma or deviation. Evidence of fresh hemorrhage in a nasal cavity or a history of epistaxis suggests a mucosal violation that is strongly suggestive of a nasal fracture. Periorbital ecchymosis should also make the physician highly suspicious that a nasal fracture has occurred. Nasal bone radiographs may be helpful in confirming the diagnosis of a nasal fracture, but may not play an important role in the decision for surgical reduction of the fracture.

Because nasal fractures heal more quickly in children than adults, the evaluation and management of a suspected nasal fracture should not be delayed. Although the occurrence of a septal hematoma is uncommon, every child with a suspected nasal fracture should be evaluated for this complication. Early drainage of a septal hematoma and treatment with antibiotic therapy are necessary to prevent abscess formation or permanent deformity of the septal cartilage. Following a drainage procedure, the nasal cavities should be packed or a through-and-through septal suture placed to prevent recurrence of the hematoma.

> ## SPECIAL CONSIDERATION:
> Because nasal fractures heal more quickly in children than adults, the evaluation and management of a suspected nasal fracture should not be delayed.

Closed reduction of a nasal fracture may be indicated if there is deviation or dislocation of the nasal bones. Although this may be performed acutely, closed reduction typically is delayed for several days following the injury so that the edema has a chance to subside. With the exception of a cooperative adolescent, closed reduction of a nasal fracture in children should be performed under general anesthesia. Oral antibiotic therapy should be considered because of the mucosal violation. Parents should be warned that a closed reduction may not restore the nose completely to its original appearance and that further nasal surgery may be necessary when the child grows older. Because of concerns of altering the cartilage growth centers, nasal surgery in the pediatric age group should be conservative, reserving more complicated cosmetic or septal reconstructive procedures for late adolescence or adulthood.

Practice Pathway 29–6 outlines the management of nasal fractures.

Practice Pathway 29–6   NASAL FRACTURE

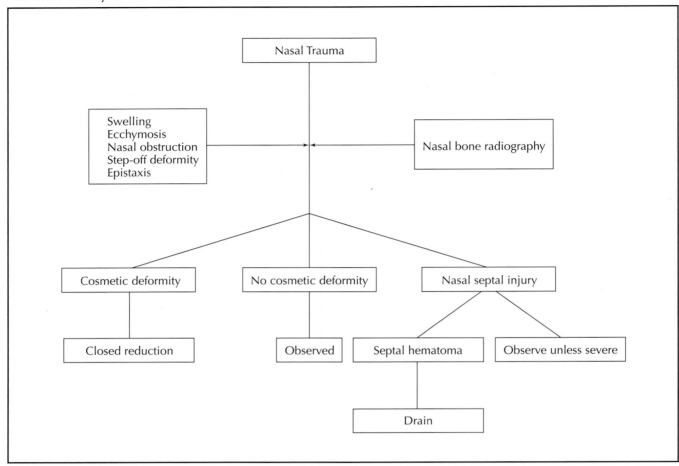

CONCLUSION

Serious maxillofacial injuries to children are relatively rare fortunately. With the continued improvement in restraining devices, the incidence should decrease further. Most mandible fractures can be treated with observation or intermaxillary fixation alone. The need for plating the mandible is unusual. In contrast, most midfacial fractures require rigid fixation to achieve an appropriate esthetic and functional result. Removal of plates remains controversial but is recommended when feasible.

REFERENCES

1. Landis SH, Murray T, Bolden S, et al. Cancer statistics, 1998. CA Cancer J Clin 1998; 48:6–30.
2. Rowe IM, Fonkalsrund EW, O'Neil JA, et al. The injured child. In: *Essentials of Pediatric Surgery.* St. Louis: Mosby, 1995.
3. Shumrick KA, Kersten RC, Kulwin DR, et al. Extended access/internal approaches for the management of facial trauma. Arch Otolaryngol Head Neck Surg 1992; 118:1105–1112.
4. Kelly KS, Manson PN, VanderKolk CA, et al. Sequencing Le Fort fracture treatment (organization of treatment for a panfacial fracture). J Craniofac Surg 1990; 1:168–178.

5. Rahn BA. Theoretical considerations in rigid fixation of facial bones. Clin Plast Surg 1989; 16:21-27.

6. Koltai PH, Rabkin D, Hoehn J. Rigid fixation of facial fractures in children. J Craniomaxillofac Trauma 1995; 1:32-42.

7. Rowe NL. Fractures of the facial skeleton in children. J Oral Surg 1967; 26:505-515.

8. Sherick DG, Buckman SR, Patel PP. Pediatric facial fractures: A demographic analysis outside an urban environment. Annf Plast Surg 1997; 38:578-84.

9. Thoren H, Iizuka T, Hallikainen D, et al. Different patterns of mandibular fractures in children. An analysis of 220 fractures in 157 patients. J Craniomaxillofac Surg 1992; 20:292-296.

10. Posnic JC, Wells M, Pron GE. Pediatric facial fractures: Evolving patterns of treatment. J Oral Maxillofac Surg 1993; 51:836-844.

11. Kallman RM, Schilli W. Plate fixation of fractures of the mid and upper face. Otolaryngol Clin North Am 1987; 20:559-572.

12. Koltai PJ, Rabkin D. Management of facial trauma in children. Pediatr Clin North Am 1966; 43: 1253-1275.

13. Eppley BL, Platis JM, Sadoue MA. Experimental effects of bone plating in infancy on craniomaxillofacial skeletal growth. Cleft Palate Craniofac J 1993; 30:164-169.

14. Yaremchuk MJ, Fiala TGS, Barker F, et al. The effects of rigid fixation on craniofacial growth of rhesus monkeys. Plast Reconstr Surg 1994; 93:1-10.

15. Wong L, Richtsmeier JT, Manson PM. Craniofacial growth following rigid fixation: Suture excision, miniplating, and microplating. J Craniomaxillofac Surg 1993; 4:234-245.

16. Hellquist R. Facial skeleton growth after periosteal resection. Scand J Plast Reconstr Surg Hand Surg Suppl 1972; 10:1-98.

17. Crocket DM, Hungo RP, Thompson RE. Maxillofacial trauma. Pediatr Clin North Am 1989; 36:1471-1494.

18. Gruss JS. Naso-ethmoid-orbital fractures: Classification and role of primary bone grafting. Plast Reconstr Surg 1985; 75:303-315.

19. Koltai PH, Wood GW. Three dimensional CT reconstruction for the evaluation and surgical planning of facial fracures. Otolaryngol Head Neck Surg 1986; 95:10-15.

20. Yasargil MG, Reichman MV, Kubik S. Preservation of the frontotemporal branch of the facial nerve using the interfascial temporalis flap for pterional craniotomy. J Neurosurg 1987; 67:463-446.

21. Tessier P. The conjunctival approach to the orbital floor and maxilla in congenital malformation and trauma. J Maxillofac Surg 1973; 1:3-7.

22. Lynch D, Lamp JC, Royster HP. The conjunctival approach for exploration of the orbital complex fractures. Plast Reconstr Surg 1974; 54:153-157.

23. Manson PN, Ruas E, Iliff N, et al. Single eyelid incision for exposure of the zygomatic bone and orbital reconstruction. Plast Reconstr Surg 1987; 79:120-126.

24. Dierks EJ. Transoral approach to fractures of the mandible. Laryngoscope 1987; 97:4-6.

25. Raveh J, Vuillemin T, Ladrach K, et al. Plate osteosynthesis of 367 mandibular fractures: The unrestructed indication for intraoral approach. J Craniomaxillofac Surg 1987; 15:244-253.

26. Norholt S, Krishnan V, Pedersen S, et al. Pediatric condylar fractures: A long term follow-up study of 55 patients. J Oral Maxillofac Surg 1993; 51:1302-1310.

27. MacArthur CJ, Donald PH, Knowles J, et al. Open reduction-fixation of mandibular fractures. A review. Arch Otolaryngol Head Neck Surg 1993; 119: 403-406.

28. Wallis A, Donald PJ. Frontal sinus fractures: A review of 72 cases. Laryngoscope 1988; 98:593-598.

29. Sykes J, Donald PJ. Frontal and nasoethmoid fractures. In: Papel ID, Nachlas N, eds. *Facial Plastic and Reconstructive Surgery*. St. Louis: Mosby Yearbook, 1992.

30. John Phillips, M.D., Department of Plastic Surgery, Hospital for Sick Children, Toronto, Canada. Personal communication.

31. Laurenzo JF, Canady JW, Zimmerman B, et al. Craniofacial growth in rabbits: Effects of midfacial surgical trauma and rigid plate fixation. Arch Otolaryngol Head Neck Surg 1995; 121:556-561.

30 Neoplasms of the Midface and Anterior Skull Base

Trevor J. McGill and Reza Rahbar

Tumors of the midface & nasopharynx were often considered inoperable because of the anatomical complexity of the structures of the skull base. However, with the advent of improved techniques in craniofacial and reconstructive surgery, a combined intracranial/extracranial approach with block removal of tumors is now possible. (Table 30–1) Immediate reconstruction with free tissue transfer using microvascular techniques may prevent sacrificing function and cosmesis. Certain important naturally occurring foramina and fissures are present within the anterior skull base which provide a conduit for tumor growth through the cranial base into the anterior and middle cranial fossa. Thus, an angio-

fibroma originating in the nasal cavity may extend through the superior orbital fissure to gain access to the middle cranial fossa.

RADIOLOGICAL IMAGING

High-resolution contrast-enhanced computed tomography (CT) and gadolinium-enhanced magnetic resonance imaging (MRI) are invaluable in defining tumors of the skull base prior to biopsy and possible surgical resection. Rhabdomyosarcoma and other small round cell neoplasms are hyper-cellular and often form large soft tissue masses that infiltrate along tissue planes, destroying bone in a predictable fashion. These tumors often appear as high density on CT scan and frequently enhance after intravenous contrast. CT is superior in detecting bone destruction, intracranial extension and vascular content of the tumor. MRI is superior at detecting soft tissue invasion and dural or brain involvement. Catheter angiography is the definitive modality for endovascular interventional therapy, especially when preoperative embolization of skull base tumors such as juvenile angiofibroma, is required.

PARAMENINGEAL RHABDOMYOSARCOMA

Rhabdomyosarcoma is the most common malignant soft tissue tumor of the head and neck in children. These tumors can occur at any anatomical site but are found most often in the head and neck (40%).[1] Rhabdomyosarcoma is a highly malignant tumor that spreads by both local extension and lymphatic and hematogenous dissemination. Like other round cell malignancies of childhood (neuroblastoma, Ew-

---

AT A GLANCE . . .

Anterior Skull Base Tumors

- Angiofibroma
- Osteoma
- Craniopharyngioma
- Olfactory Neuroblastoma
- Chordoma
- Chondrosarcoma
- Rhabdomyosarcoma
  - Embryonal
  - Alveolar
  - Undifferentiated
- Nasopharyngeal Carcinoma
  - Squamous Cell Carcinoma
  - Nonkeratinizing Carcinoma
    - A. Differentiated Nonkeratinizing Carcinoma
    - B. Undifferentiated Carcinoma

Pediatric Otolaryngology, Edited by R.F. Wetmore, H.R. Muntz, and T.J. McGill. Thieme Medical Publishers, Inc., New York © 2000.

TABLE 30–1:   Approaches to Skull Base

1. Infratemporal fossa approach
2. Transparotid temporal bone approach
3. Trans-palatal approach
4. Facial translocation approach

ing's sarcoma, primitive neuroectodermal tumors-PNET), these hypercellular tumors present as a painless mass lesion. Orbital tumors are the most common, but rhabdomyosarcoma may arise in such parameningeal sites as the nasopharynx, the nasal cavity, middle ear, mastoid, paranasal sinuses and the pterygopalatine and infratemporal fossae. These parameningeal tumors are at risk for central nervous system (CNS) extension and are associated with a poor prognosis.

SPECIAL CONSIDERATION:

Rhabdomyosarcoma is the most common malignant soft tissue tumor of the head and neck in children.

Clinical Presentation

Tumors of the anterior skull base present with symptoms that suggest involvement of surrounding structures such as the orbit or the nasal cavity. Destruction of the anterior skull base by tumors rarely produces pain. Thus the presenting clinical features may include nasal obstruction, epistaxis, proptosis, unilateral serous otitis media and symptoms of cranial nerve dysfunction.

Clinical Evaluation

A complete head and neck examination is performed, and imaging studies include CT and MRI of the primary site. All patients require histological confirmation of rhabdomyosarcoma by either a biopsy or partial or complete excision. If a frozen section is suggestive of soft tissue sarcoma, a bone marrow aspiration should be performed at the time of surgery. Further investigation includes CT of the chest with contrast, bone scan, liver and spleen scan and laboratory studies such as a CBC, platelet count, liver function studies, calcium, phosphate, serum protein analysis and CSF cytology. Immunohistochemical staining is a useful and reliable way of iden-

tifying skeletal muscle specific proteins or genes.[2] Thus, a positive staining with antibodies for actin and desmin is considered sufficient to confirm the diagnosis of embryonal rhabdomyosarcoma. Further investigation may include cytogenetic studies which have shown these small round cell tumors to have specific chromosomal abnormalities that can be useful in confirming the diagnosis and understanding their tumor biology.[4–7]

Treatment

Patients with parameningeal rhabdomyosarcoma are presumed to have metastatic disease at the time of diagnosis. Treatment includes control of the primary site and eradicating metastases. Surgery and radiation are the principle options for managing the primary site and multi-agent chemotherapy is administered to all patients.

Chemotherapy

Chemotherapy consists of vincristine (1.5 mg/M^2), actinomycin D (0.015 mg/kg per day) and cyclophosphamide (2.2G/M^2) (VAC). Radiation therapy is the primary mode for controlling local disease such as parameningeal rhabdomyosarcoma. With high-risk patients, such as those having cranial nerve involvement, extensive bone erosion and cytologically positive CSF, radiation treatment is started at the induction of the chemotherapy protocol.[8,9] Major complications of radiation therapy include arrested facial growth and radiation-induced tumors.

Surgery

The initial role of the surgeon in the management of rhabdomyosarcoma is to make the diagnosis by obtaining a biopsy. Primary control of a parameningeal rhabdomyosarcoma is rarely achieved with surgery. Thus patients with parameningeal rhabdomyosarcomas are treated with combination chemotherapy and local radiation. If patients have residual disease following 12 months of treatment, surgery may be a consideration in the management of this residual disease.

SPECIAL CONSIDERATION:

The role of surgery in the treatment of rhabdomyosarcoma is biopsy, surgical salvage and in some cases, primary resection.

Increasing sophistication in skull base surgery and reconstruction with free tissue transfer using microvascular techniques has renewed interest in surgical excision as the primary mode of therapy for parameningeal lesions.[10,11] The infratemporal fossa approach for lateral skull base lesions allows the surgeon control over major neurovascular structures and provides exposure for the resection of tumor involving the skull base, meninges and brain (see Chapter 5).

AT A GLANCE . . .

Rhabdomyosarcoma

- Location: orbit, nasopharynx, temporal bone, paranasal sinuses, or pterygopalatine and infratemporal fossae
- Signs and symptoms: nasal obstruction, epistaxis, proptosis, unilateral serous otitis media, symptoms of cranial nerve dysfunction
- Metastatic evaluation: CT of chest, CBC and platelet count, liver function tests, calcium, phosphate, serum protein analysis, CSF cytology
- Treatment: chemotherapy, surgery

ANGIOFIBROMA OF THE NOSE AND CONTIGUOUS AREAS

Angiofibroma is a benign vasoformative tumor occurring almost exclusively in adolescent males (Fig. 30-1). Originally, it was thought that this tumor originated from embryonic cartilage trapped between the basiocciput and sphenoid bones. Current opinion, based upon clinical examination and CT imaging, suggests that this tumor arises in a broad-based fashion from the postero-lateral wall of the nasal cavity surrounding the sphenopalatine foramen.

Grossly these neoplasms appear as circumscribed, bosselated, non-encapsulated tumors covered by mucosa. The gross appearance of the excised tumor is that of a firm nodular pale mass traversed by large submucosal blood vessels (Fig. 30-2). Lesions are deceptively avascular on gross inspection.

Histologically, an angiofibroma consists of two primary components, vascular and stromal ele-

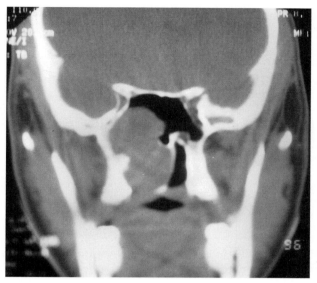

Figure 30–1: Coronal view of an angiofibroma of the nasopharynx with extension into the sphenoid sinus and destruction of the right medial pterygoid plate.

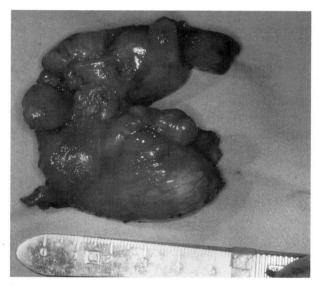

Figure 30–2: Complete specimen of angiofibroma removed intact. Note the numerous extensions into the foramina in the anterior skull base.

ments. Within the fibrous stroma there are characteristic irregular slit-like vascular channels with a ''staghorn'' appearance. These vascular channels are distributed uniformly throughout the tumor, lack contractile elements and are responsible for the tumor's capacity for massive hemorrhage following injudicious manipulation or biopsy. The origin of this tumor is important, as it helps to predict tumor growth and directs the surgical approach for tumor excision.[12-14] The specific point of origin is at the superior margin of the sphenopalatine foramen.

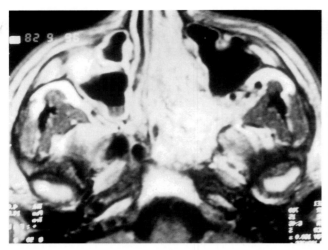

Figure 30–3: Axial view of MRI showing angiofibroma with lateral extension through the spheno-palatine foramen.

From this location the tumor may extend: (1) posteriorly into the nasopharynx; (2) anteriorly extension into the nasal cavity; and (3) laterally through the pterygopalatine fissure into the pterygomaxillary fossa along pathways of least resistance (Fig. 30–3). From the infratemporal fossa the tumor may extend anteriorly and cause bony erosion of the posterior wall of the maxillary sinus. Extension into the sphenoid, maxillary and ethmoidal sinuses, orbit, middle cranial fossa, and parasellar region is common. Session proposed staging of angiofibroma by CT as shown in Table 30–2.[12]

Clinical Presentation

The presenting features of an angiofibroma are the result of nasal obstruction. Epistaxis is the other major presenting symptom. Due to the presence of periodic nosebleeds in the population, the significance of intermittent epistaxis is often overlooked.[15] Other clinical features include hyponasal speech, facial swelling, proptosis with diplopia and/or visual field defects. Usually the symptoms have been present for 6 to 12 months before a definitive diagnosis is established.

TABLE 30–2: Staging of Angiofibroma

1A: Nose or nasopharynx
 B: Paranasal sinus
2A: Sphenopalatine foramen
 B: Pterygomaxillary fossa
 C: Infratemporal fossa
3A: Intracranial extension

Examination of the nasal cavity and nasopharynx typically reveals an ulcerated vascular lesion in the posterior nasal cavity and nasopharynx. The surface of the lesion is traversed by prominent submucosal blood vessels. Epistaxis results from the combination of local stasis, infection and superficial erosion of the mucosa over the anterior edge of the tumor. Tumor extension may enter the skull through the roof of the infratemporal fossa or via the superior orbital fissure. With intracranial extension the tumor comes to lie lateral to the cavernous sinus and anterolateral to the internal carotid artery. Tumor spread through the superior orbital fissure may result in extension into the cavernous sinus itself. These patients present with proptosis and classic signs of superior orbital fissure syndrome. Intracranial extension is usually extradural without penetration into the brain substance; however, large intracranial tumors may become adherent to the dura making surgical resection difficult. Angiofibromas do not invade the skull base by cellular infiltration, as do malignant carcinomas, but rather lead to local bone destruction through relentless expansion.

SPECIAL CONSIDERATION:

Angiofibromas do not invade the skull base by cellular infiltration, as do malignant carcinomas, but rather lead to local bone destruction through relentless expansion.

Radiological Evaluation

Computed tomography and MRI are essential in the preoperative evaluation of these tumors. CT is the best method for demonstrating the exact location and extension of tumor into the skull base. On CT these tumors are high density masses that enhance markedly; bony expansion and erosion of the skull base are commonly seen. In most cases the pterygopalatine fossa is widened, and there is anterior bowing of the posterior wall of the maxillary sinus. Extension into the paranasal sinuses, middle cranial fossa and parasellar region is common. The MRI characteristics depend upon the relative combination of vascular fibrous components and tissue edema. Contrast-enhanced T1 weighted MRI shows marked enhancement of the mass with multiple flow-related signal voids. Enhanced CT and MRI allow the surgeon to accurately stage the lesion and plan the surgical approach. Cases of angiofibroma do not require a biopsy prior to definitive resection.

Treatment

Surgical excision is considered the treatment of choice, reserving radiation therapy for intracranial tumors. Radiation therapy as a primary modality has been used in the past with some success; however, this method of treatment also raises the possibility of development of a radiation-induced tumor within the radiation field.

The surgical approach for excision of an angiofibroma provides exposure of the nasal cavity, nasopharynx, paranasal sinuses, pterygopalatine region, infratemporal fossa and skull base. The transpalatal approach has been used extensively in the past for Stage I disease. This surgical approach limits the visualization of the superolateral margin areas of the tumor and in the past may have contributed to recurrence of some tumors. A lateral rhinotomy with medial maxillectomy, ethmoidectomy and sphenoidotomy is an excellent surgical exposure for a patient with extensive Stage II disease. This incision allows excellent surgical exposure for complete removal of an extensive angiofibroma and may be combined with a lip-splitting incision to give additional lateral exposure when necessary.

In the past decade, a midfacial degloving technique has become the approach of choice for surgical resection of most tumors (Fig. 30-4). The use of intranasal and sublabial incisions avoids a facial scar while maintaining excellent surgical exposure. In larger lesions, bilateral LeFort osteotomies with a palatal drop facilitate tumor removal.[16] A medial maxillectomy and ethmoidectomy greatly enhance tumor exposure, especially in the region of the skull base. A subperiosteal elevation of the lacrimal sac and exposure of the lamina papyracea allows lateral retraction of the eye, a medial maxillectomy and ethmoidectomy. Tumor invasion of the pterygopalatine and infratemporal fossae require removal of the posterior wall of the maxillary sinus (Fig. 30-5). After exposure, the tumor should be removed as a single pedunculated vascular mass. Starting superiorly the tumor can be peeled off the endostial dura of the anterior cranial fossa. By proceeding posteriorly, tumor in the sphenoid sinus can be delivered into the nasopharynx.

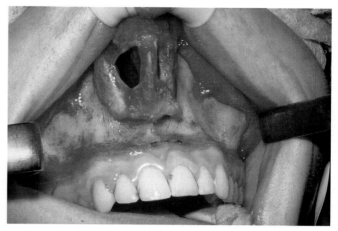

Figure 30–4:   Degloving approach to tumors of the nasopharynx.

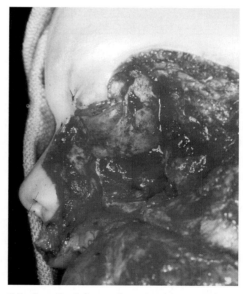

Figure 30–5:   Facial translocation approach to anterior and lateral skull base.

> ## Special Consideration:
> Midfacial degloving technique has become the procedure of choice for surgical resection of most angiofibromas.

Management of angiofibroma with intracranial extension remains controversial, despite improvements in neurosurgical technique and reduction of postoperative morbidity.[17] Skull erosion without extensive intracranial spread may not necessitate an extensive craniofacial resection. Radiation therapy is reserved for extensive intracranial extension.

AT A GLANCE . . .
Juvenile Angiofibroma

- Location: nasal cavity, nasopharynx, paranasal sinuses, orbit, middle cranial fossa
- Signs and symptoms: nasal obstruction, epistaxis, hyponasal speech, facial swelling, proptosis with diplopia/visual field defects
- Treatment: surgical excision

NASOPHARYNGEAL CARCINOMA

Nasopharyngeal carcinoma (NPC) is perhaps the most commonly misdiagnosed tumor of the head and neck.[18] NPC accounts for about 0.25% of all cancers in North America; however, it accounts for 18% of malignancies among the Chinese. Genetic susceptibility in Chinese patients has been observed in the presence of HLA-A2 and HLA-B-Sin2 loci. Consumption of nitrosamine-rich salted fish in childhood and exposure to smoke or dust inhalants also contribute to the high risk in southern Chinese.

Other etiologic factors for NPC include chronic nasal and sinus infections, exposure to Epstein Barr virus (EBV), poor hygiene and inadequate ventilation. The presence of an anti-EBV antibody profile and presence of EBV in the epithelial tumor cells support an association of EBV with NPC. Although a cause and effect relationship has not been proven, elevated EBV titers usually correlate with tumor burden and decrease with successful therapy.[19]

NPC may occur at any age; the mean age at diagnosis is 51 years. Occurring mainly in the adolescent age group, NPC accounts for one-third of nasopharyngeal neoplasms of childhood.[20] There is no sex predilection in children, but there is an increased incidence among black teenagers.[21]

Clinical Presentation

The clinical presentation of all histopathologic types of NPC is similar. Symptoms and signs include the appearance of a neck mass, hearing loss, nasal obstruction, nasal discharge, epistaxis, headache, otalgia and cranial neuropathy. Presenting signs and

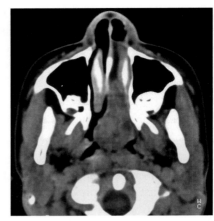

Figure 30–6: Axial CT scan of a patient with nasopharyngeal carcinoma.

symptoms are often subtle and nonspecific, leading to delay in diagnosis and frequent presentation with advanced disease. This late diagnosis often accounts for the poor prognosis.

A neck mass and hearing loss are the most common presenting signs. Cervical metastatic disease is common because the epithelium of the nasopharynx has a rich network of lymphatic channels which communicate freely across the midline, occasionally leading to bilateral cervical metastasis. The superior deep cervical lymph nodes ipsilateral to the primary site are affected first.

Tumor involvement of the lateral nasopharyngeal wall and the fossa of Rosenmuller causes eustachian tube dysfunction, serous otitis media and conductive hearing loss (Fig. 30–6). Obstruction of the choanae results in nasal congestion and chronic rhinorrhea. Epistaxis may also occur. Cranial nerve palsies and headache suggest skull base involvement, mainly through the foramen lacerum. The sixth cranial nerve is the first to become involved, leading to diplopia. Extension of disease at the skull base leads to involvement of cranial nerves III, IV, and V. Tumor in the proximity of jugular foramen may affect cranial nerves IX, X, XI, and XII.

Histopathology

NPC can be divided into different categories on the basis of the predominant histologic type. In 1978, the World Health Organization (WHO) grouped NPC into three histologic types: Type I (squamous cell carcinoma), Type II (non-keratinizing carcinoma), and Type III (undifferentiated).

WHO Type II and III tumors have a great degree of tumor pleomorphism with microscopic patterns such as spindle cell, transitional cell, lymphoepithelioma, clear cell and others. Also, their epidemiological relationship to EBV is similar. For this reason, a new classification of these tumors in 1991 is based on the presence or absence of squamous cell differentiation, namely squamous cell carcinoma and non-keratinizing carcinoma. The latter type is further subclassified into differentiated carcinoma and undifferentiated carcinoma.[22]

Diagnostic Evaluation (see Practice Pathway 30-1)

The diagnosis of NPC requires a complete physical examination. In suspected cases, the evaluation of the nasopharynx should be made with direct flexible or rigid fiberoptic examination. The gross appearance of NPC varies from a totally unidentifiable lesion to a mucosal bulge with intact epithelium to a clearly demonstrable mass with extensive involvement of the surface epithelium.

CT is valuable in evaluating parapharyngeal, retropharyngeal and skull base tumors. MRI with gadolinium is the best technique to evaluate skull base invasion, that is seen in approximately 25% of cases.[23]

Practice Pathway 30–1   NASOPHARYNGEAL CARCINOMA

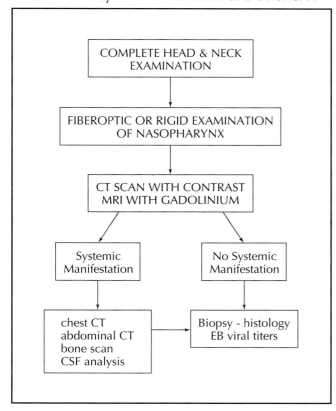

The final diagnosis is based upon the results of the biopsy.

Metastatic evaluation should include CT of the chest and abdomen and radionuclide bone scanning. Hematogenous metastases to bone and liver are the most common presentation. If there is invasion of the skull base, examination of the cerebrospinal fluid should be performed.

Immunology

Specific Epstein-Barr viral markers can be helpful in the diagnosis and clinical management of the NPC patient. Most commonly used laboratory markers are listed in Table 30–3. The precise role of the virus or cytogenetic abnormality in the pathogenesis of NPC remains unclear.

Management

Super-voltage irradiation continues to be the main treatment modality of NPC. The primary tumor and the first echelon of lymph nodes are included in the radiation field. Depending upon the extent of tumor, the radiation dosage ranges from 6500 cGy to 7000 cGy. Prophylactic radiation of the lower cervical and supraclavicular lymph nodes has shown some benefits in preventing extension of the disease.

NPC has traditionally been considered non-resectable based on its anatomic location. Radical neck dissection is seldom necessary.[24] With recent advances in craniofacial surgical technique, this is no longer true. Surgical resection of the skull base for residual or recurrent disease may be of value in selected cases (see Table 30–1).

Adjuvant chemotherapy is required in patients with disseminated systemic disease. Almost all NPC in children and adolescents is of the undifferentiated type and typically presents in stage III or IV. The overall 5-year survival of children with NPC approaches 40%.[25]

TABLE 30–3:   Epstein-Barr Viral Markers for Nasopharyngeal Carcinoma

1. Viral Cuspid Antigen (VCA)	IgA	Antibodies
	IgG	Antibodies
2. Early Antigen (EA)	IgG	Antibodies
3. Antibody-Dependent Cellular Cytotoxicity (ADCC)*		

* Prognostic indicator (not commercially available)

AT A GLANCE . . .

Nasopharyngeal Carcinoma

- Risk factors: genetic factors, consumption of nitrosamine-rich salted fish, exposure to smoke or dust inhalants, chronic nasal and sinus infections, exposure to Epstein-Barr virus, poor hygiene, inadequate ventilation

- Signs and symptoms: neck mass, nasal obstruction/discharge, hearing loss, epistaxis, headache, otalgia, cranial neuropathies

- Treatment: super-voltage irradiation, cervical node biopsy, Salvage surgery, adjuvant chemotherapy

REFERENCES

1. Robinson LI. General principles of the epidemiology of childhood cancer, In Pizzo, PA, Poplack DG (eds): *Principles and Practices of Pediatric Oncology,* 2nd Ed. Philadelphia, JB Lippincott Co, 1993.

2. Parham DM, Webber B, Holt H, et al. Immunohistochemical study of childhood rhabdomyosarcomas and related neoplasms: Results of an Intergroup Rhabdomyosarcoma Study Project. Cancer 1991; 67: 3072-3080.

3. Dodd S, Malone M, McCullough W. Rhabdomyosarcoma in children: A histological and immunological study of 59 cases. J Pathol 1989; 158:13-18.

4. Turc-Carel C, Lizard-Nacol S, Justrabo E, et al. Consistent chromosomal translocation in alveolar rhabdomyosarcoma. Cancer Genet Cytogenet 1986; 361-362.

5. Douglas EC, Valentine M, Etcubanas E, et al. A specific chromosomal abnormality in rhabdomyosarcoma. Cytogenet Cell Genet 1987; 45:148-155.

6. Barr FG, Galili N, Holick J, et al. Rearrangement of the PAX3 paired box gene in the paediatric solid tumour alveolar rhabdomyosarcoma. Nat Genet 1993; 3:113-117.

7. Davis RJ, D'Cruz CM, Lovell MA, et al. Fusion of PAX7 in FKHR by the variant t(1^w)(p36,4) translocation in alveolar rhabdomyosarcoma. Cancer Res 1994; 54: 2869-2872.

8. Pappo AS: Rhabdomyosarcoma and other soft tissue sarcomas of childhood. Curr Opin Oncol 1994; 6: 397-402.

9. Crist W, Gehan E, Ragab A, et al. The third intergroup Rhabdomyosarcoma Study: J Clin Oncol 1995; 13: 610-630.

10. McGill T. Rhabdomyosarcoma of the head and neck: an update. Otolaryngol Clin North Am 1989; 22: 631-636.

11. Healy GB, Upton L, Black PM et al. The role of surgery in rhabdomyosarcoma of the head and neck in children. Arch Otolaryng Head Neck Surg 1991; 117: 1185-1187.

12. Sessions RB, Bryan RN, Naclerio RM, et al. Radiographic staging of juvenile angiofibroma. Head Neck Surg. 1981; 3:279-283.

13. Neel HB, Whicker JH, Devine KD, et al. Juvenile angiofibroma: Review of 120 cases. Am J Surg 1973; 126:547-556.

14. Krekorian EA, Kato R: Surgical management of nasopharyngeal angiofibroma with intracranial extension. Laryngoscope 1977; 87:154-164.

15. Andrews JC, Fisch U, Valavanis A, et al. The surgical management of extensive nasopharyngeal angiofibroma with the infratemporal fossa approach. Laryngoscope 1989; 99:429-437.

16. Radkowski D, McGill TJ, Healy GB, et al. Angiofibroma: Changes in staging and treatment. Arch Otol-HNS 1996; 122(2):122-129.

17. Jones GC, DeSanto LW, Bremer JW, et al. Juvenile angiofibroma: Behavior and treatment of extensive and residual tumors. Arch Otolaryngol Head Neck Surg 1986; 112:1191-1193.

18. Scanlon PW, Devine KO, Woolner LB. Malignant lesions of the nasopharynx. Ann Otol Rhinol Laryngol 1958; 67:1005-1021.

19. Pearson G, Weiland L, Neel H, et al. Application of Epstein-Barr(EBV) serology to the diagnosis of North American nasopharyngeal carcinoma. Cancer 1983; 51:260-268.

20. Jaffe B, Jaffe N. Head and neck tumors in children. Pediatrics 1973; 51:731-740.

21. Easton JM, Levine PH, Hyams VJ: Nasopharyngeal carcinoma in the United States: a pathologic study of 177 US and 30 foreign cases. Arch Otolaryngol 1980; 106:88-91.

22. Shanmugaratnam K, Sobin L. Histological typing of tumors of the upper respiratory tract and ear. In: *International Histological Classification of Tumors,* 2nd edition. Heidelberg: Springer-Verlag, 1991.

23. Neel HB III, Taylor WF. New staging system for nasopharyngeal carcinoma: long-term outcome. Arch Otolaryng Head & Neck Surg 1989; 115:1293.

24. Dickson RI, Nasopharyngeal carcinoma: an evaluation of 209 patients, Laryngoscope 1981; 91: 333-354.

25. Baker SR, McClatchy K: Carcinomas of the nasopharynx in childhood. Otolaryng Head Neck Surg 1981; 89:555.

IV

THE ORAL CAVITY, PHARYNX, AND ESOPHAGUS

31 Structure and Function of the Oral Cavity, Pharynx, and Esophagus

Jeffrey L. Keller and Philip T. Ho

The *upper aerodigestive tract* (UADT) serves as a common pathway for the respiratory and digestive systems. Because these two systems are closely related anatomically and physiologically, precise coordination is required to allow these distinct systems to function in tandem. The unique anatomic and physiologic relationships of the oral cavity, pharynx, and esophagus are described in this chapter.

EMBRYOLOGY AND ANATOMY OF THE ORAL CAVITY

The *oral cavity* is comprised of a small outer portion, called the *vestibule,* and a large inner portion, called the *oral cavity proper.* The two are separated by the intervening alveolar ridge and teeth. The oral cavity is bounded by the lips anteriorly, the cheeks laterally, and the hard and soft palates superiorly. Its posterior boundary is an imaginary line drawn between the circumvallate papillae of the tongue and the junction of the hard and soft palates above. The embryology of the oral cavity is described with each of its component structures below.

The Lips

The *upper lip* is formed as the medial frontonasal and lateral maxillary prominences merge during weeks 6 to 8 of fetal development. Migrating, second-branchial-arch mesoderm supplies additional tissues important to the normal formation of the

upper lip. The *lower lip* is formed as the mandibular prominences merge during the fourth week of development.

The lips are comprised of the *orbicularis oris muscle,* which is surrounded by skin externally and a mucous membrane internally. The orbicularis oris muscle forms a sphincter that encircles the entire oral aperture. Numerous facial muscles insert into the orbicularis oris and contribute to the maintenance of oral competence and to facial expression. The lip extends anteriorly to the *vermilion border,* which is the junction of the lip with skin, and posteriorly to the mucous membrane of the gingivae. In the median plane, raised folds of mucous membrane, called the *labial frenula,* can be identified.

Motor innervation to the lips is supplied by branches of the facial nerve; the buccal branch innervates the upper lip, and the marginal mandibular branch innervates the lower lip. The sensory innervation of the upper lip is supplied by the *infraorbital nerve,* which is a branch of the maxillary division of the trigeminal nerve, and the lower lip is supplied by the *mental nerve,* which is a branch of the mandibular division of the trigeminal nerve.

The Cheek

The lateral wall of the oral cavity is formed by the *buccinator muscle.* The *buccal fat pad,* which may be especially prominent in children, lies between the buccinator fascia and the skin. The *buccinator fascia* is continuous with the buccopharyngeal fascia that overlies the pharyngeal musculature.

Motor innervation to the buccinator muscle is supplied by the buccal branch of the facial nerve, and sensory innervation is supplied by the second and third divisions of the trigeminal nerve.

Pediatric Otolaryngology, Edited by R.F. Wetmore, H.R. Muntz, and T.J. McGill. Thieme Medical Publishers, Inc., New York © 2000.

The Salivary Glands

The *major salivary glands* include the parotid, submandibular, and sublingual glands. These paired exocrine glands develop from stomadeal ectoderm by ingrowth of oral epithelium into the underlying mesenchyme beginning at about 6 weeks of embryologic development.

The parotid glands

The *parotid glands* are the largest of the major salivary glands and are comprised predominantly of serous-secreting cells. The parotid gland is located anteriorly and inferiorly to the auricle with a posterior extension in the subcutaneous layer, which covers the anterior portion of the sternocleidomastoid muscle. The gland extends anteriorly to overlap the masseter muscle. A component of the parotid also lies medially to the ramus of the mandible. The parotid is divided into superficial and deep lobes by the facial nerve. The parotid duct, or *Stensen's duct*, originates at the anterior border of the parotid gland, travels approximately 1.5 cm inferior to the zygoma, passes across the masseter, and pierces the buccinator muscle to enter the oral cavity opposite the upper second molar.

Blood supply to the parotid gland is through the *transverse facial artery,* which is a branch of the superficial temporal artery.

Postganglionic parasympathetic fibers from the otic ganglion travel through the auriculotemporal branch of the fifth cranial nerve to stimulate salivary secretions from the parotid gland.

The submandibular glands

The *submandibular glands* are the second largest of the major salivary glands and are comprised of mucous and serous-secreting cells. The submandibular glands arise near the midline of the floor of mouth and migrate laterally to the *submandibular triangle,* which is an area bounded by the inferior border of the mandible and the anterior and posterior bellies of the digastric muscle. A portion of the gland wraps around the deep surface of the *mylohyoid muscle,* which separates the superficial and deep lobes. The submandibular duct, or *Wharton's duct,* exits from the medial surface of the gland, crosses the floor of the mouth between the mylohyoid and hyoglossus muscles, and empties into the sublingual papillae lateral to the lingual frenulum.

The submandibular glands receive their blood supply from the facial artery, and their parasympa-

thetic innervation from the facial nerve. The preganglionic fibers leave the facial nerve through the chorda tympani, join the lingual nerve, and synapse in the submandibular ganglion. Postganglionic fibers provide stimulation to the submandibular glands.

The sublingual glands

The *sublingual glands* are the smallest of the major salivary glands and contain mucous-secreting cells. These glands develop as groups of cell buds from multiple ducts that open directly into the floor of mouth. The paired sublingual glands rest on the superficial surface of the mylohoid muscle between the hyoglossus muscle and the mandible. Approximately 12 ducts (i.e., *ducts of Rivinus*) pass from the superior border of the glands to empty into the floor of mouth. The anterior sublingual ducts sometimes unite to form a major sublingual duct, which empties into the sublingual caruncle.

Both the lingual and facial arteries provide blood supply to the sublingual glands. Parasympathetic innervation is similar to that described for the submandibular glands. Sympathetic fibers from the superior cervical ganglion are thought to supply the salivary glands as well, although their exact role remains unclear.

The Tongue

The *tongue* first appears at approximately 4 weeks gestation in the floor of the pharynx. In its earliest stage, the anterior tongue arises as two paired oval masses, known as the *lingual swellings,* and one median triangular mass, known as the *tuberculum impar.* These lateral lingual swellings grow and eventually fuse in the midline to form the anterior two-thirds of the tongue. The posterior one-third of the tongue is formed by an extensive linear swelling caudal to the tuberculum impar referred to as the *hypobranchial eminence.* In addition, third-arch mesoderm merges with the hypobranchial eminence to form the remainder of the posterior one-third of the tongue. In the process, the tuberculum impar becomes submerged by the migration and growth of tissue. The hypobranchial eminence also develops a horizontal groove, thus creating an anterior component that contributes to the posterior tongue and a posterior component that forms the epiglottis.

The division between the anterior two-thirds and the posterior one-third of the tongue corresponds to the circumvallate papillae, which forms a V shaped line. The amalgamation of the different arch structures that form the tongue accounts for its pattern of innervation. The lingual swellings are a first-arch derivative, and accordingly receive sensory innervation from the nerve of the first arch (i.e., the mandibular branch of the trigeminal [lingual] nerve). The posterior one-third of the tongue is formed largely by third-arch and fourth-arch mesoderm, and thus receives its sensory innervation from their corresponding nerves (i.e., the glossopharyngeal and vagus nerves). Both the glossopharyngeal and vagus nerves contain fibers of general sensation and taste.

The tongue is a highly-mobile, muscular organ; its anterior two-thirds are located in the oral cavity and posterior one-third is located in the oropharynx. The *sulcus terminalis* divides these two portions of the tongue. The sulcus is located on the dorsum of the tongue just posterior to the circumvallate papillae (Fig. 31–1). The anterior dorsum of the tongue is also lined with conical, filiform, fungiform, and foliate papillae; the posterior or pharyngeal portion of the tongue is lined with lymphoid tissue that forms the lingual tonsil.

The four extrinsic muscles of the tongue (i.e., the genioglossus, hyoglossus, styloglossus and palatoglossus) are important in tongue mobility. The *genioglossus* protrudes and depresses; the *hyoglossus* retracts and depresses; the *styloglossus* retracts; and the *palatoglossus* elevates the posterior portion of the tongue. The four intrinsic muscles of the tongue are supplied by branches of the hypoglossal nerve.

The Palate

The *palate* is formed by the fusion of the primary and secondary palates during the twelfth week of development. The *primary palate* is derived from the intermaxillary segment that is formed by the merging of two medial nasal swellings. The *secondary palate* forms as a result of the medial growth and fusion of the two palatal processes during weeks 7 to 12 of embryonic life. Fusion of the horizontal palatal shelves occurs initially in the midline at the anterior portion of the hard palate and proceeds posteriorly to the uvula. If the tongue rests higher in the mouth either because of a hypoplastic mandible (Pierre Robin syndrome) or a cleft lip, there is often a failure in palatal fusion, resulting in a cleft palate.[1]

SPECIAL CONSIDERATION:

If the tongue rests higher in the mouth either because of a hypoplastic mandible or a cleft lip, there is often a failure in palatal fusion, which results in a cleft palate.

The anterior two-thirds of the palate, or the *hard palate* (Fig. 31–2), separates the nasal and oral cavities; the posterior one-third of the palate, or the *soft palate,* provides a mobile barrier between the nasopharynx and the oropharynx. Proper functioning of the soft palate is essential for normal articulation and deglutition. The hard palate, which is bounded by the alveolar processes anteriorly and laterally, is comprised of the *premaxilla,* which is the palatine processes of the maxillae and the horizontal plates of the palatine bones. In young children, a suture line can often be palpated at the ultimate fusion site of the premaxillary part of the maxilla and the palatine processes. The soft palate, or *velum palatinum,* contains a membranous aponeurosis formed by an expansion of the tensor veli palatini tendon. Five muscles insert into this aponeurosis and contribute to palatal movement: tensor veli palatini, levator veli palatini, palatoglossus, pala-

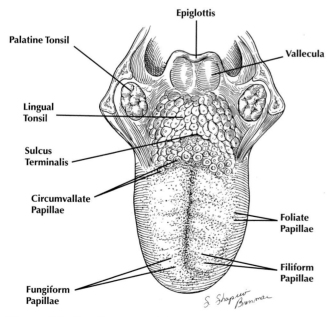

Epiglottis

Palatine Tonsil

Vallecula

Lingual Tonsil

Sulcus Terminalis

Circumvallate Papillae

Foliate Papillae

Filiform Papillae

Fungiform Papillae

Figure 31–1:   Dorsum of the tongue and palatine tonsils.

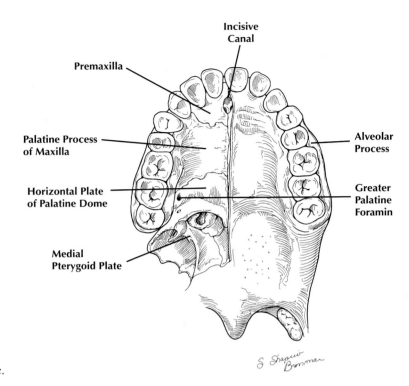

Figure 31–2:   The hard palate.

topharyngeus, and the musculus uvulae. The soft palate is continuous with the lateral pharyngeal wall through the palatoglossus and palatopharyngeus muscles, which form the anterior and posterior *tonsillar pillars,* respectively. The palatine tonsil is located in the intervening fossae between these two muscles.

Motor innervation to the muscles of the palate is through the *pharyngeal plexus.* This plexus is formed by a combination of fibers from the cranial root of the accessory nerve and the vagus nerve. The exception is the tensor veli palatini, which is supplied by the mandibular division of the trigeminal nerve. Sensory innervation to the palate is supplied by branches of the pterygopalatine ganglion. In particular, the greater palatine and nasopalatine nerves supply sensation to the hard palate, and the lesser palatine nerve supplies sensation to the soft palate.

The Mandible

The cartilage of the first pharyngeal arch consists of a dorsal component, known as the *maxillary process,* and a ventral component, known as the *mandibular process* or *Meckel's cartilage.*[2] The mesenchyme of the maxillary process gives rise to the premaxilla, maxilla, zygomatic bone, and part of the temporal bone through membranous ossification. The mandible is formed by membranous ossification of Meckel's cartilage. This cartilage extends ventrally to fuse with the cartilage of the opposite side in the floor of the pharynx.

The mandible consists of the tooth-bearing body and the superiorly-angled *ramus* (Fig. 31–3). Extending from the ramus are the *coronoid process* anteriorly and the *condylar process* posteriorly, which is separated by the mandibular notch.

The muscles most closely associated with the mandible are the muscles of mastication, which include the masseter, temporalis, and the medial and lateral pterygoids. All are innervated by branches of the mandibular division of the trigeminal nerve.

The *masseter muscle* is comprised of superficial and deep heads. The superficial portion arises on the lateral surface of the zygoma, and the deep portion arises from the inner surface of the zygoma. Both insert into the lateral surface of the ramus of the mandible. The masseter both elevates and protracts the mandible. The muscle is innervated by the masseteric branch of the mandibular nerve. The *temporalis muscle* has an extensive origin from the temporal fossa on the side of the skull and inserts into the medial ramus of the mandible and the lateral surface of the condyle. The temporalis both elevates and retracts the mandible. Two nerves usually inner-

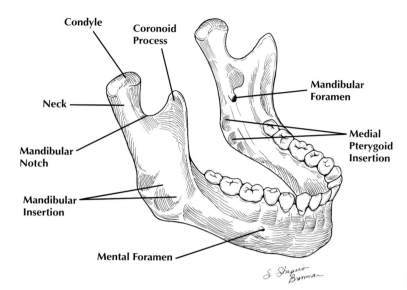

Figure 31–3:   The mandible.

vate this muscle, the anterior and posterior deep temporal nerves, which are branches of the mandibular nerve. The *lateral pterygoid muscle* arises from two heads. The superior head arises from the greater wing of the sphenoid, and the inferior head arises from the lateral surface of the lateral pterygoid plate. Both heads insert into the neck of the mandible and into the articular capsule and disk of the temporomandibular joint. The lateral pyterygoid muscle helps to protrude the mandible and to depress the chin. The lateral pytergoid is innervated by the buccal branch of the mandibular nerve. The *medial pterygoid muscle* arises from the internal surface of the lateral pterygoid plate, and inserts onto the medial surface of the ramus of the mandible. This muscle assists in elevating and protruding the mandible.

The masseter, temporalis, and medial pterygoids all act to elevate the mandible. Contraction of the masseter and medial pterygoid muscles helps to deviate the mandible to the contralateral side, and contraction of the temporalis deviates the mandible to the ipsilateral side. The lateral pterygoid muscles protract and open the jaw.

EMBRYOLOGY AND ANATOMY OF THE PHARYNX

The primitive foregut develops into the pharynx by elongation and growth between the second and seventh weeks of embryonic development. The *branchial apparatus* is the lateral extension of the foregut, which phylogenetically resembles the gill arches of a fish. There are five mesodermic arches separated by invaginations of ectoderm (i.e., clefts) and endoderm (i.e., pouches). Because the arches are of mesodermal origin, they are capable of differentiating into a variety of tissues including cartilage, bone, blood vessels, and muscle. Nerves from the overlying ectoderm grow into the adjacent arches.

The *pharynx* is a fibromuscular tube that extends from the base of skull to the inferior border of the cricoid; it serves as a common pathway for the respiratory and digestive tracts. The pharynx is divided into three components: the *nasopharynx,* which extends from the skull base to the soft palate; the *oropharynx,* which extends from the soft palate to the base of tongue; and the *laryngopharynx,* or hypopharynx, which extends from the base of tongue to the inferior border of the cricoid. The pharyngeal wall is composed of five layers; from internal to external, they are: a mucous membrane, a submucosa, a fibrous layer, a muscular layer (composed of inner longitudinal and outer circular parts), and a loose connective tissue layer. This connective tissue layer forms the *buccopharyngeal fascia,* which is continuous with the fascia overlying the buccinator muscle described previously. The longitudinal muscles of the pharynx are the palatopharyngeus, the salpingopharyngeus, and the stylopharyngeus. The circular muscles of the pharynx are the overlapping superior, middle, and inferior constrictors (Fig. 31–4).

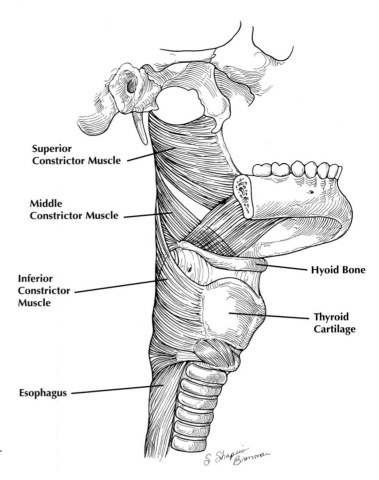

Figure 31–4: Pharyngeal constrictors.

Each constrictor inserts with the corresponding muscle of the opposite side in the pharyngeal raphe of the posterior midline. The *superior constrictor* arises from the medial pterygoid plate, called the *pterygomandibular raphe* (where the superior constrictor meets the buccinator muscle), the myelohyoid line of the mandible, and from the posterolateral portion of the tongue. The upper edge of the superior constrictor contributes to the development of *Passavant's ridge,* which is important in velopharyngeal closure.[3] The *middle constrictor* arises from the hyoid bone and lower portion of the stylohyoid ligament. The *inferior constrictor* arises from the thyroid cartilage and the cricoid cartilage. The lower fibers of the inferior constrictor lie at the junction of the pharynx and esophagus to form the *upper esophageal sphincter* (UES)

Motor innervation to all the muscles of the pharynx, except the stylopharyngeus, is supplied by the vagus nerve through the pharyngeal plexus (Fig. 31–5). The stylopharyngeus is supplied by the glossopharyngeal nerve. Sensory innervation of the pharynx is supplied largely by the glossopharyngeal nerve. The inferior pharynx also receives innervation from the vagus nerve.

EMBRYOLOGY AND ANATOMY OF THE ESOPHAGUS

The esophagus first appears at 4 weeks gestation as a small diverticulum at the ventral wall of the foregut. Between 4 to 6 weeks gestation, this diverticulum is separated into the respiratory primordium and the esophagus by the *esophagotracheal septum.* Initially, the esophagus is very short, but with the descent of the heart and lungs, it lengthens rapidly. Shortly after the formation of the esophagotracheal septum, epithelial hyperplasia completely obliterates the esophageal lumen, which slowly recanalizes. Tracheal and esophageal anomalies may

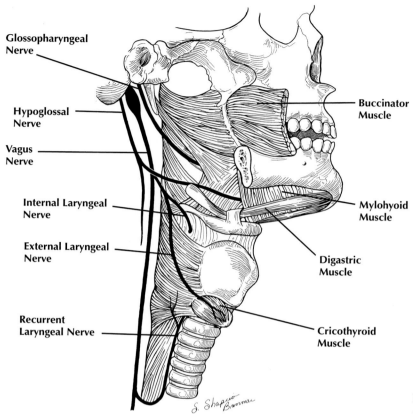

Glossopharyngeal
Nerve

Hypoglossal
Nerve

Vagus
Nerve

Internal Laryngeal
Nerve

External Laryngeal
Nerve

Recurrent
Laryngeal Nerve

Buccinator
Muscle

Mylohyoid
Muscle

Digastric
Muscle

Cricothyroid
Muscle

S. Shapiro
Brunman

Figure 31–5: Innvervation of the pharynx.

occur from faulty separation of the esophagus and trachea or from faulty recanalization.

SPECIAL CONSIDERATION:

Tracheal and esophageal anomalies may occur from faulty separation of the esophagus and trachea or from faulty recanalization of the esophageal lumen.

The *esophagus* is a muscular tube that extends from the lower border of the cricoid cartilage through the posterior mediastinum and diaphragm to the cardiac orifice of the stomach. The *cervical esophagus,* the portion which lies above the manubrium of the sternum, deviates slightly to the left of the midline and therefore projects to the left of the trachea. Anterior to the esophagus lies the *trachea;* posterior to it lies the *vertebral column,* which is covered by the prevertebral fascia and the longus

colli muscles. Anterolaterally lie the *lobes* of the thyroid gland and recurrent laryngeal nerves. The four areas of narrowing that can be found along the length of the esophagus are: the *esophageal inlet,* where the cricopharyngeus overlaps with the superior esophagus; the level of the aortic arch; the level of the left mainstem bronchus; and the *lower esophageal sphincter* (LES), where the esophagus enters the stomach.

The esophagus is comprised of four layers; from internal to external they are; mucosa, submucosa or areolar layer, inner circular, and outer longitudinal muscle. The inner circular layer is continuous with the inferior constrictor muscle above. The upper esophagus is comprised primarily of striated muscle, and the lower esophagus is comprised primarily of smooth muscle.

The blood supply to the esophagus is derived from the inferior thyroid branch of the thyrocervical trunk and from branches of the descending aorta. Innervation to the esophagus is supplied, in part, by the vagus through the recurrent laryngeal nerves and through sympathetic and parasympathetic plexus which mediate peristalsis.

AT A GLANCE. . .

Embryology of The Oral Cavity, Pharynx, and Esophagus

Oral Cavity: *Lips:* the upper lip is formed when the medial frontonasal and lateral maxillary prominences merge during weeks 6 to 8 of fetal development. The lower lip is formed as the mandibular prominences merge during the fourth week. *Cheek:* formed by the buccinator muscle. *Salivary Glands:* develop from stomadeal ectoderm by ingrowth of oral epithelium into the underlying mesenchyme beginning at about 6 weeks gestation. *Tongue:* appears at approximately 4 weeks gestation and arises from the lingual swellings and the tuberculum impar. *Palate:* formed by the fusion of the primary and secondary palates during the twelfth week of development. *Mandible:* first identified at $4^1/_2$ weeks gestation and formed by membranous ossification of Meckel's cartilage.

Pharynx: the primitive foregut develops into the pharynx by elongation and growth between the second and seventh weeks of embryonic development.

Esophagus: first appears at 4 weeks gestation as a small diverticulum at the ventral wall of the foregut. Between 4 to 6 weeks gestation, this diverticulum is separated into the respiratory primordium and the esophagus by the esophagotracheal septum.

PHYSIOLOGY OF THE UPPER AERODIGESTIVE TRACT

The oral-pharyngeal-esophageal pathway is a complex system involved in swallowing, respiration, and speech. It is only through precise neuromuscular coordination that the often contradictory functions of the UADT may occur simultaneously and safely. The physiology of these basic functions is considered in this section.

Swallowing

Traditionally, the swallowing process has been divided into three general phases that are oral, pharyn-

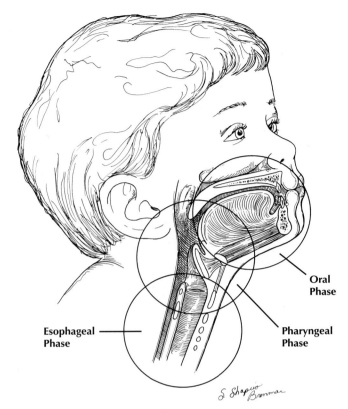

Figure 31–6:   Phases of swallowing.

geal, and esophageal (Fig. 31-6).[4] The process of *swallowing* is the passage of food through a continuous tube that is separated by a series of physiologic valves, each of which plays an important protective function. The tube consists of the mouth, pharynx, and esophagus; the valves include the lips, velum, larynx, and UES (or cricopharyngeus muscle). The process by which food passes through these valves in a coordinated fashion will be described in more detail below.

The oral phase of swallowing

The oral phase of swallowing involves the intake, breakdown, mastication, and initial movement of the food bolus. This first phase of swallowing can be further subdivided into the oral preparation and the oral transport phases.

Oral preparation involves manipulation, lubrication, and breakdown (physical and enzymatic) of the food bolus. The orbicularis oris and the buccinator muscles, both of which are innervated by the facial nerve (the seventh cranial nerve), act to compress the lips and to flatten the cheeks. These actions facilitate the retention and manipulation of food, as well as provide stabilization of food for chewing when dentition develops. The muscles of mastication (i.e., the masseter, temporalis, and medial and lateral pterygoids), which are innervated by the trigeminal nerve (the fifth cranial nerve), mobilize the mandible for food intake and chewing. Apposition of the soft palate and tongue posteriorly maintains the food bolus in the mouth and allows for nasopharyngeal respiration during the oral preparation phase of swallowing.

> ## SPECIAL CONSIDERATION:
> Apposition of the soft palate and tongue maintains the food bolus in the mouth and allows for nasopharyngeal respiration during the oral preparation phase of swallowing.

Saliva plays an important role in swallowing and digestion. The parotid gland produces predominantly serous secretions; the submandibular (submaxillary) gland produces both serous and mucous secretions; and the sublingual gland secretes mucous saliva. These major salivary glands receive both sympathetic and parasympathetic innervation. Stimulation of the glands by sympathetic fibers produces more viscous secretions. Parasympathetic stimulation provides more watery secretions.[5] Baseline salivary-flow rates range from 0.001 to 0.2 ml/min/gland, which can rise to 0.18 to 1.7 ml/min/gland with stimulation. Submandibular gland secretions predominate at rest, and parotid production predominates with stimulation.[6] The 600 to 1000 minor salivary glands that line the entire mucosal surface of the mouth and oral pharynx provide additional serous and mucous secretions. Mechanically, saliva coats and lubricates the food for improved transport. Enzymes such as amylase deoxyribonuclease (DNase) ribonuclease (RNase) and lipase begin the chemical breakdown of food.[7] Anti-infectious agents such as secretory immunoglobulin A (IgA) salivary peroxidase (i.e., thiocyanate-dependent factor), lysozyme, lactoferrin, and histatins (antifungal) prevent microbial invasion and overgrowth. The bicarbonate buffering system (pH 7.1) present in saliva helps to protect the oral and pharyngeal mucosa by lavaging and neutralizing refluxed or retained acid in the upper digestive tract.[8]

Saliva also helps to protect dentition from decay. In addition to its protective functions, saliva serves as the solvent that facilitates the passage of food and as a delivery system that enhances the taste of food.

> ## SPECIAL CONSIDERATION:
> Saliva protects the oral and pharyngeal mucosa by lavaging and neutralizing refluxed or retained acid, protects dentition from decay, and facilitates the passage of food.

At the completion of the oral preparation phase, a variety of activities occur simultaneously to mark the *oral transport phase*. Contraction of the orbicularis oris and muscles of mastication raises the intraoral pressure and propels the food bolus towards the oropharynx. The velum elevates to contact Passavant's ridge, thereby separating the nasopharynx from the oropharynx and preventing nasopharyngeal reflux. The anterior tongue elevates and sweeps the food bolus posteriorly. The lateral edges of the tongue also elevate to create a trough-effect, which further directs the food posteriorly. Finally, the posterior tongue flattens to allow for the transport of food into the oropharynx. Passage of the bolus past the anterior tonsillar pillars marks the transition from the voluntary oral phase to the largely involuntary pharyngeal phase of swallowing.

The pharyngeal phase of swallowing

The pharyngeal phase begins with the entrance of the food bolus into the oropharynx. The *pharyngeal swallow* is activated by the sensory receptors at the anterior tonsillar pillars, base of the tongue, epiglottis, and piriform sinuses, which are innervated by the fifth, ninth, and tenth cranial nerves. Although the transit time from the oropharynx to the esophagus is very short, approximately 800 msec, many important actions occur in a rapid, highly-synchronized fashion.[9]

Once the bolus reaches the oropharynx, the soft palate remains elevated in contact with the posterior pharyngeal wall, preventing nasopharyngeal reflux. This movement requires the coordinated efforts of the levator veli palatini and palatoglossus (which elevate the soft palate), the palatopharyngeus (which causes the medial movement of the pharynx), and the musculi uvulae (which causes the inversion of the soft palate). All of these muscles are innervated by the vagus nerve (tenth cranial nerve).

Several forces combine to propel the bolus through the oropharynx including: the posterior movement of the tongue; the development of a pressure gradient between the oral cavity (where there is increased positive pressure) and the pharyngeal-esophageal segment (where there is negative pressure); and the coordinated contraction of the superior, middle, and inferior constrictors. Passage of the food bolus through a relaxed cricopharyngeus marks the transition from the pharyngeal to the esophageal phase of swallowing.

Although these activities are occurring in the pharynx, a variety of protective actions also are occurring in the larynx. First, the true and false vocal folds adduct, closing off the laryngeal vestibule.[10] Second, the epiglottis deflects posteriorly to cover the laryngeal aditus and to divert food laterally into the pyriform sinuses. Third, the entire laryngeal unit elevates, immediately prior to the entrance of the food bolus into the hypopharynx. Laryngeal elevation is accomplished by contraction of the suprahyoid musculature; the process is as follows: the mylohyoid elevates the hyoid and the floor of mouth and depresses the mandible; the stylohyoid elevates the hyoid and the tongue base; the genioglossus and the hyoglossus elevate the larynx; the geniohyoid pulls the hyoid anteriorly; and the anterior belly of the digastricus raises the hyoid with a fixed mandible.[11] The superior movement of the hyoid and larynx has been reported to facilitate the opening of the cricopharyngeus.[12] In addition, activation of sensory receptors in the pharynx and anterior tonsillar pillars inhibits respiration during the swallowing process.[13]

The esophageal phase of swallowing

The *esophageal phase* involves the passage of the food bolus from the UES to the LES at the gastroesophageal junction. This passage is due to a series of nonvolitional contractions that occur throughout the length of the esophagus and that are coordinated by a complex network of reflex arcs. As soon as the bolus passes through the UES, the cricopharyngeus returns to its tonic state of contraction (from -15 mmHg to $+5$ mmHg), preventing reflux of food into the hypopharynx. In the esophagus

proximal to the bolus, the inner circular muscle contracts while the outer longitudinal muscle relaxes. In the esophagus distal to the food bolus, the circular muscle relaxes while the longitudinal muscle contracts. This creates a coordinated peristaltic wave that propels the food through the esophagus in a cranial-to-caudal fashion Contraction begins in the upper, skeletal-muscle esophagus, continues through the 4 to 8 cm transition zone (which consists of striated and smooth muscle), and finishes in the lower, smooth-muscle esophagus. The rate of esophageal peristalsis ranges from 0.8 to 2.0 cm per second in very young infants, and from 0.8 to 4.0 cm per second in older infants.[14] This primary peristaltic wave travels slower in the lower, smooth-muscle esophageal segment than in the upper segment. The esophageal phase concludes after the food bolus passes through the gastroesophageal junction and the LES returns to its tonic contraction state with pressures 15 to 30 mmHg above intragastric pressures. The diaphragmatic crura, the angle of the gastroesophageal junction, and the contraction of the diaphragm help to prevent reflux of gastric contents into the esophagus.

The three types of esophageal peristalsis that have been described are primary, secondary, and tertiary.[15-17] *Primary peristalsis,* the predominant wave of contraction described above, is initiated by the act of pharyngeal swallowing and is controlled by the central nervous system (CNS). *Secondary peristalsis* results from local distention within the esophageal lumen, which stimulates local contractions and relaxations along the esophagus. *Tertiary peristalsis* involves smooth-muscle peristalsis that is initiated in the esophagus without external neurologic input.[18]

The neurologic control of swallowing

The *swallowing center,* which is located in the reticular formation of the medulla, integrates the afferent and efferent neurologic activity. Impulses for motor control of voluntary functions, such as oral movement, speech, and breathing, originate in the inferior aspect of the precentral gyrus of the cerebral cortex and are relayed through the hypothalamus to the swallow center. The motor-neuron cell bodies are located in the nucleus ambiguus, which is separated anatomically into functional regions such as swallowing (rostral) and speech (caudal) areas. Feedback mechanisms often modify the swallow, depending on factors such as food consistency, temperature, taste, and texture. For example, a thicker food bolus can be sensed and accommodated by a longer or more intense contraction of the pharyngeal muscles during the swallow and by rapid repeated swallows following this.[19] In addition, input and relays from supramedullary pathways such as the pons, mesencephalon, and the cerebral cortex further modify swallowing behavior. During each pharyngeal swallow, for example, inhibitory signals are relayed to the respiratory centers and to the two esophageal sphincters.

The two major extrinsic neural pathways to the esophagus are the craniosacral (or parasympathetic) pathway and the thoracolumbar (or sympathetic) pathway. The pharyngeal plexus, which is comprised of fibers from the vagus, glossopharyngeal, and spinal accessory nerves, also helps to modulate pharyngeal and esophageal activity. The two enteric nervous pathways within the esophageal wall are the myenteric (or *Auerbach's*) plexus lying between the inner and outer muscle layers and the submucosal (or *Meissner's*) plexus lying within the submucosa. Although present throughout the esophagus, the enteric nervous system (ENS) plays a larger role in the lower segments of the esophagus where secondary esophageal peristalsis occurs. Activation of stretch receptors within the esophageal lumen stimulates excitatory and inhibitory neurons within the esophageal wall that coordinate esophageal contractions similar to the primary peristaltic wave described in the previous section.[4] Unlike primary esophageal peristalsis, however, these secondary peristaltic waves are local, reflex contractions that do not require pharyngeal swallows for initiation. Although the swallowing center has a minor role in mediating this secondary peristalsis, it does not initiate sequential contractions as in the upper, striated-muscle, esophageal segment.[20]

Infant Development and Swallowing

Swallowing activity begins in utero and develops throughout neonatal maturation. At 10 to 11 weeks gestation, pharyngeal swallowing of amniotic fluid is noted.[21-23] At 18 to 24 weeks, suckling is seen.[24] At 27 to 28 weeks, suckling behavior (usually single sucks with long pauses) is noted.[22] Although the ability to nipple feed develops between 32 to 37 weeks, the coordination required for breathing and swallowing usually does not develop until later. This may explain partially the difficulty premature infants often have with feeding early in life.[25] Initially, feeding occurs with a "burst-pause" pattern of swallowing that consists of 12 to 15 sucks, followed by a swallow.[26] With increasing maturity, young infants gradually develop a more deliberate feeding pattern of 2 to 3 sucks per swallow with stronger more rhythmic sucks. Pharyngeal swallows occur without interruption of the respiratory cycle.

AT A GLANCE . . .

Swallowing

Oral Phase: a voluntary phase that involves the intake, breakdown, mastication, and initial movement of the food bolus. Oral preparation involves the manipulation, lubrication, and breakdown of the food bolus, and saliva plays a major part during this phase. The oral transport phase propels the food bolus towards the oropharynx.

Pharyngeal Phase: largely an involuntary phase that begins when the food bolus enters the oropharynx. The food bolus is propelled through the oropharynx by the posterior movement of the tongue, by the development of a pressure gradient between the oral cavity and the pharyngeal-esophageal segment, and by the coordinated contraction of the superior, middle, and inferior constrictors.

Esophageal Phase: involves the passage of the food bolus from the UES to the LES. This phase is accomplished by a series of nonvolitional contractions that occur throughout the length of the esophagus.

SPECIAL CONSIDERATION:

Premature infants often may have difficulty with feeding early in life because the coordination required for breathing and swallowing does not develop until after 32 to 37 weeks gestation.

Suckling, or suckle feeding, is a swallowing behavior seen from birth to 6 months of age. This involves the tongue moving backward and forward, with the lower jaw and tongue compressing the upper jaw and palate. This response can be elicited by stroking the dorsum of the tongue.[20,22,27] Feeding consists of rhythmic and peristaltic compressions of the nipple between the tongue and hard palate, with alternating periods of negative intraoral pressure.[27] The lateral edges of the tongue rise to meet the palate, forming a trough-like configuration to facilitate central passage of the bolus.[28] Posteriorly, the tongue is apposed to the soft palate, holding the fluid in the oral cavity while respiration occurs via the nasopharynx. In infants, there is a prominent, rapid, forward movement of the posterior pharyngeal wall that initiates a prominent pharyngeal wave distally.[27] Once the food passes through the cricopharyngeus, there is closure of the UES followed by an immediate opening of the larynx and nasopharynx.

Sucking, on the other hand, involves up-and-down movement of the tongue with less mandible movement. Specialized structures, such as the pars villosa, help with feeding. The *pars villosa* is an inner ridge of specialized mucosa that consists primarily of fine villi that facilitate the sealing of the lips around a nipple. *Nonnutritive sucking* is a developmental milestone involving sucking actions with nonfeeding nipples.[29] This action involves approximately two sucks per second with no interruption of breathing. There are bursts of 30 sucks with approximately one to four swallows per burst. Though not necessarily an accurate indicator of future feeding ability, nonnutritive sucking has been associated with improved weight gain in gavage-fed infants.[30] *Nutritive sucking,* which appears at 4 to 6 months of age, is a volitional, coordinated action that involves approximately one suck per second. There is biphasic peristalsis of the tongue, with its center moving posteriorly toward the pharynx. This movement facilitates the intake of food such as milk in a bottle. The ratio of suck-to-swallow reaches 1:1, with breaths occurring between swallows. There are short periods of apnea (0.3 to 2.5 seconds) in this normal swallowing cycle. Swallows have been observed during both inspiratory and expiratory phases of respiration. When respiration is interrupted at low lung-volume states (either at end expiratory or early inspiratory phases), an extra inspiratory "swallow-breath" is elicited at the start of the next swallow.[31]

Anatomically, the infant undergoes a large number of changes that affect swallowing and respiration. During the first few months of life, the proximity of the tongue, palate, pharynx, epiglottis, and larynx make their anatomic and physiologic changes intimately related. As the infant grows, the mandible begins to enlarge, descend, and protrude. The overall profile and oral cavity space enlarges in the vertical dimension. The lips and cheeks also enlarge. The tongue, which is relatively large and occupies most of the oral cavity early in life, takes a more anterior position with growth and expansion of the oral cavity and pharynx. At birth, the larynx lies high in the neck, placing the epiglottis into contact with the soft palate. This allows the infant to breathe through the nose while sucking and swallowing. The cricoid, which is initially at the level of C-2, begins descending during the first year of life to lie ultimately at about the level of C-5 by 12 months of age.[24]

> ## SPECIAL CONSIDERATION:
> During the first few months of life, the proximity of the infant's tongue, palate, pharynx, epiglottis, and larynx make anatomic and physiologic changes intimately related.

Chewable foods are often introduced at about 7 months of age, shortly after the appearance of the deciduous teeth. Most children begin spoon-feeding and cup-drinking by the age of 4 to 6 months.[22] The enhanced coordination and strength that occurs with growth and development allow for upright-sitting, improved head and trunk control, and increased hand-to-mouth coordination. These changes set the stage for the eventual ability to self-feed. Thus, with growth and development, the volitional oral phase of swallowing undergoes a variety of maturational changes, while the basic involuntary actions of the pharyngeal and esophageal phases remain fairly stable throughout infancy and early childhood.

Infant Respiration and Airway Protection

Traditionally, infants have been considered obligate nasal breathers. During the first months of life, the oral cavity increases in size, allowing for the anterior movement of the tongue. In addition, the larynx descends inferiorly, thereby separating the epiglottis from the soft palate. The larynx reaches the level of C5 by 2 years of age, descends to the level of C6 by 5 years of age, and finally to the level of C6-C7 by 15 years of age.[32] These changes facilitate the transition from obligate nasal breathing to nasal and oral breathing.

Airway protective mechanisms can be divided into two general categories, which are mechanisms against aspiration while swallowing (or *antero-grade aspiration*) and mechanisms against reflux aspiration (or *retrograde aspiration*).[33] Most of the protective mechanisms directed at preventing an-terograde aspiration have been highlighted above in the description of the swallowing process. These mechanisms include laryngeal and nasopharyngeal closure along with laryngeal elevation. *Reflex laryn-geal closure* is a protective response that is facili-tated by mucosal receptors within the larynx, which is innervated by the superior laryngeal nerve (an afferent branch of the vagus nerve). In infants, laryn-geal stimuli, such as secretions in the larynx, results in a reflex closure of the larynx with sustained apnea.[34-36] When prolonged or poorly regulated, this laryngeal closure reflex can lead to apnea, brad-ycardia, hypoxia, or even death.[37,38] As the infant matures, however, the cough reflex replaces sus-tained apnea as the primary protective response against foreign material in and around the lar-ynx.[39,40] The infant's reflex to swallow vigorously in response to laryngeal liquids is also replaced with the cough reflex as the infant matures.[41]

Contrary to earlier beliefs, neonates and infants do not swallow and breathe simultaneously. In-stead, each swallow results in laryngeal closure and a reflex suppression of respiratory drive.[42] Studies with healthy term infants have demonstrated that minute ventilation is reduced during feeding by de-creasing breathing frequency rather than by de-creasing tidal volume.[43] As observed with sensory reflex laryngeal closure, even mildly prolonged pe-riods of hypoventilation can lead to significant apnea, bradycardia, and hypoxia in both term and preterm infants.

SPECIAL CONSIDERATION:

Neonates and infants do not swallow and breath simultaneously, and even mildly pro-longed periods of hypoventilation can lead to significant apnea, bradycardia, and hypoxia.

Gastrointestinal reflux (GER) has gained increas-ing notoriety as a clinical entity capable of affecting both the respiratory and swallowing processes. GER has been held accountable for a wide variety of problems including wheezing, recurrent pneumo-nia, stridor, laryngospasm, apnea, and respiratory failure.[44-46] Protective mechanisms directed at pre-venting retrograde or reflux aspiration include both basally-active and responsive measures. The basally-active measures include tonic contraction of the UES and LES. The LES at the gastroesophageal junc-tion maintains a basal tone of 10 to 30 mmHg over the intragastric pressure. The resting muscular tone combined with the diaphragmatic crural support and the acute gastroesophageal angle act to prevent regurgitation of gastric acid. In premature infants, however, the LES pressures are often low and the gastroesophageal angle is less acute, which predis-poses them to increased gastroesophageal reflux.[47] Immaturity of the CNS and enteric reflex mecha-nisms also contribute to aberrant LES relaxation pat-terns.[48] However, most cases of reflux resolve spon-taneously by 6 to 9 months of age.[49] The UES also maintains a basal-resting tone, although the pres-sures are lower and more variable than those of the LES.

Modifiers to the basal tone of the LES have been studied extensively. Substances that decrease LES tone include many hormones (e.g., secretin, chole-cystokinin, glucagon, and vasoactive intestinal pep-tide), neurotransmitters (e.g., dopamine, beta-ad-renergic agonists, alpha-adrenergic agonists, and anticholinergics), medications (e.g., nitrous oxide, theophylline, morphine, and diazepam), and foods (e.g., fat, chocolate, and peppermint). Other factors such as deep sleeping state and acidification of the gastric antrum also lower LES pressures. Substances that increase LES tone include gastrin, substance P, norepinephrine, acetylcholine, anticholinesterases, histamine, betanochol (muscarinic agonist), met-aclopramide, cisapride, indomethacin, and pro-tein.[48]

Responsive measures that help to prevent reflux aspiration include: *secondary esophageal peristal-sis* (which is continued esophageal peristaltic waves in response to esophageal distension from a re-tained bolus or refluxed gastric acid); the *esophago-UES contractile reflex* (which is a UES contraction in response to segmental esophageal distension); and *pharyngeal swallows* (which are repeated pha-ryngeal swallows similar to secondary esophageal peristalsis).[32] Additional protective mechanisms include the *esophago-glottal closure reflex,* which is closure of laryngeal introitus in response to abrupt esophageal distension/reflux, and the *pharyngo-UES contractile reflex,* which is increased UES tone in response to retrograde fluid. These mechanisms respond to distention of the esophagus or mechanical stimulation of the pharynx. A response known as the *esophagosalivary reflex* causes a marked increase in saliva in response to gastric acid (a low pH) in the esophagus.[50] This facilitates neutralization of acid, increased clearance of acids and food, and improved mucosal protection.

AT A GLANCE . . .
Airway Protective Mechanisms

Prevention of Anterograde Aspiration:
mechanisms include laryngeal and nasopharyngeal closure along with laryngeal elevation. At birth, the larynx lies high in the neck, placing the epiglottis into contact with the soft palate, thus allowing the infant to breathe through the nose while sucking and swallowing. During suckling (from birth to 6 months of age), the tongue is apposed to the soft palate, holding the fluid in the oral cavity while respiration occurs via the nasopharynx. During nutritive sucking (from 4 to 6 months of age), there is a biphasic peristalsis of the tongue, and its center moves posteriorly toward the pharynx. Breathing occurs between swallows and there are short periods of apnea.

Prevention of Retrograde Aspiration:
mechanisms include basally-active and responsive measures. Basally-active measures include tonic contraction of the UES and LES; Responsive measures include secondary esophageal peristalsis, esophago-UES contractile reflex, pharyngeal swallows, esophago-glottal closure reflex, pharyngo-UES contractile reflex, and esophagosalivary reflex.

Speech Development

The dramatic maturational changes that occur in the UADT influence not only deglutition and respiration, but also speech and language development. The oral cavity and pharynx modulate, articulate, and create resonance of the spoken word. Speech requires coordination of the oral cavity and pharyngeal structures, with the tongue serving as the principal mediator of articulation.

During the first months of life, the larynx, epiglottis, velum, and tongue lie in close proximity, creating a predominantly nasopharyngeal passage for breathing and sound production. After 3 to 6 months of age, growth and separation of the oral cavity and the larynx leads to oral breathing and to the acquisition of non-nasal vowel sounds.

The development of sound production during the first year of life can be divided into five general stages: phonation, cooing, expansion, canonical, and variegated babbling.[51] During the first 6 months, the infant develops nasal sounds of limited resonance. Improved velar function coupled with improved oral and laryngeal coordination allow for the production sounds involving consonants. During the second 6 months of life, there is the emergence of canonical babbling (age 6 to 8 months), with repeated sequences of genuine syllables comprised of consonants and vowels (such as "bababa," "dadada," or "mamama"). Variegated babbling is a period of "exploration" with continued use of adultlike syllables in more varied combinations.[52]

The transition from babbling to true speech occurs by the age of 18 months. Speech begins to emerge as infants learn to discriminate between sounds, to interpret words as symbols for actual objects/meanings, and to elicit their own memories in using their words. In the absence of any neurologic, developmental, or physical deficiencies, expected speech-language development includes a vocabulary of five words by the age of 18 months, 50 words by the age of 2 years, short sentences by the age of 3 years, and nearly 2000 words by the age of 4 to 5 years.[53] Although many children experience difficulties with articulation during development, less than 15% of children have difficulties beyond 5 years of age.[54] Common immature articulation patterns include *rhotacism* (which is difficulty with the letter r), *sigmatism* (which is difficulty with the letter s), omissions, substitutions, and reversals of the last-acquired consonants (i.e., th, sh, s, b, g, and f).[53] Prior to 4 years of age, there is predominantly gross language-motor skill acquisition, and from ages 4 to 11 years, there is development of more finely-coordinated language abilities.[55]

Although the precise mechanics underlying the production of speech is beyond the scope of this section, some brief discussion may be instructive to illustrate the precise coordination that is required between the lips, teeth, tongue, velum, and larynx. For example, *lingual-labial coordination* is required when producing the sounds of /y/ and /u/. This involves lip rounding and protrusion with lowering of the tongue and opening of the oral cavity.[56] *Lingual-velar coordination* is involved in the transition from lingual nasal consonant sounds (/n/) to non-nasal sounds. Nasal consonants are created by an open velum with the oral cavity occluded by the tongue (to pronounce /n/); and non-nasal vowels require elevation of the velum and lowering of the tongue. Precise coordination is needed to build up the necessary intraoral pressure for speech production. Some sounds such as /m/, /p/, and /h/ are mastered earlier in life (24 to 36 months), whereas other sounds such as /r/ and /l/ may require 32 to 48 months to acquire.[57]

REFERENCES

1. Pashley NR, Krause CJ. Cleft lip, cleft palate and other fusion disorders. Otolaryngol Clin North Am 1981; 14:125–135.
2. Sadler TW. *Langman's Medical Embryology.* Baltimore: Williams & Wilkins, 1985, p. 284.
3. Calnan JS. Modern view on Passavant's ridge. Br J Plast Surg 1958; 10:89–96.
4. Perlman AL, Christensen J. Topography and functional anatomy of the swallowing structures. In: Perlman AL, Schulze-Delrieu KS, eds. *Deglutition and Its Disorders: Anatomy, Physiology, Clinical Diagnosis, and Management.* San Diego: Singular, 1997, p. 15.
5. Garrett JR. The proper role of nerves in salivary secretion. J Dent Res 1987; 66:387–392.
6. Kontis TC, Johns ME. Anatomy and physiology of the salivary glands. In: Bailey BJ, ed. *Head and Neck Surgery—Otolaryngology.* Philadelphia: Lippincott, 1993, p. 447.
7. Kaplan MD, Baum BJ. The functions of saliva. Dysphagia 1993; 8:225–229.
8. Mandel L, Tamari K. Sialorrhea and gastroesophageal reflux. J Am Dent Assoc 1995; 126:1537–1541.
9. McConnel FMS, Cerenko D, Jackson RT, et al. Timing of major events of pharyngeal swallowing. Arch Otolargyngol Head Neck Surg 1988; 114:1413–1418.
10. Sasaki CT. Paralysis of the larynx and pharynx. Surg Clin North Am 1980; 60:1079–1082.
11. Bass NH. The neurology of swallowing. In: Groher ME, ed. *Dysphagia: Diagnosis and Management.* Boston: Butterworth-Heinemann, 1997, p. 7.
12. Jacob P, Logemann JA, Shah V, et al. Upper esopha-

geal sphincter opening and modulation during swallowing. Gastroenterol 1989; 97:1469–1478.
13. Schechter GL. Physiology of the mouth, pharynx, and esophagus. In: Cummings CW, Schuller DE, eds. *Otolaryngology—Head and Neck Surgery.* St. Louis: Mosby Yearbook, 1993, p. 816.
14. Gryboski J, Walker WA. The Esophagus. In: *Gastrointestinal Problems in Children.* Philadelphia: Saunders, 1983, p. 157.
15. Hendrix TR. Coordination of peristalsis in pharynx and esophagus. Dysphagia 1993; 8:74–78.
16. Meltzer SJ. On the causes of the orderly progress of the peristaltic movements in the oesophagus. Am J Physiol 1899; 2:266–272.
17. Meltzer SJ. Secondary peristalsis of the esophagus—A demonstration on a dog with permanent esophageal fistula. Proc Soc Exp Biol Med 1907; 4:35–37.
18. Cannon WB. Esophageal peristalsis after bilateral vagotomy. Am J Physiol 1907; 19:436–444.
19. Miller A, Bieger D, Conklin JL. Functional controls of deglutition. In: Perlman AL, Schulze-Delrieu KS, eds. *Deglutition and Its Disorders: Anatomy, Physiology, Clinical Diagnosis, and Management.* San Diego: Singular, 1997, p. 43.
20. Siegel CL, Hendrix TR. Evidence for the central mediation of secondary peristalsis in the esophagus. Bull Johns Hopkins Hosp 1961; 108:297–307.
21. Pritchard JA. Fetal swallowing and amniotic fluid volume. Obstet Gynecol 1966; 28:606–610.
22. Arvedsen JC, Rogers BT. Swallowing and feeding in the pediatric patient. In: Perlman AL, Schulze-Delrieu KS, eds. *Deglutition and Its Disorders: Anatomy, Physiology, Clinical Diagnosis, and Management,* San Diego: Singular, 1997, p. 419.
23. Tuchman DN. Dysfunctional swallowing in the pediatric patient: Clinical considerations. Dysphagia 1988; 2:203–208.
24. Moore KL. *The Developing Human: Clinically Oriented Embryology.* Philadelphia: Saunders, 1988, p. 1050.
25. Goldson E. Suck and swallow in the premature infant. Pediatr 1987; 43:96–102.
26. Wolff PH. The serial organization of sucking in the young infant. Pediatr 1968; 42:943–956.
27. Kramer SS. Radiologic examination of the swallowing impaired child. Dysphagia 1989; 3:117–125.
28. Loughlin GM, Lefton-Greif MA. Dysfunctional swallowing and respiratory disease in children. Adv Pediatr 1994; 41:135–162.
29. Tuchman DN. Cough, choke, sputter: The evaluation of the child with dysfunctional swallowing. Dysphagia 1989; 3:111–116.
30. Bernbaum JC, Pereira GR, Watkins JB, et al. Nonnutritive sucking during gavage feeding enhances growth

and maturation in premature infants. Pediatr 1983; 71:41–45.

31. Wilson SL, Thach BT, Brouillette RT, et al. Coordination of breathing and swallowing in human infants. J Appl Physiol 1981; 50:851–888.

32. Isaacson G. Developmental anatomy and physiology of the larynx, trachea and esophagus. In: Bluestone CD, Stool SE, Kenna MA, eds. *Pediatric Otolaryngology, 3rd ed.* Philadelphia: Saunders, 1996, p. 1202.

33. Shaker R. Airway protective mechanisms: Current concepts. Dysphagia 1995; 10:216–227.

34. Bartlett D. Ventilatory and protective mechanisms of the infant larynx. Am Rev Respir Dis 1985: 131(supplement):49–50.

35. Perkett EA, Vaughan RL. Evidence for laryngeal chemoreflex in some human preterm infants. Acta Paediatr Scand 1982; 71:969–972.

36. Loughlin GM. Respiratory consequences of dysfunctional swallowing and aspiration. Dysphagia 1989; 3:126–130.

37. Downing SE, Lee JC. Laryngeal chemosensitivity: A possible mechanism for sudden infant death. Pediatr 1975; 65:640–649.

38. Guilleminault C, Coons S. Apnea and bradycardia during feeding in infants weighing >2000 gms. J Pediatr 1984; 104:932–935.

39. Leith DE. The development of cough. Am Rev Respir Dis 1985; 131(supplement):39–42.

40. Miller HC, Proud GO, Berhle FC. Variations in the gag, cough and swallow reflexes and tone of the vocal cords as determined by direct laryngoscopy in newborn infants. Yale J Biol Med 1952; 24:284–291.

41. Harding R. Function of the larynx in the fetus and newborn. Ann Rev Physiol 1984; 46:645–659.

42. Shipuri CR, Martin RJ, Carlo WA, et al. Decreased ventilation in preterm infants during oral feeding. J Pediatr 1983; 103:285–289.

43. Mathew OP, Clark ML, Pronske ML, et al. Breathing pattern and ventilation during oral feeding in term newborn infants. J Pediatr 1985; 106:810–813.

44. Nielson DW, Heldt GP, Toolet WH. Stridor and gastroesophageal reflux in infants. Pediatr 1990; 85:1034–1039.

45. Arvedson J, Rogers B, Buck G, et al. Silent aspiration in children with dysphagia. Intl J Ped Otolargyngol 1994; 28:173–181.

46. Orenstein SR, Orenstein DM. Gastroesophageal reflux and respiratory disease in children. J Pediatr 1988; 112:847–858.

47. Grybowski J, Walker WA. Gastroesophageal reflux. In: *Gastrointestinal Problems in Children,* Philadelphia: Saunders, 1983, p. 30.

48. Hillemeier AC. Gastroesophageal reflux: Diagnostic and therapeutic approaches. Pediatr Clin North Am 1996; 43:197–212.

49. Hollwarth M, Uray E. Physiology and pathophysiology of the esophagus in childhood. Prog Ped Surg, 1985; 18:1–13.

50. Helm JF, Dodds WJ, Hogan WJ. Salivary response to esophageal acid in normal subjects and patients with reflux esophagitis. Gastroenterol 1987; 83:1393–1397.

51. Oller DK. The emergence of the sounds of speech in infancy. In: Yeni-Komshian G, Kavanagh J, Ferguson CA, eds. *Child Phonology, Volume 1: Production.* New York: Academic Press, 1980, p. 112.

52. Elbers L. Operating principles in repetitive babbling: A cognitive continuity approach. Cognition 1982; 2:45–63.

53. Gemelli R. Toddlerhood phase of mental development: Age 18 months to age 3 years. In: *Normal and Adolescent Development.* Washington: American Psychiatric Press, 1996 p. 211.

54. Espir MLE, Rose FC. Speech and language disorders in children. In: *The Basic Neurology of Speech and Language.* Oxford: Blackwell, 1983, p. 81.

55. Robins J, Klee T. Clinical assessment of oropharyngeal motor development in young children. J Speech Hear Disord 1987; 52:271–277.

56. Ziegler W, von Cramon D. Timing deficits in apraxia of speech. Eur Arch Psychiatr Neurol Sci 1986; 236:44–49.

57. Bernthal JE, Bankson NW. Analysis and interpretation of assessment data. In: Bernthal JE, Bankson NW, eds. *Articulation and Phonological Disorders.* Englewood Cliffs: Prentice Hall, 1993, p. 270.

32 Introduction to Disorders of the Upper Alimentary Tract

Ralph F. Wetmore

Like other areas of the head and neck, the oral cavity and oropharynx frequently require examination in children. Young children have recurrent upper respiratory infections, the signs and symptoms of which are referable to this region of the body. Oral trauma from foreign bodies and teething is common in the pediatric age group. Because the mouth and pharynx serve as the entry point for nutrition, diseases affecting these regions may have important implications for the body as a whole. Finally, the pharynx functions not only in deglutition, but also respiration; lack of coordination between these two important functions in the pharynx and larynx may have a significant impact upon the child's growth and development.

Young children are often apprehensive and how the patient is approached may determine whether the examination is successful or fraught with anxiety and frustration for the examiner, the child, and the parent. As with other pediatric examinations, placing the child on the lap of the parent or caregiver is often a good initial step. This method of examination also allows the parent to help restrain the child. The examiner also should try both verbally and physically to reassure and to prepare the child for those parts of the examination that will not cause discomfort. The child should be permitted to play or touch some of the examining instruments, especially the tongue depressor and otoscope or flashlight. Those parts of the examination that may

cause discomfort should be reserved until the end and should be accompanied by gentle but adequate restraint.

EXAMINATION OF THE ORAL CAVITY AND OROPHARYNX

As with examination of other regions of the head and neck, the examiner should begin the examination of the oral cavity and pharynx by inspecting the face for asymmetry that would suggest the presence of masses in the buccal region, in the mandible, or in the maxilla. Such masses may have an intraoral component that may be appreciated by inspection or palpation. The overall position of the mandible is also important. In the child with chronic mouth-breathing due to upper airway obstruction, the mandible will assume a position such that the mouth is always open. The presence of a partial or total facial nerve paralysis is also significant because lesions affecting the distal portion of the nerve may originate in the oral cavity.

In examining the oral cavity and oropharynx, a good light source is extremely important. A hand-held flashlight or otoscope may be sufficient for many patients; however, use of such a light source limits the examiner to one free hand. By employing either a headlight or head mirror, both hands may be free to help with restraint of the child or to hold a tongue depressor or other instruments (Fig. 32-1, 32-2). Because it may be difficult for children to hold still so that the head mirror may be utilized effectively, a headlight may be the best form of illumination.

Regions of the oral cavity and oropharynx that should be inspected include the mucosa of the lips, the buccal mucosa, the teeth and gingiva, the tongue including the ventral surface, the floor of the mouth, the palate and tonsils, and the posterior pharyngeal wall. A careful examination of the teeth

---

SPECIAL CONSIDERATION:

Parental assistance and a nonthreatening manner are the keys to the successful examination of the oral cavity and oropharynx in a child.

Pediatric Otolaryngology, Edited by R.F. Wetmore, H.R. Muntz, and T.J. McGill. Thieme Medical Publishers, Inc., New York © 2000.

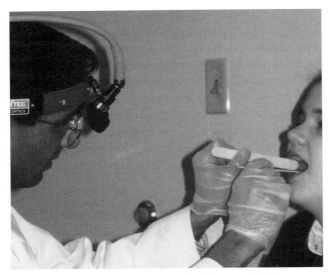

Figure 32–1: A headlight with a fiberoptic light source provides excellent illumination of the oral cavity and oropharynx.

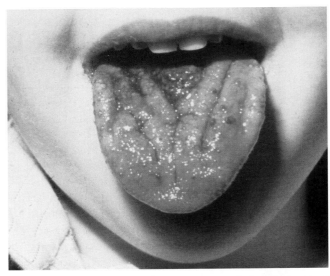

Figure 32–3: A large hemangioma of the dorsum of the tongue is readily identified by inspection.

gives an indication of the child's overall hygiene. Evidence of caries or missing teeth suggest poor dental care. The presence of excessive dental plaque and tartar often indicate infrequent dental maintenance.

The tongue should be inspected (Fig. 32-3) and, if necessary, palpated for the presence of any masses. Protrusion of the tongue allows for assessment of the hypoglossal nerve and the lateral bor-

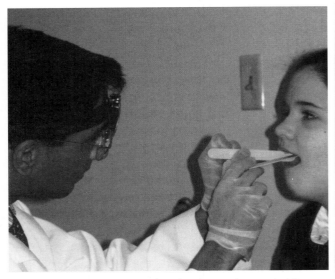

Figure 32–2: Using a head mirror that provides reflected light from an external source leaves both of the examiner's hands free to hold instruments or position the child.

ders of the tongue. By elevating the tongue with a tongue blade, the ventral surface can be examined for evidence of mucosa lesions. Fasciculation or tremor of a protruding tongue suggests other neurological problems. *Geographic tongue,* or benign migratory glossitis, appears as an irregular erythematous pattern of atrophic mucosa surrounded by slightly raised white borders. Affected areas migrate across the tongue and may be associated with complaints of a mild burning sensation.

By elevating the child's chin, effectively extending the head, the examiner can view the roof of the oral cavity (Fig. 32-4). High arching of the palate may be seen in a variety of congenital syndromes and also in patients with chronic nasal obstruction. Any masses visualized in the palate should be palpated. *Torus palatinus* is an exostosis of the hard palate and usually has no clinical significance in the pediatric age group. Vesicles or small ulcers on the soft palate are seen in a variety of viral infections of the oral cavity and pharynx. *Bifid uvula* is a common finding and usually has no clinical significance. When associated with a history of nasal regurgitation of liquids or hypernasal speech, further inspection of the junction of the hard and soft palate should be made for a submucous cleft palate. With this disorder, a V-shaped notch can be palpated along the posterior margin of the bony palate, which is an edge that is normally smooth. If the neurological supply to the palate has been compromised either peripherally in the pharyngeal neural plexus or centrally in the brainstem. The soft palate may move asymmetrically or barely at all.

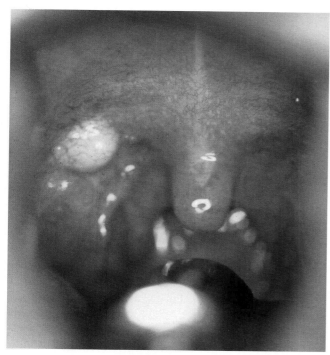

Figure 32–4: Small mucocele of the right posterior palate at its junction with the anterior tonsillar pillar.

By inserting a tongue blade into the oral cavity and depressing the tongue, the examiner can inspect the tonsillar regions and posterior pharyngeal wall. Elicitation of a gag reflex may be prevented by confining the tongue blade to the anterior two-thirds of the tongue, which is the portion of the tongue innervated by the trigeminal nerve. The posterior one-third of the tongue is innervated by the glossopharyngeal nerve, one of the nerves that mediates the gag reflex. At some point the glossopharyngeal nerve should be stimulated, which although somewhat distressing to the child, is helpful in assessing the neural control of the palate and pharynx in general. The tonsils should be inspected for size and evidence of acute or chronic infection. Erythema and tonsillar exudates indicate acute infection, whereas cryptic debris and tonsilloliths, which are small, white concretions within the tonsillar substance, are seen with chronic infection. While the tongue is depressed, the posterior pharyngeal wall can be inspected for masses or evidence of infection. Streaking of mucopurulent secretions along the posterior pharyngeal wall suggests nasal or sinus infection.

The tongue blade then may be used to retract the lips, exposing the buccal mucosa. White patches indicative of a fungal infection or bruising from dental trauma may be found in this region. By inserting

the tongue blade further into the oral cavity and retracting the buccal mucosa laterally, the examiner may be able to visualize the orifice of the parotid (Stensen's) duct, which appears as a papilla near the first maxillary molar. Evaluation of the duct and the underlying parotid gland by bimanual palpation with a gloved hand inside the mouth and the other hand over the gland is important in the assessment of masses or infection. Stones may be felt in the duct or purulent secretions may be milked from the gland.

In a similar fashion, the tongue can be elevated with a tongue blade and the floor of mouth inspected (Fig. 32–5). The orifices of the submandibular (Wharton's) ducts may be inspected and palpated for the presence of stones. Bimanual palpation of the submandibular gland with a gloved hand in the mouth and the other hand on the gland in the neck is helpful in assessing an enlarged gland or a mass within the submandibular triangle.

Lateral radiography demonstrates the oral cavity and oropharynx and is more helpful than an anterior-posterior (AP) view. The lateral neck film is most helpful for assessing masses in the region of the tongue base (i.e., lingual thyroid or vallecular cysts). The thickness of the mucosa, musculature, and lymph nodes in the posterior wall can be dem-

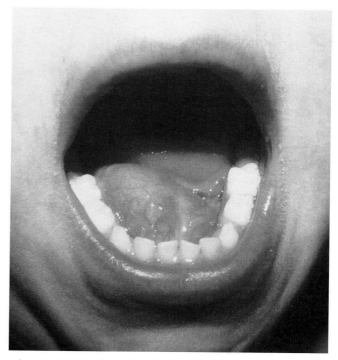

Figure 32–5: Ranula of the right floor of the mouth is identified easily by inspection.

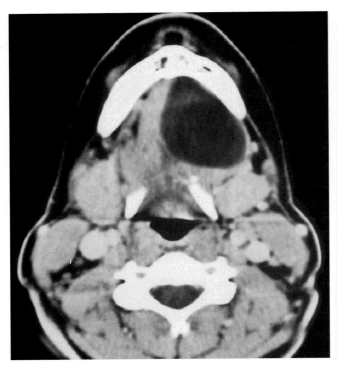

Figure 32–6: Large dermoid cyst of the floor of the mouth appears as a radiolucent area on CT.

onstrated on a lateral film. Inflammatory or neoplastic masses in the oral cavity or oropharynx are best evaluated further by computed tomography (CT) or magnetic resonance imaging (MRI) (Fig. 32-6).

EXAMINATION OF THE NASOPHARYNX

The nasopharynx is best examined by visualization. In an adolescent or older child, the nasopharynx can be examined indirectly with a nasopharyngeal mirror, although the best visualization usually is achieved with either a rigid 90 degree telescope (Fig. 32-7) or a flexible fiberoptic nasopharyngoscope (Fig. 32-8). Use of a flexible fiberoptic endoscope may be tolerated even in small children after spraying the nasal cavity with a topical decongestant and anesthetic. Endoscopic examination of the nasopharynx allows simultaneous inspection of other nasal structures, including the turbinates and meatus. At the choanae, which is the entrance to the nasopharynx from the nose, the adenoidal pad may be seen centrally and the orifices of the eustachian tubes may be seen laterally. Movement of the soft palate may also be assessed.

A lateral neck radiograph that includes the naso-

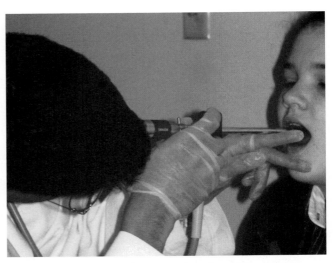

Figure 32–7: Excellent visualization of both the nasopharynx and hypopharynx can be achieved using a 90° telescope and fiberoptic light source.

pharynx still remains the best initial radiologic study to evaluate the nasopharynx for patency, nasopharyngeal masses, the size of the adenoidal pad, and any masses within the soft palate. Contrast studies to evaluate the patency of the nasopharynx (i.e., for the presence of choanal atresia) are rarely utilized today because of the superiority of CT in the evaluation of such abnormalities. Pathologies that involve the bony structures of the nasopharynx are best il-

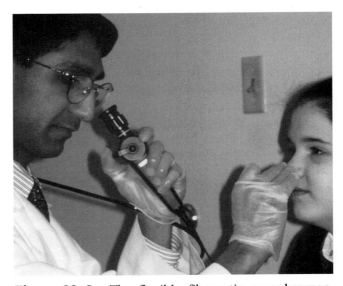

Figure 32–8: The flexible fiberoptic nasopharyngoscope can be used to examine the entire nasal airway, the nasopharynx, oropharynx, and hypopharynx. This instrument is usually well tolerated after decongesting and anesthetizing the nose.

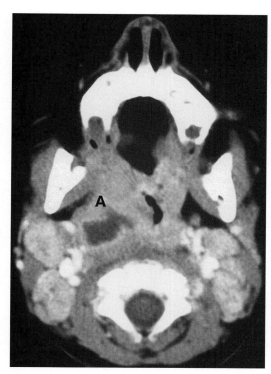

Figure 32–9: Rim-enhanced radiolucent area on CT represents an abscess (A) of the right parapharyngeal region that compromises the nasopharyngeal airway.

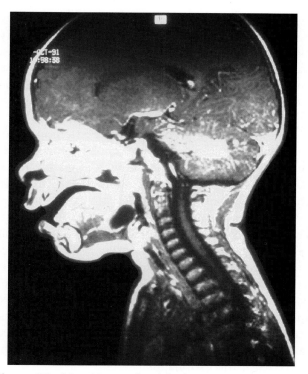

Figure 32–10: Mucocele of the base of tongue appears as a lucent area on MRI (saggital view).

lustrated by CT (Fig. 32-9), reserving the evaluation of strictly soft tissue abnormalities to MRI. MRI provides superior soft tissue detail in three planes (axial, coronal, sagittal). Because CT and MRI may complement each other, both studies may be indicated in some cases.

EXAMINATION OF THE HYPOPHARYNX

As with nasopharyngeal examination, visualization of the hypopharynx may be best accomplished by use of a flexible fiberoptic endoscope introduced through the nose, a 90 degree telescope, or a laryngeal mirror. The 90 degree telescope provides superior optics, although its use may not be tolerated as well as a small flexible nasopharyngoscope. As with the nasopharyngeal examination, use of a nasopharyngoscope requires anesthetizing and decongesting the nose. In an infant or young child, it may be necessary to administer general anesthesia in order to examine the hypopharynx. Palpation of the hypopharynx is not recommended in an awake child,

and may prove traumatic to the family, patient, and examiner.

The lateral neck radiograph remains a good screening tool for evaluation of the hypopharynx, especially for identifying masses that involve the tongue base or posterior pharyngeal wall. Both CT and MRI give superior detail; the former study should be employed if a soft tissue/bone interface requires evaluation (Fig. 32-10).

EXAMINATION OF THE ESOPHAGUS

The two major methods for evaluating the esophagus include contrast videofluoroscopy and visualization by endoscopy. The contrast study should be performed prior to any endoscopic evaluation so that anatomic abnormalities that may affect endoscopy can be identified. Contrast videofluoroscopy may demonstrate strictures, mucosal abnormalities, intrinsic masses, and radiolucent foreign bodies, especially boluses of food such as meat. Narrowing within the esophagus where foreign bodies may lodge can also be demonstrated.[1] Abnormal compression of the esophagus from a vascular ab-normality, such as an aberrant left subclavian artery, may be demonstrated. Unlike esophagoscopy, contrast studies of the esophagus show both the swallowing function and motility. Aspiration of contrast medium into the trachea may indicate laryngeal dysfunction.

Radiopaque foreign bodies may be demonstrated with AP and lateral radiography of the neck and chest (Fig. 32–11). Radiopaque foreign bodies of the esophagus can usually be distinguished from tracheal foreign bodies on these plain radiographs.

Esophageal manometry documents upper and lower esophageal sphincteric pressures and should be utilized to evaluate children with suspected esophageal motility disorders. Demonstration of gastroesophageal reflux (GER) may be performed with a pH probe that is inserted through the nose and into the esophagus. This study can measure acid reflux at various sites from the gastroesophageal junction to the level of the cricoid cartilage at the introitus of the esophagus.

Unless a foreign body requires immediate extraction, esophagoscopy should be performed after an 8 to 12 hour fast. Fasting is necessary not only for the use of general anesthesia, which may be required for rigid endoscopy, but also to allow food to pass beyond the stomach. Both rigid and flexible endoscopy may be used to perform the examination, and both have advantages and disadvantages. Flexible endoscopy may be performed under sedation, thus avoiding a general anesthetic; it also provides excellent visualization of the esophageal mucosa. On the other hand, a rigid endoscope is introduced after exposing the hypopharynx with a laryngoscope. This method, although necessitating general anesthesia, allows for better examination of the hypopharynx and upper esophagus than is possible with a flexible scope. Rigid endoscopy is safer and more effective for the dilatation of strictures and retrieval of foreign bodies, especially those with sharp edges. Following endoscopy, the child should not ingest any food or liquids for a minimum of 6 hours or until it is clear that no inadvertent injury was caused to the esophagus. Because such an injury to the esophagus is heralded by the onset of pain and fever, antipyretics should be avoided as they may mask these symptoms. A suspected perforation should be confirmed by contrast videofluoroscopy. Treatment includes restriction of food or fluids, intravenous antibiotics, and possibly surgical drainage and repair.

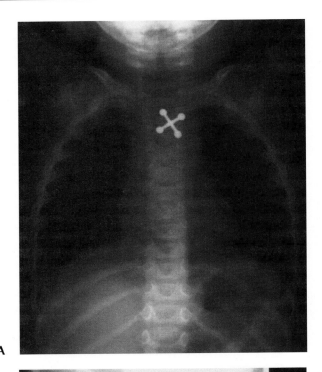

A

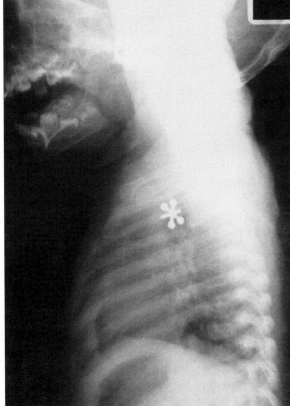

B

Figure 32–11: (A) Anterior-posterior and (B) lateral chest views illustrate a radiopaque foreign body (jack) in the mid-esophagus.

EVALUATION OF THE CHILD WITH A SORE THROAT

Sore throat is a common complaint in children, and is a frequent cause of visits to primary care physicians. Depending upon the etiology, throat pain may be acute (Practice Pathway 32-1) in some children and chronic in others. In most children, the cause of sore throat is usually infectious. Initially infection of the mucosa is usually associated with regional lymph node enlargement. Rarely, infection will spread to the deep cervical nodes. Depending upon the pathogen, pharyngitis may be nonexudative, exudative, or ulcerative. Symptoms associated with pharyngitis include otalgia from referred ear pain and dysphagia. In allergic patients, throat pain may be seen in conjunction with sneezing and allergic conjunctivitis. Nasal obstruction and postnasal drip in patients with sinusitis may cause complaints of sore throat. In some cases, gingival and dental pain may mimic throat pain.

SPECIAL CONSIDERATION:

Because of the possibility of complications, the identification of a streptococcal infection is crucial when evaluating a child with a sore throat.

Examination of the child with a sore throat should include a thorough evaluation of the head and neck.

Practice Pathway 32–1   DIAGNOSIS OF ACUTE SORE THROAT

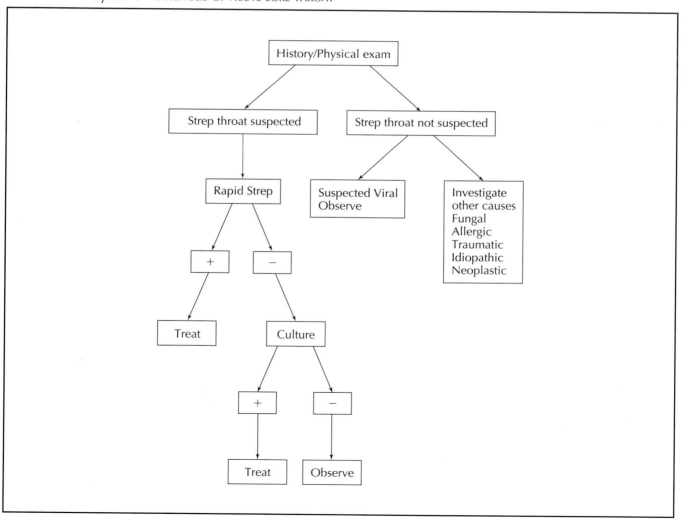

Pharyngitis is frequently associated with clinical signs of rhinitis or otitis. In children with sinusitis or infection of adenoid tissue, mucopurulent secretions may be seen to streak the posterior pharyngeal wall. With viral pharyngitis, inspection of the oropharynx may reveal vesicles on the soft palate and erythema of the tonsils. Exudative tonsillitis may be seen as the result of both viral and bacterial infection. Erythema of the larynx is common with upper respiratory infection (URI), but isolated erythema of the posterior vocal cords and the mucosa overlying the arytenoid cartilages and walls of the hypopharynx suggests GER.

Fever is not a consistent indication of the systemic involvement of a throat infection. Depending upon their size, location, and pattern, enlarged and tender lymph nodes may provide a clue to the type of infection. Bilateral nodal involvement suggests a viral etiology, whereas unilateral involvement is more commonly the result of bacterial infection. A skin rash suggestive of scarlet fever, hepatosplenomegaly associated with infectious mononucleosis, or evidence of chest infection upon auscultation are systemic signs that may help in narrowing the differential diagnosis.

Identification of the agent responsible for pharyngeal infection is best accomplished by culture. Streptococcal infection appears as hemolytic colonies if cultured on sheep blood agar plates and may be classified according to the pattern of hemolysis. Complete hemolysis is termed *beta,* partial is termed *alpha,* and absence of hemolysis is termed *gamma.* Other pathogens infecting the throat and causing complaints of sore throat may require specialized cultures for viral, fungal, or other bacterial agents.

Differential Diagnosis

Viral infection

Most episodes of *viral pharyngitis* accompany a viral URI. Symptoms include sore throat, fever, malaise, and lymphadenopathy. Responsible viral agents include rhinovirus, coronavirus, parainfluenza virus, respiratory syncytial virus, adenovirus, and influenza virus.

Primary herpetic gingivostomatitis may be caused by herpes simplex viruses types 1 or 2 (HSV-1 and HSV-2). Typically, the child complains of oral pain associated with fever and lymphadenopathy in the neck. In the primary infection, vesicles and ul-

cers may involve the lips, tongue, buccal mucosa, soft palate, and oropharyngeal mucosa. *Herpangina* is a group A coxsackievirus infection in which vesicular lesions involving the soft palate and oropharynx are accompanied by fever. *Hand-foot-and-mouth disease* is another group A coxsackie virus infection in which oral mucosal lesions are seen in association with vesicular dermatitis of the extremities.

Infection of the pharynx with the *Epstein-Barr virus* (infectious mononucleosis) is suggested by the presence of sore throat, fever, generalized lymphadenopathy, and splenomegaly. Additional signs include malaise, jaundice, and petechiae on the palate. More than 10% of atypical lymphocytes and a positive monospot test are associated with Epstein-Barr infection, although definitive diagnosis can only be confirmed with elevation of titers to the Epstein-Barr virus.

Bacterial infection

Bacterial infection of the throat may present with either acute or chronic throat pain. *Acute bacterial pharyngitis* usually involves the oropharynx, including the tonsils, but not the oral cavity. Transmission of such infections is usually either by direct contact or airborne.

Group A beta hemolytic Streptococcus pyogenes (GABHS) is a common bacterial organism that infects the throat. Fever, mucosal erythema, headache, and abdominal pain are associated symptoms. Tender, anterior cervical adenopathy correlates with streptococcal infection.[2] Factors that favor a positive streptococcal throat culture are listed in Table 32–1.[3]

TABLE 32–1: Factors Suggestive of a Positive Streptococcus Throat Culture

Autumn season
Age < 11 years
Duration < 3 days
Very sore throat
Difficult to swallow
Halitosis
Absence of cough and otitis media
Fever, myalgias, and flushed appearance
Enlarged or tender adenopathy
Erythema and tonsillar exudates

From reference 3, with permission.

Although a positive culture for GABHS in a symptomatic patient confirms streptococcal pharyngitis, a typical culture requires at least 24 hours for incubation. Culturing for *streptococcus* with both aerobic and anaerobic methods increases the rate of identification.[4] In order to identify patients with active infection who require treatment more quickly, antigen detection (rapid streptococcal) tests have been developed. Rapid streptococcal testing has been found to be more sensitive than blood agar plating. Thus, negative rapid streptococcal testing does not always need to be routinely confirmed by culture. False-positive rapid streptococcal testing may be the result of other streptococcal species, and may lead to the overdiagnosis of GABHS, although this concept is debatable.[5-7]

Elevated levels of antibodies to toxins that are produced by virulent streptococcal species, including group A, are a measure of chronic infection. Elevated antistreptolysin-O titers may identify patients with chronic infection who are susceptible to developing delayed complications such as acute rheumatic fever (ARF) and acute glomerulonephritis (AGN).

A streptococcal carrier state is defined as a child who has a positive culture for GABHS but is asymptomatic. It remains difficult to differentiate those children who are true carriers from those who are asymptomatic but who harbor active infection and are still at risk to spread disease or develop ARF or AGN.[8] Some children who are thought to be carriers may have subacute infection.[9] Even elevated antistreptolysin-O titers are not reliable for distinguishing between carriers and those with active infection.[10]

Bacteria other than GABHS may be responsible for acute pharyngitis, and these include *Haemophilus influenzae* and *groups C and G beta hemolytic streptococci.*[11] Penicillinase-producing *Staphylococcus aureus* may be responsible for penicillin treatment failures of GABHS, although this concept remains controversial.[12,13] *Mycoplasma pneumoniae,* usually a lower respiratory pathogen in children, may be a cause of pharyngitis in adolescents and adults.[14] Rarely, *Chlamydia trachomatis* may be the cause of pharyngitis.[15]

Membranous pharyngitis, or Vincent's angina, is an oropharyngeal ulcerative condition caused by a combination of *Fusobacterium necrophorum, Borrelia vincentti, Spirochaeta denticolitica,* or *Peptococcus.*[14] Children with acute epiglottitis may present with early complaints of sore throat that

progresses to stridor and fever. Fortunately, the incidence of acute epiglottitis has decreased since the introduction of the polyvalent vaccine for *Haemophilus influenzae.*[16]

Acute bacterial infection of the nose, nasopharynx, and sinuses frequently causes mucopurulent drainage along the posterior pharyngeal wall that elicits complaints of sore throat. A variety of upper respiratory pathogens may be the source of this infection. Associated symptoms include purulent nasal drainage, facial pain, nasal obstruction, and fever.

Fungal infection

Fungal infections involving the mucosa of the oral cavity and pharynx are typically seen in two populations of patients: infants and immunocompromised children. Infants may develop thrush or oral candidiasis due to irritation from bottle feeding. *Candida albicans* may also be a pathogen in immunocompromised children. Affected patients complain of dysphagia and odynophagia. Adherent white plaques are seen on involved mucosa, especially in the buccal region, and attempts to remove this plaque frequently result in bleeding. The diagnosis is confirmed by finding yeast on KOH preparations of plaque or by positive fungal cultures.

Allergic disorders

The child who is afflicted with allergy to environmental antigens frequently complains of a sore throat. These complaints may be in response to an increase in nasal secretions that are seen in allergic patients or may be the result of direct stimulation by allergens that contact the oral and oropharyngeal mucosa. It is not unusual to see erythema of pharyngeal mucosa in affected patients especially in the tonsillar regions and along the posterior pharyngeal wall. Diagnosis of allergic disorders as a cause of sore throat is difficult unless there is a response either to treatment or elimination of suspected allergens from the child's environment.

Traumatic disorders

Traumatic ulcers may involve any site on the oral mucosa, but are found frequently on the buccal mucosa secondary to chronic abrasion from neurotic habits such as cheek biting. Traumatic ulcers are usually focal and manifest a grayish-white pseudomembrane. Burns sustained from eating hot food or drink may cause ulcerative lesions and pain until healed. Pizza with hot cheese is a common offender. Corrosive burns from exposure to either alkaline or acidic substances may cause mouth or throat pain. Usually, there is evidence of a whitish eschar on the lips and tongue, and one should be suspicious of coinciding esophageal burns.

Idiopathic disorders

Recurrent *aphthous stomatitis* is probably the most common cause of oral and oropharyngeal pain, affecting 15% of the population at one time or another.[17] Aphthous ulcers afflict children more than adults.[17] The etiology remains unknown, although changes in locally-mediated immune factors that are brought on by trauma, stress, debilitating disease, or vitamin B deficiency may precipitate development of this condition. Typically, the gingival mucosa is involved with one or several small ulcers that have a grayish-white pseudomembrane, surrounded by an erythematous halo.

Behçet's syndrome is a triad of symptoms that includes recurrent aphthous ulceration causing mouth pain, uveitis and iridocyclitis, and genital ulcers. The ulcers may be shallow or deep and have a central, yellowish necrotic base.[18] The etiology of this disorder remains unknown; however, a genetic basis is suspected.

In *Reiter's syndrome,* urethritis, conjunctivitis, and arthritis may be accompanied by oral lesions. These oral ulcerations usually are superficial and transient and are associated with minimal discomfort. There is a strong association with gram-negative enteric infections.

Erythema multiforme is an acute inflammatory disorder involving the skin and mucous membranes. The most common etiologies include reactions to drugs such as phenytoin, phenobarbital, penicillin, or the sulfonamides or to infectious agents such as the Epstein-Barr virus, enteroviruses, HSV, and Mycoplasma pneumoniae.[19] The lips, anterior tongue, and floor of the mouth are usually involved with bullae formation that progresses to ulceration. The skin or mouth may be involved solely or may be associated with systemic toxicity (Stevens-Johnson syndrome).

Neoplasms

Oral neoplasms are a rare cause of throat pain in the pediatric age group. Leukemia may present with symptoms suggestive of pharyngitis. The initial ap-

pearance of lymphoma may be as unilateral enlargement of a tonsil that is associated with dysphagia, muffled speech, and throat pain. Squamous cell carcinoma may appear rarely in adolescence with sore throat or referred otalgia. Rhabdomyosarcoma or other sarcomas rarely may involve the oral cavity or pharynx, producing throat pain.

AT A GLANCE. . .
Evaluation of Sore Throat

Symptoms: throat pain, otalgia, dysphagia, postnasal drip

Signs: pharyngeal erythema, exudative tonsillitis, fever, cervical adenopathy

Diagnosis: rapid strep testing, culture

Differential Diagnosis: viral, bacterial, fungal, allergic, traumatic, idiopathic, neoplastic

---

EVALUATION OF THE CHILD WITH DYSPHAGIA

Dysphagia or difficulty in swallowing may be evident as early as the fetal period during which oral, pharyngeal, and esophageal dysfunction result in polyhydramnios.[20] Both the sucking and swallowing reflexes need to be stimulated soon after birth or their delayed development will affect deglutition for years. Both sucking and swallowing are initial oral motor skills that are followed by the more complex actions of biting and chewing.

SPECIAL CONSIDERATION:

Failure to develop normal swallowing and sucking reflexes will affect deglutition for years.

The act of swallowing can be divided into several stages, some voluntary and others involuntary, and is mediated by the action of several cranial nerves and coordinated by the brainstem (Chapter 31). Both sensory and motor functions are involved, and failure of either or both results in a poor suck reflex and failure to propel the bolus of food into the pharynx.[21] Preparation of the food bolus is a voluntary function that includes mastication and manipulation. Delivery of the bolus posteriorly into the pharynx by the tongue is also a voluntary action.[22] At this point, the remainder of the swallowing function is involuntary as the soft palate closes to seal off the nasopharynx. The bolus is then passed through the pharynx by the action of the pharyngeal musculature. At the same time, the larynx closes at the level of both the true and false vocal folds and the cricopharyngeal muscle, which comprises the upper esophageal sphincter (UES), relaxes to allow the bolus to pass into the upper esophagus.[22]

Etiology of Dysphagia

Congenital

In the infant, congenital conditions that interfere with breathing also have a profound impact on feeding. Failure to thrive in an infant who has bilateral choanal atresia is a classic example of this association. Other airway abnormalities in the newborn that affect breathing and feeding include severe laryngomalacia, laryngeal webs, subglottic stenosis, laryngeal cysts, and laryngotracheal clefts. Infants with unilateral vocal fold paralysis frequently have recurrent bouts of aspiration that interfere with swallowing. Chest abnormalities cause similar symptoms by partially obstructing either the trachea, the esophagus, or both. Arch abnormalities, such as vascular rings, congenital strictures or webs of either the trachea or esophagus, bronchogenic cysts, esophageal atresia, or tracheoesophageal fistula, may all interfere with swallowing in the newborn. Likewise, hemangiomas and lymphangiomas may interfere with pharyngeal, tracheal, or esophageal function.

Transient pharyngeal incoordination of the newborn is a symptom complex that includes increased oropharyngeal secretions, cyanosis, and choking spells.[23-26] Esophageal manometry in these infants is usually normal.[26] Improvement in symptoms occurs over a variable period of time.

Cricopharyngeal achalasia is usually congenital, but may appear from 2 to 6 months of age. Symptoms of regurgitation and aspiration result from the failure of the cricopharyngeus muscle to relax and allow food and liquids to pass into the esophagus. Other symptoms include poor eating, a congested sound in the throat, choking and coughing while eating, and nasal reflux of liquids. Symptoms are usually relieved by cricopharyngeal myotomy, surgical division of the cricopharyngeus muscle. When associated with other neurologic problems, there may be motility disorders of the entire esophagus that require more complicated treatment.[27]

Acquired

Many acquired conditions that involve the pharynx have an impact on swallowing. Trauma in the form of foreign bodies, corrosives, or other injuries to the pharynx or esophagus will interfere with swallowing. Acute infectious processes that involve the pharynx and/or mediastinum may impede swallowing temporarily. Likewise, mass lesions such as neoplasms or enlarged tonsils and adenoids may obstruct propulsion of the bolus into the pharynx. Chronic GER may result in a stricture in the region of the lower esophageal sphincter (LES). Controversy exists as to whether GER may affect the UES in the same manner.[28]

Cricopharyngeal achalasia may be seen in children of any age but is more common in its congenital form.[29] Diffuse esophageal spasm and esophageal achalasia more commonly affect the adult population but may rarely appear in adolescence. Crohn's disease may also affect the esophagus, impairing normal motility.[30] Several autoimmune disorders may impact esophageal function. Juvenile rheumatoid arthritis (JRA) affects laryngeal function and may precipitate episodes of coughing and choking. Xerostomia seen with Sjögren's syndrome may interfere with preparation of the food bolus. Scleroderma, polymyositis, and dermatomyositis may also affect esophageal motility.

Neuromuscular conditions

The onset of dysphagia is often an early sign of other neurologic dysfunction and may be seen with such symptoms as poor muscle tone, poor gag reflex, or an increase in pharyngeal secretions. Associated neurologic conditions that cause dysphagia include pharyngoesophageal dysmotility, cricopharyngeal achalasia, nasal regurgitation, and tracheal aspiration. Because the swallowing center resides within the brainstem, abnormalities such as the Arnold-Chiari malformation, bulbar poliomyelitis, and familial dysautonomia (Riley-Day syndrome) may have an impact on swallowing.

Behavioral conditions

Globus refers to complaints of a lump sensation in the throat and is a frequent cause of dysphagia in normal children, especially following an episode of choking on solid food. The sensation of globus is also a common complaint of children with GER. Psychiatric conditions that may have an impact on swallowing include anorexia nervosa, bulimia, and Munchausen syndrome.

Clinical Evaluation

Because many swallowing disorders are the result of delayed development of swallowing in the neonate and infant, a good history should include details of the early neonatal course. Prolonged intubation or other complications during the newborn period that interfered with the development of the sucking and swallowing reflexes should be identified. It is important to distinguish between dysphagia for solids or liquids. Aspiration of only liquids may be the first sign of neuromuscular problems. Liquids, on the other hand, are the last to be affected by lesions that may obstruct the esophagus.

Excessive salivation (*ptyalism*) suggests a problem with swallowing; however, this symptom also is seen with poor oral muscle control. The presence of the associated symptoms of coughing and gagging may be important in identifying the cause of dysphagia. Stridor also may be present in neonates and infants during feeding. Hoarseness is a symptom of laryngeal irritation and often is associated with GER.

Weight loss as the result of dysphagia is usually significant for a severe underlying disorder. A good nutritional assessment may help to identify the type of food that is a problem. Because the cranial nerves involved in palatal function also are part of the swallowing reflex, the presence of nasal regurgitation in the absence of an anatomic defect suggests that an underlying neurologic problem may be at the root of the dysphagia. Vomiting and the character of the vomitus are also important in determining the pathogenesis of the dysphagia.

The most important part of the physical examination is watching the patient feed. This is especially true in neonates and infants. Evidence of poor weight gain, a weak suckle, slow feeding, problems handling secretions, and oral or nasal regurgitation are also important findings. The type and consistency of food being attempted is very important, as is the relationship of breathing and eating. Chronic mouth breathing, usually the result of upper airway obstruction, interferes with the child's ability to swallow. Inspection of the dentition and tongue are important because both are involved in the formation of the food bolus.

In a child who has severe dysphagia, the clinician should look for signs of a craniofacial defect or cleft palate, which may have interfered with the development of a normal swallow at a young age. Abnormalities of the tongue, such as macroglossia, may interfere with the child's ability to eat. A good neurologic evaluation is an important part of any clinical assessment of swallowing and should include determination of the level of consciousness and cranial nerve function, specifically cranial nerves VII, IX, X, and XII.

Radiologic Evaluation

In the initial evaluation of the patient with dysphagia (Practice Pathway 32-2), both lateral neck and chest radiography serve as good screening tools. The lateral neck film demonstrates underlying problems in the upper airway that may interfere with

Practice Pathway 32–2   EVALUATION OF DYSPHAGIA

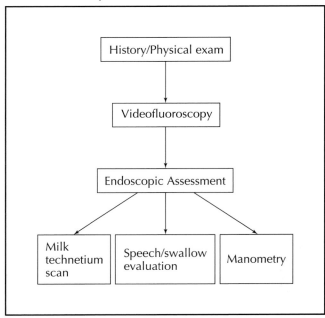

feeding. The chest radiograph provides similar information for the intrathoracic airway and may also provide evidence of acute or chronic aspiration.

Videofluoroscopy of the entire airway may be performed as part of a contrast study of the swallowing function. Airway abnormalities such as tracheomalacia, subglottic stenosis, and even unilateral vocal fold paralysis may be detected. When performing a barium swallow, the contrast study should include all phases of swallowing and not just the esophageal.[31] An important phase in the swallowing process is the formation of the liquid bolus and how it is propelled into the proximal esophagus. Aspiration of contrast into the trachea may be seen in some patients. Liquids of various consistencies can be used to determine which can be tolerated best. In patients with dysphagia for solids only, a solid food may be coated with barium to demonstrate the site of dysfunction. In infants, contrast can be instilled through a nipple. Children who are fed by nasogastric tube may be studied by pulling the tube back into the pharynx and then instilling a small amount of contrast material.

Endoscopic Evaluation

The endoscopic evaluation of the upper aerodigestive tract may be performed with either rigid or flexible endoscopes, depending on the suspected diagnosis. Rigid endoscopy permits control of the airway and easier introduction of either a bronchoscope or esophagoscope. The use of direct laryngoscopy is dependent upon general anesthesia, but permits a panoramic view of the hypopharynx and larynx. Flexible endoscopy can be performed under sedation, and may allow for study of the dynamics of swallowing.

Additional Studies

Esophageal manometry studies the dynamics of the UES and LES. Pharyngeal-esophageal sphincter incoordination may be distinguished from cricopharyngeal achalasia.[21] It may also be helpful for studying the sucking reflex in infants.[21] Manometry should not be performed at the same time as endoscopy because endoscopy may alter the readings.[21]

Use of a nuclear technetium (milk) scan may demonstrate soilage of the pulmonary tree from chronic aspiration and may also show the severity of GER. A pH probe placed into the esophagus at various levels documents the severity and frequency of reflux of acid contents from the stomach. In infants, it may be combined with a polysomnographic study to evaluate coordination between breathing and swallowing.

The clinical evaluation of the child with dysphagia should be approached by a team that includes the pediatrician, otolaryngologist, speech therapist, and radiologist. The pediatrician can assess developmental issues and the otolaryngologist can evaluate the child for structural abnormalities that interfere with feeding. The speech therapist and radiologist can work together to examine the child while he swallows contrast medium.[31] The team can then formulate a comprehensive plan for swallowing rehabilitation.

AT A GLANCE. . .
Evaluation of Dysphagia

Symptoms and Signs: coughing, gagging, ptyalism, stridor, hoarseness, nasal regurgitation, vomiting, failure to thrive

Radiologic Evaluation: lateral neck and chest radiography, videofluoroscopy

Endoscopic Evaluation: flexible or rigid esophagoscopy

Additional Studies: manometry, milk technetium scan, speech/swallow evaluation

---

REFERENCES

1. Atkins, JP, Keane WM. Esophagology. In: English GM, ed. *Otolaryngology, Vol 3*. New York: Harper and Row, 1978, p. 11–12.
2. Kaplan EL, Top FH, Dudding BA, et al. Diagnosis of streptococcal pharyngitis: The problem of differentiating active infection from the carrier state in the symptomatic child. J Infect Dis 1971; 123:490–501.
3. Douglas M, Stralnick H. A scoring system for streptococcal pharyngitis. J Fam Pract 1996; 43:537–538.
4. Schwartz RH, Hayden GF, Wientzen R. Children less than three years old with pharyngitis. Clin Pediatr 1986; 25:185–188.
5. Gerber MA, Tanz RR, Kabat W, et al. Optical immunoassay test for group A β-hemolytic streptococcal pharyngitis. JAMA 1997; 277:899–903.
6. Shulman ST. Value of new rapid tests for the diagnosis of group A streptococcal pharyngitis. Pediatr Infect Dis J 1995; 14:923–924.

7. Roe M, Kishiyama C, Davidson, et al. Comparison of Biostar Strep A OIA optical immune assay, Abbott Testpack Plus Strep A, and culture with selective media for diagnosis of group A streptococcal pharyngitis. J Clin Microbiol 1995; 33:1551–1553.

8. Kaplan EL. The group A streptococcal upper respiratory tract carrier state: An enigma. J Pediatr 1980; 97:337–345.

9. Gordis L, Lilienfeld A, Rodriguez R. Studies in the epidemiology and prevention of rheumatic fever. III. Evaluation of the Maryland rheumatic fever registry. Public Health Rep 1969; 84:333–339.

10. Gerber MA, Randolph MF, Mayo DR. The group A streptococcal carrier state: A reexamination. AJDC 1988; 142:562–565.

11. Feldman WE. Pharyngitis in children. Postgrad Med 1993; 93:141–145.

12. Bernstein SH, Stillerman M, Allerhand J. Demonstration of penicillin inhibitory by pharyngeal microflora in patients treated for streptococcal pharyngitis. J Lab Clin Med 1964; 63:14–22.

13. Quie PG, Pierce HC, Wannamaker LW. Influence of penicillin-producing staphylococci and the eradication of group A streptococci from the upper respiratory tract by penicillin treatments. Pediatrics 1966; 37:467–476.

14. Vukmir RB. Adult and pediatric pharyngitis: A review. J Emerg Med 1992; 10:607–616.

15. McMillan JA, Sandstrom C, Weiner LB, et al. Viral and bacterial organisms associated with acute pharyngitis in a school-aged population. J Pediatr 1986; 109:747–752.

16. Kessler A, Wetmore RF, Marsh RR. Childhood epiglottitis in recent years. Int J Pediatr Otorhinolaryngol 1993; 25:155–162.

17. Eversole LR. Mucosal pain disorders of the head and neck. Otolaryngol Clin North Am 1989; 22:1095–1114.

18. Moutsopoulos HM. Behcet's syndrome. In: Fouci AS, Braunwald E, Isselbacher KJ, et al., eds. *Harrison's Principles of Internal Medicine, 14th ed.* New York: McGraw-Hill, 1998, pp. 1910.

19. Frieden IJ. Hypersensitivity reactions. In: Rudolph AM, Hoffman JIE, Rudolph CD, eds. *Rudolph's Pediatrics. 20th ed.* Stamford: Appleton and Lange, 1996; p. 907.

20. Logan WJ, Bosma JF. Oral and pharyngeal dysphagia in infants. Pediatr Clin North Am 1967; 14:47–61.

21. Fisher SE, Painter M, Milmoe G. Swallowing disorders in infancy. Pediatr Clin North Am 1981; 28:845–853.

22. Jones PM. Feeding disorders in children with multiple handicaps. Dev Med Child Neurol 1989; 31:404–406.

23. Frank MM, Gatewood OM. Transient pharyngeal incoordination in the newborn. AJDC 1966; 111:178–181.

24. Macaulay JC. Neuromuscular incoordination of swallowing in the newborn. Lancet 1951; 260:1208.

25. Morgan J. Neuromuscular incoordination of swallowing in the newborn. J Laryngol 1956; 70:294.

26. Ardran GM, Benson PF, Butler NR, et al. Congenital dysphagia resulting from dysfunction of the pharyngeal musculature. Dev Med Child Neurol 1965; 7:157–166.

27. Reichert TJ, Bluestone CD, Stool SE, et al. Congenital cricopharyngeal achalasia. Ann Otol 1977; 86:603–610.

28. Sondheimer JM. Upper esophageal sphincter and pharyngoesophageal motor function in infants with and without gastroesophageal reflux. Gastroenterology 1983; 85:301–305.

29. Bishop HC. Cricopharyngeal achalasia in childhood. J Pediatr Surg 1974; 9:775–778.

30. Lenaerts C, Roy CC, Vaillancourt M, et al. Involvement in children with Crohn's disease. Pediatrics 1989; 83:777–781.

31. Griggs CA, Jones PM, Lee RE. Videofluoroscopic investigation of feeding disorders of children with multiple handicap. Dev Med Child Neurol 1989; 31:303–308.

33 Congenital Malformations of the Oral Cavity, Pharynx, and Esophagus

Glenn Isaacson

Anomalies of the human body that are present at birth are either the product of errors in embryogenesis (i.e., malformations) or the result of intrauterine events that affect embryonic and fetal growth (i.e., deformations and disruptions).[1] The more complex the formation of a structure, the more opportunities there are for malformation. As the flat embryonic plate folds and fuses to form the nose, mouth, airway, and gullet, there are many such opportunities for errors in development. These critically-timed events are reviewed in the embryology sections of Chapters 22, 31, and 42. This chapter describes some of the possible malformations of the oral cavity, pharynx, and esophagus.

MALFORMATIONS OF THE ORAL CAVITY

The Jaws

Midline union of the mandibular portions of the first branchial arches normally occurs during the fourth week of intrauterine life. This is the earliest fusion event in the face. Failed mandibular fusion may result in *mandibular clefting* (Fig. 33–1) and hypoplasia of the mandible. Retarded growth of the mandible results in *micrognathia*. Although it is only a cosmetic problem in its mild forms, micrognathia in the infant may result in neonatal upper-airway obstruction. An underdeveloped mandible results in the upward and posterior displacement of the tongue. The upward displacement inhibits the ingrowth and fusion of the secondary palatal shelves, resulting in a *cleft palate*. The posterior displacement of the tongue has been shown to be one of

the mechanisms of airway obstruction that is seen in these patients.[2] This triad of micrognathia, glossoptosis, and a U-shaped palatal cleft describes the *Robin* sequence (Fig. 33–2). Robin's sequence may occur as an isolated problem or as part of several congenital anomaly complexes and syndromes. Its designation as a "sequence" means that, unlike a syndrome, it has no single known cause. Robin's sequence may be associated with upper-airway obstruction in the neonatal period. Correct positioning of the baby in a prone position and gavage feeding are often all that are needed to allow the baby to feed and breathe. In severe cases, intervention to correct upper-airway obstruction may be life saving.[3] If a child has continuing oxygen desaturations or fails to thrive despite conservative measures, a tracheotomy often is required. Surgical maneuvers to advance the tongue, e.g. glossopany, or mandible in the infant remain controversial, although they may be successful in patients who are identified as having Sher's type 1 obstruction, in which the tongue is displaced posteriorly against the posterior pharyngeal wall.[2] Closure of the palatal defect usually is delayed for fear of worsening upper-airway obstruction.

Asymmetries of the mandible and maxilla occur in a variety of craniofacial abnormalities. *Hemifacial microsomia* (i.e., facio-auricular-vertebral spectrum) often involves the mandible as well as other components of the first and second branchial arches, including the malar eminence, parotid, and external ear. *Congenital cysts* of the maxilla may arise at fusion lines of the premaxilla and maxilla. These rarely present in infancy. By contrast, *eruption cysts,* which are associated with natal teeth may present in the newborn. Natal teeth are often the only primary dentition and should not be removed in most cases. Eruption cysts require marsupialization only when they are painful and interfere with feeding.[4]

Pediatric Otolaryngology, Edited by R.F. Wetmore, H.R. Muntz, and T.J. McGill. Thieme Medical Publishers, Inc., New York © 2000.

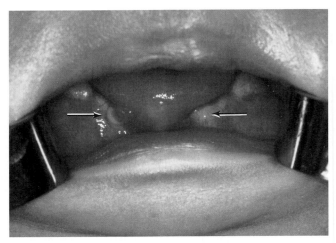

Figure 33–1: Failed mandibular fusion. Severe micrognathia was associated with these unfused hemi-mandibles (arrows).

The Lips

Fusion of the components of the upper lip occurs later in embryogenesis and is more complex than that of the lower lip. Thus, clefting anomalies of the upper lip are more common and more varied. Cleft upper lip and palate malformations are described in detail in Chapter 34. *Astomia* results from complete union of the upper and lower lips. *Microstomia* refers to the rudimentary oral aperture sometimes

seen in association with severe forms of holoprosencephaly.[5] Lateral clefting of the oral introitus leads to an asymmetric *macrostomia*. Surgical correction of this type of macrostomia requires the creation of a new oral commissure.[6]

Congenital oral synechiae can occur between the hard palate and the floor of mouth, the tongue, or the oropharynx. These are thought to arise from persistence of the buccopharyngeal membrane that separates the mouth from the pharynx in the embryo.[7]

Congenital pits of the lower lip are usually in a paramedian location. They often secrete mucous from salivary glands at their bases. They are not thought to represent fusion abnormalities, but instead are thought to arise from secondary notching of the lip epithelium. *Lip pits* may be inherited in an autosomal dominant pattern in the Van der Woude syndrome. (Fig. 33-3) This syndrome frequently includes missing teeth and a cleft lip or palate. Rarely, lip pits may communicate an ectopic parotid duct.[8]

Abnormal *labial frenula* may involve the upper or lower lips. In infancy, the maxillary labial frenulum typically extends over the alveolar ridge to form a raphe that reaches the palatal papilla. If this persists after the eruption of teeth, it may result in a spreading of the medial incisors. Similarly, if the mandibular labial frenulum extends to the interdental papilla, its traction can lead to periodontal disease and bone loss. Each type of aberrant frenulum can be treated with surgical division when clinically significant.

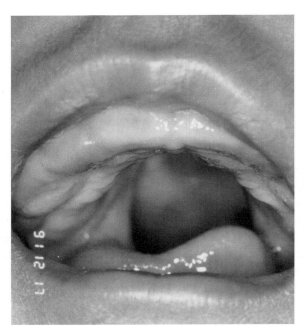

Figure 33–2: Robin sequence. A wide U-shaped palatal cleft is typical.

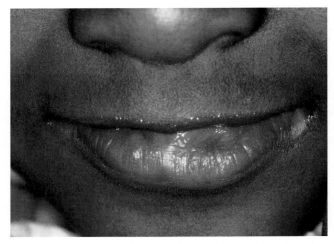

Figure 33–3: Van der Woude syndrome. Lip pits often are associated with cleft palate in this heritable disorder.

SPECIAL CONSIDERATION:

Labial and lingual frenula should be treated with surgical division when clinically significant.

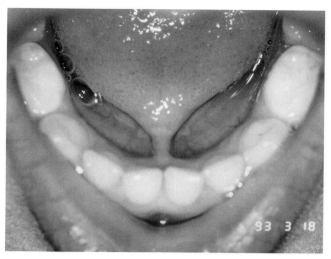

Figure 33–4: Ankyloglossia. Surgical treatment is required if a tethering frenulum prevents the tongue from reaching the upper alveolus. (Photo courtesy of Ellen S. Deutsch, MD.)

The Tongue

Macroglossia is a true excess in tongue volume and should be differentiated from *glossoptosis,* in which a normal tongue overfills a small oral cavity. Macroglossia can be further subdivided into *focal* and *generalized* varieties. Focal enlargement of the tongue is most often associated with congenital tumors, especially lymphangiomas and hemangiomas. Enlargement of half the tongue can be seen in patients with somatic hemihypertrophy. Generalized macroglossia can been seen in Beckwith-Wiedemann syndrome[9] and hypothyroidism. It also is a congenital, progressive problem in children with mucopolysaccharidoses.[10] There is debate as to whether there is true macroglossia in Down syndrome or whether the protruding tongue seen in Trisomy 21 results from poor muscular tone. Surgical reduction of tongue mass has been advocated for both cosmetic and functional reasons in children with Down syndrome.[11]

Ankyloglossia or tongue-tie is restriction of tongue movement due to a prominent lingual frenulum (Fig. 33–4). There is a widespread belief that ankyloglossia leads to speech and language delays, and strong pressure may be brought to bear on the otolaryngologist to treat tongue-ties surgically. In fact, only a small fraction of prominent lingual frenula have any effect on function. Those frenula that extend to the tip of the tongue and prevent it from reaching the upper dental alveolus are most likely to be of clinical significance. "Snipping" of a true tongue-tie may lead to scarring and worse restriction of tongue movement. Division, mobilization, and lengthening can be achieved by Z-plasty or double V-Y advancement.[12] In severe cases, a buccal mucosal graft can be used.[13]

Fissuring of the tongue can be seen concomitant with facial and/or lip edema and relapsing facial palsy in the Melkersson-Rosenthal syndrome.[14] *Median rhomboid glossitis* is not an inflammatory condition as the name implies, but an absence of papilla in the region of the embryonic tuberculum impar. *Geographic tongue* or benign migratory glossitis is a chronic, recurring disorder of the filiform papillae (Fig. 33–5). Red, slightly-depressed lesions with whitish borders characterize this benign disorder. Its cause is unknown.

Lesions of the Oral Cavity

The area of the foramen cecum is another site of predilection for oral lesions. Embryonic fusion of

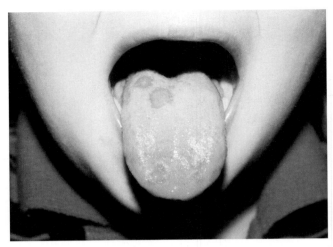

Figure 33–5: Geographic tongue. (Photo courtesy of Ellen S. Deutsch, MD.)

the anterior tongue and tongue base anlagen and the origin of the thyroglossal duct at this location present numerous opportunities for malformation. *Lingual thyroid* tissue, presenting at the foramen cecum, may represent the only thyroid gland. Radionuclide scanning can confirm the nature of this tissue as well as identify a separate, functioning thyroid gland, if present. Excision should be avoided unless the lesion causes airway obstruction.[15] If it is the only thyroid tissue, the mass of lingual thyroid can be reduced by the administration of thyroid hormone.[16] Lingual dermoid cysts[17] and mucoceles (Fig. 33–6) may present at the foramen cecum as well. Transoral, transglottic, and transhyoid approaches all have been advocated for surgical exposure.[18]

True cysts and pseudocysts of the major and minor salivary glands are among the more frequent, soft-tissue anomalies of the oral cavity. *Mucoceles* are pseudocysts of minor salivary origin. As such they lack an epithelial lining. Secretions dissect into the soft tissues surrounding the salivary gland and present as smooth swellings, most commonly in the buccal mucosa near the occlusal plane. When symptomatic these can be unroofed or marsupialized with good result. *Ranulas* are pseudocysts that are associated with the sublingual glands and submandibular ducts (Fig. 33–7). They can be congenital, probably from improper drainage of sublingual glands, or acquired from oral trauma. When large, ranulas may extend through the mylohyoid musculature of the floor of the mouth and present as a mass in the neck. Such "plunging" ranulas can be a surgical challenge since they are intimately involved with the submandibular duct and lingual nerve and lack a firm cyst wall.[19-21] Complete excision, often in continuity with the associated sublingual gland, is preferred. If this cannot be achieved, marsupialization with suture of the pseudocyst wall to the oral mucosa often is effective.

True cysts of the floor of the mouth are much less common. A primitive *foregut cyst* presenting in the floor of the mouth has been diagnosed antenatally. It was decompressed by needle aspiration at birth with subsequent surgical resection.[23] On rare occasion, a *thyroglossal duct cyst* may present in the floor of the mouth and simulate the much more commonly occurring ranula.[23]

A variety of benign congenital tumors can arise

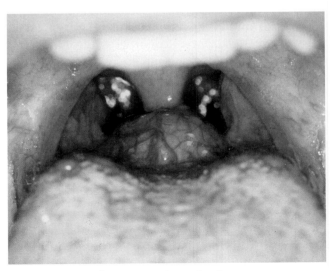

Figure 33–6: Mucocele at the foramen cecum.

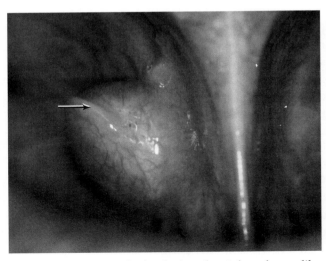

Figure 33–7: Ranula displacing the right submandibular duct (arrow).

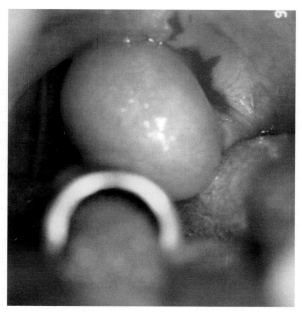

Figure 33–8: Choristoma of the tonsillar fossa. (Photo courtesy of Ellen S. Deutsch, MD.)

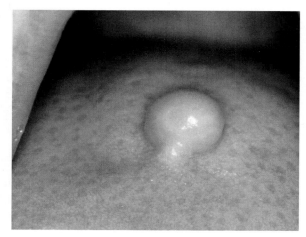

Figure 33–9: Choristoma of the tongue. (Photo courtesy of Ellen S. Deutsch, MD.)

in the oral cavity. Among the most common are teratomas and epithelial choristomas (Figs. 33–8 and 33–9). A *choristoma* is a tumor-like mass of normal cells in an abnormal location. Heterotopic gastric mucosa, enteric duplication cysts, heterotopic neural tissue, and ectopic cartilage and bone all have been reported.[24–26] *Granular cell tumors* that arise in the gnathic gingiva may be present at birth. They are uniformly benign and are treated with simple excision.

AT A GLANCE . . .

Anomalies of the Tongue and Oral Cavity

- Macroglossia
- Ankyloglossia (lingual frenulum)
- Melkersson-Rosenthal syndrome
- Median rhomboid glossitis
- Geographic tongue
- Lingual thyroid
- Lingual dermoid cysts
- Lingual mucoceles
- Ranulas
- Teratomas and epithelial choristomas
- Primitive foregut cysts/thyroglossal duct cyst
- Granular cell tumors
- Ectopic tissue

MALFORMATIONS OF THE PHARYNX

The Nasopharynx

The *nasopharynx* is an embryonic crossroad between the neural axis and the alimentary and respiratory tracts. As such, it is susceptible to a variety of malformations. Several cystic lesions of the nasopharynx have been the subject of much study and speculation.[27] The ectodermal anlage of the anterior hypophysis arises in the future nasopharynx from a diverticulum called *Rathke's pouch.*[28] Squamous-lined cysts in the midline of the nasopharynx are thought to arise from rests of this epithelium. *Thornwaldt's cysts* also are found in the midline, but are more caudal in location.[29] They are thought to arise from obstruction at *Thornwaldt's bursa,* which is a structure found at the junction of remnants of the notocord and the pharyngeal ectoderm. Prior to excision, each of these cysts must be differentiated from nasopharyngeal *cephaloceles.*[30] To rule out a cephalocele, computed tomography (CT) can confirm that the skull base is intact and magnetic resonance imaging (MRI) helps to prove that the lesion has no intracranial connection.[31] The *eustachian tube* is derived from the first branchial pouch, which arises in the pharynx and extends laterally and cephalad to contact with the first branch cleft. The pouch and cleft meet at the site of the future *tympanic membrane* and form its inner and outer layers, respectively. *First branchial pouch* cysts may present in the lateral wall of the nasopharynx.[32]

Nasopharyngeal teratomas are principally solid masses that are composed of tissues derived from all three germ layers. They may be benign or malignant. When large, teratomas can cause upper-airway obstruction in the neonate.[33] If a teratoma protrudes from the mouth, it has the potential to be diagnosed antenatally by ultrasonography. When an obstructing tumor is found, a multidisciplinary team that includes an otolaryngologist should be on hand at birth to provide the best chance of securing the airway in the critical first few minutes.[34] *Heterotopic brain* can be located in the nasopharynx, even in the absence of an encephalocele. Surgical removal, usually by a transpalatal route, has been advocated for diagnosis and relief of upper-airway obstruction.[35]

The Oropharynx

The *oropharynx* is the site of the palatine tonsils and the embryologic origin of the second branchial pouch. Second branchial cleft cysts, sinuses, and fistulae often can be tracked back to the inferior tonsillar pole during resection.[36] *Second branchial pouch cysts* may present as masses in the oropharynx.[37] Pharyngeal and pharyngolaryngeal bands rarely obstruct the upper aerodigestive tract. The associated lack of tonsillar and adenoid tissue in such cases led to a proposal that the failed formation of the second branchial pouch was the cause.[38]

The Hypopharynx

The *hypopharynx* is the source for the third and fourth branchial pouches, each arising in the pyriform sinus. Cysts of third or fourth branchial origin may present as recurrent abscesses in the neck or simulate suppurative thyroiditis. Preoperative barium esophagography or direct laryngoscopy may reveal an outpouching in the pyriform apex.[39] Failure to follow the tract all the way to the pyriform sinus may result in recurrent cervical infection. In the case of fourth branchial pouch anomalies, it may be necessary to remove a vertical strip of the posterior thyroid ala to gain adequate surgical access.[40]

Vallecular cysts may present in the hypopharynx in infancy. Aspiration or rupture of such cysts is seldom a permanent treatment. Transoral resections with cold instruments or laser as well as external transhyoid approaches have been advocated.[41]

AT A GLANCE . . .

Anomalies of the Pharynx

- Rathke's pouch cyst
- Thornwaldt's cyst
- Nasopharyngeal cephalocele
- First branchial pouch cyst
- Nasopharyngeal teratoma
- Nasopharyngeal heterotopic brain
- Second branchial cleft cysts, sinuses, and fistulae
- Second branchial pouch cysts
- Pharyngeal and pharyngolaryngeal bands
- Third or fourth branchial cysts
- Vallecular cysts

MALFORMATIONS OF THE ESOPHAGUS

The primitive gut forms during the fourth week of intrauterine life. The developing gut can be divide into three general areas: the foregut, midgut, and hindgut. The *esophagus* (like the pharynx, stomach, and lower respiratory tract) is a derivative of the foregut. The esophagus is partitioned from the trachea by the *tracheoesophageal septum.* This septum forms from two lateral tracheoesophageal folds, and gradually extends in a cranial to caudal direction as the respiratory tract lengthens and descends. The esophagus is quite short in the early embryo, but it rapidly elongates with the growing embryo during the fourth to seventh weeks. Though a complete tube from the beginning, the esophageal lumen is obliterated temporarily and recanalizes in the later part of the embryonic period.[42]

Esophageal atresia is the most common major malformation of the esophagus, affecting 1:3000 live births. Esophageal atresia usually is associated with an abnormal or fistulous connection between the esophagus and trachea. The three mechanisms that have been proposed for the origin of *tracheo-esophageal fistulae* are: (1) *epithelial occlusion,* when the esophagus fails to recanalize; (2) *intraembryonic pressure,* when pressure from the heart, great vessels, or developing lungs causes a disruption of esophageal growth; or (3) *differential growth,* when abnormalities of cellular proliferation cause the trachea to outgrow the esophagus in length. In each of these theoretical situations, the earlier the disruption, the more severe the extent of the malformation.[43]

The five general types of atresias are: (1) pure atresia; (2) esophageal atresia with proximal esophagotracheal fistula; (3) esophageal atresia with distal tracheoesophageal fistula; (4) esophageal atresia with double fistula; and (5) H-type fistula (without true esophageal atresia) (Fig. 33–10). Nearly 50% of all babies with esophageal atresia have other major malformations. Cardiovascular, other gastrointestinal, and musculoskeletal anomalies are the most common. Esophageal atresia may occur as part of the VACTERL association in 10% of cases. **V**ertebral anomalies, **A**nal malformations (i.e., imperforate anus), **C**ardiac malformations, **T**racheo**E**sophageal fistulae, **R**enal anomalies and **L**imb malformations characterize this association.[44]

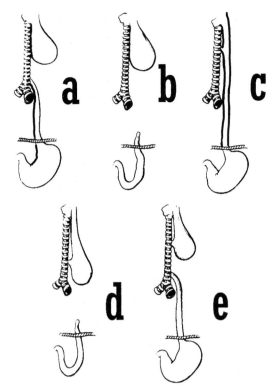

Figure 33–10:   Tracheoesophageal fistulae. (A) esophageal atresia with distal tracheoesophageal fistula. (B) pure atresia. (C) H-type fistula (without true esophageal atresia). (D) esophageal atresia with proximal esophagotracheal fistula. (E) esophageal atresia with double fistula. (Modified from Morrow SE, Nakayama DK). Congenital malformations of the esophagus. In: Bluestone CD, Stool ES, Kenna MA, eds. *Pediatric Otolarygology 3rd ed.* Philadelphia: Saunders, 1996, p. 1122.)

> ### SPECIAL CONSIDERATION:
> Nearly 50% of all babies with esophageal atresia have other major malformations.

The mortality of esophageal atresia was 100% until the 1940s when successful surgical repair was first achieved. The surgical approach to each baby must be individualized based on the severity of the primary and associated malformations. Surgery often is delayed for hours to weeks while diagnostic studies are performed. Gastrostomy and division of the tracheoesophageal fistula may be elected as a first treatment in the severely ill or premature infant. Primary repair is the treatment of choice for most patients and consists of division of the tracheoesophageal fistula and end-to-end esophageal anastomosis. Frequent, late complications of this surgery include esophageal stricture and persistent tracheomalacia.[45]

Congenital esophageal stenosis and *webs* occur most commonly in the distal third of the esophagus. They are thought to arise from incomplete recanalization of the esophageal lumen. Simple webs and fibromuscular stenosis often can be treated with dilation by esophageal bougies or hydrostatic balloon.[46] If repeated dilation is unsuccessful, resection and anastomosis may be required.

Foregut duplications complicate about 1:8000 live births. Esophageal duplications are the most common and present as round or tubular cysts, usually on the right side. They rarely communicate with the esophagus and may contain gastric mucosa. Surgical excision is the preferred treatment.

True *esophageal diverticula* are very rare. They sometimes occur in association with other esophageal structural abnormalities such as tracheoesophageal fistula. Symptoms are similar to acquired diverticula in adults with dysphagia and regurgitation being prominent.

Congenital short esophagus has been reported.

In this condition, the stomach is displaced into the thorax. Recurrent vomiting and failure to thrive may result. Surgical treatment is by Nissen fundoplication.

Motility disorders of the esophagus have been the focus of much attention in recent years. Some degree of *gastroesophageal reflux* (GER) is a normal finding in the infant.[47] With increased quantity and frequency of reflux events, a child may become very symptomatic. Esophagitis, failure to thrive, and pulmonary aspiration may all ensue. Recurrent pneumonia, sinusitis, and otitis all have been reported in association with GER.[48] The subject of GER is dealt with more extensively in Chapter 37.

Congenital cricopharyngeal achalasia repre-

Practice Pathway 33–1   CONGENITAL ESOPHAGEAL MALFORMATION

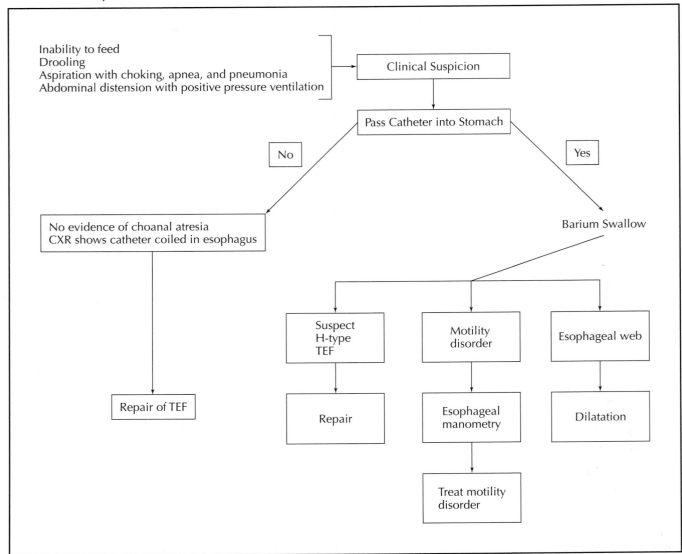

Abbreviations: CXR = chest radiograph, TEF = Tracheoesophageal fistula.

sents a failure of the upper esophageal sphincter to relax at the initiation of a swallow. Symptoms include pharyngeal dysphagia, coughing and choking with swallowing, and nasopharyngeal reflux. Achalasia is diagnosed by cine-barium esophagogram and esophageal manometry. Cricopharyngeal myotomy has been successful only partially.[49] When achalasia results from cranial nerve abnormalities associated with Chiari malformations, correction of the brainstem compression may fix the esophageal problem as well.[50] Other esophageal motility disorders have been described based on manometric criteria, including esophageal spasm and hypertensive lower esophageal sphincter.[51]

Practice Pathway 33–1 outlines the treatment for congenital esophageal malformations.

AT A GLANCE . . .
Anomalies of the Esophagus

- Tracheoesophageal fistula/esophageal atresia
- Congenital esophageal stenosis and web
- Foregut duplications
- Esophageal diverticulum
- Congenital short esophagus
- Esophageal motility disorders
- Congenital cricopharyngeal achalasia

REFERENCES

1. Jones KL. *Smith's Recognizable Patterns of Human Malformation, 4th ed.* Philadelphia: Saunders, 1988, pp. 1–9.
2. Sher AE, Shprintzen RJ, Thorpy MJ. Endoscopic observation of obstructive sleep apnea in children with anomalous upper airways: Predictive and therapeutic value. Int J Pediatr Otorhinolaryngol 1986; 11: 135–146.
3. Bull MJ, Givan DC, Sadove M, et al. Improved outcome in Pierre Robin sequence: Effect of multidisciplinary evaluation and management. Pediatrics 1990; 86:294–301.
4. Kaban LB. *Pediatric Oral and Maxillofacial Surgery.* Philadelphia: Saunders, 1990, p. 150.
5. Chervenak FA, Isaacson G, Mahoney MJ, et al. The obstetrical significance of holoprosencephaly. Obstet Gynecol 1984; 63:115–121.
6. Gray SD, Parkin JL. Congenital malformations of the mouth and pharynx. In: Bluestone CD, Stool ES,

Kenna MA, eds. *Pediatric Otolaryngology 3rd ed.* Philadelphia: Saunders, 1996, pp. 985–987.
7. Gartlan MG, Davies J, Smith RJH. Congenital oral synechiae. Ann Otol Rhinol Laryngol 1993; 102: 186–197.
8. Arriaga MA, Dindzans LJ, Bluestone CD. Parotid duct communicating with a labial pit and ectopic salivary cyst. Arch Otolaryngol Head Neck Surg 1990; 116: 1445–1447.
9. Rimell FL, Shapiro AM, Shoemaker DL, et al. Head and neck manifestations of Beckwith-Wiedemann syndrome. Otolaryngol Head Neck Surg 1995; 13: 262–265.
10. Bredenkamp JK, Smith ME, Dudley JP, et al. Otolaryngologic manifestations of the mucopolysaccharidoses. Ann Otol Rhinol Laryngol 1992; 101: 472–478.
11. Potsic WP, Cotton RT, Handler SK. *Surgical Pediatric Otolaryngology.* New York: Thieme, 1997, pp. 250–253.
12. Kaban LB. *Pediatric Oral and Maxillofacial Surgery.* Philadelphia: Saunders, 1990, pp. 131–140.
13. Godley FA. Frenuloplasty with buccal mucosal graft. Laryngoscope 1994; 104:378–381.
14. Orlando MR, Atkins JS. Melkersson-Rosenthal syndrome. Arch Otolaryngol Head Neck Surg 1990; 116: 728–729.
15. Maddern BR, Werkhaven J, McBride T. Lingual thyroid in a young infant presenting as airway obstruction; Report of a case. Int J Pediatr Otolaryngol 1988; 16:77–82.
16. Williams JD, Sclafani AP, Slupchinskij O, et al. Evaluation and management of lingual thyroid gland. Ann Otol Rhinol Laryngol 1996; 105:312–316.
17. Shaari CM, Ho BT, Shah K, et al. Lingual dermoid cyst. Otolaryngol Head Neck Surg 1995; 112: 476–478.
18. Jones JE, Healy GB. Transoral surgical management of lesion of the base of the tongue. Arch Otolaryngol Head Neck Surg 1992; 118:1350–1352.
19. Langlois NEI, Kolhe P. Plunging ranula: A case report and literature review. Hum Pathol 1992; 23: 1306–1308.
20. Matt BH, Crockett DM. Plunging ranula in an infant. Otolaryngol Head Neck Surg 1988; 99:330–333.
21. Tavill MA, Poje CP, Wetmore RF, et al. Plunging ranulas in children. Ann Otol Rhinol Laryngol 1995; 104: 405–408.
22. Citardi MJ, Traquina DN, Eisen R. Primitive foregut cysts: A cause of airway obstruction in the newborn. Otolaryngol Head Neck Surg 1994; 111:533–537.
23. Dolata Jan. Thyroglossal duct cyst in the mouth floor; An unusual location. Otolaryngol Head Neck Surg 1994; 110:580–583.
24. Batsakis JG, El-Naggar AK, Hicks MJ. Epithelial choristomas and teratomas of the tongue. Ann Otol Rhinol Laryngol 1993; 102:567–569.

25. LaBagnara J, Zauk A, Rankin L. Enteric duplications of the mouth. Otolaryngol Head Neck Surg 1992; 108:187–189.

26. Lalwani AK, Lalwani RB, Bartlett PC. Heterotopic gastric mucosal cyst of the tongue. Otolaryngol Head Neck Surg 1993; 108:204–205.

27. Nicolai P, Luzzago F, Maroldi R, et al. Nasopharyngeal cysts. Arch Otolaryngol Head Neck Surg 1989; 115:860–862.

28. Fuller GN, Batsakis JG. Pharyngeal hypophysis. Ann Otol Rhinol Laryngol 1996; 105:671–672.

29. Shank EC, Burgess LPA, Geyer CA. Thornwaldt's cyst: Case report with magnetic resonance imaging. Otolaryngol Head Neck Surg 1990; 102:169–173.

30. Chervenak FA, Isaacson G, Mahoney MJ, et al. Diagnosis and management of fetal cephalocele. Obstet Gynecol 1984; 64:86–91.

31. Kenna MA. Transsphenoidal encephalocele. Ann Otol Rhinol Laryngol 1985; 94:520–522.

32. Shidara K, Uruma T, Yasuoka Y, et al. Two cases of nasopharyngeal branchial cyst. J Laryngol Otol 1993; 107:453–455.

33. Rybak LP, Rapp MF, McGrady MD, et al. Obstructing nasopharyngeal teratoma in the neonate. Arch Otolaryngol Head Neck Surg 1991; 117:1411–1415.

34. Chervenak FA, Isaacson G, Touloukian R, et al. Diagnosis and management of fetal teratomas. Obstet Gynecol 1985; 66:666–671.

35. Anand VK, Melvin FM, Reed JM, et al. Nasopharyngeal gliomas: Diagnosis and treatment considerations. Otolaryngol Head Neck Surg 1993; 109:534–539.

36. Talaat M. Pull-through branchial fistulectomy: A technique for the otolaryngologist. Ann Otol Rhinol Laryngol 1992; 101:501–502.

37. Thaler ER, Tom LWC, Handler SD. Second branchial cleft anomalies presenting as pharyngeal masses. Otolaryngol Head Neck Surg 1993; 109:941–944.

38. Prescott CAJ. Pharyngeal and pharyngolaryngeal bands: Report of an unusual combination of congenital anomalies. Ann Otol Rhinol Laryngol 1995; 104:653–654.

39. Godin MS, Kearns DB, Pransky SM, et al. Fourth branchial pouch sinus; Principles of diagnosis and management. Laryngoscope 1990; 100:174–178.

40. Rosenfeld RM, Biller HF. Fourth branchial pouch sinus: Diagnosis and treatment. Otolaryngol Head Neck Surg 1991; 105:44–50.

41. Myers CM. Vallecular cyst in the newborn. Ear Nose Throat J 1988; 67:122–124.

42. Moore KL. The Developing Human 3rd ed. Philadelphia: Saunders, 1982, pp. 227–237.

43. Smith EI. The early development of the trachea and esophagus in relation to atresia of the esophagus and tracheoesophageal fistula. Contrib Embryol Carnegie Inst Wash 1957; 31:41–57.

44. Nguyen LT, Laberge J-M. Congenital anomalies of the esophagus. In: Tewfik TL, Der Kaloustian VM, eds. Congenital Anomalies of the Ear, Nose and Throat. New York: Oxford University Press, 1997, pp. 407–418.

45. Benjamin B, Robb P, Glasson M. Esophageal stricture following esophageal atresia repair: Endoscopic assessment and dilation. Ann Otol Rhinol Laryngol 1993; 102:332–336.

46. Myer CM, Ball WS, Bisset GS. Balloon dilatation of esophageal strictures in children. Arch Otolaryngol Head Neck Surg 1991; 117:529–532.

47. Vandenplas Y, Goyvaerts H, Helven R, et al. Gastroesophageal reflex, as measured by 24-hour pH monitoring in 509 healthy infants screened for risk of sudden infant death syndrome. Pediatrics 1991; 88:834–840.

48. Barbero GJ. Gastroesophageal reflux and upper airway disease. Otolaryngol Clin North Amer 1996; 29:27–38.

49. Reichert TJ, Bluestone CD, Stool SE, et al. Congenital cricopharyngeal achalasia. Ann Otol Rhinol Laryngol 1977; 86:603–610.

50. Putnam PE, Orenstein SR, Pang D, et al. Cricopharyngeal dysfunction associated with Chiari malformation. Pediatrics 1992; 89:871–876.

51. Perisic VN, Tomomasa T, Kuroume T, et al. Recurrent pneumonia caused by diffuse oesophageal spasm. Eur J Pediatr 1990; 150:139–140.

34 Cleft Lip and Palate

James D. Sidman and Harlan R. Muntz

*Cleft lip and palate are the most common congenital abnormalities of the head and neck. The implications for patient care are far reaching, and the patient requires surveillance by the otolaryngologist for many years. The current standard of care for these children is multidisciplinary and the typical cleft team is comprised of many specialists besides the otolaryngologist. These specialists may include the pediatrician, cleft surgeon, geneticist, oral surgeon, pediatric dentist, orthodontist, prosthodontist, speech pathologist, audiologist, nurse, genetics counselor, social worker, psychologist, and occupational therapist. Other specialists that often are consulted include an ophthalmologist, a neurosurgeon, and a physical therapist. The cleft-team approach evolved so that the child would get complete, coordinated care. The practice of only a surgeon and a pediatrician trying to provide comprehensive care to these children is no longer recognized as adequate. This chapter provides an overview of the multitude of problems that must be addressed in cleft lip or palate patients and examines the importance of team members with special areas of expertise.

SPECIAL CONSIDERATION:

A group of specialists forming a cleft palate team provides the best care for the cleft palate patient.

Cleft lip or palate is found in approximately 1:1000 white births. It is more common as well as

less common in different ethnic groups: for Japanese, the incidence is as high as 1:400 births, and for African populations, it is as low as 1:3000 births. Boys have a higher incidence of facial clefting than girls, although isolated cleft palate is found more frequently in girls. Newborns with an isolated cleft lip have unilateral involvement in 80% and bilateral in 20%. Of all cleft lip patients, 3 out of 4 have an associated cleft palate.

Currently, there is no single gene locus associated with nonsyndromic cleft lip or palate. However, many of the syndromes that have associated facial clefting have been identified genetically. These include Stickler's syndrome, velo-cardio-facial syndrome, Treacher Collins syndrome, Crouzon's syndrome and Waardenburg's syndrome. Currently, over 300 syndromes that involve facial clefting are identified.

Despite recent advances in the isolation of genes that are associated with various syndromes, at least 50% of all syndromes involving the head and neck have not been identified genetically yet. The cleft team member who routinely sees children with congenital craniofacial abnormalities often will be able to identify these children. Nonetheless, the opinion of a geneticist (preferably a geneticist with a special interest in dysmorphology) will be invaluable in diagnosing and treating these children.

Children with facial clefting often have hearing loss and middle-ear disease. This is primarily due to the link between cleft palate and chronic serous otitis media (OM) and is based in eustachian tube dysfunction that is the result of the cleft anatomy. Although there is some controversy as to the true incidence of middle-ear disease in cleft palate children, the problem is so common that it always should be assumed that a child with cleft palate has chronic otitis media with effusion (OME) until proven otherwise. Isolated cleft lip (without associated cleft palate) does not carry an increased rate of middle-ear disease or hearing loss.

All children with facial clefting should have regu-

Pediatric Otolaryngology, Edited by R.F. Wetmore, H.R. Muntz, and T.J. McGill. Thieme Medical Publishers, Inc., New York © 2000.
* Gorlin RJ, Cohen Jr MM, Levin LS; Syndromes of the Head and Neck, Oxford University Press, N.Y., 1990 pg 695.

lar audiograms to monitor hearing loss secondary to chronic middle-ear disease or sensorineural hearing loss (SNHL) associated with many craniofacial syndromes. It should be assumed that children with cleft palate who do not have a history of OM but who, on exam, have scrous otitis and conductive hearing loss (CHL) have chronic, unrecognized, middle-ear disease. These children should be treated and followed closely. Many otolaryngologists feel that virtually all children with cleft palate should have tympanostomy or pressure equalization tubes (PET) placed early in order to avoid the complications of chronic CHL and cholesteatoma formation. Older studies that were performed before the advent of PET show a cholesteatoma rate of nearly 10% in patients with cleft palate.[1] Since the popularity of PET, cholesteatoma formation in this population has decreased to less than 1%.[2]

PROBLEMS FOR THE NEONATE WITH FACIAL CLEFTING

Airway

Neonates with facial clefting often have airway management and feeding problems, and it often is difficult to distinguish the source of these two problems. Many infants with severe feeding difficulty have an unrecognized airway obstruction that can cause the feeding disorder. Coordinating an effective swallow with an obstructed airway is difficult, and the increased work of breathing in an infant with airway obstruction can result in poor weight gain due to an increased metabolic rate.

Pierre Robin sequence is the most common craniofacial abnormality associated with airway problems. It consists of the triad of micrognathia, glossoptosis, and cleft palate. Feeding difficulties often exist. It is referred to as a "sequence" because of the series of in utero events that lead to the deformity.[3,4] The small mandible causes retro- and superior displacement of the tongue. The tongue then physically obstructs fusion of the posterior palatal shelves. The position of the tongue into the palate explains the "U" shape of the Pierre Robin cleft palate versus the "V" shape of the typical cleft palate. This tongue positioning persists throughout the entire fetal period and into the neonatal period, and it can be observed easily on intraoral examination or nasal examination with the flexible nasopharyngoscope.

AT A GLANCE . . .
Pierre Robin Sequence

- Micrognathia
- Glossoptosis
- Cleft palate

Although the primary physician often notices the problem of poor feeding in Pierre Robin infants, the underlying airway obstruction can go unrecognized. Chest retractions, stridor, and poor air movement may be noted, but the true extent of the problem often is not revealed until auscultation with a stethoscope. It then becomes apparent that every second or third breath may be obstructed totally. The obstruction is the result of glossoptosis and occurs at the level of the tongue base. Prone positioning for these children may be recommended. Care must be taken not to mask chest retractions. Capillary blood gases to evaluate the carbon dioxide partial pressure (pCO_2) are very helpful in screening for hypercarbia and ineffective ventilation. Polysomnography and pulse oximetry are also helpful in determining the extent of the airway obstruction.

Treatment

Treatment of airway obstruction in Pierre Robin sequence is varied. Simple approaches involve positioning. A nasogastric tube, a nasal airway of red rubber, or a trimmed endotracheal tube placed through the nose into the hypopharynx is often effective. This artificial airway appears to push the tongue base physically forward, although it does not seem to function as a true airway through which the baby breathes. Often this airway becomes obstructed with secretions without untoward effect.

SPECIAL CONSIDERATION:

Airway management in the Pierre Robin patient is dependent on the infant's individual needs.

If positioning and a nasal airway are not beneficial, then surgical intervention must be considered. The mainstay of surgical treatment remains a tracheostomy. It usually is needed only for 4 to 12 months, after which the child is decannulated easily. Some surgeons delay decannulation until after the repair of the cleft palate in order to minimize perioperative airway complications.

Many variations of tongue-lip adhesion are used to treat glossoptosis and airway obstruction in the child with Pierre-Robin sequence.[5] Some techniques involve suturing the undersurface of the tongue to the lip, and others involve suturing it to the mandible. There are mixed reports as to the effect of this operation on feeding. Controversy exists as to whether this is truly an effective treatment for significant tongue-based airway obstruction. There is no literature to prove that children with hypercarbia, significant apnea, and failure to thrive have benefited from tongue-lip adhesion.

Recently, there have been case reports on the utilization of distraction osteogenesis of the mandible in infants with Pierre Robin sequence to bring the mandible and tongue forward.[6] Although these early reports are favorable, controlled studies with significant patient numbers are not available yet.

AT A GLANCE . . .

Management of the Pierre Robin Patient

- Observation
- Nasogastric tube
- Artificial oral or nasal airway
- Tongue-lip adhesion
- Mandibular advancement
- Tracheostomy

Feeding

Feeding a newborn with a cleft palate can be a complex problem. The difficulty arises because of the baby's inability to generate an adequate negative oral pressure. It is impossible for the baby to maintain a seal due to the cleft between the mouth and the nose, and because of this a baby with a cleft palate rarely can breast feed adequately. Maternal counseling is necessary to advise the mother who wishes to breast feed. Closer monitoring of weight gain and feeding also are necessary. Mothers should be encouraged to pump breast milk and provide this excellent form of nutrition through one of the techniques below.

Techniques

Feeding a baby with a cleft palate requires training and experience. Each hospital or cleft team should have designated experts to help parents deal with this essential but often frustrating task. A nurse, occupational or physical therapist, speech therapist, lactation consultant, or physician can serve as expert, but the involvement of the parents with feeding is essential and can provide an immediate bond between the baby and the parents. This bond can help these parents to overcome the emotional shock and guilt that they often experienced.

Nearly all techniques to feed babies with a left palate involve overcoming or supplementing the oral phase of swallowing. Enlarging the hole on the nipple of the bottle by making large cross-cuts supplements the oral phase of swallowing, allowing for a greater flow of milk into the baby's mouth when he sucks.

Other techniques involve special bottles that are soft and able to be squeezed by the caregiver. The squeezing provides a stream of milk into the baby's mouth and bypasses the need for a strong suck. The two most common cleft bottles in the United States are the Habermann feeder and the Mead-Johnson cleft bottle. Increasing the flow too much may put the child at risk of aspiration. It should be remembered that all babies with cleft palate require longer times to feed adequately and need to be burped more often because of the increased air swallowing that occurs with ineffective feeding.

Nasogastric feeding can be utilized for the first 1 to 2 weeks of a neonate's life, but should not be relied on completely. If the baby is malnourished because of poor feeding, each feeding session will be frustrating because of an uncoordinated suck and swallow secondary to the frantic attempt to achieve swallowing. In this situation, nasogastric supplementation is most effective. If the baby does not receive continuous oral stimulation, then oral aversion may result. Oral aversion in any child, with or without a cleft palate, is a very difficult problem to solve and is best dealt with by prevention.

Gastrostomy should be a last resort. Generally, it is required only in babies either with syndromes that involve significant neurologic compromise or with hypoxic brain injury. Gastrostomy should not be used to feed a child whose feeding difficulties result from airway obstruction. If the airway obstruction is treated first, and the feeding problem typically resolves.

TYPES OF FACIAL CLEFTING

Isolated Cleft Lip

Cleft lip presents in one of three forms: complete, incomplete, and microform. The *complete cleft lip* extends into the floor of the nose and is considered complete even if a bridge of tissue at the nasal sill (Simonart's band) is present. An *incomplete cleft lip* extends only part-way through the lip. A *microform cleft* only notches the vermilion, but often a muscular cleft persists.

AT A GLANCE . . .

Forms of Isolated Cleft Lip

- **Complete:** extends into the floor of the nose
- **Incomplete:** extends part of the way through the lip
- **Microform:** just notches the vermillion

Treatment

All complete cleft lips and many incomplete cleft lips involve the nose. The common deformity is flaring of the ala of the lower lateral cartilage with depression of the lower and upper lateral cartilages. The medial crus of the lower lateral cartilage is often deficient. Timing of nasal repair with a unilateral cleft lip is controversial. Some surgeons recommend performing an open rhinoplasty with repositioning of the lower lateral cartilage and medial crura at the same time as the original cleft lip repair.[7] Others only rotate the alar base at the same time as the lip repair but delay rhinoplasty until the teenage years in order to avoid scarring and interference with growth.[8]

Most surgeons repair the cleft lip between 6 and 12 weeks of age. The "rule of 10's" refers to a weight of 10 pounds, an age of 10 weeks, and a hemoglobin of 10 gms. This outmoded rule was developed before current methods of pediatric anesthesia and newborn care were available. Many physicians delay surgical repair in order to allow time for the diagnosis of other congenital anomalies, and more importantly, to allow the parents time to bond with their child. There have been a number of articles that recommend neonatal repair of cleft lip in order to take advantage, theoretically, of the healing properties of fetal collagen.[9] This hypothesis has not gained wide acceptance, and most studies have not shown a real difference in surgical results.

For the complete cleft lip, either unilateral or bilateral, some surgeons recommend a two-stage repair. The first stage is a lip adhesion in which a mucosal or skin closure is accomplished.[10] The tension provided by this closure brings the medial and lateral segments of the cleft closer together over a period of weeks. Then, the adhesion is taken down and formal muscle and skin repair of the cleft lip is accomplished.

The two most popular techniques for closure of cleft lip are the rotation-advancement flap (the *Millard repair*) and the triangular flap (the *Randall-Tennison repair*). Both techniques rely on the principle that because the medial portion of the cleft is short, tissue must be brought in laterally to augment this short medial side. The rotation-advancement flap leaves a scar that most naturally mimics the normal philtral ridge, whereas the triangular flap allows for easier closure of a wide cleft lip without undue tension. Both techniques involve rotation of the alar base into a more normal position. Neither technique utilizes closure of a coexisting alveolar cleft.

It is important to remember that, in the patient with an incomplete or microform cleft lip, the cleft may go through the muscle completely despite intact skin. If this is the case, then the repair should recreate a complete cleft-lip defect in order to close the muscle adequately and achieve symmetrical motion of the lip.

Isolated Cleft Palate

A cleft palate always involves the uvula, but the extent of soft and hard palate clefting is quite variable. Embryologic closure of the palate can be thought of as a "zipper," with the zipper closing first at the anterior hard palate, extending posteriorly to the soft palate, and ending at the uvula. The length of the cleft depends upon where the zipper stops closing.

A *submucous cleft palate* occurs when the oral mucosa is intact but the underlying palatal muscles are dehiscent. Often a transparent area (i.e., the *zona pellucida*) can be seen or a notch at the junction of the hard and soft palate can be palpated. An endoscopic nasopharyngeal examination shows notching in the soft palate that is characteristic of a submucous cleft palate.[11-13]

Treatment

Timing of cleft palate repair has changed greatly in the past 20 years. Most physicians favor earlier closure of the cleft palate in order to achieve normal speech. The current standard is closure of the entire cleft by the age of 10 to 15 months.[13a]

There are three goals involved in the closure of the cleft palate, and all are set to provide good speech results: the first obviously is to close the hole; the second is to provide adequate length to the soft palate; and the third is to achieve muscle repair that gives mobility to the soft palate through providing velopharyngeal closure.

AT A GLANCE . . .

Goals of Cleft Palate Closure

1. To close the defect
2. To provide adequate length to the soft palate
3. To achieve muscle repair that allows velopharyngeal closure

---

All techniques of cleft palate closure try to take these goals into account. Pushing the hard palate back is done in an attempt to lengthen the soft palate, but this procedure has reduced success because it scars the palate into its original position.[14] Intravelar veloplasty attempts to provide adequate mobility by achieving ideal muscle closure, but it seems no more effective than other muscle reapproximation techniques in achieving good speech results.[14a] A double-reverse Z-plasty (i.e., the Furlow technique) tries to lengthen and reapproximate the palatal muscles but carries a higher rate of fistula formation than is ideal, especially in extensive clefts of the soft and hard palate.[15]

No ideal technique of cleft palate repair exists as of yet. All have problems either with velopharyngeal insufficiency, necessitating secondary operations, or a higher rate of fistula formation.[16]

Cleft Lip with Cleft Palate

The association of a cleft lip with a cleft palate does not carry a higher percentage of feeding or airway problems than cleft palate alone. The same techniques of closure are used in both conditions. When the alveolus is cleft, attention must be directed to its alignment and eventual surgical repair. In the patient with a wide cleft lip and alveolus, realignment of the alveolus before lip repair has several advantages. First, narrowing the alveolar cleft prior to cleft lip repair aids in the lip repair by allowing less tension on the surgical closure. It also prevents rapid closure of the alveolus by the pressure of the newly closed lip, which could cause misalignment of the alveolar segments (Fig. 34-1). These points are especially pertinent in patients with a bilateral cleft lip and palate where the premaxilla is often very protrusive. Uncontrolled closure of alveolar clefts often results in the premaxilla being "locked out" in an anterior position (see Fig. 34-1). This condition leaves an unsightly protrusion of the premaxilla under the lip and a large anterior fistula in the palate. Neither of these is closed until definitive alveolar bone grafting is performed between the ages of 5 to 7 years old.

There are several techniques of presurgical orthopedics for the alveolar cleft. The techniques can be divided into two categories: surgical appliances and nonsurgical appliances. The most common surgical appliance is the Latham appliance which is screwed into the palatal segments to close the alveolar cleft gradually and to maintain position. Nonsurgical techniques include taping, bonnets with Velcro

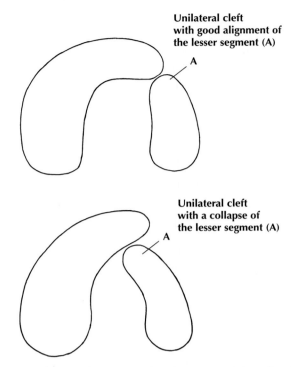

Unilateral cleft
with good alignment of
the lesser segment (A)

A

Unilateral cleft
with a collapse of
the lesser segment (A)

A

Figure 34–1: The lesser alveolar segment has the tendency to collapse causing cross bite and a skeletal deficiency on that side. (A) demonstrates a good alignment, and (B) shows the collapse.

straps, and modifications of molding appliances. Questions about facial growth, feeding concerns, and infections have been raised with surgical appliances.

Bone grafting of the alveolar cleft is performed when secondary dentition develops in order to provide normal contour and continuity of the alveolus. Donor sites include the iliac crest and calvarium. With alveolar bone grafting, closure of residual oral-nasal fistulas can be accomplished. Tooth eruption through the bone graft is well established and is to be expected. Prior to bone grafting, orthodontic expansion of the maxilla, if necessary, and proper alignment of the arch from should be accomplished as much as possible. Final correction of occlusion takes place after bone grafting in most patients.

It is common for patients with a cleft palate, with or without a cleft lip, to develop midface deficiency in the teenage years. This appears to be both genetic in basis and possibly also iatrogenic from palatal surgery. When facial growth is complete, orthodontic management with or with-

out surgical advancement of the maxilla can be accomplished to achieve normal occlusion and facial contour. Mandibular advancement is not necessary as often as maxillary advancement. When deemed necessary, however, mandibular advancement can be accomplished at the same time as maxillary advancement.

VELOPHARYNGEAL DYSFUNCTION

Incidence

Although the diagnosis of velopharyngeal dysfunction is seen most commonly in the child with a cleft palate, this speech disorder also can be seen in children with other syndromes as well as in otherwise normal children occasionally. Suspicion of velopharyngeal dysfunction should be entertained for any child who has had a cleft palate and for those with abnormal resonance, language delay, or problem with intelligibility.

Evaluation and Diagnosis

The three characteristics that describe velopharyngeal dysfunction are hypernasality, nasal emission, and nasal turbulence. *Hypernasality* is an increase in resonance. The open sphincter between the oral cavity and the nose on nonnasal phonemes allows a characteristic resonance in the nose and paranasal sinuses. *Nasal emission* is the sound of the air exploding through the nose. It is noted most on the expression of plosives where there is a high intraoral pressure. *Nasal turbulence* is the sound made when that air is forced through nasal mucous.

AT A GLANCE . . .

Characteristics of Velopharyngeal Dysfunction

- **Hypernasality:** an increase in nasal resonance with nonnasal phonemes
- **Nasal emission:** the sound of air escape through the nose
- **Nasal turbulence:** sound made when air is forced through nasal mucous

TABLE 34–1: Acceptable Utterances for The Evaluation of The Velopharynx*

pa/pa/pa
puppy
pamper
baby
sissy
sustained "s" and "sh"
Buy Bobby a puppy.
Sissy sees the sun in the sky.

---

* Note the inclusion of bilabials and fricatives with increasing complexity.

Speech quality may seem to deteriorate during an upper respiratory illness because of this sound. Velopharyngeal dysfunction may present with any of these speech symptoms in varying degrees. The severity of presentation does not indicate the gap size necessarily.

In the child with velopharyngeal dysfunction and either significant nasal airway obstruction or dysphonia, the diagnosis may be difficult. *Hyponasality,* or the reduced nasal resonance that is noted especially in the nasal phonemes of n, m, and ng, may mask the hypernasal resonance. If it is severe enough, hyponasality may stop the nasal emission and turbulence. Similarly, the severely dysphonic voice may make detection of resonance problems very difficult.

An auditory perceptual evaluation consists of having the child repeat a series of words or sounds such as those in Table 34–1. Although the focus is on the nonnasal sounds, it is wise to elicit a sample that extends from isolated phonemes to complex words and sentences, including nasal/nonnasal combinations. Sometimes the speech deteriorates with increasing complexity. The auditory perceptual evaluation should stress the appropriately-articulated phonemes because velopharyngeal dysfunction may result from articulation problems alone.

Abnormal nasal-air escape can be detected by placing a mirror beneath the nose during speech tasks. Fogging the mirror during a nonnasal phoneme suggests velopharyngeal dysfunction, even if it is masked otherwise. Another method is for the examiner to listen to the resonance with child's nose both plugged and unplugged. If there is no change in the resonance with the nose plugged, velopharyngeal dysfunction is unlikely.

> ## SPECIAL CONSIDERATION:
>
> Fogging a mirror placed under the nose during a nonnasal phoneme suggests velopharyngeal dysfunction even if it is masked otherwise.

Clearly, there must be a reasonable index of suspicion. Children with a documented cleft palate are not the only ones with velopharyngeal problems. Velopharyngeal dysfunction also can be present in other craniofacial anomalies and in children presenting with middle-ear disease or speech and language delay. Prior to adenoidectomy, it is advisable to elicit a speech sample if possible.

Once there is a determination of velopharyngeal dysfunction, further evaluation allows the prescription of a therapeutic intervention. The evaluation should allow a qualitative and quantitative description of velopharyngeal closure and ideally be recorded for team input. Two techniques that are used routinely to assist in this are: flexible fiberoptic nasopharyngoscopy and speech videofluoroscopy.

Velopharyngeal closure takes place as the velopharyngeal walls close during a speech task. Swallowing follows a different neuromuscular control, so analysis of swallowing does not describe necessarily how the sphincter closes for speech. During closure for speech, the palate, lateral walls, and posterior wall (Passavant's ridge) all may participate to some extent. Four closure patterns have been identified and described by Croft.[17] Closure of the palate predominantly towards the posterior wall is considered a *coronal* pattern. This term is used because any remaining gap at the sphincter, if present, would be in the coronal plane. Similarly, closure that has brisk lateral-wall motion but less palatal motion would be called *saggital.* If there is good motion of both the palate and the lateral walls, the closure is called *circular.* If Passavant's ridge is involved as well, the closure is called *circular with Passavant's.*

Movement of the walls can be defined numerically as a proportion of the distance traversed by one wall towards the opposite wall. It is rated from rest to maximal motion. The four numeric ratings assigned are: 1 for the palate, 1 for the posterior wall, and 1 for each of the lateral walls, as there may be asymmetry between the lateral walls.[18]

Speech videofluoroscopy requires both a speech pathologist and a radiologist who are interested in the evaluation of velopharyngeal dysfunction. As radiographic images are two-dimensional representations, the study should be done in more than one plane. Typically, there is a lateral evaluation and one or more in the anteroposterior direction or an en fas view.[18] The evaluation of these films defines the motion of the four walls. There is some limitation as to the time allowed for radiation exposure. The surgeon also must be familiar with the evaluation. As the image is presented in a two-dimensional view, the ability to orient oneself to three dimensions can be difficult.

Flexible fiberoptic nasopharyngoscopy is a tool that frequently is used by the otolaryngologist to assess velopharyngeal insufficiency, specifically the closure mechanism of the velopharynx.[13] Flexible fiberoptic endoscopy should be performed in concert by the speech pathologist and otolaryngologist. The expertise of both individuals allows the endoscopist to focus on obtaining all the necessary anatomic information while the speech pathologist directs the speech sample for the most meaningful information. Diagnostic therapy may be done at that time to see if the velopharyngeal closure may be improved by speech therapy techniques. This also has been used successfully for visual biofeedback.[19]

Both speech videofluoroscopy and flexible fiberoptic nasopharyngoscopy should be video recorded with sound for later review. This allows team members who are not present at the endoscopy to have informed and appropriate input in the clarification of diagnostic and therapeutic issues. Changes over time also can be assessed when a video is recorded.

Treatment

The above assessment lends itself to a treatment paradigm similar to the one in Practice Pathway 34–1. Because there is excellent evidence that the action of the velopharyngeal sphincter is improved with appropriate articulation,[20] early intensive articulation therapy should be started for any child with velopharyngeal dysfunction. The goal of management should be to have a normally-speaking child by the time she enters school. Instrumental assessment of difficulties must be done with at least a reasonable repertoire of consistently and appropriately articulated phonemes.

Much of the problem with speech intelligibility in these children is not actually due to velopharyngeal dysfunction, but instead is due to a problem of inappropriate articulation or what is commonly called compensatory articulations. These abnormal speech mechanisms likely are not truly compensatory because not all children with velopharyngeal dysfunction exhibit them. The child may be attempting to valve the air stream at abnormal locations. Glottal and pharyngeal stops, tongue backing, and pharyngeal and nasal fricatives all have been described. These abnormal articulations are quite noticeable even to the untrained ear. Aggressive speech therapy focused on the elimination of these articulations is essential for the normalization of speech. If the velopharyngeal dysfunction is eliminated with prosthesis or surgery but the articulation errors are not corrected the speech may remain unintelligible.

Speech therapy

Speech therapy frequently is required in children with a cleft palate. When language begins to develop, assessment of speech and language is most important. Early intervention should focus on the developing phoneme repertoire. If hypernasality, nasal turbulence, or nasal emission continues in the face of normal articulation, additional assessment should be undertaken.

Resonance therapy sessions can be helpful in some children. The attempt to use auditory biofeedback in this manner allows some children an opportunity to improve without surgery.

In the past, much of the focus of speech therapists was on strengthening the palate with nonspeech activities. Time was spent trying to blow cotton balls across the table or blow up balloons. Successful completion of these tasks was thought to be a sign that the velopharyngeal sphincter was closing. Unfortunately, even if it closed on blowing, the corollary that it would close on speech was not necessarily true. Just as the child with velopharyngeal dysfunction rarely has nasal regurgitation on feeding (suggesting a competent valve during that task), strengthening the palate for other nonspeech tasks does not necessarily help speech.

Prosthetic management

In many institutions, maxillofacial prosthodontics play a key role in the rehabilitation of speech prob-

Practice Pathway 34–1 VELOPHARYNGEAL DYSFUNCTION

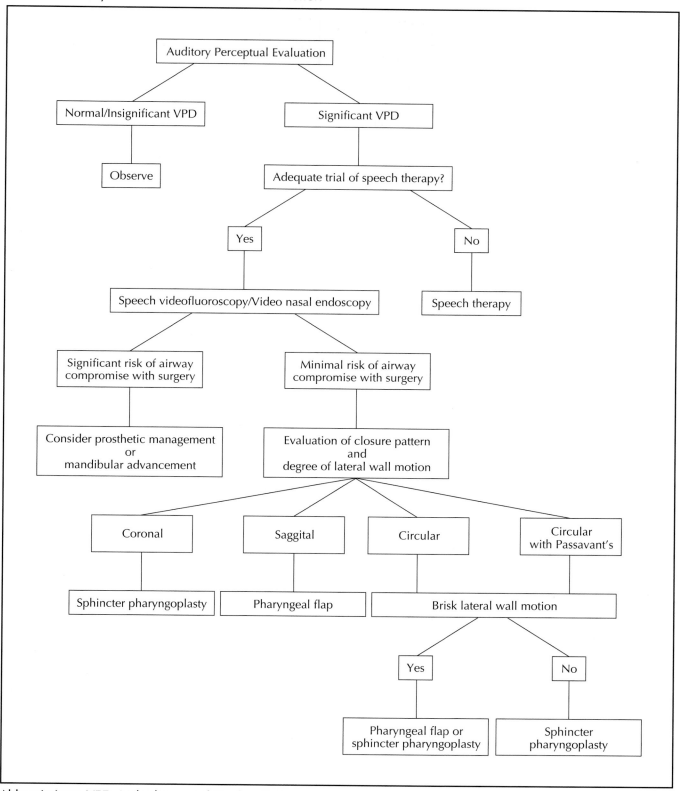

Abbreviations: VPD, Velopharyngeal Dysfunction.

lems in patients who have undergone head and neck surgery. Many of the same considerations apply to the child with velopharyngeal dysfunction. The functional defect of the palate can be addressed either by obturation or by lifting the palate to allow closure. Figure 34–2 shows how each assists in closure.

The use of prosthetics in the management of velopharyngeal dysfunction requires close cooperation between the speech pathologist, the cleft team, and the dental specialist. In the absence of such a working relationship, prosthetic management is not an option. The initial fabrication of the lift requires a maxillary impression. Bands and lugs are placed on the child's premolars. The final fitting of the prosthesis should be done with flexible fiberoptic endoscopic guidance to assure an adequate closure of the velopharynx during speech. This process is difficult without a cooperative child.

Prosthetic management is helpful in some cases of airway obstruction such as micrognathia or midface retrusion, in which surgical correction could precipitate obstructive sleep apnea (OSA). A prosthetic device may allow normalization of speech during the day at some sacrifice to nasal airway, but can be removed at night so as not to make airway obstruction worse. Prosthetic management also is helpful in those who should not undergo surgical correction because of medical contraindications.[21]

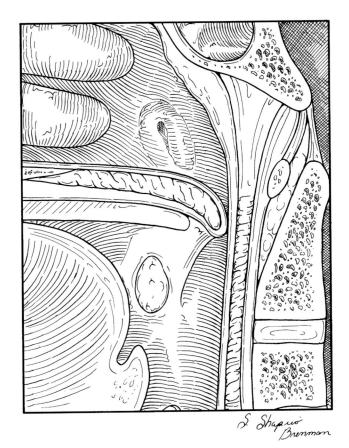

A

SPECIAL CONSIDERATION:

Prosthetic management of a palatal cleft may be helpful in some cases of airway obstruction such as micrognathia or midface retrusion: in which surgical correction could precipitate obstructive sleep apnea.

There has been some anecdotal information that the use of a prosthetic device actually stimulates the motion of the velopharyngeal sphincter, allowing reduction in the size of the obturator bulb and the amount of palatal life. Witt et al. showed no statistically significant change in pharyngeal wall motion even though some of the patients did improve.[21]

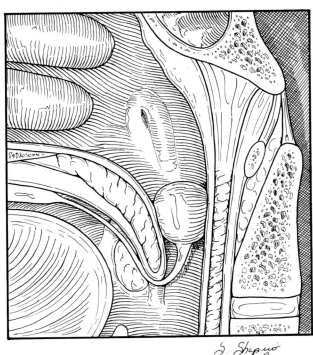

B

Figure 34–2:   A palatal lift (A) pushes the palate into an elevated position to effect closure during speech, and the obturator (B) slips into the velopharynx and permits closure of the port around the prostheses.

Often as the child passes through the mixed dentition stage, retention of the prosthesis is problematic because of tooth exfoliation. Equally, the child undergoing orthodontic maxillary expansion has difficulty because the maxilla is changing. In some cases, the prosthesis may even be counter-productive. In this age group, surgical conversion should be considered.

Surgical management

Surgical management of velopharyngeal dysfunction involves rearrangement of local tissues to obturate the velopharyngeal space (Fig. 34-3) Although some surgeons use one specific technique in all cases, the variation in closure types suggests that the surgeon should alter the technique to address the closure limitations more directly. Adjustments within each of the surgical methods can allow the procedure to be further tailored to the patient's specific closure pattern. This reemphasizes the need for accurate preoperative assessment of the closure by flexible endoscopy and/or videofluoroscopy.

Posterior Wall Augmentation. In the patient with nearly-complete closure of the velopharyngeal sphincter in either a coronal or circular pattern, the resultant defect is a small midline posterior gap. It would seem that this should close easily with the augmentation of the posterior wall by any means.

In the past, many natural and artificial substances have been inserted to increase the depth of the posterior wall to effect closure.[22-25] Many of these have been temporarily effective. The problem has been the chronic absorption of autologous implants and the inferior migration of the other implants.

The use of a rolled, superiorly-based pharyngeal flap to augment the posterior wall has been attempted. It would seem that this procedure would afford a reasonable obturation of the posterior wall and be less apt to migrate, but scar contracture and/or tissue atrophy have affected long term results adversely.[26]

Pharyngeal Flap. The *pharyngeal flap* has been the workhorse for treatment of velopharyngeal dys-

function. Essentially, a bridge is made from the posterior wall of the pharynx to the superior surface of the palate. This procedure creates a midline obturation with ports on either side for respiration. The flap has been described both inferiorly and superiorly based. The *inferiorly-based flap* tethers the palate caudally and leaves the ports lower in the pharynx. The maximal velopharyngeal sphincter activity is more superior, a position that may reduce this flap's effectiveness. The *superiorly-based flap* is currently the more commonly performed flap. It allows the port to be placed near the level of maximal velopharyngeal closure and effects a greater likelihood of closure.

The success of the pharyngeal flap is based upon the degree of lateral wall motion. As the central portion of the nasopharynx is obturated, the lateral walls must move toward the midline to effect complete closure. In the absence of lateral wall motion, closure of the ports during speech is impossible. With a wide obstructive flap, adequate intraoral pressure can be obtained, but only through sacrifice of the nasal airway. Creation of a wide flap is especially important to consider in the child with preexistent airway obstruction.

> **SPECIAL CONSIDERATION:**
>
> A posterior pharyngeal flap must be wide enough to allow closure with motion from the lateral pharyngeal walls, yet be narrow enough to maintain patency of the nasal airway.

The width of the pharyngeal flap should be tailored to the amount of lateral wall motion. The surgeon can attempt to deliver a wide, medium, or narrow flap. The vagaries of healing and scar contracture make this somewhat difficult, but such designer flaps can help reduce the overall risk of airway obstruction after flap surgery.

OSA in the immediate postoperative period can be problematic. The use of catheters to maintain an appropriately-sized port intraoperatively has been suggested.[27,28] Close observation during the night after surgery is recommended. OSA syndrome also may develop months to years later. It is important

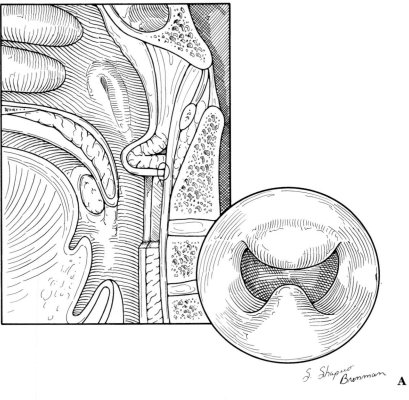

A

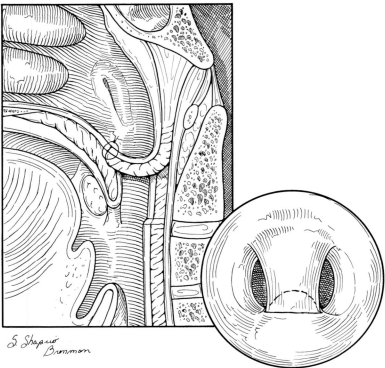

Figure 34–3: There are three common ways to obturate the velopharynx surgically. The following show a lateral and an en fas schematic of the obturation for each surgical procedure. (A) Posterior wall augmentation obturates only the posterior wall area. (B) The pharyngeal flap obturates the central portion of the velopharynx. *Figure continues.*

B

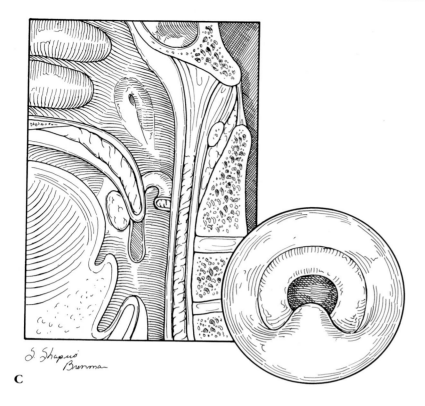

Figure 34–3: *(continued)* (C) The sphincter pharyngoplasty obturates the posterior and lateral walls.

C

to maintain a high level of suspicion and query the family frequently regarding signs and symptoms of OSA.

Sphincter Pharyngoplasty. An alternative to the pharyngeal flap, which has gained wide acceptance over the last two decades, is the *sphincter pharyngoplasty.* In this technique, the palatopharyngeus muscle and its mucosal covering are raised as a vascularized and innervated myomucosal flap. Although it was originally described by Orticochea,[29] It has undergone many changes over the years.[30] Currently, the myomucosal flap is transferred into the velopharynx to augment or obturate the lateral and posterior walls with a central port. This allows the closure of the port with minimal motion of the palate. It has been used successfully in coronal and circular closure cases. It also is effective in cases of hypotonic velopharynx in which there is little motion of the walls of the velopharynx.[31]

A tight closure still may contribute to significant airway obstruction and OSA. However, the risk is thought to be less than that with a wide pharyngeal flap. Alterations of the central port are accomplished more easily than with the bilateral port from

a pharyngeal flap. This central port may be opened or made tighter by "zipping" or "unzipping" at the connection of the flaps.[32]

AT A GLANCE . . .

Surgical Management of Velopharyngeal Dysfunction

- **Posterior Wall Augmentation:** used in patients with a nearly-complete closure of the velopharyngeal sphincter; results are usually temporary.

- **Pharyngeal Flap:** involves construction of a bridge from the posterior wall of the pharynx to the superior surface of the palate; success is based on degree of lateral wall motion.

- **Sphincter Pharyngoplasty:** the myomucosal flap is transferred into the velopharynx to augment or obturate the lateral and posterior walls with a central flap; less risk of airway obstruction and OSA.

The decision to use a particular surgery should be based on the patient's closure mechanism and not on a preconceived sense of a better method of surgery.

CONCLUSION

The care of the cleft palate child should be carried out with a team approach. Fractionation of services typically undermines the eventual outcome and often requires more frequent surgical intervention. There is no single ideal process, but each case must be considered on an individual basis. Precise documentation and team discussions help to facilitate this goal.

REFERENCES

1. Dominguez S, Harker LA. Incidence of cholesteatoma with cleft palate. Ann Otol Rhinol Laryngol 1988; 97:659–660.
2. Rood SR, Stool SE. Current concepts of the etiology, diagnosis, and management of cleft palate related otopathologic disease. Otolaryngol Clin North Am 1981; 14:865–884.
3. Robin P. A fall of the base of the tongue considered as a new cause of nasopharyngeal respiratory impairment: Pierre Robin sequence, a translation. 1923 [classical article]. Plast Reconstr Surg 1994; 93:1301–1303.
4. Sadewitz VL. Robin sequence: Changes in thinking leading to changes in patient care. [Review]. Cleft Palate Craniofac J 1992; 29:246–253.
5. Bath AP, Bull PD. Management of upper airway obstruction in Pierre Robin sequence. J Laryngol Otol 1997; 111:1155–1157.
6. Cohen SR, Simms C, Burstein FD. Mandibular distraction osteogenesis in the treatment of upper airway obstruction in children with craniofacial deformities. Plast Reconstr Surg 1998; 101:312–318.
7. McComb H. Primary repair of the bilateral cleft lip nose: A 15-year review and a new treatment plan. Plast Reconstr Surg 1990; 86:882–889.
8. Salyer KE. Early and late treatment of unilateral cleft nasal deformity. Cleft Palate Craniofac J 1992; 29:556–569.
9. Freedlander E, Webster MH, Lewis RB, et al. Neonatal cleft lip repair in Ayrshire; A contribution to the debate [see comments]. Br J Plast Surg 1990; 43:197–202.
10. Seibert RW. The role of lip adhesion in cleft lip repair. J Arkansas Med Soc 1980; 77:139–141.
11. Gosain AK, Conley SF, Marks S, et al. Submucous cleft palate: Diagnostic methods and outcomes of surgical treatment. [Review] Plast Reconstr Surg 1996; 97:1497–1509.
12. Ramamurthy L, Wyatt RA, Whitby D, et al. The evaluation of velopharyngeal function using flexible nasendoscopy. J Laryngol Otol 1997; 111:739–745.
13. D'Antonio LL, Marsh JL, Province MA, et al. Reliability of flexible fiberoptic nasopharyngoscopy for evaluation of velopharyngeal function in a clinical population. Cleft Palate J 1989; 26:217–225.
13a. Management for Cleft Lip/Palate. Huebener DV, Marsh JL. Presented at American Cleft Palate Association 4181 1997.
14. Haapanen ML. Effect of method of cleft palate repair on the quality of speech at the age of 6 years. Scand J Plast Reconstr Surg Hand Surg 1995; 29:245–250.
14b. Marsh JL, Grames LM, Holtman BI (1989) Cleft Palate Journal, 26:46-50.
15. Furlow LT Jr. Cleft palate repair by double opposing Z-plasty. Plast Reconstr Surg 1986; 78:724–738.
16. Emory REJ, Clay RP, Bite U, et al. Fistula formation and repair after palatal closure: An institutional perspective. Plast Reconstr Surg 1997; 99:1535–1538.
17. Croft CB, Shprintzen RJ, Rakoff SJ. Patterns of velopharyngeal valving in normal and cleft palate subjects: A multi-view videofluoroscopic and nasoendoscopic study. Laryngoscope 1981; 91:265–271.
18. Golding-Kushner KJ, Argamaso RV, Cotton RT, et al. Standardization for the reporting of nasopharyngoscopy and multiview videofluoroscopy: A report from an international working group. Cleft Palate J 1990; 27:337–347.
19. Witzel MA, Tobe J, Salyer K. The use of nasopharyngoscopy biofeedback therapy in the correction of inconsistent velopharyngeal closure. Int J Pediatr Otorhinolaryngol 1988; 15:137–142.
20. Ysunza A, Pamplona C, Toledo E. Change in velopharyngeal valving after speech therapy in cleft palate patients. A videonasopharyngoscopic and multi-view videofluoroscopic study. Int J Pediatr Otorhinolaryngol 1992; 24:45–54.
21. Witt PD, Rozelle AA, Marsh JL, et al. Do palatal lift prostheses stimulate velopharyngeal neuromuscular activity? Cleft Palate Craniofac J 1995; 32:469–475.
22. Wolford LM, Oelschlaeger M, Deal R. Proplast as a pharyngeal wall implant to correct velopharyngeal insufficiency. Cleft Palate J 1989; 26:119–26.
23. Denny AD, Marks SM, Oliff-Carneol S. Correction of velopharyngeal insufficiency by pharyngeal augmentation using autologous cartilage: A preliminary report. Cleft Palate Craniofac J 1993; 30:46–54.

24. Remacle M, Bertrand B, Eloy P, et al. The use of injectable collagen to correct velopharyngeal insufficiency. Laryngoscope 1990; 100:269–274.

25. Terris DJ, Goode RL. Costochondral pharyngeal implants for velopharyngeal insufficiency. Laryngoscope 1993; 103:565–569.

26. Witt PD, O'Daniel TG, Marsh JL, et al. Surgical management of velopharyngeal dysfunction: Outcome analysis of autogenous posterior pharyngeal wall augmentation. Plast Reconstr Surg 1997; 99:1287–1296.

27. Levine PA, Goode RL. The lateral port control pharyngeal flap: A versatile approach to velopharyngeal insufficiency. Otolaryngol Head Neck Surg 1982; 90:310–314.

28. Crockett DM, Bumsted RM, Van Demark DR. Experience with surgical management of velopharyngeal incompetence. Otolaryngol Head Neck Surg 1988; 99:1–9.

29. Orticochea M. A review of 236 cleft palate patients treated with dynamic muscle sphincter. Plast Reconstr Surg 1983; 71:180–188.

30. Riski JE, Serafin D, Riefkohl R, et al. A rationale for modifying the site of insertion of the orticochea pharyngoplasty. Plast Reconstr Surg 1984; 73:882–894.

31. Witt PD, Marsh JL, Grames LM, et al. Management of the hypodynamic velopharynx. Cleft Palate Craniofac J 1995; 32:179–187.

32. Witt PD, Marsh JL, Grames LM, et al. Revision of the failed sphincter pharyngoplasty: An outcome assessment. Plast Reconstr Surg 1995; 96:129–138.

35 Dental and Orthodontic Disorders

*Donald V. Huebener
and Richard J. Nissen*

The separate disciplines of pediatric dentistry and orthodontics are well known in the field of dentistry, and knowledge in these overlapping anatomic areas is also important to the medical care provider in pediatric otolaryngology. Common dental problems, such as abscessed primary or permanent teeth, developmental orofacial patterns (e.g., Class II malocclusion), and complex craniofacial deformities (e.g., Apert syndrome), necessitate an understanding of the basic diagnosis and treatment regimens that are involved in caring for simple isolated problems as well as complex multidisciplinary treatment sequences. The purpose of this chapter, therefore, is to acquaint otolaryngologists with the fundamentals of pediatric dentistry and orthodontics, in order that they may become better diagnosticians and care providers for their patients.

DENTAL GROWTH AND DEVELOPMENT

The human dentition begins development at approximately 6 weeks in utero when the *dental lamina*, the precursor of the future tooth buds, appears histologically. Tooth structures (i.e., enamel, dentin, pulp, cementum) are formed from this embryonic ectoderm and mesoderm (Fig. 35-1). Following recognizable developmental stages, the first primary tooth (*mandibular incisor*) emerges into the oral cavity between 6 and 7 months of age. Maxillary and mandibular primary teeth continue to

erupt according to specific order and sequence (Table 35-1).

The *primary dentition* consists of ten maxillary teeth and ten mandibular teeth (central incisor, lateral incisor, canine, first primary molar, and second primary molar). These teeth are represented by letters according to the diagram in Figure 35-2. As a rule of thumb, eight primary incisors should be present by 1 year of age; the remaining primary teeth should be visible in the oral cavity by approximately 2 to 2½ years of age.

At approximately 6 to 7 years of age, *mixed dentition* (some primary and some permanent teeth both present in the oral cavity at the same time) begins to appear. It is during this period (6–13 years) that the primary incisors, canines, and molars are replaced by their permanent tooth counterparts. All permanent teeth, with the exception of the permanent third molars (i.e., wisdom teeth), usually are present by 13 years of age. The permanent teeth are represented by Arabic numerals as shown in Figure 35-2.

Eruption of Teeth

The eruption of the primary teeth is a normal physiologic process. In the past, many systemic disturbances such as fever, diarrhea, irritability, and pain have been attributed to "teething." Although researchers have discounted such causal relationships, studies have shown there may be an increase in finger sucking, drooling, and daytime restlessness with the eruption of primary teeth.[1,2] In addition, a slight inflammation of the gingival tissues in the tooth eruption site may cause temporary discomfort that usually subsides in a day or so. Surgical assistance in tooth eruption by incision of overlying oral tissue generally is contraindicated.

Pediatric Otolaryngology, Edited by R.F. Wetmore, H.R. Muntz, and T.J. McGill. Thieme Medical Publishers, Inc., New York © 2000.

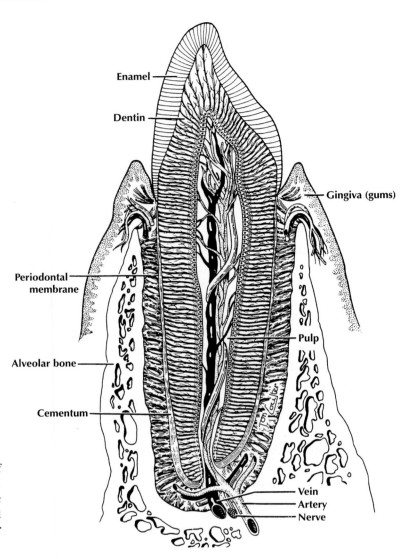

Figure 35–1: Diagrammatic representation of a mandibular incisor and its surrounding tissues. Note enamel; dentin; cementum; pulpal tissue with vein, artery, nerve, and adjacent gingival tissue; periodontal membrane; and alveolar bone.

The sequence of human primary tooth eruption in both the maxillary and mandibular arches begins with the central incisors and is followed by the lateral incisors, first molars, canines, and second molars, respectively. In contrast, the permanent dentition, which begins to erupt at 6 to 7 years, has a different sequence in the maxillary arch than in the mandibular arch. The most favorable erupting sequence in the maxillary arch begins with the first molar followed by the central incisor, lateral incisor, first premolar, second premolar, canine, and second molar, respectively. In the mandibular arch, the first molar is followed by the central incisor, the lateral incisor, canine, first premolar, second premolar, and second molar.[3] Failure of teeth to erupt in this most favorable sequence can result in factors leading to malocclusion. The eruption of the third molars, or wisdom teeth, is variable.

DENTAL CARIES

Dental caries is the most common infectious disease known to man. Although Bowen recently

TABLE 35–1:   Chronology of the Human Dentition

Tooth	Hard Tissue Formation Begins	Amount of Enamel Formed at Birth	Enamel Completed	Eruption	Root Completed
Deciduous dentition					
Maxillary					
Central incisor	4 mo in utero	Five sixths	1½ mo	7½ mo	1½ yr
Lateral incisor	4½ mo in utero	Two thirds	2½ mo	9 mo	2 yr
Cuspid	5 mo in utero	One third	9 mo	18 mo	3¼ yr
First molar	5 mo in utero	Cusps united	6 mo	14 mo	2½ yr
Second molar	6 mo in utero	Cusp tips still isolated	11 mo	24 mo	3 yr
Mandibular					
Central incisor	4½ mo in utero	Three fifths	2½ mo	6 mo	1½ yr
Lateral incisor	4½ mo in utero	Three fifths	3 mo	7 mo	1½ yr
Cuspid	5 mo in utero	One third	9 mo	16 mo	3¼ yr
First molar	5 mo in utero	Cusps united	5½ mo	12 mo	2¼ yr
Second molar	6 mo in utero	Cusp tips still isolated	10 mo	20 mo	3 yr
Permanent dentition					
Maxillary					
Central incisor	3–4 mo		4–5 yr	7–8 yr	10 yr
Lateral incisor	10–12 mo		4–5 yr	8–9 yr	11 yr
Cuspid	4–5 mo		6–7 yr	11–12 yr	13–15 yr
First bicuspid	1½–1¾ yr		5–6 yr	10–11 yr	12–13 yr
Second bicuspid	2–2¼ yr		6–7 yr	10–12 yr	12–14 yr
First molar	At birth	Sometimes a trace	2½–3 yr	6–7 yr	9–10 yr
Second molar	2½–3 yr		7–8 yr	12–13 yr	14–16 yr
Third molar	7–9 yr		12–16 yr	17–21 yr	18–25 yr
Mandibular					
Central incisor	3–4 mo		4–5 yr	6–7 yr	9 yr
Lateral incisor	3–4 mo		4–5 yr	7–8 yr	10 yr
Cuspid	4–5 mo		6–7 yr	9–10 yr	12–14 yr
First bicuspid	1¾–2 yr		5–6 yr	10–12 yr	12–13 yr
Second bicuspid	2¼–2½ yr		6–7 yr	11–12 yr	13–14 yr
First molar	At birth	Sometimes a trace	2½–3 yr	6–7 yr	9–10 yr
Second molar	2½–3 yr		7–8 yr	11–13 yr	14–15 yr
Third molar	8–10 yr		12–16 yr	17–21 yr	18–25 yr

From Kronfeld R./Bur 1935 35:18–25. Modified by Kronfeld R, Schour I./JADA 1936 26:18–32, with permission.

noted that there is a decrease in the occurrence of dental caries, it still remains the most prevalent disease affecting humans.[4] Dental caries is the result of three dependent factors: (1) presence of microorganisms (e.g., *streptococcus mutants*); (2) a fermentable substrate (e.g., sucrose); and (3) suscepti-

ble tooth structure. The microorganisms, colonizing on the tooth surface in a gelatinous substance called *plaque,* use the fermentable substrate to produce an acidic environment, thus decalcifying the inorganic part of the enamel. Once the enamel barrier of the tooth is broken, dental caries begins. If left un-

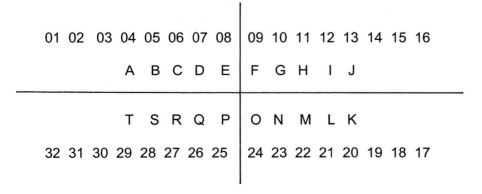

Figure 35–2: Diagrammatic representation of the primary teeth (letters) and permanent teeth (arabic numerals).

treated, dental caries can progress through the dentin into the dental pulp causing an inflammation and subsequent abscessed tooth.

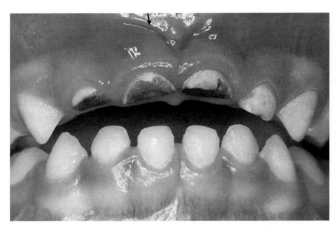

Figure 35–3: Intraoral photograph of the dentition of a 4-year-old patient. Note swelling at apex of the maxillary primary right central incisor and fistula formation.

<table>
<tr><td>

AT A GLANCE . . .

Factors Involved in the Development of Dental Caries

- Presence of microorganisms
- Fermentable substrate (e.g., sucrose)
- Susceptible tooth structure

</td></tr>
</table>

Caries in the Primary Dentition

MacDonald et al. have pointed out that in the primary dentition the sequence of caries attack follows a specific pattern: (1) mandibular molars; (2) maxillary molars; and (3) maxillary anterior teeth. Usually mandibular anterior teeth are less affected than other primary teeth.[5]

Of particular interest to healthcare providers of infants and children is the clinically-recognizable problems of *baby bottle tooth decay* (BBTD), or nursery bottle caries. It is due to prolonged feeding from a nursing bottle that contains milk or sugar-containing juice or liquid at naptime or bedtime. A similar nursing caries pattern also is observed in infants who breast-feed for prolonged periods of time.

In BBTD, there is early carious involvement of the maxillary anterior teeth and maxillary and mandibular first primary molars. The mandibular incisors are usually unaffected due to the presence of the tongue shielding them. Concern about BBTD has led care providers in both the American Academy of Pediatrics and the American Academy of Pediatric Dentistry (AAPD) to encourage discontinuance of the nursing bottle by 1 year of age.

Dental Abscess

Failure to remove dental caries and restore primary and permanent teeth to normal form and function may lead to infected pulpal tissues and subsequent *dental abscess*. Trauma to the teeth and supporting tissues also may lead to pulpal neurosis and abscess. Clinically, a dental abscess near a carious primary incisor appears as a raised, inflamed, circumscribed area of the gingival tissue as seen in Figure 35-3. A

fistulous tract may or may not be present. Radiographically, there is bone destruction and radiolucency in the bifurcation area of a primary molar (Fig. 35-4).

When permanent molars abscess, the bone destruction appears at the apex of the root, hence the term *periapical radiolucency* or *periapical abscess*. Small, chronic fistulas associated with carious teeth usually do not require antibiotic therapy unless associated with facial swelling.

TRAUMATIC INJURIES TO THE TEETH

Injuries to the primary and permanent teeth and their supporting structures require special skills in

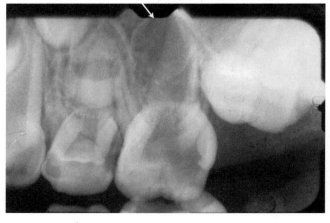

Figure 35–4: Periapical radiograph of right maxillary primary posterior teeth. Note severe caries in primary molars and periapical radiolucency in the bifurcation area of the second primary molar.

diagnosis and treatment. Traumatic injuries can be classified into four categories: (1) intrusion injuries; (2) luxation injuries; (3) fracture injuries; and (4) avulsion injuries.

Displacement of primary anterior teeth occurs frequently in children under 3 years of age. While toddlers are learning to walk and are less secure in movement, a blow to an anterior primary tooth can push part or all of the clinical crown into the maxillary alveolus. It is generally agreed that these primary teeth will reerupt into the oral cavity, and that 90% of injuries are displaced labial to the developing permanent tooth bud.[6] When the intruded primary tooth is displaced lingually or palatally, encroaching on the permanent developing tooth bud, it should be removed. Failure of a primary tooth to reerupt after intrusion may necessitate surgical removal at a later date.

Intruded displacement of permanent teeth requires gradual orthodontic repositioning if they fail to reerupt spontaneously. In severe cases of multiple intruded teeth or displacement, the care provider may elect to reposition and stabilize the luxated teeth with wire/acrylic splints. Usually displaced or intruded teeth require endodontic (root canal) therapy because the pulpal tissue becomes neurotic due to the interruption of the blood supply from the injury.

Avulsion injuries (i.e., the loss of a tooth from the tooth socket) of permanent teeth, usually one in the anterior region, require immediate replacement. Andreasen estimates that 90% of permanent teeth that were reimplanted within 30 minutes showed no discernible evidence of root resorption 2 or more years later.[7] However, 95% of teeth reimplanted more than 2 hours after avulsion, showed root resorption.[7] The prognosis for avulsed permanent teeth, therefore, is better if the tooth is reimplanted in < 30 minutes. Avulsed primary teeth usually are not reimplanted.

SPECIAL CONSIDERATION:
Avulsion injuries of permanent teeth require immediate replacement. Avulsed primary teeth usually are not reimplanted.

Stabilization of avulsed teeth with wire/acrylic splints is required for a period of 7 to 14 days. Systemic antibiotic therapy has been recommended for at least 4 days following reimplantation to reduce the incidence of inflammatory root resorption causing failure of the reimplanted tooth.[6] In general, all reimplanted teeth require endodontic therapy.

Treatment of coronal tooth fractures depends on the amount of tooth structure involved. In *Ellis I fractures* (i.e., enamel only) of primary and permanent teeth, the emergency treatment consists of smoothing the rough enamel with a rotary dental instrument. Coronal fractures of the enamel and dentin (*Ellis II*) require placement of a temporary restoration to protect exposed dentin. Coronal injuries involving the enamel, dentin, and pulpal tissue (*Ellis III*) necessitate appropriate pulpal therapy (pulp capping procedure of endodontic therapy) to ensure favorable tooth prognosis. Fractures with a favorable prognosis involving the root of a tooth require stabilization for a period of 3 months. All traumatized teeth need periapical dental radiographs to monitor healing. The ultimate choice of a restoration material for fractured teeth depends on the extent of injury and prognosis.

SPECIAL CONSIDERATION:
All traumatized teeth need periapical dental radiographs to monitor healing.

AT A GLANCE . . .
Traumatic Dental Injuries

- Intrusion injuries
- Luxation injuries
- Fracture injuries
- Avulsion injuries

PREVENTIVE DENTISTRY

Preventing dental caries requires many measures for control. The AAPD has emphasized early visits to the dentist through the Infant Oral Health Care Program.[8] Through this effort, infants are seen near the time the first tooth erupts into the oral cavity or before 1 year of age. At this visit, an oral examination is performed. Anticipatory guidance for parents centers on tooth eruption, caries, oral injuries, fluoride, toothbrushing, diet, and general oral hygiene procedures. Parents are instructed on measures for good oral health and periodicity of visits/recalls as recommended by the AAPD and major health organizations as detailed in Bright Futures.[9] The usual periodicity recommendations for infants, children and teenagers is every six months.

AT A GLANCE . . .

Effective Caries Prevention

- Fluoride treatments
- Sealants
- Appropriate eating habits
- Good oral hygiene

Effective caries prevention measures include fluoride (systemic and topical), sealants, appropriate eating habits, and the practice of good oral hygiene procedures. Research studies have shown the most effective way to reduce dental caries in the general population is through community water fluoridation. Topical fluorides (in toothpastes, mouth rinses, and professionally-applied topical fluoride treatments) increase the fluoride content on the enamel surface and assist in further preventing caries. Dietary fluoride supplements are not recommended if the fluoride content of water supplies is 0.6% ppm or more.[10] *Dental sealants* (Fig. 35–5), which are

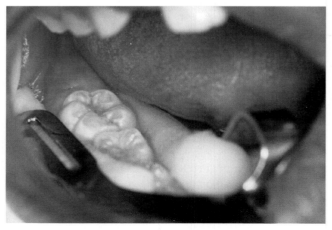

Figure 35–5: Intraoral photograph of sealant placed on mandibular right permanent first molar.

thin plastic coatings that are placed on posterior permanent molars, provide additional caries prevention in children and young adolescents. When combined with an effective oral hygiene program, these caries prevention efforts contribute to healthy teeth and supporting tissues.

OROFACIAL GROWTH AND DEVELOPMENT

Researchers continue to study how environment and genetic factors alter and affect predicted growth and development in the maxilla and mandible.[11-17] In order for this information to be of benefit and applied clinically, it is important to have a general understanding of how the maxilla and mandible change and develop in the maturing child.

At birth, the length of the cranium is 65% complete, and by the age of 5 years, about 90% of its full size.[18] The mandible is characteristically small in relation to the rest of the head at this time, but catches up to the rest of the face as the child develops. The disproportions of the skeletal facial structures decrease as the preadolescent nears puberty. In the female, skeletal growth changes in the face slowly and ceases shortly after puberty. In the male, significant changes may continue to occur well into the late teen years. The changes that affect the maxilla and mandible are of significant concern when evaluating the dental occlusion.

The growth of the maxilla and mandible is predicated by deposition and resorption of bone. The net effects of these processes create changes in the skeletal bases by way of displacement. Displacement occurs horizontally, vertically, and anterior-posteriorly relative to the cranium. It is through these mechanisms that the proportions of the face change and appear to enlarge.

The maxilla, or nasomaxillary complex, tends to grow down and forward from under the cranium. This growth is accomplished by intramembranous bone development. Ossification occurs by apposition of the bone at the sutures and by surface remodeling.[19] Bone apposition occurs on both sides of the sutures, and the peripheral borders in the maxilla continuously remodel to allow for the eruption of the developing dentition. As the palatal vault remodels, bone is removed from the floor of the nose and added to the roof of the mouth, moving the vault downward and allowing it to widen. Increases in the alveolar process are correlated closely with the eruption of teeth as well as changes seen in the mandible.

The mandible develops by both endochondral ossification as well as periosteal activity. These mechanisms allow the mandible to grow in length, creating downward and forward displacement. The growth observed is a complex process involving changes at the condyle in conjunction with significant remodeling of the body and ramus of the mandible. The body of the mandible grows by periosteal apposition of bone on its posterior surface, whereas the ramus remodels by endochondral replacement of bone at the condyle.[19] Bone also is added progressively to the external surface of the chin while the mandible remodels. This is a slow process that proceeds throughout childhood, eventually developing the chin so that it projects more prominently and appears in better proportion to the maxilla.

As the maxilla and mandible grow, it is important to note that the size of the teeth that will eventually erupt into the dental arch are preprogrammed genetically and will not change. The permanent dentition demonstrates more tooth mass than its predecessor, the primary dentition. Both the maxilla and mandible appear to get larger as the child matures; however, the arch length, or arch perimeter, does not reflect this change similarly. Hence, teeth that are crowded in a young child often remain crowded as the child matures. The perimeter of maxillary arch length slightly increases during maturation. The mandibular arch length, however, can show a great degree of variability in development. It generally remains unchanged or slightly diminishes throughout the ossification changes in the mandible. Lack of significant increases in arch length as the maxilla and mandible remodel is an important concept to note.

OCCLUSION

Classifications

In order to describe the status of the "bite" or *dental occlusion,* it is important to evaluate and categorize the relationship of the maxillary dentition relative to the mandibular dentition. An understanding of the rudimentary nomenclature used in this categorization process is necessary when evaluating patients.

In the early 1900s, Angle created the standard by which most malocclusions are categorized currently.[20] In order for Angle to classify a malocclusion, the definition of a normal occlusion had to be established. This classification system is based upon the maxillary first permanent molars and their relationship anteroposteriorly to the mandibular first permanent molars. It is, however, important to note that this system does not take into account any discrepancies in vertical or transverse planes.[21] Other alternative occlusal classification systems have been suggested, but Angle's classification of malocclusions remains the universal system used today to identify the dental relationship.

In this system, Angle described four categories by which dental occlusions can be judged. In order to apply the concepts of Angle's system, a quick review of dental molar anatomy may be helpful. Figure 35–6 demonstrates the anatomic landmarks of significance on both the maxillary and mandibular molars. These dental landmarks need to be understood in order to apply the basic principals of a dental occlusion.

Angle's *class I normal occlusion* is demonstrated in Figure 35–7. Note the mesial buccal cusp of the maxillary first permanent molar aligns in the mesial buccal groove of the mandibular first permanent molar. A class I normal occlusion and a *class I malocclusion* have the same molar relationship, but the expression "malocclusion" connotes that other teeth in either the maxillary or mandibular dental arches are malaligned. Class I malocclusions generally are indicative of good anteroposterior (AP) sym-

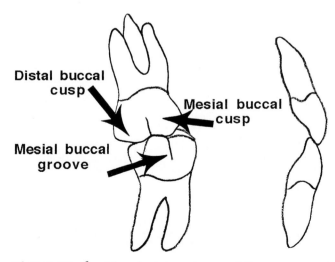

Figure 35–6: The dental anatomy of the permanent molars.

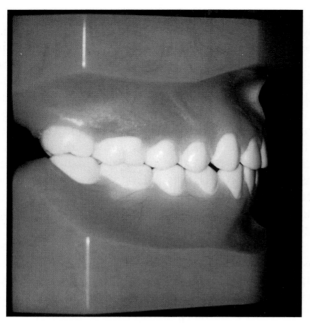

Figure 35–7: A model depicting a class I normal occlusion.

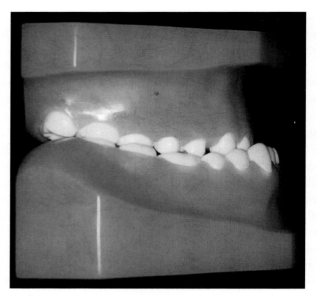

Figure 35–9: A model depicting a class III malocclusion.

metry between the maxilla and mandible, and typically, problems associated with this type of relationship pertain to unfavorable spatial tooth positioning. Common problems include dental rotations, crowding of the teeth due to lack of adequate arch length, and excessive dental spacing in between adjacent teeth.

Angle's *class II malocclusion* (Fig. 35-8) is dem-

onstrated by the mesial buccal cusp of the maxillary first permanent molar positioned mesial, or anterior, to the mesial buccal groove on the mandibular first permanent molar.

A *class III relationship* is noted by the mesial buccal cusp of the maxillary first permanent molar aligned distal to, or posterior to, the mesial buccal groove of the lower first permanent molar (Fig. 35-9). It is important to note that this system of categorizing occlusions is in reference to a permanent dentition or a developing permanent dentition known as a *mixed dentition,* which includes a combination of primary and permanent teeth. Angle's same principles of occlusion also can be applied to the primary dentition (Fig. 35-10).

In a class II or class III malocclusion, discrepancies may not relate only to a dental relationship, but also be indicative of a more severe problem involving hypo- or hyperplasia of either jaws. Technically, it is incorrect to describe a skeletal deformity as a class I, II, or III skeletal abnormality because Angle's classification system was established to describe the dentition only. However, frequently in scientific literature it is not uncommon to read the expression, "Class II or III skeletal deformity," used colloquially.

Characteristics

Angle's occlusal classifications are the most basic means by which to characterize a dental occlusal problem initially. As the occlusal relationship is

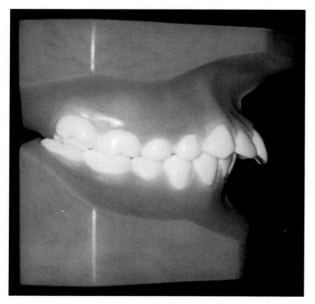

Figure 35–8: A model depicting a class II malocclusion.

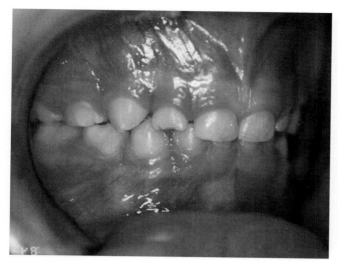

Figure 35–10: A photograph of a 5-year-old's primary dentition.

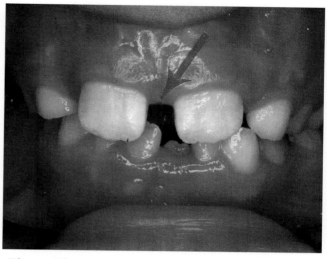

Figure 35–12: A maxillary dental diastema (arrow).

scrutinized more closely, the need for subcategories becomes necessary to describe further how the teeth relate to each other. *Incisor alignment* is a subcategory that is noted frequently when evaluating malocclusions. It is an evaluation of anterior tooth irregularities including crowding, overlapping, spacing, and dental rotations (Fig. 35–11). A severely-crowded dental arch is often synonymous with an arch length insufficiency.

Another occlusal trait that is evaluated is the presence or absence of a maxillary midline diastema. A *diastema* is a space between the maxillary central incisors. It may be demonstrated by <1 mm of dental separation, or a much larger degree of spacing (Fig. 35–12).

One common subcategory that is associated with the anterior dental relationship is *overbite* (Fig. 35–13), a term that describes the vertical component of the anterior teeth. Overbite can be defined as the vertical overlap of the incisor teeth when the posterior teeth are in contact. A *zero overbite* is known as an *edge-to-edge* relationship (Fig. 35–14), and a *negative overbite* is referred to as an *openbite* (Fig. 35–15).

Overjet describes the horizontal discrepancies of the maxillary dentition relative to the mandibular dentition (Fig. 35–16). It is defined as the horizontal overlap of the incisor teeth.

Palatal transverse discrepancies are known as *crossbites.* Crossbites also may exist in the anterior

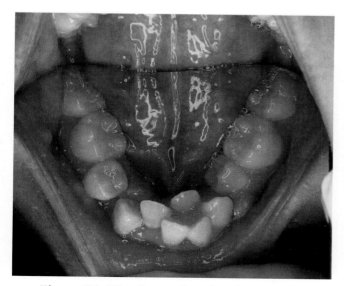

Figure 35–11: Lower dental arch crowding.

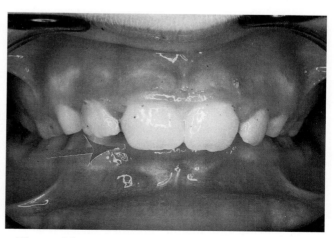

Figure 35–13: An excessive overbite relationship.

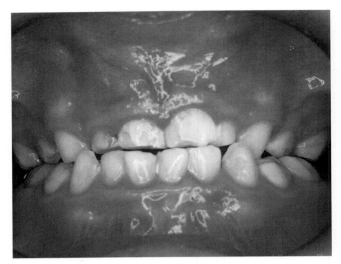

Figure 35–14: An edge-to-edge anterior dental relationship.

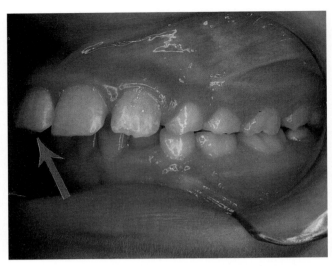

Figure 35–16: An excessive maxillary overjet relationship.

dentition creating an *underbite*. The *transverse crossbite* may be defined more precisely as unilateral, bilateral, and lingual, or less commonly seen, buccal (Fig. 35–17).

The *dental midline* describes the relationship between the midpoint of the maxillary dental arch to the midpoint of the mandibular dental arch. These midpoints are represented typically by the location of the contact of the maxillary central incisors and the contact of the mandibular central incisors (Fig. 35–18). Once this basic nomenclature is understood, the language needed to describe the orthodontic problem can be applied. Noting these additional occlusal characteristics gives the clinician

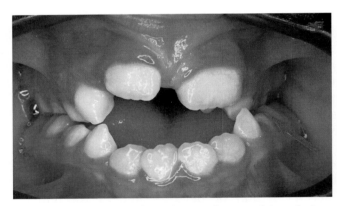

Figure 35–17: A unilateral posterior crossbite relationship.

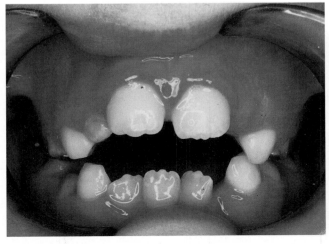

Figure 35–15: An anterior openbite dental relationship.

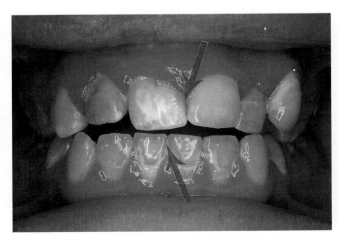

Figure 35–18: Dissimilar dental midline symmetry.

more precision in quantifying the dental relationship.

THE ORTHODONTIC CONCEPT

Historically, dental clinicians have studied and become proficient at altering the spatial relationship of teeth in the human jaws. As early as 400 B.C., scientists had written about the appearance of poorly-positioned teeth and abnormal jaw structures.[22-24] Contemporary orthodontic treatment as we know it today consists of orthopedic as well as orthodontic therapies in combination to treat the dentition and the jaws. The term *dentofacial orthopedics* is used frequently to describe tooth- or tissue-supported appliances that alter or encourage favorable changes in condylar, mandibular, and/or maxillary bone growth and remodeling. The objective of contemporary treatment is a well-proportioned face, as well as an esthetic and stable dentition. For this reason, the dental arches and the face must be evaluated in three dimensions of space: transverse, anteroposterior, and vertical. It is often through dentofacial orthopedics that it becomes possible to achieve a treatment result with the jaws in proportion to each other and to the rest of the face. Treatment to achieve a favorable outcome can be as simple as recommending the early removal of primary teeth to facilitate improved changes in arch length for the erupting permanent dentition. However, a more complicated treatment approach may be indicated utilizing fixed appliance therapy with the simultaneous wearing of an orthopedic device. Lastly, it may be necessary to recommend a more invasive procedure involving orthognathic surgery to align a dental-skeletal deformity properly. To determine which treatment approach may best serve the patient, an assessment of craniofacial features and discrepancies in spatial-dental relationships should be reviewed in conjunction with known genetic or etiologic factors. It is this evaluation that ultimately dictates the orthodontic treatment of choice for an individual patient. Contemporary

treatment no longer addresses the dentition alone, but rather the entire orofacial complex and associated supporting structures.

The Diagnosis

The orthodontic diagnosis is comprised of a combination of three sources of information: a radiographic review of orofacial structures, a clinical examination of the dentition and surrounding soft tissues, and a question and answer session pertaining to patient-familial patterns and environmental influences. Through evaluating and quantifying the dental malocclusion, the clinician is able to establish the severity of a particular problem and the urgency with which it should be addressed. The patient and parent can then be advised accordingly as to any potential adverse sequelae associated with the problem or referred to an appropriate specialist for further study and recommendations.

Radiographic Considerations

The radiographic examination is comprised routinely of a panoramic or panoral radiograph and a cephalometric film. In some instances, a full mouth series of periapical radiographs may be indicated to evaluate more closely any missing teeth or abnormal periodontal supporting structures.

Cephalometric radiographs (Fig. 35–19) may be

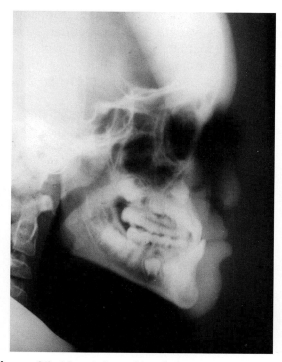

Figure 35–19:   A lateral cephalometric radiograph.

taken laterally or anterior-posteriorly. Lateral cephalograms are taken routinely during an initial exam and are important for orthodontic growth analysis, diagnosis, treatment planning, monitoring of therapy, and evaluation of final treatment outcome. An AP cephalogram may be a useful radiographic adjunct in the evaluation of skeletal asymmetries or for presurgical studies in complicated orthognathic cases. The lateral cephalograms are taken precisely so that a comparison of oral and craniofacial structures can be measured by evaluating superimposed tracings of different bony anatomic landmarks.[25] These tracings can then be studied by using a series of cephalometric appraisals including the Steiner Analysis, Ricketts Analysis, Down's Analysis, Wits Appraisal, McNamara Analysis, and other, more contemporary appraisals. Current computer imaging advances have allowed the clinician to evaluate radiographs through a process called digitization. Historically, cephalograms were hand traced. However, now digital imaging can make this process less labor intensive by way of transforming the bony landmark positions into numbers the computer can store, manipulate, and retrieve to create a computer-generated image. This image can then be evaluated through any combination of analyses or appraisals to determine potential growth trends or anticipated treatment outcomes.

A panoramic radiograph is another piece of information that may be necessary in determining the dental status of a particular patient. A panoramic radiograph (Fig. 35–20) is taken routinely to ascertain the dental maturation of a patient, rule out any neoplastic morphology, evaluate missing or supernumerary teeth, and determine if the developing dentition and supporting structures are normal and in good health.

Other additional radiographs can be taken to investigate special problems including temporomandibular joint (TMJ) disorders and congenital anomalies, but they are not taken routinely during the initial examination process. Entire books have been written on dental radiographic technique for the reader more interested in this area. See reference 26 for additional reading.

Clinical Examination

The clinical examination process consists primarily of an evaluation of the orofacial soft tissues and intraoral hard and soft tissues. The examination often is accompanied by the taking of intra- and extraoral photographs and the making of dental plaster casts to have a "study model" to analyze more closely the dentition and the status of the malocclusion. The orthodontic evaluation is primarily concerned with: (1) the documentation of the malocclusion; (2) a clinical impression of the skeletal AP relationship, which will be verified or disputed by radiographs; (3) an assessment of dental maturation, an overall appraisal of dental health, including caries, oral hygiene, periodontal status, and TMJ health; (4) pharyngeal health; and (5) orofacial musculature tone including the muscles of the tongue.

The dental examination begins by establishing the type of dentition present. It will either be a primary dentition, a permanent dentition, or a mixed dentition consisting of primary as well as permanent teeth.

Next, the occlusion is determined as noted by the Angle Classification System. The occlusal relationship will be either a class I, II, or III pattern as noted, by where the maxillary first permanent molar relates to the mandibular first permanent molar. Once the type of dentition and malocclusal relationship are established, additional occlusal characteristics can be noted such as overjet, overbite, dental spacing, dental crowding, crossbite, and openbite.

The clinician may next wish to evaluate skeletal findings and how they relate to the occlusal status. Common skeletal characteristics include excessive maxillary protrusion, mandibular skeletal retrognathia, and prognathia. As the AP discrepancy between the jaws becomes more pronounced, the dental malocclusion becomes more a consequence of the skeletal disproportionality and less of a consequence of the dental aspect of the malalignment.

If the mandible appears small or retruded, it may

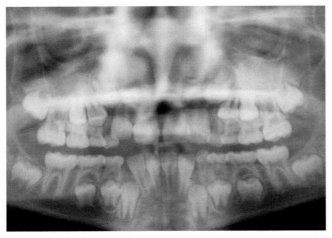

Figure 35–20:   A panoramic dental radiograph.

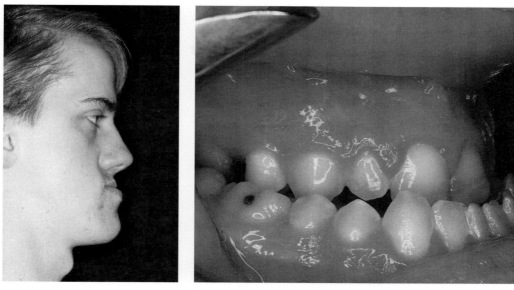

Figure 35–21:   (A and B) A patient with excessive mandibular prognathia.

be characterized as diminutive, hypoplastic, or retrognathic relative to the maxilla. The reduced definition of the mandible may be a consequence of a genetic disorder, such as that seen with Pierre Robin sequence, or may be secondary to excessive vertical maxillary growth, resulting in the displacement of the mandible down and backward. Excessive forward placement of the mandible is noted as being prognathic or protrusive. Specific skeletal features often create soft-tissue traits that mimic the underlying supporting structures. In mandibular prognathic patients (Fig. 35-21), the lower lip appears thick

and takes on a "pouty" appearance. In mandibular retrognathic patients (Fig. 35-22), the chin or lower face appears to "drop off" with little or no projection. In an excessive maxillary vertically-compromised patient (Fig. 35-23), the excessive maxillary growth tends to displace the mandible down and retruded, creating hypermentalis strain when the patient is asked to bring her lips together in occlusal rest position.

Often, in the nasopharyngeally-compromised patient, the maxilla is excessively forward or protrusive (Fig. 35-24). In evaluating these patients, it is

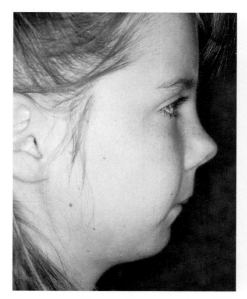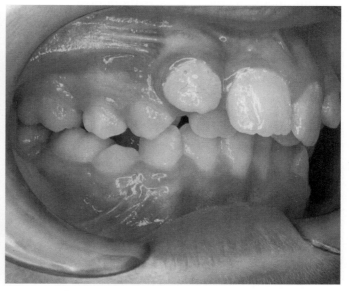

Figure 35–22:   (A and B) A patient with excessive mandibular retrognathia.

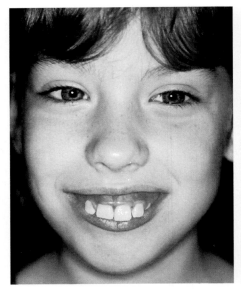
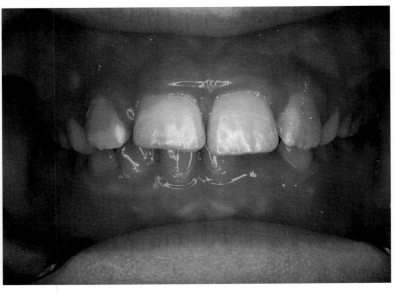

A
B

Figure 35–23:   (A and B) A patient with excessive maxillary skeletal vertical height.

incorrect to assume that the mandible is retruded, when in fact it is most likely that the maxilla is protrusive. These skeletal relationships are interdependent, and radiographic surveys are needed to determine precisely where the jaw imbalance exists or whether it is a combination of both the maxilla and mandible.

The clinical exam includes a brief check of the TMJs during routine opening and closing excursions, noting any deviations in the path of motion or any sounds made such as "pops," "clicks," or crepitus. The treatment of TMJ disorders can be enormously complicated with the involvement of many clinicians, including the dentist, orthodontist,

oral surgeon, otolaryngologist, and physical therapy specialist. The initial examination process is primarily to document normal or abnormal findings and any symptomatic associations.

The intraoral exam includes investigation of overall dental health, including an oral hygiene appraisal to note any abnormal or distinguishing characteristics associated with the gingival tissues. Healthy tissues demonstrate pink color (Fig. 35-25), and inflamed tissues appear reddish and swollen and bleed easily (Fig. 35-26).

A check of the dental tissues is indicated to note any possible caries or abnormal features in the enamel morphologic development. Any dental hard-

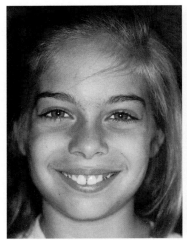
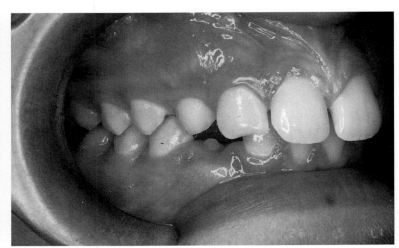

A
B

Figure 35–24:   (A and B) A patient with excessive protrusion of the maxilla.

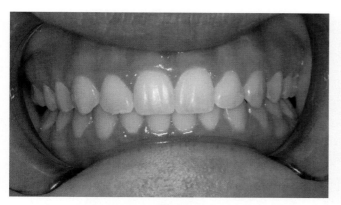

Figure 35–25: Healthy pink gingival tissues.

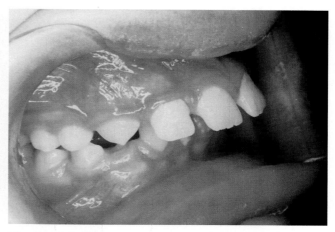

Figure 35–27: Excessive anterior maxillary dental flaring.

tissue or soft-tissue disease should be treated prior to the initiation of orthodontic treatment. Poor oral hygiene or incipient dental decay generally is exacerbated by the placement of orthodontic appliances. If the intraoral tissues are not in good health, orthodontic appliances generally are contraindicated.

Overall soft-tissue muscle tone must be assessed during the initial examination process. Flaccid oral facial musculature may be indicative of a potential openbite pattern or excessive dental spacing and flaring of the anterior incisor teeth (Fig. 35–27). Macroglossia also may mimic this dental pattern or exacerbate the condition. When the oral facial musculature is excessively tight or rigid, the opposite effect can be observed, with significant displacement of either the upper or lower incisors lingually positioned and crowded (Fig. 35–28).

The soft-tissue profile, in conjunction with underlying skeletal features, creates three characteristic facial types: convexed, straight, and concaved (Fig.

35–29). These facial types exist as subgroups of three more distinct classifications: dental malocclusions, dental-skeletal malocclusions, and craniofacial deformities. When categorizing dental malocclusions, the discrepancy between the maxillary and mandibular dentition, for argumentative purposes, may be in reference to mm of discrepancy, whereas craniofacial and dental-skeletal abnormalities may demonstrate discrepancies and asymmetries between the dental arches in excess of 1 cm.

History and Background

During the initial evaluation process, a familial history is taken to determine any relevant attributing genetic factors associated with the dental diagnosis. Parents often relate similarities between their own perceived or actual orthodontic problem and their son's or daughter's. Thus, a family background often gives the clinician insight into a potentially severe dentofacial growth problem that has yet to manifest itself clinically. Information regarding any abnormal genetic or craniofacial dysmorphology that is associated with the patient is usually revealed at this time and alerts the clinician that early treatment may be indicated.

When evaluating young patients for occlusal deviations, it is important to exclude environmental etiologic factors. A true genetic openbite pattern may require extensive orthodontic treatment in conjunction with maxillary or mandibular osteotomies to idealize the malocclusion and close the bite. If the openbite is a consequence of a nocturnal finger or thumb habit (Fig. 35–30), the malocclusion will resolve significantly by deterring the habit and

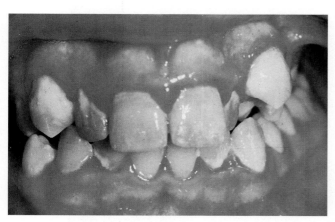

Figure 35–26: Unhealthy gingival tissues, with reddened margins and inflammation present.

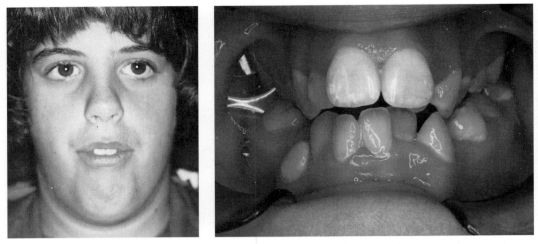

Figure 35–28: (A and B) Lower incisor crowding due to hypertonic lower lip musculature.

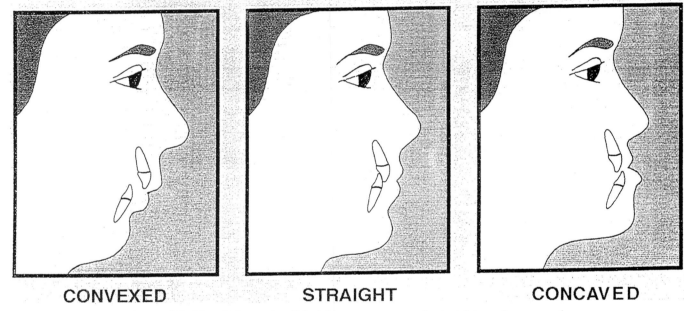

CONVEXED   STRAIGHT   CONCAVED

Figure 35–29: Schematic of facial types: convexed, straight, and concaved.

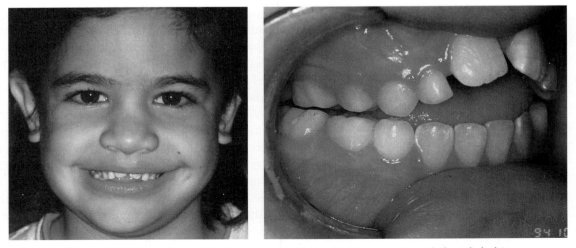

Figure 35–30: (A and B) Anterior openbite due to a nocturnal thumb habit.

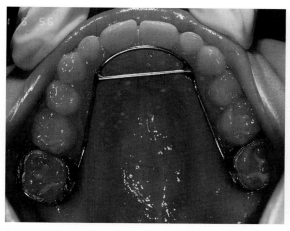

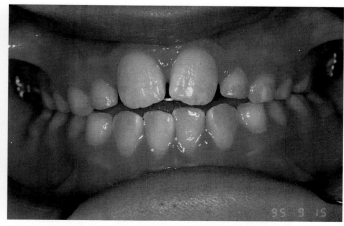

A   B

Figure 35–31:   (A and B) Resolution of openbite due to the placement of a habit appliance.

removing the environmental influence on the dentition (Fig. 35–31). Different types of orthodontic appliances are available to protect the affected anterior dentition and allow the openbite to close even if the habit persists. True environmentally-created malocclusions are best addressed at an early age before the permanent dentition has completed its eruption. Some clinicians feel interceptive care should begin prior to the eruption of the 6-year molar. Frequent environmental influences creating malocclusions include thumb or finger habits, aberrant tongue positioning, and trauma.

SPECIAL CONSIDERATION:

Environmental influences creating malocclusions include thumb or finger habits, aberrant tongue positioning (tongue thrusting), and trauma.

Aberrant tongue posturing, known as *tongue thrusting*, can be noted at rest, during active speech, and when swallowing. Such tongue posturing habits create anterior openbites or posterior lateral openbites (Fig. 35–32). Much discussion in the literature has occurred over the years as to whether the tongue creates the openbite or whether a genetic openbite exists and, as a consequence, the tongue naturally positions itself interdentally. Treatment for such problems often consists of combination therapies, including orthodontic habit appliances as well as speech therapy and articulation exercises in an attempt to retrain the tongue posturing. As the patient matures, the likelihood of altering tongue posture successfully diminishes. Without treatment, changes in skeletal and dental development are anticipated routinely with concomitant changes in soft-tissue features.

Oral Habits

During the clinical evaluation, a brief series of questions is asked to determine if there exists any acute or chronic environmental factors that may be influencing or exacerbating a dental malocclusion. These influences include: (1) the nocturnal thumb sucking habit; (2) extended or prolonged use of a pacifier; (3) aberrant swallowing patterns or speech articulation disorders in which the tongue is thrust

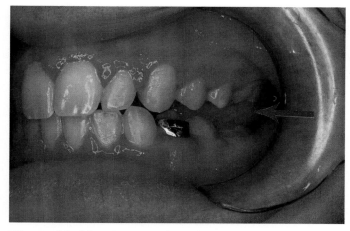

Figure 35–32:   Posterior lateral openbite due to a lateral tongue thrust habituation.

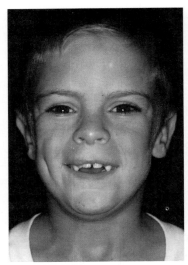
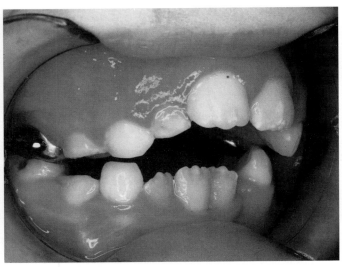

A   B

Figure 35–33: (A and B) An anterior openbite due to chronic obstructive airway disease.

forward laterally or bilabially; and (4) chronic obstructed nasal airway disease creating habitual mouth breathing tendencies. These conditions can lead to malocclusions resulting in anterior (Fig. 35-33) or lateral openbites.[26-28]

AT A GLANCE . . .

Oral Habits

- Nocturnal thumb sucking habit
- Extended or prolonged use of a pacifier
- Aberrant swallowing patterns/tongue thrusting
- Chronic nasal obstruction/habitual mouth breathing

Airway

Upper airway function often is evaluated when assessing potential factors affecting facial growth in adolescence. Incompetent nasopharyngeal airway function is believed to be a significant factor that potentially alters the growth and development of the orofacial structures.[11,12,29-34] Patients with chronic mouth breathing tendencies due to compromised nasopharyngeal patency have been shown to demonstrate clinically hypertrophic gingival tissues, protruding maxillary incisors, mandibular retrognathia, excessive vertical growth of the maxilla, developmentally-narrow maxillary trans-

verse arch width in association with high palatal vault anatomy, hypermentalis muscle activity, and often underdeveloped perioral musculature.[35-41] These findings have led to studies advocating adenoidectomies for patients demonstrating poor mandibular growth due to chronic obstructed airway pathology.[42] Conversely, other studies in the literature have challenged these findings and treatment recommendations, continuing the controversy regarding the upper airway and facial morphology.[43-45] Some otolaryngologists have even recommended partial resection of the inferior turbinates to assist with the management of aberrant dentofacial development in patients with enlarged adenoids, tonsils, or turbinate hypertrophy.[46]

SPECIAL CONSIDERATION:

Incompetent nasopharyngeal function is believed to be a significant factor in potentially altering growth and development of the orofacial structures.

Due to conflicting findings regarding upper airway obstruction and its association with poor dentofacial growth and development, it is incumbent upon the clinician to assess each patient individually to determine an appropriate treatment approach.

Trauma and familial patterns

Information relating to any history of trauma or jaw fractures is extremely important as these may significantly affect growth and development, creating asymmetries in the adolescent dentition or canting of the occlusal table. During the examination process, any traumatic episodes should be noted and further inquiry as to whether the injury was treated or allowed to heal spontaneously may be relevant. It is important to note that jaw or condylar fractures that have been treated poorly or left to heal spontaneously sometimes mimic some genetic birth defects, such as Romberg syndrome or hemifacial microsomia. If in doubt, a genetic screening evaluation may be appropriate to exclude any craniofacial implications.

An additional attributing factor that may predispose the patient to a developing malocclusion or skeletal discrepancy is racial background. Ethnicity has been shown to be a prevalent factor in occlusal trends. In 1965, the U.S. Public Health Service performed a classic epidemiologic study to examine malocclusion prevalence in children aged 6 to 11 years. Their findings revealed that 55% of the population in the United States demonstrated a class I occlusion, a class II prevalence of 35% existed, and the remaining 10% was attributed to class III occlusions.[48]

Significant differences also were demonstrated between the Caucasian and African-American populations. The African-American population demonstrated a 71% likelihood for a class I occlusion, as compared with 51% in the Caucasian group. Table 35–2 summarizes those findings.

Many investigators believe that skeletal development is regulated largely by genetic determinants and that the actual center of this control lies directly in the genes of the cells.[48] Consequently, we look like our parents. If our father has mandibular retrognathia or excessive maxillary protrusion, we cer-

tainly also may inherit these characteristics more or less prevalently. These inherited traits will then be susceptible to exaggeration or diminished expression through environmental physiologic factors.

Malocclusion and Articulation

Good articulation often is predicated upon ideal orofacial skeletal and dental anatomy. In patients with compromised orofacial structures, the ability to create normal sound production may be reduced or limited. The basic units of English speech that contribute to meaning are the 25 consonants, 14 vowels, and the prosodic elements such as melody, stress, and rhythm.[49] The lack of a specific articulation skill can be attributed to a dental malocclusion or dysmorphic jaw features. In severe malocclusions, it may be difficult or impossible to produce certain sounds. These dental abnormalities are often blamed for poor speech production, but it is important to note that some speech problems are related to neuromuscular disorders and not the dentition. Poor speech production also may be attributed to any dysmorphology in the soft-tissue anatomy of the speech organs such as that seen in macroglossia or lingual ankyloglossia.

SPECIAL CONSIDERATION:

Good articulation often is predicated upon ideal orofacial skeletal and dental anatomy. It may be necessary to correct an orthodontic problem before speech therapy can be successful.

Aberrant orofacial variations in dental and skeletal anatomy have been shown to affect the production of certain speech sounds. A lisp may be heard in the production of the sibilants /s/ and /z/ if an anterior openbite exists or if there are missing incisors. Distortion in production of the linguodental fricatives /th/, /sh/, and /ch/ can occur in a severe openbite or with missing incisors. Distortion of the labiodental fricatives /f/ and /v/ has been observed in patients with severe mandibular prognathic characteristics. These fricative consonants require very precise positioning of the organs used in speech and frequently may be produced incorrectly. Lastly, diffi-

TABLE 35–2: Prevalence of Malocclusion in Children (percent)

	Malocclusion		
	Class I	*Class II*	*Class III*
Caucasian	51.0	39.6	9.4
Black	72.0	13.6	14.4

U. S. Public Health Service Data for Children Aged 6 to 11 years (1965).

culty in the production of the linguoalveolar stops /t/ and /d/ may be related to incisor crowding.[50]

In many cases, it may be necessary to correct an orthodontic problem before speech therapy can be successful in treating the articulation disorder. It is important to note that some patients, through compensatory mechanisms and focused concentration, will be able to produce normal speech regardless of the severity of their malocclusion. Conversely, other patients possess ideal dental anatomic parameters to produce normal speech but cannot. Unfortunately, in the correction of the dental problem through the use of orthodontic appliances, most patients demonstrate further deterioration of their speech until they are able to acclimate to the appliance or until its removal.

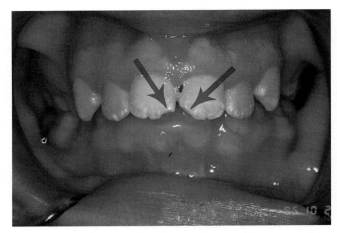

Figure 35–34: Fractured anterior maxillary central incisors due to excessive protrusion.

Timing of Treatment

Many clinical decisions are made based upon predicted growth patterns and the physiologic maturation of the patient. Psychosocial maturity also influences the timing of orthodontic intervention due to the fact that some patients simply lack the necessary social skills and age-appropriate behavior to tolerate a recommended procedure. Chronological age and dental maturation do not always coincide precisely as growth and development texts indicate. However, as a general rule, the 6-year molars are typically present or erupting by age 6 years, and the 12-year molars are anticipated by age 12 years. As discussed earlier, the physician will predict relatively consistent growth of the midface and lower face until the onset of puberty, then accelerated or a rapid growth spurt. In light of these facts, some patients may actually outgrow their clinical problem as they mature through adolescence, or conversely, be at risk for what appears to be initially a minor problem that becomes significantly more severe during the rapid growth years of pubescence. For this reason, a routine orthodontic initial evaluation often may be recommended as early as 7 years of age. Early diagnosis and treatment can guide erupting teeth into a more favorable position, preserve space for the permanent teeth, and reduce the likelihood of fracturing protruded front teeth (Fig. 35–34). Age 7 years is an ideal time for screening by an orthodontist because the posterior occlusion is established at about this time when the first molars erupt. Following the eruption of the first permanent molars, the orthodontist can evaluate the "anteroposterior and transverse" relationships of the occlusion, as well as any

functional shift. Shortly after the first permanent molars erupt, the presence of permanent incisors can be seen, and they often indicate arch length, possible crowding, habit patterns, and vertical dimension problems such as deepbite, openbite, or gummy smile. Most facial asymmetries are also likely to be apparent by age 7 years. If there is a lack of arch length (crowding) or a functional problem due to growth discrepancies, early treatment may be initiated to shorten overall treatment time, make treatment easier, and less expensive in some cases. It is important to remember that comprehensive treatment usually is not completed until all permanent teeth have completed their eruption. Consequently, the need for interceptive orthodontics must be determined on an individual basis. After a thorough diagnosis, it is determined if the benefits and opportunities significantly outweigh the time and effort involved in early treatment (Fig. 35–35). For some children, a delayed single-phase treatment still remains the best approach.

> ### Special Consideration:
>
> Early orthodontic diagnosis and treatment can guide erupting teeth into a more favorable position, preserve space for permanent teeth, and reduce the likelihood of fracturing protruded front teeth.

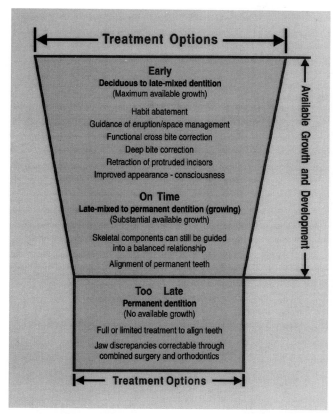

Figure 35–35: Treatment options. Courtesy O'Neil & Associates Orthodontic Marketing Resources™ 1997.[51]

Appliance Design

The armamentarium of orthodontic appliances available for use by the clinician continues to expand each year in conjunction with new advances in dental materials. As new products and appliances become more popular, what is thought of as traditional "braces" continues to evolve. Currently, there remain two basic categories of appliance design: "fixed" and "removable." *Fixed appliances* are typically tooth-supported and secured with a dental cement product or by a process known as bonding. The appliances are designed to remain firmly attached to the dentition throughout the course of treatment. *Removable appliances* are different in that they are both tooth and soft-tissue supported and, as the name implies, can be removed by the patient. The criteria for appliance selection is contingent upon many different factors. The age of the patient combined with the desired changes in dental, skeletal, and soft-tissue parameters generally dictates the appliance of choice for the treatment of a specific dental malocclusion. It is interesting to note that in societies with higher socioeconomic conditions, fixed appliance therapy tends to be more prevalent than removable treatment. This trend is not a reflection of any specific dental epidemiologic pattern, but rather attributed to the typically higher costs incurred by the patient for fixed therapy. In many instances, contrary to any socioeconomic influences, therapy including both fixed and removable appliances may be the treatment of choice indicated by the clinician.

Fixed appliances

When an adolescent proudly notes that he has just gotten braces, his enthusiasm may be in reference to an appliance as simple as a single tooth space maintainer or it may describe what is more traditionally thought of as braces, that is stainless steel brackets bonded to the permanent teeth. Braces, or more appropriately referred to as "fixed orthodontic appliances," are available in a variety of designs. Conventional orthodontic appliances (Fig. 35–36) have evolved over the years to include stainless steel brackets as well as translucent ceramic, gold-plated, lingual (on the back side of the teeth), plastic, and variations in plastic brackets (including an assortment of different colors). Traditionally, most patients and nonorthodontic clinicians equate orthodontic treatment with a combination of stainless steel brackets affixed to the labial surface of the permanent teeth in conjunction with an attached circumferential orthodontic archwire. The archwires vary in terms of different-sized diameters and shapes (rectangular or round), as well as in the actual type of metal or alloy comprising the wire. These archwires create varying tensions and pressures on the dentition, typically in force ranges of less than 150 gm. In conjuction with different wires, the use of assorted elastic chains and ties are utilized to alter the three-dimensional spatial relationships of individual teeth in the dentition. The combination of wires and elastics produces forces, interdentally causing tooth movement (Fig. 35–37). In today's changing world of orthodontics, materials have evolved from primarily stainless steel and plastics to high-tech nickel titanium alloys and ceramic composite materials. These new materials allow the expeditious movement of teeth in a cosmetic and improved esthetic format. Regardless of the newer cosmetic innovations and more expedient materials, the keys to successful treatment still lie in proper case diagnosis and the correct application of the selected orthodontic appliance.

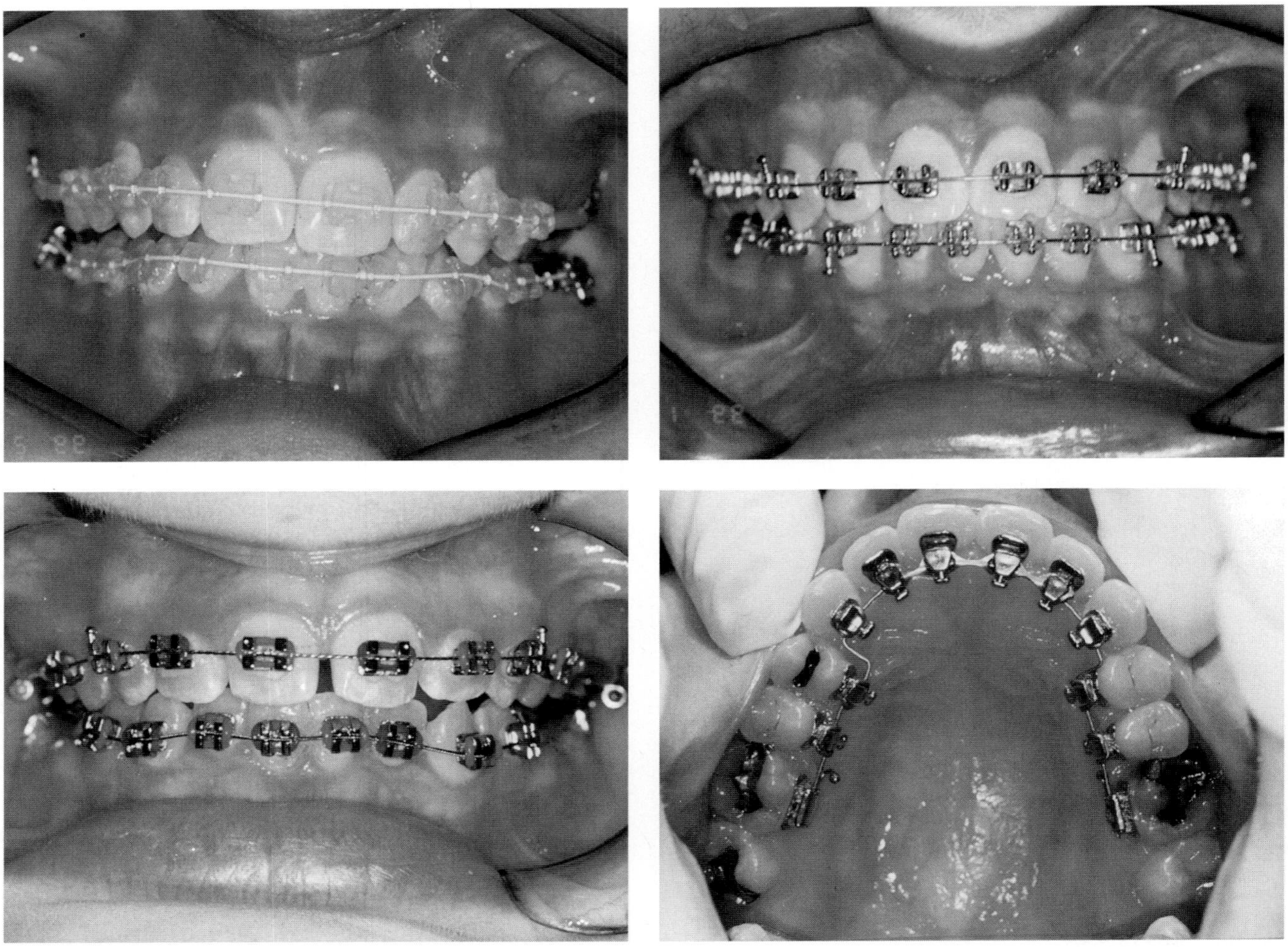

Figure 35–36:   Contemporary fixed appliances. (A) Ceramic. (B) Gold. (C) Stainless steel. (D) Lingual.

Removable appliances

Removable appliances are a group of orthodontic appliances that have many names. Historically, removable appliances are thought of as "headgears" and "retainers." Yet, many contemporary removable appliances are complicated devices designed to alter the dental skeletal anatomy in the young growing patient significantly. Removable appliances are frequently referred to clinically as "functional" or "orthopedic" appliances. Controversy continues to exist as to whether mandibular growth and midface development can be modified with functional appliance therapy. However, research continues to accumulate supporting evidence that environmental influences such as functional appliances can produce significant changes in craniofacial growth. Those changes include dental alveolar growth;[52-62] restriction of forward growth of the midface;[52,60,61,63] increased stimulation of mandibular growth;[60,63-78] redirection of condylar growth;[79-83] deflection of ramus anatomy;[73,76,78,82,84-88] changes in direction of mandibular growth;[76,77,89-96] changes in neuromuscular anatomy;[74,97-103] and adaptive changes in the glenoid fossa location.[60,64,82,103-107] This research also has demonstrated many of these anatomic and neuromuscular changes to be combined with their effects.

As the name implies, a removable appliance can be removed by the patient, and successful remova-

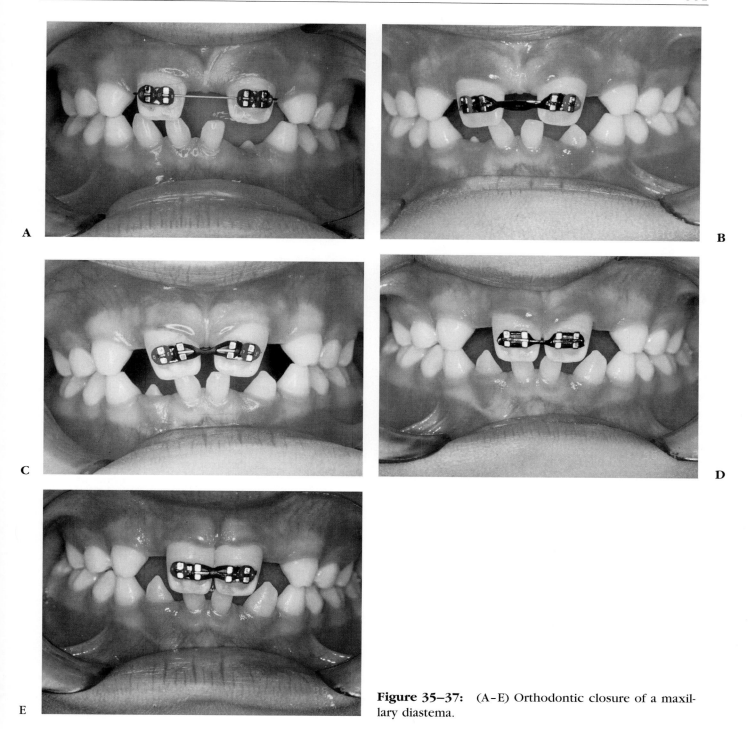

Figure 35–37:   (A–E) Orthodontic closure of a maxillary diastema.

ble appliance therapy is contingent upon good patient compliance. The more the appliance is worn by the patient, the more quickly improved changes in the malocclusion can be observed. Unfortunately, patient compliance varies. Some clinicians advocate nighttime wear of these appliances, whereas others recommend full-time wear. Historically, clinicians have recommended 24-hour-per-day compliance.

However, as the psychosocial elements of contemporary youth continue to evolve, so does the prescribed time for adequate optimal wear. Only a small percentage of today's preteen orthodontic population, as well as their parents, consider it socially acceptable to wear a headgear (Fig. 35–38) or functional appliance to school or out in public. For this reason, nighttime wear typically is advo-

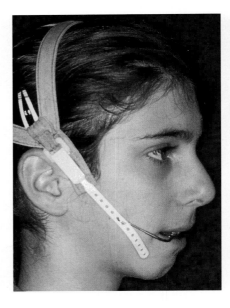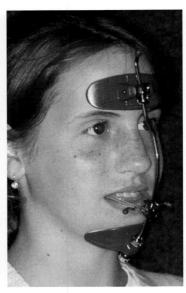

Figure 35–38: (A, B) Examples of occipital traction and protraction headgear types.

A,B

cated currently as sufficient. With this recommended prescribed wear schedule, the average length of treatment may vary from 12 to 18 months before the successful resolution of a problem can be observed. If more wear is indicated throughout the day, it requires appliance designs that do not unduly affect the patient's facial appearance or speech. Unfortunately, it is often the bulky and cumbersome appliances that have greater effectiveness in influencing dental facial growth.

Many functional appliances were introduced into North American orthodontics in the mid-1950s and have had periods of popularity and decline due to psychosocial trends in unfavorable patient response. There remains a myriad of removable appliances available for the clinician to choose from, and hybrids of current appliances continue to be developed. Entire texts have been written on appliance design, selection and application. Yet, what may be more critical to the overall success in treatment is often patient selection. Without patient compliance, a removable appliance exerts no environmental influences on orofacial development.

REFERENCES

1. Illingworth RS. Teething. Dev Med Child Neurol 1969; 11:376–377.
2. Tasanen A. General and local effects of the eruption of deciduous teeth. Ann Paedrit Fenn 1968; 14(supplement 29):1–40.
3. Moyers RE. *Handbook of Orthodontics, 4th ed.* Development of the dentition and the occlusion. St. Louis: Mosby, 1988, pp. 117.
4. Bowen WH. Dental caries: Is it an extinct disease? JADA 1991; 122(9):49–52.
5. McDonald RE, Avery DR, Storkey GK: Dental caries in the child and adolescent. In: McDonald RE, Avery DR, eds. *Dentistry for the Child and Adolescent, 6th ed.* St. Louis: Mosby, 1994, pp. 219.
6. Andreasen JO, Andreasen FM. *Essentials of Traumatic Injuries of the Teeth.* Copenhagen: Munkgaard, 1990, pp. 148.
7. Andreasen JO, Hjorting-Hansen E. Replantation of teeth. I. Radiographic and clinical study of 110 human teeth replanted after accidental loss. Acta Odontol Scand 1966; 24:263–286.
8. Infant Oral Health Care. American Academy of Pediatric Dentistry 1997–1998; 19.
9. Green M. Bright futures. Guidelines for health supervision of infants, children, and adolescents. National Center for Education in Maternal and Child Health, Arlington, 1994.
10. Fluoride. American Academy of Pediatric Dentistry 1997–1998; 19.
11. Proffit WR. Equilibrium theory revisited: Factors influencing position of the teeth. Angle Orthod 1978; 48:175–186.
12. Lowe AA. Correlations between orofacial muscle activity and craniofacial morphology in a sample of control and anterior openbite subjects. Am J Orthod 1980; 78:89–97.
13. Cheng MC, Enlow DH, Papsidero M, et al. Developmental effect of impaired breathing in the face of the growing child. Angle Orthod 1988; 53:309–320.

14. Harvold EP, Tomer BS, Vargervik K, et al. Primate experiment on oral respiration. Am J Orthod 1981; 79:359–372.

15. Solow B, Siersbaek-Nielson S, Greve E. Airway adequacy, head posture, and craniofacial morphology. Am J Orthod 1984; 86:214–223.

16. Woodside DG, Linder-Aronson S, Lundstrom A, et al. Mandibular and maxillary growth after changed mode of breathing. Am J Orthod Dentofac Orthop 1991; 100:1–18.

17. Linder-Aronson A, Woodside DG, Hellsing E, et al. Normalization of incisor position after adenoidectomy. Am J Orthod Dentofac Orthod 1993; 103:412–427.

18. Enlow DH. Introduction. *Handbook of Facial Growth.* Philadelphia: Saunders, 1975, p 6.

19. Proffit WR, Fields HW, Ackerman JL, et al. Concepts of growth and development. In: Reinhardt RW, ed. *Contemporary Orthodontics. 2nd ed.* St. Louis: Mosby, 1993, pp. 33–34.

20. Angle EH. Classification of malocclusion. D. Cosmos 1899; 41:248–264.

21. Moyers RE. Classification and terminology of malocclusion. In: *Handbook of Orthodontics for the Student and General Practitioner, 3rd ed.* Chicago: Year Book Medical, 1980, pp. 304–310.

22. Gardner BJ. Thinkers in ancient Greece. In: *History of Biology, 3rd ed.* Minneapolis: Burgess, 1972, pp. 36–40.

23. Proffit WR, Fields HW, Ackerman JL, et al. Malocclusion and dentofacial deformity in contemporary society. In: Cot L, ed. Reinhardt RW, ed. *Contemporary Orthodontics, 2nd ed.* St. Louis: Mosby, 1993, pp. 2–3.

24. Graber TM. Development of a concept. In: *Orthodontics: Principles and Practice, 3rd ed.* Philadelphia: Saunders, 1972, pp. 1–3.

25. Jacobson A. A retrognathic cephalometric technique. In: *Radiographic Cephalometry.* Carol Stream: Quintessence Publishing, 1995, pp. 39–40.

26. Proffit WR. Equilibrium theory revisited: Factors influencing position of the teeth. Angle Orthod 1978; 48:175–186.

27. Lowe AA. Correlations between orofacial muscle activity and craniofacial morphology in a sample of control and anterior openbite subjects. Am J Orthod 1980; 78:89–97.

28. Cheng MC, Enlow DH, Papsidero M, et al. Developmental effect of impaired breathing in the face of the growing child. Angle Orthod 1988; 64:419–424.

29. McNamara JA Jr. Influence of respiratory pattern on craniofacial growth. Angle Orthod 1981; 51:269–299.

30. Gross AM, Kellum GD, Franz D, et al. A longitudinal evaluation of open mouth posture and maxillary arch width in children. Angle Orthod 1994; 64:419–424.

31. Harvold EP, Tomer BS, Vargervik K, et al. Primate experiment on oral respiration. Am J Orthod 1981; 79:359–372.

32. Solow B, Siersbaek-Nielsen S, Greve E. Airway adequacy, head posture, and craniofacial morphology. Am J Orthod 1984; 86:214–213.

33. Woodside DO, Linder-Aronson S, Lundstrom A, et al. Mandibular and maxillary growth after changed mode of breathing. Am J Orthod Dentofac Orthop 1991; 100:1–18.

34. Linder-Aronson A, Woodside DG, Hellsing E, et al. Normalization of incisor position after adenoidectomy. Am J Orthod Dentofac Orthop 1993; 103:412–427.

35. Tully WJ. Abnormal functions of the mouth in relation to the occlusion of the teeth. In: Walther RP, ed. *Current Orthodontics.* Baltimore: Williams and Wilkins, 1966, pp. 1–23.

36. Linder-Aronson S. Adenoids: Their effect on mode of breathing and nasal airflow and their relationship to characteristics of the facial skeleton and the dentition. Acta Otolaryngol 1970; 265:1–132.

37. Linder-Aronson S, Aschan G. Nasal resistance to breathing and palatal height before and after expansion of the median palatine suture. Orthod Rev 1963; 14:254–270.

38. Joshi MR. A study of dental occlusion in nasal and oronasal breathers in Maharashtrian children. J All-India Dent Assoc 1964; 36:219–239.

39. Moffatt JB. Habits and their relation to malocclusion. Aust Dent J 1963; 8:142–149.

40. Harvold EP, Vargervik K, Chierici G. Primate experiments on oral sensation and dental malocclusions. Am J Orthod 1973; 63:494–508.

41. Behlfelt K, Linder-Aronson S. Craniofacial morphology in children with and without enlarged tonsils. Eur J Orthod 1990; 12:233–243.

42. Linder-Aronson, Woodside DG. Mandibular growth direction following adenoidectomy. Am J Orthod 1986; 89:273–284.

43. Kluemper GT, Vig PS. Nasorespiratory characteristics and craniofacial morphology. Eur J Orthod 1995; 17:491–495.

44. Watson RM, Warren DW, Fischer ND. Nasal resistance, skeletal classification and mouthbreathing in orthodontic patients. Am J Orthod 1968; 54:367–379.

45. Hershey HG, Stewart BL, Warren DW. Changes in nasal airway resistance associated with rapid maxillary expansion. Am J Orthod 1976; 69:274–284.

46. Meredith GM. The airway and dentofacial development. Ear Nose Throat J 1987; 66:190–195.

47. McLain JB, Proffit WR. Oral health status in the United States: Prevalence of malocclusion. J Dent Ed 1985; 49:386–396.
48. Enlow DH. Control processes in facial growth. In: Handbook of Facial Growth. Philadelphia: W.B. Saunders, Philadelphia, 1975, pp. 236–237.
49. Moyers RE. Analysis of the dentition and occlusion. In: Marshall DK, ed. Handbook of Orthodontics, 4th ed. Chicago: Year Book Medical Publishers, 1988, pp. 215–216.
50. Proffit WR, Fields HW, Ackerman JL, et al. The orthodontic problem. In: Reinhardt RW, ed. Contemporary Orthodontics, 2nd ed. St. Louis: Mosby, 1993, pp. 12–13.
51. O'Neil & Associates, Orthodontic Marketing Resources.™ 110 William Way, PO Box 2878. Williamsburg, VA, 23187, 1997.
52. Harvold EP, Vargervik K. Morphogenetic response to activator treatment. Am J Orthod 1971; 60:478–490.
53. Harvold EP. Bone remodeling and orthodontics. Eur J Orthod 1985; 7:217–230.
54. Thurow RC. Edgewise Orthodontics. St. Louis: Mosby, 1966, pp. 82–106.
55. Woodside DG. The activator. In: Graber TM, Neumann B, eds. Removable Orthodontic Appliances. Philadelphia: Saunders, 1977, pp. 269–336.
56. Wambera IC. A study of the incisal apices line inclination in various malocclusions (thesis). Toronto: Department of Orthodontics, University of Toronto, 1972.
57. Teuscher U. Direction of force application for class II, division 1 treatment with the activator-headgear combination. Studieweek, 1980, pp. 193–203.
58. Bjork A. The principle of the Andresen method of orthodontic treatment: A discussion based on cephalometric x-ray analysis of treated cases. Am J Orthod 1951; 37:437–458.
59. Trayfoot J, Richardson A. Angle Class II, division 1 malocclusion treated by the Andresen method: An analysis of 17 cases. Br Dent J 1968; 124:516–519.
60. Vargervik K, Harvold EP. Response to activator treatment in Class II malocclusions. Am J Orthod 1985; 88:242–251.
61. Pancherz H. The mechanism of Class II correction in Herbst appliance treatment. A cephalometric investigation. Am J Orthod 1982; 82:68–74.
62. Samas KV, Pancherz H, Rune B, et al. Hemifacial microsomia treated with the Herbst appliance: Report of a case analyzed by means of roentgen stereometry and metallic implants. Am J Orthod 1982; 82:68–74.
63. Woodside DG, Reed R, Doucet JD, et al. Some effects of activator treatment on the growth rate of the mandible and position of the midface. In: Cook

JT, ed. Transactions of the Third International Orthodontic Congress. St. Louis: Mosby, 1973, pp. 459–480.
64. Breitner C. Bone changes resulting from experimental orthodontic treatment. Am J Orthod Oral Surgery 1940; 26:521–547.
65. Baume LJ, Derichweiler H. Is the condylar growth center response to orthodontic therapy? An experimental study in Macaca mulatta. Oral Surg Oral Med Oral Pathol 1961; 14:347–362.
66. Charlier JP, Petrovic A, Herrmann-Stutzmann J. Effects of mandibular hyperpropulsion on the prechondroblastic zone of young rat condyle. Am J Orthod 1969; 55:71–74.
67. Stockli PW, Willert HG. Tissue reactions in the temporomandibular joint resulting from anterior displacement of the mandible in the monkey. Am J Orthod 1971; 60:142–155.
68. Elgoyhen JC, Moyers RE, McNamara JA, et al. Craniofacial adaptation to protrusive function in young rhesus monkeys. Am J Orthod 1972; 62:469–480.
69. McNamara JA. Functional adaptations in the temporomandibular joint. Dent Clin North Am 1975; 19:457–471.
70. McNamara JA. Functional determinants of craniofacial size and shape. Eur J Orthod 1980; 2:131–159.
71. McNamara JA, Carlson DS. Quantitative analysis of temporomandibular joint adaptations to protrusive function. Am J Orthod 1979; 76:593–611.
72. Hinton RJ, McNamara JA. Temporal bone adaptations in response to protrusive function in juvenile and young adult rhesus monkeys (Macaca mulatta). Eur J Orthod 1984; 6:155–174.
73. Joho JP. Changes in form and size of the mandible in the orthopaedically treated Macaca irus (an experimental study). Eur Orthod Soc Rep Congr 1968; 44:161–173.
74. Petrovic AG, Stutzmann JJ, Oudet CL. Control processes in the postnasal growth of the condylar cartilage of the mandible. In: McNamara JA, ed.: Determinants of Mandibular Form and Growth. Monograph 4, Craniofacial Growth Series. Ann Arbor: Center for Human Growth and Development, University of Michigan, 1975, pp. 101–153.
75. Pancherz H. Treatment of Class II malocclusions by jumping the bite with the Herbst appliance: A cephalometric investigation. Am J Orthod 1979; 76:423–442.
76. Altuna G. The effect of excess occlusal force on the eruption of the buccal segments and maxillary and mandibular growth direction in the Macaca monkey (thesis). Toronto: Department of Orthodontics, University of Toronto, 1979.
77. Altuna G, Woodside DG. Die Auswirkung von Ausbissblocken in Oberkiefer bei Macaca rhesus (Vor-

laufige Ergebnisse). Fortschr Kieferorthop 1977; 39:391–402.

78. Woodside DG, Altuna G, Harvold E, et al. Primate experiments in malocclusion and bone induction. Am J Orthod 1983; 83:460–468.

79. Hutchinson LG. Herbst appliance therapy in adolescent children: Stability of skeletal and dental adaptation (thesis). Toronto: Department of Orthodontics, University of Toronto, 1982.

80. Bjork A. Variations in the growth pattern of the human mandible: Longitudinal radiographic study by the implant method. J Dent Res 1963; 42:400–411.

81. Williams S, Melson B. Condylar development and mandibular rotation and displacement during activator treatment: An implant study. Am J Orthod 1982; 81:322–326.

82. Birkebaek L, Melsen B, Terp S. Alaminagraphic study of the alterations in the temporomandibular joint following activator treatment. Eur J Orthod 1984; 6:267–276.

83. Petrovic A. Control of postnasal growth of secondary cartilages of the mandible by mechanisms regulating occlusion: Cybernetic model. Trans Eur Orthod Soc 1974; 50:69–75.

84. Janzen EK, Bluher JA. The cephalometric, anatomic, and histologic changes in the Macaca mulatta after application of a continuous-acting retraction force on the mandible. Am J Orthod 1965; 51:823–855.

85. Joho JP. The effects of extraoral low-pull traction to the mandibular dentition of Macaca mulatta. Am J Orthod 1973; 64:555–577.

86. Harvold EP: Experiments on mandibular morphogenesis. In: McNamara JA, ed: *Determinants of Mandibular Form and Growth. Monograph 4, Craniofacial Growth Series.* Ann Arbor: Center for Human Growth and Development, University of Michigan, 1975, pp. 155–178.

87. Tomer BS, Harvold EP. Primate experiments on mandibular growth direction. Am J Orthod 1982; 82:114–119.

88. Harvold EP. Environmental influence on mandibular morphogenesis (abstract). Am J Orthod 1960; 46:144–145.

89. Lundstrom A, Woodside DG. A comparison of various facial and occlusal characteristics in mature individuals with vertical and horizontal growth direction expressed at the chin. Eur J Orthod 1981; 3:227–235.

90. Lundstrom A, Woodside DG. Longitudinal changes in facial type in cases with vertical and horizontal mandibular growth directions. Eur J Orthod 1983; 5:250–268.

91. Woodside DG, Linder-Aronson S. The channeliza-

tion of upper and lower anterior face heights compared to the population standard in males between ages 6 and 20 years. Eur J Orthod 1979; 1:25–40.

92. Woodside DG, Linder-Aronson S. Progressive increase in lower anterior face height and the use of posterior occlusal bite block in its management. In: Graber TM, ed. *Orthodontics: State of the Art, Essence of the Science.* St. Louis: Mosby, 1986, pp. 200–221.

93. Linder-Aronson S, Woodside DG, Lundstrom A. Mandibular growth direction following adenoidectomy. Am J Orthod 1986; 89:273–284.

94. Pearson LE. Vertical control through use of mandibular posterior intrusive forces. Angle Orthod 1973; 43:194–200.

95. Pearson LE. Vertical control in treatment of patients having backward rotational growth tendencies. Angle Orthod 1978; 48:132–140.

96. Frankel R, Frankel C. A functional approach to treatment of skeletal open bite. Am J Orthod 1983; 84:54–68.

97. McNamara JA. Neuromuscular and skeletal adaptations to altered function in the orofacial region. Am J Orthod 1973; 64:578–606.

98. Petrovic A, Stutzmann JJ. Further investigations into the functioning of the peripheral "comparator" of the servosystem (respective positions of the upper and lower dental arches) in the control of the condylar cartilage growth rate and of the lengthening of the jaw. In: McNamara JA, ed. *The Biology of Occlusal Development. Monograph 7, Craniofacial Growth Series.* Ann Arbor: Center for Human Growth and Development, University of Michigan, 1977, pp. 255–291.

99. Oudet C, Petrovic AG. Variations in the number of sacromeres in series in the lateral pterygoid muscle as a function of the longitudinal deviation of the mandibular position produced by the postural hyperpropulsor. In: Carlson DS, McNamara JA, eds. *Muscle Adaptation in the Craniofacial Region. Monograph 8, Craniofacial Growth Series.* Ann Arbor: Center for Human Growth and Development, University of Michigan, 1978, pp. 233–246.

100. Petrovic A, Stutzmann J, Oudet C. Orthopaedic appliances modulate the bone formation in the mandible as a whole. Swed Dent J Suppl 1982; 15:197–201.

101. Whetten LL, Johnston LE. The control of condylar growth: An experimental evaluation of the role of the lateral pterygoid muscle. Am J Orthod 1985; 88:181–90.

102. Sessle BJ, Woodside DG, Bourque P, et al. Effect of functional appliances on jaw muscle activity. Am J Orthod Dentofac Orthop 1990; 98:222–230.

103. Dahan J, Dombrowsky KJ, Oehler K. Static and dy-

namic morphology of the temporomandibular joint before and after functional treatment with the activator. Trans Eur Orthod Soc 1969; 45:255–274.

104. Woodside DG, Metaxas A, Altuna G. The influence of functional appliance therapy on glenoid fossa remodeling. Am J Orthod Dentofac Orthop 1987; 92: 181–198.

105. Voudouris JC. Glenoid fossa and condylar remodeling following progressive mandibular protrusion in the juvenile Macaca fascicularis (thesis). Toronto: Department of Orthodontics, Faculty of Dentistry, University of Toronto, 1988.

106. Agelopoulos GG. Long-term stability of temporomandibular joint remodeling following continuous mandibular advancement in the juvenile Macaca fascicularis: A histomorphometric, cephalometric, and electromyographic investigation (thesis). Toronto: Department of Orthodontics, Faculty of Dentistry, University of Toronto, 1991.

107. Yamin LC. Effects of functional appliances on the temporomandibular joint and masticatory muscles in Macaca fascicularis (thesis). Toronto: Department of Orthodontics, Faculty of Dentistry, University of Toronto, 1991.

Acquired Diseases of the Oral Cavity and Pharynx

Alma J. Smitheringale

A sore throat is one of the most common complaints evaluated in a pediatrician's office. There are many causative organisms—from localized viral, bacterial, or fungal infections to numerous systemic diseases, the signs and symptoms of which may involve the oral mucosa. This chapter describes common infections of the mouth and pharynx and includes oral manifestations of systemic disease.

VIRAL INFECTIONS

Table 36–1 lists the possible viral etiologies of acquired oropharyngitis.

Rhinovirus

The common cold virus is ubiquitous and is the most frequent cause of pharyngitis. This is accompanied by coryza symptoms of rhinorrhea, cough, and sneezing, but there is usually only minimal fever and lymphadenopathy compared to bacterial pharyngitis, in which the fever and lymphadenopathy are more pronounced and there is no associated rhinosinusitis nor cough.[1] Other respiratory viruses that are implicated as pathogens for pharyngitis include adenovirus, coronavirus, and some influenza viruses.[2]

Coxsackievirus

In young children, the coxsackievirus group A type 16 is the cause of *hand-foot-and-mouth disease,* which presents with fever, sore throat, and erythematous tongue, lips, and pharynx. These symp-

toms are followed 24 to 48 hours later by the appearance of vesiculopapular lesions on the palms of the hands and soles of the feet.[3] This viral process typically resolves within 7 days.

Herpangina

Herpangina also is thought to be caused by coxsackievirus groups A and B types 1 to 5 and some human enteric ECHO viruses.[4] *Herpangina* presents with flu-like symptoms, malaise, and severe throat pain. The mucosa of the soft palate, tonsils, and oral pharynx becomes erythematous. Many small clear vesicles appear and rupture to become shallow ulcers, eventually resolving in a few days.

Herpes Simplex Virus

There are two forms of herpes simplex virus (HSV) infection: a primary severe infection and a secondary recurrent infection with less morbidity. *HSV-1* affects the oral mucosa, and *HSV-2* infects the genitalia primarily.

> ### SPECIAL CONSIDERATION:
> The two forms of herpes simplex pharyngeal infection are a primary severe infection and a secondary recurrent infection with less morbidity.

Primary herpetic gingivostomatitis

Primary herpetic infection classically presents in children < 5 years. The lips, gingiva, tongue, and palate develop edema and erythema and a sharp prickling sensation. Vesicles develop and then rup-

Pediatric Otolaryngology, Edited by R.F. Wetmore, H.R. Muntz, and T.J. McGill. Thieme Medical Publishers, Inc., New York © 2000.

TABLE 36–1:   Viral Etiology of Acquired
Oropharyngitis

Rhinovirus
Coxsackievirus
Herpangina
Herpes simplex
Herpes zoster
Aphthous stomatitis
Papilloma
Infectious mononucleosis

ture into ulcers producing a desquamating grey pseudomembrane (Fig. 36–1).

These ulcers may coalesce, crust, or become secondarily infected by local bacteria. There may be associated lymphadenitis, fever, and flu-like symptoms,[5] and rarely there can be progression to disseminated herpes, skin eruptions, or meningoencephalitis. Biopsy of a vesicle shows typical intranuclear inclusion bodies. Acyclovir gives relief when applied topically or parenterally in severe systemic infections.

Secondary herpetic infection

Recurrent HSV infections erupt during episodes of fever, stress, excessive sun exposure, or any immunodeficiency state. Between exacerbations the virus remains dormant in regional neuroganglia. Herpetic eruptions are heralded by a typical tingling or burning sensation that is followed by erythema and vesicle formation. The vesicles rupture after the first day

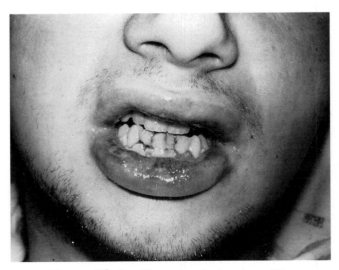

Figure 36–1:   Herpetic gingivostomatitis.

and develop into superficial ulcerations that heal spontaneously after 10 days. These lesions eventually recur in the same sites on the vermilion border of the lips as cold sores or on the oral mucosa. In infants they also may be found on the nasal vestibule and facial skin. Secondary bacterial infection with *Staphylococcus aureus* requires treatment with topical antibiotic creams.

Herpes Zoster

Shingles or *herpes zoster* presents with skin or mucosal vesicles along the distribution of the trigeminal nerve and may involve the lips and oral mucosa. The varicella (i.e., chickenpox) virus is thought to lie dormant in the sensory ganglia and erupt in an immunocompromised or stressed child. Overt chickenpox systemic infections also may involve the oral mucosa with typical vesicles that appear in crops that crust and then resolve within 10 days.

Aphthous Stomatitis

Shallow, painful aphthous ulcers may occur singly or in clusters on the oral mucosa of the tongue, soft palate, or buccal mucosa and are often recurrent. Some physicians attribute these lesions to a respiratory virus,[6] whereas it is commonly held they are either an autoimmune or a delayed hypersensitivity reaction.[7] Aphthous stomatitis is most common in teenagers and has a female preponderance. There is no vesicle formation prior to the development of ulcerations. The ulcers have a pink, raised border with a whitish center and often coalesce. They resolve in 10 to 14 days without treatment; however, in painful cases it may be helpful to apply topical anesthetic or mouthwashes and use either systemic steroids or topical steroids.[7]

Papilloma

The *human papilloma virus* (HPV) serotypes 6, 14, and 22 can infect the respiratory mucosa of the upper aerodigestive tract (UADT). Although papillomas cause the greatest morbidity in the larynx, squamous papilloma also may occur on the soft palate (Fig. 36–2), uvula, and the anterior and posterior tonsillar pillars. They produce minimal discomfort, but they should be excised with laser or cautery to avoid the risk of distal seeding into the larynx or trachea.

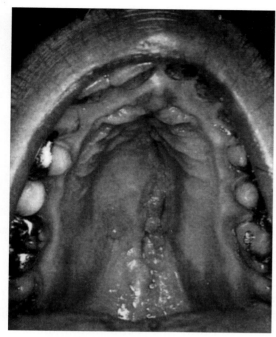

Figure 36–2: Papillomas of the palate.

roids and rarely airway management with either a nasal airway or endotracheal intubation. Generalized lymphadenopathy that may be very marked in both the anterior and posterior cervical chains and accompanying hepatosplenomegaly often suggest the diagnosis. Because of the possibility of splenic rupture, it is important to instruct the patient to avoid gymnastics or contact sports for several weeks. Occasionally, jaundice and hepatitis occur, and rarely a viral myocarditis may develop.

> ### SPECIAL CONSIDERATION:
> Rarely in cases of infectious mononucleosis, there may be airway compromise that may require airway management with either steroids or an artificial airway.

Infectious Mononucleosis

This infection is caused by the Epstein-Barr virus (EBV), and although it is most common in teenagers and college students, it also can affect young children. The tonsils become grossly hypertrophic and erythematous with a grey membrane that can be scraped off without bleeding (Fig. 36–3). Airway compromise is a possible morbidity, especially in younger children, and requires treatment with ste-

Low-grade fever, fatigue, and malaise may continue for months. Treatment includes rest, mouthwashes, good hydration, and use of corticosteroids for severe cases. Secondary bacterial infections or oral ulcerations can occur in the tonsils, and antibiotic therapy may be necessary.[8] Ampicillin, however, should not be prescribed because it may lead to a greater incidence of a cutaneous papular rash. The tonsils may remain grossly hypertrophied following a bout of infectious mononucleosis, and the

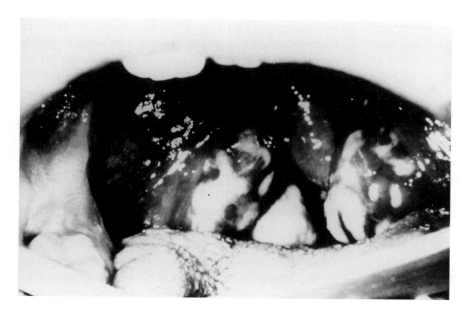

Figure 36–3: Exudative tonsillitis due to infectious mononucleosis.

TABLE 36–2:   Etiology of Acquired Oropharyngitis

Vincent's infection
    Borrelia vincentii and aerobic bacillus
Ludwig's cellulitis
    anaerobic fusobacterium and spirochete
Beta-hemolytic streptococci
Hemophilus influenzae
Neisseria gonorrhoeae
Corynebacterium diphtheriae

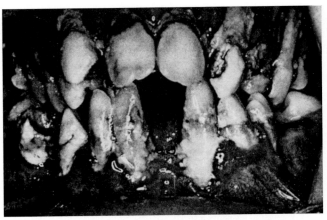

Figure 36–4:   Vincent's acute necrotizing ulcerative gingivitis.

resultant thick "hot potato voice" or sleep apnea may necessitate a tonsillectomy.[9]

SPECIAL CONSIDERATION:

In cases of infectious mononucleosis, ampicillin should not be prescribed because it leads to an increased incidence of rash.

The diagnosis of infectious mononucleosis is suggested by a positive heterophile antibody agglutination test but is confirmed by positive titers to the EBV. The blood smear typically displays many atypical lymphocytes. Infection with cytomegalovirus (CMV) may mimic EBV but is usually less severe clinically.

BACTERIAL INFECTIONS

Table 36-2 lists the possible bacterial etiologies of acquired oropharyngitis.

Gingivitis

Gingivitis with tender swelling and bleeding of the gingivae is caused by oral bacteria especially if the patient has poor oral hygiene, wears orthodontic appliances, or is immunosuppressed. It may be seen in older adolescents, especially children with Down syndrome,[10] and in chronic mouth breathers. Gingival hypertrophy is also a complication of Dilantin® therapy.

Vincent's infection or acute necrotizing ulcerative gingivitis (ANUG) is caused by an anaerobic

Borrelia vincentii spirochete and an aerobic fusiform bacillus. The interproximal gingival papillae necrotize to produce a pseudomembrane with exposure of the dental roots and loosening of the teeth (Fig. 36-4). The gingivae become very painful and hemorrhagic, and the patient presents with severe halitosis, fetid breath, malaise, and high fever. Treatment includes penicillin, local debridement of necrotic gingivae, hydrogen peroxide mouthwashes, and adequate rehydration. Rarely, lesions may spread to the soft palate and oropharynx, causing extreme odynophagia, which is a condition referred to as *Vincent's angina*.

Ludwig's Cellulitis

Sublingual space infections may extend through the mylohyoid muscle into the submandibular space, involving the entire anterior neck and the floor of the mouth and elevating the base of tongue posteriorly to the point of upper airway obstruction (UAO).[11] This type of infection is caused by gingival bacteria (i.e., anaerobic streptococci, bacteroides species, fusobacteria, and spirochetes) along with poor oral hygiene, and is often precipitated by dental extractions, especially lower molars in teenagers. It was first described by Ludwig in 1836[11] as a rapidly-progressive cellulitis that was "woody" on palpation and associated with an inability to depress the tongue. There is overlying skin erythema, pitting edema, tenderness, trismus, and high fever. Drainage of the affected region yields a brown serous fluid, not frank pus. Because elevation of the floor of the mouth with this infection may affect exposure of the larynx and impede routine intubation, fiberoptic intubation may be necessary to establish an airway. In severe cases, a tracheotomy may even be required. If inadequately treated, Ludwig's cellulitis may progress and extend into the mediastinum. Antibiotic therapy should include coverage of anaerobes including either intravenous penicillin and metronidazole or clindamycin in conjunction with surgical drainage.

> ## SPECIAL CONSIDERATION:
> If inadequately treated, Ludwig's cellulitis may progress and extend into the mediastinum.

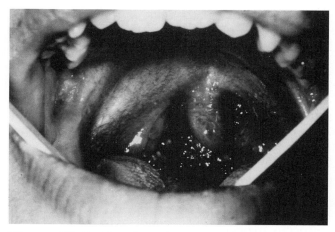

Figure 36–5: Beta-hemolytic streptococcal pharyngitis.

Anaerobic Bacterial Infections

Beta-lactamase producing bacteroides species following penicillin therapy have been implicated in the development of *tonsillitis* that may progress to frank peritonsillar abscess formation.[12,13] Foul-smelling pus is drained, and the recommended antibiotic therapy includes either clindamycin or Augmentin®.[14]

Streptococcal Pharyngotonsillitis

Pharyngotonsillitis is caused most commonly by respiratory viruses with distinguishing coryza features of rhinosinusitis, sneezing, cough, and occasional conjunctivitis. In 15 to 30% of cases, symptoms of sore throat, fever, and lymphadenopathy are more severe and are attributed to bacterial infection. The most common isolate is group A beta-hemolytic *Streptococcus pyogenes* (GABHS), which may occur in infants and children of all ages regardless of socioeconomic status (Fig. 36–5).[15,16] Systemic complications of streptococcal infection include scarlet fever, rheumatic fever, septic arthritis, and glomerulonephritis.

Scarlet fever presents as a generalized, nonpruritic, erythematous, macular skin rash that is worse on the extremities. The associated "strawberry tongue" is bright red and tender due to superficial desquamation of the papillae. Typically, the rash lasts 4 to 7 days and is accompanied by fever and arthralgias.

Rheumatic fever is rare today with only sporadic outbreaks;[17] however in the 1940s and 1950s, it was a complication that was seen in 3% of streptococcal pharyngitis infections.[18] Bacterial vegetations affect the mitral and tricuspid heart valves leading to murmurs, persisting relapsing fevers, and valvular stenosis or incompetence.

Septic arthritis with painful, hot, joint effusions is a known complication of streptococcal pharyngitis. The bacteria can be isolated by needle aspiration of the effusion. Treatment with parenteral antibiotics for at least 6 weeks is necessary to avoid osteitis, arthrodesis, and long-term morbidity from restricted range of movement.

Acute poststreptococcal glomerulonephritis (AGN) can result in 10 to 15% of those streptococcal pharyngeal infections caused by the type 12 serotype.[19]

> ### AT A GLANCE . . .
> Systemic Complications of Streptococcal Infection
> - Scarlet fever
> - Rheumatic fever
> - Septic arthritis
> - Glomerulonephritis

Etiology

Cultures from the surface of the tonsils may not always be representative of the bacteria in the core of the tonsils.[20,21] Core sampling has implicated other bacteria as pathogens of tonsillitis, notably *Streptococcus pneumoniae, Hemophilus influenzae,* and *Staphylococcus aureus.*[22] Bacteroides is the most common anaerobe isolated from tonsil tissue,[23] but it is unclear whether this has any pathogenic role in clinical pharyngitis. *Neisseria gonorrhoeae* and chlamydia also may colonize the oropharyngeal mucosa causing erythema and sore throat.

Brodsky et al. reported that the dominant core bacteria in hypertrophic tonsils was *Hemophilus influenzae* in cases where surgery was performed for obstructive symptoms.[24] On the other hand, *Streptococcus pyogenes* was found as the predominant organism in the core of tonsils excised for chronic tonsillitis.[24] Of note, an increased microbial load correlates with increased numbers of T-cells and B-cells in diseased tonsils.[25]

Therapy

In all cases of suspected bacterial tonsillitis, a throat swab should be performed for culture and sensitivity. Rapid antigen detection tests (rapid strep) may be helpful in guiding therapy until the results of the culture are known. Depending on the community, as many as 20 to 30% of all streptococcal infections in children are now beta-lactamase producing, and hence penicillin resistant.[26] In these cases, therapy with a second line antibiotic is indicated.[27] All of the *Moraxella catarrhalis* is now beta-lactamase producing, and the penicillin resistance of *Hemophilus influenzae* has risen from 7 to 40% in the past 15 years. Strains of *Streptococcus pneumoniae* that are resistant to multiple antibiotics are emerging also. When severe pharyngeal infections are not responding to penicillin, it is advisable to switch to clindamycin, vancomycin, or rifampin because there has been no demonstrable resistance to date.

> ### SPECIAL CONSIDERATION:
> In all cases of suspected bacterial tonsillitis, a throat swab should be performed for culture and sensitivity. Rapid antigen detection tests (rapid strep) may be helpful in guiding therapy until the culture results are known.

Where there have been six or more episodes of culture-proven streptococcal pharyngitis in 1 year,

it is accepted practice to recommend a tonsillectomy; however, surgical management of the asymptomatic streptococcal carrier remains a controversial issue. An estimated 15 to 20% of all school children are carriers of streptococcus in their saliva or nasal secretions, depending on their location and the season, even after adequate antibiotic therapy. These carriers may harbor infection that may then be spread to other family or school members. In some children, it may be difficult to determine whether the carrier state or an active infection exists. For this reason, it still may be reasonable to recommend a tonsillectomy even in cases in which the carrier has minimal clinical morbidity.[28] Practice Pathway 36-1 outlines the diagnosis and management of oropharyngitis.

Complications

Streptococcal tonsillitis can produce localized and disseminated suppurative complications. Peritonsillar cellulitis can progress to peritonsillar abscess (i.e., *quinsy*) (Fig. 36-6), which is characterized by drooling, trismus, "hot potato" voice, and tender lymphadenopathy. Peritonsillar infection may spread medially into the retropharyngeal space (Fig. 36-7) or laterally into the parapharyngeal space (Fig. 36-8). Either of these deep-space infections may track inferiorly into the mediastinum. Septic thrombi also may produce metastatic spread resulting in osteomyelitis, meningitis, or brain abscess. All of these conditions require intravenous antibiotic therapy, and deep-space infections require surgical drainage. If peritonsillar abscess is recurrent or associated with a history of chronic tonsillar infection, tonsillectomy may be indicated.[29]

> ### AT A GLANCE . . .
> Complications of Peritonsillar Cellulitis
> - Retropharyngeal abscess
> - Parapharyngeal abscess
> - Mediastinitis
> - Osteomyelitis
> - Meningitis
> - Brain abscess

Diphtheria

Pharyngitis caused by the pathogen *Corynebacterium diphtheriae* is very rare in North America due

Practice Pathway 36–1   DIAGNOSIS AND MANAGEMENT OF OROPHARYNGITIS

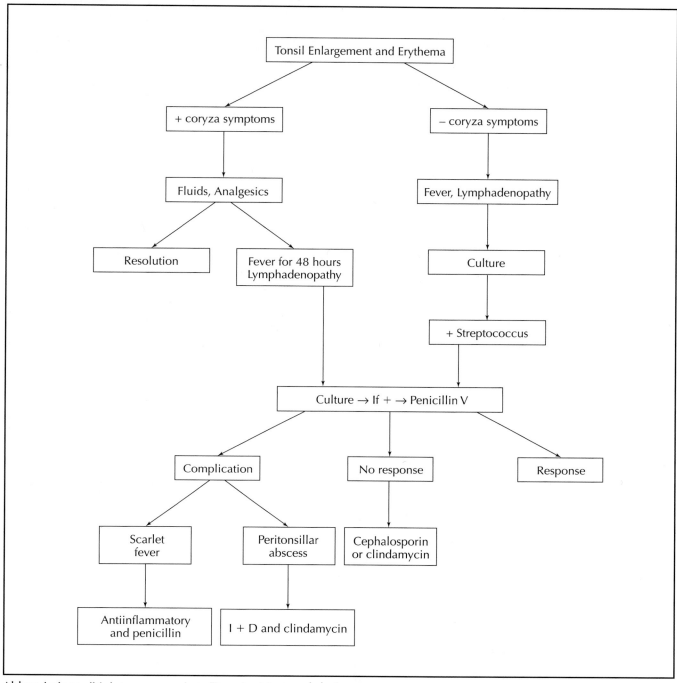

Abbreviations: IV, intravenous; I + D = incision and drainage.

to widespread immunization; however, reported cases have been seen in recent immigrants or immunosuppressed children. The onset of diphtheria is characterized by high fever and sore throat with enlarged erythematous tonsils. A necrotizing pharyngitis and fetid breath then develop and are associated with a thick yellow-grey pseudomembrane that cannot be debrided without bleeding. This membrane may involve the entire pharynx and larynx causing airway obstruction and death, unless the child is intubated or undergoes a tracheotomy. A bacterial exotoxin produced by the diphtherial infection may affect both the central nervous system (CNS) and myocardium. The diagnosis is made by

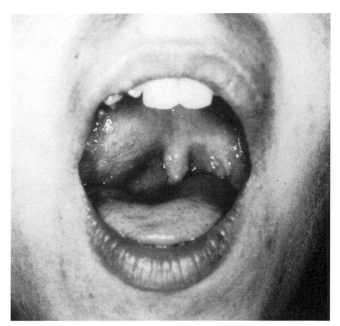

Figure 36–6: Right peritonsillar abscess with swelling of the palate and slight deviation of the uvula.

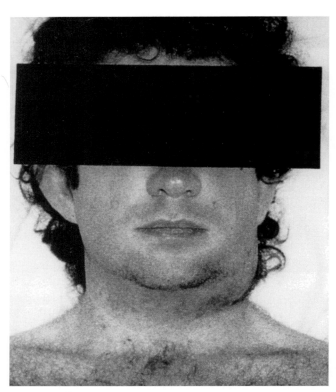

Figure 36–8: Swelling of the left neck secondary to a left parapharyngeal space infection.

identifying the diphtheroid bacteria from the membrane culture on hematoxylin and eosin stain or by blood culture.[30] Immediate treatment with intravenous penicillin and antitoxin is necessary.

> ### SPECIAL CONSIDERATION:
>
> Although diphtheria is rare in North America, reported cases have been seen in immigrants and immunosuppressed children.

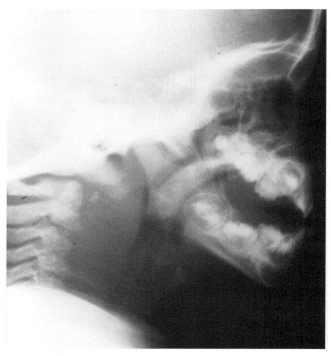

Figure 36–7: Lateral neck radiograph illustrates widening of the retropharyneal space that is consistent with a retropharyngeal abscess.

FUNGAL OROPHARYNGITIS

Oral candidiasis is common in milk-fed infants, especially those who have taken broad-spectrum antibiotics. It usually has a mild clinical presentation with the development of erythematous macules on the gingiva, soft palate, tongue, or pharyngeal mucosa and a fine white lacey membranous exudate that does not bleed with debridement. Rarely, fever or lymphadenopathy occurs. Because the oral cavity and pharyngeal mucosa are tender, the child may be irritable, may refuse to eat, and may become dehydrated. Treatment includes oral nystatin or ketoconazole.

Children who have diabetes or DiGeorge syndrome or who are immunosupressed from chemotherapy or acquired immune deficiency syndrome (AIDS) may develop severe invasive oropharyngeal and esophageal candidiasis.[31] The latter condition can be diagnosed by a distinctive lacey pattern on barium swallow. Disseminated and systemic fungal infections have a poor prognosis and require intravenous amphotericin.

ORAL MANIFESTATIONS OF SYSTEMIC DISEASE (Table 36-3)

Many systemic diseases may be diagnosed by recognizing the characteristic presentation in the oral or pharyngeal mucosa. As mentioned above, an immunosuppressed state may be heralded by oral candidiasis. Similarly, children with leukemia or AIDS may have recurrent viral infections such as pharyngitis aphthous ulcerations of the oral mucosa, bleeding ulcerative gingivitis, or recurrent herpetic ulcers of the lips and oral mucosa.[32] Angular cheilitis is com-

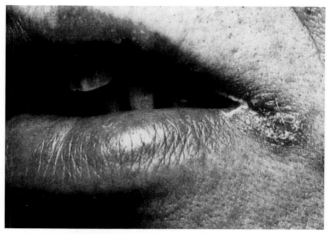

Figure 36–9: Angular cheilitis.

mon in these children, and a culture often identifies both *Pneumocystis carinii* and *Candida* (Fig. 36-9). Other oral manifestations of AIDS include hairy leukoplakia on the lateral ventral surface of the tongue (Fig. 36-10) and the purple-brown patches of Kaposi's sarcoma on the palate or buccal mucosa (Fig. 36-11). Oropharyngeal viral papillomata can occur in healthy children but are more prevalent in immunosuppressed populations.

Common childhood viral infections also may have oral manifestations. Measles (rubeola) may produce Koplik's spots on the buccal mucosa that are typical, nontender red lesions with a pale center. Varicella (i.e., chickenpox) vesicles can spread in crops to the oral mucosa and then rapidly break to form shallow ulcers. Infectious mononucleosis usually presents with tonsillar hypertrophy, membraneous exudate, and sore throat, as previously mentioned.

TABLE 36–3:   Oral Manifestations of Systemic Disease

Ulcerative Gingivitis
AIDS
Leukemia
DiGeorge syndrome
Behçet syndrome
Histiocytosis X

Bleeding Gingivitis
Hemophilia
Coagulopathies
Leukemia
Scurvy/Vitamin C deficiency

Bullous Lesions
Erythema multiforme
Stevens-Johnson syndrome
Pemphigus

Tongue Erythema
Kawasaki syndrome
Scarlet fever
Iron deficiency anemia
Vitamin B deficiency
Hemangioma

Granulomas
Tuberculosis
Wegener's granulomatosis
Leprosy

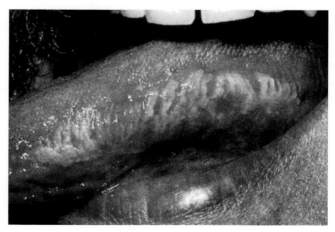

Figure 36–10: Hairy leukoplakia in a patient with AIDS.

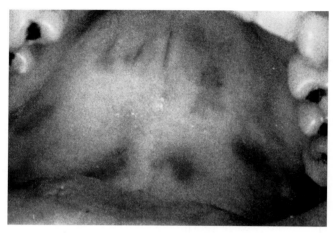

Figure 36–11:   Kaposi's sarcoma of the palate in a child with AIDS.

Behçet syndrome is characterized by ulcers of the urethra and genitalia, uveitis and iridocyclitis, and recurrent ulcers of the oral mucosa. Treatment includes systemic steroids and mouthwashes.[33] Reiter syndrome presents with arthritis, uveitis, and small white painful oral ulcers. Vitamin C deficiency or scurvy may cause bleeding ulcerative gingivitis. Vitamin B deficiency causes a smooth, red tongue. Iron deficiency anemia is manifested by a sore, red, fissured tongue and pale gingiva.

Excessive dryness of the mouth is seen with dehydration and in autoimmune diseases such as Sjögren syndrome or sarcoidosis, in which the function of the salivary glands is affected (Fig. 36–12). Bleeding of the gingiva may indicate hemophilia or other coagulopathies. Bleeding of the lips or tongue may result from chewing or self-mutilation that can occur in children with mental retardation.

Hypertrophy of the gingiva may be a sign of Dilantin® toxicity. Gingival swelling, ulceration, and bleeding, as well as loosening of teeth is also present in the childhood reticuloendothelioses such as histiocytosis X.

Erythema multiforme is nonspecific acute inflammation of the skin and mucous membranes. It may be precipitated by an infection or by a drug reaction; sulfonamides, cephalosporins, and barbiturates have been implicated. Giant vesicles develop on the lips, tongue, and gingiva that ulcerate and crust. There may be similar lesions on the nasal and conjunctival mucosa and "target" lesions on the skin. Secondary bacterial infections can ensue. Severe cases may result in Stevens-Johnson syndrome (Fig. 36–13). Treatment includes maintaining hydration, systemic steroids, and analgesics.

Kawasaki syndrome (mucocutaneous lymph node syndrome) is a disease of uncertain etiology.[34] It is characterized by 4 to 5 days of high fever and a generalized erythematous "blush" rash that seems

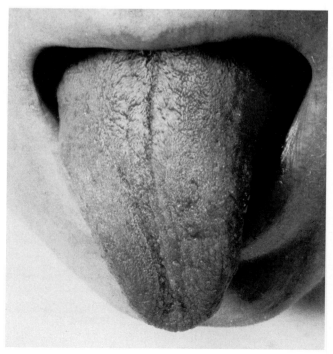

Figure 36–12:   Sicca syndrome in a child with Sjögren's syndrome.

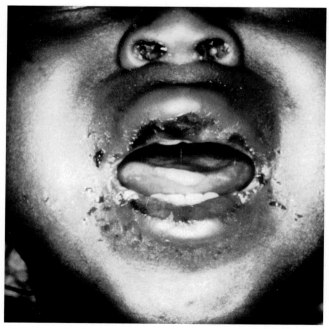

Figure 36–13:   Stevens-Johnson syndrome secondary to sulfonamide therapy.

to come and go. Typically the lips are very red and sore, and there may be intermittent joint pain.

A large tongue is a feature of Down syndrome and hypothyroidism or it may occur as a result of infiltration from hemangioma, lymphangioma, lipid dystrophies, or neurofibromatosis. Granulomatous disease in the oral mucosa is very rare in children. Tuberculous ulcers or gumma can be seen on the dorsum of the tongue or the gingiva. Wegener's granulomatosis can present with painful ulceration of the tongue and palate and may be associated with progressive avascular necrosis.

REFERENCES

1. Israel MS. The viral flora of enlarged tonsils and adenoids. J Pathol Bacteriol 1962; 84:169-176.
2. Yamanaka N, Kataura A. Viral infections associated with recurrent tonsillitis. Acta Otolaryngol (Stockh) 1984; 416:30-37.
3. Richardson H, Leibovitz A. Hand-foot-and-mouth disease in children. J Pediatr 1965; 67:6-12.
4. Healy GB. Pharyngitis. In: Cummings C, Frederickson J, Harker L, et al, eds. Otolaryngology—Head and Neck Surgery. St. Louis: Mosby, 1986, pp. 1185-1188.
5. Brunell PA. Indications for oral acyclovir in children with herpetic stomatitis. Pediatr Infect Dis J 1993; 12(11):970.
6. Cherry JD, John CL. Herpangina: The etiologic spectrum. Pediatrics 1965; 36:632-634.
7. de Asis ML, Bernstein LJ, Schliozberg J. Treatment of resistant oral aphthous ulcers in children. J Pediatr 1995; 127(4):663-665.
8. Snyderman N. Otolaryngologic presentation of infectious mononucleosis. Pediatr Clin North Am 1981; 28:1011-1016.
9. Goode RL, Coursey DL. Tonsillectomy and infectious mononucleosis—a possible relationship. Laryngoscope 1976; 86:992-995.
10. Schwartzman J, Grossman L. Vincent's ulceromembranous gingivostomatitis. Arch Pediatr 1941; 58: 515-520.
11. Spitalnic SJ, Sucov A. Ludwig's angina: Case report and review. J Emerg Med 1995; 13(4):499-503.
12. Reilly S, Timmis P, Beeden AG, et al. Possible role of the anaerobe in tonsillitis. J Clin Pathol 1981; 34: 542-547.
13. Tuner K, Nord CE. Emergence of beta-lactamase producing anaerobic bacteria in the tonsil during penicillin treatment. Eur J Clin Microbiol 1986; 5: 399-404.
14. Brook I, Yocum P, Friedman EM. Aerobic and anaerobic bacteria in tonsils of children with recurrent tonsillitis. Ann Otol Rhinol Laryngol 1981; 90:261-263.
15. Saslow MS, Jablon JM, Jenks AS, et al. Beta-hemolytic streptococci in tonsillar tissue. Amer J Dis Child 1962; 103:19-26.
16. Douglas RM, Miles H, Hansman D, et al. Acute tonsillitis in children: Microbial pathogens in relation to age. Pathology 1984; 16:79-82.
17. Veasy LG, Wiedmeier SE, Orsmond GS, et al. Resurgence of acute rheumatic fever in the intermountain area of the United States. N Engl J Med 1987; 316: 421-427.
18. Denny FW, Wannamaker IW, Brink WR, et al. Prevention of rheumatic fever: Treatment of preceding streptococcal infection. JAMA 1950; 143:151-153.
19. Bisno AC. Acute pharyngitis: Etiology and diagnosis. Pediatrics 1996; 97(6.2):949-954.
20. Surow JB, Handler SD, Telian SA, et al. Bacteriology of tonsil surface and core in children. Laryngoscope 1989; 99:261-266.
21. Brodsky L, Nagy M, Volk M, et al. The relationship of tonsil bacterial concentration to surface and core cultures in chronic tonsillar disease in children. Int J Ped Otorhinolaryngol 1991; 21(1):33-39.
22. Brook I, Yocum P, Foote PA Jr. Changes in the core tonsillar bacteriology of recurrent tonsillitis, 1977-1993. Clin Infect Dis 1995; 21(1):171-176.
23. Nord CE. The role of anaerobic bacteria in recurrent episodes of sinusitis and tonsillitis. Clin Infect Dis 1995; 20(6):1512-1524.
24. Brodsky L, Moore L, Stanievich J. The role of Haemophilus influenzae in the pathogenesis of tonsillar hypertrophy in children. Laryngoscope 1988; 98: 1055-1060.
25. Brodsky L, Moore L, Ogra PL, et al. The immunology of tonsils in children: The effect of bacterial load on the presence of B- and T-cell subsets. Laryngoscope 1988; 98:93-98.
26. van Asselt GJ, Mouton RP, van Boven CP. Penicillin tolerance and treatment failure in group A streptococcal pharyngotonsillitis. Eur J Clin Microbiol Infect Dis 1996; 15(2):107-115.
27. Gerber MA. Antibiotic resistance: Relationship to persistence of group A streptococci in the upper respiratory tract. Pediatrics 1996; 97(6.2):945-948.
28. Brook I, Leyva F. The treatment of the carrier state of group A beta hemolytic streptococci with clindamycin. Chemotherapy 1981; 27:360-367.
29. Wolf M, Kronenberg J, Kessler A, et al. Peritonsillar abscess in children and its indication for tonsillectomy. Int J Pediatr Otorhinolaryngol 1988; 16: 113-117.

30. Feigin RD, Stechenberg BW, Strandgaard BH. Diphtheria. In: Feigin RD, Cherry JD, eds. *Textbook of Pediatric Infectious Diseases.* Philadelphia: Saunders, 1987, pp. 1110–1116.

31. Flynn PM, Cunningham CK, Kerkering T, et al. Oropharyngeal candidiasis in immunocompromised children. The multicenter fluconazole study group. J Pediatr 1995; 127(2):322–328.

32. Hadfield PJ, et al. The ENT manifestations of HIV infection in children. Clin Otolaryngol 1996; 21(1): 30–36.

33. Lehner T. Pathology of recurrent oral ulceration and oral ulceration in Behçet's syndrome: Light, electron and fluorescence microscopy. J Pathol 1969; 97: 481–494.

34. Chang AC, Clark BJ III. Cardiology. In: Schwartz MW, Curry TA, Sargent AJ, et al, eds. *Pediatric Primary Care.* St. Louis: Mosby, 1997, pp. 501–502.

37 Airway Manifestations of Pediatric Gastroesophageal Reflux Disease

Andrew B. Silva

Gastroesophageal reflux (GER) is a common pediatric disorder with symptoms ranging from benign postprandial vomiting in the first year of life to failure to thrive (FTT), esophagitis, and airway obstruction. The otolaryngologist is called upon often to aid in the diagnosis and treatment of these difficult patients, especially when airway involvement is present. It is postulated that airway manifestations of GER include reflux laryngitis, stridor, pulmonary disease, apnea, acute life-threatening events (ALTE), and sudden infant death syndrome (SIDS). The purpose of this chapter is to review the relevant anatomy, physiology, and pathophysiology that is necessary to formulate an effective management plan for these complex patients.

The effects of gastroesophageal reflux disease (GERD) on the airway have been appreciated for centuries. As early as 1884, William Osler noted that GERD could exacerbate a patient's asthma, and "asthmatics learnt not to eat a large meal before bed if they were going to avoid their night-time asthma."[1] In 1934, Bray postulated that a vagally-mediated reflex that was triggered by refluxate entering the distal esophagus was involved in the pathogenesis of "difficult-to-control asthma," which is seen in some patients with GERD.[2] In 1962, Kennedy described a select group of adult patients with documented GERD and respiratory disease whose only presenting symptoms were respiratory.[3] He introduced the term *silent GERD*, which is a diagnostic challenge for the clinician. In 1993, Koufman noted that "GER-related, life-threatening airway complications are higher in children; conversely, children rarely complain of heartburn and regurgita-

tion."[4] This emphasizes the point that clinicians will have to maintain a high index of suspicion for GERD, if they are going to make the correct diagnosis in children.

DEFINITIONS

GER is defined as the retrograde passage of gastric contents into the esophagus. The pH can be acidic, basic, or neutral. GER is either physiologic (normal) or pathologic (disease). *Physiologic GER,* defined as GER, is usually asymptomatic, rarely occurs during sleep, and is frequent when the patient is in the upright position postprandially.[5] *Pathologic reflux* is symptomatic, can be recognized and quantified diagnostically, can cause pathologic changes in the upper aerodigestive tract (UADT), and is defined as GERD.

SPECIAL CONSIDERATION:

GER is the retrograde passage of gastric contents into the esophagus, and they may be acidic, basic, or neutral.

NATURAL HISTORY

Physiologic reflux, or GER is an almost universal finding in newborns; however, relatively few children require medical or surgical intervention. Brief, postprandial reflux episodes can be documented in

Pediatric Otolaryngology, Edited by R.F. Wetmore, H.R. Muntz, and T.J. McGill. Thieme Medical Publishers, Inc., New York © 2000.

almost all newborns during diagnostic testing with esophageal pH-probes.[6] The majority of these episodes go unnoticed during infancy because less than 20% of these episodes result in a visible regurgitation.[7,8]

An understanding of the natural history of reflux (i.e., when GER turns into GERD) is necessary to avoid inappropriate or unnecessary treatment. Carre reviewed the outcomes of 53 pediatric patients with hiatal hernia and reflux who did not receive any positional, medical, or surgical treatment in the mid-1900s.[9] He found that 60% of patients improved when a solid diet was achieved, 90% improved by the age of 4, 5% developed esophageal strictures, and 5% died from marasmus or pneumonia. Kibel reviewed the frequency of vomiting in 93 untreated infants.[10] He reported that 49% were still vomiting at 2 months, 6.5% at 4 months, 4.3% at 6 months, and 1% at 12 months. A common rule of thumb is that GER is usually a self-limited disease and the majority of children improve by the end of their first year of life, when they begin a solid diet. At the most, these children require positional treatment.

There is also a subset of children with persistent or difficult-to-control reflux that would benefit from early identification and treatment. Children with persistent GERD after the age of 3 are noted to have a higher rate of GER-related complications, and they often require medical or surgical intervention.[11] Carre reported a 5% mortality rate in untreated children with severe GERD.[9] Early identification and treatment of these high-risk children may avoid delayed morbidity or mortality.

Improvement in esophageal maturation and function is responsible for the resolution of reflux symptoms seen during the first year of life. The pH-probe has proven to be the most clinically relevant tool in measuring improvement. The most commonly used reflux parameters are listed in Table 37–1. The *reflux index* (RI), which is the total percentage of time that the pH is < 4, and the number of reflux

episodes > 5 minutes (which is a measure of esophageal acid clearance or, in other words, how effectively the esophagus can clear the refluxate) have proven to be the best-discriminating parameters between reflux patients and controls.[12]

A threshold pH < 4 has been used to define *acid reflux*.[13] In children, 24-hour pH-probe parameters have been used to obtain normative values for different pediatric age groups.[14,15] Vandenplas et al. screened 509 healthy infants for SIDS and reported that the RI was 13% at birth, 8% at 12 months, and averaged 10% during the first year of life.[15] The RI normalizes after the first year of life, with the RI of infants (8%) approaching that of adults (7%).[15] Esophageal acid clearance also improves during the first year of life; the number of reflux episodes that last > 5 minutes decreases while the total number of episodes remains the same.[14] The lower-esophageal-sphincter (LES) pressure has been shown to reach mature pressure levels (11.8 +/− 3.6 mmHg) by 6 to 7 weeks of life, despite the gestational age or weight.[16]

PATHOPHYSIOLOGY OF GERD

The pathogenesis of GERD is multifactorial in origin. Alterations in both the anatomic (i.e., diaphragmatic crura, phrenoesophageal ligament, gastroesophageal angle, mucosal flap valve, and intra-abdominal esophagus) and physiologic components [i.e., LES, esophageal acid clearance, epithelial resistance, and upper-esophageal sphincter (UES)] of the reflux barrier can cause GERD. The function of the *reflux barrier* is to prevent the retrograde passage of refluxate from the stomach into the esophagus or laryngopharynx. The newborn is predisposed to GERD due to a short intra-abdominal esophagus and an immature LES. The easiest way to conceptualize the pathophysiology of GERD is to follow the path of the refluxate from the stomach into the laryngopharynx.

TABLE 37–1:   Common pH-Probe Parameters

- The number of reflux episodes with pH <4
- The total recorded time that the pH is <4
- Reflux index (RI), the percentage of time the pH is <4
- The longest reflux episode
- The average esophageal acid-clearance time per episode
- The number of reflux episodes >5 minutes
- The mean duration of sleeping reflux episodes (ZMD)

SPECIAL CONSIDERATION:

The newborn is predisposed to GERD due to a short intra-abdominal esophagus and an immature lower-esophageal sphincter.

Delayed gastric emptying has been implicated in the pathogenesis of GERD because patients who experience this are predisposed to high intragastric pressures and volumes. The presence of large amounts of refluxate for longer periods of time than normal increases the risk of a reflux episode occurring, if the intragastric pressure rises above the resting LES pressure. In addition, gastric distention has been shown to trigger transient LES relaxations (TLESR) with reflux.[17] At the present time, there is still a disagreement in the literature concerning the role of gastric emptying in children with GERD.

SPECIAL CONSIDERATION:

LES relaxations are thought to play a major role in the pathogenesis of GERD.

Blaming GERD on a dysfunctional LES is misleading because there is no anatomically-distinct sphincter in the lower esophagus. Instead, there is discrete high-pressure zone in the distal 4 cm of the esophagus that is referred to as the LES. Hormonal and neural factors, the length of the intra-abdominal esophagus, abdominothoracic pressure differences, and diaphragmatic support structures can affect this area and cause reflux. Traditional thinking blames reflux on hypotonic LES, despite evidence showing that actual LES pressure correlates poorly with the presence or absence of GERD.[16]

Currently, TLESR are felt to play a major role in the pathogenesis of GERD. *TLESR are LES relaxations that occur in the absence of peristalsis, swallowing, or a normally hypotonic sphincter.* Pediatric studies document that the majority of reflux episodes in children are caused by TLESR in an otherwise normal LES.[14,18] Werlin et al. studied 27 infants with a 24-hr pH-probe and found that 34% of their reflux episodes were due to TLESR.[19] These relaxations occur more frequently in the presence of esophagitis or in a postprandial state, and they may be triggered by vagal pathways, gastric distention, or respiration.[20,21]

Swallowing plays an important role in esophageal acid clearance because it initiates a primary esophageal peristaltic wave. This wave facilitates delivery of bicarbonate-rich saliva, which neutralizes and clears the refluxate, into the distal esophagus. Experiments show that a single peristaltic wave is capable of clearing an experimentally-placed, 15-ml bolus of acid from the distal esophagus, but that it takes nine more swallows of bicarbonate-rich saliva to restore the intraluminal pH to > 4.[22] Children, especially, are prone to exposure of esophageal acid at night because they swallow less while sleeping. Esophagitis causes children with GERD not to respond to every reflux event with a swallow or peristaltic wave. They have been shown to swallow less (0.49/min) than children without GERD (3.5/min) in response to reflux events.[21] Any alterations in esophageal peristalsis or salivary flow can lead to esophagitis.

The final barrier preventing refluxate from spilling into the laryngopharynx is the UES. Traditional thinking blames pharyngoesophageal reflux (PER) an abnormally-low UES pressure.[23] Recent investigators have failed to confirm this finding.[24,25] In fact, a recent dual-sleeve manometry study demonstrated an increased UES tone in response to refluxate-induced esophageal distention; however, abrupt relaxations of the UES occurred during 54% of these episodes.[26] This resulted in PER with possible laryngeal acid exposure.

AIRWAY MANIFESTATIONS OF GERD

GERD has been implicated in the pathogenesis of reflux laryngitis,[27] stridor,[28] asthma,[29] apnea,[30] ALTE,[31] and SIDS.[32] The affects of GERD on the pediatric airway are mediated through three mechanisms: (1) macro-aspiration with chemical pneumonitis; (2) micro-aspiration with chemical pneumonitis or stimulation of laryngeal-protective reflex; (3) stimulation of an esophageal-receptor reflex responsible for causing bronchial hyperactivity. Establishing a cause and effect relationship has been difficult.

AT A GLANCE. . .

Effects of GERD on the Pediatric Airway

---

1. Macro-aspiration with chemical pneumonitis
2. Micro-aspiration with chemical pneumonitis or stimulation of laryngeal-protective reflex
3. Stimulation of esophageal reflex for bronchial hyperactivity

Laryngotracheal Complex

Reflux laryngitis

Reflux laryngitis is a well-recognized phenomenon in adults[33] and children.[34] The most common site of laryngeal injury is the glottis. Children commonly present with a hoarse voice, chronic cough, or globus sensation. Infants with laryngomalacia are especially prone to this condition because they generate high negative intrathoracic pressures during inspiration that can overcome the LES pressure resulting in reflux. This reflux, in turn, causes more laryngeal edema that results in an increased respiratory rate, even higher inspiratory pressures, and more reflux. Aggressive treatment of children with GERD can avoid these laryngeal sequelae.

Stridor

Exposure of the laryngotracheal complex to refluxate can result in edema, ulceration, granulation, posterior-glottic scarring, arytenoid fixation, subglottic stenosis, and/or obliteration of the airway. Each of these entities can result in *stridor*. Every child being evaluated for subglottic stenosis should undergo evaluation and treatment for GER prior to operative intervention.

AT A GLANCE. . .

Effects of GERD on the Laryngotracheal Complex

- Laryngeal edema
- Laryngeal ulceration
- Laryngeal granulation
- Posterior-glottic scarring
- Arytenoid fixation
- Subglottic stenosis

The first cause and effect relationship between stridor and GERD was documented by Orenstein et al. in 1983.[35] pH-Probe-documented reflux events that resulted in stridor resolved only after esophageal acid clearance, in this 9-day-old infant's pH-probe study. Nielson et al. studied seven stridorous infants with simultaneous pH-probe and cardiorespiratory testing.[36] They documented episodes of stridor and hypercarbia occurring directly after re-

flux events. Contencin et al. was able to predict the presence of GERD in children with stridor with a specificity of 83% and a sensitivity of 100% using a two-channel pH-probe when the pharyngeal pH remained < 6 for more than 1% of the study time.[37]

Pulmonary Considerations

Asthma

The relationship between GER and asthma has been known for over 50 years. Subsequently, studies have documented that GER has higher prevalence in patients with asthma, chronic obstructive pulmonary disease (COPD), and recurrent pneumonia than in the general population.[38,39] In each case, disease can be made worse by repeated insults to the tracheobronchial tree that result in inflammation and/or recurrent infection.

Asthma is by far the most common pediatric pulmonary disorder. Patients with asthma are predisposed to GER secondary to high-negative, intrapleural pressures, which are generated during inspiration from their increased work of breathing. These pressures act to amplify the gastroesophageal pressure gradient, resulting in a predisposition to reflux. Chronic hyperinflation will flatten and stretch the diaphragmatic crura as well as shorten the length of intra-abdominal esophagus, thus facilitating LES incompetence. Many of the medications used to treat asthma e.g., theophyline and beta-adrenergic agonists also will reduce the LES tone. Finally, there may be a reflex relaxation of the LES that is mediated through bronchial receptors triggered by inspiration.[40]

GERD can exacerbate asthma through two mechanisms. First, micro- or macroaspiration can cause a chronic inflammatory reaction, which can exacerbate the reactive airway disease or result in pneumonia or recurrent pneumonia with repeated episodes. Second, distal esophageal acidification can cause bronchoconstriction mediated through a vagal reflex arc. Bronchoconstriction has been induced in young asthmatic animals after tracheobronchial acid instillation.[41] Perfusion of diluted hydrochloric acid into the distal esophagus (i.e., Bernstein Test) has reproduced wheezing in asthmatics and has caused increased bronchial hypersensitivity noted during a methacholine challenge in asymptomatic patients.[42-44] In animal models, the vagal nerve section obliterates this bronchoconstrictive response. In humans, topical anesthesia or antacid neutralization of the esophagus eliminates this response.[45] Despite evidence for a vagally-mediated pathway, these studies have been criticized because microaspiration of the test acid may have caused the symptoms.[10]

Other Considerations

A direct cause and effect relationship between GERD and apnea, ALTEs, and SIDS has not been established.

Apnea

GERD can cause obstructive apnea in the presence of aspiration, altered gas exchange, and/or stimulation of the laryngeal chemoreceptor reflex.[46] *Apnea* can be a significant problem in preterm infants. The majority of prolonged apneic events in preterm infants are not related to regurgitation; however, after a regurgitation event there is a 14-fold increase in the apneic frequency.[47] The chemoreceptor reflex is felt to be the cause of this. It results from noxious stimulation of glottic superior laryngeal nerve (SLN) afferents by refluxate, and it results in apnea, bradycardia, hypotension, peripheral vasoconstriction, swallowing, and arousal with termination of the apneic event. There is evidence to show that arousal with termination of the apnea may not occur in the presence of hypoxia resulting in airway obstruction.[48] In eight healthy infants, bradycardia and apnea were recorded during distal esophageal acid perfusion.[30]

Apparent life-threatening event (ALTE)

GERD has been implicated in the pathogenesis of *ALTE,* which is defined as an apneic event during the first year of life with a combination of apnea, color change, altered muscle tone, choking, or gagging.[49] Approximately 4% of these children will go on to have a SIDS event.[50]

The reported incidence of pH-probe-documented GERD in children evaluated for an ALTE varies greatly (42 to 95%) depending on the reported series.[49,51,52] However, the incidence of GERD and sleep-related reflux is greater than controls in each case. A significant correlation also has been reported between the duration of esophageal acidification and the length of the apneic event.[52] Veereman-Wauters et al. reported that 49 of 130 infants being evaluated for an ALTE had their event within

2 hours of a feeding.[53] These 49 infants were studied with a pH-probe, and 34 had significant GERD. It is interesting to note that all 130 of these infants were considered healthy by both their parents and pediatricians prior to their ALTE. Although a direct cause and effect relationship is not established between a reflux event and an ALTE, we recommend that any child who presents after an ALTE is evaluated for GERD.[54]

Sudden infant death syndrome (SIDS)

SIDS is the leading cause of postnatal death during the first year of life and occurs in 1 to 2:1000 live births.[55] GERD and a history of a prior ALTE are risk factors for SIDS. In an animal model, Wetmore demonstrated that laryngeal instillation of acid causes obstructive apnea secondary to laryngospasm.[56] He postulated that the pathophysiology of SIDS might involve a reflex arc between SLN afferents and recurrent laryngeal nerve efferents (*obstructive apnea*) or a reflex arc involving the SLN afferents and phrenic efferents (*central apnea*).

The 24-hr pH-probe has been shown to be a useful tool in detecting children with GERD who are at high risk for developing a reflux-related death or SIDS. Jolley et al. followed 499 children with reflux for 1 year and reported a 9.1% incidence of reflux-related or SIDS deaths in infants with a type-1 reflux pattern (which is a pH-probe that demonstrates a continually high frequency of reflux episodes) and a prolonged ZMD score (see Table 37–1). In the group who underwent antireflux surgery, as compared to those who were treated medically, no deaths were reported.[32] This evidence supports aggressive surgical treatment in this select population of children with GERD.

> **SPECIAL CONSIDERATION:**
> The presentation of GERD may be atypical, and the clinician must always maintain a high index of suspicion.

HISTORY AND PHYSICAL EXAMINATION

A complete history and physical examination including a growth curve should be performed at the initial visit. Special attention should be paid to the child's birth, past medical examination, feeding, airway, and reflux history.[57] Orenstein et al.[58] has developed a 161-item questionnaire to aid in this task. Ferancha et al.[59] have identified six behaviors that are temporally associated with the onset of reflux episodes in infants: discomfort, emission of liquid or gas, yawning, stridor, stretching, and mouthing.

It is important to identify children with a tracheoesophageal fistula, esophageal atresia, colonic interposition, bronchopulmonary dysplasia, recurrent pneumonia, subglottic stenosis, or neurologic impairment. These children can be considered a "special population" because they are at a higher risk for GERD. They are more difficult to treat and have a higher morbidity and mortality because of their esophageal dismotility and/or pulmonary disease, which can be adversely affected by reflux events.

The presentation of GERD may be atypical, and the clinician must always maintain a high index of suspicion. It has been estimated that only 20% of reflux episodes actually result in a visible episode of regurgitation. This may explain why children with GERD do not present always with regurgitation. It is well known that there is a subset of children with GER whose only presenting symptoms may be airway related.

Recently, Parsons proposed that otitis media (OM) and sinusitis are atypical presentations of GERD.[60] Contencin and Nancy showed that reflux can occur to the level of the nasopharynx.[61] As well, Barbero proposed that chronic exposure of the nasal and eustachian-tube epithelium can cause edema and irritation, resulting in blocked ostia and subsequent disease or worsening of pre-existent disease. However, to date, no direct cause and effect relationship exists to support this. In medically-recalcitrant cases, a history for reflux should be elucidated. Identification and treatment of these patients should improve symptoms.[62]

Otalgia with a normal exam may be an atypical presentation of GERD. Otalgia results when PER causes hypopharyngeal irritation with referred pain. Gibson and Cochran reported a series of six infants who had been treated for recurrent OM whose only presenting sign was irritability and tugging at the ear.[63] During their work-up, all six infants were diagnosed with GERD (each infant had a normal otologic examination) after a pH-probe and/or an esophageal biopsy were performed. Each child's pattern of "recurring OM" resolved with antireflux treatment,

thus avoiding inappropriate medical or surgical otologic treatment.

Every child should have a complete physical examination including flexible nasolaryngoscopy (FFL). This allows the examiner to visualize and evaluate the upper airway directly. Identification of patients with sinusitis, adenotonsillar hyperplasia, laryngomalacia, or upper airway obstruction (UAO) will help to narrow the differential diagnosis. Evidence of laryngeal inflammation with edema and pachydermia points toward GERD.

AVAILABLE DIAGNOSTIC TESTS

Testing is not indicated for the majority of patients with reflux. It is reserved for patients with pathologic reflux in whom treatment is indicated. Since the differential diagnosis of reflux symptoms is long, it is essential to ensure that reflux is responsible for the patient's symptom complex prior to treatment. The sensitivity and specificity of a symptom-based diagnosis alone is low because 25 to 30% of the patients will be misdiagnosed.[64] The sensitivity and specificity of the most common diagnostic tests used in children with GERD are listed in Table 37–2. The diagnostic error is reduced when the diagnosis is confirmed on two separate tests.[65]

The *barium esophagram with small bowel follow-through* (BESBFT) has a low sensitivity and specificity for diagnosing reflux. The conditions of the test are not physiologic, and the patient is imaged for < 5 minutes. Thus, it is only a snapshot in time that may not reflect the patient's state of disease accurately. However, it is very useful in detecting anatomic abnormalities (e.g., TEF (tracheoesophageal fistula), vascular anomaly, gastric outlet obstruction, malrotation, and esophageal stenosis), motility disorders, and mucosal ulcers. It is useful in children who have a history that is strongly suggestive of reflux, endoscopic evidence of laryngeal inflammation, and a positive radiologic test. In these children, treatment can be initiated without pH-probe testing in selected circumstances.

The *esophageal scintiscan* (milk scan) is useful for detecting GER of any pH (acidic, neutral, or basic) in the postprandial period. Reflux commonly occurring in the postprandial period is of a higher pH and not identified on a pH-probe. In certain cases, this reflux may be responsible for the patient's respiratory symptoms. For example, a child

TABLE 37–2:   Reliability of Diagnostic Tests for GER

| Test | Jaimeson GG, Duranceau A | | Riechter JE, Castell DO | | |
	Sensitivity	Specificity	Sensitivity	Specificity	Studies Reviewed
Barium esophagram	+	+ +	40%	85%	3
Scintiscan	+ +	+ + +	61%	95%	3
pH-Probe	+ + + +	+ + + +	88%	98%	3
Endoscopy	+ +	+ + +	95%	41%	2
Biopsy	+ + +	+ + +	77%	91%	5
Lipid-laden macrophages	+ + +	unknown	N/A	N/A	N/A

Abbreviations: + + + +, excellent; + + +, good; + +, fair; +, poor.
Modified from Jaimeson GG, Duranceau A. *Gastroesophageal Reflux.* Pathogenesis, diagnosis, and therapy. Philadelphia: Saunders, 1988, p. 281, and from Richter JE, Castell DO. Ann Intern Med 1982; 97:93–103, with permission.

may reflux a neutral refluxate into the laryngeal inlet causing laryngospasm and apnea.

The scintiscan can diagnose, quantify, and calculate accurately the rate of gastric emptying. It provides an accurate, rapid, and noninvasive diagnosis while quantifying GER in a physiologic manner.[66] Delayed imaging over the lung fields 24 hours later will detect patients with pulmonary aspiration, allowing proper precautions to be taken. The sensitivity and specificity of this test is dependent on the technical expertise of the evaluating pediatric radiologist.

A single or double channel 24-hour pH study combined with either a symptom-based observation log or cardiorespiratory monitoring is the gold standard for reflux diagnosis. This allows for a temporal correlation between GER or PER with a cardiac, respiratory, or observational (stridor) event recorded during simultaneous pneumocardiography or video. The advantage of a double-channel system is having a probe located just above the gastroesophageal junction and another probe in the hypopharynx, allowing documentation of GER and PER. The patient's respiratory status (e.g., stridor, apnea, etc.) at the time of pharyngeal-acid exposure can be recorded, which allows a direct cause and effect relationship to be established.

SPECIAL CONSIDERATION:

A single or double-channel 24-hour pH study combined with either a symptom-based observation log or cardiorespiratory monitoring is the gold standard for diagnosing GER.

Varty et al. suggest that the pH study can be used to identify patients who will require surgical intervention for control of their GERD.[67] They obtained a pH study on 57 children who were failing medical management, and based on a cut-off point of >18% of the study time spent at a pH < 4, were able to predict which children ultimately would go on to require surgical intervention. Their sensitivity and specificity was 92% and 70%, respectively, for children with GERD and no concomitant illnesses. It was 80% and 86%, respectively, for children with GERD and esophageal atresia, TEF, or a neurologic disability.

The weakness of the pH study is its inability to diagnose neutral or basic reflux during the study. Attempts to overcome this during the postprandial period have included using apple juice or acidic formulas. This is not ideal because the stomach may handle these feedings differently than formula. A normal pH study does not rule out GERD and a false-negative will occur with neutral or basic refluxate, refluxate buffered by consumed milk, or an increase in salivary flow from nasogastric tube stimulation.[68]

Panendoscopy with biopsy allows for direct visualization of the mucosal lining of the UADT. An esophageal biopsy is always performed because 40% of children with a normal-appearing esophagus have histologic evidence of esophagitis.[66-69] If esophagitis exists, then an H$_2$ receptor blockers can be added to a prokinetic agent during treatment. Direct examination of the larynx allows detection of increased supraglottic vascularity, laryngeal or subglottic edema, interarytenoid pachydemia, and small lymph aggregates in the wall of the trachea, all of which are suggestive of GERD. During bronchoscopy, a bronchoalveolar lavage can be obtained.

The presence of lipid-laden macrophages has a 85% sensitivity for GERD.[70]

TREATMENT OPTIONS

The treatment for GERD must correct the anatomic or physiologic defect in the reflux barrier. Initial diagnostic testing not only identifies the defect, but it also provides a way to monitor treatment. For example, the pH-probe can differentiate between a hypersecretory state (a low pH) and a motility defect (decreased esophageal acid clearance); the former can be effectively treated with an antisecretory agent, and the latter can be effectively treated with a prokinetic agent. A follow-up study can be obtained if the patient remains symptomatic and therapy can be adjusted accordingly. This section reviews the treatment options for GERD and the rationale for the use of each. The next section, Practice Pathway, discusses a specific protocol.

Treatment can be divided into the three phases, which are outlined in Table 37–3. Phase I involves alterations in lifestyle and diet, phase II involves pharmacologic treatment, and phase III involves surgery. Every patient will not undergo an orderly stepwise escalation of his treatment. Typically, the patient with GERD responds well to less-aggressive therapy. It is important to note that many of the

TABLE 37–3: GER Treatment Levels

Level I Life style modification

- Smaller, more frequent meals
- Dietary modifications: formulas composed of medium-chain triglycerides, whey-hydrolysate, or soy, or one with a low osmolality.
- Positioning: horizontal prone or 30 degree prone position

Level II Pharmacologic treatment

- Cytoprotective agents: antacids with alginic acid, sucralfate
- H$_2$-receptor blockers: cimetidine and ranitidine
- Prokinetic agents: metaclopramide and cisapride
- Proton pump inhibitor: omeprazole

Level III Anti-reflux surgery

- Nissen Fundoplication
- Hill Gastropexy
- Belsey Mark IV

Modified from Silva, Hotaling. Advances in pediatric gastro-esophageal reflux disease. Curr Opin Otolaryngol Head Neck Surg 1994; 2:508, with permission.

drugs used for GERD are not approved by the Federal Drug Administration (FDA) in infants despite their widespread use. This underscores the need for a diagnosis prior to treatment to avoid inappropriate or unnecessary treatment.

Phase I

Lifestyle modification should be the initial form of treatment in children without life-threatening complications. This is noninvasive and lacks the side effects associated with phase II treatment. In the infant, both dietary modification and positioning may be very helpful. In the older child, avoidance of caffeine, chocolate, and carbonated beverages is helpful.

There are several modifications in the infant's formula that reduce GER. Formulas composed of medium-chain triglycerides, whey-hydrolysate, or soy, and/or a formula with a lower osmolality all promote gastric emptying resulting in less reflux.[71,72] Formulas thickened with rice cereal (15 ml in 30 ml of formula) will result in significantly less regurgitation.[73] In young children, smaller and more frequent meals will provide less material to reflux during the postprandial period. In older children, weight loss and avoidance of tight clothing will decrease reflux by reducing intra-abdominal pressure.

Body positioning is an integral component in the treatment of GERD. By having the head of the bed elevated, gravitational forces aid in preventing reflux. Originally, the seated position was recommended for infants, until the 1980s when data showed that this position actually worsened GER by increasing the intra-abdominal pressure due to bending at the waist.[74] For this reason, car seats should be avoided or at least not used in postprandial infants who have demonstrated apnea or complications with GERD. For infants with moderate reflux, car trips are best done during the fasting state in order to avoid regurgitation.

Since the 1980s, the 30 degree prone position has been preferred to the horizontal prone position. However, a recent study has demonstrated that the horizontal prone position is just as effective in reducing reflux.[75] This position is easier to use because a harness is not required to keep the child from sliding down the incline.[76]

Recently, controversy in the literature has emerged concerning the safety of prone positioning and its association to SIDS. In 1992, the American Academy of Pediatrics (AAP) announced that their official position on prone positioning and SIDS was the following: ''Based on careful evaluation of existing data indicating an association between sudden infant death syndrome (SIDS) and prone positioning for infants, the Academy recommends that healthy infants, when being put down for sleep, be positioned on their side or back.''[77] It is also known that supine positioning of an infant with GERD or obstructive sleep apnea is associated with serious airway risks; therefore, the AAP recommends that only healthy infants be placed in the supine position.

Phase II

Phase II treatment uses pharmacologic therapy with cytoprotective agents, prokinetic agents, H_2-receptor blockers, and/or proton pump inhibitors. Cytoprotective agents have the fewest side effects but require frequent dosing. This makes them most useful in the setting of symptom breakthrough during therapy, or in patients waiting for a GERD evaluation. They neutralize acidic refluxate, reduce mucosal injury, and prevent the activation of pepsin. Antacids containing alginic acid are especially helpful because they form a thick viscous foamy layer over the gastric contents, acting as an additional reflux barrier. A liquid preparation of sucralfate is now available that can effectively coat any areas of denuded esophageal mucosa with a nearly-impermeable barrier and allow healing.

The most common cause of reflux in children is altered gastroesophageal motility with TLESR. For this reason, prokinetic agents are the first-line agents used in Europe, and they are increasing rapidly in popularity in the United States. Bethanechol was one of the first agents in this class to be used; however, it has fallen out of favor because of its respiratory side effects. Metaclopramide was the next agent to become popular; it is a dopamine antagonist that increases gastric emptying, improves esophageal peristalsis, and raises the LES pressure. Its use is limited by its extrapyramidal and sedative side effects.

Cisipride is a new selective cholinergic agent that facilitates the release of acetylcholine from the myenteric plexus; it lacks the sedative and extrapyramidal side effects of metaclopramide. Cisapride has been successful in controlling reflux in both term and preterm infants.[78,79] Cisapride decreases the amount of reflux and effectively treats children with GERD and chronic respiratory disease.[78,80,81] In June of 1998, the labeling for cisapride was changed to reflect the association between its use and the occurrence of adverse cardiac events. Concern over reports of QTc interval prolongation, ventricular arrhythmias and an increasing number of drug interactions led to this revision. It is important to remember that this drug is very effective and both the North American and European Society for Pediatric Gastroenterology and Nutrition still recommend its use. They have both published medical position statements with therapeutic guidelines that should be reviewed by the reader prior to use.[82,83]

Antisecretory agents such as cimetidine, ranitidine, and famotidine (H_2-receptor blockers) have all been used to treat GERD in children. These agents competitively block one of the three receptors responsible for the parietal cells' acid secretion. They are not 100% effective because they lack any effect on the gastrin or acetylcholine receptor. Cimetidine and ranitidine are the two most commonly used. Ranitidine has the advantage with a longer half and b.i.d. dosing. Regardless of which antagonist is used, it has been noted that children require higher drug dosages (mg/kg) than adults.[84] Children are treated usually for 2 to 3 months before being re-evaluated.

Omeprazole is the strongest antisecretory agent and is classified as a proton pump inhibitor. It blocks the last step in acid production, the parietal cell potassium/hydrogen adenosine triphosphatase (ATPase) enzyme. It can block 90% of the daily acid production compared with 70% for the H_2-receptor blockers.[85] A British study demonstrated its efficacy in the treatment of severe esophagitis in 15 infants and children (including eight neurologically impaired infants) refractory to H_2-receptor blockers and prokinetic agents.[86] Because of the lack of long-term experience with this drug, the use of omeprazole is limited to patients who fail a trial with a H_2-receptor blockers.

The initial choice of therapy should include a prokinetic agent. If there is concomitant esophagitis, laryngeal irritation, and/or tracheal irritation, a antisecretory agent can be added. Children should be treated for 2 to 3 months and then re-evaluated. The medication can then be decreased gradually as they outgrow the tendency to reflux or increased, depending on their clinical response.

Because many of these medications are not FDA approved for use in infants, the use of empiric therapy (i.e., without a diagnosis) is controversial. There are some situations when therapy may be considered. Phase I therapy can be used always for patients with minor symptoms or for patients waiting for diagnostic testing. Level II therapy can be considered in the acutely-ill patient who has been admitted to the intensive care unit (ICU) with respiratory complications. A definitive diagnosis can be delayed until the patient is stable, and then the medication can be withdrawn 48 hours prior to testing.

Phase III

Surgical intervention is reserved for patients who fail aggressive medical therapy and continue to have life-threatening complications with GERD.[87] The most common surgical procedure performed is the *Nissen fundoplication*. Its goals are to restore the natural integrity of the LES, to improve the gastroesophageal-valve function, and to maintain normal deglutition. It has also been recommended in patients with feeding gastrostomies because of its tendency to exacerbate reflux by altering local anatomy and from increased intragastric pressures during rapid bolus feedings.

The anatomical basis of this repair rests on its ability to accomplish three goals: restore the competence of the cardia by increasing the length and pressure of the LES, decrease the esophageal diameter, and resist gastric distention with a 360 degree wrap.[88] The Nissen fundoplication has a 85 to 90% symptom-control rate with a 1% mortality rate.[87,89] Complications due to a failure of the wrap (persistent reflux), altered gastric emptying (dumping or delayed gastric emptying), effectiveness of the wrap (gas bloat, inability to burp or vomit, and dysphagia), and technical failures have all been noted.

PRACTICE PATHWAYS

The purpose of the initial evaluation is to determine the severity of disease (i.e., if a life-threatening airway complication is present) and the probability that the patient's symptoms are a result of GERD (a high or low level of suspicion). The initial evaluation should consist of a complete history and physical examination, FFL, BESBFT, and airway and chest radiographs. Patients with life-threatening airway complications have stridor, severe subglottic stenosis, cyanosis or apnea (often with feeding), ALTE, and/or a SIDS sibling death. Patients in the high-suspicion group have frequent regurgitation, difficulty feeding, FTT, anemia, evidence of laryngeal inflammation, and/or a positive radiologic study.

Children who do not have these are in the low-suspicion group. Depending on the degree of suspicion for GERD one of these practice pathways can be selected; however, the clinician must remember that not every child will fit neatly into a pathway, and the treatment plan may require modification (Practice Pathways 37–1, 37–2, and 37–3).

For a low level of suspicion (see Practice Pathway 37–1) phase I treatment should be instituted. If a child fails to improve, a pH-probe and/or nuclear scintiscan should be obtained. These tests are preferred to a barium esophagram because the esophagram has a low sensitivity and specificity for reflux. A positive barium study combined with a weak reflux history may result in a large number of children being treated unnecessarily with potentially dangerous drugs that are not FDA approved in infants. Patients with a diagnostic pH-probe and/or nuclear scintiscan should start phase II treatment (see Practice Pathway 37–2) only if there is still no improvement should the treatment doses be maximized and a repeat study considered. Children with difficult-to-control reflux may undergo panendoscopy and consideration for an antireflux procedure if there is no improvement.

If the clinician has a high level of suspicion for reflux and/or the child belongs in the special population group, then a pH-probe study and/or nuclear scintiscan should be done initially. If positive, patients should start phase I and II treatments simultaneously. The exception to this rule (obtaining a pH-probe study and/or nuclear scintiscan prior to medical treatment) may be the patients who you strongly believe have reflux and who have evidence of laryngeal inflammation on fiberoptic endoscopy and grossly-positive barium esophagrams. These children also benefit from simultaneous phase I and II treatments. If the child fails to improve, phase II treatment is maximized and a repeat study performed to assess progress. If the child remains refractory to treatment, panendoscopy should be performed, and consideration of an antireflux procedure should be discussed with the parents.

With life-threatening airway complications, the first priority is to evaluate the airway. The patient is admitted to an ICU and may require urgent endoscopic evaluation depending on admitting vitals. After the airway has been evaluated and/or secured, a pH-probe or nuclear scintiscan can be performed. Children with positive studies should be treated with both phase I and maximized phase II treatment plans. Treatment failures are candidates for an antireflux procedure.

Practice Pathway 37–1   SUGGESTED TREATMENT PARADIGM FOR AIRWAY SYMPTOMATIC CHILDREN WITH LOW SUSPICION FOR GERD

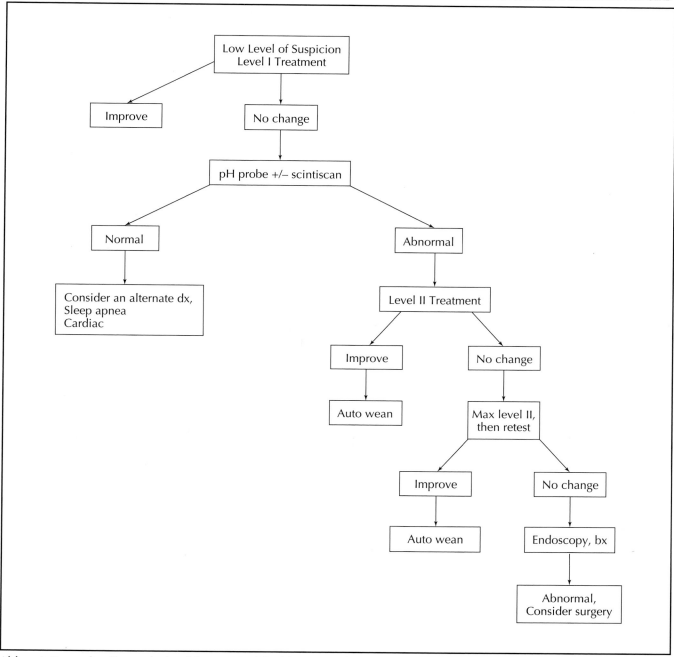

Abbreviations; dx, diagnosis; bx, biopsy. Modified from Hotaling, Silva. *Advances in Otolaryngology–Head and Neck Surgery*. St. Louis: Mosby, 1995, p. 281, with permission.

Practice Pathway 37–2   SUGGESTED TREATMENT PARADIGM FOR AIRWAY SYMPTOMATIC CHILDREN WITH A HIGH SUSPICION FOR GERD INCLUDING SPECIAL POPULATION CHILDREN

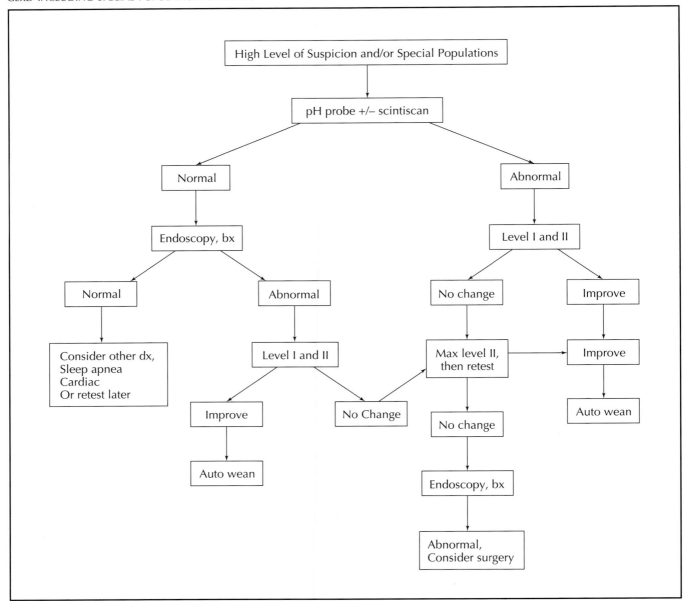

Abbreviations: dx, diagnosis; bx, biopsy Modified from Hotaling, Silva. *Advances in Otolaryngology–Head and Neck Surgery.* St. Louis: Mosby, 1995, p. 282, with permission.

Practice Pathway 37–3   SUGGESTED TREATMENT PARADIGM FOR CHILDREN WITH LIFE-THREATENING AIRWAY COMPLICATIONS OF GERD

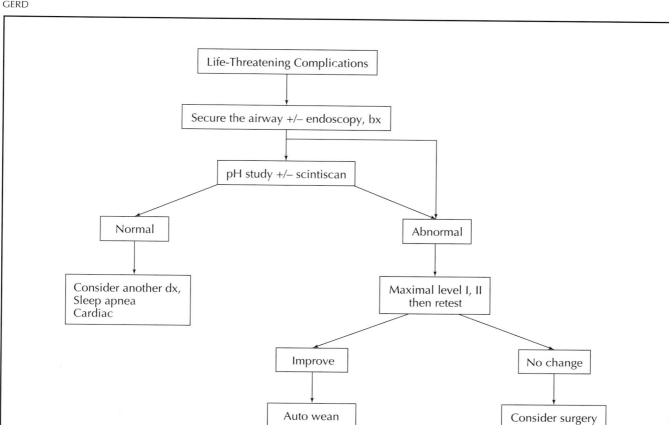

Abbreviations: dx, diagnosis; bx, biopsy Modified from Hotaling, Silva. *Advances in Otolaryngology–Head and Neck Surgery.* St. Louis: Mosby, 1995, p. 282, with permission.

Acknowledgments. I would like to thank Andrew J. Hotaling, M.D., for his help in formulating the practice pathway diagrams. He has both been an inspiration and a mentor to me during my career.

REFERENCES

1. Osler W. *The Principles and Practice of Medicine.* New York: Appleton, 1892.
2. Bray GW. Recent advances in the treatment of asthma and hay fever. Practitioner 1934; 133: 368–379.
3. Kennedy JH. "Silent" gastroesophageal reflux: An important but little known cause of pulmonary complications. Dis Chest 1962; 42:42–45.
4. Koufman JA. The otolaryngologic manifestations of gastroesophageal reflux disease (GERD). In: Myers EN, Bluestone CD, Brackmann DE, Krause CJ eds. *Advances in Otolaryngology-Head and Neck Surgery, vol 7.* St. Louis: Mosby, 1993, pp. 15–14.
5. Demeester TR, Johnson LF, Joseph GJ, et al. Patterns of gastroesophageal reflux in health and disease. Ann Surg 1976; 184:459–470.
6. Orenstein SR. Invited review: Controversies in pediatric gastroesophageal reflux. J Pediatr Gastroenterol Nutr 1992; 14:338–348.
7. Orenstein SR, Magill HL, Brooks P. Thickening of infant feeding for the therapy of gastroesophageal reflux. J Pediatr 1987; 110:181–186.
8. Paton IY, Nanayakkhara CS, Simpson H. Vomiting and gastroesophageal reflux. Arch Dis Child 1988; 63:837–836.
9. Carre IJ. The natural history of the partial thoracic stomach hiatus hernia in children. Arch Dis Child 1959; 34:344–353.
10. Kibel MA. Gastroesophageal reflux and failure to thrive in infancy. In: Gells SS, ed. *Gastroesophageal Reflux 76th Ross Conference on Pediatric Research.* Columbus: Ross Laboratories; 1979: 39–42.

11. Treem WR, Davis PM, Hyams JS. Gastroesophageal reflux in the older child: Presentation, response to treatment and long-term follow-up. Clin Pediatr 1991; 30:435–440.

12. Cucchiara S, Stiano A, Casali LG, et al. Value of 24-hr intraoesophageal pH monitoring in children. Gut 1990; 31:129–133.

13. Schindlbeck NE, Ippisch H, Klauser AG, et al. What pH threshold is best in esophageal pH monitoring? Am J Gastroenterol 1991; 86:1138–1141.

14. Vandenplas Y, Sacre-Smits L. Continuous 24-hr esophageal pH monitoring in 285 asymptomatic infants 0–15 months old. J Pediatr Gastroenterol Nutr 1987; 6:220–224.

15. Vandenplas Y, Goyvaerts H, Helven R, et al. Gastroesophageal reflux as measured by 24-hr pH monitoring in 509 healthy infants screened for risk of sudden infant death syndrome. Pediatrics 1991; 88:834–840.

16. Boix-Ochoa J. Diagnosis and management of gastroesophageal reflux in children. Surg Ann 1981; 13:123–137.

17. Cohen RM, Weintraub A, Dimarino AJ, et al. Gastroesophageal reflux during gastrostomy feeding. Gastroenterol 1994; 106:13.

18. Hebra A, Hoffman MA. Gastroesophageal reflux in children. Pediatr Clin North Am 1993; 40:1233–1256.

19. Werlin SL, Dodds WJ, Hogan WJ, et al. Mechanisms of gastroesophageal reflux in children. J Pediatr 1980; 97:244–249.

20. Boyle JT, Altschuler SM, Patterson BL, et al. Reflex inhibition of the lower esophageal sphincter (LES) following stimulation of pulmonary vagal afferent receptors. Gastroenterol 1986; 90:1353.

21. Sondheimer JM. Clearance of spontaneous gastroesophageal reflux in awake and sleeping infants. Gastroenterol 1989; 97:821–826.

22. Helm JF, Dodds WJ, Riedel DR, et al. Determinants of esophageal acid clearance in normal subjects. Gastroenterol 1983; 85:607–612.

23. Gerhardt DC, Castell DO, Winship DH, et al. Esophageal dysfunction in esophageal regurgitation. Gastroenterol 1980; 78:893–897.

24. Sondeimer JM. Upper esophageal sphincter and pharyngoesophageal motor function in infants with and without gastroesophageal reflux. Gastroenterol 1983; 85:301–305.

25. Striano A, Cucciara S, De Visia B, et al. Disorders of upper esophageal sphincter motility in children. J Pediatr Gastroenterol Nutr 1987; 6:892–898.

26. Willing J, Davidson GP, Dent J, et al. Effect of gastroesophageal reflux on upper oesophageal sphincter mobility in children. Gut 1993; 34:904–916.

27. Putnam PE, Orenstein SR. Hoarseness in a child with gastroesophageal reflux. Acta Paediatr 1992; 81:635–686.

28. Burton DM, Pransky SM, Katz RM, Kearns DB, Seid KAB. Pediatric airway manifestations of gastroesophageal reflux. Ann Otol Rhinol Laryngol 1992; 101:742–749.

29. Andze GO, Brandt ML, St Vil D, et al. Diagnosis and treatment of gastroesophageal reflux in 500 children with respiratory symptoms: The values of pH monitoring. J Pediatr Surg 1991; 26:295–300.

30. Ramet J, Egreteau L, Cruzi-Dascaloval, et al. Cardiac, respiratory, and arousal responses to an esophageal acid infusion test in near-term infants during active sleep. J Pediatr Gastroenterol Nutr 1992; 15:135–140.

31. Bethmann O, Couchard M, Ajuriaguerra M, et al. Role of gastroesophageal reflux and vagal overactivity in apparent life-threatening events: 160 cases. Acta Paediatr 1993; 389(Supplement 82):102–104.

32. Jolley SG, Halpern LM, Tunell WP. The risk of sudden infant death from gastroesophageal reflux. J Pediatr Surg 1991; 26:691–696.

33. Jacob P, Kahrilas PJ, Iterzon G. Proximal esophageal pH-metry in patients with "reflux laryngitis." Gastroenterol 1991; 100:305–310.

34. Contencin P, Maurage C, Ployet M, et al. Symposium: Gastroesophageal reflux and ENT disorders in childhood. Int J Pediatr Otorhinolaryngol 1995; 32 (Supplement):35–144.

35. Orenstein SR, Orenstein DM, Whitington PF. Gastroesophageal reflux causing stridor. Chest 1983; 84:301–302.

36. Nielson DW, Heldt GP, Tooley WH. Stridor and gastroesophageal reflux in infants. Pediatrics 1990; 85:1034–1039.

37. Contencin P, Narcy P. Gastropharyngeal reflux in infants and children–A pharyngeal pH monitoring study. Arch Otolaryngol Head Neck Surg 1992; 18:1028–1030.

38. Berquist W, Rachelefsky GS, Kadden M, et al. Gastroesophageal reflux—Associated recurrent pneumonia and chronic asthma in children. Pediatrics 1981; 68:29–35.

39. Euler AR, Byrne WJ, Ament ME, et al. Recurrent pulmonary disease in children: A complication of gastroesophageal reflux. Pediatrics 1979; 63:47–51.

40. Boyle JT, Altschuler SM, Patterson BL, et al. Reflex inhibition of the lower esophageal sphincter (LES) following stimulation of pulmonary vagal afferent receptors. Gastroenterol 1986; 90:1353.

41. Bancewicz J, Bernstein A, Pierry A, et al. Surgery for gastroesophageal reflux in asthmatic patients. Br J Dis Chest 1981; 75:320.

42. Davis RS, Larsen GL, Grunstein MM. Respiratory response to intraesophageal acid infusion in asthmatic children during sleep. J Allergy Clin Immunol 1983; 72:393–398.

43. Moote DW, Lloyd DA, McCourtie DR, et al. Increase

in gastroesophageal reflux during methacholine induced bronchospasm. J Allergy Clin Immunol 1986; 78:619-623.

44. Herve P, Denjean A, Jian R, et al. Intraesophageal perfusion of acid increases the bronchomotor response to methacholine and to isocapnic hyperventilation in asthma subject. Am Rev Respir Dis 1986; 134:986-989.

45. Mansfield LE, Stein MR. Gastroesophageal reflux and asthma: A possible reflux mechanism. Ann Allergy 1978; 41:224-226.

46. Wennergren G, Bjure J, Gertzberg T, et al. Laryngeal reflex. Acta Paediatr 1993; 389(Supplement 82): 53-56.

47. Menon AP, Schlefft GL, Thach BT. Apnea associated with regurgitation in infants. J Pediatr 1985; 106;625.

48. Lanier B, Richardson MA, Cummings C. Effect of hypoxia on laryngeal reflux apnea–implications on sudden infant death. Otolaryngol Head Neck Surg 1983; 91:597-604.

49. Newman LJ, Russe J, Glassman MS, et al. Patterns of gastroesophageal reflux (GER) in patients with apparent life-threatening events. J Pediatr Gastroenterol Nutr 1989; 8:157-160.

50. NIH Consensus Development Conference on Infantile Apnea and Home Monitoring, September 29–October 1, 1986: Consensus statement. Pediatrics 1987; 79:292.

51. Sacre L, Vandenplas Y. Gastroesophageal reflux associated with respiratory abnormalities during sleep. J Pediatr Gastroenterol Nutr 1989; 9:28-33.

52. See CC, Newman IJ, Berezine S, et al. Gastroesophageal reflux-induced hypoxia in infants with apparent life-threatening events. Am J Dis Child 1989; 143: 951-954.

53. Veereman-Wauters G, Bochner A, Caillie-Bertrand MV. Gastroesophageal reflux in infants with a history of near-miss sudden infant death. J Pediatr Gastroenterol Nutr 1991; 12:319-323.

54. McMurray JC, Holinger LD. Otolaryngic manifestations in children presenting with apparent life threatening events. Otolaryngol Head Neck Surg 1997; 116:575-584.

55. Ariagno RL, Glotzbach SF. Sudden infant death syndrome. In: Rudolph AM, ed. *Pediatrics, 19th ed.* Norwalk: Appleton and Lange, 1991, 850-858.

56. Wetmore RF. Effects of acid on the larynx of the maturing rabbit and the possible significance to the sudden infant death syndrome. Laryngoscope 1993; 103:1242-1254.

57. Sondeimer JM. Gastroesophageal reflux in children: Clinical presentation and diagnostic evaluation. Gastrointest Endosc Clin N Am 1994; 4:55-74.

58. Orenstein SR, Cohn JF, Shalaby TM, et al. Reliability and validity of an infant gastroesophageal reflux questionnaire. Clin Pediatr 1993; 32:472-484.

59. Feranchak AP, Orenstein SR, Cohn JF. Behaviors associated with onset of gastroesophageal reflux episodes in infants. Prospective study using a split-screen video and a pH-probe. Clin Pediatr 1994; 33: 654-662.

60. Parsons DS. Chronic sinusitis a medical or surgical disease? Otolaryngol Clin North Am 1996; 29(1):1-9.

61. Contencin P, Narcy P. Nasopharyngeal pH monitoring in infants and children with chronic rhinopharyngitis. Int J Pediatr Otolaryngol 1991; 22:249-256.

62. Barbero GJ. Gastroesophageal reflux and upper airway disease: A commentary. Otolaryngol Clin North Am 1996; 29(1):27-36.

63. Gibson WS, Cochran W. Otalgia in infants and children: A manifestation of gastroesophageal reflux. Int J Pediatr Otorhinolaryngol 1994; 28:213-218.

64. Costantini M, Crookes PF, Bremner RM, et al. Value of physiologic assessment of foregut symptoms in a surgical practice. Surg 1993; 114:780-786.

65. Tolia V, Calhoun JA, Kuhns LR, et al. Lack of correlation between extended pH monitoring and scintigraphy in the evaluation of infants with gastroesophageal reflux. J Lab Clin Med 1990; 115:559-563.

66. Fisher RS, Mamud LS, Roberts GS, et al. Gastroesophageal (GE) scintiscanning to detect and quantitate GE reflux. Gastroenterol 1976; 70:301-306.

67. Varty K, Evans D, Kapila L. Paediatric gastro-esophageal reflux: Prognostic indicators from pH monitoring. Gut 1993; 34:1478-1481.

68. Tovar JA, Angulo JA, Gorostiaga L, et al. Surgery for gastroesophageal reflux in children with normal pH studies. J Pediatr Surg 1991; 26:541-545.

69. Ismail-Beigi F, Horton PF, Pope CF. Histological consequences of gastroesophageal reflux in man. Gastroenterol 1970; 58:163-174.

70. Nussbaum E, Maggi JC, Mathis R, et al. Association of lipid-laden alveolar macrophages and gastroesophageal reflux in children. J Pediatr 1987; 110: 190-194.

71. Tolia V, Lin CHM, Kuhns LR. Gastric emptying using three different formulas in infants with gastroesophageal reflux. J Pediatr Gastroenterol Nutr 1992; 15: 297-302.

72. Duke JC, Sekar KC, Torres R. Does increased osmolarity increase the exposure of an infant's esophagus to reflux? Clin Res 1990; 38:50.

73. Orenstein S, Magill H, Brooks P. Thickening of infant feedings for therapy of gastroesophageal reflux. J Pediatr 1987; 110:181-186.

74. Orenstein SR, Whitington PF, Orenstein DM. The infant seat as treatment for gastroesophageal reflux. N Engl J Med 1983; 309:760-763.

75. Meyers WF, Herbst JJ. Effectiveness of positioning therapy for gastroesophageal reflux. Pediatrics 1983; 69:768-772.

76. Orenstein SR. Prone positioning in infant gastro-

esophageal reflux: Is elevation of the head worth the trouble? J Pediatr 1990; 114:184–187.

77. AAP Task Force on infant positioning and SIDS: Positioning and SIDS. Pediatrics 1992; 89:1120.

78. Malfoot A, Dab I. New insights on gastroesophageal reflux in cystic fibrosis by longitudinal follow up. Arch Dis Child 1991; 66:1339–1345.

79. Justo RN, Gray PH. Fundoplication in preterm infants with gastroesophageal reflux. J Paediatr Child Health 1991; 27:250–254.

80. Carroccio A, Iacono G, Li Voti G, et al. Gastric emptying in infants with gastroesophageal reflux: Ultrasound evaluation before and after cisapride administration. Scand J Gastroenterol 1992; 27:799–804.

81. Andze GO, Brandt ML, St Vil D, et al. Diagnosis and treatment of gastroesophageal reflux in 500 children with respiratory symptoms: The value of pH monitoring. J Pediatr Surg 1991; 26:295–300.

82. Shulman RJ, Boyle T, Colletti RB, et al. A medical position statement of the North American society for pediatric gastroenterology and nutrition: The use of cisapride in children. J Pediatr Gastroenterol Nutr 1999;28:529–532.

83. Vandenplas Y, Beli DC, Benatar A, et al. A medical position statement of the European society of paediatric gastroenterology, hepatology, and nutrition: The role of cisapride in the treatment of pediatric gastroesophageal reflux. J Pediatr Gastroenterol Nutr 1999;28:518–528.

84. Kelly DA. Do H_2-receptor antagonists have a therapeutic role in childhood? J Pediatr Gastroenterol Nutr 1994; 19:270–276.

85. Sharma BK, Walt RP, Pounder RE, et al. Optimal dose of oral omeprazole for maximal 24 hour decrease of intragastric acidity. Gut 1984; 5:957–964.

86. Gunasekaran TS, Hassal EE. Efficacy and safety of omeprazole for severe gastroesophageal reflux in children. J Pediatr 1993; 123:148–154.

87. Fung KP, Seagram G, Pasieka J, et al. Investigation and outcome of 121 infants and children requiring Nissen fundoplication for management of gastroesophageal reflux. Invest Med 1990; 13:237–240.

88. Little AG. Mechanisms of action of antireflux surgery: Theory and fact. World J Surg 1992; 16:320–325.

89. Little AG, Ferguson MK, Skinner DB. Reoperation for failed antireflux operations. J Thorac Cardiovasc Surg 1986; 91:511–517.

38 Caustic Ingestion

James W. Forsen

A *poison* is any substance, either taken internally or applied externally, that is injurious to health. *Caustic agents* comprise a subset of poisons and are defined by their ability to burn tissue. *Caustic ingestion,* as a clinical malady, relates to mucosal burns of the upper aerodigestive tract (UADT) after the intake of a caustic agent.

Despite improvements in public awareness, federal legislation, and medical management, caustic ingestion continues to be a common and controversial problem facing the otolaryngologist. Although precise numbers are not available, it is estimated that there are 26,000 ingestions of caustic agents/year in the United States.[1] A large percentage of these may go unreported. There is a bimodal distribution of patients suffering caustic ingestion. The largest group is children between the ages of 1 and 3 years, and most of these ingestions are accidental. The other large group is made up of teenagers and adults who have ingested the agent in a suicide attempt or as a suicide gesture. In this latter group, females outnumber males.[2,3] As a rule, ingestions in adults attempting suicide tend to be more severe than pediatric accidental cases.

The modern era in the management of caustic ingestion began in the first quarter of this century and was pioneered by Chevalier Jackson. In 1902, he developed a distally-lighted esophagoscope, which not only allowed for better esophageal evaluation after corrosive injury, but also for therapeutic dilatation. Because of inadequate public information and product labeling, he treated a large number of children with severe esophageal strictures that were caused by the ingestion of lye, which is an alkali. Jackson lobbied the government persistently until 1929, when the Federal Caustic Act was passed.[4] This act provided for basic warning labels to be placed on toxic and caustic substances. A subsequent decrease in the incidence of severe lye ingestions resulted. The Federal Hazardous Substance Labeling Act was passed in 1960. In the mid-1960s, with the introduction of highly-concentrated, liquid-alkaline, drain cleaners in the United States, there was a corresponding increase in the number of severe esophageal injuries after pediatric ingestions. This led to the Safe Packaging Act in 1970, which limited liquid-alkaline cleaners to concentrations <10%.

AGENTS

The management of caustic ingestion must begin with knowledge of the various agents involved and their particular potential for injury. As different products become commercially available and popular with the public, incidence rates of ingestion increase accordingly. The medical community should respond not only with treatment, but also with efforts to educate themselves, manufacturers, the public, and often, the federal government. This cycle of events is likely to continue as new classes of caustics are introduced.

Alkalis

Alkalis are base-containing products, or to put it another way, molecular substances that are able to accept a free H^+ ion. They represent the largest group of agents that are responsible for caustic ingestion, and also are responsible for the majority of esophageal injuries. However, there are no reports of death due to systemic toxicity after alkaline ingestion.[5]

Lyes are alkaline agents, which usually contain NaOH, KOH, or CaOH. They have been used for years as household and farm cleaning products and in soap making. In the United States, although liquid lyes cannot exceed a concentration of 10%, solid

Pediatric Otolaryngology, Edited by R.F. Wetmore, H.R. Muntz, and T.J. McGill. Thieme Medical Publishers, Inc., New York © 2000.

635

compounds may be much stronger. Lyes cause pain immediately upon contact with oral mucosa, and the form of the agent often limits the amount of agent ingested. Solid or granular lyes are less likely than liquid compounds to cause severe esophageal injury because they can be spit out before significant amounts are ingested. Lye injuries in the United States usually are due to drain pipe cleaners. There remains a high incidence of lye injuries in certain regions of the world such as Eastern Europe and the Middle East, where there is poor community awareness of the problem and regulations are less rigid.

Special Consideration:

Solid or granular lyes are less likely than liquid compounds to cause severe esophageal injury because they can be spit out before significant amounts are ingested.

Formerly, most household detergents were only mildly alkaline, but environmental concern led to the development of nonphosphate detergents. These latter agents contain ingredients such as silicates and carbonates that can increase the pH.[8] Experimentally, nonphosphate detergents can cause severe mucosal injury, but there are few reports of serious human esophageal injury.[7] Einhorn et al. reported eight pediatric cases of ingestion or inhalation of detergent powder that resulted in respiratory distress.[8] Four children required short-term intubation, but there were no serious sequelae. There was a reported case of hypopharyngeal stricture after ingestion of a powdered dishwashing detergent.[9] Krenzelok reported 145 ingestions of liquid dishwashing detergents with no subsequent development of esophageal injury.[10]

Hair relaxing agents are alkaline compounds that are used to straighten hair. With a pH range of 11.5 to 12.5, they have the theoretical capability of causing significant esophageal injury. In practice, however, this has not been observed.[11] These agents are prepared as creams, and this thick consistency coupled with a noxious taste limits the amount ingested. Most cases still undergo esophagoscopy.

Household ammonia in the United States is usually a low concentration that is <4%. The pH is between 9 and 12.[12] There have been case reports of esophageal injury from ammonia,[13] but these are

rare and usually are due to more concentrated solutions. A more immediate concern is the potential for laryngeal and pharyngeal edema after ammonia ingestions. This may necessitate intubation or tracheotomy.

The common use of disc batteries as power sources for devices such as hearing aids, watches, cameras, and radios began in the 1970s. Subsequently, ingestion cases began to increase, and there is now an estimated minimum incidence of 2100 cases per year in the United States.[14] Most disc batteries contain concentrated solutions of KOH or NaOH contained within heavy metal containers made of mercury, zinc, silver, nickel, lithium, or cadmium. The most frequently swallowed disc batteries are those from hearing aids (45%), and these accidents often involve children removing the battery from their own hearing aids.[14] Maves et al. demonstrated that these batteries could cause mucosal damage to a cat esophagus within 1 hour.[15] Complete perforation occurred in 4 hours. Clinical cases of esophageal stricture and perforation, and even of death, have occurred after batteries have become lodged in the esophagus. Outcome seems to be related to the size of the battery because larger ones (e.g., lithium) are more likely to resist normal passage. Injury may be due to leakage of alkaline contents, low-wattage electrical burns, or pressure necrosis. Mercuric oxide batteries have fragmented within the gastrointestinal (GI) system with subsequent elevation of blood mercury levels. No patient, however, has demonstrated mercury toxicity.[14]

Special Consideration:

Cases of esophageal stricture and perforation, and even of death, have occurred after disc batteries have become lodged in the esophagus.

Acids

Acids are substances with the ability to donate a free H^+ ion. In the United States, acids account for approximately 15% of caustic ingestions.[16] This percentage may be higher among those individuals attempting suicide. Also, ingestion of acids may be more common in other countries. For instance, Finland has banned the sale of lye products since 1969. Subsequently, acids are responsible for 25% of pediatric caustic ingestions, and cause the most severe esophageal injuries.[17] Commonly ingested acidic agents include toilet bowl cleaners, swimming pool cleaners, soldering fluxes, and rust removers. The involved acids include hydrochloric, sulfuric, phosphoric, oxallic, nitric, and others.

Bleaches

Household bleach contains sodium hypochlorite, usually in concentrations <6%. At these low concentrations, the pH is near neutral. Accordingly, ingestion of household bleach is rarely, if ever, associated with significant esophageal injury. However, swimming pool cleaners and commercial preparations may be more concentrated and, therefore, have the potential to burn.

SPECIAL CONSIDERATION:

Ingestion of household bleach is rarely, if ever, associated with significant esophageal injury.

Other

Thermal burns to the UADT are frequent, though rarely of clinical consequence. Ingestion of hot liquids, potatoes, pizza, and other foods may burn the oral cavity or pharynx, but the esophagus is usually spared. Scarring is not a common concern; however, edema of the upper airway may ensue and precipitate respiratory distress. This is seen most frequently in thermal supraglottitis after feeding a baby a bottle heated in the microwave. Differential heating may allow extremely hot formula to be given to the child.

Pill-induced esophageal injury occurs when ingested medications lodge in the esophagus. Delayed esophageal motility may affect any individual, but is more common in debilitated, dehydrated elderly patients. Antibiotics, such as tetracycline and doxycycline, account for 60% of pill-induced esophageal injuries. They may induce a local drop in pH or may cause injury due to a toxic accumulation of the drug. Antiinflammatory pills and, in particular, potassium chloride pills, may cause hemorrhage, stricture, and even death.[18]

TOXICITY

There are several factors responsible for a caustic agents' ability to produce mucosal injury. As concentration of the agent increases, so does its ability to cause damage. This was demonstrated by Krey who applied varying concentrations of NaOH to rabbit esophagi.[19] Haller and Bachman obtained similar results in cats.[20] Viscosity of the offending agent has intuitively been considered important,[20] but is not a clinically useful measurement.[5] Hoffman et al. determined that the titratable acid or alkaline reserve of an agent correlated well with its ability to injure the esophagus.[12] This correlation was even better than that seen with pH. However, in the clinical setting, titratable acid or alkaline reserve of an agent is not a value that is readily available or easily determined. In contrast, the pH of most commercially-available caustics is obtainable by contacting the local poison control center. There is a relatively good correlation between pH and the degree of injury. The critical pH that causes esophageal ulceration is 12.5. Most cases of ulceration that go on to stricture involve agents with a pH of 14, usually lyes.[5] Any patient, therefore, who ingests an alkaline agent with a pH ≥12 must be followed closely to rule out esophageal injury. There is less information regarding the critical acidic pH that is responsible for esophageal injury. In general, any acid with a pH ≤2 should be considered fully capable of causing severe damage. Finally, other factors, such as the amount ingested, the agent's form (liquid vs. solid), contact time with the mucosa, and the underlying condition of the esophagus, play some role in determining the ultimate extent of injury.

SPECIAL CONSIDERATION:

The critical basic pH that causes esophageal ulceration is 12.5. In general, any acid with a pH ≤2 should be considered fully capable of causing severe damage.

PATHOPHYSIOLOGY

Alkalis damage mucosa by way of liquefactive necrosis. The agent penetrates rapidly and deeply and continues to burn until it is diluted or neutralized by the tissue itself. Depth of burn is determined by the toxic factors already discussed.

There are three relatively distinct pathophysiologic phases to the injury. The *burn phase* causes necrosis of the superficial epithelium with possible deeper extension. Blood vessel thrombosis, fatty saponification, and infiltration of bacteria and polymorphonuclear leukocytes occur within 48 hours.[22] The mucosa initially appears erythematous or cyanotic. Between 2 and 5 days, a cast forms and later sloughs. The *reparative phase* begins approximately 5 days after ingestion. Granulation tissue forms at the periphery of the ulcer and fibroblasts deposit collagen.[6] Squamous reepithelialization begins. The *scar phase* begins between the second and third weeks. If the burn was a circumferential injury, then a stricture of the esophagus may result. The likelihood of stricture is directly related to the depth of the initial injury.

The most likely sites of injury include those where the agent may pool (such as the hypopharynx) and those where there are levels of esophageal anatomic narrowing (such as at the cricopharyngeus, the aortic arch, the left main bronchus, and the diaphragmatic hiatus. In 80% of cases of alkaline ingestion, the stomach is spared.[18] However, gastric scarring and even perforation can occur if large quantities of alkali were ingested or if the agent was highly concentrated.

AT A GLANCE . . .

Sites of Caustic Injury

- Hypopharynx
- Level of cricopharyngeus
- Level of aortic arch
- Level of left mainstem bronchus
- Level of the diaphragmatic hiatus

Acids damage mucosa by way of *coagulation necrosis,* whereby a coagulum forms at the interface between the agent and mucosa and acts to reduce further penetration of the agent into the muscle layers. The esophagus is frequently spared after strong acid exposure because of its slightly alkaline pH and the resistance of its squamous epithelium to acid.[23] The most significant complications involving acids usually occur in the gastroduodenal region, particularly near the antrum. However, if large quantities are ingested, as in patients attempting suicide, the esophagus is equally at risk.[24]

PRESENTATION

Pediatric caustic ingestion results in a constellation of signs and symptoms. Children frequently present with burns to their hands and face. The lips may be swollen and blistered. Erythema and burns to the oral cavity are relatively easy to identify. If the agent actually was swallowed, many children will display drooling and will refuse to take anything by mouth. Retching and vomiting are common after caustic ingestion. Chest and abdominal pain can be more ominous signs of severe injury and possible perforation. Stridor, wheezing, and hoarseness are indications of possible respiratory injury and compromise. Laryngeal and pharyngeal edema is not uncommon and requires rapid evaluation.

Numerous investigators have evaluated the presentation of children after caustic ingestion to determine the relationship between signs and symptoms and the degree of injury. There is a general consensus that no one particular sign or symptom is consistently predictive of the presence of significant esophageal burns. In a multicenter study, Gaudreault et al. found that vomiting, dysphagia, excessive salivation, and abdominal pain (in decreasing order) were the signs and symptoms most frequently associated with severe esophageal injury.[25] Crain et al. compared the incidence of vomiting, drooling, and stridor with esophagoscopy findings and reported that half of those patients with these signs had second or third degree burns.[26] Vergauwen et al. also found a high incidence of significant esophageal burns in patients presenting with vomiting and/or respiratory distress.[27]

It is important to note that the absence of oral cavity burns does not rule out the possibility of severe, more distal injury.[25,28] However, several groups have reported that the absence of all signs and symptoms after caustic ingestion makes the likelihood of significant esophageal injury exceedingly small.[26,29,30] In these cases, the physicians recommend no further evaluation. This is a controversial stance.

SPECIAL CONSIDERATION:

There is a general consensus that no one particular sign or symptom is consistently predictive of the significant esophageal burn. It is important to note that the absence of oral cavity burns does not rule out the possibility of severe distal injury.

CARE OF THE CAUSTIC-INGESTION PATIENT

Practice Pathway 38–1 outlines the care of the caustic-ingestion patient.

Emergency Care

Care of the pediatric caustic-ingestion patient often begins with the call of a distraught parent to an emergency room (ER). If there is suspicion of ingestion of a corrosive substance, the parent should be instructed to irrigate all contact sites and to have the child drink either milk or water. The former acts to neutralize the agent and the latter dilutes it. Giving an acid to neutralize an alkali is not recommended. Induced emesis is to be avoided, as this would provide a second opportunity for the caustic to burn the esophagus. The patient should then be brought promptly to the ER.

Once at the hospital, initial management of the caustic-ingestion patient follows ER routine. Securing an airway and cardiovascular support are priorities, although rarely necessary. A concerted effort should be made to determine the type and amount of agent ingested. If possible, it is helpful to have a family member bring in any remaining agent and the original container. The pH as well as other pertinent information can be obtained by contacting a poison control center. Interviewing witnesses to the ingestion may help determine the amount ingested and whether the patient suffered emesis, aspiration, or respiratory distress. If the ingested agent is neither toxic nor caustic and the patient is without symptoms or evidence of injury, discharge from the hospital is reasonable. All other patients require further evaluation.

After obtaining vital signs, a complete physical examination is performed with particular attention paid to the UADT mucosa. It is important to examine the patient's entire body to check for any skin burns due to spilled agent. Any obvious skin or oral cavity burns are washed with a copious amount of water. Flexible fiberoptic nasopharyngolaryngoscopy is recommended and is very helpful in detecting upper airway injury.

Intravenous (IV) access is obtained, and blood samples for a complete blood count and electrolytes are sent. If there is respiratory compromise, an arterial blood gas sample is obtained. A chest X-ray is routine and is evaluated for evidence of pulmonary edema, infiltrates, free peritoneal air, or other evidence of injury. Further abdominal films are ordered for patients with abdominal pain to rule out the possibility of viscus perforation. Gastric lavage, charcoal, and emetics are contraindicated. The passage of a nasogastric tube is controversial and usually not recommended.

There are few cases of caustic ingestion that require true emergent intervention. If there has been perforation of the esophagus or stomach, an emergent laparotomy with possible gastrectomy, esophagectomy, or esophagogastrectomy may be necessary. This is very unusual in children, and usually occurs in an adult who has ingested a large amount of a strong acid or base in an effort to commit suicide. Impending airway loss clearly requires rapid intervention. This may be seen after ingestion of very powerful caustics, after emesis with subsequent aspiration of a caustic, or after relatively mild ingestions of specific agents such as ammonia and powder detergents. These latter two compounds are rarely known to cause severe esophageal injury, but have been known to generate significant pharyngolaryngeal edema that can develop rapidly, though with delayed onset of symptoms. A high index of suspicion for potential airway injury can lead to timely intubation and avoid an urgent tracheotomy.

A final type of ingestion that requires emergent management is that involving miniature or disc batteries. A chest X-ray is mandatory to determine the position of the battery. If it is lodged in the esophagus, the patient is taken immediately to the operating room for esophagoscopy and removal. As noted earlier, esophageal injury, including perforation, can occur quickly. If the battery is detected within the stomach, then it is allowed to pass through the

Practice Pathway 38–1   CAUSTIC INGESTION

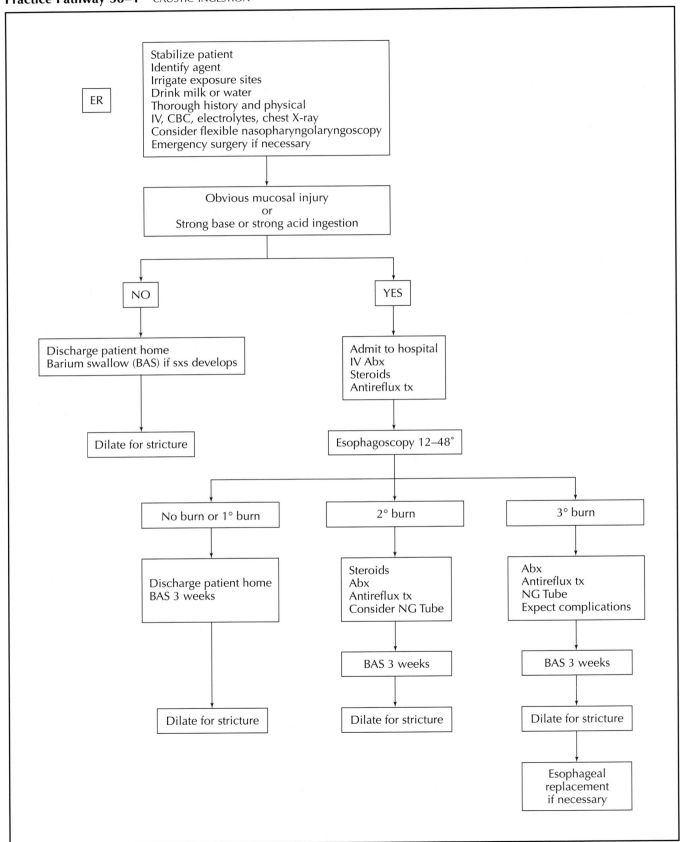

Abbreviations: IV, Intravenous; CBC, Complete Blood Count; BAS, bariums swallow; SXS, symptoms; Abx, antibiotics; tx, treatment; NG, nasogastric.

remainder of the gastrointestinal tract. Parents should monitor the child's stools for the battery. If the foreign body has not passed within 7 days or if the child develops abdominal pain, a repeat X-ray is taken. Rarely does the battery require open surgical removal, and occasionally may linger more than 2 weeks before finally being expelled. If a mercury-containing battery ruptures within the stomach or intestines, serial blood mercury levels should be followed.

Because bleach ingestions rarely are associated with significant esophageal injury, many of these patients are sent home directly from the ER. Most bleaches used in this country are weak in concentration and a large volume must be swallowed before esophageal erosion occurs. This is unlikely in cases of accidental ingestion. If there are oral cavity burns, however, these patients are investigated further. Bleach concentrations may be higher in Europe and other countries and are more likely to cause esophageal injury.

Caustic ingestion in the pediatric age group often is evidence of stress and discord within the patient's home. This sort of environment puts the child and siblings at risk for a repeat ingestion, as well as possible neglect or even abuse.[31] Treating physicians should have a low threshold for involving social services in the care of these patients and their families. Obviously, any patient who has attempted suicide with a caustic agent requires urgent psychiatric consultation and suicide precautions.

SPECIAL CONSIDERATION:

Caustic ingestion in the pediatric age group often is evidence of stress and discord within the patient's home.

Intermediate Care

Any patient who is symptomatic or has ingested a strong acid or base should be admitted for overnight hospital observation. After life-threatening issues have been addressed, attention is then directed toward evaluating and managing injury to the UADT, particularly the esophagus. The early medical management of caustic ingestion primarily is concerned with the prevention of esophageal stricture forma-

tion, and it remains controversial. Traditionally, burns have been graded according to the following criteria: (1) *first-degree burns* involve erythema and/or edema of the mucosa; (2) *second-degree burns* involve full thickness injury to the mucosa and/or submucosa, including bleb formation or ulceration; and (3) *third-degree burns* involve full thickness esophageal injury with perforation into or through the muscular layers. General clinical consensus seems to maintain that first-degree injuries require no treatment as there is little or no risk of stricture. On the other hand, third-degree burns are likely to scar and stricture regardless of medical treatment. Disagreement continues as to the efficacy of steroid use in the management of second-degree burns.

AT A GLANCE . . .
Grading of Esophageal Burns

First Degree: erythema/edema of mucosa

Second Degree: injury to mucosa and submucosa

Third Degree: full thickness injury with muscular involvement

---

Steroid therapy in the management of caustic ingestion was proposed after the work of Spain in 1950.[32] He showed that corticosteroids inhibited fibroplasia and early scar formation in mice. Haller and Bachman demonstrated that the combination of prednisolone and antibiotics decreased stricture formation after the application of lye to cat esophagi.[20] Krey also showed experimentally that antibiotics control local inflammation and granulation tissue formation to affect healing favorably.[19] Large clinical studies by Adam[33] and Hawkins et al.[34] supported the notion that steroids and antibiotics in combination were most efficacious when used to treat second-degree esophageal burns. This was challenged by a prospective, randomized study by Anderson et al. that showed no benefit from the use of steroids to treat children who have ingested a caustic substance.[35] One criticism of this study is that there was a 24-hour delay in starting the steroid regimen after the ingestion.

As there may be some benefit in reducing the early local inflammatory response and because there is little risk with short-term usage, we routinely begin steroids in cases where there is suspicion of more than a first-degree burn. We do not wait until esophagoscopy to determine whether to start steroids because there is evidence that they are more effective if given soon after the ingestion. Corticosteroids are contraindicated in cases of esophageal or gastric perforation. There is no consensus on the appropriate dosing. A single dose of dexamethasone (1 mg/kg IV, up to 25 mg) is given initially, and the need for further steroid administration is determined at the time of esophagoscopy. In these same patients, we begin broad spectrum IV antibiotics (ampicillin, 100 mg/kg/day IV q 6 hr or clindamycin, 40 mg/kg/day IV q 6 hr). The antibiotics act to decrease local bacterial colonization and the formation of granulation tissue at sites of mucosal injury. Granulation tissue predisposes to fibrosis and possible stricture. Gastroesophageal reflux (GER) is common after caustic ingestion, and the acidic irritation can act to worsen ulceration. Reflux should be treated aggressively with an H_2-receptor blocker.

SPECIAL CONSIDERATION:

We do not wait until esophagoscopy to determine whether to start steroids because there is evidence that they are more effective if given soon after the ingestion.

Definitive evaluation of the esophagus should be performed 12 to 48 hours after the injury. Evaluation prior to this interval may lead to under-diagnosis as the full extent of mucosal damage may not be evident yet. Barium swallow is not as sensitive as esophagoscopy in the diagnosis of less dramatic, but potentially clinically-relevant, esophageal burns. Therefore, the procedure of choice is esophagoscopy. According to an analysis of nine separate reports, which included a total of 1961 caustic-ingestion cases, 83% of patients underwent this procedure.[17] The timing of esophagoscopy after the ingestion is controversial. Though many clinicians

advocate waiting at least 24 hours, it is unlikely that a significant burn will be missed if the procedure is performed only 12 hours after the ingestion. This interval also will eliminates unnecessary hospital admission time for the majority of patients who fortunately will have no significant esophageal injury. Essentially every patient who has ingested a strong acid or strong base other than bleach should undergo esophagoscopy. Esophagoscopy is a low-risk and inexpensive procedure, which is very sensitive in detecting esophageal injury.

SPECIAL CONSIDERATION:

Definitive evaluation of the esophagus should be performed within 12 to 48 hours after a caustic injury of the esophagus.

There is also controversy regarding rigid versus flexible techniques. Traditionally, the latter has been more widely used by gastroenterologists and has the advantage of allowing for gastroduodenoscopy. Otorhinolaryngologists have preferred rigid esophagoscopy and, in experienced hands, the risk of perforation does not seem to be significantly higher than with the flexible scopes. After the patient is intubated, direct pharyngolaryngoscopy should always be performed. This may be followed by tracheobronchoscopy if indicated. Esophagoscopy should proceed cautiously and not distal to a visualized full-thickness burn. Flexible gastroduodenoscopy should always follow rigid esophagoscopy if there is any concern or possibility of gastric injury. If no esophageal burn is found at esophagoscopy, or if only minor first-degree burns are noted, the patient is discharged home. A barium esophagram is performed at 3 weeks postingestion.

Those patients with second-degree esophageal burns are kept in the hospital for several days. Prednisone is given (1 mg/kg b.i.d) for 2 weeks and then tapered over a period of 4 more weeks. This long course of corticosteroids is thought to decrease the collagen deposition and subsequent fibrosis that occurs during healing. Antibiotics (amoxicillin or clindamycin) are continued orally at usual dosages for

2 weeks. H$_2$-receptor blockers are given for 2 to 4 weeks. All patients should have a barium esophogram performed at 3 weeks postingestion, as this is when strictures first become evident.

For circumferential second-degree and all third-degree burns, a nasogastric (NG) tube or esophageal stent is left in place for 6 weeks. Reyes developed a silastic stent that was effective in preventing stricture formation in both cats and humans with full-thickness esophageal injuries after caustic ingestion.[36] Wijburg presented two reports of successful treatment of esophageal burns with a special silicone NG tube.[37,38] Antibiotics along with an H$_2$-receptor blocker and a prokinetic agent, such as lisapride, are used. Steroids are contraindicated in this group of patients. Severely burned patients may remain in the hospital for an extended period due to the risk from late massive hemorrhage, which can result after esophagogastric necrosis. If stricture becomes evident, serial dilations are then started.

Late Care

Serial dilations usually are performed under general anesthesia. This should begin as soon as the diagnosis of stricture is made. The procedure initially is performed several times per week and later the frequency is determined by symptoms of dysphagia. There are several different types of esophageal dilators; the most commonly used are mercury-filled bougies. Acute complications of dilation include esophageal perforation and mediastinitis; therefore, a dilator should never be forced through a stricture. Some patients can be managed for years with infrequent and effective dilations. Efficacy of the treatment is in large part determined by the degree of esophageal wall thickening.[39]

If the stricture progresses or becomes difficult to dilate using the anterograde method, then Tucker retrograde bougienage is an option.[40] This form of dilation is performed through a gastrostomy with a continuous string in the esophagus and offers several advantages. The esophagus often is dilated above a stricture and funnel-shaped below it. In addition, strictures may be multiple and lumina can be placed eccentrically. Anterograde dilation, therefore, runs the risk of creating a false passage with subsequent perforation. Retrograde bougies are safer and easier to advance in more severe or complicated strictures. Though usually done under general anesthesia, the technique can be performed outside of the operating room.

> ## SPECIAL CONSIDERATION:
>
> Anterograde dilation of an esophageal stricture runs the risk of creating a false passage with subsequent perforation; retrograde bougienage is safer and easier to perform in severe or complicated cases.

It must be remembered that patients with esophageal injury secondary to caustic ingestion are at significantly higher risk for developing squamous cell carcinoma of the esophagus. Chronic dilations actually may increase this risk, and these patients must be followed for many years. Late dysphagia can be due to stricture, tumor, or both. In a review of 2400 patients with carcinoma of the esophagus, Appelqvist found 2.6% had a history of caustic ingestion.[41] The mean age at the time of diagnosis was 48 years. Most of the lesions occurred at the level of the carina.

If esophageal stricture progresses or becomes complete, then dilation attempts must be halted and more definitive treatment sought. There are several options available for reconstruction or replacement of the esophagus. Jejunal free grafts have been used for high esophageal lesions. Colonic interposition is the procedure of choice for complete esophageal replacement, although gastric tubing or gastric pull-up procedures may be considered. If there is at least some lumen remaining within the esophagus to allow for emptying of secretions into the stomach, the esophagus may be left in situ. If this is not the case, the esophagus is removed. Although esophageal replacement usually is successful, there is a relatively high rate of complications, including stricture at anastomoses, fistulization, and persistent dysphagia.[42,43]

CONCLUSION

Pediatric caustic ingestion continues to be a significant clinical problem both in the United States and abroad. Through the concerted work of Chevalier Jackson and many others, severe esophageal burns are fortunately rare. The controversies in medical and surgical management of caustic ingestion should not obscure the reality that the best approach is through prevention, which means education of parents and the community.

REFERENCES

1. Lovejoy FH Jr. Corrosive injury of the esophagus in children. New Engl J Med 1990; 323(10):668–669.
2. Hawkins DB, Demeter MJ, Barnett TE. Caustic ingestion: Controversies in management. A review of 214 cases. Laryngoscope 1980; 90:98–109.
3. Christesen HBT. Caustic ingestion in adults—epidemiology and prevention. Clin Toxicol 1994; 32(5): 557–568.
4. Jackson C. The life of Chevalier Jackson—Autobiography. New York: MacMillan, 1938.
5. Vancura EM, Clinton JE, Ruiz E, et al. Toxicity of alkaline solutions. Ann Emerg Med 1980; 9:118–22.
6. Kikendall JW. Caustic ingestion injuries. Gastroenterol Clin North Am 1991; 20(4):847–857.
7. Lee JF, Simonowitz D, Block GE. Corrosive injury of the stomach and esophagus by nonphosphate detergents. Am J Surg 1972; 123:652–656.
8. Einhorn A, Horton L, Altieri M, et al. Serious respiratory consequences of detergent ingestions in children. Pediatrics 1989; 84(3):472–474.
9. McLear PW, Hayden RE, Muntz HR, et al. Free flap reconstruction of recalcitrant hypoparyngeal stricture. Am J Otolaryngol 1991; 12:76–82.
10. Krenzelok EP. Liquid automatic dishwashing detergents: A profile of toxicity. Ann Emerg Med 1989; 18(1):60–63.
11. Forsen JF, Muntz HR. Hair relaxer ingestion: A new trend. Ann Otol Rhinol Laryngol 1993; 102:781–784.
12. Hoffman RS, Howland MA, Kamerow HN, et al. Comparison of titratable acid/alkaline reserve and pH in potentially caustic household products. Clin Toxicol 1989; 27:241–61.
13. Klein J, Olson KR, McKinney HE. Caustic injury from household ammonia. Am J Emerg Med 1985; 3:320.
14. Litovitz T, Schmitz BF. Ingestion of cylindrical and button batteries: An analysis of 2382 cases. Pediatrics 1992; 89:747–757.
15. Maves MD, Carithers JS, Birek HG. Disc battery ingestion. Ann Otol Rhinol Laryngol 1984; 93:364–368.
16. Moore WR. Caustic ingestions. Pathophysiology, diagnosis and treatment. Clin Pediatr 1986; 25: 192–196.
17. Nuutinen M, Uhari M, Karvali T, et al. Consequences of caustic ingestions in children. Acta Paediatr 1994; 83:1200–1205.
18. Kikendall JW. Pill-induced esophageal injury. Gastroenterol Clin North Am 1991; 20(4):835–846.
19. Krey H. On the treatment of corrosive lesions in the oesophagus: An experimental study. Acta Otolaryngol 1952; 102:1–45.

20. Haller JA, Bachman K. The comparative effect of current therapy on experimental caustic burns of the esophagus. Pediatrics 1964; 34:236–245.
21. Leape LL, Ashcroft KW, Scarpelli DG, et al. Hazard to health—Liquid lye. N Engl J Med 1971; 284: 578–581.
22. Howell JM. Alkaline ingestions. Ann Emerg Med 1986; 15:820–825.
23. Maull KI, Scher LA, Greenfield LJ. Surgical implications of acid ingestion. Surg Gynecol Obstet 1979; 184:895–900.
24. Zargar SA, Kochhar R, Nagi B, et al. Ingestion of corrosive acids. Gastroenterology 1989; 97:702–707.
25. Gaudreault P, Parent M, McGuigan MA, et al. Predictability of esophageal injury from signs and symptoms: A study of caustic ingestion in 378 children. Pediatrics 1983; 71:767–770.
26. Crain EF, Gershel JC, Mezey AP. Caustic ingestions. Am J Dis Child 1984; 138:863–865.
27. Vergauwen P, Moulin D, Buts JP, et al. Caustic burns of the upper digestive and respiratory tracts. Eur J Pediatr 1991; 150:700–703.
28. Previtera C, Giusti F, Guglielmi M. Predictive value of visible lesions (cheeks, lips, oropharynx) in suspected caustic ingestion: May endoscopy reasonably be omitted in completely negative pediatric patients? Ped Emerg Care 1990; 6:176–178.
29. Christesen HBT. Prediction of complications following unintentional caustic ingestion in children. Acta Paediatr 1995; 84:1177–1182.
30. Byrne WJ. Foreign bodies, bezoars, and caustic ingestion. Gastrointest Endosc Clin N Am 1994; 4(1): 99–119.
31. Friedman EM. Caustic ingestions and foreign body aspirations: An overlooked form of child abuse. Ann Otol Rhinol Laryngol 1987; 96:709–712.
32. Spain DM, Molomut N, Haber A. Biological studies on cortisone in mice. Science 1950; 112:335–337.
33. Adam JS, Birck HG. Pediatric caustic ingestion. Ann Otol Rhinol Laryngol 1982; 91:656–658.
34. Hawkins DB, Demeter MJ, Barnett TE. Caustic ingestion: Controversies in management. A review of 214 cases. Laryngoscope 1980; 90:98–109.
35. Anderson KD, Rouse TM, Randolph JG. A controlled trial of corticosteroids in children with corrosive injury of the esophagus. N Engl J Med 1990; 323: 637–640.
36. Reyes HM, Hill JL. Modification of the experimental stent technique for esophageal burns. J Surg Res 1976; 20:65–70.
37. Wijburg FA, Beukers MM, Heymans HS, et al. Nasogastric intubation as sole treatment of caustic esophageal lesions. Ann Otol Rhinol Laryngol 1985; 94: 337–341.
38. Wijburg FA, Heymans HAS, Urbanus NAM. Caustic

esophageal lesions in childhood: Prevention of stricture formation. J Ped Surg 1989; 24:171–173.

39. Lahoti D, Broor SL, Basu PP. Corrosive esophageal strictures: Predictors of response to endoscopic dilation. Gastrointest Endosc 1956; 41:196–200.

40. Tucker JA, Turtz ML, Silberman HD, et al. Tucker retrograde esophageal dilation 1924–1974. Ann Otol Rhinol Laryngol 1974; 83(Supplement):1–35.

41. Appleqvist P, Salmo M. Lye corrosion carcinoma of the esophagus. Cancer 1980; 45:2655–2658.

42. Csendes A, Braghetto I. Surgical management of esophageal strictures. Hepatogastroenterology 1992; 39:502–510.

43. Hendren WH, Hendren, WG. Colon interposition for esophagus in children. J Pediatr Surg 1985; 20: 829–839.

39 Diseases of the Salivary Glands

Hani Z. Ibrahim and Steven D. Handler

Salivary gland diseases in children are not common. Although aspects of these disorders are similar in adults and children, there are some features that are unique to children. The otolaryngologist treating a child with a salivary gland disorder must have a knowledge of the anatomy and physiology of the major and minor salivary glands and of the inflammatory, traumatic, and neoplastic processes that can affect them in children.

BASIC SCIENCE

Embryology and Anatomy

The salivary glands develop during the sixth to eighth week of gestation. Outpouching of the ectodermal oral mucosa is followed by branching into intercalated ducts and acinar cells. The *parotid glands* are the first to form, and they travel the furthest from their point of origin in the oral mucosa to surround the facial nerve. Mesenchymal condensation around and into the major salivary glands results in the fibrous capsules and septations of these organs. Among the major salivary glands, the parotids are encapsulated last. As a result, surrounding lymphoid tissue is included within the parotid parenchyma. This fact accounts for the occurrence of clinically-apparent, intraparotid lymph nodes.

The parotid gland is the largest of the salivary glands. It is bounded by the external auditory canal (EAC) posteriorly, the zygomatic arch superiorly, the masseter muscle anteriorly, and the styloid process and muscles medially. Inferiorly, the parotid can extend over the sternocleidomastoid muscle. Demarcated by the facial nerve, the parotid is divided into a superficial and deep lobe. Therefore, prior to any surgical manipulation of the parotid gland, emphasis is placed on identifying the main trunk of the facial nerve as it leaves the stylomastoid foramen and enters the parotid parenchyma. Medial extension of parotid tissue around the mandibular ramus places parotid tissue in the parapharyngeal space. The gland is tightly encapsulated between the superficial and deep layers of the deep cervical fascia.[1] Fascial septa result in noncommunicating compartments that tend to prevent coalescence of an abscess.[2] The parotid duct (*Stenson's Duct*) leaves the gland at its anterior border just below the zygomatic arch and crosses the masseter muscle in a path to the buccal mucosa, opening opposite of the second upper molar.

> ### SPECIAL CONSIDERATION:
> Head and neck lymphadenopathy commonly can involve intraparotid lymph nodes and present as parotid masses.

The submandibular gland (*submaxillary gland*) lies in the submandibular triangle and is bound by the anterior and posterior bellies of the digastric muscle and the inferior rim of the mandible. Wrapping around the posterior margin of the mylohyoid muscle, the gland is divided into a superficial lobe and a much smaller deep lobe. Retraction of the mylohyoid muscle anteriorly provides access to the submandibular duct (*Wharton's Duct*) as well as exposure of the underlying lingual nerve, submandibular ganglion and, inferiorly, the hypoglossal nerve. The submandibular duct travels medially to open in the floor of mouth, just lateral to the lingual frenulum.

The smallest of the major salivary glands, the *sublingual gland* lies just deep to the mucosa of the floor of the mouth. Laterally, the gland is bordered by the mandible as well as the genioglossus muscle. The gland lies over the mylohyoid muscle. Approxi-

Pediatric Otolaryngology, Edited by R.F. Wetmore, H.R. Muntz, and T.J. McGill. Thieme Medical Publishers, Inc., New York © 2000.

mately ten small ducts exit the gland (*Ducts of Rivinus*) and open directly into the floor of mouth. If consolidated, these ducts form a single sublingual duct (*Bartholin's Duct*) that usually empties into the submandibular duct.[1] Throughout the oral and pharyngeal mucosa, approximately 600 to 1000 minor salivary glands drain directly into the oral and pharyngeal cavities.

The major salivary glands are supplied by both sympathetic and parasympathetic innervation. The superior cervical ganglion provides the sympathetic input that is delivered along arterial vessels to the corresponding gland. The *auriculotemporal nerve* carries postganglionic parasympathetic fibers from the otic ganglion to the parotid gland. Both the submandibular and sublingual glands receive their postganglionic fibers from the submandibular ganglion. The preganglionic fibers that supply all three major salivary glands pass through the middle-ear cavity. Fibers that supply the parotid gland form *Jacobson's nerve* along the promontory of the middle ear. Fibers that supply the submandibular and sublingual glands traverse the middle ear space with the chorda tympani.

Physiology

Saliva serves multiple important functions in the oral and pharyngeal cavities. Aside from its mechanical functions of lubrication and protection of the mucosa, saliva provides an antibacterial front based on the presence of secretory immunoglobulin A (IgA), lysozymes, and lactoferrin. Saliva also provides minerals that enhance posteruption maturation of teeth. The calcium and phosphate within saliva help counteract tooth dissolution secondary to plaque, and bicarbonate and phosphate decrease the bacterial load within plaque through pH buffering.[3] The parotid and submandibular glands are responsible for 90% of the secreted saliva. The flow rate of saliva can reach 4 ml/min under maximal stimulation.[3] The rate can be altered by numerous factors, including dehydration, systemic disease (e.g., cystic fibrosis and Sjogren's Syndrome), and neurologic disorders, as well as by numerous drugs. As for its composition, saliva initially is secreted by the acini as isotonic solution. This solution is then modified as it is transferred through the ductal system (i.e., the intercalated, striated, and excretory ducts). The degree of modification of this fluid is dependent on the salivary flow rate. Slower flow rates allow increased modification of the trans-

ported fluid and result in a more hypotonic secretion. The parotid gland has only serous-secreting acinir cells and, thus, produces thin serous saliva. The sublingual gland, on the other hand, produces thick mucous saliva. The submandibular gland has both serous and mucous cells, producing mixed saliva. Minor salivary glands can produce serous, mucous, or mixed saliva.[1]

CONGENITAL ANOMALIES

Congenital anomalies of the salivary glands include aplasia of the glands, ductal atresia, and congenital cysts. Rarest among these disorders is *congenital aplasia* of all salivary glands. The combination of xerostomia and multiple dental carries may be the only manifestation of congenital aplasia.[4] *Ductal atresia* or large *congenital cysts* may result in salivary obstruction and stasis. As expected, such anomalies become clinically evident through recurrent infections in one or more salivary glands or through the formation of cutaneous fistulae. Although cutaneous fistulae can be seen with heterotopic salivary tissue, the majority of fistulous tracts are secondary to first branchial cleft cysts in or close to the parotid gland.[4]

It may be difficult to distinguish between primary salivary gland cysts and branchial cleft cysts. Fortunately, this distinction has little bearing on the management of these cysts. Single cysts with or without fistulous tracts should be surgically excised. In managing these lesions, the surgeon must maintain a high index of suspicion for an anomalous facial nerve. Therefore, the surgeon initially should identify the facial nerve and its branches before proceeding with the excision. Glands with multiple cysts or recurrent infections should undergo total excision with facial nerve preservation.[5]

TRAUMA

Clean lacerations of salivary parenchyma require copious irrigation, debridement, and a tight layered closure to avoid the formation of seromas and fistulae. In irregular and heavily-contaminated wounds involving the parotid, the wound is debrided and irrigated, and may be allowed to granulate for several days prior to surgical layered closure. Nerve endings are marked during the initial procedure to allow for identification and reanastamosis during the delayed repair. When such wounds involve the submandibular gland, complete excision of the gland should be considered rather than surgical repair.

Lacerations anterior to the anterior border of the masseter should be inspected carefully for the presence of saliva. This may help identify injury to the parotid duct. A transected or lacerated parotid duct should be repaired primarily with interrupted fine prolene sutures over a polyethylene catheter, utilizing magnification (loupes or microscope, if available). The catheter should be kept in place (sutured to the buccal mucosa) for 2 weeks. If surgical repair is not possible, the proximal end of the duct should be ligated. This likely will lead to temporary glandular swelling followed by glandular atrophy.[6]

A *ranula* is a pseudocyst that develops in the floor of the mouth (Fig. 39-1), usually stemming from the sublingual gland.[4] Implicated in the etiology of these lesions is "inflammation and trauma of salivary ducts causing extrusion of mucus into the interstitial tissues."[4] This lesion usually presents above the mylohyoid muscle and can displace the tongue superiorly and posteriorly. If this mucus-filled cyst extends beneath the underlying mylohyoid muscle, it becomes known as a *plunging ranula*. Marsupialization is a simple treatment of a ranula but is associated with a significant rate of recurrence. Total meticulous excision of the cyst along with the ipsilateral sublingual gland has been shown to decrease the recurrence rate of these lesions.[7]

> ### SPECIAL CONSIDERATION:
> Definitive treatment of a ranula often requires excision of the affected sublingual gland.

INFECTIOUS DISEASES

Suppurative Sialadenitis

Acute bacterial sialadenitis commonly is associated with salivary stasis. It may be seen in premature newborns, as well as in chronically ill and dehydrated children.[5] Usually affecting the parotid glands, the most common causative agents are *Staphylococcus aureus, Streptococcus viridans,* and *Streptococcus pneumoniae.* Other agents include *Hemophilus influenzae* as well as anaerobes (e.g., *Bacteroides*).[8]

Signs of acute bacterial sialadenitis include fever, pain, swelling, and tenderness to palpation of the affected gland. Purulent drainage may be expressed from the duct with manual massage of the affected gland (Fig. 39-2). The majority of patients respond well to treatment with the augmented penicillin compounds, amoxicillin/clavulanate or ampicillin/sulbactam. Clindamycin serves as a good alternative for patients allergic to penicillin.[9] Oral and intravenous (IV) hydration, sialagogues (e.g., lemon drops), and massage of the affected gland toward its duct are all helpful adjuncts in the management of sialadenitis. Bacterial sialadenitis can progress to result in abscess formation within the affected gland. In such cases, incision and drainage is recommended. In the parotid gland, an abscess can point in the preauricular area or in the external ear canal; care must be taken to protect the facial nerve during the procedure.[10]

Recurrent Suppurative Parotitis

Recurrent suppurative parotitis (RSP) of childhood is a separate and common entity characterized by recurrent acute parotitis. Patients present with the

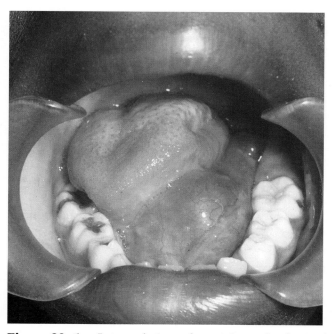

Figure 39-1: Intraoral view of a ranula on the floor of the mouth. On physical examination, this lesion was not palpable in the neck, remaining above the mylohyoid muscle.

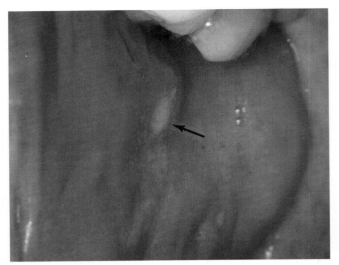
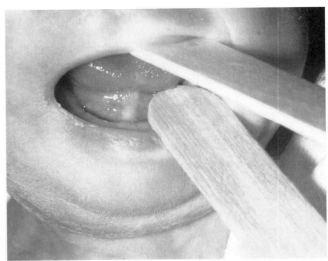

A   B

Figure 39–2: (A) Purulent fluid (arrow) expressed from the parotid duct during manual massage of the right parotid gland in a patient with acute bacterial parotitis. (B) Purulent fluid expressed from the submandibular duct in an infant with acute bacterial submandibular sialadenitis.

same symptoms and signs of acute parotitis. Although they respond well to antibiotic therapy, recurrence is seen after an interval that may vary from weeks to months or even years.[4] This disease is seen more often in males and is usually associated with a history of mumps parotitis. Poor dental hygiene, as well as chronic infection of the oral mucosa or tonsils predisposes the child to the development of RSP. Some have implicated *Streptococcus viridans* as a causative organism because it is commonly found in the ductal secretions of patients with RSP.[11] Recurrent infections of the parotid bed usually result in fibrotic tissue that adheres closely to the facial nerve. Fortunately, RSP rarely necessitates excision of the parotid gland. The majority of cases resolve spontaneously at puberty, and treatment should be as "conservative as possible, as long as possible."[4]

Granulomatous Sialadenitis

Granulomatous diseases of the salivary glands commonly involve the parotid gland. Infections such as cat-scratch disease and mycobacterium usually involve the intracapsular lymph nodes of the parotid. On the other hand, actinomycosis involves the salivary tissue itself and may be seen in both the submandibular and sublingual glands.

Cat-scratch disease is a regional granulomatous lymphadenopathy that results from skin inoculation with the gram-negative bacillus, *Branhamella*

henselae. Although 6 to 45% of patients will not have an identified skin lesion at the site of inoculation, a history of cat (or other animal) exposure in a patient with low-grade fevers and tender regional lymphadenopathy should raise suspicion of cat-scratch disease.[12] The diagnosis can be confirmed through serum testing for antibodies to the bacillus. On histologic sections of the involved lymph nodes, Warthin-Starry staining will demonstrate the intracellular bacillus. Treatment includes antibiotics (erythromycin or trimethoprim-sulfamethoxazole) as well as symptomatic care.

Mycobacterial cervical adenitis is known as *scrofula.* This can involve intraparotid nodes and is commonly seen in children 16 to 36 months old. Nontuberculous (atypical) mycobacteria account for the majority (>90%) of scrofula in children. Organisms in this class of mycobacteria include *Mycobacterium (M.) avium-intercellulare, M. scrofulaceum, M. kansasii, M. fortuitum, and M. haemophilum.*[13] The infectious organisms are ubiquitous throughout the environment and are found in water, soil, and milk.[14] They enter the body through minor intraoral mucosal trauma (e.g., teething, cuts), and settle into regional lymph nodes. The slow growing, nontender (in contradistinction to other causes of cervical adenitis), firm mass progresses to develop a violaceous hue of the overlying skin (Fig. 39–3). The lesions most commonly arise in the preauricular or submandibular area. Skin breakdown and suppurative drainage are often seen. Because cultures can

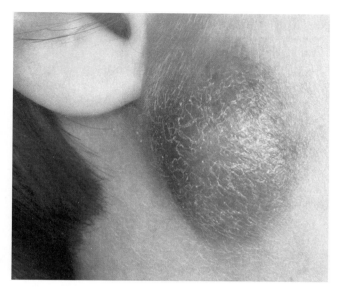

Figure 39–3: Characteristic violaceous hue of skin overlying an atypical mycobacterial lesion involving a right intraparotid lymph node. (From Handler SD, Myer CM. *Ear, Nose and Throat Disorders in Children*. Toronto: B.C. Decker, 1998, with permission.)

take up to 6 weeks to finalize, the initial diagnosis usually is based on exclusion of other causes as well as clinical suspicion.[11] As opposed to *M. tuberculosis,* atypical mycobacteria are associated with a negative tuberculosis contact history, unilateral cervical adenitis, a negative or weakly-positive purified protein derivative (PPD) skin test, and a normal chest X-ray. A contrasted magnetic resonance imaging (MRI) study has been recommended by Nadel et al.[15] because of its superior soft-tissue delineation that shows such features as stranding of subcutaneous fat, thickening of the overlying dermal layer, obliteration of tissue planes, and heterogeneity within the mass. Necrosis within the mass demonstrates a multichambered appearance. Rarely, with the progression of necrosis, these loculations can coalesce into a single large "cold abscess." Treatment is total excision; or curettage of the necrotic lesion is recommended if it lies close to vital structures such as the facial nerve. Recurrence is common, especially after incomplete excision or incision and drainage of lesions.

M. tuberculosis accounts for <10% of scrofula in children. Constitutional symptoms are commonly associated with *M. tuberculosis* infection. When a child is suspected of having *M. tuberculosis* disease, HIV testing is recommended and treatment (using isoniazid and rifampin, as well as pyrazinamide for the first 2 months) is initiated until cultures are final.

If *M. tuberculosis* infection is confirmed by cultures, treatment is recommended for a 6-month course.[13]

AT A GLANCE . . .

Scrofula

Incidence: Second only to benign reactive lymphoid hyperplasia, granulomatous disease is frequently the underlying source of neck masses in children. Scrofula (primarily nontuberculous mycobacteria) is the most common cause of cervical granulomatous disease. Organisms enter the body through minor intraoral mucosal trauma (e.g., teething), and settle into regional lymph nodes. Infections commonly afflict children 16–36 months in age.

Symptoms and Signs: A slow-growing, nontender, firm mass (most commonly found in the preauricular or submandibular area) progresses to develop a violaceous hue of the overlying skin. Skin breakdown and suppurative drainage are seen often.

Diagnosis: Because cultures can take up to 6 weeks to finalize, the initial diagnosis usually is based on exclusion of other causes as well as clinical suspicion. Nontuberculous (i.e., atypical) mycobacteria are associated with a negative tuberculosis contact history, unilateral cervical adenitis, a negative or weakly-positive PPD skin test, and a normal chest X-ray. A contrasted MRI study contributes to the diagnosis.

Treatment: Treatment is based on total excision or curettage of the necrotic lesion when it lies close to vital structures such as the facial nerve. Recurrence is common, especially after incomplete excision or incision and drainage.

Less commonly, *actinomycosis* involves the salivary gland parenchyma and usually results from intraoral trauma or dental manipulation followed by retrograde ductal migration of the organism.[11] *Actinomyces israelii* is the most commonly implicated species and is found within the parotid gland more than the other major salivary glands. Presentation includes a painless, indurated mass in the absence of systemic symptoms. Cutaneous fistulae are seen in 61% of infected patients.[16] Anaerobic cultures as well as sulfur granules on staining confirm the diagnosis. A 6-course of IV penicillin (erythromycin in the penicillin-allergic patient) followed by a 6-course of an oral antibiotic is the mainstay of treatment.[17]

AT A GLANCE . . .
Infectious Diseases

Suppurative Sialadenitis: usually seen in premature newborns, the chronically ill, and dehydrated patients; symptoms include fever, pain, swelling, and tenderness to palpation of the affected gland; treatment is with antibiotics.

Recurrent Suppurative Parotitis: characterized by recurrent acute parotitis; symptoms are the same as those of acute parotitis; seen more often in males and associated with a history of mumps parotitis; treatment is with antibiotics; most cases resolve spontaneously at puberty.

Granulomatous Sialadenitis:
Cat-scratch disease: a regional granulomatous lymphadenopathy; treatment is with antibiotics.
Mycobacterial cervical adenitis: also know as scrofula, it involves intraparotid nodes and is commonly seen in children 16–36 months old.
Actinomycosis: usually results from intraoral trauma or dental manipulation followed by retrograde ductal migration of the organism; treatment is with IV penicillin and a 6-month course of oral antibiotics.

Viral Sialadenitis: associated with coxsackievirus A, echoviruses, influenza A, cytomegalovirus, and mumps virus; symptoms include a low-grade fever, chills, headaches, and malaise; treatment is supportive, with a soft bland diet and pain control.

Viral Sialadenitis

Viral sialadenitis is associated with certain sialadenotropic viruses such as coxsackievirus A, echoviruses, influenza A, cytomegalovirus and, most commonly, the mumps (i.e., paramyxovirus) virus. Although 30% of mumps cases remain subclinical, epidemic parotitis (i.e., mumps) is the most common cause of parotid swelling.[8,18] Transmitted through salivary droplets and after a 2- to 4-week incubation period, the infection is manifested by prodromal symptoms of low-grade fever, chills, headaches, and general malaise. Shortly afterwards, swelling is seen to involve the parotid glands and, occasionally, the other major salivary glands. This infection may last as long as 10 to 14 days. The diagnosis may be confirmed with serologic identification of antibodies to the mumps' S and V antigens.[8] The peak incidence of infection is seen in children 4 to 6 years old. Infection usually provides permanent immunity. Infants under 1 year of age are usually immune to infection, secondary to maternal antibodies. Treatment of acute mumps is supportive, with a soft bland diet and pain control. Childhood immunization has proved very effective in preventing mumps parotitis.

Complications of mumps are rare. They are seen more commonly with postpubertal infection. Orchitis (with ensuing sterility if both testes are involved) meningoencephalitis, sudden deafness, pancreatitis, and chronic obstructive sialadenitis may complicate an acute mumps infection.[8]

SYSTEMIC DISEASE

Salivary gland enlargement is the common denominator of systemic metabolic, endocrine, and autoimmune disorders that affect the salivary glands. Both obesity and starvation, as well as diabetes and hypothyroidism, are associated with fatty infiltration of the salivary glands, more noticeably in the parotid gland. Ingestion of copper, mercury, bismuth, and lead, as well as injections of iodine-containing compounds, can lead to diffuse enlargement of the salivary glands.[5] *Cystic fibrosis* (CF) contributes to variable alterations of the salivary secretions and, through an unknown mechanism, is associated with enlarged submandibular glands.

Sjögren's syndrome is characterized by xerostomia, keratoconjunctivitis sicca, and connective tissue disease, and is associated with diffuse nontender enlargement of the major salivary glands (Fig. 39-4). Biopsy of minor salivary glands shows lymphocytic infiltration with glandular atrophy.[7] In the absence of systemic manifestations, symmetrically painless swelling of the major salivary glands is known as *Mikulicz's syndrome.*

Children with the *human immunodeficiency virus* (HIV) initially can manifest this infection with salivary gland enlargement. Most commonly seen

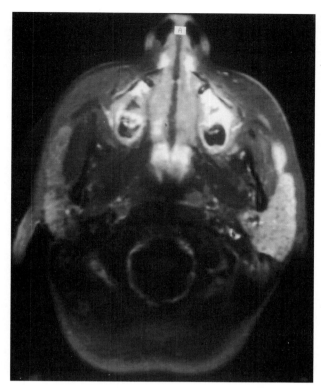

Figure 39–4: Axial computed tomographic image showing bilateral enlargement of parotid glands in a patient with Sjogren's syndrome.

in the parotid gland, multiple lymphoproliferative cystic lesions can develop bilaterally. These lesions are epithelial-lined and filled with macrophages and lymphocytes in serous fluid. A dense lymphoid infiltrate with germinal centers surrounds these cysts. With the diagnosis of HIV infection, identification on MRI of multiple cystic lesions in the parotid provides a presumptive diagnosis of HIV-associated lymphoepithelial cysts. Clinical management through clinical observation is recommended.[2] Patients with HIV also have a propensity to develop solid lesions of the salivary glands such as intraglandular lymphadenopathy, infectious processes, and HIV-related malignancies (e.g., lymphoma).

TUMORS

Of all salivary gland tumors, <5% occur in children. Histologically, the distribution of the various tumor types is distinct from that seen in adults. Classified as epithelial and nonepithelial (i.e., mesenchymal)

(Table 39–1), major salivary gland tumors in the pediatric population are dominated by benign mesenchymal lesions, namely hemangiomas. Among the epithelial lesions, there is a higher proportion of malignant lesions in comparison to that seen in adults. The parotid gland is seven times more likely to be involved with a neoplasm than the submandibular gland.[19]

Benign Tumors

In children, benign tumors of the salivary glands are most commonly hemangiomas, followed by pleomorphic adenomas and lymphangiomas. The benign mesenchymal lesions are primarily the vasoformative tumors (91%): hemangiomas and lymphangiomas. These lesions are seen predominantly in neonates and infants. They rarely are diagnosed in children above 10 years of age. On the other hand, the benign epithelial lesions, largely composed of pleomorphic adenomas (92%), are seen more commonly in children over 10 years of age.[19]

Hemangiomas of the salivary glands often are diagnosed at or shortly after birth. These vascular lesions may or may not involve the overlying skin. Found more commonly in females and on the left side, these lesions can show an increase in size during the neonatal period but, for the most part, involute spontaneously by the age of 2.[19] Fifty percent of parotid hemangiomas are associated with other cutaneous hemangiomas (Fig. 39–5).[20] The diagnosis is made based on history and physical examination. MRI (Fig. 39–6) may be needed to differentiate a parotid hemangioma without overlying skin involvement from a lymphangioma. Given their tendency for spontaneous regression after the first few years of life, asymptomatic salivary gland hemangiomas usually are managed by close observation. Complicating factors such as rapid growth rate, intralesional hemorrhage, infection, platelet sequestration, high-output cardiac failure, and/or psychosocial difficulties may require therapeutic intervention. First-line medical therapy is systemic or intralesional corticosteroids that help to induce involution of these benign lesions. Interferon alpha-2A has been used with some success in lesions failing to respond to steroid therapy. Surgical excision is indicated for unresponsive lesions, especially those resulting in airway or visual compromise. Preoperative arteriography with possible embolization

TABLE 39–1: Distribution of Salivary Gland Tumors in Children

Tumor Type	Total No.	Perinatal	1–11 mo	1–10 y	10–16 y	Not Stated
Benign Epithelial						
Pleomorphic adenoma	81	1	1	27	52	
Embryoma	2	2				
Warthin's tumor	2					2
Cystadenoma	2					2
Basal cell adenoma	1	1				
Malignant Epithelial						
Mucoepidermoid carcinoma	60		1	26	31	2
Acinic cell carcinoma	22			7	15	
Undifferentiated carcinoma	10	2	1	5	2	
Adenocarcinoma	8		1	4	3	
Adenoid cystic carcinoma	6			1	5	
Squamous cell carcinoma	4			1	3	
Benign Mesenchymal						
Hemangioma	96	28	49	16	1	2
Lymphangioma	20			1		19
Neurogenic	7				1	6
Lipoma	2					2
Fibromatosis	3			3		
Malignant Mesenchymal						
Sarcoma	18			2		16
Total	344	34	53	93	113	51

Adapted from Luna MA, Batsakis JG, El-Naggar AK. Salivary gland tumors in children. Ann Otol Rhinol Laryngol 1991; 100:869–871.

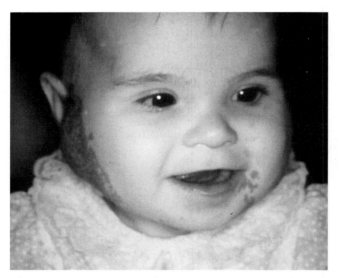

Figure 39–5: Perioral hemangiomas seen in this patient with a large right parotid hemangioma. (From Handler SD, Myer CM. *Ear, Nose and Throat Disorders in Children.* Toronto: B.C. Decker, 1998, with permission.)

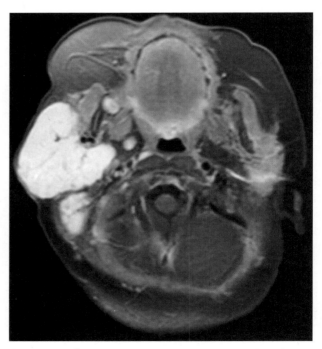

Figure 39–6: T1-weighted, fat suppressed, enhanced MRI of a parotid hemangioma. Note the characteristic reticulated pattern of the hemangioma with dark flow voids that represent vessels within the lesion.

of primary feeding vessels may facilitate surgical excision.

Lymphangiomas also are noted soon after birth. These soft, compressible, lymphatic malformations may increase in size secondary to accumulation of lymphatic fluid, infection, or intralesional bleeding. Most importantly, these lesions rarely involute. In contradistinction to many parotid hemangiomas, these lesions usually do not involve the overlying skin. Physical examination (Fig. 39-7) along with MRI (Fig. 39-8) can help distinguish these lesions from hemangiomas without overlying skin involvement. Surgical excision is the primary mode of treatment.[21] Complete resection should be attempted only if this does not threaten nearby vital structures. Residual tumor can be left behind and excised in staged procedures should the lesion progress in size.

Pleomorphic adenoma in children is treated in a fashion similar to that in adults. Fine needle aspiration is performed less commonly given the higher risk of malignancy in a solid tumor of the salivary glands in a child. Surgical excision of the tumor with a cuff of normal glandular tissue by way of a superficial parotidectomy with facial nerve preservation (or total submandibular gland excision) is the recommended procedure.

Of note, *embryomas* are rare benign epithelial

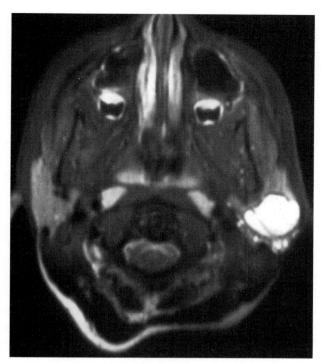

Figure 39–8: T2-weighted MRI of lymphangioma of the parotid region. Note the bright cystic space divided by darker septations.

tumors diagnosed primarily in the first year of life. Malignant transformation has been quoted to be as high as 25% in these lesions and, therefore, surgical excision is recommended.[19]

Malignant Tumors

In children, the most common malignant tumor of the salivary glands is *mucoepidermoid carcinoma*, followed by *acinic cell carcinoma* and *sarcoma.* These lesions primarily involve the parotid gland. Similar to the benign tumors, the mesenchymal lesions (i.e., sarcoma) are diagnosed most commonly in the perinatal period, and the epithelial tumors (i.e., mucoepidermoid and acinic cell) usually are diagnosed in children older than 10 years of age. As in adults, facial nerve weakness and neck adenopathy are seen more often with malignant lesions of the parotid gland. Treatment, regardless of the tumor grade, involves superficial or total parotidectomy (depending on the tumor location) with facial nerve preservation, if possible. Postoperative radiation therapy usually is given to patients with high-grade malignancy, local metastatic spread, and/or residual tumor after surgical excision. *Rhabdomyosarcoma* is the most common sarcoma affecting the

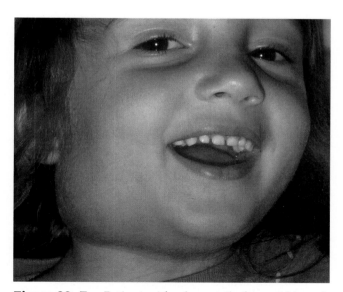

Figure 39–7: Patient with a large tail of parotid lymphangioma. Note the absence of skin discoloration that helps to differentiate this lesion from a hemangioma. (From Handler SD, Myer CM. *Ear, Nose and Throat Disorders in Children.* Toronto: B.C. Decker, 1998, with permission.)

salivary glands in children. It is best treated with surgical excision followed by radiation therapy and chemotherapy if distal spread is known or suspected.

DROOLING

Drooling (or *sialorrhea*) is a common problem in neurologically-impaired children, given the lack of coordinated control of the orofacial and head and neck muscles. Drooling may be associated with hypersecretion of saliva (e.g., teething, mucous membrane irritants, parasympathomimetic or sympatholytic drugs, rabies, etc.), but is usually a result of the inability of the child to manage a normal amount of saliva. There may be less frequent swallowing because of poor motor control and there is usually reduced sensory awareness of saliva, which normally stimulates a swallow to occur. In some cases, the degree of drooling is so excessive that it causes significant health and social problems. Constant wetness of the chin and perioral areas can lead to skin irritation, chapping, malodor, and secondary infection. Once these problems occur, the continuing drooling makes them extremely difficult to control.[22]

Social problems associated with drooling are numerous. The child's clothing is constantly wet and must be changed frequently by the caregivers. Bibs and napkins often are utilized in an effort to keep the child's clothing as dry as possible. Dribbled saliva can soil communication aids such as books and computers, as well as the clothing of the caregivers. Parents usually are aware and concerned about this problem. Often, the higher-functioning child may be cognizant of and embarrassed by this problem and may actually initiate the investigation into treatments available for the drooling.[23]

Management

Most investigators advocate a team approach in the management of the drooling child.[23] The members of the team may include a speech–language pathologist, an occupational therapist, a physical therapist, a psychologist, an otolaryngologist, a plastic surgeon, a developmental pediatrician, a neurologist, and a pediatric dentist. Input from these specialists and others as indicated should be sought in the man-

agement of this difficult problem. Practice Pathway 39–1 outlines the management for sialorrhea.

> ## SPECIAL CONSIDERATION:
>
> The management of the child with drooling (sialorrhea) requires a team approach. Treatment options include medication, facilitation of oromotor and swallowing skills, and surgical intervention.

Nonsurgical

Although drooling can improve spontaneously as neuromuscular control improves with age, some children may require intervention of some type. Conservative management strategies should be attempted first. These include development of oral motor skills and swallowing function through feeding therapy, oral facilitation exercises, and the development of stable, upright positioning of the head and trunk. Increasing awareness of saliva may help to encourage more frequent swallowing as well as the need to wipe the face.

Medical management is considered when more conservative approaches are not successful. Management of drooling with anticholinergic drugs can reduce the amount of saliva produced but may result in undesirable side effects, such as dry mouth, restlessness, blurred vision, sedation, urinary retention, or constipation.[24]

Surgical

Surgical management of the child with drooling should be considered when conservative measures have been unsuccessful in eliminating or reducing the severity of the problem. Referral for surgical management rarely is made before the child is 6 years of age.

Up to 70% of the daily output of 1 to 1.5 l of saliva is produced by the two submandibular glands. Operations to treat drooling fall into two major categories: those intended to reduce the total amount of saliva produced and those designed to change the point of entry of saliva into the oral cavity/oropharynx so that swallowing of saliva is facilitated.[23] Tympanic neurectomy and section of the

Practice Pathway 39–1   DROOLING (SIALORRHEA)

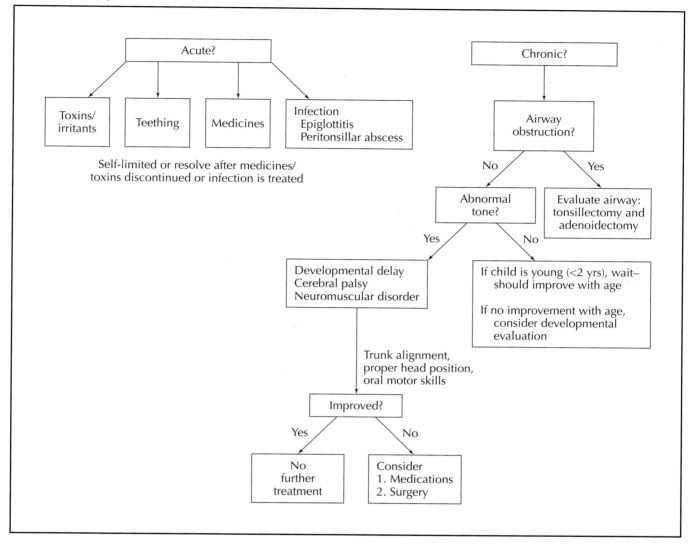

chorda tympani nerve are procedures intended to sever the parasympathetic innervation to the parotid gland and the submandibular gland, respectively. Although these procedures may have some initial success in reducing salivary secretions, the production of saliva often returns to normal within 6 months, presumably from regeneration of neural fibers. In addition, the morbidity of these procedures can be quite significant and can include tympanic membrane perforation and loss of taste.

Wilkie first popularized surgical treatment of sialorrhea with bilateral parotid duct transposition (to the tonsillar fossae), followed by submandibular gland excision, if needed.[25] Many variations of salivary gland surgeries have been described since then, and these procedures involve some or all of

the following: excision of submandibular glands, rerouting of submandibular and/or parotid ducts, ligation of parotid ducts, and excision of the sublingual glands. All of these procedures result in dramatic improvement in the patient's symptoms and social activities. Complications of surgical intervention are minor and include temporary cheek swelling, ranula formation, or obstruction of the transpositioned duct. The reduced salivary production after these procedures is often thicker than preoperatively, but this usually poses no problem to the child. Occasionally, additional fluids are required during eating.

Because saliva has a protective function in maintaining dental hygiene and preventing dental caries, early investigators who performed treatment directed at reducing the amount of saliva were concerned about the possibility of increased dental caries secondary to decreased salivary flow around the teeth. Daily postoperative fluoride treatments were recommended in some of the earlier studies. However, even without special dental care, the number of dental caries has not increased in this population.[22]

AT A GLANCE . . .
Drooling

Pathogenesis: lack of coordinated control of the orofacial and head and neck muscles

Adverse Effects: skin irritation, chapping, malodor, secondary infection, and social problems

Management: *Nonsurgical:* development of oral motor skills and swallowing function, anticholinergic drugs; *Surgical:* tympanic neurectomy, section of the chorda tympani nerve, bilateral parotid duct transposition

---

REFERENCES

1. Kontis TC, Johns ME. Anatomy and physiology of the salivary glands. In: Bailey BJ, ed. *Head & Neck Surgery—Otolaryngology.* Philadelphia: Lippincott, 1993, pp 447–454.
2. Seibert RW. Diseases of the salivary glands. In: Bluestone CD, Stool SE, Kenna MA, eds. *Pediatric Otolaryngology.* Philadelphia: Saunders, 1996, pp. 1093–1107.
3. Rice DH. Salivary gland physiology. Otolaryngol Clin North Am 1977; 10:273–285.
4. Seifert G, Mieblke A, Haubrich J, et al. *Diseases of Salivary Glands.* Stuttgart: Georg Theime Verlag, 1986, pp. 63–70.
5. Yeh S. The salivary glands. In: Ballenger JJ, ed. *Diseases of the Nose, Throat, Ear Head & Neck.* Philadelphia: Lea & Febiger, 1991, pp. 308–311.
6. Olson NR. Traumatic lesions of the salivary glands. Otolaryngol Clin North Am 1977; 10:345–350.
7. Wenig B. Non-neoplastic lesions of the oral cavity, nasopharynx, tonsils and neck. In: *Atlas of Head and Neck Pathology.* Philadelphia: Saunders, 1993, pp. 105–112.
8. Rice D. Diseases of the salivary glands. Non-neoplastic. In: Bailey BJ, et al, eds. *Head & Neck Surgery—Otolaryngology.* Philadelphia: Lippincott, 1993, pp. 475–483.
9. Fairbanks D. *Antimicrobial Therapy in Otolaryngology—Head & Neck Surgery,* 8th Ed. Alexandria: American Academy of Otolaryngology—Head & Neck Surgery Foundation, 1996, p. 68.
10. Morgan DW, Pearmen K, Raafat F, et al. Salivary disease in childhood. Ear Nose Throat J 1989; 68: 155–159.
11. Kane WJ, McCaffrey T. Infections. In: Cummings CW, Fredrickson JM, Harker LA, et al, eds. *Otolaryngology—Head and Neck Surgery.* St. Louis: Mosby-Year Book, 1993, pp. 1008–1017.
12. Suskind DL, Handler SD, Tom LWC, et al. Nontuberculous mycobacterial. Clin Pediatr 1997; 36: 403–409.
13. Rosenfeld RM. Cervical adenopathy. In: Bluestone CD, Stool SE, Kenna MA, eds. *Pediatric Otolaryngology.* Philadelphia: Saunders, 1996, pp. 1512–1524 Vol. 2.
14. Wolinsky D. Nontuberculous mycobacteria and associated disease. Am Rev Respir Dis 1979; 119: 107–159
15. Nadel D, Bilaniuk L, Handler S. Imaging of granulomatous neck masses in children. Int J Pediatr Otorhinolaryngol 1996; 37:151–162.
16. Littlejohn MC, Bailey BJ. Granulomatous diseases of the head and neck. In: Bailey BJ, et al, eds. *Head & Neck Surgery—Otolaryngology.* Philadelphia: Lippincott, 1993, pp. 173–186.
17. Hensher R, Bowerman J. Actinomycosis of the parotid gland. Br J Oral Maxillofac Surg 1985; 23: 128–134.
18. Morgan DW, Pearman K, Raafat F, et al. Salivary disease in childhood. Ear Nose Throat J 1989; 68: 155–159.
19. Luna MA, Batsakis JG, El-Naggar AK. Pathology consultation: Salivary gland tumors in children. Ann Otol Rhinol Laryngol 1991; 100:869–871.
20. White AK. Salivary gland disease in infancy and childhood: Non-malignant lesions. J Otolaryngol 1992; 21: 422–428.
21. McGill TJ, Mulliken JB. Vascular anomalies of the head and neck. In: Cummings CW, Fredrickson JM, Harker LA, et al, eds. *Otolaryngology–Head and Neck Surgery.* St. Louis: Mosby-Year Book, 1993, pp. 333–346.
22. Crysdale WS. Drooling. In: Gates G, ed. *Current Therapy in Otolaryngology: Head & Neck Surgery.* B. C. Decker, Hamilton, Ontario, 1994, pp. 426–429.
23. Solot CB. Promoting function: Communication and feeding. In: Dormans JP, Pellegrino L, eds. *Caring for Children with Cerebral Palsy.* Baltimore: Paul H. Brookes Publishing, 1997, pp. 347–370.
24. Lew KM, Younis RT, Lazar RH. The current management of sialorrhea. Ear Nose Throat J 1991; 70: 99–105.
25. Wilkie TF. The problem of drooling in cerebral palsy: A surgical approach. Can J Surg 1967; 10:60–67.

40 Traumatic Injuries to the Oral Cavity and Pharynx

Dwight T. Jones

Penetrating injuries of the oropharynx occur almost exclusively in children. They are not uncommon injuries. Busy urban children's hospitals report on average approximately four cases a week. Most of these can be evaluated and treated in the emergency room without the need for hospital admission. In certain instances, however, depending upon the type of object causing the injury and the location of impact, certain other diagnostic tests and evaluations are required to ensure that no other serious injury has occurred.

PRESENTATION AND EVALUATION

Injuries to the oropharynx occur most commonly in children in the 3- to 5-year age group. These children are usually toddlers who, because of their oral developmental stage, naturally are placing objects in their mouths a good deal of the time. Because of their age, they are prone to running and falling, subsequently impaling the foreign object somewhere in the oropharynx. Most children present to the emergency room in hemodynamically-stable condition, with a history of spitting up small amounts of blood prior to their arrival. The oral foreign object usually has been removed by the parents.[1]

The type of foreign object that causes injury is similar in most cases. It is usually a long cylindrical object with a pointed tip. In a recent review of 77 cases, wooden and metal sticks, plastic toys, and ballpoint pens comprised the majority of items involved. Although injury can occur anywhere in the

oral cavity, the area most commonly involved is the posterior oropharynx or the superior tonsillar region.[1] Other common sites include the dorsum of the tongue and the palate. Because of the size and type of foreign body, the injury commonly appears as a simple puncture wound or contusion. Larger lacerations can occur, depending on the type and area of impact, but these are much less common.

> **SPECIAL CONSIDERATION:**
> Although an oropharyngeal injury can occur anywhere in the oral cavity, the area most commonly involved is the posterior oropharynx or the superior tonsillar region.

It is important on initial presentation for the examiner to obtain a comprehensive history regarding the type of foreign body, angle of impact, force of impact, and amount of blood loss. A thorough examination of the oral and pharyngeal cavities should follow. If the child is uncooperative, the examination should be completed in the operating room so that proper assessment of the wound and area of injury can be completed. Although most injuries are usually minor lacerations that require little or no care, the main concern in all cases should be to determine that the injury did not occur in the lateral peritonsillar region, leading to subsequent contusion or laceration of the internal carotid artery (ICA). The incidence of such an injury and ensuing neurologic sequelae [e.g., cerebrovascular accident (CVA)] is uncommon, but its devastating outcome demands that a high level of suspicion be maintained in evaluating any child with an oropharyngeal injury.[2]

Pediatric Otolaryngology, Edited by R.F. Wetmore, H.R. Muntz, and T.J. McGill. Thieme Medical Publishers, Inc., New York © 2000.

Practice Pathway 40–1 MANAGEMENT OF WOUNDS TO THE ORAL CAVITY AND PHARYNX

```
                            ┌──────────────────────┐
                            │ Oropharyngeal Injury │
                            └──────────────────────┘
                  ┌──────────────────┐        ┌──────────────────┐
                  │ Tongue/Midline   │        │ Lateral palate   │
                  │ palate           │        │ Lateral pharynx  │
                  └──────────────────┘        └──────────────────┘

      ┌──────────────┐   ┌──────────────┐
      │ Small puncture│  │ Large        │        ┌──────────────────┐  ┌────────────────────┐
      │ or laceration │  │ laceration   │        │ Unlikely vascular│  │ Suspected vascular │
      └──────────────┘   └──────────────┘        │ injury           │  │ injury             │
                                                 └──────────────────┘  └────────────────────┘

                    ┌──────────────┐
                    │ Consider CT if│
                    │ palatal injury│
                    └──────────────┘

      ┌──────────────┐   ┌──────────────┐         ┌──────┐
      │ Observe; oral│   │ Surgical     │         │ MRA  │
      │ antibiotics  │   │ closure;     │         └──────┘
      └──────────────┘   │ oral         │
                         │ antibiotics  │
                         └──────────────┘         ┌──────────────────┐   ┌──────────────────────┐
                                                  │ Observe with     │   │ MRA; carotid         │
                                                  │ neurologic checks│   │ arteriography        │
                                                  └──────────────────┘   └──────────────────────┘

                                                               ┌──────────────┐
                                                               │ Anticoagulate│
                                                               └──────────────┘

                                                                    ┌────────────────┐
                                                                    │ Surgical repair│
                                                                    └────────────────┘
```

Abbreviations: MRA, Magnetic Resonance Angiography.

MANAGEMENT

The management of wounds to the oral cavity and pharynx depends on the location, size, and depth of penetration (Practice Pathway 40-1). Again, a complete history is important to discern the type of foreign body involved and the mechanism of injury.

Tongue

Lacerations and punctures to the tongue are frequently minor and may require no treatment or very limited debridement and cleansing with saline. Because of the rich vascular supply, simple tongue wounds may be accompanied by a history of notable bleeding. Large wounds, even up to 2 cm, tend to heal well by secondary intention. Larger gaping wounds with ragged borders may require debridement and surgical closure. Depending on the age and cooperation of the patient and the size and location of the laceration, this closure may need to be performed under general anesthesia. Absorbable suture material placed several mm from the wound edge helps secure the freshened edges. Up to 50% of the lateral portion of the tongue may be lost without causing noticeable effect on the quality of speech as long as the tip of the tongue is intact. Good oral hygiene facilitates healing. Use of oral antibiotics should be considered if the oral mucosa has been violated.

> **SPECIAL CONSIDERATION:**
>
> Large wounds of the tongue tend to heal well by secondary intention.

Palate

Injuries to the soft palate occur less often than to other areas. The junction between the soft and hard palate is the most common location for injury, and most commonly, a "trap-door" type of injury occurs. This injury usually begins on the surface of the hard palate and extends back to the soft palate. Bleeding can be brisk, but is usually self-limited. Most of these injuries occur in the midline or near the midline, but careful inspection is required to ensure that no injury has occurred in the lateral soft-palate area.

> **SPECIAL CONSIDERATION:**
>
> The most common location of a palatal injury is at the junction between the hard and soft palate.

Most injuries to the palate heal without intervention, if the edges of the wound are in close proximity. Trap-door or large lacerations that are contaminated with dirt or foreign matter should be debrided, cleaned, and closed (Fig. 40-1). Deeper wounds that involve the lateral soft palate should be managed as described in the next section. Concerns about injury to the hard palate can be assessed by computed tomography (CT). Again, because of the plentiful blood supply, wounds in this region usually heal without difficulty or need for major surgical intervention.

Lateral Oropharynx

Injuries to the lateral oropharynx are some of the most common that occur in children. Because of the close proximity to the ICA, it is an area that presents the most risk in terms of major sequelae. Although rare, injuries to the ICA can occur either through contusion or direct laceration, and any child presenting with injury to this region of the mouth must be evaluated thoroughly for this possible complication.[1]

Children with an injury to the ICA may present like most other patients with an oropharyngeal injury and may not have experienced extensive bleeding (Fig. 40-2). In nearly all cases, the wound is a puncture type and little bleeding has occurred or bleeding may have been brisk for only a very short period of time and then ceased. Even objects that have not caused a significant laceration, but have resulted in severe blunt trauma (e.g., a toothbrush), can cause ICA contusion and subsequent neurologic impairment. On the other hand, a severe palatal injury does not necessarily indicate that the ICA has been damaged.

Although neurologic signs can develop immediately following a lateral pharyngeal injury, the more common feature is a "lucid Interval" during which there is a delayed onset of neurologic symptoms; symptoms may occur anywhere from 3 to 24 hours following injury.[2,3] This delay probably represents the time that is necessary for the development of a thrombus or propagation of an intimal tear. Neurologic symptoms can vary from aphasia to contralateral hemiplegia, depending upon the severity of the injury to the vessel. Showering of small emboli is seen occasionally.[4,5]

> **SPECIAL CONSIDERATION:**
>
> After a lateral pharyngeal injury, there may be a "lucid interval" of up to 24 hours before neurologic symptoms appear.

Occasionally, patients present to the emergency room with the foreign body still embedded in the soft tissue of the oral cavity. If the site of the puncture is the lateral pharyngeal wall, plain radiographs of this area may determine the depth of penetration

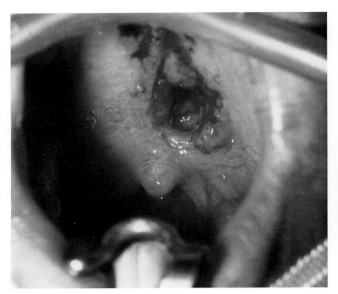
A

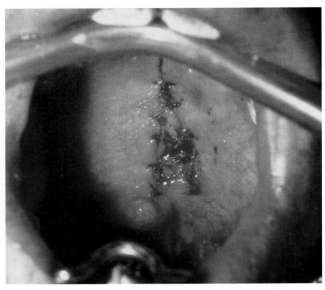
B

Figure 40–1: (A) This ''through-and-through'' laceration of the soft palate occurred when a child fell while running with a pencil in her mouth. Adenoid tissue in the nasopharynx may be visualized through the defect. (B) View of the soft palate after surgical closure of the defect in the operating room with an absorbable suture.

but are seldom useful in determining if the ICA is injured. If the depth of the injury is unclear or it is questionable whether a foreign body is still present, CT or magnetic resonance imaging (MRI) may provide additional information. Objects still embedded in this region are removed more safely in the operating room under general anesthesia, allowing for control of potential ICA bleeding.

Children with small puncture wounds that do not require surgical intervention may be discharged from the emergency room with instructions to return at the first sign of irritability or a change in baseline mental status. Parents must be told exactly what to look for and how often to check their children over the next 48 hours, including waking them from sleep at night. In the infant or mentally handicapped patient, neurologic assessment might be difficult and hospitalization should be considered for the next 24 to 48 hours. Patients with large, open, exposed wounds or in whom a deeply-penetrating wound is suspected should be managed in the operating room setting. Exploration, cleaning, and debridement of the wound can be performed. A loose closure in a layered fashion with coverage of an exposed CA (carotid artery) should allow proper healing.

The evaluation of suspected ICA injury remains controversial. In cases of highly-suspected injury (laceration or contusion) the diagnosis should be

confirmed with carotid angiography.[3,4] Carotid arteriography should be performed by a vascular or neuroradiologist who is familiar with the pediatric patient. Although carotid angiography has risks and complications that can be significant, the risk of a CVA due to a CA injury far outweighs those of angiography. It is important to evaluate the CA for laceration, intimal tears, and frank thrombosis. Any of these findings can lead to severe neurologic complications and/or death. Magnetic resonance angiography (MRA) may demonstrate thrombosis of the CA or a traumatic arteriovenous malformation, but may not identify other vascular injuries such as an intimal tear.

If the diagnosis of a thrombosis is established, anticoagulation should be considered, although this mode of therapy remains controversial. Prior to beginning anticoagulation, it is important to rule out intimal tears of the CA because anticoagulation in this setting can lead to further dissection and extension of the injury.[5]

SPECIAL CONSIDERATION:

In cases of traumatic CA thrombosis, anticoagulation is controversial but should be considered in selected cases.

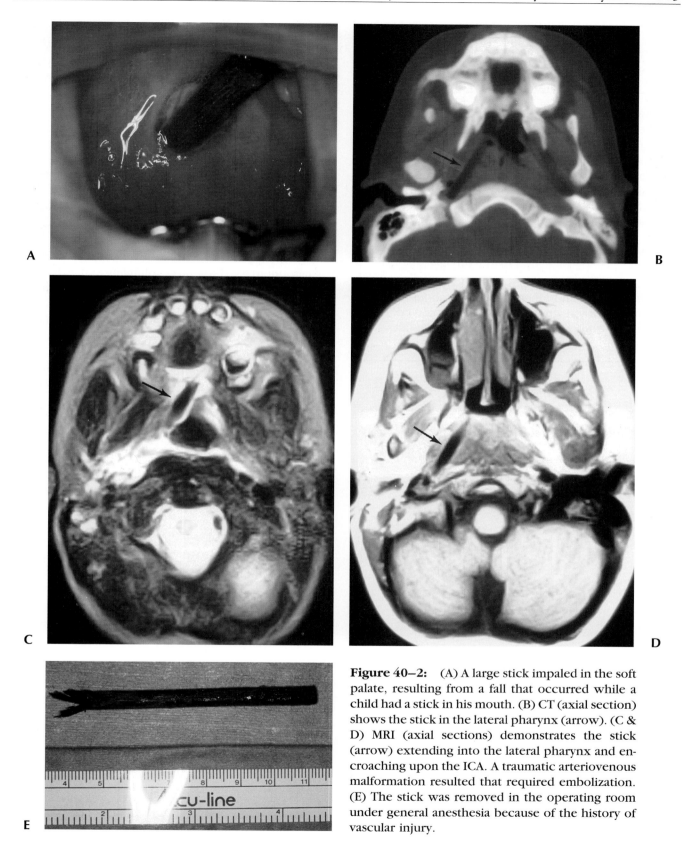

Figure 40–2:   (A) A large stick impaled in the soft palate, resulting from a fall that occurred while a child had a stick in his mouth. (B) CT (axial section) shows the stick in the lateral pharynx (arrow). (C & D) MRI (axial sections) demonstrates the stick (arrow) extending into the lateral pharynx and encroaching upon the ICA. A traumatic arteriovenous malformation resulted that required embolization. (E) The stick was removed in the operating room under general anesthesia because of the history of vascular injury.

AT A GLANCE . . .

Management of Oral Cavity and Pharyngeal Wounds

Tongue: wounds are usually minor and require little treatment other than debridement and cleansing with saline; most wounds heal well, but larger wounds may require surgical closure.

Palate: these injuries most commonly occur between the soft and hard palate; most injuries heal without intervention.

Lateral Oropharynx: this injury presents the most risk because of the proximity of the CIA, and all children who have injury to this part of the mouth must be evaluated thoroughly for possible complications; radiographs, CT, and MRI should be used to obtain further information about the location of a foreign object; objects should be removed in the operating room under general anesthesia.

CONCLUSION

Most oropharyngeal injuries can be managed conservatively with observation alone or in conjunction with oral antibiotics. The otolaryngologist should always be cognizant of more severe injury to the neurovascular structures of the parapharyngeal space, which are located just lateral to the oropharyngeal cavity.

REFERENCES

1. Radkowski D, McGill TJ, Healy GB, et al. Penetrating trauma of the oropharynx in children. Laryngoscope 1993; 103:991-994.
2. Hengerer AS, DeGroot TR, Rivers RJ, et al. Internal carotid artery thrombosis following soft palate injuries: A case report and review and 16 cases. Laryngoscope 1984; 94:1571-1575.
3. Bicherstaff ER. Etiology of acute hemiplegia in childhood. Br Med J 1964; 2:82-87.
4. Higgins GL, Meredith JT. Internal carotid artery thrombosis following penetrating trauma of the soft palate: An injury of youth. J Fam Pract 1991; 32:316-322.
5. Pitner SE. Carotid thrombosis due to intraoral trauma: An unusual complication of a common childhood accident. N Engl J Med 1966; 274(14):764-767.

41 Neoplasms of the Oral Cavity, Pharynx, and Upper Alimentary Tract

Laurie A. Ohlms

Neoplasms of the upper aerodigestive tract are rare in children. Benign tumors are the most common, accounting for over 90% of such lesions.[1,2] A wide variety of tumors, both congenital and acquired, can arise in the oral cavity, pharynx, and esophagus. The otolaryngologist must be familiar with these neoplasms and be prepared to approach each patient with a systemic evaluation and treatment plan.

EVALUATION

The initial evaluation of the child with an oral cavity or pharyngeal neoplasm begins with a careful history. It is important to document the onset of symptoms, change in size of the lesion, and the presence of pain, bleeding, inflammation, or ulceration. Any problems with speech, swallowing, or respiration also should be noted.

A full head and neck examination should be performed. Direct inspection of the oral cavity and oropharynx is usually possible in the infant or child. The flexible nasopharyngolaryngoscope allows closer evaluation of a hypopharyngeal tumor. The size and color of the mass should be noted, and the examiner also should assess whether the mass is fixed, tender, mucosal or submucosal, ulcerated, or infected.

The history and physical examination alone may establish the diagnosis, as with a hemangioma. For other lesions, radiographs provide additional helpful information. Screening dental radiographs often initially identify lesions of the mandible and maxilla.

Computed tomography (CT) and magnetic resonance imaging (MRI) scans may be indicated for large tumors and for preoperative surgical planning. A biopsy is then indicated to establish the diagnosis so that proper treatment can be instituted.

ORAL CAVITY

Over 90% of pediatric oral cavity tumors are benign.[3] These lesions may be seen at any time throughout childhood, from birth to adolescence, and have an equal incidence in males and females. Vascular lesions, such as hemangiomas, are most common in children under 6 years of age, whereas odontogenic tumors are more common in older children.[1] Oral cavity neoplasms can be divided into two groups—soft tissue lesions and bony jaw tumors that involve the mandible and maxilla.

Benign Soft Tissue Oral Cavity Neoplasms

Hemangiomas

Hemangiomas of the oral cavity frequently involve the lips, cheeks, or tongue. These lesions usually are not present at birth, but grow rapidly during the first few months of life as a result of endothelial proliferation.[4] Proliferation usually ceases around 12 months of age, and the hemangioma gradually involutes over the next 5–7 years. Mucosal hemangiomas are raised and red (Fig. 41–1), whereas submucosal lesions appear blue or purple. Often, a careful history and physical examination establishes the diagnosis. Conservative management with close observation is appropriate for most small, asymptomatic hemangiomas, as these lesions spontaneously

Pediatric Otolaryngology, Edited by R.F. Wetmore, H.R. Muntz, and T.J. McGill. Thieme Medical Publishers, Inc., New York © 2000.

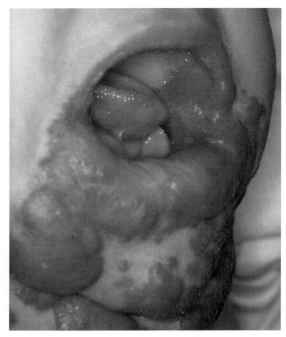

Figure 41-1: Hemangioma involving the buccal mucosa and tongue as well as the face and neck in an infant.

involute after the first year of life. Larger hemangiomas may cause pain, bleeding, or airway obstruction. Therapy begins with corticosteroids, and 30–60% of hemangiomas respond to oral steroids.[5] Some hemangiomas can be treated with a carbon dioxide laser to relieve symptoms of airway obstruction.[6,7] Interferon alfa-2A also has been used successfully to treat large life-threatening hemangiomas that are unresponsive to conventional steroid or laser therapy.[8,9]

SPECIAL CONSIDERATION:

A careful history and physical examination often will establish the diagnosis of a benign, vascular, oral cavity lesion in a young child, thus avoiding the need for radiographs.

Vascular malformations

Unlike most hemangiomas, other vascular oral cavity lesions are present at birth. A *vascular malformation* develops as a result of abnormal blood and lymphatic vessel morphogenesis. The lesion is pres-

ent at birth and grows commensurately with the child.[10,11] The malformation may expand or increase in size after trauma, infection, or hormonal changes (e.g., puberty, pregnancy). Thirty-five percent of vascular malformations are associated with skeletal abnormalities, usually secondary changes in the size and shape of nearby bones, such as the mandible.[10]

Malformations are subdivided by the type of vessel involved; they can be capillary, venous, arterial, or lymphatic malformations. Combined malformations consist of a combination of abnormal vessel types, such as the *arteriovenous malformation* (AVM). Capillary, venous, and lymphatic malformations are low-flow lesions, whereas arterial malformations and AVMs are high-flow lesions. The type of malformation usually can be established by physical examination or with the guidance of MRI scans.[12]

Management of the vascular malformation depends on the vessel type. *Lymphatic malformations* often involve the oral cavity, usually the tongue and floor of mouth. Mucosal disease of the tongue may have a "fish egg" appearance (Fig. 41-2). Lymphatic malformations of the tongue may enlarge dramatically in the presence of infection. Upper respiratory infections (URI) should be treated promptly in these children to minimize swelling of the lymphatic malformation. Long-term growth of these lesions may lead to malocclusion and bony overgrowth of the mandible. The primary treatment

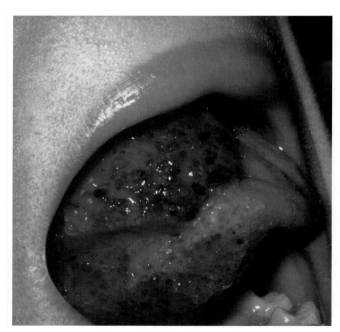

Figure 41-2: Lymphatic malformation of the tongue in an adolescent male.

of a lymphatic malformation of the oral cavity remains surgical excision. Some lymphatic malformations of the tongue may be amenable to laser therapy to debulk or decrease the size of the lesion. The optimal time of surgery is debatable; some authors recommend excision when the child is 18–24 months old.[2] Preoperative or perioperative tracheotomy may be necessary for airway control in those children with larger lesions. The goal of treatment is complete excision when possible, preserving normal function and structures. Larger lymphatic malformations may require planned, staged, serial excisions.

Venous and arterial malformations require a different approach. The vascular nature of these lesions makes excision difficult because of bleeding. The neodymium yttrium aluminum garnet (Nd: YAG) laser can treat some venous malformations.[11] The goal remains complete removal of the lesion while preserving normal anatomy. Sclerotherapy has also been successful in treating venous malformations of the lips, tongue, and other oral cavity sites. The sclerosing agent (ethanol or sodium tetradecyl sulfate) is injected directly into the lesion with fluoroscopic guidance. Potential complications include necrosis of surrounding normal tissues and neural injury.[11,12] Multiple injections may be necessary for large venous malformations.

AVM are high-flow vascular lesions, which make surgical excision difficult. Incomplete excision of an AVM may lead to increased collateral flow and enlargement of the malformation. Embolization of these lesions by a skilled interventional radiologist is often the best course of treatment.

Unlike hemangiomas, vascular malformations do not undergo spontaneous involution. Their growth potential continues throughout the patient's life. Therefore, the goal of treatment is often to restore function (e.g., voice, airway, swallowing) with partial excision or ablation. Long-term follow-up of these children is essential.

Practice Pathway 41–1 illustrates the major diagnostic and treatment differences between hemangiomas and vascular malformations. The diagnosis can usually be made after a careful history and physical examination, with the help of an MRI scan when necessary. When the diagnosis remains uncertain, a biopsy is indicated.

Miscellaneous neoplasms

Mucoceles are common oral cavity lesions. These painless, soft, smooth masses may be found on the tongue, on the floor of the mouth, and in the

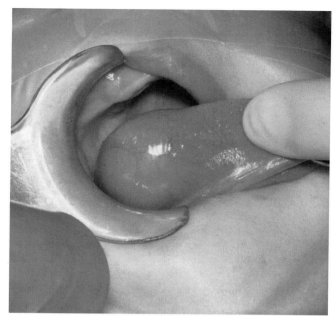

Figure 41–3:   Mucocele involving the tongue.

vallecula (Figs. 41–3, 41–4, and 41–5), and occasionally cause airway obstruction. A floor of the mouth mucocele may be called a *ranula,* appearing as a mucosal-covered, translucent blue or white cystic mass. It is usually caused by obstruction of a sublingual gland duct. A CT scan may help define the extent of the ranula and rule out extension into

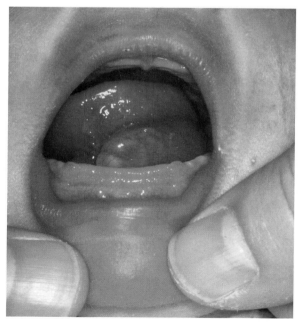

Figure 41–4:   Mucocele on the floor of the mouth in a newborn. This lesion resolved with simple aspiration.

Practice Pathway 41–1   DIAGNOSIS AND MANAGEMENT OF ORAL CAVITY VASCULAR LESIONS

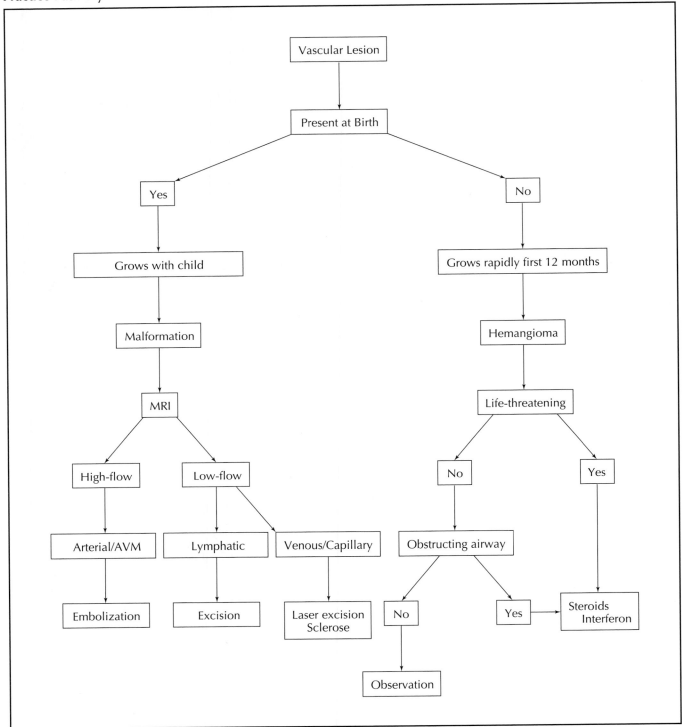

A
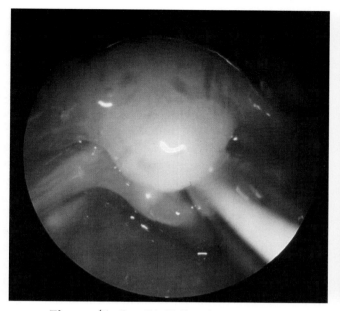
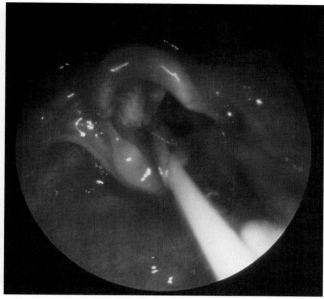
B

Figure 41–5:   (A) Vallecular mucocele causing stridor and feeding difficulty in a newborn. The mucocele displaces the epiglottis in this view. (B) Endoscopic view after marsupialization of the vallecular mucocele.

the neck (i.e., a plunging ranula). Treatment involves excision of the lesion or marsupialization when complete excision is not possible.

A variety of benign epithelial neoplasms can be found in the oral cavity. *Squamous papillomas* of the oral cavity are usually small, localized, slow-growing lesions involving the palate, tongue, and lips. Treatment is local excision, often with a laser.[6] Recurrence is unusual, except in the rare case of florid oral papillomatosis. The *white sponge nevus* is a rare familial form of oral mucosal epithelial hyperplasia. The lesion may appear at birth or later in childhood. A diffuse, white thickened mucosal growth may involve the lips, the floor of the mouth, buccal mucosa, or tongue. This benign lesion is asymptomatic and usually requires no treatment.[2] *Dermoids,* usually found in the anterior floor of mouth, may be present at birth or develop later in childhood. Twenty percent of all head and neck dermoids are found in the oral cavity.[2] Treatment is local excision. *Choristomas,* which are normal tissue in an abnormal location, also can be seen in the oral cavity. Oral cysts containing gastric mucosa may occur on the tongue and the floor of the mouth in young children. Treatment is complete excision.

Tumors of fibrous tissue origin, known as *desmoids* or *fibromatosis,* are thought to arise from the musculoaponeuroses. These benign, but locally aggressive, lesions may erode or invade bone. Be-

cause of a high recurrence rate, wide local excision is required.

Failure of normal embryonic descent of the developing thyroid gland may result in a rest of thyroid tissue at the base of tongue known as a *lingual thyroid.* The mass appears as a globular, red, smooth or lobulated, midline mass between the foramen cecum and the vallecula. Symptoms include dysphagia, dyspnea, muffled voice, and occasional hemorrhage.[13] In 70% of patients, lingual thyroid represents the only functioning thyroid tissue. Evaluation includes nuclear medicine thyroid scans to document the functional status of the mass and to look for functioning thyroid tissue elsewhere in the neck. Treatment of symptomatic masses begins with suppressive thyroid hormone therapy. If symptoms persist, surgery is indicated. Excision with postoperative thyroid hormonal replacement or autotransplantation of thyroid tissue to a suitable skeletal muscle bed is performed.[13]

Granular cell tumors may occur throughout the body; in the oral cavity, they often involve the tongue (Fig. 41–6). Also known as granular cell myoblastoma or Abrikosov's tumor, these lesions are now thought to represent a benign proliferation of peripheral neurogenic elements of the Schwann cell.[14] The granular cell tumor appears as a firm submucosal nodule. A congenital granular cell tumor, located on the alveolar ridge, is called *epulis of the*

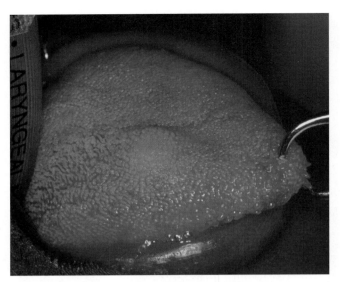

Figure 41–6:   Granular cell tumor of the midportion of the tongue.

newborn. Histologically, half of these neoplasms show pseudoepitheliomatous hyperplasia of the overlying epithelium and may be confused with carcinoma. After complete excision, recurrence is rare.

Neural tumors of the oral cavity are rare. Multiple neuromas of the lips or tongue can be seen in *multiple endocrine neoplasia syndrome type II,* associated with pheochromocytoma, medullary carcinoma of the thyroid, and hyperparathyroidism. *Neurofibromas* may occur as solitary lesions or in patients with neurofibromatosis type 1. The plexiform type may be especially difficult to control locally.[2]

Malignant Soft Tissue Oral Cavity Neoplasms

Malignant neoplasms of the oral cavity are quite rare in children. *Rhabdomyosarcoma* is the most frequent soft tissue malignancy in childhood and the most common sarcoma of the head and neck in children.[15,16] This embryonic, malignant neoplasm of skeletal muscle usually occurs in the head and neck between the ages of 2 and 6 years. In the oral cavity, the most common sites of involvement are the tongue, palate, and cheeks. The child presents with a rapidly growing mass, often with ulceration and bleeding, which suggests a malignant process. Metastatic disease may be present at the time of diagnosis; lung and bone metastases are most common. Treatment for rhabdomyosarcoma is determined by the primary site of involvement. Surgery is usually reserved for diagnostic biopsy; complete excision

is performed only for small lesions when it is possible to avoid functional or cosmetic defects. Combination chemotherapy and radiation therapy are the mainstay of treatment for most oral cavity rhabdomyosarcomas.[16]

Other oral cavity sarcomas reported in the pediatric population include *fibrosarcoma, leiomyosarcoma, angiosarcoma,* and *Kaposi's sarcoma.*[17-19] The patient usually develops a bulky, infiltrating submucosal mass. Treatment consists of a combination of surgery, radiation, and chemotherapy. Prognosis is fair to poor.

Epidermoid carcinoma is extremely rare in children. Reported cases include squamous cell carcinomas of the tongue, lips, and palate.[2,20,21] In these very young patients who have no history of tobacco or alcohol exposure, such tumors may be related to genetic factors or immunodeficiency.[21] There are isolated reports of oral squamous cell carcinoma developing in organ transplant survivors who are immunosuppressed.[22] These rare neoplasms are staged and treated like similar tumors in adults. Pediatric tumors tend to be more aggressive, with more virulent behavior and poorer prognosis.[21]

Other malignant neoplasms of the oral cavity include rare cases of *neuroblastoma, melanoma, lymphoma, mucoepidermoid carcinoma, adenoid cystic carcinoma,* and *hemangiopericytoma* (Fig. 41–7).[2,23] These tumors are treated like similar neoplasms at other anatomic sites.

AT A GLANCE. . .

Soft Tissue Neoplasms of the Oral Cavity

Benign: hemangioma, vascular lesions, mucocele, epithelial neoplasms, desmoid, lingual thyroid, granular cell tumors, neural tumors.

Malignant: rhabdomyosarcoma, other sarcomas, epidermoid carcinoma, melanoma, lymphoma, mucoepidermoid carcinoma, adenoid cystic carcinoma, hemangiopericytoma.

Benign Tumors of the Gingiva and Jaws

A wide variety of benign lesions arise from the gingival soft tissues and from the mandible and maxilla. Lesions arising from the mandible or maxilla are di-

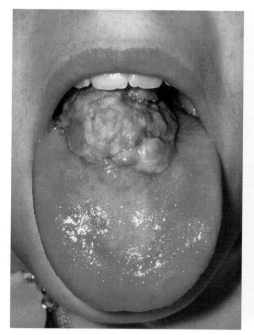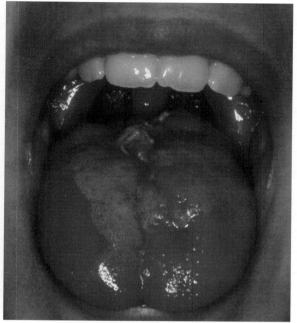

A   B

Figure 41–7: (A) Hemangiopericytoma of the tongue in a young girl. (B) Intraoral view after excision via midline glossotomy.

vided into odontogenic and nonodontogenic tumors, based upon the cell type of origin.

Gingival tumors

Benign gingival tumors include *peripheral giant cell reparative granuloma,* which is a sessile reddish mass of vascular connective tissue (Fig. 41–8). The lesion may arise after local trauma, and has a tendency to bleed easily. Treatment is by exicision or curettage. *Pyogenic granuloma* also represents an exuberant soft tissue response to relatively minor local trauma. This soft pedunculated growth has a smooth red surface and bleeds easily. Histology shows numerous small capillaries and the lesion may be confused with hemangioma. Treatment is local excision. *Epstein pearls* are small keratin cysts seen on the alveoli or palate of newborns. These cysts usually exfoliate within a few weeks.[2] *Melanotic neuroectodermal tumor* of infancy develops in the first 6 months of life as a mass on the anterior maxilla, near the junction of the globular and maxillary processes. The infant presents with facial swelling and nasal obstruction. Physical examination reveals a firm nontender mass of the alveolar ridge and palate. Dark pigment may be noted. Histologic evaluation will demonstrate islands of pigmented epithelium in a dense fibrous stroma.[24] Recurrence is unusual after complete local excision.

Odontogenic tumors

Odontogenic tumors comprise a diverse group of lesions that arise from the jaw tissues associated with tooth formation, including the early precursors of dental development, such as the *ameloblast,*

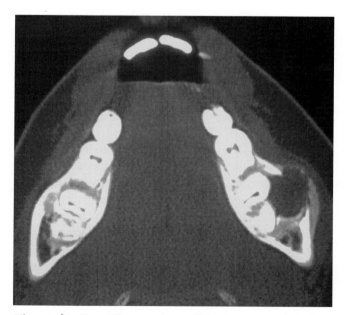

Figure 41–8: CT scan of mandible demonstrating giant cell reparative granuloma with a characteristic radiolucent appearance.

which is associated with enamel formation, and the *odontoblast,* which leads to dentin formation. A wide variety of nonneoplastic odontogenic cysts may occur;[14] however, this Chapter's scope does not permit discussion of these cystic lesions. Selected odontogenic neoplasms that may be seen in children are discussed here.

SPECIAL CONSIDERATION:

Odontogenic tumors arise from tissues involved with tooth formation, including the ameloblast (enamel formation) and the odontoblast (dentin formation).

In children, odontogenic tumors can occur at any age. Small lesions initially may be noted on routine dental examination. Larger lesions may interfere with tooth eruption, leading to an absent tooth in a child without a history of extraction. Secondary infection and swelling due to bony expansion also may be seen. Some odontogenic tumors are diagnosed on routine, intraoral-screening, dental radiographs. Many of these lesions have similar radiographic appearances, necessitating biopsy for diagnosis.

There are several biopsy techniques for jaw lesions. Aspiration is a simple method that may be accomplished with local anesthesia in an older, cooperative child. If straw-colored fluid is obtained, a benign, cystic lesion is likely. Purulent fluid indicates an infectious process, and bloody or serosanguinous fluid may suggest a vascular malformation. No aspirate usually indicates a solid neoplasm and the need for an open biopsy. In children, both excisional and incisional biopsies will most likely require general anesthesia. *Excisional biopsy* is useful for small lesions that are readily accessible and can be removed without violating adjacent structures. *Incisional biopsy* is indicated for very large or aggressive tumors, so that an accurate diagnosis can be made before choosing definitive treatment.

Most odontogenic lesions are benign and minimally aggressive. The goals of therapy are to remove all abnormal tissue and prevent recurrence, while preserving normal structure and function. Odontogenic tumors can be treated by a variety of surgical techniques. *Enucleation* involves local removal of the lesion itself. *Curettage* removes 1 to 2 mm of the bony wall after the tumor is enucleated. Curettage is accomplished by hand or with the use of rotary instrumentation. *Resection* requires osteotomy through uninvolved bone adjacent to the lesion, without disruption of the tumor. *Marginal resection* of a mandibular tumor allows preservation of a portion of the border of the mandible, avoiding a continuity defect. *Partial resection* removes a full-thickness portion of the involved bone. *Composite resection* includes removal of the tumor along with adjacent bone, soft-tissue, and lymph nodes, and is usually reserved for malignant neoplasms.[25]

Ameloblastoma is a benign odontogenic neoplasm that usually involves the mandible (Fig. 41-9). The patient presents with a soft swelling in the mouth. Radiographs show a multicystic, osteolytic and expansile lesion.[2] Treatment is complete excision. The *myxoma* is also thought to be of odontogenic origin. Two-thirds of these tumors are seen in patients 10 to 29 years of age, presenting with a large, painless, facial mass and loosened teeth.[24] The most frequent site of involvement is the posterior mandible. The myxoma is a locally aggressive tumor and requires marginal or en bloc resection.[25] The *odontogenic adenomatoid tumor* (also known as *adenoameloblastoma*) is usually seen in patients less than 20 years of age. Two-thirds of these lesions occur in females, and appear as a painless swelling in the anterior maxilla that is associated with an impacted tooth. Recurrence is rare after enucleation. An *odontoma* is actually a hamartoma that is derived from functional ameloblasts and odontoblasts, and it forms enamel and dentin in an abnormal pattern. These lesions can be found in all locations in the jaw, and are frequently associated with dentigerous cysts. Treatment is enucleation.[25]

Nonodontogenic tumors

Nonodontogenic tumors of the mandible and maxilla do not arise from dental precursors. These lesions include the *hemorrhagic bone cyst* (also known as a solitary or traumatic bone cyst). This idiopathic cavity usually forms in the posterior mandible of males in the second decade. The tumor may cause painless swelling or be discovered on routine dental radiographs, where it appears as a radiolucent lesion that expands the bony cortex.[2] The cavity is thought to develop after local trauma. Treatment is by surgical obliteration of the cavity.[25]

Aneurysmal bone cysts occur most commonly in

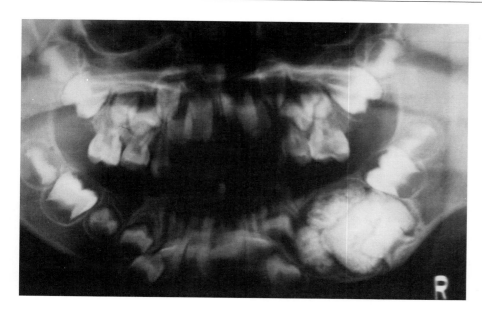

Figure 41–9: Ameloblastoma of the right mandible just anterior to the molars (Panorex).

females, in the vertebral column and long bones. In the head and neck, the mandible is most often involved. The patient presents with a localized area of swelling and pain. Radiographically, the lesion is radiolucent with a multilocular, honeycombed appearance. Histologically, the aneurysmal bone cyst consists of fibrous connective tissue, stroma, and multiple vascular spaces. Brisk hemorrhage frequently occurs during surgical removal. Rapid enucleation is recommended, using bone wax or packing to control bony bleeding. Recurrence is rare.

Eosinophilic granuloma (or *Langerhan's cell histiocytosis*) may involve the mandible or maxilla. The patient presents with swelling; painful, ulcerative, gingival lesions; and loosened teeth. Radiographs demonstrate osteolytic lesions that may be circumscribed or diffuse.[24] A complete evaluation is indicated to rule out systemic disease. Treatment of the jaw lesions includes curettage and low-dose radiation therapy.

Fibrous dysplasia of the maxilla and mandible is usually monostotic, and not associated with the stigmata of Albright's syndrome (Fig. 41–10). The lesion consists of hamartomatous replacement of bone with collagen, fibroblasts, and osteoid.[2] The process is usually unilateral, involving the maxilla more often than the mandible. Lesions grow rapidly from early childhood to adolescence. Maxillary lesions may expand into the canine fossa and zygomatic areas causing cheek swelling or proptosis. Conservative subtotal resection is indicated for children with cosmetic deformity, pain, or functional problems with vision or chewing.

Cherubism is a familial developmental process in which the bone is replaced by fibrous tissue. Symmetric enlargement of the mandible begins early in childhood, resulting in a rounded face with a "cherublike" appearance. Bony enlargement ceases around 10 years of age, followed by regression after puberty. Surgical reshaping of affected areas for cosmesis may be appropriate in some patients.

Central giant cell reparative granuloma occurs in the mandible and maxilla of young patients, usually 10 to 20 years of age. A firm ill-defined nontender mass may cause facial asymmetry. Treatment is with curettage or resection. *Tori,* exophytic be-

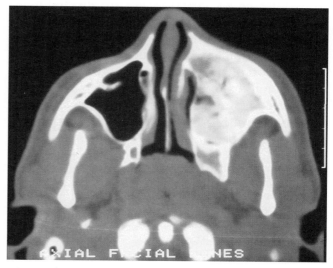

Figure 41–10: CT scan illustrating fibrous dysplasia of the left maxilla involving most of the left maxillary sinus.

nign bony overgrowths usually at the midline of the hard palate, occur in 20% of the population, and are often noted first at puberty. Occasionally, tori are found on the lingual aspect of the mandible in the premolar region. Most tori are asymptomatic and do not require treatment.

AT A GLANCE...

Benign Neoplasms of the Gingiva and Jaws

Benign gingival tumors: peripheral giant cell reparative granuloma, pyogenic granuloma, Epstein pearls, melanotic neuroectodermal tumor of infancy

Benign odontogenic tumors: ameloblastoma, myxoma, adenomatoid tumor, odontoma

Benign nonodontogenic tumors: hemorrhagic bone cyst, aneursymal bone cyst, eosinophilic granuloma, fibrous dysplasia, cherubism, central giant cell reparative granuloma, torus

---

Malignant Tumors of the Gingiva and Jaws

Malignant jaw tumors are quite rare. Symptoms suggestive of a malignant process include rapid growth of the mass, loosening and displacement of teeth, soft tissue ulceration, pain, paresthesias, and trismus. These rare lesions include *sarcoma, carcinoma,* and *malignant fibrous histiocytoma. Burkitt's lymphoma* may also involve the jaws, usually around the age of 3 years. Males are affected more often than females, and the maxilla is involved twice as often as the mandible. This osteolytic tumor grows very rapidly with frequent systemic spread. Left untreated, most patients die within 4 to 6 months. Aggressive chemotherapy achieves initial remission in over 90% of patients, but relapse is common. Surgical debulking may improve prognosis in some patients.[2]

PHARYNX (OROPHARYNX AND HYPOPHARYNX)

Children rarely develop neoplasms of the oropharynx and hypopharynx. Benign tumors include *hemangioma, lipoma, fibrous histiocytoma, papil-*

loma, pleomorphic adenoma, neurofibroma, and *fibromatous polyp.* Such tumors are treated like similar lesions in other anatomic sites.

Malignant pharyngeal tumors are quite unusual in children. *Rhabdomyosarcoma* of the pharynx is usually of the embryonal type; treatment includes combination chemotherapy and radiotherapy. In the head and neck, *lymphoma* usually involves the cervical nodes, although extranodal disease may also occur. Pediatric patients infected with the human immunodeficiency virus (HIV) are at increased risk for the development of lymphoma.[26] *Oropharyngeal lymphoma* may arise in the structures of Waldeyer's ring or from the posterior pharyngeal wall. Symptoms include difficulty swallowing, snoring, and a muffled voice. Physical examination reveals a bulky enlarging oropharyngeal mass or asymmetric tonsil enlargement. Excisional biopsy will establish the diagnosis. In a child undergoing tonsillectomy, asymmetric tonsils should be sent separately for pathologic evaluation. If lymphoma is suspected, the specimen should be delivered fresh in saline to the pathologist. Touch preparation and special T- and B-cell studies can be performed if indicated.[27] Once the diagnosis of lymphoma is established, a metastatic workup is performed. Treatment includes radiotherapy for localized disease, and chemotherapy is added for systemic disease.

ESOPHAGUS

Primary esophageal tumors are uncommon in children. There are isolated reports of aggressive respiratory papillomatosis invading the esophagus and causing obstruction. Childhood esophageal adenocarcinoma is rare, but has been reported to occur in the setting of *Barrett's esophagus* (mucosal dysplasia). Endoscopic surveillance is recommended for patients with Barrett's esophagus to allow early detection of possible malignant change.[28] Seven percent of patients with esophageal carcinoma have a history of caustic ingestion in childhood. After caustic ingestion, there is a 1000-fold increase in the incidence of esophageal carcinoma.[29] The interval between injury and the development of squamous cell carcinoma varies between 13 and 70 years; therefore, life-long follow up is essential in these patients.[30]

REFERENCES

1. Sato M, Tanaka N, Sato T, Amagasa T. Oral and maxillofacial tumours in children: A review. Br J Oral Maxillofac Surg 1997; 35:92-95.
2. Gonzales C. Tumors of the mouth and pharynx. In: Bluestone CD, Stool SE, Kenna MA, eds. *Pediatric Otolaryngology.* Philadelphia: Saunders, 1996, p. 1108.
3. Bhaskar SN. Oral tumors of infancy and childhood. J Pediatr 1963; 63:195-210.
4. Mulliken JB, Glowacki J. Hemangiomas and vascular malformations in infants and children: A classification based on endothelial characteristics. Plast Reconstr Surg 1982; 69:412-422.
5. Enjolras O, Riche MC, Merland JJ, Escande JP. Management of alarming hemangiomas in infancy; A review of 25 cases. Pediatr 1990; 85:491-498.
6. Crockett DM, Healy GB, McGill TJI, Friedman EM. Benign lesions of the nose, oral cavity, and oropharynx in children: Excision by carbon dioxide laser. Ann Otol Rhinol Laryngol 1985; 94:489-493.
7. Sie KCY, McGill T, Healy GB. Subglottic hemangioma: Ten years experience with the carbon dioxide laser. Ann Otol Rhinol Laryngol 1994; 103:167-172.
8. Ezekowitz RAB, Mulliken JB, Folkman J. Interferon alfa-2a therapy for life-threatening hemangiomas of infancy. N Engl J Med 1992; 326:1456-1463.
9. Ohlms LA, Jones DT, McGill TJI, Healy GB. Interferon alfa-2a therapy for airway hemangiomas. Ann Otol Rhinol Laryngol 1994; 103:1-8
10. Kaban LB, Mulliken JB. Vascular anomalies of the maxillofacial region. J Oral Maxillofac Surg 1986; 44:203-213.
11. Ohlms LA, Forsen J, Burrows PE. Venous malformation of the pediatric airway. Int J Pediatr Otorhinolaryngol 1996; 37:99-114.
12. Burrows PE, Fellows KE. Techniques for management of pediatric vascular anomalies. In: Cope C, ed. *Current Techniques in Interventional Radiology.* Philadelphia: Current Medicine, 1995, p. 12.
13. Gray SD, Parkin JL. Congenital malformations of the mouth and pharynx. In: Bluestone CD, Stool SE, Kenna MA, eds. *Pediatric Otolaryngology.* Philadelphia: Saunders, 1996, p. 985.
14. van der Waal I, Snow GB. Benign tumors and tumor-like lesions of oral cavity and oropharynx. In: Cummings CW, Fredrickson JM, Harker LA, et al., eds. *Otolaryngology-Head and Neck Surgery.* St. Louis: Mosby Year Book, 1993, p. 1237.
15. Kodet R, Fajstavr J, Kabelka Z, Koutecky J, Eckschlager T, Newton WA Jr. Is fetal cellular rhabdomyoma an entity or a differentiated rhabdomyosarcoma? A study of patients with rhabdomyoma of the tongue and sarcoma of the tongue enrolled in the intergroup rhabdomyosarcoma studies I, II, and III. Cancer 1991; 67:2907-2913.
16. Cole RR, Cotton RT. Pediatric malignancies. In: Bailey BJ, Johnson JT, Kohut RI, et al., eds. *Head and Neck Surgery-Otolaryngology.* Philadelphia: Lippincott 1993, p. 1388.
17. Beeson WH, Singer MI, Lingeman RE. Congenital fibrosarcoma in the oral cavity. Laryngoscope 1980; 90:1336-1343.
18. Wanebo HJ, Koness RJ, MacFarlane JK, Eilber FR, Byers RM, Elias EG, et al. Head and neck sarcoma: A report of the head and neck sarcoma registry. Society of Head and Neck Surgeons Committee on Research. Head Neck 1992; 14:1-7.
19. Lack EE. Leiomyosarcomas in childhood: A clinical and pathologic study of 10 cases. Pediatr Pathol 1986; 6:181-197.
20. Frank LW, Enfield CD, Miller AJ. Carcinoma of the tongue in a newborn child: Report of a case. Am J Cancer 1936; 26:775-777.
21. Son YH, Kapp DS. Oral cavity and oropharyngeal cancer in a younger population. Review of literature and exerience at Yale. Cancer 1985; 55:441-444.
22. Lee YW, Gisser SD. Squamous cell carcinoma of the tongue in a nine-year renal transplant survivor: A case report with a discussion of the risk of development of epithelial carcinoma in renal transplant survivors. Cancer 1978; 41:1-6.
23. Perez-Atayde AR, Kozakewich HW, McGill T, Fletcher JA. Hemangiopericytoma of the tongue in a 12-year-old child: Ultrastructural and cytogenetic observations. Hum Pathol 1994; 25:425-429.
24. Dehner LP. Tumors of the mandible and maxilla in children. I. Clinicopathologic study of 46 histologically benign lesions. Cancer 1973; 31:364-384.
25. Larsen PE, Hegtvedt AK. Odontogenesis and odontogenic cysts and tumors. In: Cummings CW, Fredrickson JM, Harker LA, et al., eds. *Otolaryngology-Head and Neck Surgery.* St. Louis: Mosby-Year Book, 1993, p. 1414.
26. Willard CC, Foss RD, Hobbs TJ, et al. Primary anaplastic large cell (KI-1 positive) lymphoma of the mandible as the initial manifestation of acquired immunodeficiency syndrome in a pediatric patient. Oral Surg Oral Med Oral Pathol Oral Radiol Endod 1995; 80:67-70.
27. Ward RF. Head and neck tumors in children. In: Healy GB, ed. *Common Problems in Pediatric Otolaryngology.* Chicago: Year Book Medical Publishers, 1990, p. 349.
28. Hassall E, Dimmick JE, Magee JF. Adenocarcinoma in childhood Barrett's esophagus: Case documentation and the need for surveillance in children. Am J Gastroenterol 1993; 88:282-288.
29. Appelqvist P, Salmo M. Lye corrosion carcinoma of the esophagus—a review of 63 cases. Cancer 1980; 45:2655-2658.
30. Hopkins RA, Postlethwait RW. Caustic burns and carcinoma of the esophagus. Ann Surg 1981; 194:146-148.

V

THE LARYNX, TRACHEA, AND UPPER AIRWAY

42 Structure and Function of the Upper Airway

Orval E. Brown

This chapter focuses on the structure and function of the larynx and trachea, including anatomy, aspects of embryology, and development of the airway, physiology, and host defenses.

Although rather simple in structure, the larynx has complex interrelationships and functions, including respiration, protection of the airway during swallowing and from foreign matter, and phonation. As our understanding of the larynx and airway advances, how these structures and their functions develop and relate are becoming better elucidated.

LARYNGEAL ANATOMY

Structural Framework

The structural framework of the larynx consists of both bone (specifically the hyoid bone) and the major cartilages, including the thyroid, cricoid, epiglottic, and arytenoids (Fig. 42-1). The *hyoid bone* serves as the superior attachment of the larynx, as the thyrohyoid membrane and strap muscles insert on it. The hyoid bone consists of a midbody and the paired greater and lesser cornu. The hyoid is derived embryologically from the second and third branchial arches; the lesser cornu is derived from the second branchial arch; and the greater horn and midbody are derived from the third branchial arch.[1]

The *cartilaginous tissues* of the larynx are composed of hyaline cartilage, with the exception of the epiglottis which is composed of elastic cartilage. Elastic cartilage also is found at the tip of the vocal process and at the superior portion of the arytenoid cartilage from the vocal process to the apex.[2] These cartilages developed from the fourth, fifth, and sixth branchial arches. The *cricoid cartilage* is the only complete cartilaginous ring in the airway. This is often described as a signet ring with the narrow arch positioned anteriorly and the broad posterior arch serving as the framework for the cricoarytenoid joints and cricothyroid joints. The cricoid cartilage stabilizes the larynx and provides the foundation for its essential functions.

The *thyroid cartilage* is a V-shaped structure consisting of lateral lamina and paired superior and inferior horns. The thyroid notch forms the laryngeal prominence, and the thyroid cartilage articulates with the cricoid via the cricothyroid joints. This joint facilitates motion, acting similarly to a hinge between the cartilages.

The *epiglottis* is a cartilaginous structure that is composed mostly of elastic cartilage that is attached to the thyroid cartilage at its most inferior portion and to the tongue base at its anterior midportion.

The *arytenoid cartilages* consist primarily of hyaline cartilage, but do contain some elastin. They articulate on the superior surface of the posterior arch of the cricoid cartilage via the cricoarytenoid joints (Figs. 42-2 and 42-3). The arytenoids consist of a concave base, a muscular process that projects laterally, and a vocal process that projects anteriorly. The corniculate cartilages and cuneiform cartilages are small, paired cartilages at the apex of the arytenoids, just lateral to the posterior commissure.

The larynx has two pairs of synovial joints: the *cricoarytenoid joints* and the *cricothyroid joints*. These joints have a synovial membrane that lines the joint cavity as well as joint capsules bound by ligaments of elastic and collagen fibers. Both these joints are susceptible to arthritic problems, but the cricoarytenoid joint is involved more commonly.

Soft Tissue

The structural framework of the larynx serves to support the surrounding soft tissue, which includes

Pediatric Otolaryngology, Edited by R.F. Wetmore, H.R. Muntz, and T.J. McGill. Thieme Medical Publishers, Inc., New York © 2000.

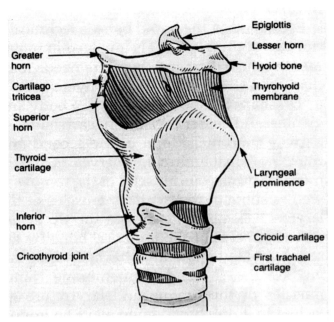

Figure 42–1: Oblique view of the larynx. (From Blitzer A, Brin MF, Sasaki CT, et al. *Neurologic Disorders of the Larynx.* New York: Thieme, 1992, p. 4, with permission.)

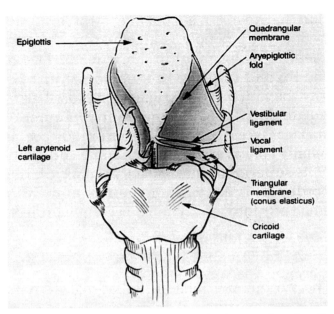

Figure 42–3: Posterior view of the larynx showing fibroelastic membrane attachments. Arytenoid cartilage on right moved laterally to demonstrate membrane attachments to the ligaments. (From Blitzer A, Brin MF, Sasaki CT, et al. *Neurologic Disorders of the Larynx.* New York: Thieme, 1992, p. 5, with permission.)

the laryngeal mucosa, the quadrangular and triangular membranes, and the laryngeal musculature.

The *mucosal lining* of the upper airway consists primarily of pseudostratified ciliated columnar epithelium (i.e., respiratory epithelium). However, because the larynx is exposed to forces caused by

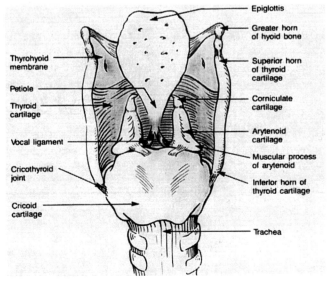

Figure 42–2: Posterior view of the larynx. (From Blitzer A, Brin MF, Sasaki CT, et al. *Neurologic Disorders of the Larynx.* New York: Thieme, 1992, p. 4, with permission.)

swallowing, phonation, and cough, strong mucosa is required in certain areas. These areas are lined with stratified squamous epithelium, and include the covering of the true vocal cords, the laryngeal surface of the aryepiglottic folds, the arytenoids, and the lingual surface of the epiglottis. Squamous epithelium also covers the piriform sinuses laterally on each side of the larynx and extends posteriorly into the esophageal introitus. The other areas, including the subglottis, the ventricle, and the laryngeal vestibule, are lined with respiratory epithelium.

The respiratory epithelium of the larynx has abundant compound tuboalveolar glands that are exocrine glands. These are mucus glands and are usually branched with small narrow funnel-shaped ducts that extend to the mucosal surface and produce secretions rich in immunogloblin A (IgA). These glands are absent on the free edges of the vocal cords. These secretions provide a mucus blanket, which is transported by the cilia, and also provide lubrication for the vocal cords.

The mucosa covers the musculature and the internal membranous structure of the larynx. The *quadrangular membrane* is superior, paired, and begins at the aryepiglottic fold and descends inferiorly to

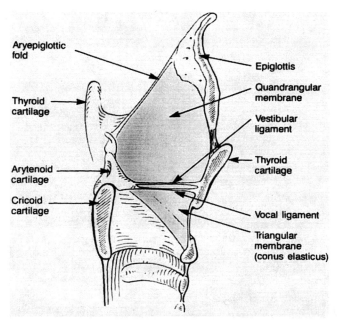

Figure 42-4: Midsagittal cut of the larynx showing the fibroelastic membrane attachments. (From Blitzer A, Brin MF, Sasaki CT, et al. *Neurologic Disorders of the Larynx.* New York: Thieme, 1992, p. 5, with permission.)

the level of the vocal ligament (Figs. 42-4 and 42-5). The *triangular membrane* is located inferiorly and also is known as the *conus elasticus.* This membrane is attached inferiorly to the cricoid cartilage and superiorly to the thyroid cartilage at the

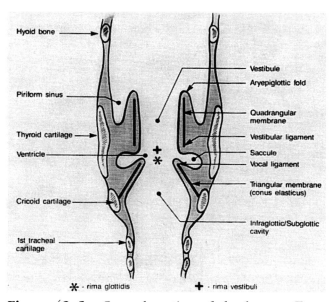

Figure 42-5: Coronal section of the larynx. (From Blitzer A, Brin MF, Sasaki CT, et al. *Neurologic Disorders of the Larynx.* New York: Thieme, 1992, p. 6, with permission.)

level of the vestibular ligament. These membranes are separated at the level of the laryngeal ventricle.

The musculature of the larynx consists of extrinsic and intrinsic muscles and the classification may vary depending on the author (Fig. 42-6). In general, the *cricothyroid muscle* is considered the extrinsic muscle of the larynx, whereas the intrinsic muscles consist of two groups. One set of intrinsic muscles is associated with the quadrangular membrane and consists of the *thyroarytenoid, thyroepiglottic,* and *aryepiglottic muscles.* The *vocalis* is associated with the thyroarytenoid muscle. These muscles act to provide closure of the larynx. The thyroarytenoid muscles approximate the false vocal cords, and the aryepiglottic muscle closes the vestibule. The second set of intrinsic muscles includes the *posterior* and *lateral cricoarytenoid* and *interarytenoid muscles* and are associated with the arytenoid cartilages. The posterior cricoarytenoid arises from the posterior aspect of the cricoid lamina in a broad fan-shaped fashion. The lateral cricoarytenoid muscle is smaller and arises from the anterior aspect of the cricoid arch. It inserts on the muscular process of the arytenoid. The interarytenoid or arytenoid muscle arises from the posterior and lateral aspect of the arytenoid and inserts on the opposite arytenoid cartilage. The action of these muscle groups to open the airway during maximal inspiration is complex.[3,4]

Blood Supply

The blood supply of the larynx originates superiorly via the *superior laryngeal artery* and inferiorly via the *inferior laryngeal artery.* The superior laryngeal artery branches from the superior thyroid artery, which branches from the external carotid artery. Rarely, the superior thyroid artery branches from the common carotid. The superior laryngeal artery enters the larynx at the thyrohyoid membrane and supplies the superior larynx in the distribution of the quadrangular membrane. The inferior laryngeal artery is derived from the inferior thyroid artery, which is a branch of the thyrocervical trunk. This artery enters the larynx along the inferior border of the thyroid cartilage and supplies the inferior larynx in the distribution of the conus elasticus. There are complex anastomoses between the inferior and superior laryngeal arteries in the endolarynx. The venus drainage follows a similar pattern with the *superior laryngeal vein* and *inferior laryngeal vein* paralleling their respective arteries.

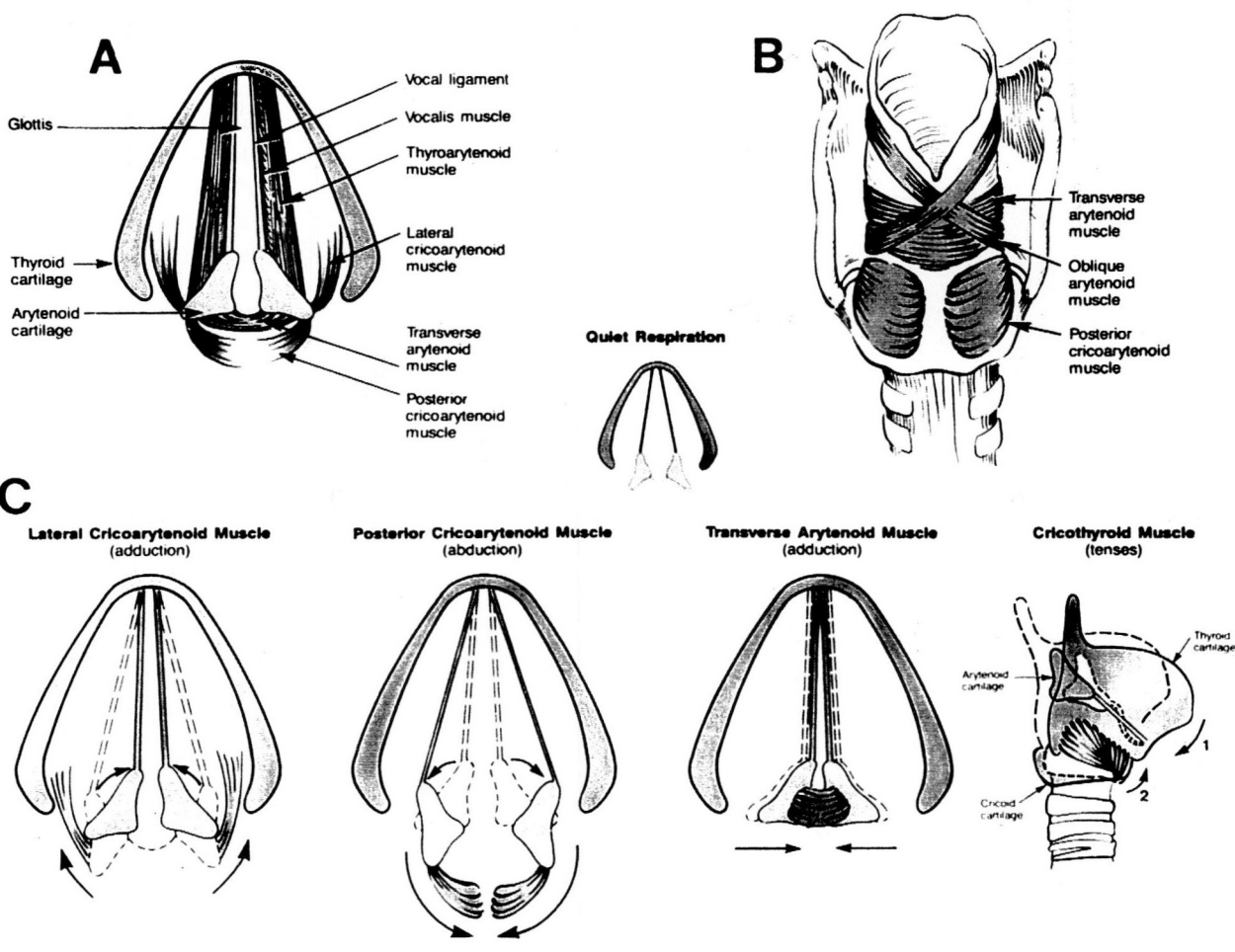

Figure 42–6:   (A and B) Intrinsic muscles of the larynx and (C) the movement of the vocal cords caused by their contraction. Dashed lines indicate position of vocal cords and arytenoid cartilages before movement caused by contraction of the muscles (arrows). Solid lines indicate position of vocal cords and arytenoid cartilage after contraction. Under cricothyroid muscle, 1 and 2 indicate possible movements of cartilages. (From Blitzer A, Brin MF, Sasaki CT, et al. *Neurologic Disorders of the Larynx.* New York: Thieme, 1992, p. 7, with permission.)

The larynx is rich in lymphatics, except on the free edge of the vocal cords. The lymph capillaries drain into nodes that are compartmentalized into a superficial and deep system. The *superficial lymph vessels* are located within the laryngeal mucosa, whereas the *deep vessels* are located within the submucosa and deeper tissues. The vocal cords serve as a dividing boundary between the inferior and superior drainage of the laryngeal lymphatics. The vessels follow the course of the superior and inferior thyroid arteries, in a similar pathway to the venus drainage.

The lymphatics within the mucosal or the superficial layer communicate freely between the right and left sides of the larynx; however, the submucosal or deep lymphatics have separate right and left distribution, and there is little or no communication between the two sides of the larynx. There is also a medial drainage of the deep submucosal lymphatics that appears at the cricothyroid membrane and passes into the anterior tracheal lymph nodes.

Nerve Supply

The innervation of the larynx originates in the central nervous system (CNS) in the nucleus ambiguus, retrofacial nucleus, and the dorsal motor nuclus of the tenth cranial nerve. The motor neuron cell bodies of the recurrent laryngeal nerve arise from the nucleus ambiguus, which is located in the upper medulla and is adjacent to respiratory motor neurons in the brainstem. These respiratory motor neurons control the diaphragm and other respiratory musculature. The cell bodies of the nucleus ambiguus are divided into two sections, between which there is little or no overlap. The innervation of the posterior cricoarytenoid, lateral cricoarytenoid, and interarytenoid muscles is located in the caudal half of the nucleus ambiguus. The posterior cricoarytenoid neurons are located medially, and the thyroarytenoid group are located laterally. The motor neuron bodies of the lateral cricoarytenoid and interarytenoid muscles are between these two motor neuron pools.

These motor neurons produce axonal processes that contribute to the vagus nerve and also the cranial portion of the eleventh cranial nerve; however, all innervation is carried by the vagus nerve, which is inferior to the jugular foramen. The *vagus nerve* gives off two branches to innervate the larynx: the superior and recurrent laryngeal nerves. The *superior laryngeal nerve* consists of an external and internal laryngeal nerve. The *external laryngeal nerve* innervates the cricothyroid muscle and the inferior constrictor muscle of the pharynx. The *internal laryngeal nerve* only receives sensation from the supraglottic larynx. The innervation of the larynx is distributed in a unilateral fashion from the respective vagus nerve, with the exception of the interarytenoid muscle, which is the only muscle with bilateral innervation. The *recurrent laryngeal nerve* enters the larynx posteriorly paralleling the inferior laryngeal artery. This nerve supplies the intrinsic muscles of the larynx and sensory fibers to the inferior larynx as well.[1,2]

Cell bodies of sensory fibers from the supraglottic larynx, which are carried by the internal branch of the superior laryngeal nerve, are located in the nodose ganglion and project to the vagus nerve into the medulla where they synapse with the nucleus ambiguus, nucleus solitarius, and nucleus dorsomedialis. Cell bodies of the vagus nerve from the recurrent laryngeal nerve, which transmit sensation from the subglottic larynx, project to the nucleus solitarius and nucleus ambiguus.

The larynx also is innervated with adrenergic and cholinergic (autonomic) fibers from the superior cervical ganglia and the vagus nerve. These fibers contain various neuropeptides and neurotransmitters and are involved in glandular secretion and neurovascular control of small blood vessels.

AT A GLANCE . . .

Laryngeal Anatomy

Laryngeal Cartilage: *Unpaired:* thyroid, cricoid, epiglottis. *Paired:* arytenoid, corniculate, cuneiform

Laryngeal Joints: cricoarytenoid, cricothyroid

Laryngeal Muscles: *Extrinsic:* cricothyroid. *Intrinsic:* thyroarytenoid (includes vocalis), thyroepiglottic, and aryepiglottic; posterior cricoarytenoid, lateral cricoarytenoid, and interarytenoid

Laryngeal Membranes: quadrangular, triangular

Laryngeal Blood Supply: superior laryngeal artery (from external carotid via superior thyroid artery), inferior laryngeal artery (from thyrocervical trunk via inferior thyroid artery)

Laryngeal Nerve Supply: *Superior laryngeal nerve:* the external laryngeal nerve innervates cricothyroid and the internal laryngeal nerve receives sensation from the supraglottic larynx. *Recurrent laryngeal nerve:* innervates the intrinsic laryngeal muscles and receives sensation from the inferior larynx

---

TRACHEAL ANATOMY

The trachea and bronchi consist of C-shaped rings that are open posteriorly. In the peripheral airways, the cartilage is less prominent. The cartilages are connected by smooth muscles between the cartilaginous rings, which can contract to change the diameter of the airways. The cartilages are connected by membranous and fibrous soft tissue that provides flexibility to the airway. The trachea and bronchi are lined by respiratory epithelium, but in the smaller airways, this epithelium becomes more cuboid and contains less cilia. There are no cilia in the smaller airways. Goblet cells frequently are found in this mucosa and produce a thin layer of mucus; these cells are controlled by the parasympathetic system. Mucociliary transport removes inhaled particles and other secretions in the airway. The sensory innervation of the trachea is via the vagus nerve and ascends superiorly as previously described.[1,2]

LARYNGEAL FUNCTION

The laryngeal functions are complex and involve respiration, swallowing, and phonation. The larynx coordinates its function with the pharynx and esophagus for competing objectives in the pharynx (that is, airway versus food passage and communication). The development of the larynx in primitive animals reveals that the first and most primitive function was protection of the lower airway. The lungfish has a primitive sphincter that allows respiration with air and protection from water. Air is drawn through the sphincter to inflate the lungs and is relaxed to allow air to escape during exhalation.[5] Amphibians have a more highly-developed larynx with a cartilage skeleton. Dilator as well as constrictor muscles of the larynx are present.

Respiration

The larynx functions in breathing and ventilation both as a sphincter and an active organ of respiration. The larynx regulates airflow, and through a complex set of reflexes, the level of laryngeal movement (adduction and abduction) varies. The *posterior cricoid arytenoid* (PCA) muscle contracts with each inspiration just prior to activation of the diaphragm. The level of this activity, which widens the airway, varies between slight motion during quiet breathing and more active inspiration during maximal airflow. Occlusion of the upper airway is a potent generator of dilation of the upper airway by the PCA and also has the effect of increasing diaphragmatic force. The diaphragm is modulated partially by laryngeal airflow sensors that feed back to the CNS and coordinate the diaphragm and other accessory muscles of respiration.

Protective Functions

Protective functions of the larynx include *cough,* which expels mucus and is important to protect the tracheobronchial tree from foreign bodies. Cough can be in response to stimulation of the larynx or other receptors in the airway. The cough reflex usually is suppressed during sleep. Cough begins with deep inspiration, followed by tight closure of the true vocal cords. Diaphragmatic contraction along with contraction of the chest wall muscles produces pressure in the airway followed by a sudden opening of the true vocal cords, resulting in a rapid outflow of air.

Other reflexes of the larynx respond to stimulation by foreign matter, such as foreign bodies or toxins. These cause a strong closure reflex of the larynx, which protects the airway. Laryngospasm represents a prolonged closure reflex.[1-4]

Speech

Human speech is a coordinated process that consists of three components, including phonation, resonance, and articulation. During *phonation,* the vocal cords generate sound by vibration. *Resonance* is the distribution of these vibrations to the remainder of the upper airway. *Articulation* is the shaping of the sound within the oral cavity. The role of the larynx in phonation requires that there is adequate breath support, that the edges of the vocal folds are aligned, and that the vocal fold has the proper mucosal and muscular function to control the shape and tension of the vocal folds. Vibration of the folds is a very complex function with the vocal fold mucosal vibration pattern varying in many ways. A previous theory of vocal fold function by Husson held that each vibratory cycle was caused by a separate nerve impulse relating to a vibration of the vocal fold.[1] This neurochronaxic theory has been disproved, and now it is accepted that the aerodynamic properties that affect the tissues of the vocal folds produce sound. This means that the vocalis muscles do not move the vocal folds, but instead act to alter the sound by adjusting their length, tension, and mass.

The current model of vocal fold function (myoelastic aerodynamic theory) requires that the mucosa vibrate over the underlying vocal ligament of the vocalis muscle during phonation. This action is possible because the muscosa is separated by a specialized connective tissue that allows this to occur. The most superficial layer of the muscosa is made up of fibers of collagen and elastin and is known as *Reinke's space.* The intermediate layer is composed of elastic fibers and the deep layer is composed of collagen fibers. These intermediate and deep layers form the *vocal ligament.*

Phonation is produced by vibration of the mucosa over the vocalis structures (i.e., the ''bodycover'' concept of phonation). The pattern of mucosal vibration varies with register and pitch and occurs as a wave in the mucosa. Different regions of this mucosa vibrate differently with pitch. The vibratory wave begins at the inferior vocal cord and moves superiorly. As the superior edges of the vocal cord separate, the inferior edges are closing. Bernoulli effects of airflow on the inferior vocal fold accelerate closure. This theory was advanced by Ishizaka as the "two-mass model" theory.[3,6]

Swallowing

The larynx functions during swallowing to protect the airway. This protection is done by closure and elevation of the larynx. The strap muscles elevate the larynx during swallowing, which brings the airway up and out of the way of the passage of the food bolus. The food bolus divides at the epiglottis, which folds down at the time of swallowing and helps to prevent entrance of food into the airway. The pressure for folding down the epiglottis in the adult is about 16 gm.[7] Closure of the larynx involves three levels. Closure is maintained by the true vocal folds, then by the false vocal folds and arytenoids, and finally by the epiglottis and aryepiglottic folds. Probably the most important level of closure is the arytenoids and false vocal folds. This closure is maintained for only a fraction of a second as the bolus passes and then opens quickly. At this instant the cricopharyngeus muscle relaxes and the bolus passes into the esophagus. The cricopharyngeus then contracts again to prevent reflux of the food bolus.

AT A GLANCE . . .

Laryngeal Function

Respiration: Dilator of the airway during maximal inspiration; Closure and cough reflexes
Phonation: Generator of sound
Swallowing: Closure and elevation of the larynx during swallowing

---

EMBRYOLOGY AND DEVELOPMENT OF THE LARYNX AND TRACHEA

Prenatal life is divided into an embryonic stage, which includes the first 8 post-ovulatory weeks, and a fetal stage, which extends from the eighth week until birth. These weeks have been divided arbitrarily into 23 Carnegie stages. The first week corresponds to stages one through four; the second week to stages five and six; the third week to stages seven to nine; the fourth to fifth weeks correspond to stages 10 to 15; and the fifth through eighth weeks represent stages 16 through 23.

Tucker et al. have investigated the embryology of the larynx extensively.[7-12] Prior to stage eight, there is no evidence of a respiratory system or foregut. The median pharyngeal groove appears during stage nine, which indicates the beginning of the respiratory system and includes the future larynx. At stage 10 the laryngotracheal sulcus appears and the pulmonary primordia also appear. The tracheoesophageal septum appears at stage 12. The right and left lung primordia are definitive by stage 13, and definitive parts of the larynx such as the arytenoids and the epithelial lamina of the larynx are seen at stage 14. At stage 17 the epiglottis can be identified, cricoid condensation begins to appear, and laryngeal vestibular outgrowths develop. At stage 18 the thyroid lamina is seen, and at stage 19 (at approximately 48 days) the epiglottis assumes a concave shape. At stage 23 (at approximately 57 days) most laryngeal structures are present and reasonably well formed. By stage 23 the epithelium of the larynx is similar to that of the esophagus and respiratory tube.[13] This epithelium is pseudostratified columnar and shows cilia over parts of the larynx including the epiglottis. The larynx is already innervated by the recurrent laryngeal nerve near the sagittal cleft of the vestibule. Silver impregnated receptors of sensory innervation at this stage also have been observed. At stage 23 the infrahyoid and most of the major laryngeal muscles are present, and the innervation follows essentially that of the adult pattern. The vocalis muscle is present for the first time.

As fetal development progresses, in the third month the thyroid lamina fuse anteriorly, and the laryngeal ventricle develops between the true and false vocal cords. By the fifth month, fibroelastic cartilage is present in the epiglottis, and in the sixth month the epithelium changes as gland formation occurs in the ventricles. By the eighth month the epiglottis assumes its omega-shaped contour.

There are several controversies regarding the early development of the human larynx. Traditionally, it is thought that the laryngeal primordium develops from the cranial end of the laryngotracheal sulcus. This region develops from the ventral wall of the foregut in the area of the fourth pharyngeal pouch. The caudal end of this region eventually becomes the trachea and lungs. An epithelial lamina forms with the pharyngoglottic duct on its dorsal border, ultimately becoming the laryngeal vestibule that is continuous with the infraglottic cavity at stage 21. There is one theory that the epithelial lamina is a primary structure and represents the primordium of the laryngeal cavity; however, Zaw-Tun proposes that the epithelial lamina plays no part in the development of the laryngeal primordium.[14] Sanudo and Domenech-Mateu theorize that there are two structures, the epithelial septum and the epithelial lamina, that contribute to the development of the laryngeal cavity.[15] The epithelial septum also contributes to the laryngotracheal septum, but the epithelial lamina probably has no effect on this morphogenesis.

The trachea and esophagus develop and are separated by what is thought to be an ascending tracheoesophageal septum. Zaw-Tun has suggested that this hypothesis is in error and that the trachea actually arises from cephalad as a diverticulum and grows caudally.[14] In their studies of Carnegie stage twelve embryos, Sutliff and Hutchins think that the normal growth of the tracheoesophageal sulcus is directed by a saddle-shaped catenoidal sulcal fold of this sulcus.[16] The development of the septum is dependent on this fold, and abnormalities of the tracheoesophageal septum may lead to such developmental errors as tracheoesophageal fistula (TEF) and posterior laryngeal clefts.

Etiologic studies of the vocal cord in fetuses and infants have identified the *macula flava,* which is an area of fibroblasts, elastic, and collagenous fibers, that influences the growth and maturation of the vocal folds.[17,18] The macula flava have been found in an immature form in 24-week fetuses at the anterior and posterior ends of the fetal vocal folds.[15] These structures are essential to the proper development and growth of the vocal ligament. The adult macula flava is a dense mass of fibrous tissue, but the fibrous tissue is much less dense in newborns.[17]

Fetal breathing has been identified by Lopez and Cajal[19] and by Isaacson and Birnholz.[20] Ultrasound studies have noted diaphragmatic and laryngeal movements in second and third trimester fetuses. These diaphragm movements have been coordinated with inspiratory and expiratory flow of amniotic fluid. Opening and closing of the fetal glottis has been found to precede the onset of inspiratory flow by 100 m sec and can be associated with up-

ward displacement of the larynx, which may represent fetal swallowing. Fetal breathing is most likely essential to proper pulmonary development. When fetal breathing is impaired, such as with oligohydramnios, pulmonary maldevelopment and hypoplasia results. As in adults, fetal inspiration is likely an active process resulting from diaphragmatic and chest wall muscular retraction, and expiration is caused by passive recoil of the chest wall. During the second or third trimester fetal breathing has become more mature, and the laryngeal coordination reflexes have developed. At birth, the larynx has been prepared by fetal breathing for the transition to air breathing.

At birth, the neonatal larynx is different in structure from that of the adult. The larynx is situated higher in the neck relative to the adult larynx. The cricoid is at a level with the fourth cervical vertebra and the tip of the epiglottis with the first cervical vertebra. Having the larynx more cephalad permits simultaneous suckling and respiration due to apposition of the epiglottis and the soft palate. The distance between the hyoid and the thyroid cartilage is very small. The aryepiglottic folds are thicker, and the arytenoids are relatively larger. All of these differences help to protect the child's airway during swallowing. The length of the vocal cord in a normal neonate is 7 mm, and the subglottis has a normal diameter of 4 to 5 mm, forming the narrowest part of the airway.[20,21]

As the child grows, the larynx gradually descends in the neck.[22-25] At age 2 years, the cricoid descends to the level of the fifth cervical vertebra and is opposite C6 or C7 by the teenage years. The gap between the thyroid cartilage and hyoid increases. Growth of the larynx is rapid until age 3 years or so and then slows. This growth is identical for both sexes until puberty. The relationship of the vocal fold to the cartilages remains constant during growth, with the anterior commissure located at the vertical midline of the thyroid cartilage. With growth of the larynx, there is a lowering of the pitch.

During the teenage years, sexual dysmorphism of the larynx is notable.[26] The pubertal male larynx is significantly larger, and the thyroid eminence is more prominent in the male. The vocal cords in both sexes reach their adult length by puberty; however, the male vocal fold length has increased more than two times that of the female. The pattern of ossification of the laryngeal cartilages reveals no sex differences. Ossification begins in the second decade of life but is more commonly present in persons over 20 years of age. The process of ossification begins in the inferior portion of the thyroid cartilage and extends superiorly. At the same time ossification of the cricoid cartilage begins in the posterior aspect and spreads inferiorly and anteriorly. The cornicula and cuneiform cartilages usually do not ossify.[27]

The newborn trachea is soft and six times more compliant than that of the adult. In studies of the tracheal wall, the transverse muscle fibers are arranged uniformly, but the longitudinal smooth muscle varies throughout the entire tracheal length. Muscle is present more frequently in the lower half of the trachea, which functions to preserve stability of the tracheal lumen.[28,29]

Tracheal growth progresses throughout childhood into puberty. The length of the trachea changes from approximately 4 cm in neonates to approximately 12 cm in adults. After puberty, the C-shaped cartilage rings do not expand, so tracheal growth is the result of tracheal muscle and ligaments. There is no difference in tracheal growth between boys and girls, and the tracheal diameter remains constant over the length of individual tracheas.[30,31]

Reed et al. described an anterior angulation change of 9.9 degrees in the pediatric trachea.[32] This point of inflection was found to lie below the sternal notch in children < 2 years and grew above the notch in older children. The superior limb of the trachea was angled anteriorly in relation to the inferior limb.

The larynx functions with complex neuromuscular mechanisms to protect the airway; however, the protective functions in neonates and infants seem to work less efficiently. The cough reflex is less effective in patients under 6 months of age, and the laryngeal closure reflex, which is protective of the larynx from foreign bodies and food, is also less effective. Infants respond to stimulus of fluid in the pharynx with obstructed breathing, apnea, and swallowing. Cough is less common. Occasionally, prolonged apnea and laryngospasm can occur with these stimuli. Usually, laryngospasm results in hypoxia and hypocarbia, which causes the airway to reopen. However, in children with immature control of reflexes, prolonged laryngospasm may result in severe asphyxia, an event that may play a role in sudden infant death syndrome.[32-36] The coordination of breathing and swallowing is imperfect in this stage of maturation, and aspiration may result in cyanosis and bradycardia when young infants are feed-

ing. Eichenwald et al. reported that the diaphragm and posterior cricoarytenoid muscle coordination is disrupted frequently in newborn infants.[35] This incoordination indicates that the maturation of the respiratory reflexes is immature and not as effective in newborn infants as it is in adults. In some patients, aminophylline may effect improvement.[32-35]

AT A GLANCE . . .

Differences between Neonatal and Adult Larynx

1. Larynx higher in neonate than adult.
2. Distance between hyoid and thyroid cartilage is small.
3. Aryepiglottic folds are thicker.
4. Arytenoid cartilages are relatively larger.
5. Ossification of the laryngeal cartilages does not begin until second decade of life.

REFERENCES

1. Graney DO, Flint PW. Anatomy. In: Cummings CW, et al., eds. *Otolaryngology Head and Neck Surgery, 3rd ed.* New York: Mosby, 1998, pp. 1823.
2. Sato K, Kurita S, Hirano M, et al. Development of elastic cartilage in the arytenoids and its physiologic significance. Ann Otol Rhinol Laryngol 1990; 99: 363–368.
3. Woodson CE. Laryngeal and pharyngeal function. In: Cummings CW, et al., eds. *Otolaryngology Head and Neck Surgery, 3rd ed.* New York: Mosby, 1998, pp. 1834–1894.
4. Kirchner JA. Physiology of the larynx. In: Paparella MM, et al., eds. *Otolaryngology.* Philadelphia: Saunders, 1991, pp. 333–342.
5. Bartlett D. Respiratory functions of the larynx. Physiol Rev 1989; 69:33–357.
6. Ishizaka K, Flanagan JL. Synthesis of voiced sounds from a two-mass model of the vocal cords. Bell Syst Tech J 1977; 51:1233–1235.
7. Fink BR, Martin RW, Rohrmann CA. Biomechanics of the human epiglottis. Acta Otolaryngol (Stockh) 1979; 87:554–559.
8. Tucker JA, Tucker GF. Some aspects of fetal laryngeal development. Ann Otol Rhinol Laryngol 1975; 87: 49–55.
9. O'Rahilly R, Tucker JA. Early development of the larynx in staged human embryos. Part 1: Embryos of the first five weeks (to stage 15). Ann Otol Rhinol Laryngol 1973; 82:3–27.

10. Müller F, O'Rahilly R, Tucker JA. The human larynx at the end of the embryonic period proper. I. The laryngeal and infrahyoid muscle and their innervation. Acta Otolaryngol (Stockh) 1981; 91:323-336.

11. Tucker J, Vidic B, Tucker GF, et al. Survey of the development of laryngeal epithelium. Ann Otol Rhinol Laryngol 1976; 85(5 supplement):3-16.

12. Tucker JA, O'Rahilly R. Observations on the embryology of the human larynx. Ann Otol Rhinol Laryngol 1972; 81:520-523.

13. Montgomery PA, Stafford ND, Stolinski C. Ultrastructure of human fetal trachea: A morphological study of the luminal and glandular epithelia at the midtrimester. J Anat 1990; 173:43-59.

14. Zaw-Tun HA, Burdi AR. Reexamination of the origin and early development of the human larynx. Acta Anat (Basel) 1985; 122:163-184.

15. Sanudo JR, Domentech-Mateu JM. The laryngeal primordium and epithelial lamina. A new interpretation. J Anat 1990; 171:207-222.

16. Sutliff KS, Hutchins GM. Septation of the respiratory and digestive tracts in human embryos: Crucial role of the tracheoesophageal sulcus. Anat Res 1997; 238:237-247.

17. Campos Banales ME, Perez Pinero B, Rivero J, et al. Histologic structure of the vocal fold in the human larynx. Acta Otolaryngol (Stockh) 1995; 115:701-704.

18. Sato K, Hirano M. Histologic investigation of the macula flava of the human newborn vocal fold. Ann Otol Rhinol Laryngol 1995; 104(7):556-562.

19. Lopez R, Cajal C. Description of human laryngeal functions and phonation. Early Human Dev 1996; 45:63-72.

20. Isaacson G, Birnholz JC. Human fetal upper respiratory tract function as revealed by ultrasonography. Ann Otol Rhinol Laryngol 1991; 100(9 pt 1):743-747.

21. Isaacson G. Developmental anatomy and physiology of the larynx, trachea and esophagus. In: Bluestone CD, et al., eds. *Pediatric Otolaryngology, 3rd ed.* Philadelphia: Saunders, 1996, pp. 1202-1219.

22. Pracy R. The infant larynx. J Laryngol Otol. 1983; 97:933-947.

23. Magripes Y, Laitman JT. Developmental change in the position of the fetal human larynx. Am J Phys Anthropol 1987; 72:463-472.

24. Roche AF, Barkla DH. The level of the larynx during childhood. Ann Otol Rhinol Laryngol 1965; 74:645-654.

25. Hudgins PA, Siegel J, Jacobs I, et al. The normal pediatric larynx on CT and MR. AJNR 1997; 18:239.

26. Schwartz DS, Keller MS. Maturational descent of the epiglottis. Arch Otolaryngol Head Neck Surg 1997; 123:627-628.

27. Kahane JC. A morphological study of the human prepubertal and pubertal larynx. Am J Anat 1978; 151:11-20.

28. Hately W, Evison G, and Samuel E. The pattern of ossification in the laryngeal cartilages: A radiologic study. Brit J Radiol 1965; 38:585-591.

29. Wailoo M, Emery JL. Structure of the membranous trachea in children. Acta Anat 1980; 106:254-261.

30. Griscom NT, Wohl Me, Fenton T. Dimensions of the trachea to age 6 years related to height. Pediatr Pulmonol 1989; 6:186-190.

31. Wailoo MP, Emery JL. Normal growth and development of the trachea. Thorax 1982; 37:584-587.

32. Reed JM, O'Connor DM, Myer CM. Magnetic resonance imaging determination of tracheal orientation in normal children: Practical implications. Arch Otolaryngol Head Neck Surg 1996; 127:605-608.

33. Thach BT. Neuromuscular control of upper airway patency. Clin Perinatol 1992; 19:773-788.

34. Carlo WA, Kosch PC, Bruce EN, et al. Control of laryngeal muscle activity in pre-term infants. Pediatr Res 1987; 22:87-91.

35. Eichenwald EC, Howell RG, Kosch PC, et al. Developmental changes in sequential activation of laryngeal abductor muscle and diaphragm in infants. J Appl Physiol 1992; 73:1425-1431.

36. Sasaki CT. Development of laryngeal function etiologic significance in sudden infant death syndrome. Laryngoscope 1979; 3:420-438.

43 Radiologic Evaluation of the Upper Airway

Joan K. Zawin

Radiologic evaluation of the pediatric airway is a challenging but integral component of the diagnostic and therapeutic management of children with respiratory distress. Children must not be treated as miniature adults. Rather, certain modifications in radiologic techniques such as beam collimation, pulse-fluoroscopy, immobilization devices, and sedation should be employed judiciously in order to obtain diagnostic studies in a timely and safe fashion.

In this chapter, the radiologic techniques that are available for the evaluation of the pediatric airway are reviewed, and emphasis is placed on their appropriate clinical applications.

STANDARD RADIOGRAPHS OF THE NECK

Technique

Frontal and lateral radiographs of the neck are usually the first imaging study obtained to assess the upper airway. These exposures should be made at the end of inspiration, with the head and neck extended and held in a true lateral position.[1,2] Whenever possible, the child should be seated in the upright position with a gonad shield in place. Infants can be placed in a specially-designed immobilization chair, and a supportive chin strap may be used to prevent hyperflexion and resultant occlusion of the airway by the chin at the level of the hyoid bone.[3] This precaution is particularly important when radiographing hypotonic infants, such as those with Down syndrome, or children with congenital structural abnormalities that predispose them to airway

compromise, such as those with mucopolysaccharidoses.[4] Although children with respiratory difficulty are usually most comfortable in the upright position, diagnostic radiographs of the upper airway can be obtained in the supine position,[5-7] and may be the only feasible option when dealing with neonates and critically-ill children.

Radiographs of the upper airway should include all structures between the nasopharynx and the carina (Fig. 43–1).[3,5] A high kilovoltage, collimated, filtered, magnification technique should be employed.[8] This technique not only results in a reduction of the dose of ionizing radiation, but also provides a more detailed view of the airway by increasing the contrast between air and surrounding bones and soft tissues. Hence, these modifications are most useful in improving airway detail on frontal radiographs of the neck when all of these structures overlap (see Fig. 43–1B). If there is clinical suspicion of foreign-body aspiration, a low kV technique also should be obtained to improve visibility of faintly radiopaque foreign bodies.[3] The radiologic evaluation of such a child can be expanded to include frontal and lateral chest radiographs, bilateral decubitus views of the chest, and/or airway fluoroscopy as needed (vide infra).

SPECIAL CONSIDERATION:

A high kV, collimated, filtered, magnification technique results in a reduction of the dose of ionizing radiation and provides a more detailed view of the airway.

Lateral Radiographs

A properly-obtained lateral radiograph of the neck is the most useful projection for the evaluation of

Pediatric Otolaryngology, Edited by R.F. Wetmore, H.R. Muntz, and T.J. McGill. Thieme Medical Publishers, Inc., New York © 2000.

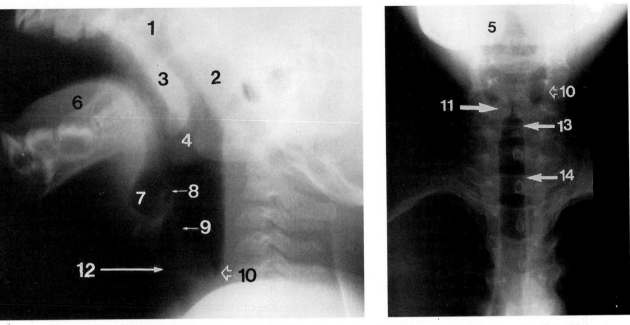

Figure 43–1:   Normal lateral (A) and frontal (B) radiographs of the neck. 1, nasopharynx; 2, adenoids; 3, palate; 4, palatine tonsils; 5, lateral tonsillar tissue; 6, tongue; 7, vallecula; 8, epiglottis; 9, aryepiglottic folds; 10, pyriform sinus; 11, vocal cords; 12, laryngeal ventricle; 13, subglottic airway; 14, cervical trachea.

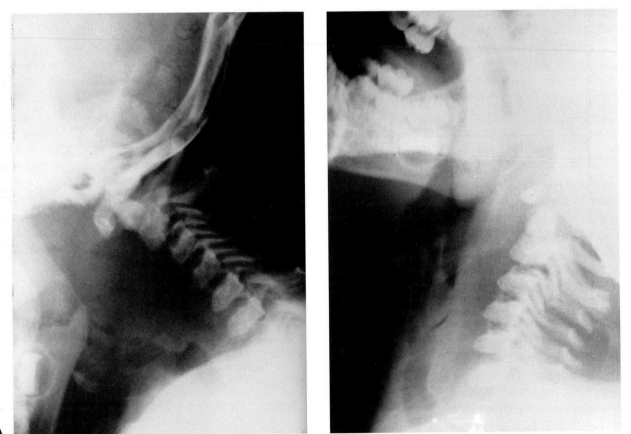

Figure 43–2:   Prevertebral "pseudomass." Obtaining lateral radiographs of the airway with the head and neck in flexion (A) causes apparent thickening of the prevertebral soft tissues, resulting in a "pseudomass." A repeat radiograph obtained with the head and neck extended (B) shows normal prevertebral soft tissues with disappearance of the "pseudomass."

the nasopharynx, oropharynx, and supraglottic structures (see Fig. 43-1A).[1,7,9] However, films obtained with improper technique can be quite misleading. Exposures that are made with the head and neck flexed result in anterior buckling of the airway, causing spurious thickening of the prevertebral soft tissues and the creation of a retropharyngeal "pseudomass" (Fig. 43-2). Similarly, exposures made during expiration or during swallowing obscure the supraglottic structures (Fig. 43-3).[1-3,10]

More often than not, the lateral radiograph of a child's neck includes the skull base, occiput, and maxillary antra. As with all radiologic studies, every structure on an image must be evaluated carefully, with all abnormalities noted and correlated with the child's symptomatology. Examples of such serendipitous findings include: wormian bones and/or an enlarged, "cherry," sella in children with hypothyroidism;[11] a small midface and craniosynostosis in children with Apert syndrome[12] and lytic calvarial

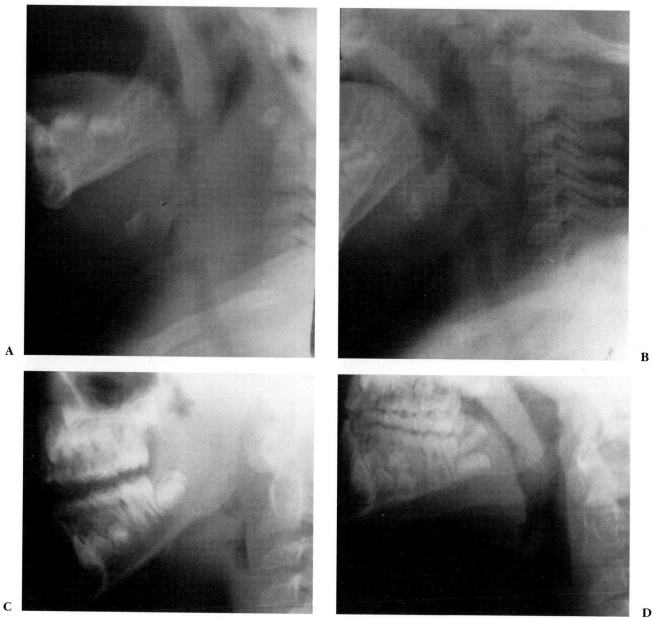

Figure 43-3: Suboptimal lateral neck radiographs. Lateral neck radiographs obtained at expiration (A) also cause the creation of a prevertebral "pseudomass" due to the normal expiratory buckling of the airway. This "pseudomass" disappears during inspiration (B). Lateral radiographs obtained during swallowing (C) obscure the supraglottic structures, which are well delineated with proper technique (D).

or mandibular lesions suggesting leukemia, neuroblastoma, or Langerhans' cell histiocytosis (Fig. 43-4).[13] Examples of other unexpected, but pertinent, findings include soft-tissue masses or radiopaque foreign bodies in the nose or nasopharynx (Fig. 43-5) and air-fluid levels overlying the maxillary antra-suggesting unilateral or bilateral acute bacterial maxillary sinusitis (Fig. 43-6).

The nasopharynx

The structures located above the soft palate are delineated best radiographically on a lateral view.[5] The main focus of interest in this region is the posterior-superior nasopharynx, where the adenoids develop. Radiographically-visible adenoidal tissue should never be seen in neonates but should be noted routinely in full-term infants >6 months of age.[14] Posterior nasopharyngeal masses in a child <1 month of age are abnormal and must never be attributed to benign adenoidal hypertrophy. In such cases, the differential diagnosis should include teratoma, hemangioma, neuroblastoma, and basilar encephalocele.[5,9,14,15] Absence of posterior nasopharyngeal adenoidal tissue in a child >6 months of age who has had no prior surgery is also abnormal and indicates an immunodeficient state (Fig. 43-7).[13,14]

> ## SPECIAL CONSIDERATION:
>
> Structures located above the soft palate are delineated best on a lateral view.

The normal adenoidal tissue, which can extend inferiorly into the retropharyngeal region, reaches its largest size relative to the size of the nasopharynx in children 3 to 5 years of age,[1,16] which explains why the nasopharyngeal airway seems compromised most often in this age group. Initially, the adenoidal tissue has a convex, somewhat lobular contour with gradual development of the normal adult concave contour over time.[16] Although the adenoids may be enlarged due to neoplastic involvement, most cases of adenoidal hypertrophy are due to bacterial or viral infections (Fig. 43-8),[9,17] and may or may not be accompanied by lateral pharyngeal tonsillar enlargement. The degree of enlargement often is assessed in a gestalt fashion, but pub-

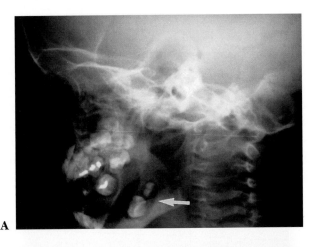

A

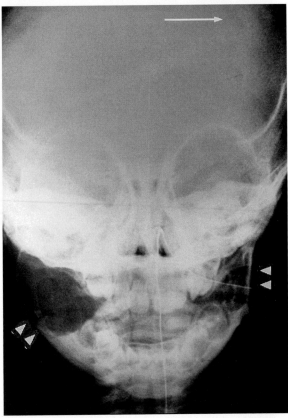

B

Figure 43–4: Unsuspected lytic mandibular lesions. (A) Lateral radiograph of the airway demonstrates the presence of "floating teeth" (arrow). This radiolucency surrounding the teeth suggests the diagnosis of Langerhans' cell histiocytosis in this 4-year-old boy. (B) Frontal radiograph of the airway shows large bilateral lytic mandibular lesions (arrowheads) in another child subsequently diagnosed with Langerhans' cell histiocytosis. A small left calvarial lytic lesion also is noted (thin arrow).

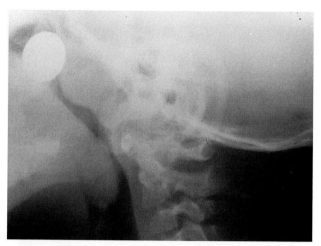

Figure 43–5: Unsuspected foreign body in nose. Lateral radiograph of the airway obtained to assess adenoidal size shows not only the enlarged adenoids, but also a coin in the nose—an unexpected dividend.

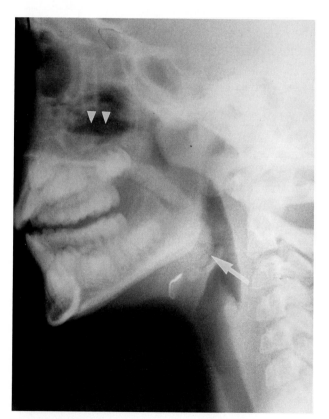

Figure 43–6: Unsuspected sinusitis. Lateral radiograph of the airway obtained in an 8-year-old girl with a soft-tissue mass along the posterior tongue that obliterated the vallecula air space (arrow), and which proved to be the lingual thyroid. An air-fluid level is noted incidentally in the region of the maxillary antra (arrowheads), indicating acute bacterial sinusitis. A Waters view is needed to determine which maxillary sinus is involved. Note paucity of pretracheal soft tissue in this child without any normally-positioned thyroid tissue present.

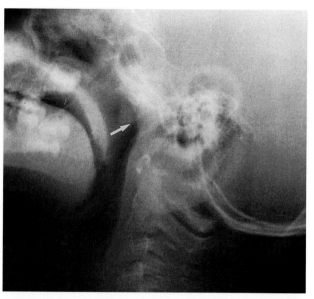

Figure 43–7: Absence of adenoidal tissue. Lateral radiograph of the neck of a 2-year-old boy with repeat upper respiratory tract infections demonstrates minimal, if any, posterior nasopharyngeal soft-tissue density in the expected region of the adenoids (arrow). Subsequent biochemical evaluations confirmed the diagnosis of agammaglobulinemia.

lished standards and more precise methods of adenoidal measurement, such as the adenoidal: nasopharyngeal ratio,[18] are available. Lateral films obtained for the assessment of adenoidal size should be obtained with the mouth closed and not during swallowing.[1,6,19] This allows for maximum aeration of the nasopharynx and prevents erroneous overestimation of adenoidal size relative to the size of the nasopharynx.[19]

SPECIAL CONSIDERATION:

Lateral films obtained to assess adenoidal size should be taken with the mouth closed and not during swallowing to avoid overestimation of adenoidal size relative to the size of the nasopharynx.

The mouth and oropharynx

Structures of the mouth, including the palate, uvula, tongue, lingual tonsils, vallecula, and mandible, are delineated well on lateral radiographs of the neck

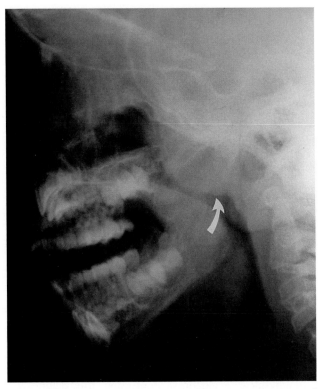

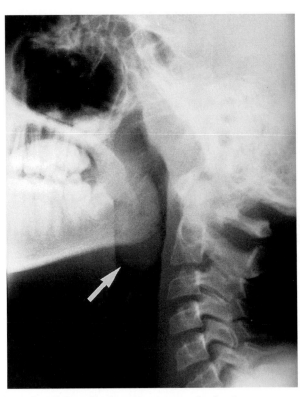

A   B

Figure 43–8: Adenoidal and tonsillar hypertrophy. Lateral radiographs demonstrate marked enlargement of the posterior nasopharyngeal–adenoidal tissue (A) (curved arrow) and palatine tonsils (B) (arrow) in two children with mononucleosis.

(see Fig. 43–1A). The micrognathia present in children with Pierre Robin sequence and Treacher Collin's syndromes can be identified readily and distinguished from the macroglossia seen in children with Beckwith-Wiedermann syndrome, congenital hypothyroidism, and the rare cases of lingual neo-

plasms, vascular malformations, or fibromatosis (Fig. 43–9).[9,11,12] In the latter instance, definitive evaluation of the extent of tumor or fibrous infiltration of the tongue and oral cavity requires cross-sectional imaging such as computed tomography (CT) or magnetic resonance imaging (MRI).[20,21]

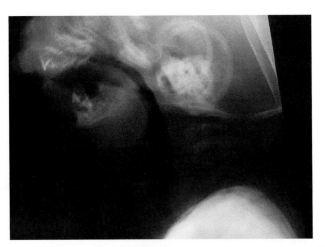

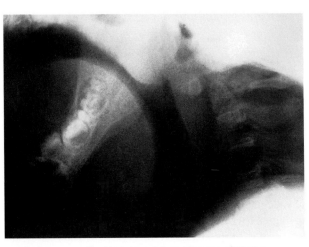

A   B

Figure 43–9: Disproportionate mandibular and lingual size contributing to upper airway obstruction. (A) Lateral radiograph demonstrates micrognathia in a 2-month-old with Pierre Robin sequence. This appearance is distinguished easily from (B) the macroglossia seen on a lateral radiograph of a 1-year-old with Beckwith-Wiedermann syndrome.

The neck and larynx

Every lateral radiograph of the neck should be assessed for maintenance of the normal vallecula airspace. The differential diagnosis for masses that may partially or completely obliterate the vallecula airspace in children is reviewed in Table 43-1.[5,7,9,13] Due to the critical location of these masses, even small lesions can displace the epiglottis posteriorly and inferiorly, thereby occluding the airway. In most instances, these masses are indistinguishable based on their radiographic appearance (Fig. 43-10). Exceptions include teratoma, which may contain characteristic calcifications,[15] and lingual thyroid unaccompanied by additional, normally-located thyroid tissue (see Fig. 43-6). In the latter instance, a paucity of pretracheal soft tissue density sometimes can be appreciated on the lateral radiograph.

The most urgent circumstance in which a lateral radiograph of the neck is obtained in pediatric patients involves cases of suspected acute bacterial epiglottitis.[2,5,13,22] In many instances, radiographs are not obtained prior to intubation. If, however, there is some uncertainty as to the diagnosis, a lateral radiograph of the neck can be obtained with minimal manipulation of the child, as immediate airway occlusion is an ever present danger. Obtaining the lateral radiograph in the upright position is most efficacious because a child with acute epiglottitis is usually most comfortable sitting with his head extended and neck flexed. This radiograph can be done with portable equipment in the emergency room. Alternatively, a higher quality film can be obtained in the radiology department, providing the child is accompanied by trained medical personnel

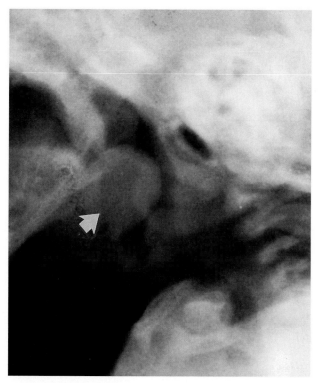

Figure 43–10: Obliteration of the vallecula air-space. Lateral radiograph of a 1-month-old with respiratory distress reveals a soft-tissue mass at the base of the tongue obscuring the vallecula air-space (arrow). This was resected and found to be an epiglottic mucous retention cyst.

who are appropriately equipped to act in the event of acute airway occlusion.[6,7,9]

> **SPECIAL CONSIDERATION:**
> Acute bacterial epiglottitis is the most urgent circumstance in which a lateral radiograph of the neck is obtained in pediatric patients.

The classic radiographic finding in acute epiglottitis is the "thumb" sign.[13,22] Normally, the epiglottis is quite thin in the anteroposterior (AP) dimension, resembling a little finger (see Fig. 43-1A), whereas the abnormal, inflamed epiglottis appears shorter and has an increased AP dimension, resembling a thumb (Fig. 43-11).[22] The enlarged epiglottis narrows or obliterates the vallecula air-space and is associated with marked thickening of the aryepiglottic folds,[23] distention of the hypopharyngeal air-

TABLE 43–1: Vallecular Masses in Children

Infectious/inflammatory
  Abscess
  Hypertrophied lingual tonsils
Traumatic
  Foreign body
  Hematoma (especially in hemophiliacs)
Neoplastic
  Teratoma
  Lingual masses—fibromas, neurofibromas, hemangiomas
Congenital
  Mucous retention cyst
  Ectopic thyroid
  Thyroglossal duct cyst

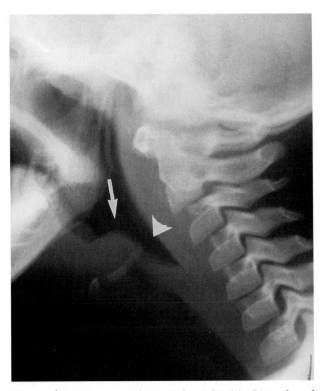

Figure 43–11:   Acute bacterial epiglottitis. Lateral neck radiograph of a toxic-appearing 4-year-old with acute respiratory distress shows a very swollen epiglottis, resembling a "thumb" (arrow). There is accompanying thickening of the aryepiglottic folds (arrowhead) and mild hypopharyngeal distention.

way, and straightening or reversal of the normal cervical lordosis (see Fig. 43–11). In 25% of cases, there is accompanying subglottic edema and airway narrowing, which may be suspected on the lateral view but is appreciated best on an AP view (Fig. 43–12).[24] The differential diagnosis of epiglottic enlargement in children is extensive Table 43–2 and includes caustic ingestion, radiation therapy, hemorrhage, granulomatous disease, sarcoidosis, and angioneurotic edema.[5,7,9,13,25,26] The so-called "omega" or *U-shaped epiglottis* is an asymptomatic anatomic variant that appears large on lateral radiographs due to the presence of full, infolding lateral folds.[7,13] Unlike most pathologic processes involving the epiglottis, this entity is not accompanied by thickening of the normal, violin-string thin, aryepiglottic folds.

Whereas most pathologic processes affecting the supraglottic structures involve enlargement of normal structures or the presence of abnormal structures, occasionally the abnormality is the absence of a normal structure. This may be quite difficult to detect, especially if the abnormality is very rare or is asymptomatic. An example of such a situation is congenital absence of the epiglottis (Fig. 43–13).[27] Alternatively, abnormal ossification of normal structures, such as the stylohyoid ligament (Fig. 43–14), can occur and may be asymptomatic or associated with dysphagia, the *Eagle syndrome*.[28]

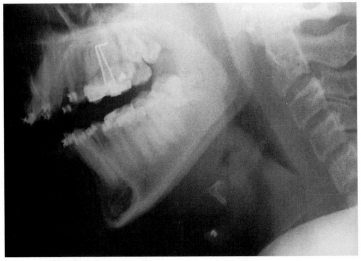

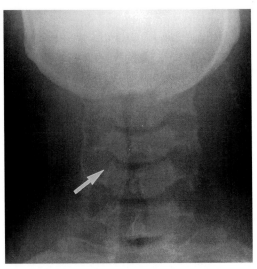

A   B

Figure 43–12:   Laryngeal edema following radiation therapy to the head and neck. Lateral neck radiograph of a teenager with nonHodgkin's lymphoma who was treated with chemotherapy, radiation therapy, and bone marrow transplantation (A) shows the classic enlargement of the epiglottis and aryepiglottic folds that is indistinguishable from that seen in acute bacterial epiglottitis. Frontal radiograph of this teenager (B) demonstrates edematous symmetric subglottic narrowing (arrow), which mimics the classic radiographic appearance of viral croup as well (see Figs. 43–16 and 43–25).

TABLE 43–2: Causes of Epiglottic Enlargement in Children

Infectious
  Acute bacterial epiglottitis (*Hemophilus influenzae* type B is the most common pathogen)
  Granulomatous disease (Mycobacteria tuberculosis)
Traumatic
  Caustic ingestion
  Radiation
  Foreign-body ingestion/implantation
  Hemorrhage (special concern in children with coagulopathies and bleeding dyscrasias)
Congenital
  Omega epiglottis
  Mucous retention cyst
  Lymphangioma
Other
  Angioneurotic edema
  Anasarca
  Sarcoidosis
  Stevens-Johnson syndrome
  Neoplasms (lymphoma, neurofibroma)

The vocal cords, subglottic structures, and cervical trachea are delineated well on lateral radiographs of the neck (see Fig. 43-1A). In order to distend this portion of the airway in children with an indwelling tracheotomy tube, transient occlusion of the artificial airway usually is required.[3] Abnormal tracheal cartilage calcifications,[29-32] foreign bodies, and masses in these portions of the airway

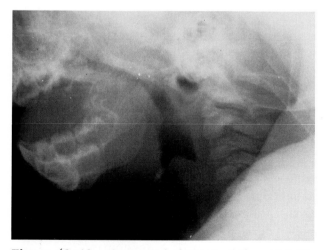

Figure 43–13: Congenital absence of the epiglottis. Lateral neck radiograph of a 7-month-old boy with absence of the epiglottis and aryepiglottic folds, which are observations that may not be made in an asymptomatic child.

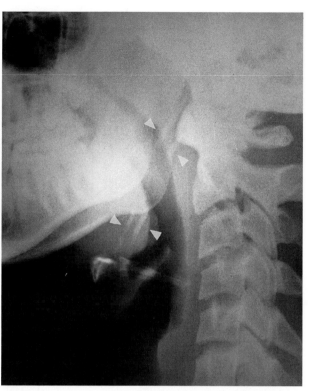

Figure 43–14: Eagle syndrome. Lateral radiograph of the neck of a 16-year-old girl with dysphagia demonstrates bilateral discontinuous ossification of the stylohyoid ligaments (arrowheads). These ossified ligaments lie on either side of the pharynx and limit the amount of pharyngeal distention during swallowing, thus causing the sensation of "food getting stuck" in the throat.

can be detected radiographically, particularly when they are surrounded by air (Fig. 43-15). Some masses have common locations such as recurrent laryngeal papillomas on the true vocal cords[7,33] and subglottic hemangiomas along the posterior or lateral wall of the subglottic airway.[7,13] Granulation tissue, subglottic stenosis, and tracheomalacia related to prolonged intubation tend to develop along the posterior wall of the glottis and subglottic airway where the endotracheal tube compresses and traumatizes the mucosa.[5,34] Similarly, after removal of a tracheotomy tube, granulomas and stenosis often are seen along the antero-superior stomal margin and at the level of the tip of the artificial airway.[35] However other masses such as the plaques seen with membranous laryngotracheobronchitis (LTB),[36] are more nonspecific in appearance and location and can be simulated by mucous strands/collections on a standard radiograph. A repeat lateral radiograph following coughing or airway fluoroscopy may be required to distinguish markedly-mobile mucous from fixed pathology.

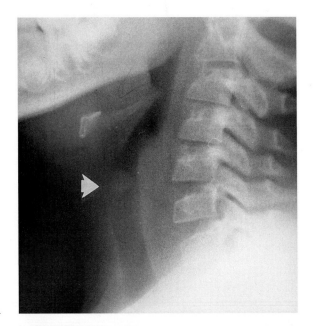

A

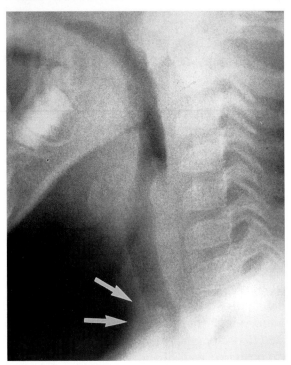

B

Figure 43–15: Tracheal granulation tissue. Lateral radiograph of the neck (A) shows a subglottic granuloma (arrowhead) following prolonged intubation. A similar view in another child who had a tracheotomy (B) demonstrates a soft-tissue mass along the anterior wall of the cervical trachea at the site of the old stoma (arrows).

Although the diagnosis of acute viral LTB (i.e., croup) usually can be made clinically, frontal and lateral radiographs of the neck often are obtained to exclude epiglottitis and other causes of stridor. Although the frontal radiograph of the neck offers

the clearest evidence of the subglottic narrowing found in LTB, the lateral view provides numerous supportive findings. On a properly obtained inspiratory, nonrotated lateral radiograph of the neck, these children have a normal-appearing epiglottis and aryepiglottic folds, marked distention of the hypopharyngeal airway, and accompanying haziness and swelling of the glottis/subglottic structures (Fig. 43-16).[13,37,38] Due to the presence of the inexpandable, complete cricoid cartilage ring, inflammatory mucosal and submucosal subglottic edema obstructs the airway at this level. During inspiration, negative intraluminal pressures are created in the cervical trachea distal to the obstructed subglottis causing it to collapse. Conversely, if a lateral radiograph of the neck is obtained during expiration in children with LTB, there will be distention of the trachea below the level of the obstructed, edematous subglottic airway.[38] These dynamic changes in cervical tracheal diameter are not specific for LTB, but also are seen with other causes of obstruction at the level of the glottis such as bilateral vocal cord paralysis (VCP),[39] laryngeal webs (which may tether the vocal cords),[5,7,9] and abnormally, thickened vocal cords (which can be seen in children with storage diseases or multiple papillomas).[4,33]

SPECIAL CONSIDERATION:

The frontal radiograph of the neck offers the clearest evidence of the subglottic narrowing that is found in LTB and the lateral view provides numerous supportive findings.

Pretracheal and prevertebral soft-tissue abnormalities and their associated compression or displacement of the neighboring larynx and pharynx can be evaluated only on lateral radiographs obtained with proper technique (Fig. 43-17).[3,10] Abnormal soft-tissue thickness, air collections, radiopaque foreign bodies, and calcifications can be detected, suggesting the presence of idiopathic or posttraumatic retropharyngeal abscesses (Fig. 43-18) or neoplasms such as neuroblastoma[40] or teratomas.[15]

Published standards for the expected normal prevertebral retropharyngeal soft-tissue thickness exist for children, and usually are based on a comparison of this thickness to the anterior-posterior width of

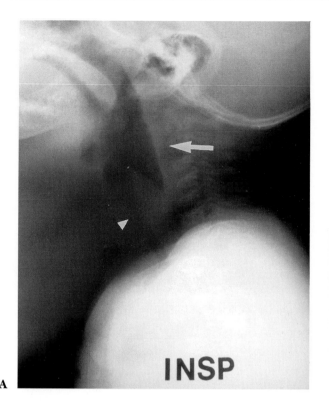

A   INSP

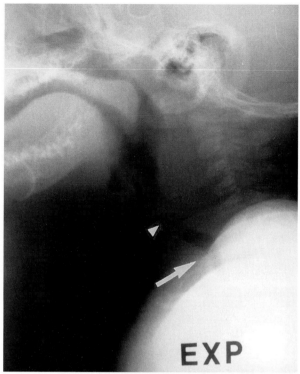

B   EXP

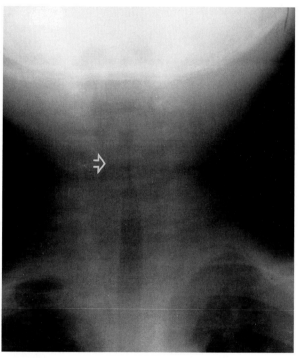

C

Figure 43–16: Dynamic airway changes in viral croup. Inspiratory (A) and expiratory (B) lateral neck radiographs of an infant with viral croup. Both demonstrate the classic "haziness" of the edematous vocal cords and subglottic airway (arrowheads). With inspiration, there is distention of the hypopharynx, whereas the cervical trachea distends during expiration (arrows). The frontal radiograph (C) confirms the presence of the classic "steeple" sign (open arrow) in this 8-month-old with croup.

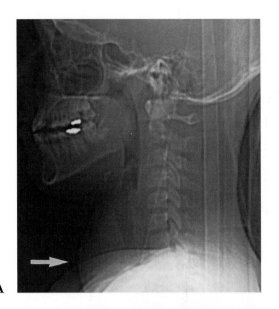

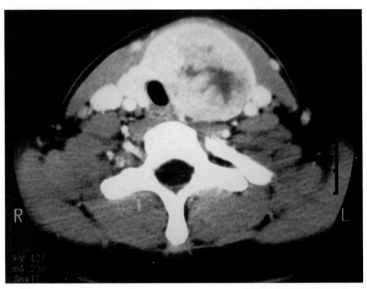

A

B

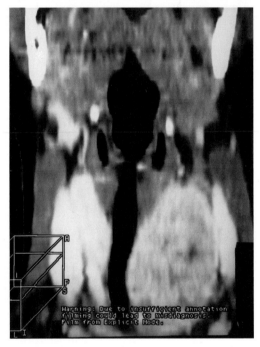

C

Figure 43–17: Pretracheal mass. Digital lateral CT scout film (A) shows the presence of a large pretracheal mass (arrow), subsequently proven to be thyroid carcinoma. Axial contrast-enhanced CT image (B) demonstrates a partially-necrotic mass involving the left lobe of the thyroid gland, compressing and displacing the trachea to the right. A coronal reformatted CT image (C) provides additional information regarding the tumor's relation to the airway and neurovascular bundles.

a neighboring cervical vertebra, usually C4. Normal prevertebral soft-tissue AP thickness gradually decreases as the child grows older and should not exceed ¾ times the AP dimension of C4 in infants, or more than 3 mm in older children.[41,42]

These standards cannot be accepted as hard and fast rules in all cases because many ill children are unable to cooperate, and prevertebral inflammatory processes are often accompanied by reversal of the normal cervical lordosis due to paravertebral muscle spasm. In such cases, one of the most reliable, albeit somewhat subjective, signs of prevertebral space-occupying pathology is the loss of the normal step-

off between the air-filled pyriform sinuses and the upper airway,[13] resulting in an abnormal, straight vertical air-soft tissue interface in the prevertebral region (Fig. 43–19).

SPECIAL CONSIDERATION:

One of the most reliable signs of prevertebral space-occupying pathology is the loss of the normal step-off between air-filled pyriform sinuses and the upper airway.

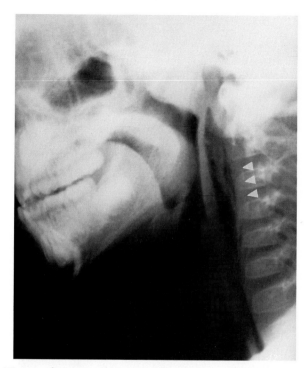

Figure 43–18: Posterior pharyngeal perforation. Lateral neck radiograph shows abnormal, irregular retropharyngeal air collections (arrowheads) in a 4-year-old who fell while running with a toothbrush in her mouth, suffering a posterior pharyngeal perforation.

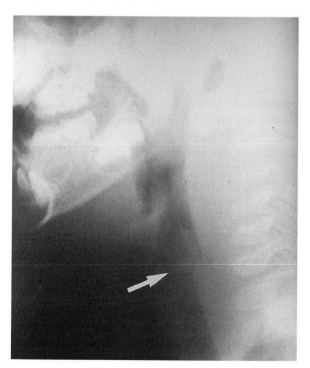

Figure 43–19: Retropharyngeal abscess. Lateral radiograph of the neck demonstrates markedly-increased prevertebral soft-tissue thickness that anteriorly displaces and compresses neighboring air-filled structures. This results in the obliteration of the normal step-off seen between the pyriform sinuses and the larynx (arrow).

TABLE 43–3: Retropharyngeal Masses in the Pediatric Population

*Infectious***
  Cellulitis with edema
  Lymphadenopathy
  Abscess
Traumatic
  Foreign body (with associated posterior pharyngeal perforation)
  Instrumentation (intubation, endoscopy, nasogastric tube insertion)
  Hematoma +/− cervical spine injury
Neoplastic
  Lymphangioma
  Hemangioma
  Neurofibroma
  Neuroblastoma
  Lymphoma
Congenital
  Ectopic thyroid (retropharyngeal goiter)
  Branchial cleft cyst
Other
  Hypothyroidism (congenital myxedema)
  Angioneurotic edema
  Lymphadenopathy associated with Langerhans' cell histiocytosis

**Always assess cervical spine for unsuspected diskitis and/or osteomyelitis

Although the differential diagnosis for retropharyngeal space-occupying pathology is lengthy (Table 43–3)[9,11,13,17,41] one of the most common entities is the retropharyngeal abscess, which usually results from local or lymphatic spread of nasopharyngeal or inner ear infections. Occasionally, foreign-body or iatrogenic perforation of the posterior pharyngeal wall may be the cause of the retropharyngeal abscess.[2,37] Advanced retropharyngeal infections usually extend across the midline, causing thickening of the prevertebral soft tissues and anterior displacement of the airway with loss of the normal step-off between the pyriform sinuses and the airway. Because these infections begin in the bilateral paramedian lymph nodes, early retropharyngeal infections may not cause these classic radiographic signs and may cause only a subtle soft-tissue "double density" on the lateral neck radiograph (Fig. 43–20). In such cases, further imaging with contrast enhanced CT is usually necessary.[43]

Finally, the differential diagnosis for prevertebral soft-tissue fullness should include foreign bodies lodged in the cervical esophagus, particularly those that have inflamed or perforated the anterior esoph-

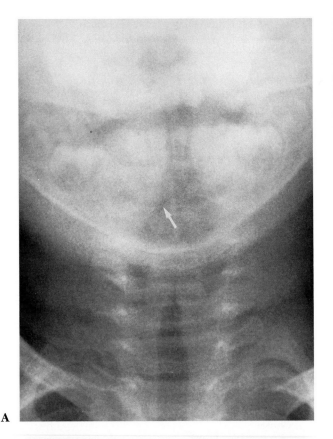

A

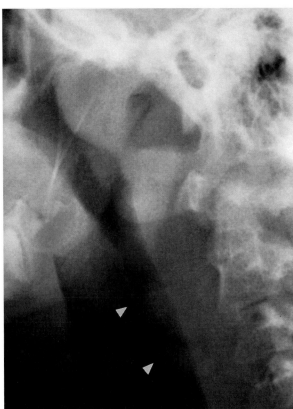

B

C

Figure 43–20:   Peritonsillar abscess with ipsilateral retropharyngeal extension. Frontal radiograph of the neck (A) shows asymmetric enlargement of the tonsillar tissue along the lateral pharyngeal walls, suggesting a right tonsillar abscess (arrow). Although the lateral radiograph (B) does not show the classic obliteration of the step-off between the pyriform sinuses and the larynx that is seen with retropharyngeal abscesses, there is a subtle soft tissue "double density" (arrowheads) projected along the posterior pharyngeal wall. Image for the subsequent contrast-enhanced CT scan (C) confirms the presence of a rim-enhancing right tonsillar abscess (small square) that extends caudally to the retropharyngeal space, but remains well to the right of midline. This causes the subtle "double density" seen on the lateral radiograph. The obliteration of the step-off between the pyriform sinuses and larynx is not seen on the lateral radiograph until the infectious process crosses the midline.

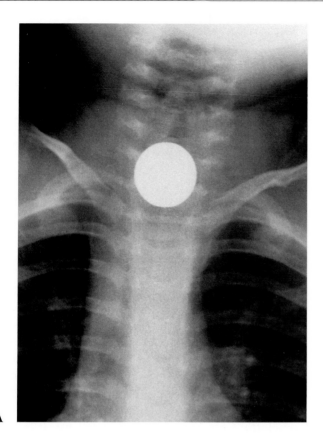

A

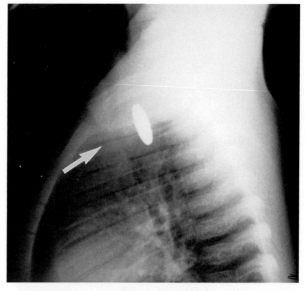

B

C

Figure 43–21: Coin in esophagus. Frontal (A) and lateral (B) radiographs of the neck demonstrate the classic alignment of a coin lodged in the esophagus, in this case at the thoracic inlet. The child ingested the coin several days earlier, accounting for the inflammatory soft-tissue fullness between the trachea and the esophagus (arrow). A follow-up esophagram (C) was performed to exclude esophageal perforation, injecting low osmolality aqueous contrast then barium through a nasoesophageal catheter. Although no leak was found, the tracheal narrowing and retrotracheal inflammatory changes were noted (arrowhead).

ageal wall and caused retrotracheal inflammation with anterior displacement and narrowing of the cervical trachea and resultant stridor (Fig. 43–21).[2,35,44,45] In addition, the cervical spine must be evaluated since traumatic injuries, neoplastic disease, and infectious processes involving the vertebra and/or disk spaces may be associated with fullness of the retropharyngeal soft tissues due to the presence of hematoma, tumor, or abscess respectively (Fig. 43–22).

Frontal (AP) Radiographs

A well-centered AP radiograph of the neck should include all structures between the mandible and carina. The nares, nasopharynx, and proximal main stem bronchi usually are included in the field of view in infants and small children (see Fig. 43–1B). This projection reveals any narrowing and/or displacement of the airway in the coronal plane, as well as the unilateral or bilateral nature of intratracheal or extratracheal pathology, including separate

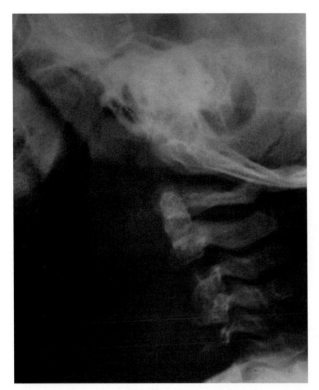

Figure 43–22: Cervical diskitis and osteomyelitis. Lateral radiograph of the neck in an inconsolable infant reveals the presence of classic retropharyngeal soft-tissue findings consistent with the presence of a retropharyngeal abscess. The radiograph also reveals the etiology of this abscess—an infection involving the C3 and C4 vertebral bodies and intervening disk space. The cervical kyphosis reflects loss of disk space and vertebral body height, as well as paravertebral muscle spasm.

delineation of each pyriform sinus (a common place for foreign bodies to lodge) (Fig. 43-23).[35] If the X-ray beam is angled caudally,[8] if the child's head is hyperextended, or if her mouth is opened, the occipital bones no longer obscure the oropharynx and any asymmetry of the lateral pharyngeal tonsillar tissue can be appreciated (see Fig. 43-20A).

The frontal radiograph of the neck is essential for evaluation of vocal cord contour and motion, the laryngeal ventricle, and the subglottic airway. The tips of the pyriform sinuses are projected on either side of the vocal cords, at approximately the level of C4.[1] Vocal cord granulation tissue and papillomas may be detected, appearing as nonspecific soft-tissue densities outlined by air.[33,34] A film obtained during inspiration or sniffing should demonstrate normal, symmetric abduction of the vocal cords, whereas films obtained during breath-holding, swallowing, phonation, or a Valsalva's maneuver should reveal adduction of the cords (Fig. 43-24).[3,46,47]

Whereas vocal cord motion can be assessed by obtaining AP radiographs of the neck during different phases of respiration, airway dynamics are best evaluated with airway fluoroscopy (vide infra), particularly in very young children.[1,39]

SPECIAL CONSIDERATION:

The frontal radiograph of the neck is essential for the evaluation of vocal cord contour and motion, the laryngeal ventricle, and the subglottic airway.

But perhaps the most common indication for obtaining an AP radiograph of the upper airway is for the evaluation of children with stridor, in whom subglottic stenosis is suspected. In this situation, a frontal film obtained with the vocal cords adducted is preferred, as the configuration and caliber of the subglottic airway is delineated clearly by air outlining the under-surface of the horizontal true vocal cords and the lateral vertical walls of the airway at the level of the cricoid cartilage, thus producing the

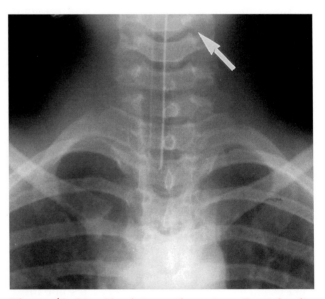

Figure 43-23: Tooth in pyriform sinus. Frontal radiograph of the neck was obtained in this 14-year-old boy in the recovery room immediately following tonsillectomy and adenoidectomy. The anesthesiologist who ordered the film was relieved when the tooth that was knocked out during intubation was found in the left pyriform sinus (arrow).

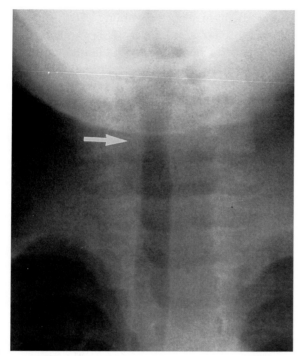

A

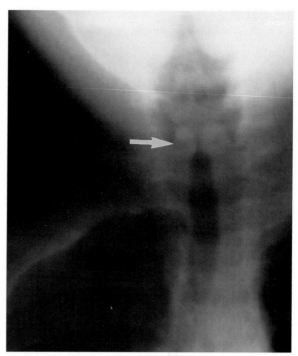

B

Figure 43–24: Vocal cord motion. Frontal radiographs of the neck obtained during inspiration (A) then phonation (B) reveal symmetric abduction then adduction of the vocal cords respectively (arrows).

normal "squared-off" configuration of this portion of the airway (see Figs. 43-1B and 43-24B).[1,9,13] Symmetric or asymmetric loss of this "squared" configuration due to subglottic airway narrowing of at least 1 cm in length[38] suggests the presence of congenital or acquired subglottic stenosis (Table 43-4.[5,7,13,24,34,48]

The most common cause of stridor in children is viral LTB.[5,6] The classic AP radiographic finding in

TABLE 43–4: Subglottic Narrowing in Children

Infectious
   Laryngotracheobronchitis (usually viral etiology)
   Epiglottitis (25% have subglottic extension of inflammation)
Traumatic
   Prolonged intubation (granulation tissue, acquired retention cysts, tracheomalacia)
   Burns (aspiration of caustic chemical, severe gastroesophageal reflux with aspiration, radiation)
Congenital
   Abnormal cartilage (elliptical cricoid)
   Soft-tissue abnormalities (membranes, webs, mucous retention cyst)
Neoplastic
   Subglottic hemangioma
   Recurrent laryngeal papillomas

LTB is symmetric effacement of the normal subglottic "squared:shoulders" appearance due to inflammatory edema that compromises airway caliber at the level of the inexpandable complete cartilaginous cricoid ring.[34] This radiographic appearance has been likened to a "sharpened pencil"[6] or a funnel but is referred to most commonly as the "steeple" sign (Fig. 43-25).[7,9,13] Occasionally, children with LTB have asymmetric subglottic edema and narrowing.[6,48] Conversely, the "steeple" sign is not specific for LTB and can be seen with other entities such as subglottic hemangioma,[49] congenital subglottic stenosis,[49] acute epiglottitis,[24] and as a sequel to prolonged intubation.[19] If the segment of subglottic narrowing is quite long and/or more inferiorly located than expected, an elliptical cricoid should be considered,[34,50,51] with diagnostic confirmation made endoscopically.

In neonates with stridor or very young children with clinical episodes resembling recurrent or intractable LTB, subglottic hemangioma should be considered.[6,34,51] Classically, these hemangiomas are found on the posterior or lateral walls of the airway and produce asymmetric subglottic narrowing on the AP radiographs (Fig. 43-26).[9,52] The clinician must recognize, however, that a significant percentage of these children will have symmetric

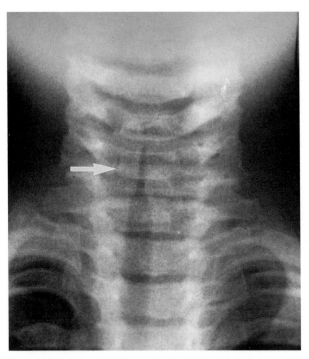

Figure 43–25: Viral croup. Frontal radiograph of the neck of a 21-month-old with a "barking cough" demonstrates the classic "steeple" sign seen with LTB (arrow).

subglottic narrowing resembling LTB.[49] In addition, asymmetric subglottic narrowing can be seen with other entities such as congenital and acquired mucous retention cysts, laryngeal papillomas, granulation tissue, and LTB.[6,49,50] Congenital and acquired cervical tracheal masses such as polyps, infectious membranes,[36] granulation tissue, and neoplasms[53] also can be identified on AP radiographs of the neck, particularly if they cause airway narrowing in the coronal plane.

SPECIAL CONSIDERATION:

In neonates with stridor or very young children with clinical episodes resembling recurrent or intractable LTB, subglottic hemangioma should be considered.

The cervical and intrathoracic portions of the trachea should be of uniform caliber, with slight deviation away from the aortic arch.[1,19] This tracheal deviation is accentuated during expiration (Fig.

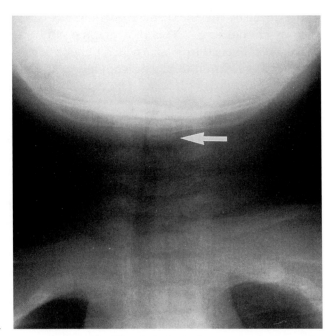

A

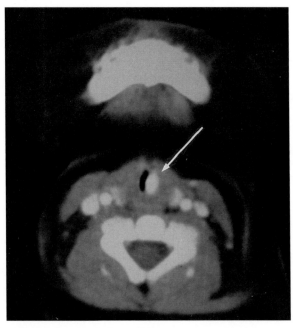

B

Figure 43–26: Subglottic hemangioma. Frontal neck radiograph in an infant with recurrent episodes of "LTB" (A) demonstrates asymmetric narrowing of the subglottic airway due a soft-tissue mass along the left lateral wall of the airway (wide arrow). Because additional pathology was suspected, a contrast-enhanced CT (B) was performed and showed a uniformly-enhancing mass along the left side of the airway (thin arrow) consistent with a subglottic hemangioma.

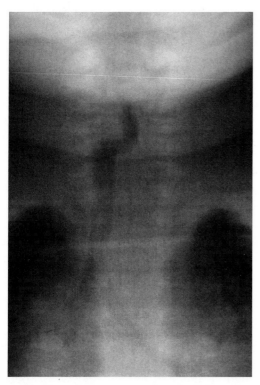

Figure 43–27: Expiratory tracheal buckling and deviation to the right in a child with a left aortic arch.

43–27) and is toward the right, away from the left aortic arch, in the majority of the population. A trachea that is completely midline is a significant and abnormal finding, suggesting a double aortic arch (Fig. 43–28).[54] Tracheal deviation in the coronal plane also can be caused by neighboring soft-tissue or vascular masses of the neck or superior mediastinum. Although follow-up sonography and additional cross-sectional imaging is usually necessary in these cases (vide infra), the structures on either side of the trachea on the frontal neck radiograph must be evaluated carefully for asymmetric or abnormal soft-tissue densities, calcifications, radiopaque foreign bodies, and abnormal gas collections (Fig. 43–29). Similarly, osseous abnormalities must not be overlooked, as they can relate directly or indirectly to a child's respiratory symptoms (see Fig. 43–4B).

SPECIAL CONSIDERATION:

Tracheal deviation in the coronal plane can be caused by neighboring soft-tissue or vascular masses of the neck or mediastinum.

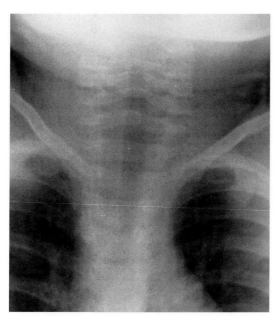

A

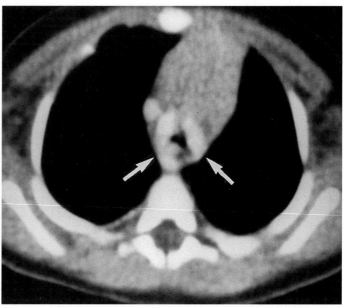

B

Figure 43–28: Double aortic arch. Frontal radiograph (A) demonstrates the presence of a midline trachea in a 1-month-old with respiratory distress. This is never a normal finding and should suggest the possibility of a vascular ring. Follow-up contrast-enhanced CT image (B) documents the presence of a double aortic arch. The right and left aortic arches (arrows) surround the trachea and confine it to a midline position.

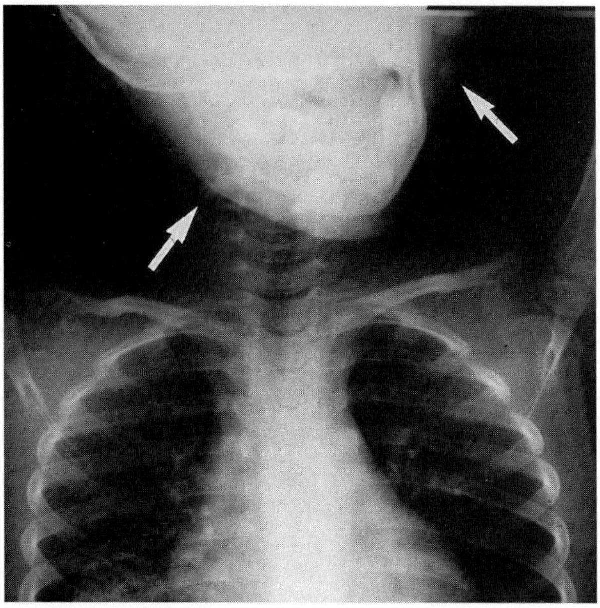

Figure 43–29: Tuberculosis. Frontal CXR of a girl with a positive tuberculin skin test, shows a partially-calcified, right, parenchymal density and right hilar lymph node calcifications. These findings are consistent with healed foci of prior tuberculous infection—the so-called Ranke's complex. Bilateral calcified cervical lymph nodes (arrows) are present also, indicating the infection extended into the neck as well.

AT A GLANCE . . .

Radiographs of the Neck

Lateral Radiographs: most often used to evaluate the nasopharynx, oropharynx, and supraglottic structures; images usually include the skull base, occiput, and maxillary antra; especially useful for imaging the posterior-superior nasopharynx, the structures of the mouth (palate, uvula, tongue, lingual tonsils, vallecula, and mandible), and those of the neck (the vocal cords, subglottic structures, and cervical trachea). *Indications:* epiglottitis, laryngotracheobronchitis, soft-tissue abnormalities.

Frontal Radiographs: a well-centered radiograph should include all structures between the mandible and carina; the nares, nasopharynx, and proximal main stem bronchi usually are included on the frontal radiographs of infants and small children; used to evaluate vocal cord contour and motion, the laryngeal ventricle, and the subglottic airway. *Indications:* stridor, laryngotracheobronchitis, tracheal deviation

Finally, the visualized portions of the pulmonary apices must be evaluated, as unsuspected pathology such as apical pneumothorax, parenchymal consolidation, and vascular congestion may be a contributing factor, if not the actual cause, of the child's respiratory distress. Apical herniation of the lung, usually due to congenital weakness or absence of Sibson's fascia in children,[55] presents as a painless, intermittent mass at the base of the neck. A frontal radiograph of the neck obtained during expiration or a Valsalva's maneuver will show the radiolucent, inflated, apical lung segment herniating into the base of base of the neck (Fig. 43-30), with occasional deviation of the trachea to the contralateral side.[55] This appearance is classic and should obviate further radiologic evaluation.

CHEST RADIOGRAPHS

Although a comprehensive review of pediatric chest radiography is beyond the scope of this chapter, a systematic approach to chest X-ray (CXR) interpretation and a working knowledge of the different projections available and their clinical applications are required for all physicians treating children with respiratory distress. Frontal and lateral CXRs usually are obtained at end-inspiration, with the child sitting or standing.[9] Frontal CXR of neonates and critically-ill children can be obtained in the supine position and supplemented with cross-table lateral chest radiographs, either in the radiology department or at the bedside. These cross-table lateral views are most useful in confirming the position of support tubes and catheters, as well as the presence of small, anteriorly-located mediastinal and pleural air collections.[56]

Although expiratory films are useful for detecting diffuse and focal postobstructive air trapping and tiny pneumothoraces,[13,57] spurious enlargement of the cardiac silhouette, buckling/bowing of the trachea, and crowding of the bronchovascular markings (particularly at the lung bases and perihilar regions) may be mistaken for actual pathology by the inexperienced reader (Fig. 43-31). Inspiratory radiographs are needed for accurate assessment of heart size and pulmonary vascularity, alveolar consolidations (e.g., pneumonia, atelectasis, pulmonary edema, hemorrhage) (Fig. 43-32), interstitial disease (e.g., peribronchial thickening, reticular, nodular, miliary patterns), and parenchymal masses/

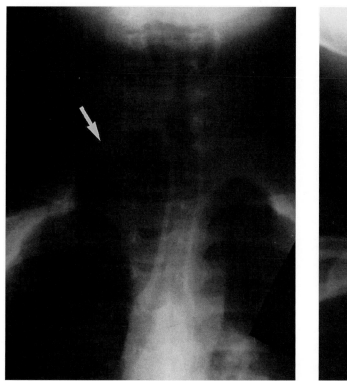
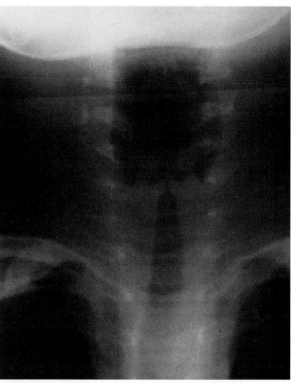

A   B

Figure 43–30: Transient apical lung herniation—a normal variant. Frontal radiograph obtained during a Valsalva's maneuver (A) shows upward herniation of the right pulmonary apex (arrow), which displaces the trachea to the left. A second film obtained immediately afterwards at rest (B) shows that the herniated apical segment of the right lung returns to the chest cavity and the trachea returns to midline.

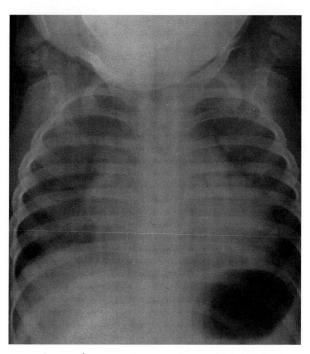
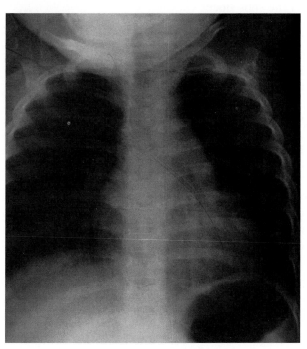

A   B

Figure 43–31: Inspiratory versus expiratory frontal chest radiographs. Affect of inspiratory effort on frontal chest radiograph findings. Frontal chest radiograph obtained at expiration (A) creates the impression of cardiomegaly, vascular congestion, and bibasilar consolidations/atelectasis. A second film obtained moments later at end-inspiration (B) is completely normal without any cardiovascular or pulmonary pathology.

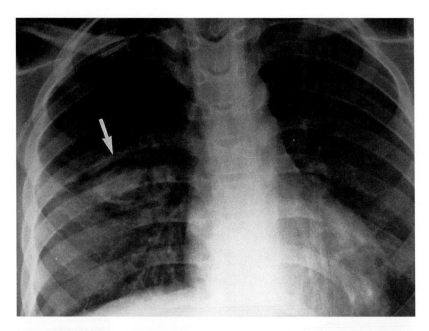

A

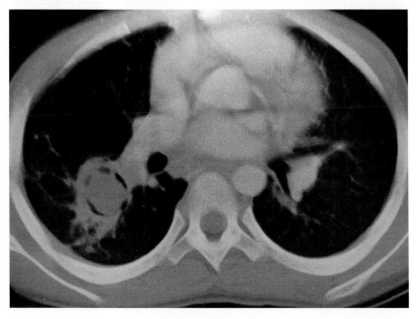

B

Figure 43–32: Invasive aspergillosis. A frontal CXR (A) of a 15-year-old with acute lymphocytic leukemia following several courses of chemotherapy and bone marrow transplantation demonstrates the presence of a right lobe parenchymal density that has a lucent rim (arrow). An image from the subsequent chest CT scan filmed at lung window and level settings (B) confirms the presence of a right lower lobe consolidation with peripheral cavitation. This peripheral cavitation is characteristic of invasive aspergillosis, which causes pulmonary parenchymal infection and then infarction due to its angio-invasive behavior.

cavities (e.g., primary and metastatic neoplasms, abscesses, pneumatoceles, granulomata, arterial-venous malformations.[9,13,58] Due to the hyparterial location of the left main stem bronchus, the left hilum is normally at or just above the level of the right hilum.[59] Any deviation from this arrangement is abnormal and suggests volume loss or a space-occupying process (Fig. 43-33).

On a normal upright frontal CXR obtained at an adequate degree of inspiration, vascular markings should be symmetric and confined to the medial 2/3 of the lungs, with the vessels more numerous and larger at the bases.[54] Abnormally increased or decreased pulmonary arterial circulation, pulmonary

SPECIAL CONSIDERATION:

The left hilum is normally at or just above the level of the right hilum, and any deviation from this is abnormal, suggesting volume loss or a space-occupying process.

venous congestion, and vascular asymmetry are important radiographic findings, suggesting congenital or acquired heart disease (Fig. 43-34), which may be an unsuspected cause of a child's respiratory

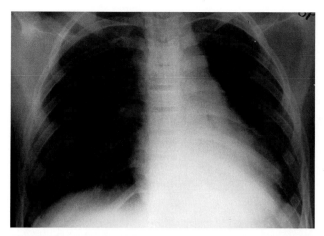

Figure 43–33: Left lower lobe atelectasis. Frontal CXR in an asthmatic child demonstrates left lower lobe consolidation that obliterates the left hemidiaphragm and is associated with downward displacement of the left hilum, indicating left lower lobe atelectasis.

distress. Hence, cardiac size, position, and orientation must be assessed as well.

The two most common vascular rings, double aortic arch and right aortic arch with aberrant left subclavian artery and left ligamentum arteriosum,[60] also are associated with classic findings on frontal and lateral CXR. The findings noted on the lateral film include increased retrotracheal soft-tissue fullness, anterior tracheal bowing, and tracheal narrowing.[61] Tracheal indentations, the location of the aortic arch(es), and descending thoracic portion should be noted on the frontal view.[61] Because the location

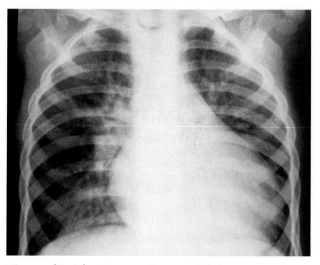

Figure 43–34: Ventricular septal defect. Frontal CXR of a 2-year-old with respiratory distress demonstrates the classic cardiomegaly and pulmonary over-circulation characteristic of left-to-right intracardiac shunts.

of the aortic arch usually is obscured by the thymus in infants and young children,[13] any deviations in tracheal position or the presence of a midline trachea on the frontal CXR are important observations in suggesting the possibility of a vascular ring.[60,61]

In up to 30% of children under the age of 2 years, there is an indentation along the anterior wall of the proximal intrathoracic trachea noted on lateral CXR, just below the thoracic inlet (Fig. 43–35). This indentation is caused by the brachiocephalic artery, the origin of which arises slightly more to the left of midline in young children as compared to adults.[62] Usually, this finding is asymptomatic.[62,63] If the child does have stridor, additional cross-sectional imaging, such as CT or MRI, is needed to exclude definitively other intrathoracic causes of stridor and to define mediastinal and vascular anatomy further.

Focal stenosis, abnormal airway dilatation (e.g., bronchiectasis), intraluminal masses, abnormal calcifications, radiopaque foreign bodies, and abnormal branching patterns involving the tracheobronchial tree can be diagnosed, or at least suspected, on the chest radiograph. In the pediatric population, most aspirated foreign bodies are not radiopaque and lodge in the bronchi.[64]

If aspiration occurs while the child is supine, the foreign body typically enters the right upper lobe bronchus; aspiration occurring in the erect position usually results in the foreign body entering the bronchus intermedius, the right middle bronchus, or the lower lobe bronchus.[65]

The spectrum of CXR findings with foreign-body aspiration include atelectasis distal to a bronchus that is completely occluded by a foreign body, postobstructive air trapping and oligemia distal to a partially-obstructing foreign body (Fig. 43–36), and occasionally air leaks such as pneumothorax and pneumomediastinum.[64] Coins that are lodged within the trachea can be distinguished easily from those in the esophagus by their orientation on the CXR. Due to the incomplete nature of normal tracheal cartilaginous rings, coins in the trachea align in the sagittal plane, whereas those in the esophagus align in the coronal plane (see Fig. 43–21).[2]

SPECIAL CONSIDERATION:

Due to the incomplete nature of normal tracheal cartilaginous rings, coins in the trachea align in the sagittal plane and those in the esophagus align in the coronal plane.

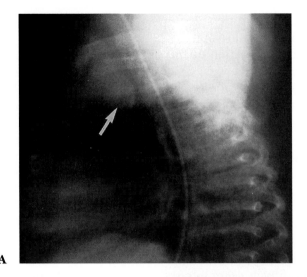

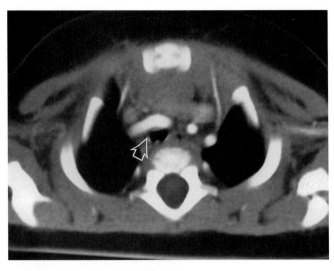

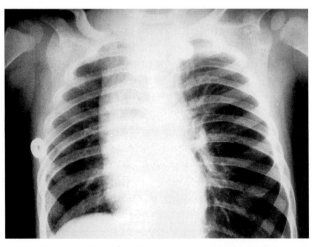

Figure 43–35: Brachiocephalic artery impression along the anterior tracheal wall. A lateral CXR (A) in an 8-month-old girl with suspected pneumonia shows the commonly-seen anterior impression along the anterior tracheal wall just below the thoracic inlet (arrow) caused by the brachiocephalic artery. This finding is seen in up to 30% of children under 2 years of age and is usually asymptomatic. Axial (B) and sagittal reformatted (C) contrast-enhanced CT images confirm mild deformity of the right anterolateral tracheal wall by the brachiocephalic artery as it crosses from left to right (open arrows).

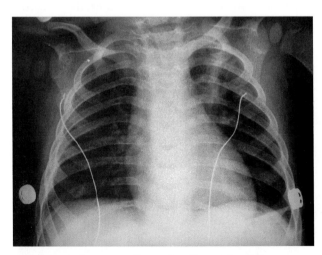

Figure 43–36: Postobstructive air trapping due to an aspirated peanut. Frontal radiograph of the chest in a 1-year-old with a sudden "choking" episode (A) shows hyperinflation of the left lung, which is hyperlucent, oligemic, and displaces the heart to the right. These are classic findings of postobstructive air trapping on the left that is caused by an endobronchial mass or foreign body that is large enough to occlude the intrathoracic airway during expiration only. Follow-up radiograph after bronchoscopic removal of the peanut from the left main stem bronchus (B) shows minimal subsegmental atelectasis in the left upper lobe and the heart now in the normal midline position.

Esophageal foreign bodies may be radiopaque, such as coins, and they most commonly lodge at the thoracic inlet.[45,64] These foreign bodies also can be located at the level of the aortic arch, the left main stem bronchus, the gastroesophageal sphincter, or proximal to a stricture.[9,35,64] Acutely, these foreign bodies may compress the airway due to their size and/or associated dilatation of the esophagus.[45] If, as is often the case, the child is initially asymptomatic, long-standing esophageal foreign bodies can compromise the airway by causing compressive tracheomalacia or retrotracheal inflammatory masses and mediastinitis if they perforate through the esophageal wall.[45,65]

The visualized portions of the upper abdomen should be evaluated for evidence of intestinal obstruction or perforation. As well, abnormally-positioned esophageal catheters, probes, and feeding tubes (Fig. 43-37) must be noted, as they may be responsible for, or contribute to, the child's respiratory problems. Similarly, congenital and acquired osseous abnormalities such as scoliosis, pectus deformities, and rib fusions can cause respiratory compromise.[66] Some syndromes, such as thanatophoric dysplasia (Fig. 43-38), are associated with such severely abnormal development of the bony thorax

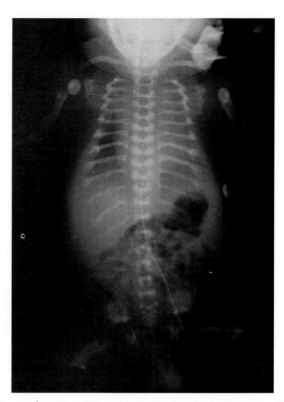

Figure 43–38: Thanatophoric dysplasia. Frontal radiograph of a newborn with thanatophoric dysplasia demonstrates the classic radiographic findings, including a long narrow trunk with very short ribs, severe platyspondylisis, and marked shortening and bowing of the long bones. The underdeveloped bony thorax results in severe respiratory distress and death shortly after birth.

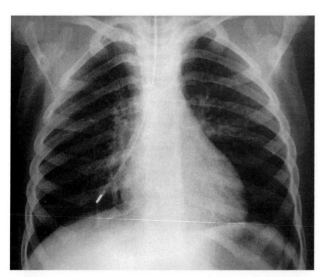

Figure 43–37: Esophageal pH-probe inadvertently placed in the airway. Frontal CXRs are obtained routinely following pH-probe placement to insure that they are located appropriately 3-5 cm above the gastroesophageal junction. In this girl, the pH-probe is not in the expected midmediastinal position, but rather overlies the lower right lung. This indicates that the pH-probe has entered the right main stem bronchus instead of the esophagus.

and hence the lungs that these neonates are usually stillborn or expire very shortly after birth.[67]

But perhaps the most crucial part of the evaluation of any CXR involves the identification and localization of indwelling artificial airways. Two orthogonal views of the chest are required to state definitively that an endotracheal tube is in the airway (Fig. 43-39). In most clinical circumstances, the tip of the endotracheal tube should be midway between the thoracic inlet and the carina. If the tip advances into a main stem bronchus, the contralateral main stem bronchial lumen is occluded, resulting in variable degrees of atelectasis in the contralateral lung (Fig. 43-40). The position of the endotracheal tube tip does, however, change with movement of the head and neck. With flexion, the tip moves caudally and with extension or lateral rotation it moves cranially.[68] Whereas the amount of such endotracheal tube movement is usually insignificant in children and adults, it can be quite significant in neonates and infants.

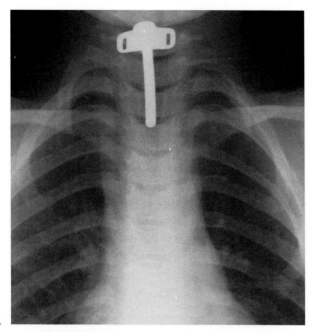
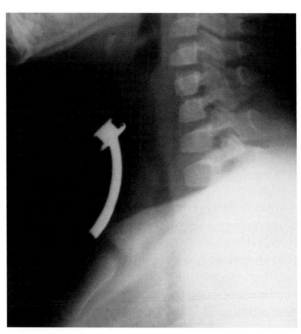

A   B

Figure 43–39: Artificial airway position. The indwelling tracheotomy tube appears to be in the desired position on the frontal CXR (A). However, the tube actually is positioned in the soft tissues anterior to the airway—a finding that can be detected only on the lateral radiograph (B) in this case.

Two supplemental radiographic techniques that are available for evaluation of the chest are: (1) *decubitus views,* and (2) *inspiratory-expiratory frontal CXR.* Normally, the dependent hemithorax on a decubitus view contains a deflated lung and an elevated hemidiaphragm, while the nondependent lung is maximally inflated.[5,57,59] Hence, decubitus views can be used to detect postobstructive air trapping in the dependent lung,[69] and to distinguish normal prominent bronchovascular markings from true parenchymal consolidations (the latter persisting in the nondependent lung).[70,71] Decubitus views also are used to document and quantify a free-flowing pleural effusion in the dependent hemitho-

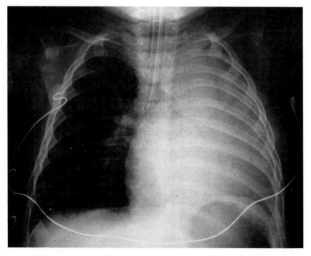
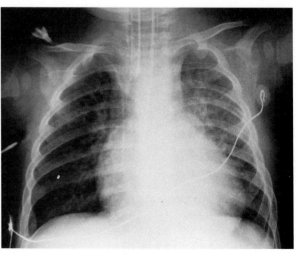

A   B

Figure 43–40: Abnormal endotracheal tube positioning. Initial frontal CXR (A) in this child shows the inadvertent placement of the endotracheal tube down the right main stem bronchus. The sidewall of the tube has occluded the orifice of the left main stem bronchus, resulting in atelectasis of the left lung. Repeat CXR following repositioning of the tube (B) shows partial reinflation of the left lung.

rax and to detect small pneumothoraces in the non-dependent hemithorax.[57,70,71]

In children who are able to cooperate, paired inspiratory–expiratory frontal CXRs can be used to detect postobstructive air trapping when foreign-body aspiration is suspected. Small pneumothoraces are also more noticeable on the expiratory CXR.[57]

AT A GLANCE . . .

Chest Radiographs

Expiratory Radiographs: used to detect diffuse and focal postobstructive air trapping and tiny pneumothoraces.

Inspiratory Radiographs: needed for accurate assessment of heart size, pulmonary vascularity, alveolar consolidations, interstitial disease, parenchymal masses/cavities.

Indications: focal stenosis, abnormal airway dilatation, intraluminal masses, abnormal calcifications, radiopaque foreign bodies, intestinal obstruction or perforation, identification and localization of indwelling artificial airways, and abnormal branching patterns involving the tracheobronchial tree.

AIRWAY FLUOROSCOPY

Airway fluoroscopy is a noninvasive way of documenting dynamic changes in airway caliber and position during different phases of respiration with the ability to correlate these changes with audio abnormalities. These examinations can be videotaped, and immobilization devices[7,9] can be used to minimize the child's exposure to ionizing radiation. *Lateral fluoroscopy* is used to document the inspiratory nasopharyngeal and oropharyngeal collapse in the sleep apnea lab,[5,19] the inspiratory anterior and inferior buckling of the aryepiglottic folds and the downward bending of the epiglottis seen with laryngomalacia,[1,5-7,35] and the excessive expiratory collapse of the intrathoracic trachea in children with congenital or acquired tracheomalacia.[6,34]

Frontal fluoroscopy is used to assess the motion of the vocal cords[3,5,7] and hemidiaphragms.[3,72] In addition, *anterior fluoroscopy* is used as a supplemental technique for evaluating children suspected of foreign-body aspiration, in whom standard CXRs, decubitus views, and inspiratory–expiratory views are equivocal.[9,59] Normally, the heart and mediastinum remain in the midline during all phases of respiration.[59] If these structures shift, for example to the left during inspiration and return to midline during expiration, the presence of complete blockage of

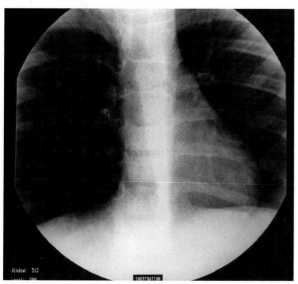
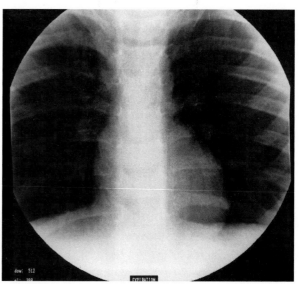

A   B

Figure 43–41: Fluoroscopic findings immediately following aspiration of a bead. Inspiratory (A) and expiratory (B) frontal spot radiographs obtained during chest fluoroscopy show inspiratory shift of the heart and mediastinum to the left with return of these structures to the midline with expiration. This indicates that the bead is preventing air from entering at least a portion of the left lung during inspiration. If the foreign body is not detected immediately, eventually the air distal to the bead is reabsorbed, resulting in left-sided atelectasis.

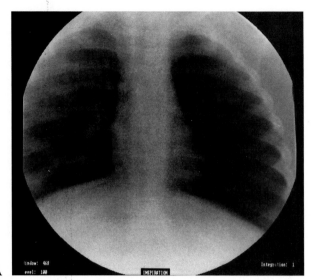
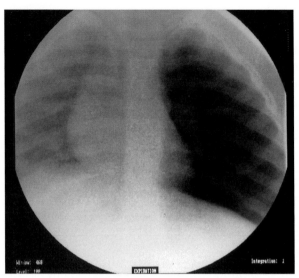

A   B

Figure 43–42:   Fluoroscopic findings indicating foreign-body postobstructive air trapping. Inspiratory (A) and expiratory (B) frontal spot images from a chest fluoroscopy study show the heart and mediastinum in a normal midline position during inspiration but shifted to the right during expiration by a hyperlucent, hyperinflated left lung, indicating the presence of postobstructive air trapping on the left. At bronchoscopy a bead was removed from the left main stem bronchus.

a portion of the airway on the left with eventual ipsilateral postobstructive atelectasis is suggested (Fig. 43–41). Alternatively, if the heart and mediastinum shift, for example to the right during expiration, the presence of partial obstruction of a portion of the airway on the left with resulting postobstructive air trapping should be suggested (Fig. 43–42).[59]

SPECIAL CONSIDERATION:

Anterior fluoroscopy is a supplemental technique used to evaluate children with suspected foreign-body aspiration in whom radiographs are equivocal.

CONTRAST STUDIES

This section provides a brief outline of the clinical uses and indications of esophagrams, speech and rehabilitative swallow studies, bronchograms, fistulograms, and sinograms. Whereas the latter two categories usually require sedation, the esophagrams and rehabilitative swallow studies require use of the appropriate immobilization device. All rehabilitative swallow studies and some esophagrams are

performed with the child upright. Pulse oximetry and warming lights should be used when studying a neonate or any child with intermittent apneic spells or cyanosis (Fig. 43–43).

Esophagram

The indications for esophagrams in children are quite numerous.[9,73] Each study should include assessment of esophageal peristalsis, luminal diameter, distensibility, and mucosal integrity. Intraluminal lesions such as tumors, webs, varices, and foreign bodies may be detected (Fig. 43–44). Although the esophagram is commonly referred to as a "barium swallow," water-soluble contrast is used for selected studies, such as those performed after recent esophageal surgery or when there is a possible esophageal foreign body with its inherent risk of associated perforation due to mucosal friability.[2,9,35] Despite the high cost, nonionic aqueous contrast agents are used in such cases, as they are associated with a lower risk of chemical pneumonitis and pulmonary edema if accidentally aspirated. If there is no leakage of the nonionic aqueous contrast, a more detailed examination is then performed utilizing the more radiopaque and palatable barium.

In current practice, the esophagram is the examination of choice for the initial documentation and subsequent follow-up evaluations of esophageal strictures and their response to attempted dilata-

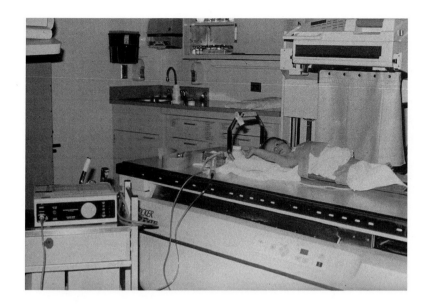

Figure 43–43: Pediatric fluoroscopy suite. In addition to radiographic equipment, a properly-equipped room should contain warming lights, restraining devices, a pulse oximeter, wall suction, and oxygen, all of which should be readily available for immediate use as needed.

tions (Fig. 43-45).[74,75] Regions of esophageal narrowing, which may be due to intrinsic or extrinsic causes, should be studied in two orthogonal planes, preferably straight AP and lateral because certain pathologic processes, such as vascular rings, produce characteristic patterns of extrinsic esophageal indentations.[6,60] For example, the large posterior and right lateral esophageal indentations can be seen with both a double aortic arch and a right aor-

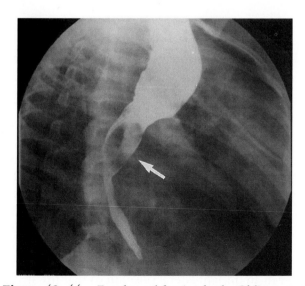

Figure 43–44: Esophageal foreign body. Oblique spot radiograph from a barium esophagram in a 2-year-old with history of esophageal atresia repair shows a filling defect in the midesophagus (arrow) that is consistent with a food bolus stuck above a long distal esophageal stricture. The stricture reflects the child's ongoing severe gastroesophageal reflux (a common problem in children with a history of esophageal atresia).

tic arch with aberrant left subclavian artery and left ligamentum arteriosum (Fig. 43-46), whereas a pulmonary sling causes characteristic, but nonspecific,[76] anterior esophageal and posterior tracheal indentations on the lateral esophagram.

An esophagram is often part of the work-up of children with failure to thrive or repeat respiratory tract infections, especially involving the right upper lobe. Such infiltrates in young children suggest ongoing aspiration either due to abnormal swallowing function, gastroesophageal reflux (GER), and/or abnormal tracheoesophageal communications.[13] The initial esophagram in such children must include an evaluation of the stomach, duodenum, and proximal jejunum in order to exclude distal pathology such as pyloric stenosis or intestinal malrotation. If primary GER is noted, the radiologist should document the amount of oral contrast administered, the level to which the reflux occurred, the promptness with which it was cleared, and the presence of accompanying aspiration and/or cough reflex.

When studying a child for possible tracheoesophageal fistula (TEF), the entire airway from glottis to carina must be kept in the fluoroscopic field of view, with the child in a right lateral or anterior oblique position. In this way, contrast entering the airway due to aspiration can be distinguished from that passing through a TEF, and the level of the TEF can be documented (Figs. 43-47 and 43-48). If the standard esophagram is normal and a TEF is suspected still, a nasoesophageal tube can be inserted with its tip positioned just below the level of the carina. Utilizing the aforementioned patient positions and fluoroscopic field of view, thin barium is

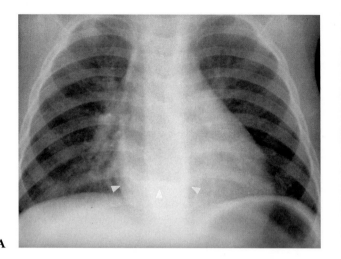

A

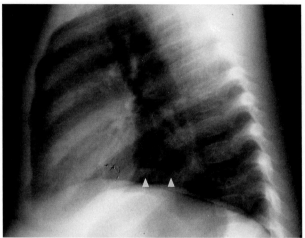

B

Figure 43–45: Tracheobronchial remnant. Frontal (A) and lateral (B) chest radiographs of a 1-year-old girl with history of multiple respiratory tract infections demonstrate the presence of a posterior mediastinal air-fluid level (arrowheads), suggesting distal esophageal obstruction. Subsequent esophagram (C) reveals a short, nondistensible, distal esophageal stricture (arrow). Following unsuccessful attempts at dilatation, surgical resection of a cartilaginous ring surrounding the distal esophagus was performed.

C

injected as the esophageal catheter is slowly withdrawn (see Fig. 43–48). Occasionally, even this technique fails to delineate an existing TEF due to occluding mucous or debris. Hence, if clinical suspicion remains high despite a prior normal esophagram, these procedures may need to be repeated at another sitting.

Speech and Rehabilitation Swallow Studies

Rehabilitation swallow studies, also known as *modified barium swallow studies,* involve dynamic assessment of the preoral, oral, pharyngeal, and esophageal phases of swallowing,[77,78] and can be performed at all ages. A detailed clinical history of

feeding patterns and pathology should be obtained first, so that the examination is tailored to the child's specific needs. The studies, which provide diagnostic and therapeutic information, are conducted by a speech pathologist with the radiologist providing fluoroscopic and interpretive assistance. The child is placed in the appropriate-size immobilization chair in an upright lateral position so that the structure and function of the oral cavity, entire pharynx, and cervical esophagus can be assessed.[79] Video and audio recordings of the fluoroscopic examination are made as various consistencies and textures of liquids and foods, which approximate the child's usual diet, are mixed with barium and then administered. The utensil or nipple used for feeding, the

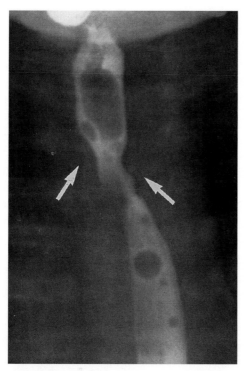
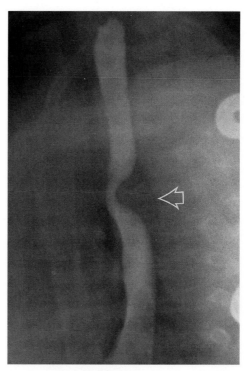

A   B

Figure 43–46: Double aortic arch. Frontal spot film from a barium esophagram (A) shows the bilateral extrinsic esophageal impressions caused by the larger right and smaller left aortic arches (arrows). The lateral view (B) shows the classic large posterior esophageal indentation (open arrow) at the site of the union of the two aortic arches.

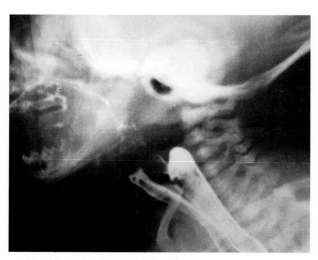

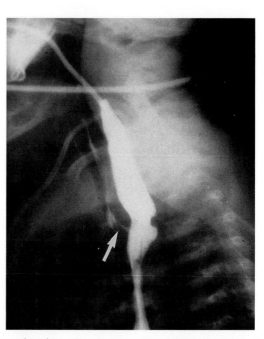

Figure 43–47: Laryngotracheal cleft. Lateral esophagram in a 1-month-old with recurrent episodes of pneumonia demonstrates a large amount of contrast in the airway entering at the level of the glottis. Subsequent endoscopy confirmed the presence of a laryngotracheal cleft.

Figure 43–48: Tracheoesophageal fistula. Lateral spot radiograph obtained while thin barium was slowly injected through an esophageal catheter demonstrates the presence of a TEF (arrow), which classically is referred to as an "H-shaped" fistula. This abnormality is more appropriately referred to as "N-shaped" fistula because the tracheal opening of the TEF is at a higher level than the posterior esophageal opening.

head and neck positioning, and the degree of chin support are varied and their effects on the child's ability to protect the airway during swallowing are determined.[78,80]

The child's ability to form a bolus, initiate a swallow, occlude the nasopharyngeal airway, and protect the lower airway are evaluated. Lingual, palatal, and pharyngeal motion and coordination are assessed also. Abnormal findings include nasopharyngeal reflux, laryngeal penetration (i.e., contrast beneath the epiglottis, but above the vocal cords), and frank aspiration (i.e., contrast reaching or passing distal to the glottis) (Fig. 43–49). But perhaps the

most significant observation is the identification of aspiration that is not accompanied by a normal cough reflex and hence was not suspected by the child's caregiver.[78] If the initial swallows are normal, repeat fluoroscopic evaluation should be performed at the end of the child's normal-size feeding to detect fatigue aspiration.[35]

Video fluoroscopy is used also to evaluate children with speech disorders, such as hypernasality.[81] Fluoroscopy is performed in the lateral, anterior, and basal projections with a small amount of intranasal barium occasionally administered.[3,81] Palatal motion, occlusion of the nasopharynx, and lateral

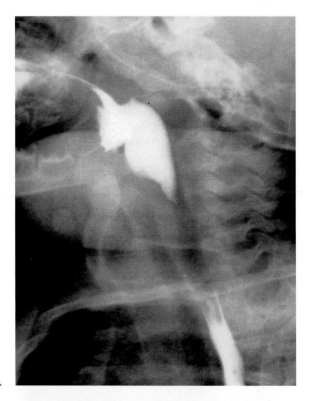

A

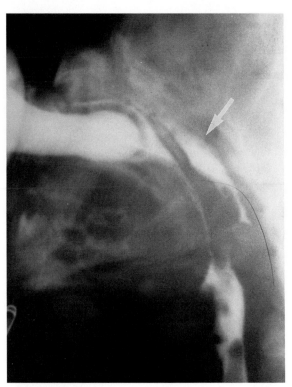

B

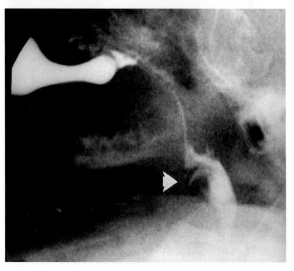

C

Figure 43–49: Normal and abnormal swallows. A lateral image during a normal swallow (A) shows how the epiglottis protects the glottis and how the palatal and posterior pharyngeal structures occlude the nasopharyngeal airway. Similar views of a rehabilitation swallow study performed in a neurologically-impaired child (B and C) demonstrate nasopharyngeal reflux (arrow) and penetrations (arrowhead) (i.e., contrast reaching but not passing through the glottis).

pharyngeal wall motion are assessed as the child repeats a variety of phrases. Clearly, the child must be able to cooperate if a diagnostic study is to be obtained without the use of excessive radiation.

SPECIAL CONSIDERATION:

If initial swallows during a swallow study are normal, repeat fluoroscopic evaluation should be performed at the end of the child's normal-size feeding to detect fatigue aspiration.

Bronchography

In the past, contrast studies of the tracheobronchial tree were performed to evaluate children with focal air trapping, atelectasis, and bronchiectasis. These examinations required the use of general anesthesia, and were accompanied by the risk of acute respiratory compromise and pulmonary edema.[3] With the advent of sophisticated cross-sectional imaging and bronchoscopic techniques, few if any indications for bronchography exist at the present time. One such indication is in children with complex tracheo-bronchial stenosis and malformations such as those that accompany a pulmonary sling.[76] Long regions of stenosis, complete tracheal rings, and abnormal carinal position and morphology (the so-call ''inverted T'' sign) (Figs. 43-50 and 43-51) commonly accompany this vascular ring, and are associated with variable degrees of over- or underinflation of the lungs.[50,76]

But perhaps the most common current indication for the instillation of contrast into the tracheobronchial tree is for the localization, measurement, and subsequent balloon dilatation and/or placement of endobronchial stents in children with bronchial stenosis (Fig. 43-52).[34,82] These procedures require the combined efforts of the departments of radiology, otolaryngology, and anesthesiology, and are performed with low-osmolality water-soluble contrast agents, which are cleared rapidly from the lung and which are associated with a reduced risk of chemical pneumonitis and pulmonary edema.

SPECIAL CONSIDERATION:

Low-osmolality water-soluble contrast agents are cleared rapidly from the lungs and are associated with a reduced risk of chemical pneumonitis and pulmonary edema.

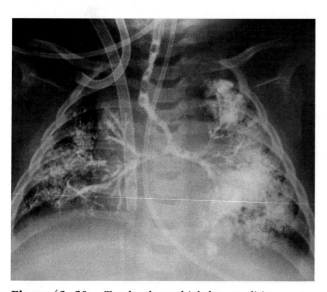

Figure 43–50: Tracheobronchial abnormalities accompanying a pulmonary sling. Contrast study of the airway in a boy with a pulmonary sling demonstrates marked narrowing of the distal trachea, low-lying carina, and horizontally-oriented narrow main stem bronchi—the ''inverted T'' sign. Follow-up surgery confirmed the presence of complete tracheal rings.

AT A GLANCE . . .

Indications for Contrast Studies

Esophagram: esophageal strictures, children with failure to thrive or repeat respiratory infections, and tracheoesophageal fistula

Speech and Rehabilitation Swallow Studies: used to evaluate preoral, oral, pharyngeal, and esophageal phases of swallowing, and children with speech disorders

Bronchography: children with complex tracheobronchial stenosis and malformations such as those that accompany a pulmonary sling; the localization, measurement, and subsequent balloon dilatation and/or placement of endobronchial stents in children with bronchial stenosis

Fistulograms and Sinograms: used to evaluate cutaneous fistulas and sinuses; also used for parotid and submandibular sialograms

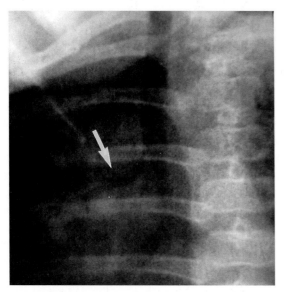
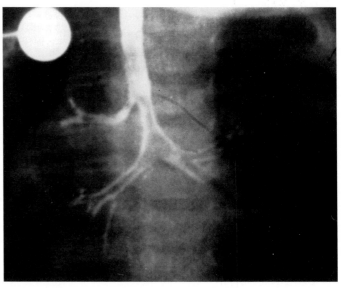

A   B

Figure 43–51: Epitracheal bronchus. Oblique spot film from a fluoroscopic airway evaluation (A) suggests the presence of an epitracheal bronchus (arrow). Follow-up bronchogram (B) confirms that the right upper lobe bronchus arises from the trachea above the level of the carina.

Fistulograms and Sinograms

These examinations are performed readily in the fluoroscopy suite. Sedation may be needed in children who cannot cooperate.[74,83] Utilizing sterile technique, the cutaneous opening is cannulated with a 27-gauge sialogram catheter. Low-osmolality aqueous contrast is then injected under fluoroscopic observation, with spot radiographs obtained in multiple projections (Fig. 43–53). A similar procedure is followed when performing sialograms in the pediatric population.

STANDARD TOMOGRAPHY

Tomography involves the use of relatively-high doses of radiation, and it is quite difficult to perform in children due to rapid respiratory rates and an inability to cooperate fully.[3] This modality has been replaced by CT and MRI for evaluating the pediatric airway and surrounding structures. Presently, the only indication for standard tomography of the neck is the evaluation of the cervical spine (Fig. 43–54).

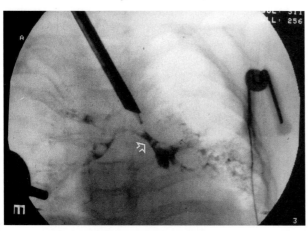
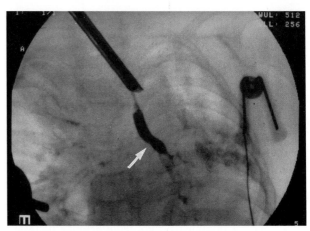

A   B

Figure 43–52: Balloon dilatation of bronchial stenosis. Preliminary bronchogram (A) demonstrates stenosis of the left main stem bronchus (open arrow). A catheter is passed through the bronchoscope (B) and balloon dilatation of the stenosis is performed. The "waisting" in the mid portion of the balloon (arrow) indicates a small segment of residual narrowing.

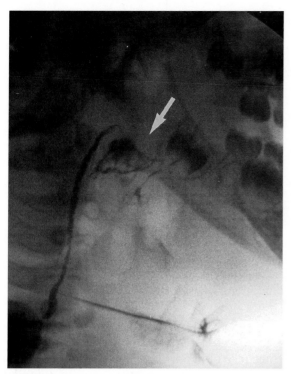

Figure 43–53: Branchial fistula. A 27-gauge sialogram catheter was used to cannulate a tiny draining cutaneous opening along the right sternocleidomastoid muscle. The injected contrast ascends in the fistulous tract and ultimately opacifies the posterior oropharynx (arrow).

ULTRASONOGRAPHY

Ultrasonography is an increasingly popular imaging modality for the evaluation of the neck,[84,85] mediastinum,[86] pleural space,[87] and diaphragm.[9,84] This technique is particularly useful in pediatric radiology because it can be performed portably and without the use of ionizing radiation or sedation. Furthermore, Doppler capability allows the radiologist to qualify and quantify the arterial and venous flow in a structure without the use of intravenous contrast. Although ultrasonography is used to assess diaphragmatic[88] and occasionally vocal cord motion,[89] the primary indication for it in pediatric otolaryngology is the detection and characterization of neck masses. The location, size, vascularity, and composition (i.e., solid, cystic, and calcified components) of a mass can be determined with real-time scanning in multiple planes. Some of the most common indications for neck sonography in children include torticollis/fibromatosis coli (Fig. 43-55),[90] lymphadenopathy, and lesions involving the thyroid gland (Fig. 43-56) and its embryologic remnants, such as thyroglossal duct cysts.[91-93]

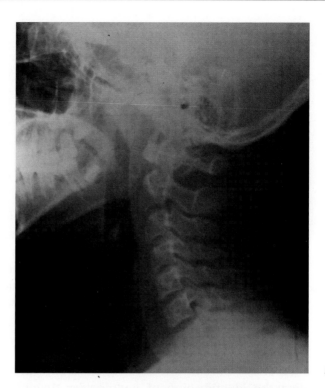

A

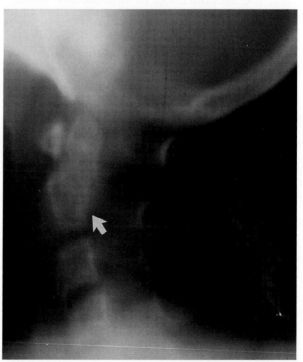

B

Figure 43–54: Cervical spine fracture. Lateral radiograph of the neck (A) of a 13-year-old with neck pain shows effacement of the normal 'step-off'' between the pyriform sinuses and the airway. The responsible fracture through the base of the dens is a subtle finding, but is clearly seen on a lateral tomogram (B) (arrow).

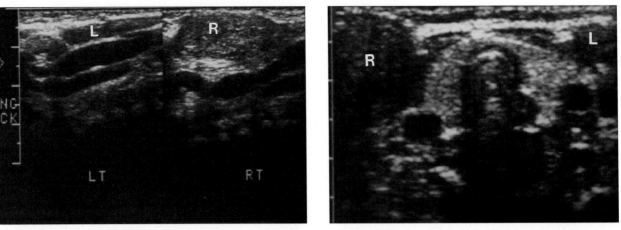

A   B

Figure 43–55: Fibromatosis coli. Longitudinal (A) and transverse (B) scans of the neck of a six-week-old baby with torticollis demonstrate fusiform enlargement of the right sternocelidomastoid muscle (R) as compared to the normal left (L). Injury to the muscle during vaginal delivery may result in this abnormality, which spontaneously resolves with time.

Mediastinal ultrasonography is a noninvasive method of assessing thymic tissue in children,[86] including the identification of multilocular thymic cysts, which are found in a small percentage of children with human immunodeficiency virus (HIV) infection.[94,95] If such thymic cysts are found, the neck should be evaluated for coexistent lymphadenopathy, and the parotid glands should be scanned for the presence of hypoechoic, lymphoepithelial cysts that also can develop in HIV-positive children.[96] Other indications for ultrasonography include assessment of vascular patency,[97] fluid collections and masses in the pleural space,[87] and guidance for percutaneous biopsies, aspirations, and drainages.[98]

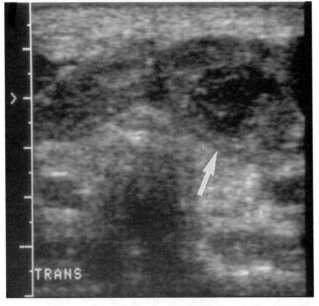

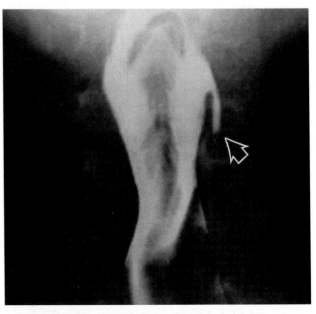

A   B

Figure 43–56: Pyriform sinus tract fistula. Transverse sonographic image of the thyroid gland (A) in a 13-year-old girl with recurrent neck infections demonstrates a complex, fluid-filled mass in the left lobe (arrow) that is consistent with a thyroid abscess. Following antibiotic therapy, a barium swallow (B) confirms the presence of a pyriform sinus tract fistula (open arrow), which is a remnant of the third or fourth branchial apparatus. The barium study should be delayed until after the acute infection has resolved; otherwise, the sinus tract may not be delineated due to occlusion by exudate or compression by surrounding inflammation.

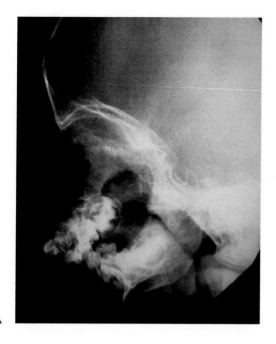

A

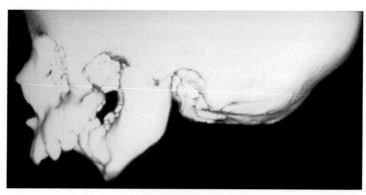

B

Figure 43–57: Nager syndrome. Lateral neck radiograph (A) demonstrates the classic facial deformities, including micrognathia, seen with this syndrome. Now, CT scanning with 3D-reconstructions (B) are used for preoperative planning.

COMPUTED TOMOGRAPHY

Computed tomography (CT) involves the rapid acquisition of sequential axial, and in some cases direct coronal, images of the neck and chest. Now, coronal, sagittal, and three-dimensional (3D) reconstructions are obtained easily with the new helical scanners (Fig. 43-57).[99] Noncontrast scans allow for the detection of calcification and acute hemorrhage (Fig. 43-58), and those obtained following the administration of 2 to 4 cc/kg low-osmolality aqueous contrast provide improved soft-tissue contrast due to the variable vascularity and enhancement patterns of neighboring structures. The ability to view the images at different window and level settings also improves spatial resolution, and the ability to measure a structure's Hounsfield units provides information regarding tissue composition.

Unlike ultrasonography, CT cannot be done portably, it utilizes ionizing radiation, it may require intravenous access, and it is more expensive. Although scanning time has been greatly reduced since the introduction of helical CT scanners, image quality is still very susceptible to motion artifacts, necessitating the use of sedation in uncooperative and very young children.[99] In children who are being evaluated for respiratory problems, the risk:benefit ratio for sedation must be considered, as it is often preferable to obtain a diagnostic CT study that has some motion artifact rather than administer sedation and risk acute respiratory failure. If seda-

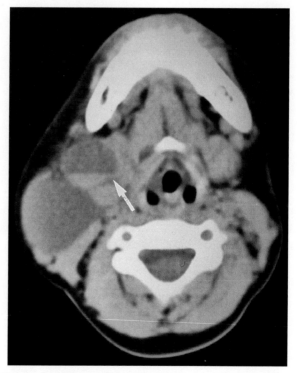

Figure 43–58: Hemorrhage into a venous–lymphatic malformation. Noncontrast-enhanced CT scan performed in a 6-year-old with a rapidly-enlarging right neck mass demonstrates the presence of multiple fluid-fluid levels (arrow) in a predominately-cystic neck mass. The high attenuation dependent layer is hemoglobin, indicating acute hemorrhage. These blood components are much easier to detect on noncontrast CT images.

tion is deemed necessary, it is prudent to have the appropriate personnel and artificial airways present in the CT suite.

SPECIAL CONSIDERATION:

In children who are being evaluated for respiratory problems, the risk:benefit ratio for sedation must be considered, as it is often preferable to obtain a diagnostic CT study that has some motion artifact than administer sedation and risk acute respiratory failure.

CT provides a detailed depiction of normal and abnormal cross-sectional anatomy of the neck and

chest, including the axilla, osseous structures, spinal canal contents, and pulmonary parenchyma. CT is the gold standard for evaluation of the pulmonary parenchyma and lung masses,[100] with high-resolution techniques further improving the depiction of interstitial, small airway, and air-space diseases (see Fig. 43-32).[101-103] Helical CT that has the ability to reconstruct the data in multiple planes also has replaced standard tomography and bronchography in the evaluation of the tracheobronchial tree, including depiction of branching patterns,[99,104] luminal masses and stenosis (Fig. 43-59),[105-108] and causes of extrinsic compression such as vascular rings (see Fig. 43-28) and mediastinal masses.[9,109]

CT has replaced choanography in the evaluation of choanal atresia[110,111] because it clearly depicts the membranous or bony nature of the atresia as well as the associated bony deformities. Prior to the examination, nasal secretions must be suctioned because the CT attenuation value of mucous is often

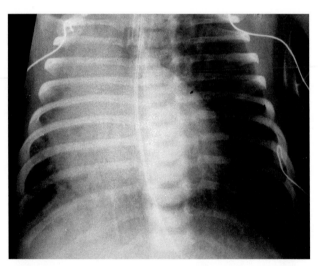

A

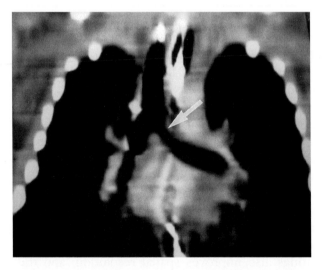

B

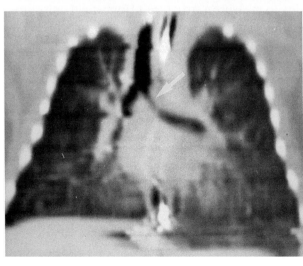

C

Figure 43–59: Congenital stenosis of the left main stem bronchus. Frontal CXR of a 6-day-old girl (A) shows overinflation of the left lung with shift of the heart and mediastinum to the right. Axial contrast-enhanced CT images show no extrinsic cause for this stenosis. The coronal reformatted images filmed at soft-tissue (B) and lung (C) windows show the extent of the intrinsic bronchial narrowing (arrows).

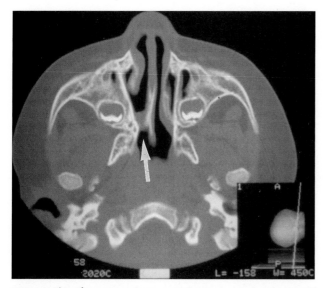

Figure 43–60: Membranous choanal atresia. Axial CT image demonstrates a persistent soft-tissue attenuation membrane obstructing the posterior right nasal cavity (arrow). Suctioning of both nasal cavities is essential before scanning because mucous can be mistaken for a membrane and can prevent accurate determination of an existing membrane's thickness.

identical to that of the membranous form of choanal atresia (Fig. 43–60). Vascular, solid, and cystic neck and mediastinal masses are delineated well on CT, and this modality is particularly useful in evaluating retropharyngeal infections.[85] Early in the development of tonsillar and retropharyngeal abscesses, there is lymphadenopathy and abnormal paramedian and/or midline retropharyngeal soft-tissue attenuation material consistent with a phlegmon (Fig. 43–61).[43] Surgical drainage should not be attempted at this time, but should be delayed until the inflammatory process matures and a well-defined, rim-enhancing infected fluid collection is seen.

MAGNETIC RESONANCE IMAGING

Magnetic resonance imaging (MRI) is being used increasingly to study children with congenital heart disease,[112] vascular compression of the airway (Figs. 43–62 and 43–63),[113-115] and soft-tissue masses of the neck and chest (Fig. 43–64).[85,116] These images have excellent tissue contrast and spatial resolution

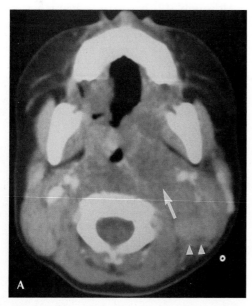
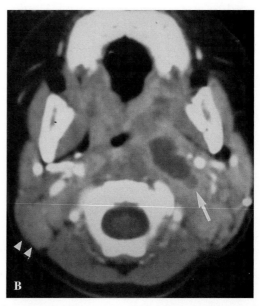

Figure 43–61: Evolution of tonsillar and retropharyngeal infection. Initial contrast-enhanced CT scan (A) of a child with fever and respiratory distress reveals a poorly-defined soft-tissue attenuation inflammatory mass in the left tonsillar and retropharyngeal spaces (arrow) that is consistent with a phlegmon. Follow-up scan 2 days later (B) shows maturation of the infectious process with a rim-enhancing, exudate-filled abscess (arrow) now seen in the same region. Note accompanying bilateral posterior cervical lymphadenopathy (arrowheads).

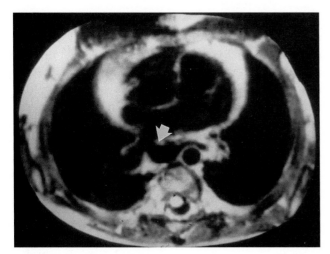

Figure 43–62: Pulmonary artery sling. Axial T1-weighted spin echo MRI demonstrates anomalous origin of the left pulmonary artery from the right pulmonary artery (arrow). The sling around the airway is created as the left pulmonary artery passes between the trachea and the esophagus as it crosses from right to left to supply the left lung.

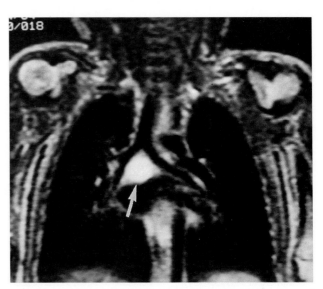

Figure 43–64: Mediastinal bronchogenic cyst. Coronal T2-weighted SE image shows a round, high signal, subcarinal mass (arrow) consistent with a bronchogenic cyst. This foregut malformation was not compressing the airway and was asymptomatic.

and can be obtained in multiple planes without having to move the child. This is particularly useful when studying the skull base, nasopharynx, tongue, and the floor of the mouth (Fig. 43–65).[20,21,43,85] Different pulse sequences are used to determine tissue composition, and intravenous gadolinium can be administered to assess tissue vascularity. Flow-

sensitive sequences, including CINE, are available to study blood flow in the heart, great vessels, and peripheral circulation.[115,117] MRI is also the premier modality for bone marrow imaging and is the only imaging technique with enough spatial resolution to visualize complete tracheal rings.[113]

Although MRI has many advantages, small calcifi-

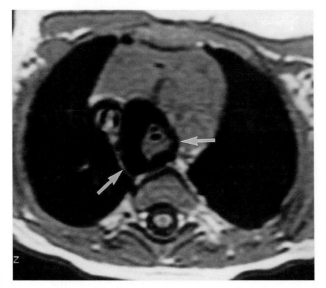

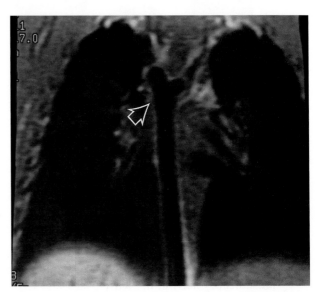

A   B

Figure 43–63: Double aortic arch. Axial (A) T1-weighted SE MRI shows both aortic arches surrounding the trachea (arrows). The T1-weighted SE coronal MRI (B) nicely demonstrates the posterior union of the two arches (open arrow).

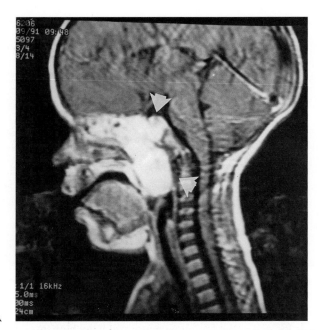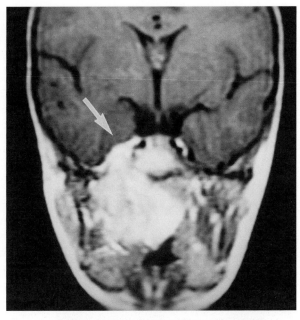

A   B

Figure 43–65: Rhabdomyosarcoma. Sagittal (A) and coronal (B) postgadolinium T1-weighted SE imaging of the head and neck of a 3-year-old girl reveal a large enhancing (i.e., vascular) mass in the posterior nasopharynx (arrowheads), which invades the skull base, displaces the right temporal lobe (arrow), and is in close proximity to the cavernous sinus.

cations and foreign bodies may be overlooked easily, and the amount of time needed to perform a sequence precludes evaluation of the pulmonary parenchyma due to respiratory motion artifacts. These examinations are also expensive and rather long, typically lasting 45 to 60 minutes. Children usually require sedation, especially if cardiac and respiratory gating are added for optimal evaluation of the chest. Hence, despite the availability of MRI-compatible pulse oximeters and cardiac monitors, MRI may not be possible in children with a compromised respiratory status who are not intubated. Also, as with CT, artifacts are created by indwelling metallic hardware. In fact, children with pacemakers and those with indwelling ferromagnetic hardware should never be scanned with MRI.

NUCLEAR MEDICINE

This section briefly reviews the scintigraphic studies available to evaluate children with suspected thyroid pathology or respiratory distress.

Thyroid Imaging

Thyroid imaging studies are used for localization and functional assessment of ectopic thyroid tissue,

and to study children with thyroid masses or abnormal levels of thyroid hormone.[118] In order to lessen the radiation dose to the thyroid, technetium 99m or iodine[123] are the radionuclides used in children. Iodine[131] is, however, used to treat certain children with hyperthyroidism or metastatic thyroid carcinoma.[118]

Interpretation of these examinations requires a working knowledge of thyroid embryology.[119] The presence of lingual thyroid tissue can be suspected on a lateral radiograph of the neck and confirmed with a noncontrast CT scan where lingual thyroid tissue is of high attenuation due to its intrinsic iodine content (Fig. 43–66). Although additional pretracheal thyroid tissue can be detected similarly on CT, a radionuclide study is still needed to determine the function of all of the thyroid tissue present.

Gastroesophageal Reflux Studies

Gastroesophageal reflux (GER) studies involve administering a small dose of technetium 99m sulfur colloid (5 uCi/ml) mixed with a volume of formula or milk that is consistent with the child's usual feeding.[120] Because the entire radiation dose to the child is contained within this mixture, the child can be placed under the gamma camera for prolonged observation without additional radiation exposure.

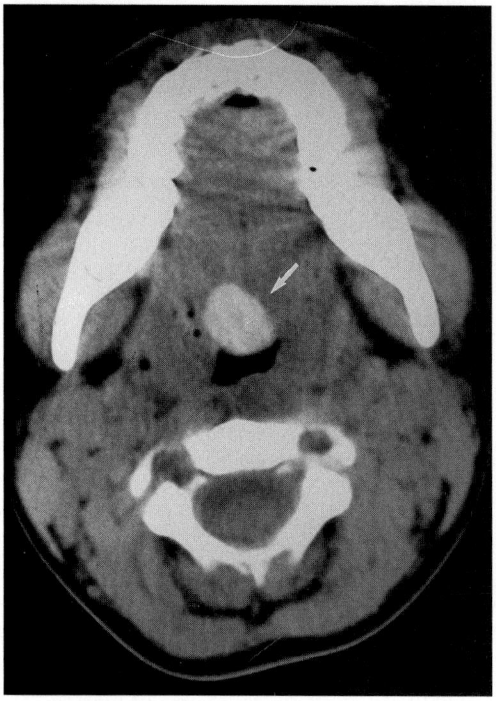

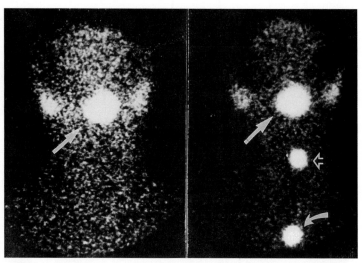

A

B

Figure 43–66: Lingual thyroid. Image from a noncontrast-enhanced CT scan of the same patient as Figure 43-6 (A) shows a posterior lingual mass that is characteristic of a lingual thyroid. The mass is located at the foramen cecum and has a high attenuation, presumably due to its iodine content. Preoperative iodine[123] study (B) includes images without markers (left) and images with markers (right) at expected level of thyroid (open arrow) and suprasternal notch (curved arrow). This shows that the only area of uptake is at the tongue (arrows), proving the lingual thyroid is the only functioning thyroid tissue present.

Hence, these studies have a high sensitivity for the detection of GER. Although nuclear GER studies can assess the frequency and severity (level) of the reflux episodes over the period of observation, spatial resolution is very poor (Fig. 43-67). Hence, this examination should be preceded by an upper gastrointestinal (GI) series in order to exclude anatomic causes of GER, such as gastric outlet obstruction, duodenal stenosis, and intermittent midgut volvulus due to intestinal malrotation. Simultaneous evaluation of esophageal transit and gastric emptying can be performed with only slight modification in technique.[119,120]

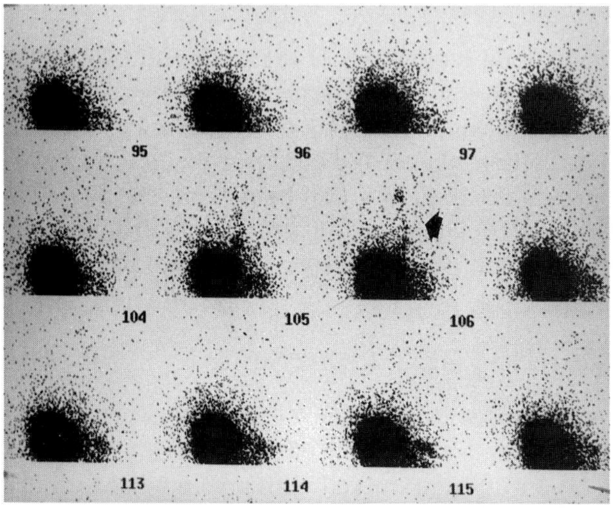

Oral Aspiration Studies (Salivagrams)

Oral aspiration studies usually are performed in neurologically-devastated children who suffer repeat episodes of aspiration pneumonia despite gastrostomy tube feedings and fundoplication, and who therefore are suspected of aspirating their saliva. The child is placed under the gamma camera, and computer images are obtained every 30 seconds as a small amount of technetium 99m sulfur colloid (approximately 300 uCi in 100 ul) is placed in the child's mouth.[120] Radiopharmaceutical that appears immediately in one or both lungs confirms ongoing aspiration of saliva (Fig. 43-68). If most of the material enters the stomach, the period of observation can be extended to assess for ongoing GER. As with the nuclear GER studies, the nuclear salivagrams are

Figure 43–67: Nuclear GER study. Following the ingestion of technetium 99m sulfur colloid mixed with a standard feeding, sequential images of the chest and abdomen reveal at least 2 episodes of reflux reaching the proximal esophagus (arrow).

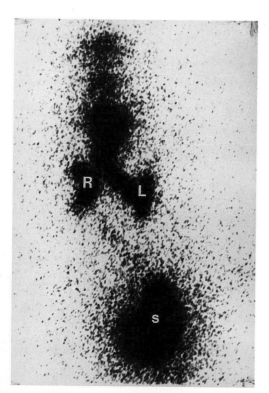

Figure 43–68: Nuclear oral aspiration study. An image obtained immediately after a small amount of technetium 99m sulfur colloid is put in the child's mouth shows prompt entry of the radionuclide into both lungs (R, L), which is consistent with aspiration of oral secretions (S = stomach).

very sensitive and involve only a very small dose of radiation. Due to poor spatial resolution, these studies should be preceded by a barium study to exclude the presence of a laryngeal cleft or TEF.

AT A GLANCE . . .

Indications for Nuclear Medicine

Thyroid Imaging: localization and functional assessment of ectopic thyroid tissue, and to study children with thyroid masses or abnormal levels of thyroid hormone

Gastroesophageal Reflux Studies: to detect GER; should be preceded by an upper GI series to exclude anatomic causes of GER

Oral Aspiration Studies: performed in neurologically-devastated children who suffer repeat episodes of aspiration pneumonia despite gastrostomy tube feedings and fundoplication

---

INTERVENTIONAL RADIOLOGY

A comprehensive review of interventional radiology is well beyond the scope of this chapter. Along with continued advances in cross-sectional imaging techniques, diagnostic and therapeutic procedures are being performed increasingly in children. These studies include preoperative embolization of vascular neoplasms such as nasopharyngeal juvenile angiofibroma (Fig. 43–69),[74,121] injection of liquid sclerosing agents to shrink vascular malformations,[122] balloon dilatation of esophageal[75,123] and tracheobronchial stenosis see (Fig. 43–52),[82] and most recently the placement of endotracheal metallic stents.[34] Almost all of these studies require sedation of the children and, therefore, should be performed only in an angiography suite that is equipped with the appropriate personnel and equipment.

SPECIAL CONSIDERATION:

Almost all interventional radiology studies require sedation and should be performed only in an angiography suite that is equipped with the appropriate personnel and equipment.

Biopsies, aspiration, and drainage procedures may be performed under fluoroscopic, sonographic, or CT guidance.[74,98] Although radiologists at some institutions offer fluoroscopically-guided foley catheter removal of esophageal foreign bodies,[5,124] the safety of this technique is controversial and the availability of the procedure remains limited.

CONCLUSION

Numerous radiologic techniques are available for the evaluation of the pediatric airway. Despite the addition of more sophisticated imaging modalities, properly-performed radiographs of the neck and chest remain the mainstay in the work-up of children with respiratory distress. When ordering any

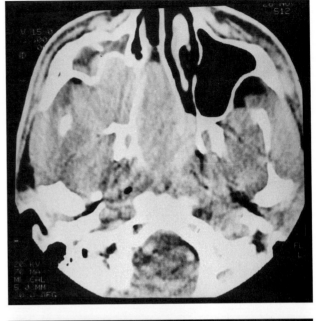

Figure 43–69: Juvenile nasopharyngeal angiofibroma. Axial CT image (A) of a 7-year-old boy with epistaxis reveals the presence of a large nasopharyngeal mass that deforms, rather than destroys, the posterior wall of the right maxillary sinus. This is a finding commonly seen with these benign, locally-invasive tumors. Preoperative angiography was performed. Injection of the internal maxillary branch of the right external carotid artery (B) illustrates the vascular nature of this mass. In order to facilitate resection, embolization with Gelfoam™ was performed (C) just prior to surgery.

A

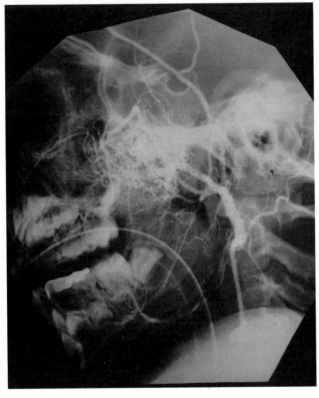

B

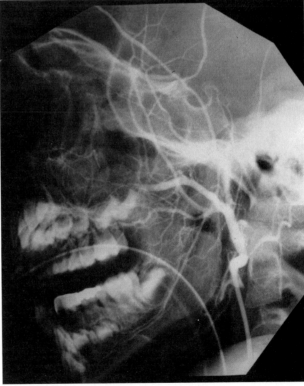

C

radiologic study, the physician always must prioritize maintenance of the child's airway and oxygenation. Communication between otolaryngologists and radiologists is essential to ensure that the appropriate study is selected in a given clinical situation and that it is performed in an efficacious and safe manner.

SPECIAL CONSIDERATION:

Properly-performed radiographs of the neck and chest remain the mainstay in the work-up of children with respiratory distress.

REFERENCES

1. Dunbar JS. Upper respiratory tract obstruction in infants and children. AJR 1970; 109:227-246.
2. Edwards DK. The child with stridor. In: Hilton S, Edwards DK, eds. *Practical Pediatric Radiology, 2nd ed.* Philadelphia: Saunders, 1994, pp. 45-84.
3. Poznanski AK. *Practical Approaches to Pediatric Radiology.* Chicago: Year Book, 1976, pp. 241-258.
4. Shapiro J, Strome M, Crocker AC. Airway obstruction and sleep apnea in Hurler and Hunter syndromes. Ann Otol Rhinol Laryngol 1985; 94:458-461.
5. Macpherson RI, Leithiser RE. Upper airway obstruction in children: An update. Radiographics 1985; 5:339-376.
6. Strife JL. Upper airway and tracheal obstruction in infants and children. Radiol Clin North Am 1988; 26:309-322.
7. John SD, Swischuk LE. Stridor and upper airway obstruction in infants and children. Radiographics 1992; 12:625-643.
8. Joseph PM, Berdon WE, Baker DH, et al. Upper airway obstruction in infants and small children. Radiology 1976; 121:143-148.
9. Hedlund GL, Griscom NT, Cleveland RH, et al. Respiratory system. In: Kirks DR, Griscom NT, eds. *Practical Pediatric Imaging—Diagnostic Radiology of Infants and Children, 3rd ed.* Philadelphia: Lippincott-Raven, 1998, pp. 619-819.
10. Sneed WF, Miller RH, Mintz AA. Retropharyngeal pseudomass. South Med J 1984; 77:528-530.
11. Taybi H. Metabolic disorders. In: Taybi H, Lachman RS, eds. *Radiology of Syndromes, Metabolic Disorders, and Skeletal Dysplasias, 4th ed.* St. Louis: Mosby Year Book, 1996, pp. 537.
12. Taybi H. Syndromes. In: Taybi H, Lachman RS, eds. *Radiology of Syndromes, Metabolic Disorders, and Skeletal Dysplasias, 4th ed.* St. Louis: Mosby Year Book, 1996, pp. 1.
13. Swischuk LE. *Imaging of the Newborn, Infant, and Young Child, 4th ed.* Baltimore: Williams and Wilkins, 1997, pp. 678-892.
14. Capitanio MA, Kirkpatrick JA. Nasopharyngeal lymphoid tissue. Radiology 1970; 96:389-391.
15. Smimiotopoulos JG, Chiechi MV. Teratomas, dermoids, and epidermoids of the head and neck. Radiographics 1995; 15:1437-1455.
16. Jeans WD, Fernando DCJ, Maw AR, et al. A longitudinal study of the growth of the nasopharynx and its contents in normal children. Br J Radiol 1981; 54:117-121.
17. Starshak RJ, Wells RG, Sty JR, et al. *Diagnostic Imaging of Infants and Children-Volume II.* Gaithersburg: Aspen, 1992, pp. 255-353.
18. Fujioka M, Young LW, Girdany BR. Radiographic evaluation of adenoidal size in children: Adenoidal—nasopharyngeal ratio. AJR 1979; 133:401-404.
19. Schlesinger AE, Hernandez RJ. Radiographic imaging of airway obstruction in pediatrics. Otolaryngol Clin North Am 1990; 23:609-637.
20. Smoker WRK. Oral cavity. In: Som PM, Curtin HD, eds. *Head and Neck Imaging, 3rd ed.* St. Louis: Mosby, 1996, pp. 488-544.
21. Kassel EE, Keller MA, Kucharczyk W. MRI of the floor of the mouth, tongue, and oropharynx. Radiol Clin North Am 1989; 27:331-351.
22. McCook TA, Kirks DR. Epiglottic enlargement in infants and children: Another radiologic look. Pediatr Radiol 1982; 12:227-234.
23. John SD, Swischuk LE, Hayden CK, et al. Aryepiglottic fold width in patients with epiglottitis: Where should measurements be obtained? Radiology 1994; 190:123-125.
24. Shackelford GD, Siegel MJ, McAlister WH. Subglottic edema in acute epiglottitis in children. AJR 1978; 131:603-605.
25. McHugh K, deSilva M, Kiham HA. Epiglottic enlargement secondary to laryngeal sarcoidosis. Pediatr Radiol 1993; 23:71.
26. Masip MJ, Esteban E, Alberto C, et al. Laryngeal involvement in pediatric neurofibromatosis: A case report and review of the literature. Pediatr Radiol 1996; 26:488-492.
27. Reyes BG, Arnold JE, Brooks LJ. Congenital absence of the epiglottis and its potential role in sleep apnea. Ann Otol Rhinol Laryngol 1994; 30:223-226.
28. Lorman JG, Biggs JR. The Eagle syndrome. AJR 1983; 140:881-882.
29. Goldbloom RB, Dunbar JS. Calcification of cartilage in trachea and larynx in infancy associated with congenital stridor. Pediatrics 1960; 26:669-673.
30. Capitanio MA, Kirkpatrick JA. Upper respiratory tract obstruction in infants and children. Radiol Clin North Am 1968; 6:265-277.
31. Andersen PE, Justesen P. Chondrodysplasia punctata. Report of two cases. Skeletal Radiol 1987; 16:223-226.
32. Tamburrini O, Bartolomeo-DeIuria A, Di Guglielmo GL. Chondrodysplasia punctata after warfarin. Case report with 18-month follow-up. Pediatr Radiol 1987; 17:323-324.
33. Bauman NM, Smith RJH. Recurrent respiratory papillomatosis. Ped Clin North Am 1996; 43:1385-1401.
34. Lesperance MM, Zalzal GH. Assessment and man-

agement of laryngotracheal stenosis. Pediatr Clin North Am 1996; 43:1413–1427.

35. Bowen A, Ledesma-Medina J, Fujioka M, et al. Radiologic imaging in otorhinolaryngology. Pediatr Clin North Am 1981; 28:905–939.

36. Han BK, Dunbar JS, Striker TW. Membranous laryngotracheobronchitis (membranous croup). AJR 1979; 133:53–58.

37. Kushner DC, Harris GBC. Obstructing lesions of the larynx and trachea in infants and children. Pediatr Clin North Am 1978; 16:181–194.

38. Currarino G, Williams B. Lateral inspiration and expiration radiographs of the neck in children with laryngotracheitis (croup). Radiology 1982; 145:365–366.

39. Williams JL, Capitanio MA, Turtz MG. Vocal cord paralysis: Radiologic observations in 21 infants and young children. AJR 1977; 128:649–651.

40. Abramson SJ, Berdon WE, Ruzal-Shapiro C, et al. Cervical neuroblastoma in eleven infants—a tumor with favorable prognosis. Clinical and radiologic (US, CT, MRI) findings. Pediatr Radiol 1993; 23:253–257.

41. McCook TA, Felman AH. Retropharyngeal masses in infants and young children. Am J Dis Child 1979; 133:41–43.

42. Swischuk LE, Smith PC, Fagan CJ. Abnormalities of the pharynx and larynx in childhood. Semin Roentgenol 1974; 9:283–300.

43. Hudgins PA, Jacobs IN, Castillo M. Pediatric airway disease. In: Som PM, Curtin HD, eds. Head and Neck Imaging, 3rd ed. St Louis: Mosby Year Book, 1996, pp. 545–611.

44. Smith PD, Swischuk LE, Fagan CJ. An elusive and often unsuspected cause of stridor or pneumonia—the esophageal foreign body. AJR 1974; 122:80–89.

45. Macpherson RI, Hill JG, Othersen HB, et al. Esophageal foreign bodies in children: Diagnosis, treatment, and complications. AJR 1996; 166:919–924.

46. Curtin HD. Larynx. In: Head and Neck Imaging, 3rd ed. St Louis: Mosby Year Book, 1996, pp. 612–707.

47. Gray SD, Smith ME, Schneider H. Voice disorders in children. Pediatr Clin North Am 1996; 43:1357–1384.

48. Holinger LD, Toriumi DM, Anandappa EC. Subglottic cysts and asymmetrical subglottic narrowing on neck radiograph. Pediatr Radiol 1988; 18:306–308.

49. Cooper M, Slovis TL, Madgy DN, et al. Congenital subglottic hemangioma: Frequency of symmetric subglottic narrowing on frontal radiographs of the neck. AJR 1992; 159:1269–1271.

50. Chen JC, Holinger LD. Congenital tracheal anomalies: Pathology study using serial macrosections and

review of the literature. Pediatr Pathol 1994; 14:513–537.

51. Mancuso RF. Stridor in neonates. Ped Clin North Am 1996; 43:1339–1356.

52. Sutton TJ, Nogrady MS. Radiologic diagnosis of subglottic hemangioma in infants. Pediatr Radiol 1973; 1:211–216.

53. Breyer RH, Dainauskas JR, Jensik RJ, et al. Mucoepidermoid carcinoma of the trachea and bronchus. The case for conservative resection. Ann Thorac Surg 1980; 29:197–204.

54. Strife JL, Bisset GS III, Burrows PE. Cardiovascular system. In: Kirks DR, Griscom NT, eds. Practical Pediatric Imaging—Diagnostic Radiology of Infants and Children, 3rd ed. Philadelphia: Lippincott-Raven, 1998, pp. 511–618.

55. McAdams HP, Gordon DS, White CS. Apical lung hernia: Radiologic findings in six cases. AJR 1996; 167:927–930.

56. Edwards DK. The newborn with respiratory distress. In: Hilton S, Edwards DK, eds. Practical Pediatric Radiology, 2nd ed. Philadelphia: Saunders, 1994, pp. 9–43.

57. Edwards DK. The child who wheezes. In: Hilton S, Edwards DK, eds. Practical Pediatric Radiology, 2nd ed. Philadelphia: Saunders, 1994, pp. 85–111.

58. Alford BA, McIlhenny J, Jones JE, et al. Asymmetric radiographic findings in the pediatric chest: Approach to early diagnosis. Radiographics 1993; 13:77–93.

59. Felson B. Chest Roentgenology, Philadelphia: Saunders, 1973, pp. 185–250.

60. Mandell VS, Braverman RM. Vascular rings and slings. In: Fyler DC, ed. NADAS Pediatric Cardiology. Philadelphia: Hanley and Belfus, 1992, pp. 719.

61. Pickhardt PJ, Siegel MJ, Gutierrez FR. Vascular rings in symptomatic children: Frequency of chest radiographic findings. Radiology 1997; 203:423–426.

62. Strife JL, Baumel AS, Dunbar JS. Tracheal compression by the innominate artery in infancy and childhood. Radiology 1981; 139:73–75.

63. Swischuk LE. Anterior tracheal indentation in infancy and early childhood: Normal and abnormal. AJR 1971; 112:12–17.

64. Donnelly LF, Frush DP, Bisset GS III. The multiple presentations of foreign bodies in children. AJR 1998; 170:471–477.

65. Cotton E, Yasuda K. Foreign body aspiration. Pediatr Clin North Am 1984; 31:937–941.

66. Donnelly LF, Bisset GS III. Airway compression in children with abnormal thoracic configuration. Radiology 1998; 206:323–326.

67. Lachman RS. Skeletal dysplasias. In: Taybi H, Lachman RS, eds. Radiology of Syndromes, Metabolic Disorders, and Skeletal Dysplasias, 4th ed. St Louis: Mosby Year Book, 1996, pp. 745.

68. Donn SM, Kuhns LR. Mechanism of endotracheal tube movement with change of head position in the neonate. Pediatr Radiol 1980; 9:37-40.

69. Capitanio MA, Kirkpatrick JA. The lateral decubitus film: An aid in determining airtrapping in children. Radiology 1972; 103:460-462.

70. Kaufman AS, Kuhns LR. The lateral decubitus view: An aid in evaluating poorly defined pulmonary densities in children. AJR 1977; 129:885-888.

71. Prewitt LH, Sane SM. Lateral decubitus radiograph of the chest in pediatric radiology—An additional use. Minn Med 1979; 62:423-426.

72. Chen IY, Armstrong JD II. Value of fluoroscopy in patients with suspected bilateral hemidiaphragmatic paralysis. AJR 1993; 160:29-31.

73. Buonomo C, Taylor GA, Share JC, et al. Gastrointestinal tract. In: Kirks DR, Griscom NT, eds. *Practical Pediatric Radiology—Diagnostic Radiology of Infants and Children, 3rd ed.* Philadelphia: Lippincott-Raven, 1998, pp. 821-1007.

74. Towbin RB, Ball WS. Pediatric interventional radiology. Radiol Clin North Am 1988; 26:419-440.

75. Mihailovic T, Perisic VN. Balloon dilatation of cricopharyngeal achalasia. Pediatr Radiol 1992; 22:522-524.

76. Döhlemann C, Mantel K, Vogl TJ, et al. Pulmonary sling: Morphological findings. Pre- and postoperative course. Eur J Pediatr 1995; 154:2-14.

77. Dodds WJ, Stewart ET, Logemann JA. Physiology and radiology of the normal oral and pharyngeal phases of swallowing. AJR 1990; 154:953-963.

78. Wright RER, Wright FR, Carson CA. Videofluoroscopic assessment in children with severe cerebral palsy presenting with dysphagia. Pediatr Radiol 1996; 26:720-722.

79. Ott DJ, Pikna LA. Clinical and videofluoroscopic evaluation of swallowing disorders. AJR 1993; 161:507-513.

80. Jones B. The tailored examination of the dysphagic patient. Appl Radiol 1995; 2:27.

81. Stringer DA, Witzel MA. Velopharyngeal insufficiency on videofluoroscopy: Comparison of projections. AJR 1986; 146:15-19.

82. Jaffe RB. Balloon dilation of congenital and acquired stenosis of the trachea and bronchi. Radiology 1997; 203:405-409.

83. Egelhoff JC, Ball WS, Koch BL, et al. Safety and efficacy of sedation in children using a structured sedation program. AJR 1997; 168:1259-1262.

84. Fernbach SK, Feinstein KA. Selected topics in pediatric ultrasonography—1992. Radiol Clin North Am 1992; 30:1011-1031.

85. Vazquez E, Enriquez G, Castellote A, et al. US, CT, and MR imaging of neck lesions in children. Radiographics 1995; 15:105-122.

86. Wernecke K, Diederich S. Sonographic features of mediastinal tumors. AJR 1994; 163:1357-1364.

87. Wernecke K. Sonographic features of pleural disease. AJR 1997; 168:1061-1066.

88. Diament MJ, Boechat MI, Kangarloo H. Real-time sector ultrasound in the evaluation of suspected abnormalities of diaphragmatic motion. J Clin Ultrasound 1985; 13:539-543.

89. Garel C, Hassan M, Legrand I, et al. Laryngeal ultrasonography in infants and children: Pathological findings. Pediatr Radiol 1991; 21:164-167.

90. Crawford SC, Harnsberger HR, Johnson L, et al. Fibromatosis coli in infancy: CT and sonographic findings. AJR 1988; 151:1183-1184.

91. Wadsworth DT, Siegel MJ. Thyroglossal duct cysts: Variability of sonographic findings. AJR 1994; 163:1475-1477.

92. Lim-Dunham JE, Feinstein KA, Yousefzadeh DK, et al. Sonographic demonstration of a normal thyroid gland excludes ectopic thyroid in patients with thyroglossal duct cyst. AJR 1995; 164:1489-1491.

93. Lucaya J, Berdon WE, Enriquez G, et al. Congenital pyriform sinus fistula: A cause of acute left-sided suppurative thyroiditis and neck abscess in children. Pediatr Radiol 1990; 21:27-29.

94. Leonidas JC, Berdon WE, Valderrama E, et al. Human immunodeficiency virus infection and multilocular thymic cysts. Radiology 1996; 198:377-379.

95. Avila NA, Mueller BU, Carrasquillo JA, et al. Multilocular thymic cysts: Imaging features in children with human immunodeficiency virus infection. Radiology 1996; 201:130-134.

96. Soberman N, Leonidas JC, Berdon WE, et al. Parotid enlargement in children seropositive for human immunodeficiency virus: Imaging findings. AJR 1991; 157:553-556.

97. Nazarian GK, Foshager MC. Color doppler sonography of the thoracic inlet veins. RadioGraphics 1995; 15:1357-1371.

98. Klein JS, Schultz S, Heffrer JE. Interventional radiology of the chest: Imaged-guided percutaneous drainage of pleural effusions, lung abscesses, and pneumothorax. AJR 1995; 164:581-588.

99. Frush DP, Siegel MJ, Bisset GS III. Challenges of pediatric spiral CT. Radiographics 1997; 17:939-959.

100. Shady K, Siegel MJ, Glazer HS. CT of focal pulmonary masses in childhood. RadioGraphics 1992; 12:505-514.

101. Kuhn JP. High-resolution computed tomography of pediatric pulmonary parenchymal disorders. Radiol Clin North Am 1993; 31:533-551.

102. Moon WK, Kim WS, Kim IO, et al. Diffuse pulmonary disease in children: High-resolution CT findings. AJR 1996; 167:1405-1408.

103. Seely JM, Effman EL, Müller NL. High-resolution CT of pediatric lung disease: Imaging findings. AJR 1997; 168:1269–1275.

104. Shipley RT, McLoud TC, Dedrick CG, et al. Computed tomography of the tracheal bronchus. J Comput Assist Tomogr 1985; 9:53–55.

105. Griscom NT, Whol MEB. Dimensions of the growing trachea related to age and gender. AJR 1986; 146:233–237.

106. Griscom NT. CT measurement of the tracheal lumen in children and adolescents. AJR 1991; 156: 371–372.

107. Quint LE, Whyte RI, Kazerooni EA, et al. Stenosis of the central airways: Evaluation by using helical CT with multiplanar reconstructions. Radiology 1995; 194:871–877.

108. Lee KS, Yoon JH, Kim TK, et al. Evaluation of tracheobronchial disease with helical CT with multiplanar and three-dimensional reconstruction: Correlation with bronchoscopy. RadioGraphics 1997; 17:555–567.

109. Meza MP, Benson M, Slovis TL. Imaging of mediastinal masses in children. Radiol Clin North Am 1993; 31:583–604.

110. Slovis TL, Renfro B, Watts FB, et al. Choanal atresia: Precise CT evaluation. Radiology 1985; 155: 345–348.

111. Carpenter BLM, Merten DF. Radiographic manifestations of congenital anomalies of the airway. Radiol Clin North Am 1991; 29:219–240.

112. Choe YH, Kim YM, Han BK, et al. MR imaging in the morphologic diagnosis of congenital heart disease. RadioGraphics 1997; 17:403–422.

113. Simoneaux SF, Bank ER, Webber JB, et al. MR imaging of the pediatric airway. RadioGraphics 1995; 15:287–298.

114. Newman B, Meza MP, Towbin RB, et al. Left pulmonary artery sling: Diagnosis and delineation of associated tracheobronchial anomalies with MR. Pediatr Radiol 1996; 26:661–668.

115. Berlin SC. Magnetic resonance imaging of the cardiovascular system and airway. Pediatr Clin North Am 1997; 44:659–679.

116. Donnelly LF, Strife JL, Bisset GS III. The spectrum of lower airway compression in children: MR imaging. AJR 1997; 168:59–62.

117. Rebergen SA, Niezen RA, Heibing WA, et al. CINE gradient-echo MR imaging and MR velocity mapping in the evaluation of congenital heart disease. Radiographics 1996; 16:467–481.

118. Palitiel HJ, Larsen R, Treves ST. Thyroid. In: Treves ST, ed. *Pediatric Nuclear Medicine, 2nd ed.* New York: Springer-Verlag, 1995, pp. 135–148.

119. Fogelman I, Maisey MN, Clarke SEM. *An Atlas of Clinical Nuclear Medicine, 2nd ed.* St Louis: Mosby, 1994.

120. Heyman S. Gastroesophageal reflux, esophageal transit, gastic emptying, and pulmonary aspiration. In: Treves ST, ed. *Pediatric Nuclear Medicine, 2nd ed.* New York: Springer-Verlag, 1995, pp. 430–452.

121. Davis KR. Embolization of epistaxis and juvenile nasopharyngeal angiofibromas. AJR 1987; 148: 209–218.

122. Maynar M, Reyes R, Pulido-Duque JM, et al. Vascular procedures in the pediatric age group. In: Castañeda-Zúñiga WR, Tadavarthy SM, eds. *Interventional Radiology, 2nd ed.* Baltimore: Williams and Wilkins, 1992, pp. 717.

123. Maynar M, Guerra C, Reyes R, et al. Dilation of esophageal strictures. In: Castañeda-Zúñiga WR, Tadavarthy SM, eds. *Interventional Radiology, 2nd ed.* Baltimore: Williams and Wilkins, 1992, pp. 1230.

124. Harned RK III, Strain JD, Hay TC, et al. Esophageal foreign bodies: Safety and efficacy of foley catheter extraction of coins. AJR 1997; 168:443–446.

44 Communication Disorders

Howard C. Shane, Dorothy M. Brown,
Kara B. Kelley-Corley, Hope E. Dickinson, Kara Fletcher,
Arden Hill, Marnie S. Millington, Sarah N. Quinn,
and Geralyn Harvey-Woodnorth

An understanding of human communication and its disorders is central to sound clinical practice in otolaryngology. As most disorders of human communication are related directly to structures and processes evaluated and treated routinely by the otolaryngologist, the evaluation, treatment, and prevention of communication disorders should be viewed as vital parts of the otolaryngologist's clinical and research roles. The structures of the larynx, pharynx, and the oral nasal cavity, for example, are a routine part of the otolaryngologist's examination and are related to the production of voice, resonance, and speech sounds. Because otolaryngologists treat the structures that are responsible for hearing acuity and auditory processing, they have a direct influence on a child's language growth and development.

Otolaryngologists who care for children on a regular basis should interact with speech-language pathologists. These interactions occur routinely around the treatment of children with voice, language, and articulation disorders, as well as around the management of children who are hearing impaired or deaf. These professional interactions address treatment considerations and diagnostic issues. For example, detailed information about the nature of a vocal pathology that is provided by the otolaryngologist should help to set the stage for the treatment regimen carried out by the speech-language pathologist. Similarly, the improvement of hearing status increases the chances that a language-based communication deficit will be avoided and helps to form the foundation for successful communication therapy.

The otolaryngologist may reduce the possibility of a communication disorder by treating an underlying medical condition, thus serving a preventative role in respect to these disorders. For example, a mild-to-moderate hearing loss related to otitis media (OM) may underlie a child's speech and language problems, but because of the otolaryngologist's appropriate treatment of this condition it may be possible for the child to be protected from the communication problems that are associated with temporary hearing loss.

This chapter briefly examines human communication with an emphasis on disorders. It takes a traditional view of communication disorders and categorizes them according to disorders that are related to speech, language, voice, feeding and swallowing, and fluency. With the possible exception of disorders related to fluency, the practicing otolaryngologist who cares for children often will have a direct role in diagnosis and treatment of the disorders or the disorder categories that are outlined. Each section is organized to provide an overview of the communication difficulty and is followed by typical diagnostic procedures and treatment principles and practices.

Pediatric Otolaryngology, Edited by R.F. Wetmore, H.R. Muntz, and T.J. McGill. Thieme Medical Publishers, Inc., New York © 2000.

DISORDERS OF SPEECH

Speech is the end product of a complex sequence of events that involves cognition, symbolization, motor planning, and articulation. *Phonology* is a general term that refers to all aspects of the study of speech sounds, including speech perception and production as well as the cognitive and motor aspects of speech. *Articulation* is the motor aspect of the production of speech and, as such, is part of phonologic development.[1] In order to learn to speak, a child must learn both the physical movements required as well as the organizational aspects of his native speech-sound system.

Phonologic processes affect sound change within a word. The sounds and sound patterns of different languages can differ in several ways, including the sounds that are available for use, the permissible ordering of these sounds, and the rules that operate on the sounds. A *phonologic rule* (also called a phonologic process or pattern) is a formal expression of a regularity that occurs in the phonology of a language or in the phonology of an individual speaker. Such rules, or processes, affect sound change within a word.

Speech development begins in the newborn period and follows an orderly pattern through the early school years. Although there is considerable variation from child to child, there are several identifiable developmental stages. The roots of adult speech can be found in infant vocalizations. Infants from different backgrounds all progress through the same stages of development at approximately the same ages.[1] Even infants with identified disabilities that affect speech and language (e.g., developmental disabilities or hearing loss) pass through the earliest stages of speech development.[2] These earliest stages are similar in all infants because the earliest vocalizations are determined by the size and shape of the infant vocal tract and the changes occurring therein.[1] By the time children are in the early elementary school years, speech should be adult-like, with no sound errors or missing sounds from their repertoire.[3] The stages of speech development are:

- **The Newborn/Stage 1:** This stage is known as the *phonation stage.* From birth to the first month of life, most infants' sounds are reflexive and vegetative, with cries and partial vowel sounds predominating.[4] Most sounds are nasalized. Coughs, burps, grunts, and sighs are also common.[3] At the end of the first month, cries begin to become dif-

ferentiated (i.e., distinct cries for hunger, pain, etc.).[3]

- **2 to 3 Months/Stage 2:** This sometimes is referred to as the "coo" or "goo" stage. There is a definite start and stop to oral movements,[5] and babies begin to have greater control over phonation. Laughter and "cooing" with open vowel sounds emerge.[4,6] Some back and middle vowel sounds and back consonants with incomplete resonance are heard.[5] Sounds continue to be nasalized.

- **4 to 6 Months/Stage 3:** This is known as the *expansion* or *exploration stage.* Babies begin to increase their vocal repertoire and now engage in "vocal play."[3] Babies gain greater control over parts of the vocal mechanism, including the tongue.[5] Prolonged periods of vocalizations and strings of sounds begin to emerge. More labial than back sounds are now present. Babies begin to "babble," with strings of sounds consisting of at least one consonant and one vowel. Consonant-vowel (CV) and vowel-consonant (VC) strings are now most common. "Raspberry" sounds, growls, squeals, friction noises, and yells also are heard.[1] A contrast in pitch and amplitude begins to occur.

- **7 to 9 Months/Stage 4:** This stage is characterized by the emergence of repetitive syllable productions, known as *reduplicated babbling.*[5] Vocalizations in CV syllables begin to sound increasingly like the child's native language. There is an increase in lip control and the consonant repertoire is restricted to labial and alveolar plosive sounds (e.g.,/m/, /n/, /p/, /t/, /d/, and /j/). Long strings of reduplicated CV syllable babble are common now (e.g., "bababababa") with a peak in babbling at about 8 months.[3] By 10 months, the baby often produces long strings of babble with intonation similar to adult language.

- **10 to 12 Months/Stage 5:** This stage is defined by the use of "variegated babble" and "jargon." The baby is now able to elevate the tongue tip. The baby continues to produce long strings of babble and now produces CV syllables with a variety of consonants and vowels.[6] The consonant repertoire increases, with a predominance of the phonemes /m, v, b, p/. Different syllable shapes (e.g., CV, VC, CVC, CCV) emerge, with CV syllables predominating. Intonation patterns similar to the adult language are heard. Variegated babble with varied intonation patterns make up "jargon" and parents often comment that their child now speaks in her "own language."

The stages beyond the first year are:

- **First Words Stage:** First true words emerge somewhere around 12 months,[3] and are primarily CV, VC, CVCV in syllable shape.[5] Most first words are one syllable or fully or partially reduplicated syllables (e.g., "baba," "mommy"). Closed syllables (i.e., CVC) also are seen, but less frequently. First words typically are composed of labial and alveolar stops (i.e., /p, b, t, d/), nasals (i.e., /m, n/), and glides (i.e., /w, j/).[1] There is variability in the acquisition of first words, with some babies not producing a true first word for several months.
- **16 months to 2 years:** A rapid expansion of vocabulary occurs beginning around 18 months. At this age, a child's speech should be understood approximately 25 percent of the time.[3] A decrease in speech intelligibility may occur due to the child's increasing length of utterance. Verbal productions now become increasingly stable and more closely resemble the adult form.[1] By 2 years of age the child has acquired the speech sounds /p, h, w, m, n, b, k, g/.[5]
- **2½ to 3 years:** A child should be understood 60 to 75 percent of the time.[3] By 36 months the child has acquired /d, f, j, t, n, s/ and all vowels.[5]
- **4 years:** The child has acquired /r, l, θ, d/.[5] The average Standard American English (SAE) speaker produces the majority of speech sounds correctly,[7] and is intelligible 100% of the time.[3]
- **6 to 8 years:** The child has acquired sibilant sounds, fricatives, and consonant blends.[5] By age 7 years, a child's speech should be developed fully and resemble the adult native language, although longer words may continue to present difficulty.[3]

Phonological Processes to Simplify Speech

Children simplify speech in various ways. Phonological processes describe the differences between the sounds a child produces and the sounds present in the standard adult production.[3] Phonological processes are systematic simplifications used to restructure an adult word form (Macken, MA & Ferguson, CA in Weiss, Gordon, & Lillywhite, 1987, chapter "Later Phonological Development".) They are developmental in nature and are appropriate at particular ages. In addition to rule-based simplifications, a child may exhibit other sound errors. Errors of distortion (e.g., a "lisp") do not occur in typical development and may, therefore, reflect a speech disorder related to the oral structure or function.

Factors Adversely Affecting Speech Development

There are myriad risks for delayed or disordered speech development. Structural anomalies may include those involving dentition (e.g., malocclusion, missing teeth, dental arch anomalies), lips (e.g., cleft lip), palate (e.g., unilateral or bilateral cleft palate), tongue (e.g., ankyloglossia, macroglossia), velum (e.g., velopharyngeal incompetence), and nasopharynx (e.g., hypertrophied tonsils or adenoids). Other risks include hearing loss (conductive or sensorineural); early childhood injuries, diseases and infections; oral motor delays/disorders; cognitive and linguistic deficits; and environmental and psychosocial difficulties.[3,8,9]

AT A GLANCE . . .

Factors Affecting Speech Development

- Anatomic (dentition, lips, palate, tongue, velum, nasopharynx)
- Hearing loss
- Early childhood injuries, diseases, and infections
- Oral motor delays
- Cognitive and linguistic deficits
- Environmental and psychosocial difficulties

Referral to a speech-language pathologist should be considered when a child has an identified risk, has not reached developmental milestones within expected time frames, has poor speech intelligibility, or has frustration related to communication failure. Any of the above may indicate the presence of an articulation disorder, a phonologic disorder, or a motor speech disorder.

AT A GLANCE . . .

Referral to Speech-language Pathologist

- Child with an identified risk
- Failure to reach developmental milestones
- Poor speech intelligibility
- Frustration secondary to communication failure

Articulation deficits are motoric in nature and result from difficulties in the movement of oral articulators. A lisped production of /s/ is motoric and results from incorrect tongue placement. *Motor-speech disorders* are also motoric in nature. *Dysarthrias* result from deficits in the execution of movement, in which errors are the product of weak, slow, uncoordinated, articulator movement.[10] *Developmental apraxias* of speech result from deficits in motor programming. Although the child's articulators are adequate in strength, speed, range of motion, and coordination, errors result when the child is forced to sequence speech sounds for the purpose of volitional speech.[11] *Phonologic disorders* are linguistic in nature and result from the application of an inappropriate speech production rule. Disorders occur when the child creates an atypical rule, as in the atypical deletion of initial consonants such as 'abbit' for 'rabbit,' or when a developmentally-appropriate simplification is produced when it is no longer developmentally appropriate.[1]

Assessment and Management of Speech Disorders

Assessment of a child's speech includes both parent interview and a direct diagnostic assessment. When children present with speech deficits, the reported concern often is reduced speech intelligibility, which causes the parents' inability to understand their child's speech and their need to act as translator for their child. Information relating to the child's prenatal, birth, health, developmental, educational, and family histories should be collected. The above information allows for the development of hypotheses regarding the child's speech diagnosis and the nature of the speech deficit, as well as identification of optimal treatment approaches and techniques to facilitate improvement in speech intelligibility.

Following parental interview, the speech evaluation includes direct assessment of the child's speech. The assessment procedure depends to some extent on the information obtained through the interview, and typically consists of both standardized and nonstandardized measures. *Standard measures* compare aspects of the child's speech to same-age peers using a normative curve as referent. This information relates to articulatory accuracy and the presence and pervasiveness of phonologic processes using individual words or words in sentences in response to picture or object stimuli. During the

diagnostic process, the accuracy of the production of each speech sound across initial, medial, and final positions in words is assessed.

Nonstandardized assessment can provide information regarding the nature of the speech deficit, and this information can help the therapist to comment on prognosis for treatment and to make recommendations regarding the focus of treatment. A nonstandardized assessment is the collection of a speech sample for later analysis. Samples are phonetically transcribed and different types of information regarding sound inventory and error type are collected.

Speech intelligibility tasks are another important assessment tool. These tasks can be administered and judged in a variety of different formats, with the result being an estimate of connected speech intelligibility. *Structural-functional exams* and *motor-speech exams* are administered to determine the adequacy of oral articulators in the production of both nonspeech and speech sequences. The structural-functional exam assesses the structure and function of the articulators (e.g., lips, tongue, teeth, jaw, velum) and determines their adequacy based on a series of tasks designed to assess the parameters of movement. The speech-language pathologist uses the results from this measure to assist in the diagnosis of a dysarthria and/or developmental apraxia of speech. If the contribution of a dysarthria is found to be significant to the child's overall speech intelligibility, a speech subsystem assessment is then conducted. This examination uses perceptual methods to assess the relative contribution of respiration, phonation, resonation, and articulation processes to the child's overall speech impairment. Results from this measure provide the focus for treatment.[12] The motor-speech exam is administered to evaluate how the articulators produce speech sounds in sequences of increasing length and phonetic complexity. It assesses the child's ability to imitate speech sequences accurately as the temporal interval between clinical stimulus and the child's response increases. The results from this measure assist considerably in the diagnosis of developmental apraxias of speech and provide information regarding treatment targets.

Stimulability testing is the final step in a speech evaluation. The procedures used help to determine which therapeutic techniques facilitate improvements in speech performance. The nature of the errors affects treatment approaches.

When the assessment is completed, a model for

intervention is personalized for the child. Choosing a treatment program and developing specific targets for remediation depend on the variables previously outlined. Speech therapy can be delivered in individual or group settings. Individual therapy is often necessary for children with severe speech deficits, as well as for those with concomitant language delays. If children present with other issues such as distractibility or decreased attention, individual therapy also may prove to be most beneficial. Group therapy is an appropriate choice when a therapist is treating several children with similar abilities and deficits.

The amount of speech therapy and its duration are a consideration when implementing treatment. Factors to consider include: the age, the motivation of both child and caregivers, attention span, the severity and nature of the speech deficit, and concomitant communicative deficits.

Parent training should be incorporated into therapy whenever possible. Faster gains are more likely to occur when therapy is administered in both clinical and home environments. Supportive, motivated, and willing parents can be highly beneficial to a child's speech development.

DISORDERS OF LANGUAGE

Although most children appear to acquire language almost effortlessly, approximately 8 to 12% of children will have language delays during their preschool years.[13] Given the complexities of language development, it is remarkable that more children do not have delays. Delays can be evident in expressive language alone and may affect vocabulary usage, utterance length, and syntactical abilities. When delays are isolated to expression, underlying issues of phonologic ability or sound production may be contributory. Of greater concern are delays that affect both comprehension (receptive language) and expression. Approximately 5% of children under the age of 5 years[13] can be described clinically as *specific language impaired* (SLI) which means that there are language difficulties that are not associated with any other specific cognitive deficit. Children with receptive and expressive language delays or disorders may have difficulty understanding directions and questions in addition to having reduced spoken output. This can lead to difficulties in the social use of language, which is known also as *prag-*

matics. Although the etiology of such delays rarely can be determined definitively, familial history of developmental language disorders and/or earlier history of middle-ear pathology are possible contributory factors. An even smaller percentage of children may have comprehension difficulties with apparently-intact expressive language skills, raising the strong suspicion of an underlying central auditory processing disorder.

SPECIAL CONSIDERATION:

Although most children appear to acquire language almost effortlessly, approximately 8 to 12 percent of children will have language delays during their preschool years.

Assessment and Management of Language Disorders

When children have language delays, hearing loss is the first disorder to be excluded. Of note, children with fluctuating hearing loss secondary to OM are the largest group of children with hearing loss. When a preschool-aged child is suspected of having delays in language development, a comprehensive evaluation is essential. A speech and language evaluation including a hearing assessment should be arranged. When comprehension difficulties are suspected, full cognitive assessment with a developmental psychologist is critical. A *full cognitive assessment* is necessary to determine whether a child's language difficulties are characteristic of a global or pervasive developmental disorder or are representative of a specific language impairment or learning disorder. U.S. federal law mandates availability of assessment and intervention for children with suspected delays through either local early intervention programs (birth to 3 years) or through the public schools from age 3 to 22 years. (In some states a separate community agency provides services for children from birth to 5 years.) Most pediatric hospitals also have comprehensive developmental assessment teams through which diagnoses and recommendations for intervention can be made. Children found to have significant language delays or disorders are then eligible for intervention services through public programs. For the preschool-aged child this typically includes placement in a specialized or integrated preschool with speech and language therapy provided at the school. Depending upon the needs of the child and family, language intervention also can be obtained through hospital-based or private speech and language practitioners.

Many children identified as having language delays during their preschool years show significant resolution of these difficulties by grade one. Although the most recent research offers conflicting results,[14,15] a number of these children have significant ongoing language difficulties. Such difficulties are classified as a language learning disorder when they are significant enough to affect academics and are clearly discrepant with a child's overall cognitive functioning. Children who by grade one continue to have difficulties in language comprehension and/or production are clearly at risk for academic difficulty, particularly as they approach the language dependent task of learning to read. Children with more subtle language or auditory processing difficulties who have problems comprehending spoken language may be thought mistakenly to have a primary attention deficit and/or a behavioral problem. A comprehensive assessment is, therefore, extremely important for accurate treatment.

Assessment for the school-age child who is suspected of having a language learning disorder should include a speech and language evaluation, in addition to cognitive and educational assessment with a learning specialist. The speech and language pathologist assesses various aspects of language function including vocabulary, syntax, comprehension, discourse, written language, verbal memory, and retrieval skills. Hearing assessment for children 7 years and older should include a central auditory processing battery completed by an audiologist. Children with language learning disorders have difficulties in various aspects of central auditory processing (e.g., auditory closure, figure-ground listen-

ing, short-term auditory memory, processing rate, etc.). Determining a child's specific strengths and weaknesses is essential to developing an optimal intervention plan. For some children, their learning difficulty may be highly specific to one aspect of auditory processing (e.g., sound discrimination), although more general oral language functions may be spared. For these children, decoding for reading may be particularly troublesome.

Assessment teams are available both through a child's school and through hospital or private settings. (Central auditory processing testing typically is done in a hospital or private audiology setting.) A child who is identified as having a language learning disorder is eligible for services through the public school. A team of professionals should be gathered and an individual education plan (IEP) should be written to address the child's needs and to determine appropriate services. If parents question the outcome of a school assessment or plan, they have the right to an outside assessment. Most children identified as having language learning disorders benefit from some degree of support throughout their school years.

DISORDERS OF VOICE

Voice problems in children are well documented, with reported occurrence ranging from 6 to 23% in school-age children.[16-18] There are a number of etiologies for voice disorders in children. These include trauma, iatrogenic causes, neurologic problems, neoplasms, congenital anomalies, infectious diseases, inflammation, behavioral patterns, and psychogenic causes.[19]

AT A GLANCE . . .

Etiology of Voice Disorders

- Trauma
- Iatrogenic causes
- Neurologic problems
- Neoplasms
- Congenital anomalies
- Infectious diseases
- Inflammation of the upper respiratory tract
- Behavioral patterns
- Psychogenic causes

The otolaryngologist often interacts with speech-language pathologists regarding voice disorders related to phonation and resonance. The following information addresses voice problems that are related to phonation. *Disorders* in voice production can present as a disruption across the vocal parameters of quality, pitch, and/or loudness. *Deviations* in voice quality are commonly categorized as hoarseness/roughness, breathiness, tension, tremor, strain/strangle, interruption in voicing, and diplophonia.[20] Abnormalities in the quality, or tone, of the voice are most common in children.[21] Pitch abnormalities may be manifested by an inappropriately high or low pitch for a child's age and gender, monopitch, pitch breaks, or reduced pitch range.[22] Abnormality in loudness is characterized by too loud a voice, too soft a voice, monoloudness, or difficulty with control of loudness variation. Severity of the voice problem can range from mild

AT A GLANCE . . .

Deviation in Voice Quality

- Hoarseness/roughness
- Breathiness
- Tension
- Tremor
- Strain/strangle
- Interruption in voicing
- Diplophonia

to severe. The presence of a voice disorder may interfere with speech intelligibility and may affect how a child is perceived by family, teachers, and peers.[23]

Assessment and Management of Voice Disorders

Management of children who present with voice problems requires an assessment, determination of a diagnosis, and development and implementation of a treatment plan. This necessitates a multidisciplinary approach and is often accomplished through the joint efforts of the pediatrician, otolaryngologist, and the speech-language pathologist. In some settings, the otolaryngologist and speech-language pathologist complete a comprehensive medical and behavioral assessment at the same time. This is optimal as it allows for efficient utilization of resources with enhanced opportunity for communication between the professionals and family. Other professionals across many disciplines are concerned with the voice and also may be involved in the management of the child with voice problems. These professionals include neurologists, teachers, psychologists, social workers, school nurses, singing instructors, and audiologists.

The speech-language pathologist's evaluation of a child with a voice disorder includes: (1) acquisition of pertinent background information; and (2) assessment of the child's voice. Background information to be obtained includes a review of the otolaryngologist's laryngeal diagnosis and medical treatment plans, as well as any data available regarding alterations in laryngeal structure and/or function. In addition, the speech-language pathologist considers general medical history and collects voice symptom history, voice use history, and any relevant information regarding psychosocial factors.

Perceptual and instrumental assessments of voice production are routine components of the voice evaluation. Whereas completion of structured tasks may not be possible with infants and toddlers, the majority of preschool and school-age children comply with a variety of structured tasks that can result in an adequate sample of vocal production. Tasks that are used routinely in many clinical settings include sustained production of isolated vowels, sustained production of /s/ and /z/, counting, sentence imitation, oral reading or recitation of a nursery rhyme, and a spontaneous speech sample. If standard elicitation techniques are adapted to include clinician models, practice trials, and visual cues, thorough assessment may be completed successfully even with young children.[24]

Instrumental measures including videostroboscopy, acoustic analysis, aerodynamic procedures, and electroglottography should be conducted as part of the pediatric voice evaluation whenever possible. The availability of instrumentation and voice laboratories across the country has increased with recent advances in technology, and instrumental procedures are being used successfully now with children.[25-28] Utilization of instrumentation allows clinicians to visualize vocal cord movements during speech tasks and to obtain repeatable objective measures of pertinent acoustic, aerodynamic, and physiologic parameters. This information provides an objective means for measuring change following management, either therapeutic or surgical, and provides a permanent record of the visual images and data.

The results from the voice assessment aid the clinician in making a decision about whether voice therapy is appropriate and, if so, what the intervention strategies and anticipated outcome might be. The goal of voice therapy varies from child to child, depending on the nature of their problem. The general goal, however, is to help each individual achieve the best voice possible to meet his communicative needs. Voice therapy with children should emphasize education, vocal hygiene, and behavioral therapy techniques. Information regarding the etiology of the voice problem, its nature, and maintenance factors should be imparted directly in a manner that is appropriate to the child's developmental age. Understanding can be aided through the use of visual images, such as video-endoscopic recordings, models, or line drawings. It is helpful to keep information sessions with children brief and to repeat the presentation numerous times.

SPECIAL CONSIDERATION:

The general goal of voice therapy is to help each individual achieve the best voice possible to meet her communicative needs.

Vocal hygiene is aided by maintenance of good hydration through adequate daily consumption of water and elimination of caffeine. Provision for quiet activities can be implemented on a regular basis in order to reduce the amount of talking, and other modifications, such as a reduction of background noise, are also helpful. Improved vocal use, such as quiet voice, is sometimes accomplished with young children through systematic verbal praise for incidental use of the target voice and actively ignoring the undesirable behavior. Elimination of vocal abuses, such as production of sound effects, yelling, and production of squeaky voices, is best addressed through implementation of behavioral therapy techniques that are directed at teaching use of alternative, more appropriate, vocal productions. Other therapy techniques that are appropriate for children and their indication for use with different physiologic conditions are described in the literature.[20,22,29]

It is beneficial to approach behavioral treatment with children as a dynamic process. Incorporation of age-appropriate play activities that provide opportunities for functional use of the target behaviors is one means of doing this. Play activities also can bridge the gap between therapy and the child's routine daily interactions and aid in generalization of learned skills across settings. In addition, motivation and incentive for good vocal use can be shaped through implementation of point systems, charts, or stickers to reward use of the target behaviors. Children benefit from external support to change their vocal habits, and the inclusion of teachers, parents, or other caregivers in therapy fosters carryover of therapy procedures to different settings and aids in the achievement of desired results.

AUGMENTATIVE AND ALTERNATIVE COMMUNICATION

In the past two decades there has been a rapid growth in the use of supplemental communication strategies for children with severe expressive communication disorders. The use of *augmentative or alternative communication* (AAC) strategies and techniques has the potential to assist such children when their communication deficit is either of a temporary or permanent nature. *Temporary AAC* use benefits the children who require supplemental support until surgical or spontaneous recovery, maturation, and/or training makes this support no longer necessary. There are some children, on the other hand, who will always need a supplemental system to increase speech intelligibility or enable effective communication. The term *augmentative* is used because it implies that speech communication has not been abandoned and that other methods are meant to augment or supplement speech. An *alternative communication approach* has a somewhat more negative connotation as it suggests that speech itself is likely to be replaced. The latter term usually is reserved for persons who are experiencing a progressive speech loss due to regressive neurologic conditions such amyotrophic lateral sclerosis (ALS) or myotonic dystrophies. In either case, the goal of augmentative and alternative communication is communication by the most effective means possible at any given time.

The growth of AAC is due to three interrelated forces. These include:

1. An ideological shift in societal values, which encourages movement away from the large institutional placements for persons with severe expressive deficits to more community-based facilities.
2. Technological improvement that has greatly expanded the opportunities for persons with severe expressive disorders. The microprocessor has provided a powerful tool that allows a person, regardless of physical disability, to control a computer, use a computer voice, and independently formulate and express ideas and information.
3. Government inducements that, in the past decade, have given persons with severe expressive speech deficits the benefit of U.S. federal legislation that insures individualized education in the least restrictive public education setting (i.e., PL 94–142). Additionally, improved public policy around the use of assistive technology (i.e., Technology Act of 1988) and provisions for improved access in entertainment, transportation, and industry (i.e., Americans with Disabilities Act) have been legislated.

Two primary forms of AAC, referred to as aided and unaided approaches, have been used effectively with persons experiencing severe expressive speech deficits. The first approach involves the use of some tangible electronic or nonelectronic device that serves as the aid to communication. With the availability of more sophisticated, electronic options (microprocessor-based) and a growing body of literature on positive outcomes, aided communi-

cation approaches are enjoying a rapid increase in usage. An unaided approach, on the other hand, refers to the use of strategies that require only what is part of the normal human body for communication. These would include speech, gestures, facial expression, signs, and any consistent behaviors that can be interpreted meaningfully. It is becoming more widely recognized that unaided communication in the form of sign language can be highly successful for persons who can hear but who experience a severe expressive communication problem related to an etiology other than hearing loss.

Individuals who benefit from an AAC intervention include those with a wide range of etiologies covering the entire age span. The three primary reasons a person is introduced to an AAC approach are: (1) severe motor impairment (affecting motor speech production); (2) severe language disorder including severe auditory processing; and (3) significant cognitive deficit. Persons experiencing either acquired or congenital disorders fall within these boundaries.

AT A GLANCE . . .

Children Requiring Augmentative and Alternative Communication

1. Those with severe motor impairment
2. Those with severe language disorder
3. Those with significant cognitive deficit

The evaluation process for possible implementation of an AAC method generally involves a team evaluation. The specific elements of an evaluation typically include assessment of general motor and motor speech capabilities, language and cognitive skills, and sensory deficits. The evaluation attempts to determine the basis of the severe communication deficit and then whether speech therapy alone or in combination with an augmentative approach is the optimal strategy.

The introduction of either an aided or unaided communication strategy seems to have a positive, rather than a detrimental, affect on speech development. Although families are often reluctant to introduce an AAC system for fear that the child may give up on spoken communication, the reverse seems to be the case. There is no definitive explanation for the growth in speech of some individuals who are given AAC systems, but it is postulated that the positive changes may be related to an overall lessening of pressure to talk or reduced frustration associated with effective communication through other means.

The otolaryngologist plays an important role as a team member in the management of a child who uses an AAC strategy. This role falls into four categories:

- **Saliva Management:** Drooling can be detrimental to a child's development of social interactions (with or without an AAC method). In addition, it can have a negative effect on the operation of an electronic keyboard or communication aid. Surgical and pharmacologic procedures are generally the options of choice to manage drooling for the patient with a severe expressive communication impairment.
- **Vocal Cord Management:** Vocal intensity is in part related to vocal cord integrity. It is essential to know the status and function of the vocal cords before making the decision about whether to introduce voice therapy or to use an assistive vocal amplifier to increase vocal loudness.
- **Hearing Loss Management:** The nature and degree of hearing loss impacts the decision to select an aided or unaided AAC approach. In addition, the type of symbol set used on an aided system (e.g., pictured signs or graphic symbols) is related to hearing status and the patient's potential to benefit from synthetic voice output generated from a computer.
- **Airway and "Talking Trach" Management:** The successful application of a "talking trach" such as a Passey-Muir valve (Passey-Muir, Inc., 4521 Campus Drive, Suite 273, Irvine, CA 92612) can eliminate the need for introducing a full blown AAC system.

AT A GLANCE . . .

Role of the Otolaryngologist in ACC Management

- Saliva management
- Vocal cord management
- Hearing loss management
- Airway management

In some institutions, patients who will be unable to speak temporarily following surgery are provided with a unique opportunity to have their voices recorded preoperatively and made available to them postoperatively.[30] By using small hand-held communication devices, these children can communicate until they are able to speak again.

DISORDERS OF FLUENCY

Fluency refers to the forward flow of speech, reflecting many aspects of timing, organization, and coordination. Rate, rhythm, intonation, and stress also contribute to the perceived fluency of speech. *Dysfluency* refers to any interruption in the flow of speech, and includes repetitions (e.g., "r..r..r.. right"), prolongations (e.g., "mmmmommy"), and blocks of airflow during speech production.

Research has shown strong evidence that fluency disorders are familial, with roughly two-thirds of cases reporting a family history of stuttering. There is a higher incidence in male and first-degree relatives.[31] Although studies have determined no significant differences in the environmental factors of families with people who stutter and those who do not,[32] studies of monozygotic and dizygotic twins with identical environments have been inconclusive in terms of a purely genetic etiology.[33] Such evidence suggests that fluency disorders arise from an interaction of genetic and environmental factors.

A certain amount of dysfluency is considered developmental, and about 4% of children between the ages of 2 and 5 years go through a period of typical dysfluency that coincides with rapid growth in expressive language acquisition. Such typical disruptions in the fluency of speech include revisions, single syllable word repetitions (e.g., "I-I-I-I went"), and interjections (e.g., well, um, uh), with no greater than 10 dysfluencies per 100 words.[34] Roughly 1 percent of children who exhibit developmental dysfluency continue to have a long-term fluency disorder.[35]

SPECIAL CONSIDERATION:

Roughly 1% of children who exhibit a developmental dysfluency continue to have a long-term fluency disorder.

Pediatric fluency disorders are classified typically into four levels: borderline stuttering, beginning stuttering, intermediate stuttering, and advanced stuttering.[34] Diagnosis of a fluency disorder in the preschooler can be difficult because characteristics can shift from "normal" dysfluencies to borderline stuttering over short periods of time. This shifting may reflect changes in expressive language demands, social-emotional situations (arrival of a sibling, beginning of school, etc.), and parent-child relationships. Children who exhibit *borderline stuttering* typically have higher rates of dysfluent words, repetitions, and prolongations than a child who exhibits "normal" dysfluent speech.[34] Children who exhibit borderline stuttering also tend to have little awareness of their dysfluencies and stutter in a "relaxed" manner.

The child who exhibits *beginning stuttering* is between 2 and 8 years of age and has begun to respond to typical dysfluencies with tension that is often visible. This child's dysfluent speech is characterized by rapid irregular syllable repetitions, an accompanying rise in pitch, and the onset of blocking.[34] Secondary behaviors, such as eye blinking or head nods, often emerge during this phase, and are postulated to result from the muscular effort that is generated in response to the anticipation of difficulty.[33] Awareness and frustration related to speech difficulty are present at the moments of dysfluency, but dysfluent speech continues to be episodic.

Children who exhibit *intermediate stuttering* are typically between 6 and 13 years of age, and are distinguishable from those of the previous phase primarily by their fear of stuttering and avoidance behaviors.[34] Core behaviors continue to include repetitions and prolongations, but blocking emerges as the most frequent type of dysfluency. Blocking is often accompanied by tension at various points along the articulatory tract (e.g., laryngeal tension, jaw clenching). In addition to visible secondary behaviors, such as head nods and limb movements, children who exhibit intermediate stuttering begin to avoid words by using substitutions, circumlocutions, and postponements.[36] Fear of specific situations such as speaking in front of the classroom often results in avoidance behaviors (e.g., incomplete assignments, class absences), and these children may suffer from a negative self-image.

The *advanced stage of stuttering* is characterized primarily by dysfluency that has persisted into adolescence and adulthood. The primary core behavior continues to be blocks that are longer in duration and accompanied by increased articulatory tension. The adolescent who exhibits advanced stuttering often has built an extensive repertoire of avoidance behaviors and may suffer from intense emotional reactions related to the presence of dysfluent speech.[34] The range of presenting behaviors can vary greatly among individuals.

AT A GLANCE . . .
Levels of Fluency Disorders

Borderline stuttering: can be difficult to diagnose; child has higher rates of dysfluent words, repetitions, and prolongations than a child who exhibits "normal" dysfluency.

Beginning stuttering: children between ages 2 to 8 years; rapid irregular syllable repetition, rise in pitch, and onset of blocking. Secondary behaviors emerge.

Intermediate stuttering: children between ages 6 to 13 years; distinguished from beginning stuttering by fear and avoidance behaviors; blocking most frequent type of dysfluency.

Advanced stuttering: characterized by dysfluency that has persisted into adolescence and adulthood.

Assessment and Management of Fluency Disorders

The assessment of fluency disorders is not remarkably different from other speech and language evaluations. Testing consists of two general components: (1) information gathering regarding attitudes, feelings, beliefs, and history related to the presenting problem; and (2) objective and subjective assessment of speech fluency and related behaviors (e.g., articulation, vocal quality, language skills).[37] The speech-language pathologist gathers an extensive case history (preferably prior to the evaluation), interviews the child's parent, and observes child-parent interaction. Speech samples are collected from a variety of different settings (e.g., spontaneous speech, automatic speech, picture description, reading tasks) to assess the effect of communicative pressure on the fluency of speech. The speech-language pathologist analyzes the data to determine the pattern of dysfluent speech, frequency of dysfluencies, situational fluctuations, and presence of secondary behaviors. Formal speech and language tests are administered to determine if any concomitant speech or language disorders are present.

Treatment techniques vary according to age and severity of disorder, but typically consist of four approaches: (1) modification of the environment; (2) modification of the child's behavior/attitude; (3) remediation of concomitant speech and language disorders; and (4) direct modification of dysfluent speech.[38] Intervention may include indirect (e.g., environmental modification via parent counseling) and direct (e.g., specific attempts to modify speech production) strategies. Two specific direct intervention approaches include: (1) *stuttering modification therapy* during which the person who stutters is taught to stutter more fluently; and (2) *fluency shaping therapy,* the goal of which is to replace stuttering instances with fluent speech.[34] In the pediatric population, initial therapy typically focuses on modification of environmental factors. Extensive family involvement is suggested for the maximum benefit of intervention.

AT A GLANCE . . .

Treatment of Fluency Disorders

- Modification of environment
- Modification of child's behavior/attitude
- Remediation of concomitant speech and language disorders
- Direct modification of dysfluent speech

DISORDERS OF FEEDING & SWALLOWING

Successful feeding is essential for adequate growth and development. Feeding refers to the process by which a child ingests food. This process is dependent upon the feeding environment, the parent-child interaction, the child's oral-motor skill development, and the child's comfort and safety with food. Factors that may contribute to feeding difficulty include: (1) difficulty with bottle or breast feeding; (2) gagging; (3) hypersensitivity of the oral cavity; (4) hyposensitivity of the oral cavity; (5) gastroesophageal reflux (GER); and (6) difficulty with the acquisition of developmental feeding skills.

Assessment and Management of Swallowing Disorders

The pediatric swallow is evaluated in four phases: (1) the oral preparatory phase; (2) the oral initiation phase; (3) the pharyngeal phase; and (4) the esophageal phase. In the *oral preparatory phase* the clinician evaluates how well a child orients to the food source, receives the food mass (commonly referred to as a bolus), contains the bolus, prepares the bolus, and propels the bolus within the oral cavity. In the *oral initiation phase,* the clinician assesses the timeliness and coordination of the initiation of the swallow, looking for adequacy of tongue base retraction, presence of nasopharyngeal reflux, and premature spillage into the hypopharynx. During this phase, obstructive dysphagia may be diagnosed due to tonsillar and adenoidal hypertrophy. In the *pharyngeal phase* of the swallow, the adequacy of laryngeal elevation, epiglottic deflection, pharyngeal peristalsis, and laryngeal closure are assessed. Potential anatomic landmarks where food can collect during this phase include the vallecula, the pyriform sinuses, and the posterior pharyngeal wall. During the final phase of the swallow, the *esophageal phase,* the adequacy of cricopharyngeal relaxation for accommodating movement of the bolus into the esophagus is assessed. Objective assessment of the esophagus should be performed with a barium swallow study when concerns arise either about esophageal anatomy or motility of the bolus through the esophagus. Aspiration of the bolus may occur before, during, or after the swallow is triggered, depending upon the phase and severity of involvement. There is a high incidence of silent aspiration in children with neurologically-based dysphagia.[39] Therefore, instrumental assessment should be considered for comprehensive evaluation of swallow function.

SPECIAL CONSIDERATION:

There is a high incidence of silent aspiration in children with neurologically-based dysphagia.

Clinical indicators of possible swallowing dysfunction that warrant further assessment by an experienced feeding and swallowing specialist are listed in Table 44–1.

AT A GLANCE . . .

Phases of Pediatric Swallowing

- Oral preparatory phase
- Oral initiation phase
- Pharyngeal phase
- Esophageal phase

Initial assessment of possible dysphagia typically begins with the clinical or bedside evaluation. This subjective assessment involves comprehensive intake of medical and feeding histories, a thorough oral peripheral examination, and observation of the child during mealtime.

There are instrumental tools designed to assess pediatric swallow function. Videofluoroscopic swallow study, also referred to as a modified barium swallow study, provides objective assessment of the physiology of the swallow by evaluating the safety and efficiency of each swallow phase. This study is conducted while the child is appropriately positioned for feeding and offered foods within her current diet repertoire. Contraindications for this study would include: (1) the need for suction to maintain airway patency; (2) severe oral aversion; (3) current illness; or (4) respiratory distress. In a fiberoptic endoscopic evaluation of swallowing (FEES), a flexible endoscopic tube attached to a light source is inserted into the nasopharynx and the swallow is viewed from above. Using this technique, prema-

TABLE 44–1: Indicators of Possible Swallowing Dysfunction

Recurrent upper respiratory infections

Frequent episodes of coughing, choking, or gagging

Fluctuating temperatures of unknown origin

Change in phonatory or respiratory quality during or after feeding

Nasopharyngeal reflux

Fatigue during feeding

Difficulty coordinating respiration and swallowing during bottle or breast feeding

Apnea, bradycardia, or decrease in oxygen saturation levels associated with feeding

Inadequate weight gain

Diagnosis of presumed asthma

Weak or deteriorating voluntary cough

Difficulty passing solid foods into the hypopharynx

---

ture spillage of boluses into the pharynx, bolus residue, subglottic aspiration, and laryngeal penetration can be detected. This study can be performed at the bedside and requires no radiation. Ultrasound is an imaging modality that also is utilized for assessment of feeding and swallowing. The oral preparatory phase can be examined in the unstimulated state with no enhancing material necessary. The pharyngeal phase cannot be viewed directly, and therefore laryngeal penetration and aspiration cannot be observed. Aspiration can be suspected based on the findings of the oral phase and full excursion of the hyoid bone by observing the hyoid shadow.

AT A GLANCE . . .

Evaluation of Pediatric Swallowing

- Videofluoroscopic swallow study
- Fiberoptic endoscopic evaluation of swallowing (FEES)
- Ultrasound assessment

There are numerous potential factors affecting feeding and swallowing function in the pediatric population. These include neurogenic impairments, prematurity, anatomic defects, cardiopulmonary status, traumatic brain injury, and sensory processing issues. Management of feeding and swallowing dysfunction can vary greatly depending on the phase and severity of involvement. Management strategies may include, but are not limited to:

1. Positioning changes
2. Diet modifications (i.e., texture changes, alterations in viscosity of liquids)
3. Supplemental feedings (i.e., nasogastric-tube (NG-tube), gastrostomy tube (G-tube), jejunostomy-tube (J-tube)
4. Intervention to assist in texture progression, tube weaning, developmental feeding skill acquisition, and/or normalizing oral sensitivity
5. Secretion management

Managing the child with feeding and swallowing issues requires the input of many pediatric specialists. Some of those specialists who make up a dysphagia team include: a speech pathologist, a gastroenterologist, an otolaryngologist, a nutritionist, a pulmonologist, and a radiologist. It is the input from these specialists that promotes a feeding program that is both safe and successful to maximize growth and development.

CONCLUSION

Communication disorders in the pediatric population are associated with a number of interrelated conditions and factors. The otolaryngologist encounters children with such deficits on a continuous basis. It is essential that the practitioner recognize these relationships, the importance of referral if problems are suspected, and the role she plays on the team that diagnoses and treats these disorders.

REFERENCES

1. Stoel-Gammon C, Dunn C. *Normal and Disordered Phonology in Children.* in Weiss et al. Austin: PRO-ED, 1985.
2. Locke JL. Clinical phonology: The explanation and treatment of speech sound disorders. J Speech Hear Discord 1983; 48(4)339-341.
3. Weiss CE, Gordon ME, Lillywhite HS. *Clinical Management of Articulatory and Phonologic Disorders, 2nd ed.* Baltimore: Williams & Wilkins, 1987.
4. Stark RE. Features of infant sounds: The emergence of cooing. J Child Lang 1978; 5(3):379-390.
5. Owens RE Jr. *Language Development: An Introduction, 4th ed.* Allyn and Bacon, Needham MA 1996, pp. 67-106.
6. Oller, D. (1978) Infant Vocalization and the Development of Speech. *Allied Health and Behavior Sciences.* 1, 523-549.
7. Sander EK. When are speech sounds learned? J Speech Hear Discord 1972; 37(1):55-63.
8. Schwartz RG. In: Shames GH, Wiig EH, Secord WA, eds. *Human Communication Disorders, 4th ed.* New York: Merrill, 1994, pp. 251-263.
9. Bernthal R, Bankson N. *Articulation and Phonological Disorders, 3rd ed.* Englewood NJ: Prentice-Hall, 1993, pp. 162-215.
10. Yorkston K, Beukelman D, Bell K. *Clinical Management of Dysarthric Speakers.* Boston: Little, Brown, 1988, pp. 2.
11. Crary MA. *Developmental Motor-Speech Disorders.* San Diego: Singular, 1993, pp. 27-28.
12. Strand EA. Treatment of motor speech disorders in children. Seminars in Speech and Language 1995; 16(2):126-138.
13. Castrogiovanni, A. (1999) "Communication Facts" Information Publication American Speech Hearing Association (ASHA) Rockville, MD.
14. Paul R. Clinical implications of the natural history of slow expressive language development. Am J Speech Lang Pathol 1996, 5(2):22-25.
15. Nippold MA, Schwarz IE. Children with slow expressive language development: What is the forecast for school achievement. Am J Speech Lang Pathol 1996, 5(2):22-25.
16. Senturia BH, Wilson FB. Otorhinolaryngologic findings in children with voice deviations: Preliminary report. Ann Otol Rhinol Laryngol 1968; 77: 1027-1042.
17. Silverman EM, Zimmer CH. Incidence of chronic hoarseness among school-age children. J Speech Hear Dis 1975; 40:211-215.
18. Yairi E, Currin LH, Bulia N, et al. Incidence of hoarseness in school children over a 1-year period. Journal of Communication Disorders 1974; 7:321-328.
19. Cohen SR, Thompson JW, Geller KA, et al. Voice change in the pediatric patient: A differential diagnosis. Ann Otol Rhinol Laryngol 1983; 92:437-443.
20. Colton RH, Casper JK. *Understanding Voice Problems: A Physiological Perspective for Diagnosis and Treatment.* Baltimore: Williams & Wilkins, 1996, pp. 13-20; 270-316.
21. Gray SD, Smith ME, Schneider H. Voice disorders in children. Pediatr Clin North Am 1996; 43(6): 1357-1384.
22. Wilson DK. *Voice Problems in Children, 3rd ed.* Baltimore Williams and Wilkins, 1987, pp. 3-8; 162-268.
23. Ruscello D, Lass N, Podbesek J. Listener's perception of normal and voice disordered children. Folia phoniatica 1988; 40:290-296.
24. Champley EH, Andrews ML. The elicitation of vocal responses from preschool children. Language, Speech, and Hearing Services in Schools 1993; 24: 146-150.
25. Chait DH, Lotz WK. Successful pediatric examination using nasoendoscopy. Laryngoscope 1991; 101: 1016-1018.
26. Lotz WK, D'Antonia LL, Chait DH, et al. Successful nasoendoscopic and aerodynamic examinations of children with speech/voice disorders. Int J Pediatr Otorhinolaryngol 1993; 26(2):165-172.
27. Zajac DJ, Farkas Z, Dindzans LJ, et al. Aerodynamic and laryngographic assessment of pediatric vocal function. Pediatr Pulmonal 1993; 15:44-51.
28. Zajac DJ, Linville RN. Voice perturbations of children with perceived nasality and hoarseness. Cleft Palate J 1989; 26:226-232.
29. Boone DR, McFarlane SC. *The Voice and Voice Therapy, 4th ed.* Englewood Cliffs, NJ: Prentice Hall, 1988, pp. 103-182.

30. Costello JC. Communication beyond words: AAC communication options for patients with trachs. Paper given at Dispelling the fear of tracheostomies: Care in the 90's; Boston, MA, September, 1995.

31. Ambrose NG, Yairi E, Cox N. Genetic aspects of early childhood stuttering. J Speech Hear Res 1993; 36: 701–706.

32. Cox N, Seider RA, Kidd K. Some environmental factors and hypotheses for stuttering in families with several stutterers. J Speech Hear Res 1984; 27: 543–548.

33. Bloodstein O. *A Handbook on Stuttering, 4th ed.* Chicago: The National Easter Seal Society, 1987.

34. Peters TJ, Guitar B. Stuttering: An Integrated Approach to Its Nature and Treatment. Baltimore: Williams & Wilkins, 1991, pp. 71–107.

35. Guitar B, Conture E. The child who stutters: To the pediatrician. Stuttering Foundation of America, Publication No. 23, 1991.

36. Van Riper C. *The Nature of Stuttering, 2nd ed.* Englewood Cliffs, NJ: Prentice-Hall, 1982.

37. Conture EG. *Stuttering, 2nd ed.* Englewood Cliffs, NJ: Prentice-Hall, 1990, pp. 83–84.

38. Riley GD, Riley J. Evaluating stuttering problems in children. Journal of Childhood Communication Disorders 1982; 6(1):15–25.

39. Arvedson J, Rogers B, Buck G, et al. Silent aspiration prominent in children with dysphagia. Int J Pediatr Otorhinolaryngol 1994; 28:173–181.

45 Disorders of the Voice

Roger C. Nuss

In the past, the hoarse voice in certain children has generally been attributed to "screamer's nodules." The general advice given to these children was that they would possibly "grow out of it" with physical and emotional maturation, growth of the larynx, and changes in vocal demands. Voice therapy was offered, but frequently delivered by a speech pathologist with little experience in voice disorders. Perhaps understandably, children, parents, and clinicians would often feel frustrated by a lack of progress.

It has become apparent over the past decade that this simplistic view of pediatric voice disorders does a disservice to both affected children and their families. Otolaryngologists, speech language pathologists, and other professionals with an interest in pediatric voice disorders are becoming increasingly sophisticated and experienced in the evaluation, diagnosis, and management of voice problems in children. This is beginning to have an effect, with noticeably improved short-term outcomes as well as long-term prognosis for the hoarse child.

The identification of children with voice disorders is not always straightforward. One must have an understanding of the wide range of "normal" children's voices at different ages in order to separate out pathologic childhood voice problems. In addition, optimal management of the hoarse child requires an appreciation of the wide spectrum of causes of voice disorders.

Evaluation of hoarse children is best done by a multi-disciplinary team in the setting of a voice laboratory.[1] An experienced speech language pathologist performs subjective evaluations of voice quality. Voice recordings and electroglottography are noninvasive and well-tolerated by most children. Aerodynamic measurements provide a better understanding of subglottal pressure and airflow. Strobo-scopic videolaryngoscopy affords the best opportunity to make an accurate diagnosis of vocal fold pathology.

Recommended therapy for childhood voice disorders is evolving. Traditionally, voice therapy was the mainstay of conservative management options. Presently, it is recognized that effective voice therapy must be delivered by a speech and voice clinician who has special training and expertise in voice disorders. Not all speech pathologists in the public school systems have this background. The diagnosis and management of medical conditions that aggravate voice disorders is increasingly recognized as an important component of therapy for the hoarse pediatric patient. Surgical management of children with vocal fold pathology is becoming increasingly sophisticated and is following many of the innovations developed in the field of adult phonomicrosurgery.

DEFINITIONS, INCIDENCE

There is a fairly wide spectrum of "normality" in children's voices, which in itself varies with age, sex, and pubertal development. Subjectively, parents, teachers, pediatricians, and speech language pathologists may all have a different set of criteria upon which they evaluate a particular child. Thus, a parent's assessment of the child's voice may not be at all congruous with the pediatrician's judgment.

Objective assessments of a child's voice include measurement of fundamental frequency, range, loudness, and perturbation characteristics. Speech language pathologists with a special interest and expertise in voice disorders are able to combine their experience with objective measures of children's voices with their subjective assessment of a child's voice quality. They perhaps are best able to characterize a child's voice as hoarse/disordered or falling within the normal range.

Pediatric Otolaryngology, Edited by R.F. Wetmore, H.R. Muntz, and T.J. McGill. Thieme Medical Publishers, Inc., New York © 2000.

Practice Pathway 45–1 EVALUATION OF THE VOICE

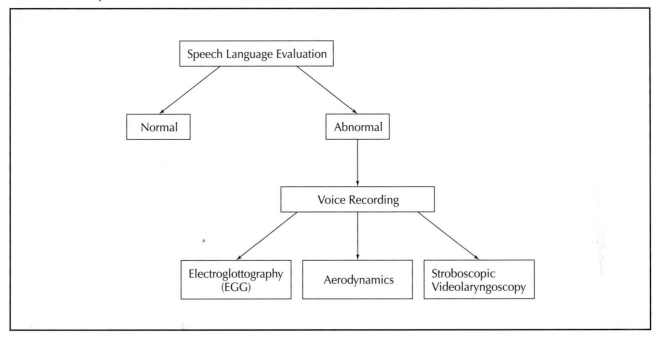

There have been several attempts to describe the incidence of voice disorders or hoarseness among various populations of children. There is a wide variation in the reported incidence, which may represent different populations studied or varying definitions used for "hoarseness." Most studies have reported an incidence of hoarseness among school aged children of 18–23%, with males more frequently affected than females.[2–6] Interestingly, there was no significant difference in the incidence of hoarseness in child singers.[7] Several studies have reported a lower incidence of voice disorders, in the range of 4 to 7%, in children growing up in a more rural community[8,9] and have suggested a higher incidence in children living in a city environment or visiting a summer camp program.[4,9] Contrary to some generalized notions, not all children outgrow this problem. A longitudinal study of 203 hoarse children revealed persistent voice disorders in 35% at one year, and roughly 9% at four years after diagnosis.[10]

IDENTIFICATION OF CHILDREN WITH VOICE DISORDERS

The child with a disordered vocal quality may be recognized and brought to attention by many differ-

ent concerned individuals, including parents, schoolteachers, speech therapists, friends, pediatricians, and otolaryngologists. These various "referral sources" have different backgrounds, knowledge, and experience in identifying and treating childhood voice disorders. For instance, the child's parents may have a knowledge of laryngeal cancer and wish to rule out this unlikely cause of hoarseness in their own child. The schoolteacher sees that the dysphonic child has difficulty with communication and intelligibility and hopes to prevent learning and socialization problems. School speech pathologists may be working with a child on his/her articulation, but recognize that voice quality is an important issue that may limit progress. Finally, pediatricians and otolaryngologists may identify vocal fold nodules as the most common cause of hoarseness in children, but wish to rule out such problems as laryngeal papillomas, scarring or immobility secondary to prolonged intubation and other less common problems.[11] No matter where the referral process originates, it is important to recognize why a child is being sent in for evaluation, and what information can realistically be provided. This information is quite valuable in tailoring the voice evaluation in a manner so that the primary question at hand may be answered.

Voice disorders in children are increasingly recognized as a barrier to successful academic achievement and socialization in the school environment.[12] Attention is now being directed toward younger children with voice issues, in an effort to correct these problems before they result in other school difficulties.

ETIOLOGY OF VOICE DISORDERS

Voice disorders in children may be categorized as falling into one or more of the following groups: congenital, acquired/traumatic, infectious/inflammatory, central or peripheral neuromotor, and neoplastic (Table 45–1). These categories are not exclusive, and a particular child may have several contributing factors to her dysphonic voice quality. For example, evaluation of the preschooler with hoarseness may reveal bilateral vocal fold nodules, arytenoid erythema and mucosal hyperplasia, and supraglottic compression. These findings may suggest not only evidence of aggressive voice use, but also laryngeal manifestations of gastroesophageal reflux and vocal hyperfunction. Optimal management relies on identifying all contributing factors in a child's voice disorder. Congenital causes of voice disorders include laryngomalacia, glottic webs, subglottic or supraglottic cysts, and vocal fold paresis or palsy. In addition, vocal fold nodules and sulcus deformities may sometimes be identified even in the neonate, seemingly prior to any opportunity for "voice abuse" or trauma. Vascular malformations within the larynx may also present with a weak or absent cry and airway obstruction during the newborn period.

Acquired and traumatic causes of hoarseness in children are most frequently associated with "voice abuse" and hyperfunction. It is of course rather subjective to describe typical childhood voice use as normal in those with no voice disorder, and as "abuse" in children with hoarseness and vocal fold nodules. Presently, there is no objective means of measuring the quantity and quality of childhood voice use. Typical lesions associated with excessive use and poor vocal hygiene include vocal fold nodules, polyps, vocal fold hemorrhage and varix, as well as Reinke's edema. Laryngeal trauma may also occur from blunt neck trauma and laryngeal fracture, traumatic endotracheal intubation with arytenoid dislocation or avulsion of a vocal ligament. Smoke exposure as well as thermal inhalation injury

may affect vocal function. Irradiation of the neck for treatment of childhood malignancies may create a dry and chronically inflamed larynx and associated poor vocal quality. Finally, gastroesophageal reflux is felt to frequently contribute to many types of voice disorders and is associated with posterior laryngeal edema and mucosal hyperplasia.

Most infectious causes of pediatric voice disorders are temporary, including typical acute viral laryngitis, caused by a parainfluenza virus. However, the setting of acutely inflamed and hyperemic vocal folds may predispose a child to developing more chronic laryngeal changes if voice use is not subdued during such periods of active inflammation. Bacterial infections of the larynx are less common, but may lead to airway compromise and the need for careful inpatient monitoring and treatment. Systemic autoimmune illnesses, including juvenile rheumatoid arthritis and relapsing polychondritis, may also affect the larynx and be a cause of varying hoarseness.

> **SPECIAL CONSIDERATION:**
> The evaluation and treatment of stridor or any airway compromise takes precedence over the evaluation of a voice disorder.

Neurologic causes of voice disorders may result in a unilateral or bilateral vocal fold paresis or palsy. Central nervous system processes most commonly seen include hydrocephalus, intraventricular hemorrhage, and Arnold-Chiari malformation. Peripheral neurologic causes of vocal fold palsy most frequently include surgical trauma, presumed "stretch" injury during birth, and recurrent laryngeal nerve neuropraxia related to cardiac or great vessel abnormalities.

> **SPECIAL CONSIDERATION:**
> The accurate diagnosis of a vocal fold palsy is best done while a child is fully awake, and not under the effects of any general anesthetic or amnestic agent.

TABLE 45-1:   Etiologies of Voice Disorders in Children

Genetic
  Achondroplasia
  Diastrophic dwarfism[32]
  William's syndrome
  Cri du chat syndrome
  Lysozymal storage diseases[33]
Congenital
  Laryngomalacia
  Laryngeal atresia
  Glottic and subglottic webs[34]
  Posterior laryngeal cleft
  Sulcus vocalis[35,36]
  Laryngocele
  Supraglottic or glottic mucous retention cyst
  Tracheoesophageal fistula
  Vascular malformations
  Vocal fold immobility
Infectious
  Viral
    Influenza
    Parainfluenza
    Herpes simplex
    Human papilloma virus
    Varicella
    Coxsackie
    Epstein-Barr virus[37]
    Others
  Bacterial
    S pneumoniae
    S aureus
    H influenzae, type B
    Diphtheria
    Rhinoscleroma
    Actinomycosis
    M tuberculosis
    Others
  Fungal[38]
    Blastomycosis
    Histoplasmosis
    Coccidiodomycosis
    Aspergillosis
    Others
Inflammatory
  Chronic laryngitis
  Allergic laryngitis[39]
  Rheumatoid arthritis
  Relapsing polychondritis
Neoplasia
  Benign
    Laryngeal papilloma
    Hemangioma
    Supraglottic and glottic cysts
    Neurofibroma
    Chondroma
    Granular cell tumor[40]
    Others
  Malignant
    Squamous cell carcinoma
    Rhabdomyosarcoma[41]
    Other sarcomas
    Leukemia
    Lymphoma
    Neuroblastoma

Trauma
  Laryngeal fracture[42,43]
  Traumatic intubation
    Arytenoid dislocation[44]
    Intubation granuloma
    Vocal ligament avulsion
  Foreign body
  Smoke exposure
  Gastroesophageal reflux[24,45]
  Recurrent laryngeal nerve injury
  Penetrating neck wound
  Irradiation
  Thermal inhalational injury
  Spontaneous pneumomediastinum[46]
Vocal abuse
  Vocal hyperfunction
  Vocal fold nodules
  Reinke's edema
  Vocal fold polyps
  Vocal fold hemorrhage/varix
Neurologic
  Supranuclear
    Hemorrhage
    Hydrocephalus
    Anoxic encephalopathy
    Metabolic storage diseases
    Multiple sclerosis
    Neoplasms
    Viral encephalitis
  Nuclear
    Arnold-Chiari malformation
    Pseudobulbar palsy
    Meningomyelocele
    Guillain-Barre syndrome
    Bulbar poliomyelitis
  Peripheral
    Trauma (birth, surgical, blunt)
    Cardiac or great vessel abnormalities
    Mediastinal disease
    Myasthenia gravis
    Neoplasms
    Toxins
    Meningitis
    Polyneuritis[47]
    Chemotherapy
Other
  Dehydration[48]
  Puberphonia
  Conversion dysphonia[49]
  Psychogenic dysphonia[50]

Adapted from Cohen et al[31].

Benign neoplasms of the larynx in children include hemangiomas, other vascular malformations, and papillomas. Recurrent respiratory papillomatosis, caused by the Human papilloma virus, is truly a chronic viral infection of the larynx but is often considered and treated as a recurrent benign neoplasm. Malignancies of the larynx are uncommon in children, but they do occur and serve as a reminder that any suspicious lesion in a child's larynx requires biopsy. Squamous cell carcinoma and rhabdomyosarcoma would be the most frequent lesions in this uncommon group of malignancies.

EVALUATION TECHNIQUES

Complete pediatric voice evaluation, like that of an adult, has several important components that may be best performed by a team approach, including a pediatric otolaryngologist and a speech-language pathologist with special expertise in voice disorders. At times, involvement of a gastroenterologist, a pulmonologist, and a psychologist may be helpful. Voice evaluations are geared toward providing the maximal information possible while minimizing a child's fears and anxieties about his visit. The voice evaluation begins with the least invasive and threatening components, progresses to slightly more invasive testing, and is completed by stroboscopic videolaryngoscopy. By the time this procedure is performed, there hopefully is a good rapport between the child and the clinicians, with a better chance for successful completion of the examination. As may be suspected, the pediatric voice evaluation is more time and labor intensive than the corresponding examination in adults.[13] However, this is necessary if useful information is to be obtained.

The speech-language pathologist initially evaluates the dysphonic child, in order to obtain a perceptual evaluation of a child's voice quality.[14] Children's voices are judged on the basis of hoarseness, coarseness, harshness, pitch, range, loudness, breathiness, nasality, and intelligibility. Additionally, neck muscle tension and strained voice quality are noted.[15,16] Voice recordings are next performed on a high quality digital audiotape. Sustained vowels as well as connected speech are recorded, using a standard format and a standard reading passage. These voice recordings are analyzed with commercially available software, with resulting descriptions of fundamental frequency (pitch), sound pressure level (loudness), range, frequency perturbation (jitter), and intensity perturbation (shimmer).

Electroglottography (EGG) is a fairly nonthreatening test that most children will tolerate.[17] It provides an indirect assessment of vocal fold contact during phonation using surface electrodes to measure changes in electrical impedance of the neck. The glottal cycle results in a duty cycle of electrical impedance changes picked up by electrodes. In addition to allowing for the calculation of fundamental frequency and jitter, it also provides a measure of the degree of vocal hyperfunction ("pressed" EGG signal) or incomplete glottal closure. Derived values of open quotient and closed quotient reflect the percentage of the vocal cycle that the vocal folds are apart or in contact with each other.

Aerodynamic assessment involves the indirect measurement of glottal airflow rate, subglottic air pressure, and glottal resistance to airflow. The device includes a pneumotachograph mounted in a facemask and a translabially placed catheter coupled to a pressure transducer. Meaningful data is generally obtained in the cooperative older child. Such information is especially helpful in instances of a breathy voice quality and suspected vocal fold paresis or palsy.

Stroboscopic videolaryngoscopy is the most invasive component of pediatric voice evaluation, but also the most informative. It may be successfully accomplished in children as young as three years of age, with cooperation on the part of the child.[18] This examination requires skill, patience, and reassurance on the part of the examiner. Typically, the child is introduced to the fiberoptic scope, allowed to feel it and look through the scope. Connecting the fiberoptic laryngoscope to a CCD camera and video monitor creates a good opportunity for the child to have some fun with the apparatus. The procedure is explained to the child and the parents or guardian, and consent is obtained to proceed with this examination. Adequate decongestion and anesthesia is important to improve a child's ability to cooperate. The nasal passage is decongested with 0.05% oxymetazoline. After waiting a few minutes, 1% lidocaine is applied to the nasal passage either in spray form, by dropper, or by placing a soaked cotton ball into the nasal passage. The entire fiberoptic laryngoscopy examination is videotaped for later review and analysis. Laryngeal function is analyzed for degree of supraglottic compression, arytenoid movement, vocal fold motion, vocal fold edge smoothness or irregularity, glottal closure, mucosal wave, phase symmetry of vocal fold vibration, and presence of swelling or secretions suggestive of other medical conditions aggravating the voice disorder. The stroboscopy flash timing may be triggered by either a contact microphone held against a patient's neck or by the electroglottography signal.

SPECIAL CONSIDERATION:

Fiberoptic laryngeal examinations in children are best performed with videotape recording. This allows for a quicker exam, improved diagnostic accuracy, and a record of findings for future comparison.

The information obtained through these five components of a pediatric voice evaluation require data analysis, interpretation, and video review in order to accurately diagnose a child's voice disorder and any contributing factors, as well as make appropriate recommendations for treatment and therapy. In addition, the storage of this information in a voice data bank is especially helpful for later retrieval of information and comparison with future voice evaluations. This will provide the best mechanism for objective outcome analysis and serve as a resource for clinical investigations.[19,20]

AT A GLANCE . . .

Evaluation Techniques

- Subjective evaluation: assessment of hoarseness, coarseness, harshness; pitch, range, loudness; breathiness, nasality; intelligibility; neck muscle tension, straining
- Voice recordings: sustained vowels, connected speech; maximal phonation time; fundamental frequency; loudness (sound pressure level); range; frequency and intensity perturbation
- Electroglottography: fundamental frequency; open quotient, closed quotient
- Aerodynamics: glottal airflow, subglottic air pressure, glottal resistance
- Stroboscopic videolaryngoscopy: supraglottic compression, arytenoid movement, vocal fold movement, vocal fold irregularity or smoothness, glottal closure, mucosal wave, phase symmetry, mucous secretions, contributing medical conditions

---

THERAPY

Therapy of voice disorders in children will frequently require a multi-faceted approach. Voice therapy is the backbone of conservative management of pediatric voice disorders. This is not to say that it is ineffective; rather, much can be gained from therapy when the cause of a child's hoarseness is identified and specific steps are taken to correct the problem. In the past, referral of a dysphonic child for speech and voice therapy frequently resulted in a "generic" approach, with basic recommendations made regardless of the nature of the underlying voice problem. This is changing, as clinicians' diagnostic skills improve and therapy is more specifically tailored to the cause of the voice disorder. As a result, we may expect greater success in correction of many childhood voice disorders including vocal fold nodules and hyperfunction.[21] Improved voice quality is possible even with significant laryngeal scarring from surgery, if the voice clinician has an opportunity to visualize and understand the nature of a child's laryngeal anatomy and function.

Vocal therapy is extremely important to help identify and unload potentially harmful vocal habits and misuse. Therapy also reinforces the concept of vocal hygiene with children and their families and helps to foster a positive approach toward changing long-standing voice habits. Motivated children are able to comprehend and incorporate techniques such as diaphragmatic/abdominal breathing, coordination of respiration and phonation, periods of voice rest, elimination of abusive behavior, and hydration strategies.

Certain voice disorders are best treated and sometimes cured with voice therapy alone. Certain "functional" dysphonias seen in children, including conversion dysphonia, psychogenic aphonia, and puberphonia may be managed with short courses of intensive therapy. The results are sometimes excellent, though relapses are not uncommon. Underlying structural disease of the larynx must first be ruled out.

Medical therapy for systemic disease processes may have a large impact on voice disorders in children. A review of medical conditions, medications, and treatments is important in order to understand their role in a child's voice problem [Table 45-2]. Environmental allergies may predispose a child to vocal fold edema as well as trauma due to coughing

TABLE 45–2: Medical Conditions Which May Exacerbate Voice Disorders

- Gastroesophageal reflux disease
- Asthma, cough, use of inhaled corticosteroids
- Environmental allergies, use of anti-histamines
- Cystic fibrosis, cough, use of inhaled DNase
- Sinusitis, post-nasal drip, throat clearing
- Hypothyroidism
- Juvenile rheumatoid arthritis

and sneezing. Antihistamine medications may have a significant drying effect in the larynx, further exacerbating laryngeal pathology. Asthma and related cough may cause vocal fold injury. Inhaled steroids are becoming increasingly popular for management of chronic asthma and are quite effective in reducing a child's reliance on other medications. However, there has been concern raised about these medications and possible atrophy of the vocalis muscle and/or the superficial lamina propria and resulting dysphonia.[22]

Aerosolized recombinant human DNase I has been found to be quite effective in patients with cystic fibrosis to break up thick viscous DNA material making up secretions in the airway. This medication has been found to reduce the risk of respiratory tract exacerbations and improve pulmonary function. However, dysphonia has been found to be a reported side effect of this medication, manifested by the development of vocal fold edema. This side effect may be only transient.[23]

Gastroesophageal reflux disease (GERD) is common in children and may play a direct role in the development of chronic hoarseness.[24] Laryngeal findings may include posterior laryngeal edema and erythema, mucosal hyperplasia, true vocal fold edema, and mucous stranding. Prominent lymphoid follicles may also be associated with GERD. Unfortunately, this is still a rather subjective diagnosis on the part of the examining clinician. Objective measures such as 24-hour pH monitoring, esophagoscopy and biopsy, and manometry are not entirely sensitive or specific for the diagnosis of clinically significant GERD causing voice disturbance. Based on the level of concern, empiric treatment of GERD may be entertained. This may include such basic instructions as avoidance of snacks before bedtime, elevation of the head of bed, avoidance of caffeine and excessive citrus, and avoidance of large meals before exercising or singing, when intra-abdominal pressure is increased. Over-the-counter antacid medications may also be recommended. With rising concern of the role of GERD, prokinetic drugs (cisapride), H_2-receptor antagonists, and proton-pump inhibitors (omeprazole) may be considered.[25] In children, these medications are most frequently prescribed in consultation with a gastroenterologist.

Surgical management of pediatric voice disorders is an evolving field. Much can be learned from the application of phonomicrosurgical techniques used in the adult population.[26,27] Surgery may be the preferred treatment for certain selected laryngeal lesions, including intubation granulomas and supraglottic cysts. Vocal fold nodules, however, are still most appropriately managed in the pediatric age group with an initial trial of voice therapy and treatment of any co-existent medical problems. If underlying vocal abuse and hyperfunction can be eliminated, either through therapy or with a child's emotional and physical maturation, microsurgical resection of vocal fold nodules may be considered.[28] Successful long-term outcome after resection of nodules requires careful screening and on-going involvement with voice therapy both pre- and postoperatively.

A vocal fold palsy in a child will typically result in a weak and breathy voice quality, as well as a feeling of dyspnea with exercise. This condition may also predispose a child for aspiration and feeding difficulties.[29] Medialization laryngoplasty may be a useful procedure in such children. This technique has been successfully used in children as young as six years of age with a congenital unilateral vocal fold palsy. As might be expected, the voice results are not an immediate "cure" but gradually improve over a period of months with ongoing therapy. In children, there is the additional concern of adequate medialization of the paralyzed vocal fold, but also compromise of the glottic airway with the potential for stridor with exercise.

The surgical management of laryngeal papillomas is also evolving.[30] Traditional methods of laser ablation of all visible papillomas in the larynx may lead to excessive thermal damage and resulting scarring of the superficial lamina propria and vocal ligament. The application of phonomicrosurgical techniques including the submucosal injection of a 1:75,000 saline:epinephrine solution may allow for adequate hemostasis in addition to more precise excision of the laryngeal papillomas without mechanical or thermal trauma to underlying structures.

```
┌─────────────────────────────────────────┐
│           AT A GLANCE . . .               │
│           Treatment Modalities            │
│  ───────────────────────────────          │
│                                            │
│  • Voice therapy: vocal hygiene and abuse │
│    reduction, hydration, increase/decrease │
│    glottal closure, decrease muscular      │
│    tension, respiration, easy onset,       │
│    improve coordination of respiration     │
│    and phonation, resonance/voice          │
│    placement, decrease ventricular         │
│    phonation, raise/lower pitch,           │
│    increase/decrease loudness, lower       │
│    laryngeal placement, reinforce reflux   │
│    treatment                               │
│                                            │
│  • Medical therapy: hydration;             │
│    environmental allergies, allergic       │
│    rhinitis, (avoidance of anti-           │
│    histamines, use of intranasal steroid   │
│    sprays), asthma (inhaled steroid        │
│    preparations), gastroesophageal reflux  │
│    disease [basic GERD precautions,        │
│    antacids, prokinetic drugs (cisapride), │
│    H₂-receptor antagonists, proton-        │
│    pump inhibitors (omeprazole)]           │
│                                            │
│  • Surgery - indications: conservative     │
│    excision of benign lesions, "cold"      │
│    techniques, microlaryngeal instruments; │
│    avoidance of laser on true vocal folds; │
│    submucosal infusion technique),         │
│    management of laryngeal papillomas,     │
│    medialization laryngoplasty (careful    │
│    patient selection, airway issues),      │
│    management of laryngeal fracture        │
└─────────────────────────────────────────┘
```

CONCLUSION

We often remind ourselves that children are not simply "little adults." Children with voice disorders do require a specialized approach in order to make accurate perceptual assessments of voice quality and to obtain reliable objective measures of voice parameters. Stroboscopic videolaryngoscopy can be safely and comfortably carried out even in young children, but the examination takes time, patience, and a gentle touch. We will begin to see the benefits of comprehensive voice evaluations in children, as our diagnostic ability improves and allows for more effective treatment recommendations. Voice therapists working with children are becoming more sophisticated in their treatment approach, although careful outcome analysis will be needed in the future to demonstrate this effect. Phonosurgical techniques that have been used in the dysphonic adult population will also have value as we explore their role in the management of pediatric voice disorders.

REFERENCES

1. Gray SD, Smith ME, Schneider H. Voice disorders in children. Pediatr Clin North Amer 1996; 43(6): 1357-1384.
2. Baynes RA. An incidence study of chronic hoarseness among children. J Speech Hear Disord 1966; 31(2): 172-176.
3. Silverman EM. Incidence of chronic hoarseness among school-age children. J Speech Hear Disord 1975; 40:211-215.
4. Casper M, Abramson AL, Forman-Franco B. Hoarseness in children: Summer camp study. Int J Pediatr Otorhinolaryngol 1981; 3(1):85-89.
5. Maddern BR, Campbell TF, Stool S. Pediatric voice disorders. Otolaryngol Clin North Amer 1991; 24(5): 1125-1140.
6. Sederholm E, McAllister A, Dalkvist J, Sundberg J. Aetiologic factors associated with hoarseness in ten-year-old children. Folia Phoniatr Logop 1995; 47(5): 262-278.
7. Bonet M, Casan P. Evaluation of dysphonia in a children's choir. Folia Phoniatr Logop 1994; 46(1): 27-34.
8. Leeper HA, Leonard JE, Iverson RL. Otorhinolaryngologic screening of children with vocal quality disturbances. Int J Pediatr Otorhinolaryngol 1980; 2(2): 123-131.
9. Milutinovic Z. Social environment and incidence of voice disturbances in children. Folia Phoniatr Logop 1994; 46(3):135-138.
10. Powell M, Filter MD, Williams B. A longitudinal study of the prevalence of voice disorders in children from a rural school division. J Commun Disord 1989; 22(5):375-382.
11. Reilly JS. The "singing-acting" child: the laryngologist's perspective—1995. J Voice 1997; 11(2): 126-129.
12. Hirschberg J, Dejonckere PY, Hirano M, Mori K, Schultz-Coulon HJ, Vrticka K. Voice disorders in children. Int J Pediatr Otorhinolaryngol 1995; 32 (Suppl):S109-S125.
13. Lotz WK, d'Antonio LL, Chait DH, Netsell RW. Successful nasoendoscopic and aerodynamic examinations of children with speech/voice disorders. Int J Pediatr Otorhinolaryngol 1993; 26(2):165-172.
14. De Bodt MS, Van de Heyning PH, Wuyts FL, Lambrechts L. The perceptual evaluation of voice disorders. Acta Otorhinolaryngol Belg 1996; 50(4): 283-291.
15. Kane M, Wellen CJ. Acoustic measurements and clinical judgement of vocal quality in children with vocal nodules. Folia Phoniatr Logop 1985; 37(2):53-57.
16. Ruscello DM, Lass NJ, Podbesek J. Listeners' perceptions of normal and voice-disordered children. Folia Phoniatr Logop 1988; 40(6):290-296.

17. Zajac DJ, Farkas Z, Dindzans L, Stool SE. Aerodynamic and laryngographic assessment of pediatric vocal function. Pediatr Pulmonol 1993; 15(1):44-51.

18. D'Antonio L, Chait D, Lotz W, Netsell R. Pediatric video nasoendoscopy for speech and voice evaluation. Otolaryngol Head Neck Surg 1986; 94(5): 578-583.

19. Smith ME, Marsh JH, Cotton RT, Myer CM 3d. Voice problems after pediatric laryngotracheal reconstruction: videolaryngostroboscopic, acoustic, and perceptual assessment. Int J Pediatr Otorhinolaryngol 1993; 25(1):173-181.

20. MacArthur CJ, Kearns GH, Healy GB. Voice quality after laryngotracheal reconstruction. Arch Otolaryngol Head Neck Surg 1994; 20(6):641-647.

21. Ramig LO, Verdolini K. Treatment efficacy: voice disorders. J Speech Lang Hear Res 1998; 41(1): S101-116.

22. Hanania NA, Chapman KR, Kesten S. Adverse effects of inhaled corticosteroids. Am J Med 1995; 98(2): 196-208.

23. Shak S. Aerosolized recombinant human DNase I for the treatment of cystic fibrosis. Chest 1995; 107 (Suppl.)(2):65S-70S.

24. Gumpert L, Kalach N, Dupont C, Contencin P. Hoarseness and gastroesophageal reflux in children. J Laryngol Otol 1998; 112(1):49-54.

25. Olafsdottir E. Gastro-oesophageal reflux and chronic respiratory disease in infants and children: treatment with cisapride. Scand J Gastroenterol 1995; 30 (Suppl.):32-34.

26. Bouchayer M, Cornut G. Microsurgical treatment of benign vocal fold lesions: indications, technique, results. Folia Phoniatr Logop 1992; 44(3-4):155-184.

27. Kass ES, Hillman RE, Zeitels SM. Vocal fold submucosal infusion technique in phonomicrosurgery. Ann Otol Rhinol Laryngol 1996; 105:341-347.

28. Benjamin B, Croxson G. Vocal nodules in children. Ann Otol Rhinol Laryngol 1987; 96(5):550-553.

29. Levine BA, Jacobs IN, Wetmore RF, Handler SD. Vocal cord injection in children with unilateral vocal cord paralysis. Arch Otolaryngol Head Neck Surg 1995; 121(1):116-119.

30. Nuss RC. Management of pediatric laryngeal papillomatosis. Oper Tech Otolaryngol Head Neck Surg 1998; 9(4):210-213.

31. Cohen SR, Thompson JW, Geller KA, Birns JW. Voice change in the pediatric patient. A differential diagnosis. Ann Otol Rhinol Laryngol 1983; 92:437-443.

32. Heuer RJ, Sataloff RT, Spiegel JR, Jackson LG, Carroll LM. Voice abnormalities in short stature syndromes. Ear Nose Throat J 1995; 74(9):622-629.

33. Papsin BC, Vellodi A, Bailey CM, Ratcliffe PC, Leighton SE. Otologic and laryngologic manifestations of mucopolysaccharidoses after bone marrow transplantation. Otolaryngol Head Neck Surg 1998; 118(1):30-36.

34. Cohen SR. Congenital glottic webs in children. A retrospective review of 51 patients. Ann Otol Rhinol Laryngol Suppl 1985; 121:2-16.

35. Itoh T, Kawasaki H, Morikawa I, Hirano M. Vocal fold furrows. A 10-year review of 240 patients. Auris Nasus Larynx 1983; 10 Suppl:S17-S26.

36. Ford CN, Inagi K, Bless DM, Khidr A, Gilchrist KW. Sulcus vocalis: a rational analytical approach to diagnosis and management. Ann Otol Rhinol Laryngol 1996; 105:189-200.

37. Di Girolamo S, Anselmi M, Piccini A, De Lauretis A, Passali D. Aspecific membranous laryngitis after infectious mononucleosis. Int J Pediatr Otorhinolaryngol 1996; 34(1-2):171-174.

38. Hass A, Hyatt AC, Kattan M, Weiner MA, Hodes DS. Hoarseness in immunocompromised children: association with invasive fungal infection. J Pediatr 1987; 111(5):731-733.

39. Huang SW, Kimbrough JW. Mold allergy is a risk factor for persistent cold-like symptoms in children. Clin Pediatr 1997; 36(12):695-699.

40. Conley SF, Milbrath MM, Beste DJ. Pediatric laryngeal granular cell tumor. J Otolaryngol 1992; 21(6): 450-453.

41. Kato MA, Flamant F, terrier-Lacombe MJ, Habrand JL, Schwaab G, Luboinski B, Valteau-Couanet D, Lemerle J. Rhabdomyosarcoma of the larynx in children: a series of five patients treated in the Institut Gustave Roussy. Med Pediatr Oncol 1991; 19(2):110-114.

42. Bent JP 3d, Silver JR, Porubsky ES. Acute laryngeal trauma: a review of 77 patients. Otolaryngol Head Neck Surg 1993; 109(3):441-449.

43. Ford HR, Gardner MJ, Lynch JM. Laryngotracheal disruption from blunt pediatric neck injuries: impact of early recognition and intervention on outcome. J Pediatr Surg 1995; 30(2):331-334.

44. Sataloff RT, Bough ID Jr, Spiegel JR. Arytenoid dislocation: diagnosis and treatment. Laryngoscope 1994; 104(11):1353-1361.

45. Putnam PE, Orenstein SR. Hoarseness in a child with gastroesophageal reflux. Acta Paediatrica 1992; 81(8):635-636.

46. Walsh-Kelly C, Kelly KJ. Dysphonia: an unusual presentation of spontaneous pneumomediastinum. Pediatr Emer Care 1986; 2(1):26-27.

47. Parano E, Pavone L, Musumeci S, Giambusso F, Trifiletti RR. Acute palsy of the recurrent laryngeal nerve complicating Epstein-Barr virus infection. Neuropediatrics 1996; 27(3):164-166.

48. Yurdakok K, Ozmert E. Hoarse cry: a sign of dehydration. Lancet 1995; 346(8985):1306.

49. Koufman JA, Blalock PD. Classification and approach to patients with functional voice disorders. Ann Otol Rhinol Laryngol 1982; 91(4):372-377.

50. Schalen L, Andersson K, Eliasson I. Diagnosis of psychogenic dysphonia. Acta Otolaryngol Suppl 1992; 492:110-112.

46 Introduction to Disorders of the Upper Airway

Gerald B. Healy

An understanding of the developmental anatomy of the upper aerodigestive tract (UADT) is essential for the clinician who treats patients with disorders of this anatomic region. Generally, the upper airway is considered to include the nasal cavity, nasopharynx, oropharynx, hypopharynx, larynx, tracheobronchial tree, and esophagus. The major portion of embryologic development in this region takes place between the third and eighth fetal week. Most true developmental anomalies of this area usually have their origin during this essential period of organogenesis.

The UADT is also intimately related to the derivatives of the dorsal ventral aorta, which explains the potential for congenital vascular anomalies to produce upper airway pathology.

The pediatric airway demonstrates many unique features. For example, the larynx is located significantly higher in the infant than in the adult, with the inferior margin of the cricoid cartilage residing at approximately the level of the second cervical vertebra in the newborn. This descends to the level of the seventh cervical vertebra in the adult. In the normal infant, the larynx is more anterior and superior in the neck than in the adult. This elevated position brings the epiglottis and palate into close proximity, thus making the child a necessary nose breather in the first few weeks to months of life. The fact that the infant is an obligate nose breather during this time has potential clinical significance for various congenital abnormalities of the nasal airway.[1]

Both the larynx and the trachea of the newborn infant differ greatly in size from their adult counterparts. The glottic opening of the newborn measures approximately 7 mm in the anteroposterior dimen-

sion with a posterotransverse dimension of 4 mm. The tracheal diameter varies from approximately 3 mm in the premature infant to about 25 mm in the adult.

SPECIAL CONSIDERATION:

The larynx is located significantly higher in the infant than in the adult, with the inferior margin of the cricoid cartilage residing at the level of the second cervical vertebra in the newborn.

EVALUATION AND DIAGNOSIS

Newborns and infants presenting with noisy breathing can offer a challenging diagnostic dilemma for both the primary care physician and the consulting otolaryngologist. Normal respiration does not produce audible sounds. Infants with anomalies of the aerodigestive tract (ADT) present with stridor and/or feeding difficulties. Noisy breathing usually is produced by the partial obstruction of air passage into and out of the respiratory system. These noises may be loud or soft and high or low pitched, depending on the type and extent of the obstruction and the resulting flow dynamics. Documenting the time in the respiratory cycle and the quality of the stridor may give valuable diagnostic clues to determine the level of airway pathology.

Patient evaluation begins by obtaining a precise and detailed history from the parents or other care givers. A careful history may point to the diagnosis in more than 80% of cases. The speed with which the diagnostic evaluation is undertaken obviously is dictated by the patient's general condition. In cases

Pediatric Otolaryngology, Edited by R.F. Wetmore, H.R. Muntz, and T.J. McGill. Thieme Medical Publishers, Inc., New York © 2000.

where severe respiratory obstruction is present, an ideal evaluation may not be possible.

In addition to a careful history, a detailed physical examination of the airway must be undertaken. This usually begins by applying a stethoscope to the neck and chest of the infant to document the stridor as well as the phase of respiration in which it is occurring. Because infants with airway obstruction may have an accelerated respiratory rate, the examiner's ear may be fooled without the aid of a stethoscope in the determination of the phase of respiration in which the stridor is most pronounced.

Purely inspiratory stridor usually indicates lesions in the more superior part of the airway, and lesions occurring distal to the vocal cords usually demonstrate a pronounced expiratory component. Biphasic stridor most commonly points to lesions of the subglottic airway, although glottic pathology occasionally may present this way.

It is critical to analyze the quality of the stridor carefully, as this also may be useful in identifying specific anatomic locations of the pathologic process. Sonorous, inspiratory stridor frequently results from lesions in the nose or nasopharynx. Inspiratory stridor that is high pitched is commonly secondary to pathology at the supraglottic level.

Stridor that is intense and persistent may indicate an acute process, such as inflammation, trauma, or a foreign body. This is especially true in children who have been well and healthy up to the onset of symptoms. Changes in the severity of stridor also may be an important historic detail. Stridor that increases gradually over time may indicate a lesion that is expanding, such as a congenital cyst or a neoplasm such as papilloma. Symptoms that change with position may also offer another diagnostic clue. Infants with high-pitched, inspiratory stridor secondary to supraglottic pathology may improve in the prone position. Hyperextension of the neck and thrusting of the chin to a more forward (or "sniffing") position frequently indicates an effort by the patient to straighten the airway (as may be seen when extrinsic vascular compression of the trachea is present).

It is critically important to take a feeding history. Newborns, who are obligate nose breathers, may have significant feeding difficulties in the presence of obstructing lesions of the nasal cavity or nasopharynx. Lesions that impact the pharynx or supraglottic larynx are more likely to cause feeding difficulty than are lesions of the intrinsic airway. Exceptions to this may be seen in those patients with vascular anomalies that compress both the trachea and the esophagus. Those patients who have a true communication of the trachea and esophagus, such as a tracheoesophageal fistula, also have obvious feeding difficulties. An associated cough may point to an anatomic communication between the esophagus and trachea or an inadequate neurologic pathway, as is seen in vocal cord paralysis.

After completing a thorough history, the UADT is then investigated. The three major areas of investigation include physical examination, radiographic examination, and endoscopic confirmation. Practice Pathway 46-1 outlines the evaluation of stridor.

Physical Examination

Careful observation of the patient is critical before initiating a hands-on examination. The examiner should note the patient's level of consciousness, position, color, and respiratory rate, as well as the presence or absence of retraction.

The patient's general physical condition is noted, including the presence or absence of congenital anomalies in the head and neck area, craniofacial malformations, and mass lesions. The skin is observed carefully for the presence or absence of any evidence of hemangiomas. The patient's color should be observed to determine the level of oxygenation. Circumoral pallor or cyanosis may be the first sign of hypoxia. However, this finding does not represent a respiratory problem necessarily as it also may be seen in patients with cardiac anomalies.

The patient's position should be observed. Infants with pathology of the supraglottic larynx prefer the prone position, whereas lesions of the intrinsic larynx or trachea may not be relieved by changes of position.

SPECIAL CONSIDERATION:

Infants with pathology of the supraglottic larynx prefer the prone position, where lesions of the intrinsic larynx or trachea may not be relieved by changes in position.

The actual examination begins with careful auscultation of the neck and chest. This helps the examiner to identify the phase and quality of the stridor and determine if there is evidence of associated pulmonary pathology. The quality of the patient's cry

Practice Pathway 46-1   STRIDOR

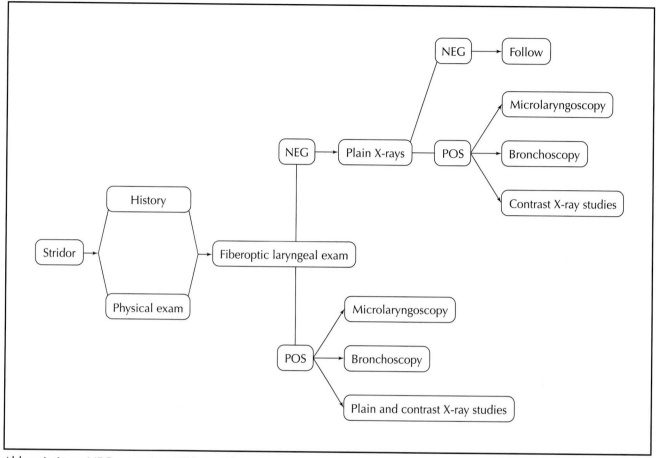

Abbreviations: NEG, negative; POS, positive.

and the presence or absence of cough should be noted. The lack of cry may indicate significant glottic pathology, such as a congenital web.

Normal functions such as nasal respirations and swallowing are evaluated next. It is critical to ascertain nasal airflow in the newborn infant. Numerous methods of assessing patency of the nasal airway are available. These include passing nasal catheters or holding a small nasopharyngeal mirror in front of the nares. Frequently, patients with supraglottic or oropharyngeal obstruction or esophageal anomalies have difficulty swallowing secretions; in these cases, drooling may be an important diagnostic clue.

The examination should be performed with extreme caution. Gentle manipulation of the oral cavity and mandible can help determine whether oropharyngeal obstruction is present. Pulling the tongue or jaw forward may give relief to patients with pathology in this anatomic location. The patient should not be agitated or excited, especially if evidence of hypoxia is already present.

Careful palpation of the neck should be undertaken to determine the location of the trachea. The examiner should keep in mind that the trachea may be located slightly to the right of the midline in the newborn. Deviation also may occur with respiration, as the mediastinum shifts secondary to overinflation or under-inflation of one lung. Lesions in the mediastinum or in structures adjacent to the trachea, such as the thyroid, may produce fixed deviations of the trachea. Large congenital anomalies involving the neck, such as lymphatic malformations, may cause extrinsic compression of the hypopharynx or trachea. These lesions usually are readily apparent on examination.

When these phases of the examination are completed, a reasonable differential diagnosis should be formulated. This process should then determine the next step in the evaluation. Those patients demonstrating mild symptoms and minimal distress may allow immediate visualization in the nursery or office setting. This can be completed with the use of flexible fiberoptic instrumentation. These patients also may tolerate a planned systematic radiologic assessment. In those patients with significant airway obstruction, a rigid examination in the operating room is usually more appropriate. A concomitant radiologic assessment may not be feasible in these severe cases, but this determination must be left to the clinical judgment of the examiner.

The advent of flexible fiberoptic instrumentation, including laryngoscope and bronchoscope, has allowed a more rapid confirmation of a differential diagnosis. This instrumentation also gives important information as to the neurologic status of the larynx, as well as the dynamic function of the hypopharynx and supraglottis. These functions must be assessed in the unsedated and unanesthetized patient. Small diameter flexible instruments are somewhat limited in terms of optics, however. This limitation produces a diminished depth of field, and thus subtle lesions such as tracheoesophageal fistula or laryngeal cleft may be overlooked. Video and photographic documentation should be available to the examiner and such recordings may allow future review of pathology. These examinations should be undertaken only in settings where appropriate resuscitative equipment is available.

Patients undergoing flexible fiberoptic laryngoscopy should be placed in a semi-sitting position to bring the larynx more anterior and to permit better visualization of the glottic structures. Endoscopic examination of the esophagus may be useful, but should only be undertaken where appropriate airway protection can be provided.

SPECIAL CONSIDERATION:

Patients undergoing flexible laryngoscopy should be placed in a semi-sitting position to bring the larynx more anterior and to permit better visualization of the glottic structures.

Radiologic Evaluation

Patients with airway distress or stridor should undergo a thorough radiologic assessment of the upper airway, chest, and esophagus if the clinical situation permits. This evaluation includes both anteroposterior (AP) and lateral films of the neck and chest. Inspiratory and expiratory films should be obtained if possible. Fluoroscopy is frequently useful in answering questions regarding the constancy of any finding seen on static radiography. Fluoroscopy with contrast should be strongly considered in any patient suspected of aerodigestive pathology. This study defines vascular compressions, fistulae between the trachea and esophagus, and neurologic difficulties that lead to aspiration or discoordination of the pharynx during swallowing. Computed tomography (CT) is not especially helpful in identifying lesions of the upper airway. The only exception to this is in cases of suspected choanal atresia or stenosis where CT may be extremely useful in planning correction. Magnetic resonance imaging (MRI) is more useful in defining lesions of the upper airway. This is especially true in cases of vascular anomalies that compress the trachea or esophagus.[2]

Endoscopic Evaluation

Endoscopic evaluation remains the most definitive way of establishing a diagnosis in any patient suspected of having a congenital or acquired anomaly of the UADT. It requires cooperation, diligence, precision, and skill. The cooperation must be with other members of the endoscopic team, which includes the endoscopist, anesthesiologist, and radiologist. Adequate and appropriate instrumentation must always be available, including a complete selection of rigid and flexible laryngoscopes, bronchoscopes, and esophagoscopes. Magnifying telescopes together with still and video cameras must be available for documentation.

The use of endoscopy may vary from one examiner to another. At one end of the spectrum are those physicians who feel the airway can be evaluated with an AP and lateral soft tissue X-ray of the neck, an AP and lateral chest X-ray, and a barium esophagogram. This evaluation usually is coupled with a flexible fiberoptic examination of the nose, nasopharynx, supraglottic, and glottic regions. At the other end of the spectrum are those physicians who would use a complete radiographic examination coupled with a flexible examination of the structures mentioned above and a rigid endoscopic evaluation of the larynx, tracheobronchial tree, and esophagus. Whichever method is employed, all procedures should be undertaken in a safe setting with appropriate resuscitative equipment available. Complete evaluation of the entire ADT is mandated because there may be more than one congenital lesion in the region. Approximately 18% of patients have simultaneous lesions affecting different areas of the airway.[3] Topical anesthesia is useful when the patient is evaluated either awake or under general anesthesia. Lidocaine (0.5%) is used for this purpose in the nasal cavity, hypopharynx, and larynx.

If complete evaluation under general anesthesia is entertained, the following methodology should be considered. Examination begins with the awake infant in the semi-sitting position with the head stabilized. A flexible fiberoptic laryngoscope is passed through each side of the nasal cavity to examine the patency of the nasal airway. The evaluation is then continued into the nasopharynx where anatomy and patency as well as function, are evaluated. The examination proceeds to the level of the hypopharynx and supraglottic larynx where dynamic function and mobility of the vocal cords are assessed. This evaluation is useful in determining the presence of lesions such as laryngomalacia or vocal cord paralysis.

Induction of general anesthesia is then undertaken using a mask ventilation technique, with positive pressure to assist the respiratory effort when necessary. Time must be taken to achieve an appropriate depth of anesthesia. The patient must be deep enough to negate laryngeal reflexes but also should be allowed to breath spontaneously. If a fixed obstruction is present, a longer time for induction may be necessary.

After an appropriate level of anesthesia is reached, the larynx is visualized and 0.5% lidocaine is applied topically. Appropriate oximeter and electrocardiogram (EKG) leads are attached and an intravenous (IV) line is inserted. Endoscopy can usually begin safely at this point.

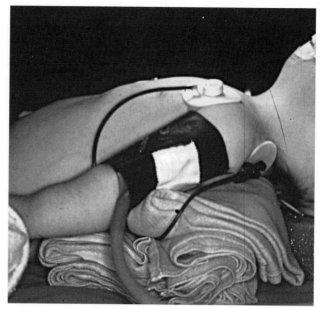

Figure 46–1: Recommended position for endoscopic evaluation of the airway.

SPECIAL CONSIDERATION:

During endoscopy in young infants, it may be necessary to flex the head forward in order to allow the more anteriorly placed larynx to achieve a more posterior position for clear visualization.

The patient's shoulders are elevated and the head is raised so that it is somewhat hyperextended (Fig.

46–1). In young infants, it may be necessary to flex the head forward in order to allow the more anteriorly placed larynx to achieve a more posterior position for clear visualization. The gingiva or teeth are protected and a laryngoscope is inserted to inspect the oropharynx, hypopharynx, and larynx. A magnifying telescope is valuable at this stage for documentation and magnification. The supraglottic, glottic, and subglottic structures can be evaluated with this instrumentation. The tip of the laryngoscope should be inserted carefully into the posterior commissure to rule out the possibility of laryngeal cleft.

The patient should continue to breath spontaneously. Oxygenation may be assisted by placing a small catheter into the nose and into the hypopharynx for appropriate insufflation of oxygen and anesthetic gas. Careful monitoring of the oximeter is mandatory and if the oxygen saturation drops, the laryngoscope should be removed and mask ventilation continued until appropriate oxygenation is achieved. If it is necessary to establish an airway for safe oxygenation, an appropriate size bronchoscope can be inserted carefully. A magnifying telescope is inserted through the bronchoscope for better visualization of the tracheobronchial tree (Fig. 46–2). If oxygenation appears to be adequate, a bronchoscopic telescope may be inserted alone, and spontaneous respiration may continue to oxygenate the patient adequately. This is an acceptable technique but requires extreme skill, diligence, and the coop-

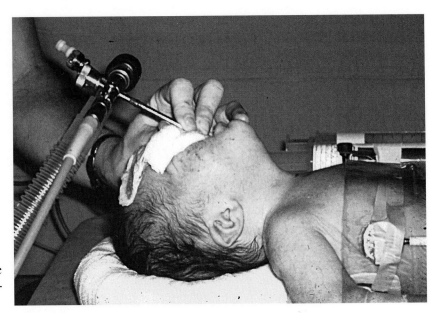

Figure 46–2: Bronchoscopy for the establishment of an airway in a compromised infant.

eration of both the anesthesiologist and the endoscopist.

Flexible bronchoscopic equipment may be used in young infants in light of the availability of small diameter bronchoscopes that allow ventilation. The depth of field of these instruments is, however, somewhat limited, and thus they do not offer the same visibility as rigid instrumentation.

AT A GLANCE . . .

Evaluation of Disorders of the Upper Airway

History: questions that should be asked include if stridor changes with position, if it has increased over time, and if the newborn experiences difficulty feeding.

Physical: the patient's level of consciousness, position, color, and respiratory rate, as well as the presence or absence or retraction should be noted; physical should include auscultation of the neck and chest, evaluation of respiration and swallowing, gentle manipulation of the oral cavity and mandible, and palpation of the neck.

Radiologic Evaluation: AP and lateral films of the neck and chest on inspiration and expiration, fluoroscopy, CT (limited), and MRI.

Endoscopic Evaluation: rigid and flexible laryngoscopes, bronchoscopes, and esophagoscopes; magnifying telescopes together with still as well as video cameras for documentation.

After completing the examination of the larynx and tracheobronchial tree, the airway is secured and the esophagus evaluated. This may be done by either rigid or flexible instrumentation.

At the completion of the examination, the endoscopist must decide whether the airway can maintain ventilation without assistance or whether an artificial airway must be placed, either in the form of an endotracheal tube or a tracheotomy tube. This assessment is made on the basis of degree of obstruction, the nature of the pathology, and the endoscopist's clinical judgment.

ANOMALOUS CONDITIONS

The more common anomalous conditions that affect the UADT are listed in Table 46–1.

Nose

Patients presenting with choanal atresia or stenosis frequently demonstrate significant respiratory distress at birth. This is especially true in bilateral cases where severe cyanosis and distress occur if the mouth is closed. The patient's symptoms usually are relieved either by crying or the placement of an oral airway. Stenosis of the anterior nasal cavity also may precipitate the same symptoms. Diagnosis is established by careful nasal examination and CT (Fig. 46–3).

Severe nasal septal deformity may be present in

TABLE 46-1: Common Congenital Anomalies of the Aerodigestive Tract

Nose/Nasopharynx
  Choanal atresia
  Choanal stenosis
  Septal deformity
  Turbinate hypertrophy
  Masses (glioma, encephalocele, adenoid hyperplasia), even in
    newborn
Oral/Oropharynx
  Macroglossia
  Craniofacial deformity (Apert, Pierre Robin)
  Masses and cysts (thyroglossal, lingual thyroid, lymphatic mal-
    formation)
  Neurologic deficit
Larynx
  Supraglottic
    Laryngomalacia
    Cysts
    Neoplasm (hemangioma, lymphatic malformation)
    Cleft (bifid epiglottis)
    Web
  Glottic
    Web (anterior and posterior) and atresia
    Neurologic dysfunction
    Stenosis
    Cleft
  Subglottic
    Cysts
    Hemangioma
    Stenosis
    Web
    Cleft
Trachea
  Tracheoesophageal fistula
  Tracheomalacia
  Vascular compression
  Congenital stenosis (complete ring)
  Hemangioma
  Cyst
  Agenesis
  Tracheal bronchus
Esophagus
  Tracheoesophageal fistula
  Vascular decompression
  Duplication

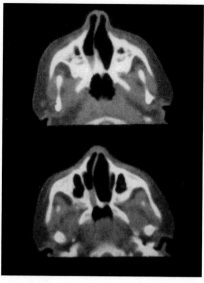

Figure 46-3: CT scan of choanal atresia.

Oropharynx

The vallecula and the base of tongue region are the most common areas affected by congenital anomalies of the oropharynx in newborns and infants. Lesions in this area include thyroglossal duct cyst, vallecular cyst, and lingual thyroid. (Fig. 46-5).

Larynx

Supraglottis

The most common anomaly of the supraglottic larynx in the newborn is *congenital flaccid larynx* (i.e., *laryngomalacia*). This condition results in

the newborn. This can be secondary to birth trauma and can induce significant respiratory distress (Fig. 46-4). In those cases where distress is present, repositioning of the septum should be undertaken immediately. In other cases, repositioning may take place any time during the newborn period.

A variety of masses may impact respiration in the newborn or older child. Conditions such as adenoid hypertrophy, encephalocele, and nasal glioma may be present. Careful examination of the nasal cavity is required to rule out these lesions. A topical decongestant should be applied to complete this exam in a thorough manner.

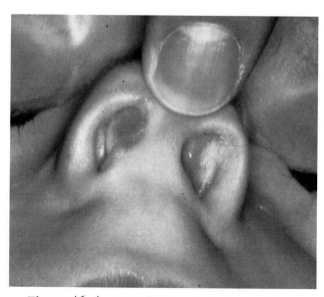

Figure 46-4: Septal deformity in the newborn.

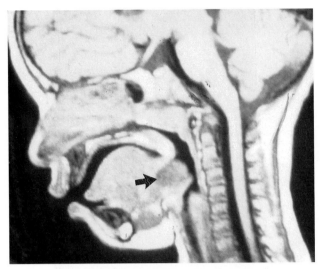

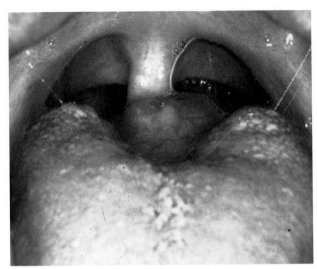

A   B

Figure 46–5:   (A) MRI of lingual thyroid in the base of tongue region (arrow). (B) Intraoral presentation of lingual thyroid.

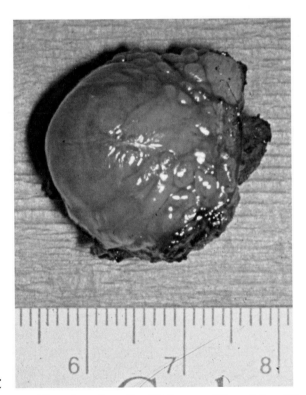

C

Figure 46–5: Continued   (C) Resected lingual thyroid.

flaccidity and incoordination of the supraglottic cartilage and mucosa of the arytenoids, aryepiglottic folds, and epiglottis. These patients are frequently asymptomatic at birth, but gradually develop symptoms in the first few weeks of life. The diagnosis must be made while observing the functioning larynx in the awake state. In severe cases, intervention

may be necessary in the form of epiglottoplasty or tracheotomy.

Benign neoplasms also may present in the supraglottic area within the first few days or weeks of life. The most common lesions are vascular malformations such as hemangioma, lymphatic malformation, or vascular malformation. Often the full dimension of these lesions may not be appreciated for several weeks or months after birth. Premature intervention may prove unrewarding in the long term and should only be undertaken in cases where severe distress is present. In some lesions such as hemangiomas, spontaneous resolution frequently occurs after the first year of life.

Glottis

Vocal cord paralysis may present unilaterally or bilaterally (see Fig. 46–5). Unilateral lesions are usually idiopathic in nature and often self-limited. In these patients, there is frequently hoarseness or a weakened cry but rarely airway distress. Those patients with bilateral paralysis may have a normal cry but demonstrate significant airway distress with biphasic stridor. Chest radiography extremely important in the evaluation of these patients to rule out mediastinal or cardiac anomalies. In those cases where bilateral paralysis is present, a thorough neurologic examination and an imaging study of the brain are required to rule out lesions such as hydrocephalus or the Arnold-Chiari malformation. Trache-

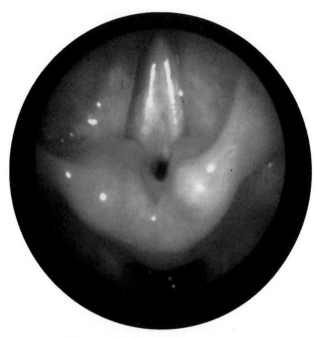

Figure 46–6: Severe glottic web.

otomy may be necessary, especially where significant airway distress is present.

Glottic Webs commonly affect the anterior portion of the glottis. Webs may be of variable thickness and may extend into the subglottic space for a varying distance (Fig. 46-6). These patients usually present with aphonia. Therapy is dictated by the amount of stridor present. If 50% or more of the glottis is occupied by the web, then treatment usually is required.

Subglottis

Congenital Stenosis usually occurs secondary to a deformity of the cricoid cartilage. A subglottis with an anterior-posterior diameter of <4 mm is usually indicative of this lesion. Severe cases may require immediate intervention with the placement of a tracheotomy. Anterior cricoid decompression (i.e., cricoid split) may be considered in selected cases.

Subglottic hemangioma usually manifests itself during the first few weeks of life. These patients frequently develop biphasic stridor sometime after the third week of life that worsens with exertion or agitation. Some feeding difficulty may be present. Many patients have an associated cutaneous hemangioma. In patients with severe symptomatology, treatment is directed toward decompression of the subglottic space.

Trachea

Tracheomalacia

Tracheomalacia may occur either in a primary or secondary form. *Primary tracheomalacia* is a rare entity resulting from a congenital deformity of the supporting tracheal rings. Patients may present with varying degrees of respiratory distress. Clinically, the patients exhibit expiratory stridor secondary to collapse of the anterior tracheal wall against the soft posterior tracheoesophageal septum. Both cases are self-limited, but in severe cases it may be necessary to place a tracheotomy to stent the trachea during development.

Secondary tracheomalacia occurs as a result of extrinsic compression, as may be seen in vascular anomalies or secondary to surgical intervention, such as tracheoesophageal fistula repair. Symptoms are similar to those seen in primary tracheomalacia. Patients may present with reflex apnea and recurrent pneumonitis secondary to their chronic obstruction. Therapy should be directed toward the correction of the underlying lesion.

Tracheoesophageal fistula may occur in various forms. The most common variety involves proximal esophageal atresia with the distal esophagus communicating with the trachea. A more subtle form is the "H" type, in which small communication exists between the upper trachea and the upper third of the esophagus.

These patients usually present with feeding difficulties and aspiration soon after birth. This lesion can be extremely subtle and require observation by the radiologist and the endoscopist. Management involves surgical correction in all cases.

Vascular anomalies

The trachea and esophagus enjoy an intimate relationship with the great vessels during embryologic development. This increases the potential for malformation, however. These anomalies may either completely surround the esophagus and trachea, producing obstruction, or compress the anterior wall of the trachea alone.

The most common lesions include anomalous subclavian artery, double aortic arch, right aortic arch, and innominate artery compression (Fig. 46-7). Surgical correction usually is required to eliminate this problem.

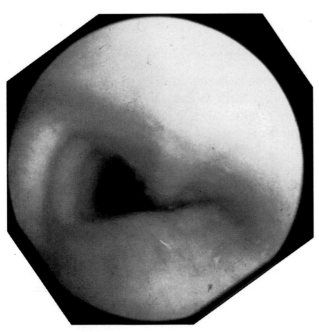

Figure 46–7: Innominate artery compression of the trachea.

Tracheal stenosis

Congenital tracheal stenosis is usually secondary to complete tracheal rings occurring either segmentally or throughout the entire tracheobronchial tree. Management should be conservative, if possible, but severe cases may require aggressive surgical intervention.

EVALUATION OF COUGH AND HOARSENESS

Cough

The *cough response* is one of the fundamental protective mechanisms of the respiratory system. Coughing serves two functions: it removes secretions from the airway and expels foreign material from the respiratory system. The stimulus to cough usually is related to one of four factors, which include chemical irritation, mechanical obstruction, thermal stimulation, and inflammation.

Multiple factors are necessary for the generation of a cough response. These include: (1) an intact sensory apparatus; (2) an appropriate afferent and efferent pathway to and from the central nervous system (CNS); (3) an intact central processing mechanism to insure adequate timing and distribution of neuromuscular activity; and (4) an adequate muscu-

loskeletal system. Traditionally, the four phases of cough production are inspiratory, contractive, compressive, and expulsive. The cough reflex becomes increasingly stronger with age, obviously being weakest in the premature infant.[4]

The evaluation of a patient with cough begins with an accurate history. The age of the child in question may become critically important in determining the cause of cough. Coughing in the newborn is unusual and may suggest a significant pathology, including congenital anomalies or pneumonia. Coughing associated with feeding may suggest tracheoesophageal fistula, reflux, or an aortic arch anomaly. A mechanical obstruction such as a foreign body is a possibility in any age group.

SPECIAL CONSIDERATION:

Coughing in the newborn is unusual and may suggest a significant pathology, including congenital anomalies or pneumonia.

It is critical to identify the specific features and timing of the cough. This includes an assessment of the quality, the duration, and the productivity. The quality of the cough may identify an anatomic site of origin. For example, a barking cough may indicate subglottic pathology. The timing of the cough also may be helpful in ascertaining a diagnosis. For example, cough occurring at night may be secondary to gastroesophageal reflux or chronic sinusitis, whereas cough related to physical exercise may indicate asthma. The duration of the cough also may provide important diagnostic clues. Persistent cough usually indicates a chronic condition such as bronchitis or asthma, whereas episodic coughing may indicate a self-limiting condition such as a respiratory infection. A productive cough usually is indicative of inflammation, and a nonproductive cough may point to a fixed lesion.

A careful physical examination may provide some diagnostic clues. The general appearance of the patient should be assessed carefully. Patients who exhibit growth delay may have a chronic underlying pulmonary condition. Patients with significant allergic problems may have tell-tale signs in the nasal cavity or hypopharyngeal area. Careful auscultation of the chest in all phases of respiration should be undertaken, noting the symmetry of respiration, as well as the presence or absence of wheezing, rales, or rhonchi.

The ears should be carefully examined also, as impacted cerumen or hairs growing in the ear canal may stimulate Arnold's nerve leading to recurrent coughing. The nasal cavity and nasopharynx may provide clues of chronic rhinitis, sinusitis, or polyps. Nasal polyps in children <10 years of age are almost pathognomonic for cystic fibrosis (CF).

A careful laryngeal examination should be undertaken to evaluate the patient for congenital anomalies such as laryngeal cleft, vocal cord paralysis, or tell-tale signs of reflux laryngitis.

The overall evaluation should also include a chest X-ray and contrast radiographs where indicated. These would be especially valuable in patients where aspiration is suspected. In cases where the clinical history may point to unusual causes, specialized laboratory evaluations may be indicated. These would include evaluation for CF, allergy, tuberculosis, and the immotile cilia syndrome. The causes of coughing are multiple and varied but those related to the upper airway are outlined in Table 46-2.

AT A GLANCE . . .

Cough

Pathogenesis: usually a response to chemical irritation, mechanical obstruction, thermal stimulation, or inflammation.

Evaluation: identify the quality, timing, duration, and productivity of the cough; physical examination should include auscultation of the chest; examination of the ears, larynx, nasopharynx, and nasal cavity; and a chest X-ray and contrast radiographs where indicated.

Differential Diagnosis: pulmonary conditions, allergies, cystic fibrosis, laryngeal cleft, vocal cord paralysis, reflux laryngitis, tuberculosis, immotile cilia syndrome.

Hoarseness

Hoarseness may be defined as an altered voice quality that also may include an alteration of the cry in

TABLE 46-2: Causes of Coughing Related to the Upper Airway

Adenoiditis
Allergy
Foreign body
Pharyngitis
Congenital cysts
Laryngeal cleft
Laryngotracheal bronchitis
Cystic fibrosis
Tuberculosis
Gastroesophageal reflux
Chronic sinusitis
Immotile cilia syndrome
Kartagener's syndrome

infancy. It is caused by an abnormality of the structure and/or function of the vocal cords.

The intensity of the voice varies with subglottic pressure against glottic resistance. Pitch and timber are influenced by the length and tension of the vibrating vocal cords. The shape of the free margins of the vocal cords also determine voice quality. The failure in one or more of these areas usually results in a coarse or hoarse vocal quality.

The evaluation of hoarseness begins with a careful history that includes age of onset, rate of progression, and association with any events such as trauma, surgery, or infection. A careful cardiac and respiratory history also must be taken as pathology in these areas also can lead to dysfunction of the recurrent laryngeal nerve with secondary vocal cord paralysis.

Physical exam includes a careful examination of the general well-being and condition of the patient. The skin also is evaluated carefully for lesions such as hemangioma or others similar that may have a laryngeal component. A thorough neurologic examination should be undertaken. Precise auscultation of the neck and chest is required. Whenever feasible, flexible fiberoptic laryngoscopy should be attempted in order to evaluate the dynamic function and anatomic configuration of the vocal cords. More specific testing, such as voice evaluation and stroboscopy, may be considered if adequate cooperation of the patient can be achieved.

Radiographs of the neck and chest should be considered in patients where a definite cause cannot be found by laryngoscopy or in those patients where cooperation is limited. Fluoroscopy also may be of value. Recently, ultrasound has been utilized to evaluate vocal cord motion, and it can be quite help-ful in determining vocal cord function, especially in infants. The ultimate evaluation should include direct laryngoscopy under general anesthesia in those cases where a definite diagnosis cannot be achieved by the methods outlined above.[5]

SPECIAL CONSIDERATION:

The ultimate evaluation of hoarseness should include direct laryngoscopy under general an-esthesia in those cases where a definite diag-nosis cannot be achieved by other methods.

The causes of hoarseness are numerous and in-clude congenital, neurogenic, neoplastic, inflamma-tory, and traumatic possibilities. A differential diag-nosis of hoarseness in children is included in Table 46-3.

AT A GLANCE . . .

Hoarseness

Pathogenesis: abnormality in the structure and/or function of the vocal cords.

Evaluation: age of onset, rate of progression, and association with trauma, surgery, or infection should be documented; physical includes evaluation of the skin, auscultation of the neck and chest, neurologic evaluation, and flexible fiberoptic laryngoscopy.

Differential Diagnosis: congenital, neurogenic, neoplastic, inflammatory, and traumatic possibilities.

TABLE 46-3: Differential Diagnosis of Hoarseness in Children

Congenital
  Laryngomalacia
  Glottic web
  Vocal cord sulcus
  Laryngocele
  Mucous retention cyst
  Lymphatic malformation
  Hemangioma
  Cri du chat syndrome
Neurologic
  Vocal cord paralysis
Traumatic
  Vocal cord nodules
  Hematoma
  Laryngeal fracture
  Arytenoid dislocation
Neoplasm
  Papilloma
  Neurofibroma
  Carcinoma
Inflammatory
  Laryngitis
  Laryngotracheitis
  Supraglottitis

REFERENCES

1. Tucker JA, Tucker GF. Some aspects of fetal laryngeal development. Ann Otol Rhinol Laryngol 1975; 84:49-55.
2. Myer CM III, Auringer ST, Wiatrak BJ. Magnetic reso-nance imaging in the diagnosis of innominate artery compression of the trachea. Arch Otolaryngol Head Neck Surg 1990; 116(3):314-316.
3. Friedman EM, Vastola AP, McGill TJ, et al. Chronic pediatric stridor: Etiology and outcome. Laryngo-scope 1990; 100(3):227-280.
4. Holinger LD, Sanders AD. Chronic cough in infants and children. An update. Laryngoscope 1991; 101:596-605.
5. Cohen SR, Thompson JW, Geller KA, et al. Voice change in the pediatric patient: A differential diagno-sis. Ann Otol Rhinol Laryngol 1983; 92:437-443.

47 Congenital Anomalies of the Larynx and Trachea

C. Anthony Hughes, and Michael E. Dunham

Congenital airway anomalies (CAAs) usually present with respiratory or feeding symptoms in the neonate or infant. Most anomalies affect the larynx and comprise greater than 85% of the stridor cases in children <2.5 years of age.[1] Given the potential sequelae of upper airway obstruction in this age group, clinicians managing these children should have an organized approach to diagnosis and treatment. Intervention for CAAs varies from simple observation to extensive airway reconstruction. This chapter gives an overview of the most common CAAs, and emphasizes diagnostic and therapeutic principles and pathways.

EVALUATION AND MANAGEMENT OF CONGENITAL AIRWAY ANOMALIES

Diagnosis

Most children with a CAA present with *stridor*. The evaluation focuses on the distinction between self-limited lesions and conditions that are life-threatening. The evaluation progresses from noninvasive to invasive studies that are guided by the suspected risk to the airway. Practice Pathway 47–1 outlines the diagnosis for stridor.

> ### SPECIAL CONSIDERATION:
> The evaluation of a child with a suspected congenital laryngeal or tracheal anomaly should focus on the distinction between self-limited lesions and conditions that are life-threatening.

The initial interview with the family includes a detailed history covering various aspects of respiratory function, phonation (cry), and feeding. Any history of stridor is characterized by its quality, intensity, duration, and exacerbating factors. Stridor should be differentiated from stertor or pulmonary wheezing and characterized as inspiratory, expiratory, or biphasic. Other important characteristics include severity (the parents' assessment), progression, cyanosis, and sleep disturbances. A history of recurrent spitting-up, dysphasia, feeding intolerance, or aspiration can be associated with gastroesophageal reflux (GER), laryngeal cleft, or vocal fold paralysis. The quality of the cry is also helpful. A weak cry may point to vocal fold paralysis, whereas a strong cry with only inspiratory stridor is more consistent with a supraglottic lesion.

The initial physical exam includes head and neck inspection, pulmonary auscultation, and a survey of the skin for cutaneous lesions. The clinician should observe how changes in the child's position affect the quality and intensity of the stridor and note any drooling or feeding difficulties.

High-voltage, soft-tissue, anterior-posterior and lateral airway films may help localize the lesion. A barium esophagogram can detect external compression or a tracheoesophageal fistula (TEF). Computed tomography (CT) or magnetic resonance imaging (MRI) is useful in defining vascular anomalies including vascular rings, pulmonary artery slings, or aberrant innominate artery.

When assessing the child with stridor, it is important to confirm the diagnosis visually. For some lesions, this can be established in the office with flexible fiberoptic laryngoscopy (FFL). Office FFL should be performed in children for whom operative endoscopy under general anesthesia is not indicated currently. Suspected laryngomalacia is the usual indication. The endoscopist performs the exam with an assistant holding the child's head while she is

Pediatric Otolaryngology, Edited by R.F. Wetmore, H.R. Muntz, and T.J. McGill. Thieme Medical Publishers, Inc., New York © 2000.

Practice Pathway 47–1   DIAGNOSTIC PATHWAY FOR CONGENITAL STRIDOR

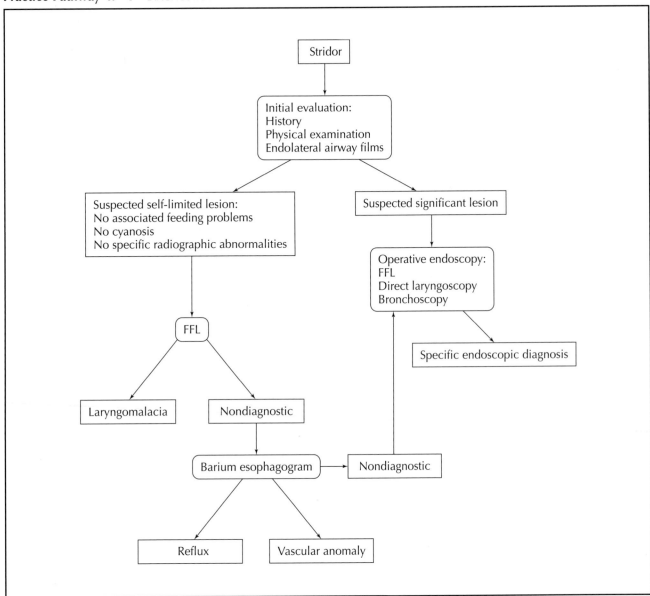

Abbreviations: FFL, Flexible Fiberoptic Laryngoscopy.

restrained. A few drops of topical lidocaine (2%) can provide topical anesthesia in children >1 year of age.

With the initial history and physical and radiographic findings, the diagnostic pathway branches depending on the severity of the lesion. If a significant CAA is suspected, operative endoscopy under general anesthesia is indicated. The most important diagnostic tool used to evaluate airway lesions in children is endoscopy.[2] Prior to anesthesia, an awake flexible endoscopy is performed to assess cord mobility. When possible, the anesthesiologist should maintain spontaneous ventilation during general anesthesia. Topical lidocaine applied to the larynx and trachea supplements the general anesthetic. The larynx can be sized using endotracheal tubes and checking for appropriate leak pressures.[3]

SPECIAL CONSIDERATION:

The most important diagnostic tool used to evaluate airway lesions in children is endoscopy.

Treatment

Initial treatment for most CAAs includes maintaining an airway and safe feeding. Ancillary procedures such as tracheotomy and gastrostomy tube placement may be necessary before the underlying lesion is repaired definitively. Children presenting with significant distress should be evaluated in the operating room where there is the ability to perform a tracheotomy if required. Once a safe airway is established, the surgeon can proceed with further diagnostic or operative interventions. Treatment then becomes a matter of managing the specific underlying condition.

CONGENITAL ANOMALIES OF THE LARYNX AND TRACHEA

Laryngomalacia

Laryngomalacia is the most common cause of stridor in infants. Presenting symptoms include inspiratory stridor and feeding difficulties. Apnea is rare and the infant's cry is usually normal. On fluoroscopic examination, the supraglottic structures may be seen to collapse. During awake flexible endoscopy, the epiglottis may be omega-shaped and appear to fold posteriorly with inspiration. The cuneiform cartilages are prominent and prolapse into the glottis with inspiration (Fig. 47–1).

The onset of stridor is usually within the first few weeks of life, and consists of an intermittent fluttering inspiratory noise. It is louder with supine positioning, crying, or agitation. In some patients, it is louder during sleep. The severity of the stridor typically worsens with growth and increasing oxygen demands and then slowly resolves between 6 and 18 months of age.[4]

Infants with gastroesophageal reflux disease (GERD) may be affected more severely by laryngomalacia. Airway symptoms often are improved with antireflux precautions and medications. Central neurologic disorders associated with neuromuscular coordination difficulties are likely to exacerbate laryngomalacia in affected infants.

Awake flexible laryngoscopy confirms the diagnosis. If the history is severe enough to warrant operative evaluation for associated lesions, FFL evaluation should be postponed until the time of bronchoscopy.

Most cases of laryngomalacia can be managed with simple reassurance and observation (Practice Pathway 47-2). Occasionally, home monitoring is helpful when the parents are anxious about caring for the infant at home. In cases where the symptoms of laryngomalacia are severe and result in airway distress, apnea, or failure to thrive, *epiglottoplasty* (a surgical procedure that involves division of the aryepiglottic folds) may prevent the need for a tracheostomy or alternative modes of feeding.[5]

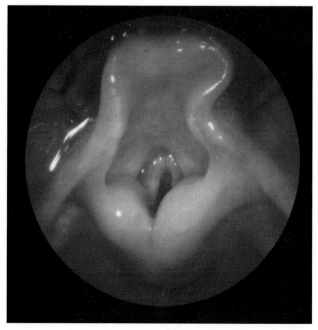

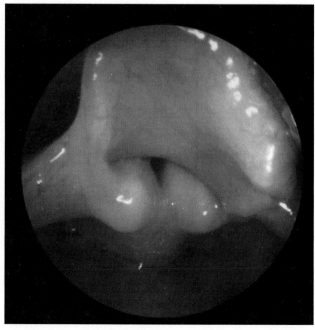

A   B

Figure 47–1:   (A) Laryngomalacia on expiration, and (B) on inspiration.

Practice Pathway 47–2   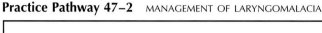 MANAGEMENT OF LARYNGOMALACIA

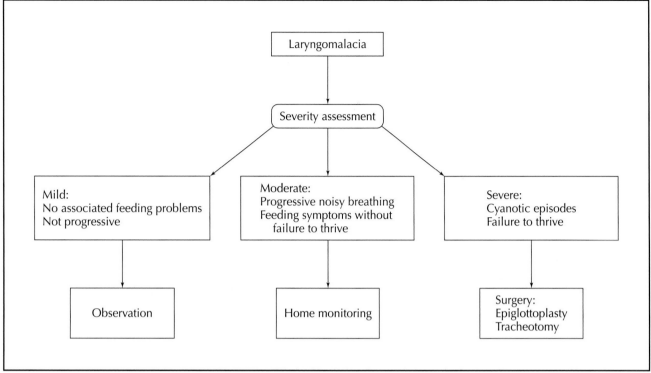

Vocal Fold Paralysis

Vocal fold paralysis (VFP) is the second most common laryngeal anomaly in neonates after laryngomalacia. VFP accounts for approximately 10% of all congenital laryngeal lesions. Most bilateral abductor VFP cases in infants are congenital, and approximately half of these patients have additional anomalies.[6,7] When VFP is diagnosed in an infant, central or acquired cases must be ruled out. Arnold-Chiari malformation is the most common cause of bilateral VFP in newborns. In this condition, VFP probably results from brainstem compression and stretching of the vagal nerve rootlets due to caudal displacement of the brainstem or cerebellum into the foramen magnum. Other less common acquired causes of bilateral VFP in infants include laryngeal neoplasm and birth trauma.

Children with congenital bilateral VFP usually present with respiratory compromise. Stridor may be inspiratory or biphasic. The voice or cry is weak and breathy in unilateral paralysis, but may be normal in bilateral cases. Aspiration and/or feeding difficulties often are present and may be the only presenting symptoms leading to an endoscopic evaluation for diagnosis. The diagnosis is made by FFL exam in the office or operating room. Vocal fold mobility should be assessed while the patient is awake without topical anesthesia to the larynx.

Other preoperative studies that may be helpful include chest radiography, lateral and AP airway films or fluoroscopy, and a barium swallow. CT or MRI may be helpful in the diagnosis of central nervous system (CNS) lesions. Infants suspected of having GERD should undergo a pH-probe.

Treatment for VFP is designed to stabilize the airway, provide for feeding and adequate nutrition, and avoid complications related to aspiration (Practice Pathway 47-3). Surgical intervention may include tracheotomy for airway stabilization, especially in bilateral cases. Most surgeons defer further surgical attempts to establish an airway in cases of bilateral VFP until the patient is 4 to 5 years of age. At that time, transverse cordotomy and arytenoidec-

Practice Pathway 47-3   MANAGEMENT OF VOCAL FOLD PARALYSIS

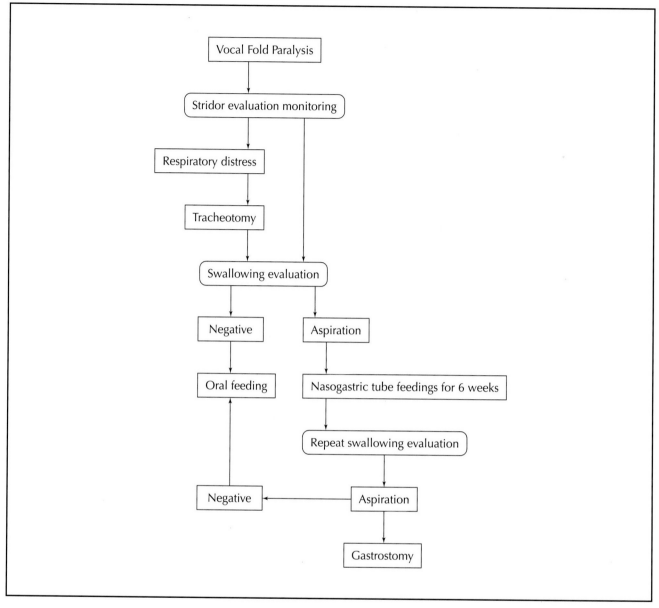

tomy can been used to improve the airway and promote decannulation.[8-10] Unfortunately, aspiration with pulmonary complications is common in children with VFP, and feeding by long-term nasogastric intubation or gastrostomy often is required.

Cri du Chat Syndrome[11]

Cri du chat syndrome is a rare and unusual syndrome in which affected infants present with a characteristic high-pitched cry that resembles the mewing of a cat. The laryngeal findings include an incomplete closure of the posterior glottis that suggests paralysis of the interarytenoid muscle. This syndrome is the result of a partial deletion of chromosome 5, and is associated with mental retardation, microcephaly, characteristic facies, and congenital heart disease. In spite of the laryngeal incompetence, affected children do not have respiratory distress or significant aspiration.

Laryngeal Cysts, Webs, Laryngoceles, and Clefts[12,13]

These congenital morphologic anomalies of the larynx usually present at or shortly after birth with signs of respiratory compromise and feeding difficulties. *Laryngoceles* are air-filled dilations of the

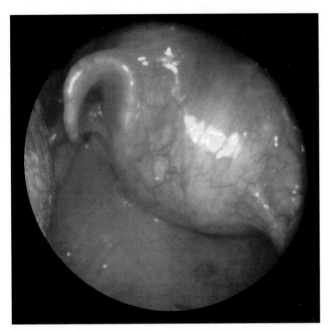

Figure 47-2:   Endoscopic appearance of a lateral saccular cyst.

laryngeal saccule that communicate with the laryngeal ventricle. Internal laryngoceles arise in the anterior ventricle and extend posteriorly and superiorly to the false vocal fold and aryepiglottic fold. External laryngoceles extend cephalad through the thyrohyoid membrane.

Saccular cysts may appear clinically identical to laryngoceles but should be distinguishable on endoscopy. Saccular cysts are fluid-filled and lack communication with the airway. Anterior saccular cysts are mucosal-covered and protrude between the false and true vocal folds. Lateral saccular cysts extend into the false vocal fold and aryepiglottic fold (Fig. 47-2). CT may be helpful in determining the extent of these lesions (Fig. 47-3).

Surgical treatment of laryngoceles, if required, consists of endoscopic marsupialization. Saccular cysts may respond to endoscopic marsupialization, but usually require removal of the entire cyst lining. Definitive therapy may require tracheotomy and excision through a laryngofissure approach with postoperative stenting (Fig. 47-4).

> ### SPECIAL CONSIDERATION:
>
> Whereas laryngoceles can be treated with endoscopic marsupialization, saccular cysts usually require removal of the entire cyst lining through a laryngofissure approach.

Laryngeal webs present with respiratory compromise that is dependent on the size and location

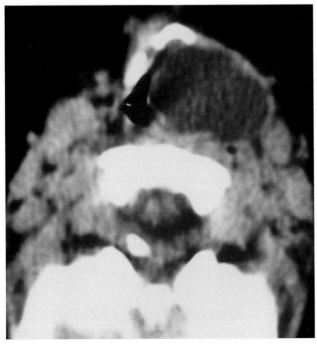

Figure 47-3:   CT scan of the neck demonstrating an extensive saccular cyst.

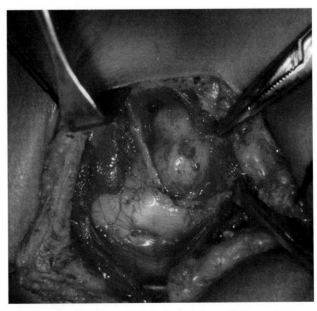

Figure 47-4:   Transcervical excision of a lateral saccular cyst.

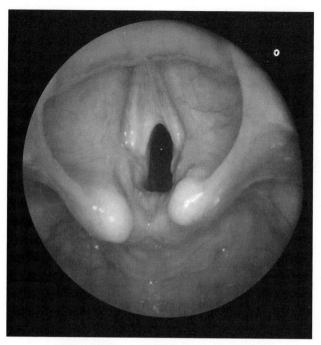

Figure 47–5: Congenital laryngeal web.

tory and may be associated with a barking cough. Many children have a history of recurrent croup. The diagnosis is suggested by subglottic narrowing noted on airway films and is confirmed by endoscopy. If symptoms are severe, the condition may require anterior laryngotracheal decompression (i.e., anterior cricoid split) or laryngotracheal reconstruction with a cartilage graft. Tracheostomy may be necessary in severe cases.

SPECIAL CONSIDERATION:

Congenital subglottic stenosis usually is associated with a small or malformed cricoid cartilage.

of the web. Most webs are located anteriorly (Fig. 47-5). Thin webs can be lysed endoscopically, whereas thick webs require laryngofissure with stenting. Posterior glottic webs are more difficult to remedy and have a higher recurrence rate.

Laryngeal clefts are rare anomalies that present with signs of stridor and aspiration.[14] An esophagogram may show spillage of contrast material from the upper esophagus into the trachea. The diagnosis is made by suspension microlaryngoscopy with direct palpation and measurement of the posterior glottis (Figs. 47-6 and 47-7). Type I lesions are confined to the level of the interarytenoid space above the level of the vocal folds. Type II lesions represent a partial cricoid cleft. Type III and IV lesions transverse the cricoid completely.[15] Type II or III clefts usually require an anterior thyrotomy or lateral pharyngotomy approach with multiple-layer closure.

Congenital Subglottic Stenosis

Congenital subglottic stenosis usually is associated with a small or malformed cricoid cartilage, with or without thickening of the underlying submucosal layer. Clinically, the diagnosis is considered when a 4-mm scope or age-appropriate-sized endotracheal tube cannot pass through the subglottic larynx in an infant who has not been intubated previously.[16] Most children present with symptoms of upper airway obstruction. The stridor is biphasic or inspira-

Laryngeal Hemangioma

Hemangiomas are proliferative endothelial lesions that are found commonly on the skin of infants. Rarely, these lesions may affect such organ systems as the brain or liver or may be so extensive as to cause arteriovenous shunting that results in congestive heart failure. *Laryngeal hemangiomas* typically are found in the subglottis and may occlude the airway in one of two forms. Typically, subglottic hemangiomas may develop in the submucosa of the posterior subglottis, forming a mass lesion that impinges on the airway in a posterior to anterior direction. In other cases, the lesion may spread in a circumferential pattern, causing narrowing of the subglottic airway. Cutaneous hemangiomas are found in 50% of patients with a subglottic hemangioma, so a high index of suspicion should be maintained in any infant who presents with progressive biphasic stridor during the first few months of life. In addition to stridor, affected infants may present with a "barking" cough, intermittent respiratory distress, hoarseness, and failure to thrive. The diagnosis of a subglottic hemangioma may be suggested on a lateral neck radiograph; however, confirmation should be made endoscopically. Lesions should not be biopsied because of the risk of bleeding. Treatment includes observation, corticosteroids, laser excision, open excision through a laryngofissure, and tracheostomy. This topic is discussed more extensively in Chapter 55.

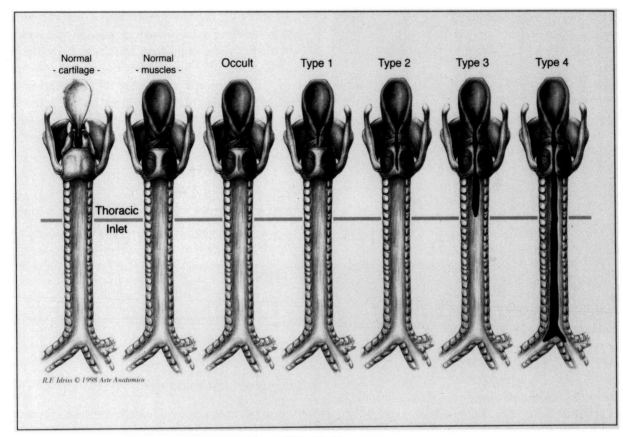

Figure 47-6:   Classification of laryngeal clefts.

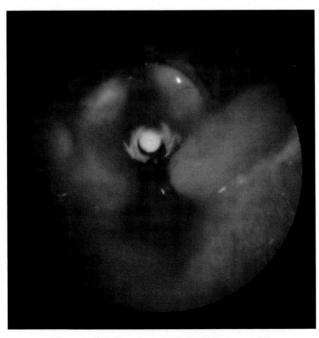

Figure 47-7:   Laryngeal cleft (type III).

Tracheoesophageal Fistula

Five major types of TEF have been recognized (See Chapter 33). The most common form of TEF is the *type III anomaly* consisting of an upper esophageal pouch with distal tracheal-esophageal fistula (Fig. 47-8). The opening into the trachea is immediately proximal to the carina along the posterior wall. *H-type* fistulas are direct communications between the esophagus and trachea in the lower cervical area.

Symptoms appear at birth with respiratory compromise and aspiration. Associated congenital anomalies include heart disease, visceral malrotations, and genitourinary abnormalities. The fistula may be diagnosed with direct contrast injection and fluoroscopy. H-type fistulas are often diagnosed endoscopically (Fig. 47-9). The diagnosis and localization of the fistula tract can be confirmed with the passage of a small ureteric catheter through the tracheal opening. Surgical correction usually is performed shortly after birth through a thoracotomy approach (Fig. 47-10). Postoperative respiratory difficulties may occur due to tracheomalacia at the site of the repair, vocal fold paralysis, recurrent or

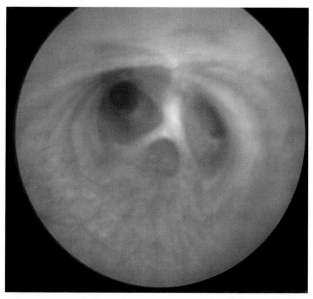

Figure 47–8:   Tracheoesopheageal fistula (type III), tracheal opening.

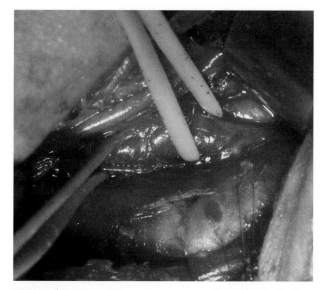

Figure 47–10:   Cervical exposure of an H-type tracheoesophageal fistula.

secondary fistula, or previously undiagnosed laryngeal cleft.

Congenital Tracheal Stenosis[18,19]

Congenital tracheal stenosis usually results from complete tracheal rings. These anomalies vary from short segmental lesions to involvement of the entire trachea (Fig. 47-11). With segmental stenosis, sections of narrowed trachea may interrupt sections

of normal caliber trachea. A funnel-shaped stenosis results in a progressive narrowing of the trachea in a distal direction. The most severe form results in tracheal atresia or agenesis that is not compatible with life. It is not unusual for tracheal stenosis to be associated with other anomalies that may affect the tracheal airway, such as pulmonary artery sling. Diagnosis of tracheal stenosis is confirmed by bronchoscopy, and treatment depends upon the severity

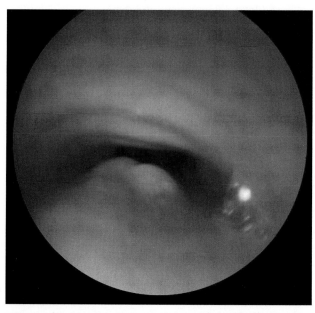

Figure 47–9:   Tracheoesopheageal fistula (H-type), tracheal opening.

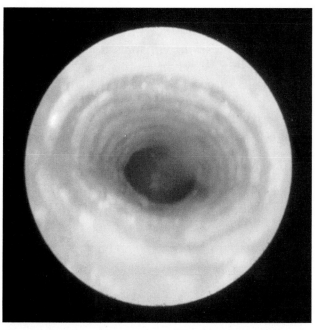

Figure 47–11:   Congenital tracheal stenosis with complete tracheal rings.

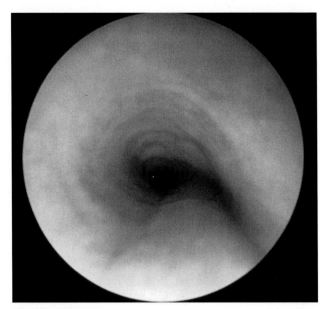

Figure 47–12: Aberrant innominate artery compression of the trachea.

of stenosis. Because stenotic segments appear to grow faster than normal surrounding trachea, asymptomatic or mildly-symptomatic children may be treated by observation alone. Most patients with symptomatic tracheal stenosis require tracheoplasty through a thoracotomy approach with or without the use of cardiopulmonary bypass.

Vascular Rings and Tracheal Compression[20]

Tracheal compression by vascular anomalies presents with symptoms that mimic primary tracheomalacia. Endoscopy, however, demonstrates distal tracheal compression with pulsation. An esophogram may show external esophageal compression suggesting a vascular ring. CT or MRI confirms the diagnosis in most cases. Since the advent of magnetic resonance angiography (MRA), angiography often is not indicate for confirmation. The aberrant innominate artery has a characteristic endoscopic appearance with pulsatile compression of the right anterolateral wall of the trachea (Fig. 47–12). This gives the tracheal lumen a triangular appearance.

SPECIAL CONSIDERATION:

Tracheal compression due to a vascular anomaly presents with symptoms that mimic primary tracheomalacia.

Pulmonary artery sling usually presents with progressive respiratory distress. The anomaly results when the left pulmonary artery arises from the right, encircles the trachea, and passes between the trachea and esophagus. The vessel compresses the right lower trachea and right main bronchus. Pulmonary artery sling often is associated with congenital tracheal stenosis and complete tracheal rings. The double aortic arch and right arch with left ligamentum arteriosum completely encircle the trachea and esophagus. Symptoms are usually present at birth and include biphasic stridor exacerbated by feeding. Children with vascular anomalies respond well to surgical correction; however, segmental tracheomalacia may result at the site of the compression, and it is not unusual for stridor and feeding difficulties to persist after surgery. Practice Pathway 47–4 outlines the management for vascular tracheal compression.

AT A GLANCE . . .

Congenital Laryngeal and Tracheal Anomalies

Laryngeal
  Laryngomalacia
  Vocal fold paralysis
  Laryngeal cysts
  Laryngeal webs
  Laryngeal clefts
  Laryngocele
  Congenital subglottic stenosis
  Subglottic hemangioma

Tracheal
  Tracheoesophageal fistula
  Congenital tracheal stenosis
  Vascular rings
  Primary tracheomalacia

CONCLUSION

With the exception of laryngomalacia, the incidence of most congenital and tracheal anomalies is rare. Most infants with these disorders present with stridor, respiratory distress, and often feeding difficulties. Direct airway endoscopy is the primary method by which these lesions are evaluated. Once

Practice Pathway 47–4   MANAGEMENT OF VASCULAR TRACHEAL COMPRESSION

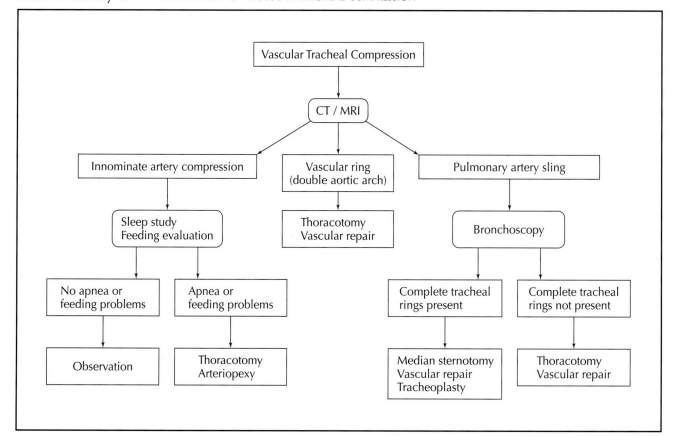

diagnosed, the goals of treatment include the establishment of long-term airway stability and an adequate feeding route. Most of these congenital laryngeal anomalies have a significant impact upon the patient's ability to thrive, and surgical correction usually is required.

REFERENCES

1. Zalzal GH. Stridor and airway compromise. Pediatr Clin North Am 1989; 36:1389–1402.
2. Holinger LD. Diagnostic endoscopy of the pediatric airway. Laryngoscope 1989; 99:346–348.
3. Myer CM III, O'Connor DM, Cotton RT. Proposed grading system for subglottic stenosis based on endotracheal tube sizes. Ann Otol Rhinol Laryngol 1994; 103:319–323.
4. Holinger LD. Etiology of stridor in the neonate, infant, and child. Ann Otol Rhinol Laryngol 1980; 89: 397–400.
5. Holinger LD, Konior RJ. Surgical management of severe laryngomalacia. Laryngoscope 1989; 99: 136–142.
6. Holinger LD, Holinger PC, Holinger PH. Etiology of bilateral abductor vocal cord paralysis–A review of 389 cases. Ann Otol Rhinol Laryngol 1976; 85: 428–436.
7. Grundfast KM, Harley E. Vocal cord paralysis. Otolaryngol Clin North Am 1989; 22:569.
8. Ossoff RH, Duncavage JA, Shapshay SM, et al. Endoscopic laser arytenoidectomy revisited. Ann Otol Rhinol Laryngol 1990; 99:764–771.
9. Ejnell H, Mansson I, Hallen O, et al. A simple operation for bilateral vocal cord paralysis. Laryngoscope 1984; 94:954–958.
10. Kashima HK. Bilateral vocal fold motion impairment: Pathophysiology and management by transverse cordotomy. Ann Otol Rhinol Laryngol 1991; 100:717–721.
11. Ward PH, Engel E, Nance WE. The larynx in the cri-du-chat syndrome. Laryngoscope 1968; 78:1716–1733.
12. DeSanto LW, Devine KD, Weiland LH. Cysts of the larynx—Classification. Laryngoscope 1970; 80: 145–176.

13. Holinger LD, Barnes DR, Smid LJ. Laryngocele and saccular cysts. Ann Otol Rhinol Laryngol 1978; 87: 675–685.

14. Benjamin B, Inglis A. Minor congenital laryngeal clefts: Diagnosis and classification. Ann Otol Rhinol Laryngol 1989; 98:417–420.

15. Moungthong G, Holinger LD. Laryngotracheoesophageal clefts. Ann Otol Rhinol Laryngol 1997; 106: 1002–1011.

16. Healy GB. Subglottic stenosis. Otolaryngol Clin North Am 1989; 22:599–606.

17. Tsai JY, Berkery L, Wesson DE, et al. Esophageal atresia and tracheoesophageal fistula: Surgical experience over two decades. Ann Thoracic Surg 1997; 64: 778–783.

18. Dunham ME, Holinger LD, Backer CL, et al. Management of severe congenital tracheal stenosis. Ann Otol Rhinol Laryngol 1994; 103:351–356.

19. Manson D, Filler R, Gordon R. Tracheal growth in congenital tracheal stenosis. Pediatr Radiol 1996; 26: 427–430.

20. Backer CL, Ilbawi MN, Idriss FS, et al. Vascular anomalies causing tracheoesophageal compression. J Thorac Cardiovasc Surg 1990; 97:725–731.

48 Vocal Cord Paralysis

Andrew L. de Jong and Ellen M. Friedman

> Untold thousands of infants have asphyxiated because of bilateral abductor paralysis—the cyanosis being attributed to a persistent foramen ovale or failure of respiration to start.
> Chevalier Jackson, 1937[1]

For a long time, *vocal cord paralysis* (VCP) has been recognized as a significant cause of stridor and hoarseness in children. The earliest written report of childhood VCP was published in Guy's Hospital Reports in 1882. Taylor reported a 12-year-old girl with a diagnosis of hysterical catalepsy and inspiratory stridor. Laryngoscopy revealed the vocal cords to be "close together."[2] In 1953, Clerf reviewed a series of 293 patients, 10% of whom had congenital cord paralysis.[3] W. F. Goff analyzed 229 cases of VCP in 1979. He was the first to divide the etiology of VCP into congenital and acquired.[4]

VCP can affect any or all of the normal laryngeal functions of respiration, voice production, or deglutition. The manifestations of VCP vary greatly with age, however. Today, the otolaryngologist has become central in establishing the definitive diagnosis and in managing laryngeal pathology in neonates, infants, and children.

This chapter describes the approach to the child with VCP, the various etiologies for VCP, and the management strategies for it. Unilateral and bilateral VCP are discussed with emphasis on their distinct presentation, evaluation, and treatment decisions in the pediatric patient.

EPIDEMIOLOGY

VCP, unilateral or bilateral, accounts for approximately 10% of all congenital laryngeal lesions.[5] It is second in frequency only to laryngomalacia as a cause of neonatal stridor.[6] Due to difficulties in making the diagnosis, the previously reported incidence of VCP in the literature may not represent the true number of children with it. Now, flexible laryngoscopy and enhanced anesthetic techniques allow otolaryngologists to make this diagnosis more accurately. With these technical advances and improved infant survival rates, the actual incidence of VCP may need to be reexamined. VCP manifests early in life, and is without gender predilection.[6,7,8] The majority is recognized before the age of 2.[7] Cohen et al. reported 100 children with VCP, 58% of whom presented within the first 12 hours of birth.[8]

> **SPECIAL CONSIDERATION:**
>
> Unilateral or bilateral vocal cord paralysis accounts for approximately 10% of all congenital laryngeal lesions, most of which are associated with other congenital anomalies.

Isolated unilateral or bilateral VCP is rare in the pediatric age group. Usually, it is only one manifestation of a multisystem anomaly. Although most frequently associated with central nervous system (CNS) malformations, VCP can be seen in conjunction with other congenital anomalies such as cardiovascular or pulmonary malformations.[9] A higher incidence of other associated laryngeal malformations such as clefts or stenosis also has been reported.[5,6,10]

NEUROANATOMY

A thorough understanding of laryngeal neuroanatomy is important when evaluating a child with VCP. The neuromuscular pathways of the larynx have been well defined.[10-13] *Cortical function re-*

Pediatric Otolaryngology, Edited by R.F. Wetmore, H.R. Muntz, and T.J. McGill. Thieme Medical Publishers, Inc., New York © 2000.

lates to the formulation of speech and language and not to direct laryngeal muscular innervation, which is controlled at the subcortical level. Extensive interhemispheric connections between cortical areas also are involved in speech production. Thus, unilateral lesions of the cerebrum rarely affect individual vocal cord motion.

Corticobulbar fibers connect the cortex to the brainstem. These fibers descend through the internal capsule to synapse on motor neurons in the nucleus ambiguus within the medulla (Fig. 48-1).[13] The *nucleus ambiguus* serves as the relay station for laryngeal function. Although there is some crossover, the ipsilateral nucleus ambiguus receives visceral efferent fibers that provide unilateral motor innervation of the larynx. Sensory input transmitted through the nucleus ambiguus helps form the afferent arc of the laryngeal protective reflexes (i.e., coughing and vomiting). Lower motor neurons leave the nucleus ambiguus and travel laterally within the midbrain. From here, the lower motor neurons exit the brainstem between the olive and pyramid as a series of rootlets (see Fig. 48-1). The roolets are divided between the vagus (i.e., the tenth cranial nerve) and the spinal accessory (i.e., eleventh cranial nerve) nerves. The majority of the lower motor neurons travel briefly with the spinal accessory nerve.

The *vagus nerve,* the largest and most widely-distributed cranial nerve, initially exits the skull base and consists of parasympathetic and afferent fibers. The superior (i.e., jugular) and inferior (i.e., nodose) ganglia are the sensory ganglia of the vagus nerve and are located within the petrous temporal bone. Below the nodose ganglia, the vagus nerve is joined by motor neurons from the nucleus ambiguus that were associated with the eleventh cranial nerve. As the vagus nerve exits the skull base through the jugular foramen; it immediately starts branching. Small nerve branches are distributed to the pharyngeal constrictor muscles as well as the muscles of the soft palate. Disorders involving midbrain function, therefore, potentially can cause more serious laryngeal dysfunction than cerebral injuries. Such lesions can affect all of the three essential laryngeal functions of breathing, phonation, and deglutition.

Caudal to the nodose ganglia, the vagus nerve branches to form the *superior laryngeal nerve* (SLN), which then divides into an internal and an external branch (see Fig. 48-1). The main trunk of the vagus nerve continues a parallel descent within the carotid sheath through the neck and into the thorax on both sides. Once in the chest, the course differs for the right and left nerves. On the right side, the tenth cranial nerve branches again to form the right *recurrent laryngeal nerve* (RLN). It loops below the subclavian artery and turns in a posterior-superior direction, ascending towards the larynx in the tracheoesophageal groove. On the left side, the vagal trunk extends further into the chest before branching. The left RLN is formed at the level of the aortic arch. Traversing below the ligamentum arteriosum, it then ascends towards the larynx in the tracheoesophageal groove. Both RLN then enter the larynx at the cricothyroid joint (see Fig. 48-1).

Sensation and motor function for each side of the larynx are supplied by three nerves, all of which are branches of the vagus nerve. The SLN divides into the internal and external branches. The internal branch provides sensation to the endolarynx, and the external branch provides innervation to the cricothyroid muscle. All remaining intrinsic laryngeal muscles are innervated by the RLN (Table 48-1).

ETIOLOGY

VCP is a sign not a diagnosis, and a thorough search for the underlying cause is essential in every case.

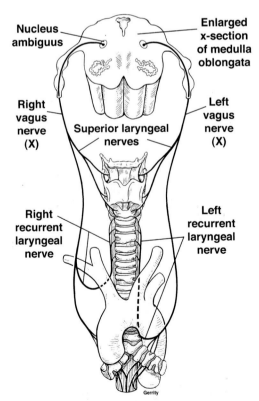

Figure 48-1: Courses of the left and right vagus nerves.

TABLE 48–1: Intrinsic Laryngeal Musculature

Muscle	Innervation	Vocal Cord Action
Cricothyroid	SLN	Adduction, Tensor
Interarytenoid	RLN	Adduction
Lateral cricoarytenoid	RLN	Adduction
Posterior cricoarytenoid	RLN	Abduction
Thyroarytenoid	RLN	Adduction, Tensor

Abbreviations: SLN, Superior Laryngeal Nerve; RLN, Recurrent Laryngeal Nerve.

Children are subject to some of the same causes of VCP as adults, namely surgical trauma and neoplasms. But these common reasons for VCP in adults are not the most common causes in children. An idiopathic or a neurologic etiology remains the most common factor in children.[7]

Traditionally VCP in children has been divided into two broad categories: congenital and acquired. Each group accounts for approximately one half of the cases.[7,9,10] Alternatively a systems approach to the problem offers a thorough survey and allows the otolaryngologist to formulate a complete differential diagnosis (Table 48-2). Table 48-3 summarizes the etiologies of VCP.

Central Nervous System

CNS anomalies are implicated in pediatric VCP in 25 to 35% of cases.[7,14] CNS involvement is almost always the result of brainstem pathology. Supranuclear etiologies are rare causes of VCP because of the extensive interhemispheric connections of the laryngeal efferent neural pathways.

The most common CNS congenital anomaly that is implicated in VCP is the *Arnold-Chiari malfor-mation* (ACM). Typically, it is associated with bilateral VCP. Some physicians feel that any infant born with an ACM and a high-pitch, inspiratory stridor has bilateral VCP until proven otherwise.[13]

There are two forms of ACM. *Type I ACM* involves an isolated caudal displacement of the cerebellum without an associated meningomyelocele. *Type II ACM,* which often is associated with a meningomyelocele, manifests caudal displacement of the cerebellum and brainstem. Although both types are associated with VCP, Type II is implicated more commonly.[15-17] The pathogenesis of bilateral VCP in ACM patients is thought to be secondary to traction on the vagus nerve by caudal displacement of the cerebellum and/or brainstem (although many physicians indicate that this is an oversimplification of what is probably a complex, multifactorial process).[7,18-21] The complex nature of the respiratory problems in ACM patients cannot be overemphasized. These children often have a concomitant central respiratory problem, and may continue to experience respiratory difficulties even after tracheotomy is performed.[13]

Less frequent CNS causes of VCP include leukodystrophy, encephalocele, hydrocephalus, and cerebral or nuclear dysgenesis.[14,20-24] Central neural degenerative diseases such as syringomyelia or syringobulbia can be associated with bilateral VCP.[23,24] *Amyotrophic lateral sclerosis* (ALS), occasionally presenting in the second decade of life, also may manifest as unilateral or bilateral vocal cord involvement.[11] Neural injury secondary to perinatal hypoxia also must be considered as a cause of VCP. Rarely, bilateral VCP has been attributed to a cortical stroke.[25]

TABLE 48–2: Signs and Symptoms of VCP

Clinical Finding	
Unilateral VCP	*Bilateral VCP*
+	+ +
−	+
−	+
+	−
+	−
+/−	+/−
+/−	+/−
+/−	+/−

Abbreviations: +, finding present; −, finding not present; +/−, variable presence of finding.

AT A GLANCE . . .

Central Nervous System Causes of VCP

- Arnold-Chiari malformation
- Leukodystrophy
- Encephalocele
- Hydrocephalus
- Cerebral or nuclear dysgenesis
- Syringomyelia/syringobulbia
- Amyotrophic lateral sclerosis
- Perinatal hypoxia
- Cortical stroke

TABLE 48–3:   Etiology of VCP

Etilogy	Unilateral VCP (example)	Bilateral VCP (example)
CNS	infrequent	common (ACM)
PNS	infrequent	common (Myasthenia gravis)
Trauma	common (thoracic surgery, ETT)	infrequent
Neoplasm	common (skull base tumor)	infrequent
Inflammatory	infrequent	infrequent (Guillian-Barré)
Cardiovascular anomaly	common (VSD)	infrequent
Metabolic	infrequent (chemotherapy)	infrequent
Genetic	infrequent	infrequent
Idiopathic	common	common

Abbreviations: CNS, central nervous system; PNS, peripheral nervous system; ACM, Arnold-Chiari malformation; ETT, endotracheal intubation; VSD, ventricular septal defect.

Peripheral Nervous System

Peripheral neuropathic and progressive neurologic disorders also may affect vocal cord function in children. Myasthenia gravis, although usually a disorder of young adults, can affect infants and children.[26,27] Vocal cord involvement can be a rare manifestation of myasthenia gravis. However, when this occurs, there is usually bilateral cord immobility.[10] Myotonic dystrophy, Werdnig-Hoffman disease (i.e., infantile muscular atrophy), benign congenital hypotonia, and Charcot-Marie-Tooth disease all have been implicated in pediatric VCP.[6,10]

AT A GLANCE . . .

Peripheral Nervous System Causes of VCP

- Myasthenia gravis
- Myotonic dystrophy
- Werdnig-Hoffman disease
- Benign congenital hypotonia
- Charcot-Marie-Tooth disease

Trauma

Although direct or surgical trauma to the vagus or RLN is a common cause of VCP in adults, it is a rare cause of VCP in children. Surgical trauma involving the vagus nerve and its branches is most common after thoracic surgical procedures that involve the heart or great vessels.[20,23] Zhar and Smith reported a frequency of 8.8% of left VCP after patent ductus

arteriosus ligation.[28] Traumatic VCP is usually unilateral, although unilateral and bilateral VCP have been reported following tracheoesophageal fistula repair.[8] Posterior fossa trauma, as well as closed head injuries, also are known causes of bilateral VCP.[29,30]

Trauma from instrumentation of the larynx and hypopharynx can cause transient or permanent VCP. Unilateral and bilateral VCP is a well-documented complication of endotracheal intubation; it usually is associated with cuffed endotracheal tubes in adults.[31-33] Transient bilateral VCP after laryngeal mask airway (LMA) insertion has been reported.[34]

Birth trauma, which is often associated with unilateral paralysis, may be a potential source of injury. A history of difficult delivery, forced traction, or neck torsion during delivery have been implicated in VCP.[6,8] Abnormal cervical traction due to unusual intrauterine positioning is another possible etiologic factor.

Neoplasia

Tumors and congenital neoplasms of the skull base, neck, or mediastinum are an uncommon source of VCP in children. Unilateral VCP is more common when a neoplasm is the underlying cause, although bilateral VCP also has been reported.[6] In these situations, the VCP is a slow, progressive process that initially affects one side. Thyroid malignancy and benign thyroid hyperplasia can affect vocal cord function, but these are rare in children.[35]

Inflammatory Causes

Viral, bacterial, and granulomatous conditions have been implicated in pediatric VCP. Various encephalopathies (e.g., Reye's syndrome), poliomyelitis, diphtheria, rabies, tetanus, syphilis, and botulism have been reported as causing VCP in children.[2,5, 6,36,37] Fortunately, many of these diseases are rare today because of the use of antibiotics and immunization programs. Guillain-Barré syndrome continues to be associated with pediatric VCP. This demyelinating neuropathy rarely affects laryngeal function, but may involve both vocal cords.[38]

AT A GLANCE . . .

Inflammatory Causes of VCP

- Viral encephalopathies
- Poliomyelitis
- Diphtheria
- Rabies
- Tetanus
- Syphilis
- Botulism
- Guillain-Barré syndrome

Cardiovascular Anomalies

Congenital anomalies of the cardiovascular system frequently are associated with VCP. Left VCP is more common than right VCP. Because of its longer course and closer proximity to the heart, the left recurrent nerve is more vulnerable than the right in cases of congenital heart disease or cardiac surgery. Ventricular septal defect, tetralogy of Fallot, and cardiomegaly have been associated with VCP. Abnormalities of the great vessels including vascular rings, double aortic arch, and patent ductus arteriosus all have been implicated in laryngeal paralysis.[5,6,39]

Metabolic Causes

Unilateral and bilateral VCP has been reported in association with hypokalemia and organophosphate poisoning.[40,41] Vincristine-induced recurrent VCP has been well documented. The paralysis is dose-related and resolves slowly over a 4- to 6-week period after discontinuing the medication.[42,43]

Genetic Causes

Familial bilateral VCP is related to X-linked and autosomal-recessive inheritance patterns. The number of cases is small.[42-46]

Idiopathic Causes

In many studies, idiopathic paralysis ranks as the first or second most common cause of VCP in children, accounting for 36 to 47% of the cases in a variety of series.[8,9,14,28] Idiopathic VCP may represent a viral neuropathy similar to Bell's palsy or sudden sensorineural hearing loss (SNHL); however, such a link remains difficult to prove.

SIGNS AND SYMPTOMS

Any or all of the normal laryngeal functions (i.e., voice, respiration, or deglutition) may be abnormal in the pediatric patient with VCP. The signs and symptoms may be subtle, going unnoticed for months or being attributed to recurrent croup or asthma.[47] The most common manifestation of VCP unilateral or bilateral, in children is stridor (see Table 48–2).[6-9,14] Ineffective cough, aspiration, recurrent pneumonia, and feeding difficulties can be associated with unilateral or bilateral VCP. Respiratory distress is more severe in cases of bilateral VCP. Consistent stridor, cyanosis, and apnea are frequent findings in these cases.[7] Voice and cry may, in fact, be virtually normal in children with bilateral VCP. Children with unilateral VCP frequently have changes in phonation, hoarseness, dysphonia, or an abnormal cry.[7]

DIAGNOSTIC EVALUATION

The initial concern in any child with suspected VCP is airway stability. Extensive diagnostic evaluations should be deferred until the airway is stabilized or secured. Any child with severe stridor and respiratory compromise is best evaluated in the operating suite. The operating room should have appropriately-sized bronchoscopic equipment and the necessary resuscitation and emergency supplies. In those instances when respiratory distress is not a primary concern, a thorough unhurried evaluation may be undertaken.

The evaluation of a child with suspected VCP begins with a thorough history and physical examination, including an understanding of the quality of the voice or cry, the presence and severity of the stridor, and any associated feeding difficulties. A weak cough or a history of aspiration or recurrent pneumonia can be additional clues that point toward the larynx as a source of the child's problems. Any history of surgical or accidental trauma, including birth and surgical procedures involving the posterior fossa, thorax, or neck, must be elicited. Associated medical conditions or congenital anomalies, such as neurologic disorders or congenital heart disease, must be investigated. The initial physical examination centers on a survey of the stigmata of associated congenital anomalies. Associated findings that are pertinent to the severity or degree of the respiratory compromise such as intercostal retractions and respiratory rate should be documented.

Various methods have been used and reported in the literature to document VCP. Methods such as cinefluoroscopic examination, ultrasound, pulmonary function tests, and direct laryngoscopy under general anesthetic were frequently used to evaluate laryngeal function in children.[5-7,13,45-49] For a variety of reasons, these methods have proven unsatisfactory. During visualization of the vocal cords, rigid laryngoscopy may result in distortion of the larynx due to poor placement of the metal blade. This technique may lead to a misdiagnosis of VCP.[7,49,50] With the introduction and wide availability of flexible endoscopic equipment, flexible laryngoscopy in the awake patient has become the cornerstone for diagnosis of pediatric VCP. The vast majority of children with VCP are diagnosed accurately using this technique alone.[7] Nevertheless, flexible laryngoscopy can be challenging in the very young child with copious secretions, rapid respiration, narrowed epiglottis, or anterior-appearing larynx. In such cases, there may be a role for some of the previously mentioned techniques.

SPECIAL CONSIDERATION

Use of a rigid laryngoscope may lead to misdiagnosis of VCP due to distortion of the larynx by the laryngoscope blade.

Flexible laryngoscopy has several advantages over other methods of laryngeal evaluation in the pediatric patient. Flexible nasopharyngoscopy provides a dynamic view of the upper respiratory tract with minimal distortion. Other advantages of flexible laryngoscopy include the fact that it is a relatively safe and well tolerated in all age groups. Flexible nasopharyngoscopy also can be performed at the bedside or in the office setting and does not require a general anesthetic.

AT A GLANCE . . .

Advantages of Flexible Laryngoscopy

1. Provides dynamic view of larynx with minimal distortion
2. Relatively safe
3. Well tolerated
4. No need for general anesthesia

The clinical findings of VCP obligate the otolaryngologist to search for an underlying cause. In neonates, infants, and young children with suspected VCP, the focus and work-up differs from that required for adults. Compared to adults, in whom attention is directed to the neck and lung apices, the focus in children is on the brainstem and mediastinum as well as any potential etiologic factors elicited in the initial history and physical examination.[13] For cases in which the etiology is not apparent, the entire course of the efferent laryngeal nerves should be imaged. This should include computerized tomography (CT) or magnetic resonance imaging (MRI) with special attention to the brain, the brainstem, and the thorax. These imaging studies may demonstrate congenital anomalies of the brainstem, such as ACM, or of the mediastinum (Fig. 48–2).

Swallow function studies and cinefluoroscopy remain important components in the evaluation of children with VCP. These studies are important for two reasons: first, swallow function studies can provide evidence of subtle neurologic disorders that are associated with an abnormal swallowing mechanism and that also may be related to abnormal vocal cord function[13]; and second, a barium swallow may provide valuable information about the afferent laryngeal nerve input, revealing evidence of laryngeal

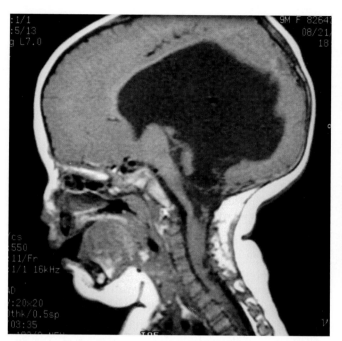

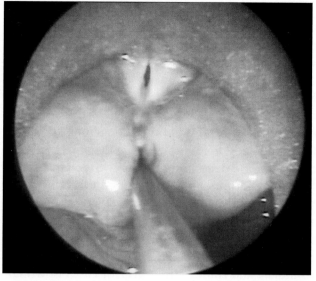

Figure 48–3: Photograph of the larynx of an infant who was referred with bilateral VCP. Direct laryngoscopy revealed an interarytenoid web. The laryngeal probe is placed posterior to the web.

Figure 48–2: *T1*-weighted sagittal midline MRI. The image shows an ACM type II with a dysplastic cervical-medullary junction extending into the mid-cervical region. Marked hydrocephalus also is present.

penetration of barium or aspiration. Additionally, a barium swallow also may document an associated mediastinal anomaly, such as a vascular ring.

Although flexible laryngoscopy has become invaluable in the diagnosis of pediatric VCP, rigid laryngoscopy and bronchoscopy continue to play a significant role in the identification of associated airway anomalies and unknown etiologies of VCP after noninvasive work-up has been completed. The diagnosis of idiopathic VCP requires the exclusion of underlying systematic conditions, occult neoplasm, or associated anomalies. Direct laryngoscopy is also critical in cases involving endolaryngeal trauma or endotracheal intubation. Unilateral or bilateral VCP must be differentiated from cricoarytenoid fixation or posterior glottic stenosis, both of which can mimic VCP (Fig. 48-3). Direct laryngoscopy allows close visual inspection and palpation of the arytenoid cartilage and the posterior glottis. This examination can best be performed under general anesthesia with spontaneous ventilation.[7,49,50] Appropriate anesthetic technique is critical in order to allow complete assessment of the child's airway. In difficult cases, confirmation of unilateral or bilateral VCP may require laryngeal electromyography. In contrast to adults, this diagnostic procedure in

children usually is performed under a general anesthetic at the time of the endoscopy.

MANAGEMENT

Factors that influence management decisions include etiology of the paralysis, prognosis for recovery, unilateral or bilateral involvement, and the severity of symptoms or associated conditions. These factors must be evaluated in conjunction with the goals of any intervention. Treatment goals in children with VCP include: (1) establishing and maintaining a safe and stable airway; (2) obtaining or preserving intelligible speech; and (3) swallowing without aspiration. A conservative approach with close observation may be indicated as the initial management step for children with VCP.

AT A GLANCE . . .

Treatment Goals for Vocal Cord Paralysis

- Establish/maintain safe airway
- Obtain/preserve speech
- Swallowing without aspiration

Since management strategies vary depending on the child's underlying condition, a global assessment of the child is essential. For example, a child with a progressive neuromuscular disease may require more aggressive initial management, as there is little potential for recovery from the paralysis. In other cases, the VCP may resolve with treatment of the underlying condition or congenital anomaly. One well-known example is the timely treatment of ACM or the decompression of hydrocephalus.[5,6,13,28] Many authors suggest that children with a meningomyelocele, ACM, and bilateral VCP not undergo an invasive airway procedure, such as tracheotomy, until a ventricle peritoneal shunt or posterior fossa decompression procedure is performed.[8,9,13,51] Grundfast and Harley stress that for cases in which the potential for airway improvement is good the airway should be secured with nasal tracheal intubation for at least 4 weeks prior to considering tracheotomy.[13]

Spontaneous resolution of unilateral or bilateral VCP is a much more frequent occurrence in the pediatric population. The reported rate of recovery varies within the literature from 16 to 64 percent.[6-9,14] Recovery has been noted from 6 weeks to 5 years after the initial diagnosis.[6-9,14] In the management of children, observation for one year is essential before any decision is made concerning irreversible laryngeal procedures. Practice Pathway 48-1 outlines the management for VCP.

Unilateral VCP

The management of unilateral VCP in children and adults differs greatly. Children adjust well to persistent, unilateral VCP with little sequelae. Unilateral VCP usually results in a weakened cry, but generally these children are able to maintain an adequate airway. Additional stresses such as trauma, vigorous activity, or an upper respiratory infection (URI) may not be well tolerated. Nevertheless, surgical intervention rarely is required in cases of unilateral VCP in infants or children. It is uncommon for a child with unilateral VCP to require a tracheotomy unless there are significant associated upper airway anomalies or evidence of chronic aspiration.[20,52]

Unilateral VCP rarely contributes to long-term voice quality problems in children. Laryngeal augmentation procedures and thyroplasty techniques, therefore, rarely are indicated in infants and young children. When unilateral VCP contributes to poor voice production, the treatment of choice remains speech therapy.[13,53]

Bilateral VCP

Children with bilateral VCP frequently require surgical intervention. The airway is markedly compromised, usually resulting in stridor and respiratory distress. Most physicians agree that tracheostomy is necessary in over 50 percent of these cases.[5] This position recently was challenged by Zhar and Smith who followed four neonates with bilateral VCP for an average of 6 months without airway intervention.[9] Fifty-two infants and children with bilateral VCP were followed by deGaudemar et al. for an average of 4 years and only 19 percent required tracheotomy.[14] Thus, expectant management without an artificial airway may be indicated more often than previously thought.

When indicated, the initial surgical procedure of choice is tracheotomy. Tracheotomy remains the least-aggressive surgical management step and the gold standard for the treatment of pediatric bilateral VCP. It is a potentially reversible procedure, allowing time for potential spontaneous laryngeal recovery. It also maintains a stable airway that affords an unobstructed view of the larynx for sequential reevaluation of vocal cord function. Once a tracheotomy is performed, repeat examinations are necessary to detect spontaneous return of laryngeal function or to plan further intervention. Serial endoscopic examination of these patients should be performed at 1- to 2-month intervals to detect return of laryngeal function. Because of the various factors involved (including the variable time interval for spontaneous recovery) the length of follow-up required before further surgical intervention is considered in children is difficult to determine. Approximately 50 percent of children that need a tracheotomy for VCP require cannulation for more than 3 years.[7,8] Most physicians recommend waiting at least 12 months before an irreversible lateralization procedure is attempted.[7,8] Laryngeal electromyography (EMG) can provide prognostic information about laryngeal nerve function and the potential for nerve recovery.[10,54]

Practice Pathway 48–1   SUSPECTED VOCAL CORD PARALYSIS

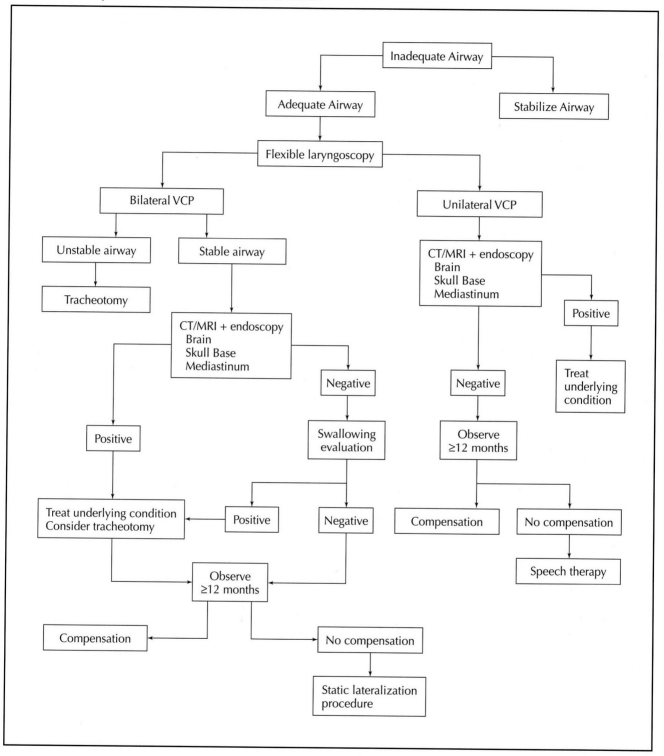

When it is determined that there is insufficient return of laryngeal function, a myriad of surgical approaches to enhance the paralyzed larynx can be considered. All procedures must be judged in terms of their effect on the three cardinal functions of the larynx. The position of the paralyzed vocal cords influences the type of procedure. In adults, peripheral causes of VCP that result in the vocal cords in abduction are most common. In this situation, vocal cord medialization or augmentation techniques are useful. In children, on the other hand, central causes of VCP are the most common etiologies. These problems result in the vocal cords being in a position of adduction. Lateralization methods, therefore, play an important role in cases of pediatric VCP. The primary goals of lateralization techniques are the establishment of an adequate airway and the maintenance of a serviceable voice. These procedures should not be considered until the child has been followed for an extended period of time, which may allow for spontaneous laryngeal recovery. When indicated, management strategies can be divided into two broad categories of static or vocal cord lateralization techniques and dynamic or reanimation techniques.

Static or lateralization procedures

Static procedures improve airway patency by enlarging the glottic aperture. This can be accomplished either by excising laryngeal tissue (vocal cord and/or the arytenoid cartilage) or by fixation techniques that rely on mechanical lateralization of the vocal cord. Static techniques often employ both tissue removal and mechanical lateralization methods simultaneously, as in the Woodman procedure.[55] Surgical widening of the glottis must balance voice and airway patency issues. The family must be made fully aware of this trade-off prior to consenting for surgery. In adults, cordectomy or arytenoidectomy may be performed through various external approaches, including a lateral cervical approach, translaryngeal approach, or laryngofissure.[55-60] In 1939, King described *arytenoidpexy,*

in which the arytenoid cartilage was displaced outwardly and the omohyoid muscle was transposed to help maintain the lateral position.[61] *The Woodman procedure,* first introduced in 1946, was the culmination of the extralaryngeal approach to bilateral VCP. The procedure, a modification of the King technique, included removal of a portion of the arytenoid with suture anchorage of the posterior vocal cord to the posterior cornu of the thyroid cartilage.[55] By the 1950s, the Woodman procedure had become the most common operation for bilateral VCP in adults and was performed occasionally in children.[62,63] The external approach in children or adults is problematic. It requires precise suture placement and can be complicated by excessive scar tissue formation. Scar tissue formation can be a significant concern in the pediatric airway because of the smaller glottic dimensions. External lateralization techniques are associated with a 20 to 40 percent decannulation failure rate.[64-67]

The carbon dioxide (CO_2) laser was introduced for the endolaryngeal management of bilateral VCP by Eskew and Bailey in 1983.[64] Using a canine model, they found that the laser provided an easy and safe method of enlarging the glottic lumen. Ossoff et al. were the first to report the clinical application of this technique.[65] Successful decannulation was reported in 10 of 11 adult patients with bilateral VCP. Minimal dysphonia was noted after laser arytenoidectomy in these patients. Various physicians have reported excellent decannulation rates with minimal compromise in voice quality using this endoscopic technique.[66-68] A more recent approach to the endoscopic restoration of an adequate airway is *endolaryngeal laser partial cordectomy with or without arytenoidectomy.* Various methods have been described with results similar to that accomplished with laser arytenoidectomy.[69-71] Eckel et al. prospectively compared 18 adults undergoing laser subtotal cordectomy to 10 adults undergoing laser arytenoidectomy, and comparison of decannulation rate, phonation, and respiratory function between these groups showed that both methods were equally effective and reliable.[72]

Laser arytenoidectomy and cordectomy are excellent techniques in adults. The results are less clear when this method is used in children.[13,14,73] One major problem is the size constraint of the pediatric larynx relative to the adult larynx. It can be difficult to determine the proper balance between airway patency and voice issues in children. Ossoff et al. noted a higher rate of late failures in children compared to adults because of scar tissue formation and the smaller glottic diameter in children.[66] Bower et al. reviewed the surgical treatment results of 30 children with bilateral VCP.[74] Nineteen children underwent external arytenoidectomy, 12 children had laser arytenoidectomy, and one child underwent a Woodman procedure. Decannulation was successful in 84 percent of the children after an external laryngeal approach compared with 56 percent of those undergoing laser arytenoidectomy. No significant difference in voice quality was noted between groups and aspiration was not encountered.

An alternative method, using the CO_2 laser, is *endolaryngeal vocal process resection*. First described in children by Bigenzahn and Hoefler, this method is a minimally-invasive procedure.[73] The vocal process of the arytenoid cartilage is vaporized, creating a posterior-glottic triangular defect and separation of the vocal cord from the arytenoid cartilage. After wound healing, the glottic airway becomes enlarged. Bilateral procedures also can be performed in select cases with minimal voice compromise.[73]

New efforts for static medialization in children using *CO② laser ventriculotomy* have shown promise. Based on the adult technique described by Kashima,[75] this procedure has been used successfully in a small number of pediatric patients. Friedman et al. have used the CO_2 laser to resect a triangular portion of the posterior true and false vocal cord.[76] This technique relies on extending the endolaryngeal incision laterally to the level of the thyroid cartilage (Fig. 48–4). The incision is made immediately anterior to the vocal process with approximately $\frac{1}{4}$ to $\frac{1}{3}$ of the posterior vocal cord removed.

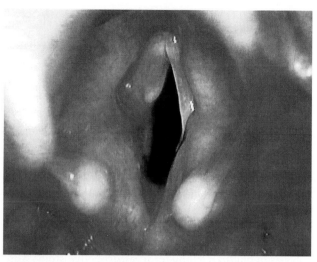

Figure 48–5:   Photograph of the larynx of a child with bilateral VCP 3 months after CO_2 laser ventriculotomy. Note patency of the glottic aperture.

This procedure allows improved respiratory function, minimal change in voice quality, and no reported problems with aspiration (Fig. 48–5).

Reanimation techniques

Laryngeal reinnervation has been considered the ideal form of rehabilitation for bilateral VCP. Methods that have been described include phrenic nerve to RLN anastomosis, phrenic nerve to posterior cricoarytenoid muscle, and omohyoid nerve-muscle pedicles.[77-79] Almost all of the work with reinnervation of the larynx has been performed in animal models or in adults. Limited data is available involving pediatric patients with VCP. In 1986, Tucker addressed pediatric laryngeal reinnervation in 30 patients under the age of 5 and reported a success rate of 50 percent.[53] Electrical stimulators or laryngeal pacing are being explored.[80,81] Although recent data suggest that this may be a useful technique in both adults and children someday, it remains experimental.[82] Given the established superior success rates of extralaryngeal and endolaryngeal approaches, reinnervation techniques remain a theoretical and experimental approach to bilateral VCP in children.

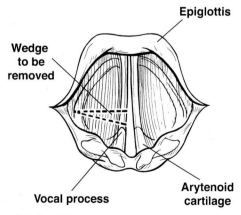

Figure 48–4:   Schematic representation of CO_2 laser endolaryngeal technique for vocal cord lateralization (ventriculotomy). The incision is carried laterally to the laryngeal surface of the thyroid alar cartilage.

REFERENCES

1. Jackson C, Jackson CL. *The Larynx and Its Diseases.* Philadelphia: W. B. Saunders, 1937.

2. Cavanagh F. Vocal palsies in children. J Laryngol Otol 1955; 69:399–418.

3. Clerf LH. Unilateral vocal cord paralysis. JAMA 1953; 151:900–903.

4. Goff WF. Vocal cord paralysis. Gen Pract 1969; 40: 79–84.

5. Dedo DD. Pediatric vocal cord paralysis. Laryngoscope 1979; 89:1378–1384.

6. Holinger LD, Holinger PC, Holinger PH. Etiology of bilateral abductor vocal cord paralysis. Ann Otol Rhinol Laryngol 1976; 85:428–436.

7. Rosin DF, Handler SD, Potsic WP, et al. Vocal cord paralysis in children. Laryngoscope 1990; 100: 1174–1179.

8. Cohen SR, Birns JW, Geller KA, et al. Laryngeal paralysis in children a long-term retrospective study. Ann Otol Rhinol Laryngol 1982; 91:417–424.

9. Zhar RIS, Chen AH, Behrendt DM, et al. Incidence of vocal fold paralysis in infants undergoing ligation of patent ductus arteriosus. Ann Thorac Surg 1966; 61:814–816.

10. Rothschild MA, Bratcher GO. Bilateral vocal cord paralysis and the pediatric airway. In: Myer CM, ed. *The Pediatric Airway.* Philadelphia: Lippincott, 1995, pp. 133–150.

11. Gacek RR, Malmgran LT. Laryngeal motor innervation: Central. In: Blitzer AB, Brin MF, Fahn S, et al. eds. *Neurologic Disorders of The Larynx.* New York: Thieme; 1992, pp. 29–35.

12. Willatt DJ, Still PM. Vocal cord paralysis. In: Paparella MM, Shumrick DA, Gluckman JL, et al. eds. *Otolaryngology.* Philadelphia: Saunders; 1991, pp. 2289–2306.

13. Grundfast KM, Harley E. Vocal cord paralysis. Otolaryngol Clin North Am 1989; 22:569–597.

14. de Gaudemar I, Roudaire M, Francois M, et al. Outcome of laryngeal paralysis in neonates: A long-term retrospective study of 113 cases. Int J Pediatr Otorhinolaryngol 1996; 34:101–110.

15. Kirsch WM, Duncan BR, Black FO, et al. Laryngeal palsy in association with meningomyelocele, hydrocephalus and the Arnold-Chiari malformation. J Neurosurg 1968; 218:207–214.

16. Oren J, Kelly DH, Todres ID, et al. Respiratory complications in patients with myelodysplasia and Arnold-Chiari malformation. Am J Dis Child 1986; 140: 221–224.

17. Papasozomenos S, Rossessmann U. Respiratory distress and Arnold-Chiari malformation. Neurology 1981; 31:97–100.

18. Sieben RL, Hamida MB, Shulman K. Multiple cranial nerve deficits associated with Arnold-Chiari malformation. Neurology 1971; 21:673–681.

19. Bluestone CD, Delerme AN, Samuelson GH. Airway obstruction due to vocal cord paralysis in infants with hydrocephalus and meningomyelocele. Ann Otol Rhinol Laryngol 1972; 81:778–783.

20. Gentile RD, Miller RH, Woodsen GE. Vocal cord paralysis in children 1 year of age and younger. Ann Otol Rhinol Laryngol 1986; 95:622–625.

21. Cotton RT, Richardson MA. Congenital laryngeal anomalies. Otolaryngol Clin North Am 1981; 14: 203–218.

22. Fitzsimmons JS. Laryngeal stridor and respiratory obstruction associated with meningomyelocele. Arch Dis Child 1965; 40:687–688.

23. Zager EL, Ojeimann RG, Poletti GE. Acute presentation of syringomyelia. J Neurosurg 1990; 72: 133–138.

24. Willis WH, Weaver DF. Syringomyelia with bilateral vocal cord paralysis. Arch Otolaryngol 1968; 87: 42–44.

25. Holinger PH. Clinical aspects of congenital anomalies of the larynx, trachea, bronchi and esophagus. J Laryngol Otol 1961; 75:1–44.

26. Stuart WD. Otolaryngologic aspects of myasthenia gravis. Laryngoscope 1965; 75:112.

27. Fairley JW, Hughes M. Acute stridor due to bilateral vocal cord paralysis as a presenting sign of myasthenia gravis. J Laryngol Otol 1992; 106:737–738.

28. Zhar RIS, Smith RJH. Vocal fold paralysis in infants twelve months of age and younger. Otolaryngol Head Neck Surg 1996; 114:18–21.

29. Myer CM, Fitton CM. Vocal cord paralysis following child abuse. Int J Pediatr Otorhinolaryngol 1988; 15: 217–220.

30. Pfenninger J. Bilateral vocal cord paralysis after severe blunt head injury: A case of failed extubation. Crit Care Med 1987; 15:701–702.

31. Nutinen J, Karja J. Bilateral vocal cord paralysis following general anesthesia. Laryngoscope 1981; 91: 83–86.

32. Brandwein M, Abramson AL, Shikowitz MJ. Bilateral vocal cord paralysis following endotracheal intubation. Arch Otolaryngol Head Neck Surg 1986; 112: 877–882.

33. Cavo JW. True vocal cord paralysis following intubation. Laryngoscope 1985; 95:1352–1358.

34. Inomata S, Nishikawa T, Suga A, et al. Transient bilateral vocal cord paralysis after insertion of a laryngeal mask airway. Anesthesiology 1995; 82:787–788.

35. Godwin JE, Miller KS, Hoang KGG, et al. Benign thyroid hyperplasia presenting as bilateral vocal cord paralysis complete remission following surgery. Chest 1991; 99–1029.

36. Cannon S, Ritter FN. Vocal cord paralysis in postpoliomyelitis syndrome. Laryngoscope 1987; 97: 981–983.

37. Thompson JW, Rosenthal P, Camilon FS. Vocal cord paralysis and superior laryngeal nerve dysfunction in

Reye's syndrome. Arch Otolaryngol Head Neck Surg 1990; 116:46-48.

38. Panosian MS, Quatela VC. Guillain-Baré syndrome presenting as acute bilateral vocal cord paralysis. Otolaryngol Head Neck Surg 1993; 108:171-173.

39. Benjamin B. Congenital disorders of the larynx. In: Cummings CW, ed. *Otolaryngology—Head and Neck Surgery 2 ed.* New York: Mosby, 1992, pp. 1831.

40. Moralee SJ, Reilly PG. Metabolic stridor bilateral vocal cord abductor paralysis secondary to hypokalemia? J Laryngol Otol 1992; 106:56-57.

41. Aiuto LA, Paulakis SG, Boxer RA. Life-threatening organophosphate induced delayed polyneuropathy in a child after accidental chlorpyrifos ingestion. J Pediatr 1993; 122:658-660.

42. Grundfast KM, Milmoe G. Congenital hereditary bilateral abductor vocal cord paralysis. Ann Otol Rhinol Laryngol 1982; 91:564-566.

43. Gacek RR. Hereditary abductor vocal cord paralysis. Ann Otol Rhinol Laryngol 1976; 85:90-93.

44. Isaacson G, Moya F. Hereditary congenital laryngeal abductor paralysis. Ann Otol Rhinol Laryngol 1987; 96:701-704.

45. Tucker HM. Congenital bilateral recurrent nerve paralysis and ptosis: A new syndrome? Laryngoscope 1983; 93:1405-1407.

46. Koppel R, Friedman S, Fallet S. Congenital vocal cord paralysis with possible autosomal recessive inheritance: Case report and review of the literature. Am J Med Genetics 1996; 64:485-487.

47. Randolph C, Lapey A, Shannon DC. Bilateral abductor paralysis masquerading as asthma. J Allergy Clin Immunol 1988; 81:1122-1125.

48. Bogaard JM, Pauw KH, Versprille A, et al. Maximal expiratory and inspiratory flow-volume curves in bilateral vocal cord paralysis. Orl J Otorhinolaryngol Relat Spec 1987; 49:35-41.

49. Benjamin B. Technique of laryngoscopy. Int J Pediatr Otorhinolaryngol 1987; 13:299-313.

50. Grundfast K, Harley E. Vocal cord paralysis. Otolaryngol Clin North Am 1989; 22:569-597.

51. Holinger PC, Holinger LD, Reichert TJ, et al. Respiratory obstruction and apnea in infants with bilateral abductor vocal cord paralysis, meningomyelocele, hydrocephalus and Arnold-Chiari malformations. J Pediatr 1978; 92:368-373.

52. Swift AC, Rogers J. Vocal cord paralysis in children. J Laryngol Otol 1987; 101:169-171.

53. Tucker HM. Vocal cord paralysis in small children: Principles in management. Ann Otol Rhinol Laryngol 1986; 95:618-621.

54. Parnes SM, Satya-Murti S. Predictive value of laryngeal electromyography in patients with vocal cord paralysis of neurogenic origin. Laryngoscope 1985; 95:1323-1326.

55. Woodman DG. A modification of the extralaryngeal approach to arytenoidectomy for bilateral abductor paralysis. Arch Otolaryngol 1946; 43:63-65.

56. Amedee RG, Mann WJ. A functional approach to lateral fixation in bilateral abductor cord paralysis. Otolaryngol Head Neck Surg 1989; 100:542-545.

57. Thornell WC. Intralaryngeal approach in arytenoidectomy in bilateral abductor vocal cord paralysis. Trans Am Acad Ophthalmol Otolaryngol 1949; 53:631-635.

58. Downey WL, Keenan WG. Laryngosfissure approach for bilateral abductor paralysis. Arch Otolaryngol 1968; 88:513-516.

59. Helmus C. Microsurgical thyrotomy and arytenoidectomy for bilateral recurrent laryngeal nerve paralysis. Laryngoscope 1972; 82:491-503.

60. Geterud A, Ejnell H, Stenborg R, et al. Long-term results with a simple surgical treatment of bilateral vocal cord paralysis. Laryngoscope 1990; 100:1005-1008.

61. King BT. A new and functioning respiratory operation for bilateral abductor cord paralysis: Preliminary report. JAMA 1939; 112:814-823.

62. Woodman DG. Bilateral abductor paralysis: A survey of 521 cases of arytenoidectomy via the open approach as reported by 90 surgeons. Arch Otolaryngol 1953; 58:150-153.

63. Priest RE, Ulvestad HS, Van De Water F, et al. Arytenoidectomy in children. Ann Otol Rhinol Laryngol 1960; 69:869-881.

64. Eskew JR, Bailey BJ. Laser arytenoidectomy for bilateral vocal paralysis. Otolaryngol Head Neck Surg 1983; 91:294-298.

65. Ossoff RH, Sissen GA, Duncavage JA, et al. Endoscopic laser arytenoidectomy for the treatment of bilateral vocal cord paralysis. Laryngoscope 1984; 94:1293-1297.

66. Ossoff RH, Duncavage JA, Shapshany SM, et al. Endoscopic laser arytenoidectomy revisited. Ann Otol Rhinol Laryngol 1990; 99:764-771.

67. Lim RY. Laser arytenoidectomy. Arch Otolaryngol Head Neck Surg 1985; 111:262-263.

68. Crumley RL. Endoscopic laser medial arytenoidectomy for airway management in bilateral laryngeal paralysis. Ann Otol Rhinol Laryngol 1993; 102:81-84.

69. Holm AF, Wonters B, Van Averbeek JJM. CO_2 laser cordectomy for bilateral vocal cord paralysis. Lasers Med Science 1989; 4:93-96.

70. Dennis DP, Kashima H. Carbon dioxide laser posterior cordectomy per treatment of bilateral vocal cord paralysis. Ann Otol Rhinol Laryngol 1989; 98:930-934.

71. Eckel HE. Microlaryngoscopic laser vocal fold lateralization for the treatment of bilateral vocal cord paral-

ysis—techniques and results. Laryngol Rhinol Otol (Stuttg) 1991; 70:17–20.

72. Eckel HE, Fhumfart M, Vossing M, et al. Cordectomy versus arytenoidectomy in the management of bilateral vocal cord paralysis. Ann Otol Rhinol Laryngol 1994; 103:852–857.

73. Bigenzahn W, Hoefler H. Minimally invasive laser surgery for the treatment of bilateral vocal cord paralysis. Laryngoscope 1996; 106:791–793.

74. Bower CM, Choi SS, Cotton RT. Arytenoidectomy in children. Ann Otol Rhinol Laryngol 1994; 103:271–278.

75. Dennis DP, Kashima H. Carbon dioxide laser posterior cordectomy for treatment of bilateral vocal cord paralysis. Ann Otol Rhinol Laryngol 1989; 98:930–934.

76. Friedman EM. Personal communication.

77. Tucker HM. Nerve-muscle pedicle reinnervation of the larynx: Avoiding pitfalls and complications. Ann Otol Rhinol Laryngol 1982; 91:440–444.

78. Crumley RL. Phrenic nerve graft for bilateral vocal cord paralysis. Laryngoscope 1983; 93:425–428.

79. Colledge L, Ballance C. Surgical treatment of paralysis of vocal cord and paralysis of diaphragm. Br Med J 1927; (1):553–559.

80. Broniatowski M, Kaneko S, Nose Y, et al. Laryngeal pacemaker II: Electronic pacing of reinnervated posterior cricoarytenoid muscles in canine. Laryngoscope 1985; 95:1194–1198.

81. Broniatowski M, Tucker HM, Kaneko S, et al. Laryngeal pacemaker Part I. Electronic pacing of reinnervated strap muscles in the dog. Otolaryngol Head Neck Surg 1986; 94:41–44.

82. Sanders I. Electrical stimulation of laryngeal muscle. Otolaryngol Clin North Am 1991; 24:1253–1274.

49 Management of Foreign Bodies

Harlan R. Muntz

When Chevalier Jackson returned from England after a prolonged preceptorship with Sir Morell MacKensie, specialization of the medical profession in the United States was not common practice, even though the treatment of diseases of the upper aerodigestive tract (UADT) needed a specialist.[1] At the turn of the century, foreign bodies caused an enormous amount of morbidity and mortality in this country. Esophageal foreign bodies resulted in a slow agonizing death from starvation. Airway foreign bodies killed through decreased ventilation and infection. Much of the early development of otorhinolaryngology and indeed the development of modern medical instrumentation was by bronchoesophagologists in an attempt to find better ways to remove foreign bodies safely.

This chapter is unusual as all head and neck foreign bodies are addressed together. Even though the location may vary, many of the principles of safe removal have similarities. Vegetable matter, small toys or parts of toys, or other things found in the house, garden, and playground can be placed in the ear canal, nose, or mouth. Many children go through phases when everything is placed in the mouth. Multiple foreign bodies or recurrent episodes of foreign-body placement are not unusual.

In the United States, there has been an attempt to assist the public with the protection of young children from the dangers of small parts.[2] Toys that are small or that easily fragment into small pieces carry a greater danger for aspiration, ingestion, and choking. Certain toys are marked as unsuitable for children under 3 years old. These recommendations are based on the three-dimensional size of the pieces

and the potential for them to lodge in the upper airway.[3]

Education is of prime importance in the prevention of foreign-body episodes. Even if a parent buys age-appropriate toys for his child, an additional risk exists with either a sibling's toys or, more often, vegetable matter. Arjmand et al demonstrated that the lack of an identifiable primary care provider increased the risk of a foreign body in the aerodigestive tract (ADT).[4] Parental awareness of the potential dangers is the key to the reduction of incidence, although even in the educated and caring family not all foreign-body episodes will be prevented.

PRINCIPLES FOR REMOVAL

The retention of a head and neck foreign body occurs when the size or shape of the object allows its entry but not egress. In the ear canal and nose, the foreign body may have been inserted by the child even with discomfort. The isthmus of the ear canal or the narrowing of the nasal cavity at the level of the inferior turbinate can act as a limitation for further progress of the foreign body, but it also can deter removal. The esophagus can dilate to allow rather large objects to traverse, but the object may become trapped once esophageal spasm occurs. Natural areas of esophageal narrowing occur at the cricopharyngeus, the thoracic inlet, the cardiac border, and the gastroesophageal sphincter. The airway is narrowed at the vocal cords, subglottis, and bronchi. The shape and size of the foreign body determines its eventual location. Large or irregularly-shaped ingested objects may lodge in the pharynx. A sharp object, such as a fish bone, may pierce the mucosa and be retained at any point along the upper alimentary tract (UAT).

Pediatric Otolaryngology, Edited by R.F. Wetmore, H.R. Muntz, and T.J. McGill. Thieme Medical Publishers, Inc., New York © 2000.

The narrowed or sharp end of a foreign body usually trails, i.e. follows behind, the blunt or rounded end as it enters the orifice. If the sharp end were to enter first, contact with the mucosa would cause retention of the object or the object would tumble, allowing the sharp end to trail. Although this allows the foreign body easy entry, removal is hindered because the sharp end frequently catches in the mucosal wall, precluding removal. Disimpaction of the sharp end and sheathing it in an endoscope prevents it from catching in the mucosa. In the esophagus and tracheobronchial tree, puncture or laceration can result in pneumothorax or pneumomediastinum and mediastinitis. In the ear and nose, pain and bleeding also may result. Pushing the foreign body further may cause distal injury to delicate areas, such as the bronchial mucosa or tympanic membrane (TM). An esophageal foreign body, on the other hand, may be pushed into the stomach, and the sharp end turned for removal through the esophagus; a large foreign body may be left in the stomach for removal through a gastrostomy. Many small esophageal foreign bodies or food items can be left in the stomach and allowed to digest or to pass through the remainder of the gastrointestinal tract to be eliminated with the stool. Pushing a nasal foreign body into the nasopharynx

can lead to aspiration into the larynx or trachea and should be discouraged.

Successful foreign-body removal is dependent upon careful attention to detail. The foreign body should be exposed adequately. Improved visualization utilizing xenon light sources, telescopes, and the operating microscope have resulted in a reduction of the morbidity and mortality that was seen during Jackson's era. For removal of any foreign body, proper selection of a forceps is critical and the use of visual and tactile sensation is fundamental.

Forceps

In preparation for removal of any foreign object, the clinician should analyze its size, shape, and texture. It is always helpful to have another, similar object to study and practice grasping. Attention to the sharp points and edges, to the possibility of breakage with extraction (thus leading to multiple foreign bodies), and to the actual size and smoothness of the object are clues in selecting the best forceps. Forceps are available in a variety of sizes and forms. The clinician should be familiar with most of them and have many available in the event of a difficult extraction.

Over the years, numerous foreign-body forceps have been invented. In the early 1900s, most reports of episodes involving foreign bodies were focused on the development of new and better forceps for specific problems. Chevalier Jackson was known to perform endoscopy and, after assessing the situation, proceed to the shop to create a forceps for that specific foreign-body problem. Developing new forceps at a moment's notice is beyond the scope of today's otolaryngologist, but fortunately, a large assortment of foreign-body forceps are available from instrument companies.

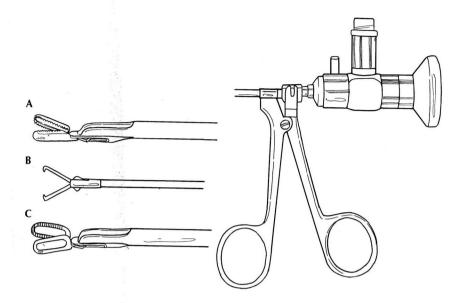

A

B

C

Figure 49–1: Three types of foreign-body forceps. (A) Alligator. (B) Rotational. (C) Globular grasping.

Most foreign-body forceps can be categorized into four types. The *alligator type* opens its straight jaws to grasp the foreign body; it usually has serrations to add friction. A *globular grasping forceps* surrounds the object with curved blades. A *rotational forceps* allows free movement of an object so that it may tumble, allowing the point to trail. A *hollow object forceps* opens within the lumen of a cylinder for removal (Fig. 49-1).

Serrated alligator forceps grasp the foreign body with significant tension, and the serrations increase the friction, allowing the foreign body to be extracted. Alligator forceps work well in the removal of some vegetable matter, irregular hard objects, and disks. They also are useful for the sharp point of a pin or needle. Round and highly-polished foreign bodies can slip easily with these forceps.

Round objects pose difficulty during extraction. Serrated forceps may slip off the object, or may crush it if it is soft. A *peanut forceps* is an excellent example of a globular grasping forceps that can be used for almost any spherical object. The distal end of the forceps must go beyond the equator of the mass and cradle it for removal. This prevents crushing, in the case of a nut or seed, and allows retention within the forceps.

Rotational forceps are useful in extracting pins, needles, tacks, and nails. Impaction of the sharp point within the tracheal or esophageal mucosa can preclude removal or cause severe injury. If the dimensions of the foreign body are such that it can rotate within the lumen, the object can be grasped. As the foreign body and endoscope are being re-

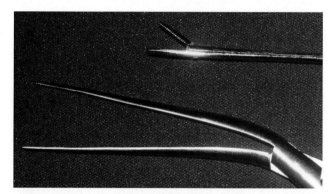

Figure 49–2: Hartman's forceps are used for round and irregular objects in the nose and ear because they allow a wider opening than the alligator type forcep.

moved, the impacted point allows the foreign body to tumble, placing the sharp point distally and preventing further injury or impaction on removal.

A cylinder in the bronchus is a very difficult foreign body to remove. Hollow object forceps, which were devised by Jackson, address this problem. The serrations are located on the outside of the forceps. The jaws are introduced into the opening of the foreign body, and as the forceps are opened, the foreign body is grasped from the inside. Grasping the edge of a hollow foreign body may allow removal, but often the opposite side catches the mucosa and makes removal difficult.

Standard forceps made for bronchoesophagology, are too large for removal of foreign objects in the ear canal or nose. When trying to remove a foreign body from the ear canal or the nose, *Hartman's forceps* (Fig. 49-2) or short alligator forceps often can grasp the object readily. The action of the alligator jaws makes it less useful for large foreign bodies. On the other hand, a Hartman's forceps opens from the area of the handle, allowing the jaws to extend widely around large and round objects.

In the ear canal, the rigidity of the wall prevents the forceps from opening larger than the canal, necessitating the use of wire loops or right-angle picks in the removal of a foreign body. Extending the loop or pick beyond the foreign body may allow easy extraction. Care must be taken, especially in a struggling child, to avoid injury to the distal TM.

Visualization

Adequate visualization of the foreign body is of utmost importance. Most surgeons are very visually oriented, and good visualization should improve success and decrease complication. The earliest esophagoscopes were introduced with an "olive" or obturator. The scope was inserted blindly above the foreign body, and then removal was attempted.

During the early years of bronchoesophagology, debates focused on the relative merits of proximal or distal illumination. Initially, the light source directed light down the shaft of the endoscope. With the invention of the incandescent bulb, a small carrier ending in the light bulb allowed distal light. Later, fiberoptic light rods were introduced that avoided the obstruction of the light by the forceps and placed visualization nearer to the foreign body.

A light source should be selected for its production of abundant light. Because the view through an endoscope is from reflected light, an insufficient light source frequently makes it difficult to see the object or important anatomy. The use of *optical forceps* has allowed both distal illumination and better visualization of foreign bodies. These forceps bring the object visually closer and allow removal of the object based on sight more than feel.

In the ear canal, use of the *operative microscope* allows excellent lighting and visualization of the foreign body and frees both hands for manipulation of instruments. Although many continue to use a headlight or mirror for removal of a nasal foreign body, the use of the operating microscope simplifies this process as well. If needed, the introduction of a nasal or ear speculum into the vestibule can improve visualization by retraction of the lower lateral cartilages.

In most cases, it is best to use the largest but shortest appropriate endoscope to remove a foreign body. When the working distance between the hand and the foreign body is shorter, the forceps are more stable and it is easier to complete the technically difficult task. A variety of lengths in endoscopes and forceps should be available to the clinician.

It is important for the child to be prepared adequately for the procedure at hand. At the turn of the century, all foreign-body extractions were done while the patient was awake or under local anesthesia. Today, removal of almost all esophageal and endobronchial foreign bodies is performed under general anesthesia, which allows airway control. Ear and nasal foreign bodies often are removed in the office without any anesthesia. The child who cannot be restrained in the office setting may need conscious sedation or general anesthesia during removal.

REMOVAL OF FOREIGN BODIES

Practice Pathway 49–1 outlines the management for foreign-body removal.

Ear Foreign Bodies

Foreign bodies within the external ear canal are not usually emergencies. Live insects are very disturbing to a child, and if they cannot be removed, they should at least be killed until elective removal can be accomplished. Wet beans may swell and make removal more difficult at a later time. If the child exhibits nystagmus or complains of vertigo, there is a good possibility of injury to the cochlea or vestibular labyrinth, and removal with exploration of the middle ear for fistula should be performed. If a TM perforation is detected after a foreign body is removed, audiometry should be performed to assure that no damage has been done to the ossicles or inner ear.

If a foreign body cannot be removed easily by the emergency room physician or pediatrician, referral to an otolaryngologist is necessary. Multiple attempts usually are painful to the child, and the resultant fear and struggle may reduce the likelihood of a successful removal by the specialist even with use of the operating microscope and appropriate instrumentation.

Using an operating microscope improves visuali-

Practice Pathway 49–1   MANAGEMENT OF FOREIGN BODIES

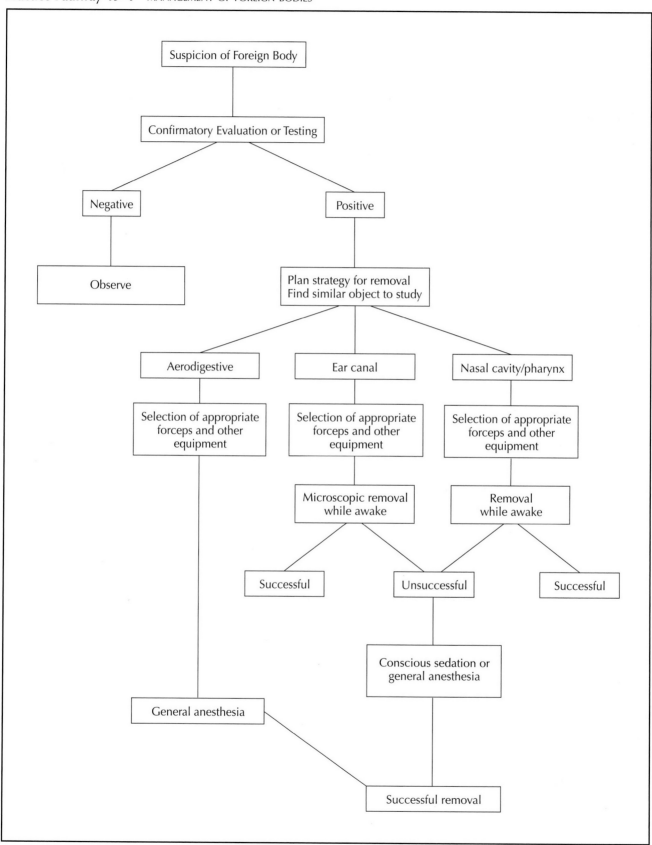

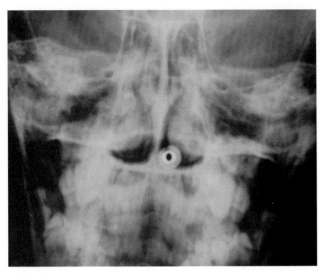

Figure 49–3: An AP radiograph of the head shows a rivet under the inferior turbinate of the left nasal cavity.

zation and the chance for retrieval. The patient should be restrained by parents or medical staff to avoid unnecessary injury to the ear canal and TM. In the uncooperative child, the otolaryngologist should consider the use of conscious sedation or general anesthesia.

Nasal Foreign Bodies (Figs. 49-3 and 49-4)

If a nasal foreign body dislodges into the airway, a simple problem can become life threatening be-

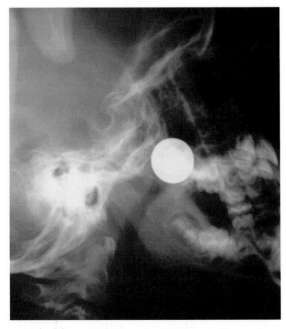

Figure 49–4: Lateral neck radiograph demonstrates a coin in the nasopharynx.

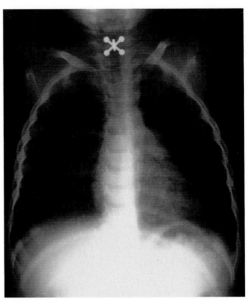

Figure 49–5: A (posterior-anterior) radiograph of the chest reveals a jack in the hypopharynx.

cause the object can become lodged in the larynx or tracheobronchial tree. Because of this, the acute placement of a nasal foreign body should be evaluated carefully and removed if possible. Frequently, however, the nasal foreign body is discovered because of long-standing purulent rhinorrhea. In these cases, the foreign body is unlikely to dislodge and move to the lower airway where it can be removed electively. Most nasal foreign bodies can be removed in the office setting when the child is restrained. Conscious sedation carries a greater airway risk if the laryngeal reflexes are decreased by the sedation. General anesthesia is rarely necessary. Flexible or rigid endoscopy can be helpful in locating the foreign object and in determining its shape and structure, thereby assisting in plans for its removal.

Few forceps are made specifically for the nose. Most ear forceps can be used in the anterior nose. Long Hartman's forceps are often sufficient. Wire loops, polyp snares, alligator forceps, and even Fogarty balloons also have been used.

Epistaxis may result from mucosal damage. After removal of the foreign body, the epistaxis should be treated.

Oral Cavity to Hypopharynx Foreign Bodies (Fig. 49-5)

A foreign body in the oral cavity or pharynx may increase the risk of airway compromise. A large foreign body often presents with choking and vomiting. In the case of acute airway obstruction, an attempt may be made in the field to remove the object with a finger swipe. Care should be taken not to push the foreign body distally, causing complete obstruction.

In small children, a common cause of death from foreign-body aspiration is choking on a piece of hot dog. It is common because hot dogs are a common staple in childrens diets. If the child bites off a large piece or the parent fails to cut the hot dog into small enough pieces, it may become lodged in the hypopharynx or at the cricopharyngeus and obstruct the airway. If the child survives to the hospital, the removal should be approached with great care. A ventilating bronchoscope should be available in the event of complete obstruction.

Other objects that can cause foreign-body aspiration are latex balloons and fish bones. Small children should not be allowed to play with latex balloons because they can pop and the pieces can become lodged in the airway. The result is immediate airway obstruction and potential death.[5] Fish bones also may become lodged in the pharynx, usually at the base of the tongue or vallecula but sometimes as caudal as the pyriform sinus. Because they are small, almost translucent and not radio-opaque, detection is often difficult. The Buffalo fish, from the central Mississippi River area, is one of the few exceptions to this as it is radio-opaque.

Flexible endoscopy and/or mirror examination can help locate the small foreign body in the pharynx. If a foreign-body sensation persists, direct laryngoscopy should be performed to identify an embedded or difficult-to-visualize object.

Esophageal Foreign Bodies (Fig. 49–6)

Esophageal foreign bodies are not uncommon. Children often put objects into their mouths while playing and inadvertently swallow them. Large objects may become lodged in the esophagus. Esophageal spasm can retain the foreign body, even if it is relatively small. The child may present with discomfort, dysphagia, drooling, or even airway compromise. Infants on a liquid or soft diet may remain asymptomatic for some time. A high index of suspicion of a foreign-body ingestion always should be maintained.

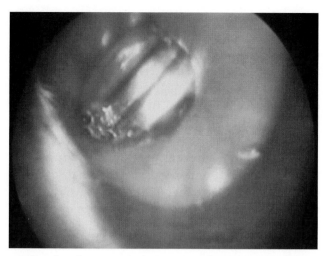

Figure 49–6:   View through a Storz-Hopkins esophagoscope illustrates three coins in the proximal esophagus.

If the child presents with airway distress, the esophageal foreign body should be considered an

---

SPECIAL CONSIDERATION:

A high index of suspicion of a foreign-body ingestion or aspiration always should be maintained.

---

emergency and endoscopic removal performed without delay. Similarly, if the object has sharp edges and there is risk of esophageal perforation, removal should be emergent. The disk battery is a special circumstance. In this case, the esophagus may perforate within hours.[6] Because there may be a delay in the detection and emergency room evaluation, there should be no delay in the endoscopic removal. If transmural burns are noted at endoscopy, the child should be treated for severe caustic ingestion.

SPECIAL CONSIDERATION:

A disk battery in the esophagus is a special case, which like the sharp esophageal foreign body, necessitates immediate removal.

The child with a smooth esophageal foreign body, minimal dysphagia, and no airway distress can be considered an urgent case. If the child is observed through a sleep cycle, there is at least some chance that the foreign body may pass due to a reduction of the esophageal spasm. The use of smooth muscle relaxants has been tried with minimal success.

The debate continues as to what is an acceptable and safe method for esophageal foreign-body extraction. The removal of radiopaque smooth discs (e.g., coins) from the esophagus by radiology has been recommended by some. Coins can be removed from the esophagus by passing a ballooned catheter beyond the foreign body under fluoroscopic guidance. The balloon is inflated and then removed, pulling the coin out with the catheter. Although there have been no documented severe complications of removal of a coin in this way, there are a number of objections. Some of these are that the airway is not protected, that the disk may be dislodged from the esophagus and find its way to the larynx or nasopharynx, and that the assumption must be made that the radiopaque object is the only foreign body. If there were an additional unseen object, the catheter may cause damage to the esophageal wall. The foreign body must have been swallowed recently. If the object has been present for several days, there may be ulceration of the esophageal wall and granulation tissue, which increases the risk of esophageal perforation. The removal procedure usually is done with the child awake and restrained in the Trendelenburg position. Some question whether this procedure is actually less traumatic to the child than undergoing a general anesthetic.

Flexible fiberoptic endoscopy (FFE) has been very useful in the diagnosis of diseases of the UAT. At the turn of the century, even gastroscopy was performed with a rigid endoscope. The introduction of the FFE has greatly improved our ability to diagnose and treat many diseases. The flexible esophagoscope usually is used with the child under conscious sedation. However, if an FFE is used for foreign-body extraction under sedation, the airway is not secured. Also because few effective foreign-body forceps are available for fibroptic scopes, there are limitations to the use of FFE for foreign-body extraction.

The availability of a variety of sized rigid endoscopes and the multiplicity of forceps designed for foreign-body retrieval make rigid endoscopy the treatment of choice. The airway is protected with an endotracheal tube while the child is under general anesthesia. The presence of multiple foreign bodies is assessed easily, as is the finding of radiolucent foreign bodies. Assessment of the entire esophagus as well as the hypopharynx and larynx can be accomplished readily.

Rigid esophagoscopy always should be performed with gentleness and finesse. The tissues are damaged easily by forceful manipulation. A rent in the mucosa alone is healed easily. Damage through the muscular wall can result in scar formation and stricture, not to mention the complication of mediastinitis. This rare complication can be fatal if there is a delay in discovery or if overwhelming infection is not treated aggressively. Pneumomediastinum and pneumothorax can require a chest tube. An esophageal laceration should be treated by an open repair.

Tracheobronchial Foreign Bodies (Figs. 49-7-49-9)

Foreign bodies of the airway carry the risk of sudden asphyxiation. They should be considered an emergency unless they have been present for quite some time. The child with a positive history for an airway foreign body should have endoscopy even in the face of negative radiographs and physical exam. Frequently, there is no suggestive history. Findings on chest radiograph or chest auscultation may suggest

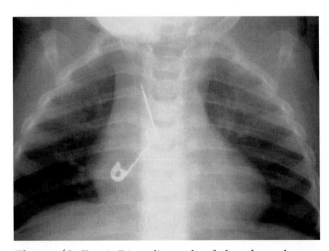

Figure 49–7: A PA radiograph of the chest demonstrates an open safety pin in the right mainstem bronchus.

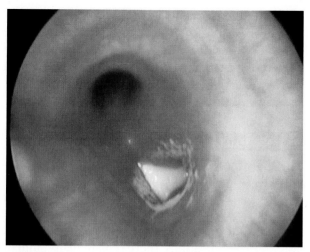

Figure 49–9: View through a Storz-Hopkins broncho-scope reveals a peanut in the right mainstem bronchus.

the diagnosis. A high level of suspicion must be present or these children may suffer significant respiratory complications, including chronic infection and fistula formation.

The most-commonly inhaled foreign bodies are vegetable matter. In the United States, peanuts and popcorn seeds are very common. Children should not be allowed seeds and nuts in their diet until their teeth are present to adequately chew them (around the age of 4 years). Seeds and nuts are lightweight and are aspirated easily if the child suddenly inhales. Additional common objects that are aspirated include raw vegetables and hard candies.

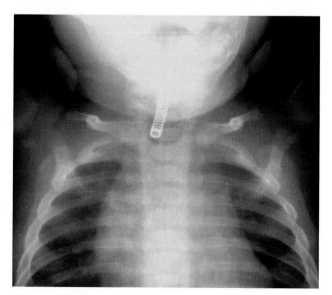

Figure 49–8: A PA radiograph of the chest shows a spring caught in the larynx.

These are radiolucent and their location can only be suspected by physical exam and the suggestion of hyperinflation or consolidation on chest radiograph. Seeds and nuts are best removed with a globular grasping forceps (peanut forceps), whereas raw vegetables such as carrots should be removed easily with an alligator forceps. If the type of foreign body is unknown, a selection of foreign-body forceps should be available. Careful attention to forceps selection is essential in the airway. A partial airway obstruction can become a complete obstruction very quickly. The foreign body must be controlled at all times. Prompt atraumatic removal is the goal.

A large foreign body may be retained at the subglottis. The triangular shape of the glottis can make extraction difficult. Most frequently, the object may be manipulated through the space, but it is important to remember that it also may be removed through a tracheotomy. The foreign body can be pushed from the subglottis to the stoma and removed. The neck and trachea are allowed to heal, and no tracheotomy tube is necessary unless the airway is compromised by edema.

The use of FFE for removal of a foreign body in the tracheobronchial tree is fraught with risk because the airway is not controlled. Though the patient may be given oxygen, ventilation for the child cannot be assumed. The forceps that are available for use through an FFE channel are very limited. The size of the forceps is also limited as the working channel is usually much smaller than the light-carrying cable. For this reason, FFE should not be considered for use in the routine removal of airway foreign objects in children. The exception may be a pin or needle in the distal airway. The rigid endoscope may not be able to visualize these distal foreign bodies. The combined use of a rigid endoscope for ventilation and an FFE to traverse the smaller distal airway can give the advantages of both instruments. An alternative will be the use of a biplanar fluoroscopy to assist in locating the foreign body.

SPECIAL CONSIDERATION:

Systemic corticosteroids and topical epinephrine are two medications that may help in the removal of certain foreign bodies.

Care must be taken to avoid injury to the tracheal and bronchial mucosa. Even a small rent can contribute to a pneumothorax when using positive pressure ventilation. Granulation tissue may be present with a chronically-retained foreign body. Preoperative treatment with high-dose steroids may reduce the inflammation and facilitate removal. Topical epinephrine at the time of retrieval also can reduce bleeding and edema. Fracture of the foreign body can cause a single object to become multiple foreign bodies. For this reason, care must be taken not to crush the foreign body when trying to remove it. Occasionally, a swollen seed or bean may need to be divided in order for it to be able to traverse the larynx.

CONCLUSION

Removal of a foreign body is a complicated process requiring diligence and planning by the surgeon. Although each location in the head and neck has specific considerations for urgency of removal and potential complications, there remain many similarities in the planning process and actual removal. Adequate exposure, good visualization, and selection of the appropriate endoscope and forceps for removal are necessary in every case. Great satisfaction can be obtained from a successful removal that prevents further injury and morbidity.

REFERENCES

1. Jackson C. *The Life of Chevalier Jackson.* pp. 1–38. MacMillian Company, New York, 1938.
2. Reilly JS, Walter MA. Consumer product aspiration and ingestion in children: Analysis of emergency room reports to the National Electronic Injury Surveillance System. Ann Otol Rhinol Laryngol 1992; 101: 739–741.
3. Rimell FL, Thome A Jr, Stool S, et al. Characteristics of objects that cause choking in children. JAMA 1995; 274:1763–1766.
4. Arjmand EM, Muntz HR, Stratmann SL. Insurance status as a risk factor for foreign body ingestion or aspiration. Int J Pediatr Otorhinolaryngol 1997; 42:25–29.
5. Ryan CA, Yacoub W, Paton T, et al. Childhood deaths from toy balloons. Am J Dis Child 1990; 144: 1221–1224.
6. Maves MD, Carithers JS, Birck HG. Esophageal burns secondary to disc battery ingestion. Ann Otol Rhinol Laryngol 1984; 93:364–369.

50 Infectious and Inflammatory Disorders of the Larynx and Trachea

Kathleen C.Y. Sie

Infectious and inflammatory disorders of the larynx and trachea are common in infants and children because of their developing immune systems and increased exposure to a wide variety of pathogens. Some disease entities such as laryngotracheobronchitis (LTB), (i.e., croup), are very common and result in minimal morbidity. Others such as epiglottitis and recurrent respiratory papillomatosis (RRP) cause significant morbidity and even some mortality. The effects of some of these airway diseases, epiglottitis for example, have been diminished by new medical advances [e.g., *Hemophilus influenzae* type B (HIB) vaccine], however RRP continues to afflict patients in spite of a better understanding of this disease process. The future may hold new challenges as old foes such as tuberculosis come back to haunt us.

Often, diseases of the laryngotracheal region can be diagnosed with a detailed patient history given by the parent and a careful physical examination. Radiologic studies may be necessary to establish the diagnosis in some cases, wheres other children may require endoscopic examination of the entire airway, including culture or biopsy in order to confirm the physician's suspicions. This chapter reviews the common infectious and inflammatory diseases of the larynx and trachea, but also includes less common but significant disorders that may have an impact upon a child's health.

CLINICAL EVALUATION

In assessing the child with an airway abnormality the history should be directed to determine the de-

gree of airway obstruction, duration of symptoms, and associated illnesses or exposures. Symptoms are generally due to airway compromise that results in noisy breathing, signs of accessory respiratory muscle use such as retractions, and possibly color change. Related symptoms include cough, a change in voice, feeding difficulties, failure to thrive, and disturbed sleep. Past medical history, including immunization status, is important. Parents also should be asked specifically about the possibility of foreign-body aspiration (see Chap. 49).

When evaluating the infant or child with symptoms and signs of airway obstruction, it is important to examine the patient thoroughly. After noting the child's vital signs, including temperature and heart and respiratory rates, the examination should begin with a careful inspection of the child. The initial purpose of this inspection is to determine the severity of the child's illness so that appropriate therapy can be promptly instituted if he has an unstable airway. Much also can be learned by watching the child breathe and listening to the sounds of her breathing. Stridor or noisy breathing should be assessed with the unaided ear as well as with a stethoscope placed over the patient's airway. Characterization of the stridor relative to the phase of respiration (i.e., inspiratory, expiratory, or biphasic) may be helpful in localizing the site of involvement. The patient's neck and chest wall should be observed to assess the degree of accessory respiratory muscle use. The lung fields should be auscultated for decreased breath sounds or wheezing suggestive of an infiltrate, foreign body, or reactive airway disease.

In general, the diagnosis of a child presenting with airway symptoms often can be made based on the history and physical examination alone. Other

Pediatric Otolaryngology, Edited by R.F. Wetmore, H.R. Muntz, and T.J. McGill. Thieme Medical Publishers, Inc., New York © 2000.

tests such as pulse oximetry, radiographs of the neck and/or chest, and blood studies may provide supportive information regarding the patient's overall status or the diagnosis. In some cases, flexible laryngoscopy may be helpful in assessing the child's larynx; however, care must be taken to avoid unnecessary procedures in the patient with an acutely-inflamed larynx, especially in those with suspected epiglottitis, to avoid further swelling or acute airway obstruction (AAO). Cultures or biopsies of the involved areas may be required to confirm a diagnosis. Tests that are specific to certain diagnoses are mentioned in the appropriate sections that follow.

The immediate management of these patients de-

Practice Pathway 50–1   INFECTIOUS AND INFLAMMATORY DISORDERS OF THE LARYNX AND TRACHEA

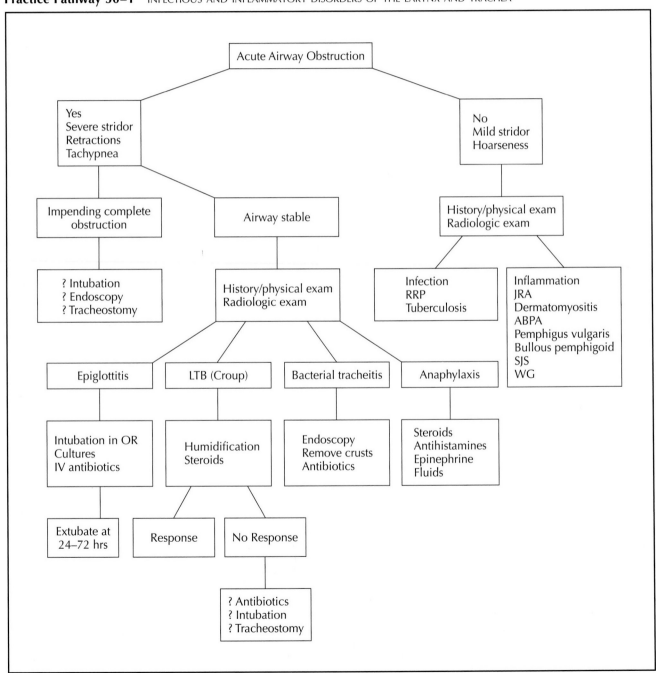

Abbreviations: OR, Operating Room; IV, Intravenous; LTB, Laryngotracheobronchitis; RRP, Recurrent Respiratory Papillomatosis; JRA, Juvenile Rheumatoid Arthritis; ABPA, Allergic Bronchopulmonary Aspergillosis; SJS, Stevens-Johnson Syndrome; WG, Wegener's granulomatosis

pends upon the degree of airway obstruction at the time of presentation (Practice Pathway 50-1). In general, patients with significant airway obstruction need to be admitted to the hospital and carefully monitored. In patients with more severe airway obstruction, securing the airway may be necessary before further evaluation ensues.

With this general approach in mind, the specific types of infectious and inflammatory disorders of the pediatric airway are described below.

AT A GLANCE . . .

Symptoms of Airway Obstruction

- Noisy breathing/stridor
- Retractions
- Color change/cyanosis
- Cough
- Feeding problems
- Failure to thrive
- Sleeping abnormalities

INFECTIOUS DISORDERS OF THE LARYNX AND TRACHEA

Table 50-1 lists both the infectious and inflammatory disorders of the larynx and trachea.

Laryngotracheobronchitis (Viral Croup)

Laryngotracheobronchitis (LTB) is the most common cause of upper airway obstruction (UAO) in patients between 6 months and 6 years of age.[1,2] The clinical spectrum of LTB is quite broad: some patients have the characteristic barking cough without stridor, whereas others may have cough and significant airway obstruction. Patients with LTB present with a prodromal upper respiratory infection (URI) that is associated with barking cough, hoarseness, and biphasic stridor. This particular form of croup may involve the entire glottis, not just the subglottis. In addition, the infection may extend further into the trachea and bronchi. The most common viral agents implicated are parainflu-

TABLE 50–1: Infectious and Inflammatory Disorders of the Larynx and Trachea

Infectious
Laryngotracheobronchitis (Croup)
Epiglottitis
Bacterial tracheitis
Recurrent respiratory papillomatosis (RRP)
Diphtheria
Mucocutaneous candidiasis
Other viral illnesses (e.g., herpes simplex, varicella)
Tuberculosis
Histoplasmosis
Inflammatory
Juvenile rheumatoid arthritis (JRA)
Dermatomyositis
Allergic bronopulmonary aspergillosis (ABPA)
Pemphigus vulgaris (PV)
Bullous pemphigoid
Stevens-Johnson syndrome
Anaphylaxis
Hereditary angioedema
Wegener's granulomatosis

enza and influenza viruses. These patients most commonly present between 1 and 3 years of age.

The diagnosis of LTB usually is confirmed by the history and physical examination. Anterior-posterior (AP) and lateral neck radiographs may provide support for this diagnosis. On the AP view, a "steeple sign" refers to the characteristic subglottic narrowing of the airway seen in children with croup (Fig. 50-1). Narrowing also may be identified on the lateral radiograph. The diagnosis of LTB should be based primarily on clinical history and physical examination, as the radiographic findings are neither sensitive nor specific.

Children with mild forms of LTB may be cared for at home with humidification and, in some cases, use of oral corticosteroids. In the emergency room or hospital setting, treatment may include humidification, inhaled racemic epinephrine, and corticosteroids.[1,3-5] Patients with LTB should respond to therapy in 24 to 48 hours. The role of empiric antibiotic therapy to treat associated bacterial infection is controversial. Laryngoscopy, bronchoscopy, and intubation should be reserved for patients with severe airway obstruction. If at all possible, intubation should be avoided in these patients. Because of the inflamed subglottis, intubated children may be at risk for acquired subglottic stenosis. If intubation is

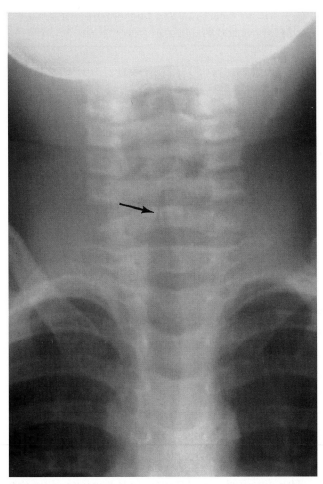

Figure 50–1: Soft-tissue radiograph of the neck taken in the AP projection demonstrates subglottic narrowing (arrow) of the tracheal air column (Photograph courtesy of Andrew F. Inglis, Jr., M.D.).

required, it is helpful to obtain a culture from the subglottis to rule out concomitant bacterial tracheitis. Careful attention should be paid to the amount of leak around the tube. If the leak cannot be maintained, consideration should be made to downsizing the endotracheal tube or performing a tracheotomy. The need for tracheotomy is rare with LTB.

Many children have a history of recurrent croup. Those children with persistent airway symptoms between episodes of croup, failure to thrive, or exercise intolerance should undergo elective laryngoscopy and bronchoscopy between episodes of acute infection to rule out underlying anatomic abnormalities that may require intervention. Also, infants <6 months of age with a history of croup should be examined carefully. These patients may have an anatomic lesion, most notably subglottic hemangioma, that may be causing their symptoms.

> **SPECIAL CONSIDERATION:**
> Infants <6 months of age with a history of croup should be evaluated for an anatomic lesion (e.g., a subglottic hemangioma) that may be causing their symptoms.

Spasmodic croup refers to abrupt onset of barking cough with or without stridor and hoarseness. These patients usually have no prodromal illness and awaken in the middle of the night with the acute onset of the characteristic cough. The distinction between spasmodic croup and LTB is primarily a clinical one. LTB is a viral illness, whereas factors such as a change in environmental temperature, allergy, or gastroesophageal reflux (GER) may contribute to the development of spasmodic croup. In general, children presenting with symptoms of spasmodic croup have a milder degree of airway obstruction and usually can be treated as outpatients with supportive measures such as humidification. On occasion, these patients may have more significant airway involvement, necessitating the use of corticosteroids; they rarely require hospitalization for observation or racemic epinephrine treatments.

> **SPECIAL CONSIDERATION:**
> Children presenting with spasmodic croup have a milder degree of airway obstruction and usually can be managed as outpatients with supportive measures.

Epiglottitis

Epiglottitis is an acute bacterial infection involving the supraglottic larynx and should be more aptly labeled *supraglottitis*. Young children between 2 and 7 years of age are most commonly affected, and generally present with rapid onset of airway distress with no history of URI. By the time patients present for medical attention, they are generally toxic in appearance and have high fever, tachycardia, and inspiratory stridor. They often are found sitting in

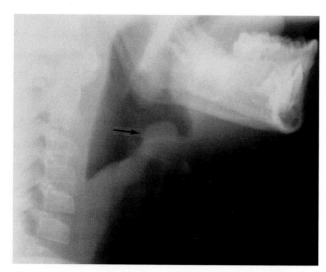

Figure 50–2: Soft-tissue radiograph of the neck taken in the lateral projection demonstrates the widened epiglottic shadow seen with acute epiglottitis (arrow).

the "sniffing" position in an effort to maintain their airway. These children are usually quite anxious, realizing that their airway is significantly compromised.

When epiglottitis is suspected, intraoral examination should be deferred or performed only if equipment is available to secure the airway immediately. The patient should be taken to the radiology suite for a lateral neck radiograph only if accompanied by a team of physicians who can secure the airway. Excessive manipulation of the child and his airway should be avoided to minimize the risk of acute exacerbation of airway obstruction. The classic radiographic finding is the widening or "thumbprinting" of the epiglottic shadow (Fig. 50-2).

SPECIAL CONSIDERATION:

When acute epiglottitis is suspected, intraoral examination should be deferred or performed only if equipment and personnel are available to secure the airway immediately.

Most institutions secure the airway in either the emergency department or operating room with an airway team that includes an anesthesiologist and airway surgeon. To avoid precipitating AAO, the patient should be allowed to sit up while anesthesia

is induced. The induction of anesthesia may be prolonged because of the limited gas exchange. Once the child is asleep, direct laryngoscopy is performed and the patient is intubated (Fig. 50-3). Cultures of the epiglottis may be taken after the airway is secured. Blood cultures should be taken while the child is anesthetized.

The intubated child is transferred to the intensive care unit. In general, these patients require intubation for 24 to 72 hours. Depending on the type of sedation employed, most children do not require ventilatory support. Several parameters can be used to determine the optimal time for extubation, including daily laryngoscopy to assess the status of the epiglottis and the presence of an air leak around the endotracheal tube. Upon extubation, the child is observed in the hospital for at least another 24 to 48 hours. Positive blood cultures may necessitate a longer period of intravenous (IV) antibiotic therapy.

Hemophilus influenzae type B (HiB), which is a pleomorphic, coccobacillary, gram-negative organism that is capable of aerobic and anaerobic growth, is the most common organism causing acute epiglottitis in children. The type B strains are unique in their antigenic capsule. The nontypable strains of *Hemophilus influenzae* are unencapsulated and primarily cause mucosal infections as opposed to the invasive infections that are characteristic of HiB. The infection is thought to spread hematogenously, and patients often have positive blood cultures.[6]

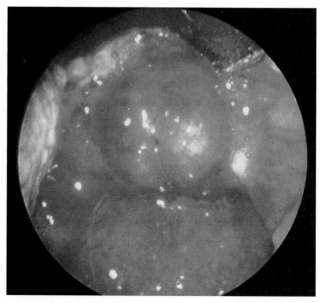

Figure 50–3: Endoscopic appearance of an acutely-inflamed epiglottis in a patient with epiglottitis.

Empiric antibiotic therapy using ceftriaxone, cefuroxime, or cefotaxime should be instituted. With the introduction of the HIB vaccine, epiglottitis is now more commonly associated with nontypable *Hemophilus influenzae* and other organisms. Antibiotic therapy should be tailored to the pathogenic organism, and the duration of antibiotic therapy is determined by the clinical response.

The incidence of epiglottitis has dropped significantly in the United States as a result of routine immunization of young children with the HiB vaccine. The earliest form of the HiB vaccine was introduced in late 1990 and was ineffective for children under 2 years of age. However, the newer conjugated form is effective in children as young as 2 months of age. The ability to immunize infants as young as 2 months of age has changed the morbidity of invasive *Hemophilus* infections significantly in this country.[7,8] Now, epiglottitis in the postvaccine era usually is caused by other organisms and is more common in the adult population.

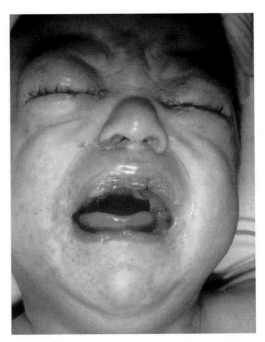

Figure 50–4: Appearance of a patient with measles (Photograph courtesy of Scott C. Manning, M.D.).

SPECIAL CONSIDERATION:

The incidence of epiglottitis has dropped significantly in the United States as a result of routine immunization of young children with the HIB vaccine.

Despite the virtual elimination of invasive HIB infection, it is important for physicians to understand the management issues surrounding patients with epiglottitis to avoid disastrous outcomes.

Bacterial Tracheitis

Bacterial tracheitis may occur as a primary infection with a history of URI or as a complication of another infection.[9,10] Bacterial tracheitis has been associated with measles, varicella, and even viral croup. The most common organisms isolated are *Staphylococcus aureus,* group A beta-hemolytic *Streptococcus, Moraxella catarrhalis,* and *Hemophilus influenzae.*

Generally, these patients present with fever, stridor, and brassy cough. They are commonly toxic and may have the characteristic findings of an asso-

ciated illness (e.g., measles) (Figs. 50–4 and 50–5).[11]

The diagnosis is made on direct endoscopic inspection of the subglottic and tracheal airway. Characteristic findings include purulent debris with pseudomembranes and mucosal ulceration. Cultures of the involved areas should be taken, although they are often nondiagnostic. Blood cultures

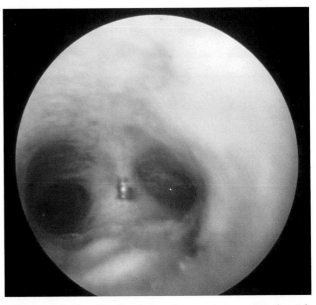

Figure 50–5: Tracheal involvement associated with measles (Photograph courtesy of Scott C. Manning, MD.).

also may be helpful. Empiric antibiotic therapy should be broadly directed against both gram-positive and gram-negative organisms until culture results are available.

Establishment of an airway with endotracheal intubation, or rarely tracheotomy, is required often. Ideally, airway control should be obtained in the operating room. At that time, laryngoscopy and bronchoscopy should be performed. Bronchoscopy may be therapeutic, as well as diagnostic, allowing debridement of the secretions and crusts from the trachea.

> ## SPECIAL CONSIDERATION:
>
> In a child with bacterial tracheitis, bronchoscopy may be therapeutic (i.e., debriding of crusts) as well as diagnostic.

Recurrent Respiratory Papillomatosis

Human papilloma virus (HPV) is a subfamily of the family Papovaviridae, a nonenveloped deoxyribonucleic acid (DNA) virus. Papillomaviruses cause epithelial infections involving either cutaneous or mucosal sites, and are classified by the species of origin and the genetic similarity to other viruses within the same species. Both adult-onset and juvenile-onset RRP are caused by HPV-6 and HPV-11, which are viruses that also are found in the genital tract. These two types of HPV are associated with the rare cases of dysplasia or malignant transformation of papillomatous lesions. Perinatal transmission is thought to account for most cases of RRP in children.

Affected children, usually between 2 and 5 years of age, present with stridor or voice changes. The classic clinical triad involves the first-born child who was delivered vaginally of a teenage mother. Rare cases of children delivered by cesarean section have been described. Males are affected more often than females. The mothers often are noted to have active genital condylomata.

There is some evidence that diagnosis under 6 months of age portends a poor prognosis.[12] Generally, the lesions continue to proliferate and ultimately "burn out" after several years. It is controversial whether viral typing prognosticates the severity of airway obstruction.[13,14]

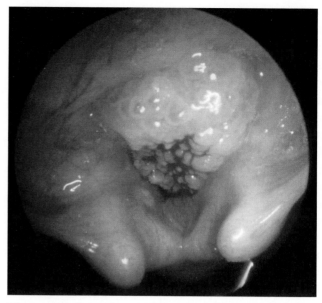

Figure 50–6: Large papillomatous lesion involving the base of the epiglottis and both false vocal cords.

The diagnosis of RRP is made upon endoscopy with observation of the characteristic lesions (Fig. 50–6). Because any region of the upper aerodigestive tract (UADT) can be involved laryngoscopy, bronchoscopy, and careful inspection of the oro- and nasopharynx should be performed (Fig. 50–7).

The primary goal of treatment is to prevent airway obstruction while the lesions are in the prolifer-

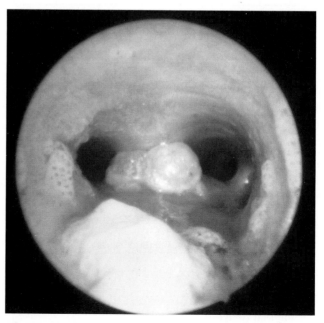

Figure 50–7: Recurrent respiratory papillomas of the trachea (Photograph courtesy of Andrew F. Inglis, Jr., MD.).

ative phase and minimize complications of therapy. Routine microlaser laryngoscopy to debulk the obstructive lesions periodically is the mainstay of therapy. The main complication of management of these children involves airway stenosis. Risk factors for airway stenosis include involvement of the posterior glottis and a prolonged period of frequent endoscopic procedures.[15] Although the carbon dioxide (CO_2) laser is used most commonly, the argon laser has been used for lower airway lesions.[16] Other therapeutic modalities have included photodynamic therapy, systemic interferon therapy,[17-19] methotrexate,[20] and most recently, indole therapy.[21] Several treatments, including isotretinoin[22] and acyclovir[23,24] have been controversial. Intralesional injection of cidofovir has been advocated.[25] The multitude of therapeutic approaches attests to the inadequacy of any single treatment option. Tracheotomy should be avoided in the management of the papillomas if at all possible; however, tracheotomy is occasionally necessary for the management of the sequelae of therapy.

SPECIAL CONSIDERATION:

The primary goal of treatment in a child with RRP is to prevent airway obstruction and minimize complications of therapy.

Despite the strong association of RRP with vaginal delivery in mothers with active condylomata, the incidence of infection is sufficiently low that there are no formal recommendations for cesarean section in these patients.[26,27]

AT A GLANCE . . .

Factors Favoring RRP

- First born child
- Teenage mother
- Vaginal delivery
- Male sex
- Mothers with genital warts

Others

Other types of bacterial infections may cause airway symptoms, although the primary site of infection may not involve the larynx or trachea. For example, *Corynebacterium diphtheriae* produces a pharyngolaryngeal pseudomembrane that may result in noisy breathing. This organism also produces an exotoxin that causes multiple cranial neuropathies including involvement of the recurrent laryngeal nerves (RLN) with resultant stridor.

Other mucosal infections involving the hypopharynx and glottis may present with stridor. These infections include mucocutaneous candidiasis, herpes simplex, and varicella.

Unusual Infections Involving the Pediatric Airway

Tuberculosis

Laryngeal tuberculosis, caused by *Mycobacterium tuberculosis,* is very rare in the United States. However, tuberculosis has become more common in recent decades in relation to an increased population of immunocompromised patients. Affected children may present with severe pharyngitis associated with mucosal ulceration and membrane formation. The infection is most likely to spread hematogenously and may be associated with abdominal tuberculosis. Unlike adults, children with laryngeal tuberculosis usually do *not* have pulmonary involvement.[28-30]

SPECIAL CONSIDERATION:

Unlike adults, children with laryngeal tuberculosis usually do not have pulmonary involvement.

Diagnosis requires laryngoscopy and bronchoscopy with biopsy of the inflamed area. The specimen should be sent for both culture and pathologic examination. Diagnosis is confirmed by isolating acid-fast bacilli from culture or biopsy material, along with the classic histologic findings of caseating granulomas. Mycobacterial organisms are notoriously fastidious and often require many weeks to identify using routine culture techniques. The introduction of molecular methods of microbial identification has facilitated diagnosis of tuberculous infections. Polymerase chain reaction (PCR) is used to amplify the DNA present, and DNA probes can then be used to identify the organism definitively. These techniques can be used on cultured organisms and clinical specimens, as well as in fixed-tissue specimens. Antibiotic susceptibility testing is recommended for all specimens positive for *Mycobacterium tuberculosis.* Susceptibility testing is important for public health reasons as well as patient management. A positive reaction to tuberculin purified protein derivative skin tests provides further support for the diagnosis of tuberculous infections.

Treatment of laryngeal tuberculosis includes establishment of a safe airway followed by medical therapy. Principles of treatment for tuberculosis include: (1) a high rate of spontaneous mutation; (2) a potential for recurrence if the treatment course is inadequate; and (3) drug resistance that is usually the result of noncompliance. Antituberculous regimens include at least two agents and are administered for 6 to 12 months. Isoniazid, rifampin, ethambutol, and streptomycin are first-line agents. Triple-drug therapy and longer courses of treatment may be required for resistant organisms. Patients are at greatest risk for recrudescence of infection within 12 months after completion of therapy. Antibiotic management should be overseen by public health staff in an effort to maximize compliance, minimize the risk of drug resistance, and monitor patients for drug toxicity.[31]

Tuberculous lesions that cause obstructive symptoms also may be found in the trachea or mainstem bronchi. These lesions generally represent infection of the paratracheal or parabronchial lymph nodes eroding into the large airways. Bronchoscopy with biopsy and culture is required for diagnosis, and treatment is with antituberculous medications.

Histoplasmosis

Dimorphic fungus, which can cause laryngeal lesions, is confused easily with squamous cell carcinoma. Biopsy and special staining is required for diagnosis. Treatment includes prolonged administration of amphotericin B.

INFLAMMATORY DISORDERS OF THE LARYNX AND TRACHEA

For a list of these inflammatory disorders, please see Table 50-1.

Juvenile Rheumatoid Arthritis

Juvenile rheumatoid arthritis (JRA) is an autoimmune disease that classically presents with fevers and joint pain. Chronic joint involvement includes inflammation of the synovial lining of joint spaces that may cause damage to the articular surfaces and surrounding soft tissues.

Children may present with the symptoms of JRA at any age, although infants under 1 year of age are rarely affected. There are five subgroups of JRA based on the serology, number of joints involved, and presence of systemic symptoms, and each has been described well. The systemic signs that may be associated with JRA include fever, hepatosplenomegaly, abdominal pain, lymphadenopathy, rash, pericarditis, pleuritis, leukocytosis, anemia, and occasionally, disseminated intravascular coagulopathy.

Children with JRA may present with airway obstruction related to involvement of the cricoarytenoid joint. *Cricoarytenoid arthritis* is rare but should be considered, particularly in patients with known JRA presenting with UAO. Patients with JRA also may develop *bronchitis obliterans* related to their primary disease. Patients with bronchitis obliterans may have markedly impaired pulmonary function without radiographic abnormalities. The diagnosis is made during laryngoscopy and bronchoscopy. Treatment of both of these airway manifestations of JRA involves aggressive medical management of the underlying disease. The rheumatologist generally oversees the management of these patients.

The etiology of JRA is unclear, although there is some evidence that affected children have circulating autoantibodies. The role of these antibodies in the pathogenesis of this disease remains unclear. Diagnosis is primarily based on the clinical findings. Supportive laboratory tests include rheumatoid factor (RF), antinuclear antibodies (ANA) and erythrocyte sedimentation rate (ESR). Whereas the RF is almost always positive in adults with rheumatoid arthritis, this is much less true in children. Laboratory testing may be most important in ruling out other possible causes of joint pain in children (e.g., Lyme disease, inflammatory bowel disease, or septic arthritis).

SPECIAL CONSIDERATION:

Whereas the RF is almost always positive in adults with rheumatoid arthritis, this is much less true in children.

Treatment of JRA includes high-dose corticosteroids, antiinflammatory medications, and cytotoxic agents such as methotrexate, gold injections, and antimalarials. Physical therapy is an important intervention to preserve and maintain joint function, although this is not helpful in the management of cricoarytenoid involvement. Immunotherapy has been advocated recently, although its benefits remain unclear.[32] Chronic pain, joint deformities, and visual defects related to iridocyclitis may occur. The overall prognosis for children with JRA is good; most children do not develop significant disability related to the disease.

AT A GLANCE . . .

Systemic Signs of JRA

- Fever
- Hepatosplenomegaly
- Abdominal pain
- Lymphadenopathy
- Rash
- Pericarditis
- Pleuritis
- Leukocytosis
- Anemia/DIC (Disseminated intravascular coagulopathy)

Dermatomyositis

Dermatomyositis (DMS) is an inflammatory disease of striated muscles and skin. The inflammation is characterized by obliterative vasculitis involving the small vessels. This disease typically involves the proximal limb and trunk muscles; the palatal and respiratory muscles also may be involved. The characteristic cutaneous manifestations of DMS include "heliotrope hue," which is a violaceous erythema of the upper lids, and erythematous macules and papules over the extensor surfaces of the joints, especially the small joints of the hands. This vasculitis also may involve the gastrointestinal tract or the pharyngeal and supraglottic mucosa.

Diagnosis of DMS includes the presence of the clinical symptoms, which are proximal muscle weakness, rash, elevated muscle enzymes, and characteristic findings on electromyogram (EMG). Mus-

cle biopsy may confirm the diagnosis and is important in distinguishing DMS from other forms of myositis. The diagnostic findings on pathologic section include fiber necrosis, variation in fiber size, endothelial swelling, and occlusive vasculitis.

The pathogenesis of this disease is unknown, although infection has been implicated as a contributing factor.

DMS generally is responsive to medical management with high-dose corticosteroids. Azathioprine, methotrexate, hydroxychloroquine, and cyclosporine have all demonstrated some benefit. These adjunctive agents may be useful in a steroid sparing capacity.[32]

Allergic Bronchopulmonary Aspergillosis

The three major groups of pulmonary aspergillosis are invasive, noninvasive, and *Aspergillus* sensitivity syndromes [e.g., extrinsic asthma, extrinsic allergic alveolitis, and allergic bronchopulmonary aspergillosis (ABPA)]. *ABPA* usually occurs in atopic and asthmatic patients. Children with ABPA may present with fever, unilateral wheezing, and focal radiographic findings suggestive of foreign-body aspiration. Findings that support the diagnosis of ABPA include a history of reactive airway disease, intermediate *Aspergillus* skin reactivity, increased serum immunoglobulin E (IgE) eosinophilia, *Aspergillus* precipitating antibodies, increased immunoglobulin G (IgG) IgE–*Aspergillus* antigen complexes, and proximal bronchiectasis. Confirming the diagnosis can be difficult.

Patients with ABPA may develop a mucus plug, which creates a cast of the lower airways, causing focal signs. Patients may expectorate spontaneously a mucus plug, or bronchoscopy may be required to extract the plug. Histologic examination of the plug reveals casts of eosinophils and also may demonstrate fungal elements. Occasionally, the diagnosis of ABPA is made by finding the characteristic cast of the lower airway when bronchoscopy is performed to rule out a foreign-body aspiration (Fig. 50–8).

The treatment of choice is corticosteroids. Response to therapy can be followed with serial chest radiographs and serum IgE levels. Clinical response should be detectable within 2 months of initiating therapy. This disease is primarily allergic in etiology, and therefore antifungal treatment has not been effective.[33]

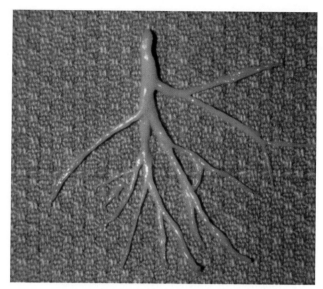

Figure 50–8: Cast of the airway endoscopically removed from a patient with allergic bronchopulmonary aspergillosis (Photograph courtesy of Andrew F. Inglis, Jr., MD.).

AT A GLANCE . . .

Types of Pulmonary Aspergillosis

- Invasive
- Noninvasive
- Aspergillus sensitivity syndromes

Pemphigus Vulgaris

Pemphigus vulgaris (PV) is seen occasionally in children. This is a serious chronic intraepidermal bullous dermatosis with autoantibodies directed against antigens on the epidermal cell surfaces. This disease may affect cutaneous or mucosal surfaces. The supraglottic mucosa may be involved, causing symptoms of UAO. In general, patients with airway involvement have cutaneous manifestations of the disease. Patients with widespread disease are at risk for electrolyte disturbances and infection.

Patients with active PV generally have a positive *Nikolsky's sign* (i.e., blister formation by displacement of perilesion skin by friction). Diagnosis is made on biopsy of the bullous lesions, showing suprabasilar acantholysis. Direct immunofluorescence shows deposition of both IgG and C3 (Complement 3) in the epidermal intercellular spaces. Circulating autoantibodies are present in most patients.

Treatment depends upon the severity of disease. Mild cases may respond to topical corticosteroids applied to the areas of involvement. More widespread disease generally is responsive to systemic corticosteroids.[34]

Bullous Pemphigoid

Bullous pemphigoid is an autoimmune disorder that is characterized by tense subepidermal lesions and that is seen primarily in the elderly population. However, cases have been reported in infants as young as 2 months of age. Most childhood cases occur before the age of 8 years.

The lesions are tense blisters arising on an urticarial base or on normal skin. The blisters heal without scarring. Mucosal involvement is more common in children than in adults. The supraglottis may be involved, causing symptoms of UAO.

Diagnosis is made by the presentation of the clinical lesions and histologic findings of subepidermal bullous lesion with a dermal eosinophilic inflammatory infiltrate. Immunofluorescence shows linear deposition of IgG and C3 on the basement membrane.

Treatment includes systemic corticosteroids. Sulfones (i.e., dapsone, sulfapyridine) have been used also.[34]

SPECIAL CONSIDERATION:

The diagnoses of pemphigus vulgaris or bullous pemphigoid may be suspected clinically but are confirmed by biopsy.

Stevens-Johnson Syndrome

Stevens-Johnson Syndrome (SJS) is a form of erythema multiforme. The syndrome is characterized by severe erythema multiforme with bullous formation, extensive mucosal erosions, and marked constitutional symptoms. This disease is more common in children than adults, and most commonly affects children in the second decade of life. SJS is preceded commonly by a febrile illness that includes headache and malaise. The mucocutaneous lesions erupt rapidly and quickly turn into tender blisters. The blisters rupture, leaving potentially-large denuded areas. Significant mucosal involvement is typical. Complications of SJS are common and include sepsis, electrolyte disturbances, and pneumonia.

The onset of SJS is thought to be an immune response to a precipitating factor, such as drugs, mycoplasma, or herpes simplex infection. It is postulated that the inciting agent localizes at the mucocutaneous junction and a cell-mediated immune response causes the tissue damage.

The course of this disease process generally lasts 3 to 4 weeks. Treatment is generally supportive with wound care, fluid resuscitation, and avoidance of corticosteroids. With aggressive medical care of any complications that arise, the prognosis for these patients is good. Long-term sequelae are related to scarring from the mucosal lesions.[34]

Anaphylaxis

Allergic reactions are categorized into four major classes: (1) *anaphylactic reactions* (type I); (2) *cytotoxic reactions* (type II); (3) *toxic immune complexes* reactions (type III); and (4) *delayed-type hypersensitivity reactions* (type IV). Although the latter three types of allergic responses may contribute to the pathophysiology of some of the other diseases described in this chapter, the anaphylactic reaction (type I) is the allergic response that is associated with allergic angioedema causing airway obstruction. This response is mediated by IgE antibodies and is related to urticaria, hay fever, allergic rhinitis, and allergic asthma. The onset of anaphylactic reactions may be sudden, requiring immediate treatment. The patient may have a tingling sensation followed by pallor, weakness, pruritus, urticaria, nausea, vomiting, diarrhea, palpitations, wheezing, stridor, cyanosis, and hypotension. The type I reaction includes the "late" allergic responses, including airway obstruction, that appear several hours after exposure to the allergen. Most of these types of allergic reactions result from exposure to a systemic allergen, such as foods or medications. Insect stings also may evoke this reaction.

Treatment of an acute episode of anaphylaxis, which includes airway obstruction, should include establishment of an adequate airway and medical management of the allergic reaction. Medical management of anaphylaxis should include immediate administration of epinephrine, antihistamines, and fluid resuscitation. Corticosteroids also may be beneficial in this setting, although the onset of action is longer than the other agents mentioned.

Prevention of subsequent episodes is critical. Identification of the allergen is important in order to implement avoidance measures. Allergy testing in patients with a history of anaphylaxis must be performed with extreme care to avoid an anaphylactic reaction to the allergen. This testing should be performed at least 1 month after the anaphylactic event in order to avoid false-negative results related to a refractory period.[35]

AT A GLANCE . . .

Mechanisms of Hypersensitivity

Types:
Anaphylactic reaction (type I): associated with allergic angioedema and is mediated by IgE antibodies; related to urticaria, hay fever, allergic rhinitis, and allergic asthma
Cytotoxic reaction (type II): IgC or IgM reacts with components of the cell membrane causing complement activation.
Toxic immune complex reaction (type III): antigen-antibody complexes cause tissue injury, serum sickness
Delayed hypersensitivity reaction (type IV): T-cell mediated response; contact allergies

Symptoms and Signs: pallor, cyanosis, weakness, pruritus, urticaria, nausea, vomiting, diarrhea, palpitations, wheezing, stridor, and hypotention

Treatment: epinephrine, antihistamines, fluid resuscitation, corticosteroids

---

Hereditary Angioedema

Hereditary angioedema is a defect of the complement system in which the patient has a deficiency of functional C1 (Complement 1) inhibitor. Clinically, hereditary angioedema is characterized by transient, localized, nonpitting edema, without associated urticaria, erythema, or pain. Often, there is an inciting event, usually trauma. In the head and neck, the oral mucosa and occasionally the larynx typically are involved. The episodes generally last 2 to 3 days and gradually remit. Clinical manifestation of the disease may occur as early as 2 years of life. The severity of the episodes increases with age.

Affected patients may have decreased levels of C1 inhibitor or may have normal levels on serology (C1 inhibitor) with impaired function. Both forms are autosomal dominant, with 10% of cases thought to result from spontaneous mutation.

The diagnosis is made when the patient with the characteristic clinical picture has complement levels drawn. During an acute episode, there are decreased C2 (Complement 2) and C4 (Complement 4) levels, as well as decreased total complement levels. In the convalescent phase of the disease, the C4 level is low and the C3 (Complement 3) level is normal. In approximately 85% of cases, C1INH levels will be low; in the remaining 15%, the levels will be normal although the activity may be decreased. The diagnosis can be confirmed on complement activation tests.

Treatment of patients with angioneurotic edema involves avoidance of precipitating factors and supportive measures. It is important that the child and family understand the association of an inciting event with the onset of symptoms. Children with airway involvement should have their airway stabilized in the routine manner (i.e., intubation or tracheotomy for severe airway obstruction). Danazol has been used in adults to prevent acute episodes, however because of its androgenic effects it is not recommended for use in children. Epinephrine may be helpful in treatment of the edema, although corticosteroids and antihistamines are not useful generally. Epsilon-aminocaproic acid (EACA), a plasminogen activation inhibitor, may be useful for prophylaxis during dental or surgical procedures.[36]

Wegener's Granulomatosis

Wegener's granulomatosis (WG) is a necrotizing vasculitis causing granulomatous lesions of the respiratory mucosa, lungs, and kidneys. The eyes, skin, nervous system, and heart may be involved also. Although the classic otolaryngologic manifestations of the disease involve the nasal mucosa, the larynx and subglottic airway also may be involved.[37-40]

SPECIAL CONSIDERATION:

Although the classic otolaryngologic manifestations of WG involve the nasal mucosa, the larynx and trachea also may be involved.

The clinical presentation of these patients is variable, as the disease may involve a number of different systems. Rarely, these patients may present with

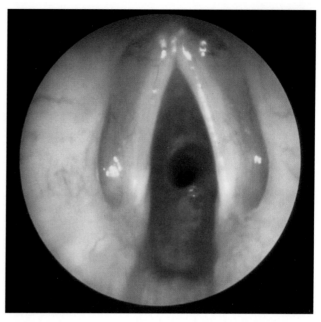

Figure 50–9: Subglottic narrowing in a patient with Wegener's granulomatosis.

AAO as a result of laryngeal or subglottic involvement. More commonly, a patient with known WG develops symptoms of airway involvement. Any patient with known WG and symptoms localized to the airway should undergo laryngoscopy and bronchoscopy (Fig. 50–9). Diagnosis is made by histologic findings of granulomatous vasculitis and laboratory tests that measure the presence of serum cytoplasmic antineutrophil cytoplasmic antibodies (cANCA).

Treatment of patients with WG includes trimethoprim-sulfamethoxazole for localized disease. Systemic disease requires treatment with corticosteroids and cytotoxic agents, primarily cyclophosphamide. Patients with AAO may require airway management until response to medical management is obtained. cANCA levels may be used to monitor response to therapy.

SUMMARY

Children are afflicted frequently by infectious and less commonly by inflammatory diseases of the airway. Often the diagnosis of these disorders can be made on clinical examination alone, although direct laryngoscopy and bronchoscopy with culture or biopsy may be required in some cases. The treatment of most of these diseases is medical and results in a significant reduction in morbidity.

REFERENCES

1. Skolnik NS. Treatment of croup. A critical review. Am J Dis Child 1989; 143(9):1045-1049.
2. Baugh R, Gilmore BB. Infectious croup: a critical review. Otolaryngol Head Neck Surg 1986; 95:40-466.
3. Geelhoed GC. Croup. Pediatr Pulmonol 1997; 23: 370-374.
4. Yates RW, Doull IJ. A risk-benefit assessment of corticosteroids in the management of croup. Drug Saf 1997; 16:48-55.
5. Klassen TP, Rowe PC. Outpatient management of croup. Curr Opin Pediatr 1996; 8:449-452.
6. Wurtele P. Acute epiglottitis: Historical highlights and perspectives for future research. J Otolaryngol 1992; 21(Supplement 2):1-15.
7. Force RW, Lugo RA, Nahata MC. Haemophilus influenzae type B conjugate vaccines. Ann Pharmacother 1992; 26:1429-1440.
8. Madore DV. Impact of immunization on Haemophilus influenzae type B disease. Infect Agents Dis 1996; 5:8-20.
9. Rabie I, McShane D, Warde D. Bacterial tracheitis. J Laryngol Otol 1989; 103:1059-1062.
10. Labay M, et al. Membranous laryngotracheobronchitis: A complication of measles. Intensive Care Med 1985; 11:326-327.
11. Manning S, et al. Measles: An epidemic of upper airway obstruction. Otolaryngol Head Neck Surg 1991; 105:415-418.
12. Chipps BE, et al. Respiratory papillomas: Presentation before six months. Pediatr Pulmonol 1990; 9: 125-130.
13. Rimell FL, et al. Pediatric respiratory papillomatosis: Prognostic role of viral typing and cofactors. Laryngoscope 1997; 107:915-918.
14. Gabbott M, et al. Human papillomavirus and host variables as predictors of clinical course in patients with juvenile-onset recurrent respiratory papillomatosis. J Clin Microbiol 1997; 35:3098-3103.
15. Perkins JA, Inglis AF, Richardson MA. Iatrogenic airway stenosis with recurrent respiratory papillomatosis. Arch Otolaryngol Head Neck Surg 1998; 124:281-287.
16. Bergler W, et al. Treatment of recurrent respiratory papillomatosis with argon plasma coagulation. J Laryngol Otol 1997; 111:381-384.
17. Healy GB, et al. Treatment of recurrent respiratory papillomatosis with human leukocyte interferon. Results of a multicenter randomized clinical trial. N Engl J Med 1988; 319:401-407.
18. Kashima H, et al. Interferon alfa-n1 (Wellferon) in juvenile onset recurrent respiratory papillomatosis: Results of a randomized study in twelve collaborative institutions. Laryngoscope 1988; 98:334-340.
19. Leventhal BG, et al. Randomized surgical adjuvant trial of interferon alfa-n1 in recurrent papillomatosis. Arch Otolaryngol Head Neck Surg 1988; 114: 1163-1169.
20. Avidano MA, Singleton GT. Adjuvant drug strategies in the treatment of recurrent respiratory papillomatosis. Otolaryngol Head Neck Surg 1995; 112: 197-202.
21. Coll DA, et al. Treatment of recurrent respiratory papillomatosis with indole-3-carbinol. Am J Otolaryngol 1997; 18:283-285.
22. Eicher SA, Taylor CLD, Donovan DT. Isotretinoin therapy for recurrent respiratory papillomatosis. Arch Otolaryngol Head Neck Surg 1994; 120: 405-409.
23. Kiroglu M, et al. Acyclovir in the treatment of recurrent respiratory papillomatosis: A preliminary report. Am J Otolaryngol 1994; 15:212-214.
24. Morrison GA, Evans JN. Juvenile respiratory papillomatosis: Acyclovir reassessed. Int J Pediatr Otorhinolaryngol 1993; 26:193-197.
25. Snoeck R, et al. Treatment of severe laryngeal papillomatosis with intralesional injections of cidofovir. J Med Virol 1998; 54:219-225.
26. Kosko JR, Derkay CS. Role of cesarean section in prevention of recurrent respiratory papillomatosis-Is there one? Int J Pediatr Otorhinolaryngol 1996; 35:31-38.
27. Kashima HK, Mounts P, Shah K. Recurrent respiratory papillomatosis. Obstet Gynecol Clin North Am 1996; 23:699-706.
28. Ramadan HH, Wax MK. Laryngeal tuberculosis. A cause of stridor in children. Arch Otolaryngol Head Neck Surg 1995; 121:109-112.
29. Elias JAC, et al. Tuberculosis presenting as laryngeal stridor in a child. J Infect 1988; 16:61-64.
30. du PA, Hussey G. Laryngeal tuberculosis in childhood. Pediatr Infect Dis J 1987; 6:678-681.
31. Toossi Z, Ellner J. Tuberculosis and leprosy. In: Gorbach S, Bartlett J, Blacklow N, eds. *Infectious Diseases.* Philadelphia: Saunders, 1998, pp. 1505-1513.
32. Tucker L, Miller L, Schaller J. Rheumatic disorders. In: Stiehm E, ed. *Immunologic Disorders in Infants and Children,* Philadelphia: Saunders, 1996, pp. 742-793.
33. Pfaff J, Taussig L. Pulmonary disorders. In: Stiehm E, ed. *Immunologic Disorders in Infants and Children.* Philadelphia: Saunders, 1996, pp. 659-696.
34. Morrison L, Hanifin J. Dermatologic disorders. In: Stiehm E, ed. *Immunologic Disorders in Infants and Children.* Philadelphia: Saunders, 1996, pp. 644-658.
35. Pearlman D, Bierman C. Allergic disorders. In: Stiehm E, ed. *Immunologic Disorders of Infants and Children.* Philadelphia: Saunders, 1996, pp. 603-643.
36. Kamani N, Douglas S. Disorders of the mononuclear

phagocytic system. In: Stiehm E, ed. *Immunologic Disorders of Infants and Children.* Philadelphia: Saunders, 1996, pp. 469–509.

37. O'Devaney K, et al. Wegener's granulomatosis of the head and neck. Ann Otol Rhinol Laryngol 1998; 107: 439–445.

38. DeRemee RA. Wegener's granulomatosis. Curr Opin Pulm Med 1995; 1:363–367.

39. Matt BH. Wegener's granulomatosis, acute laryngotracheal airway obstruction and death in a 17-year-old female: Case report and review of the literature. Int J Pediatr Otorhinolaryngol 1996; 37:163–172.

40. Leavitt RY, Fauci AS. Less common manifestations and presentations of Wegener's granulomatosis. Curr Opin Rheumatol 1992; 4:16–22.

51 Infant and Pediatric Apnea

Ralph F. Wetmore

While the adverse effects of airway obstruction at night have been described in the medical literature for well over 100 years, the last 3 decades have produced an explosion of information about disordered respiration during sleep. Perhaps the most famous description of a sleep disorder was that penned by Sir William Osler[1] in 1906 in his treatise *The Principles and Practice of Medicine,* in which he graphically described the association between hypersomnolence and obesity, a condition that he compared to the fat boy, Joe, a character in Charles Dicken's *The Posthumous Papers of the Pickwick Club.*

In 1959, Cole and Alexander[2] described a clinical correlation between obesity, chronic hypoventilation, and pulmonary hypertension. Subsequently, Menashe et al.[3] reported the development of cor pulmonale and hypoventilation due to adenotonsillar hypertrophy in two children. The presence of airway obstruction and *apnea,* the temporary cessation of breathing, have become well recognized throughout pediatric medicine. Apnea has been implicated in the pathogenesis of sudden infant death syndrome (SIDS) and in the identification of obstructive sleep apnea (OSA) in children, which is a condition that is clinically distinct from the adult disorder and has assumed greater importance in the past two decades. This chapter is divided into two major sections, one discussing the abnormalities of respiration in the neonate and infant, and the other reviewing OSA in children through adolescence.

DEFINITIONS

The basic definitions of the three major classes of apnea remain identical in the adult, child, and infant. *Central apnea* (CA) is the complete cessation of breathing without respiratory effort. *Obstructive apnea* (OA) is the lack of airflow due to airway obstruction while respiratory efforts continue. The combination of obstructive and central elements defines *mixed apnea* (MA). However, despite the similar definitions, one of the major problems that has faced the study of apnea in infants and children is the mistaken impression that adult criteria for normal and abnormal sleep can be applied to the infant and pediatric populations.

Apnea in Neonates and Infants

All three types of apnea may be found in neonates and infants and must be distinguished from periodic breathing. *Periodic breathing* is defined as events of regular respiration of up to 20 seconds that are followed by apneic periods of no longer than 10 seconds, which occur at least three times in succession.[4] Periodic breathing in preterm infants is usually not of clinical significance, although rarely it may cause upper airway obstruction.[5,6] *Significant apnea* (central, obstructive, or mixed) in neonates and infants includes episodes of greater than 20 seconds of duration, or episodes of less than 20 seconds if accompanied by bradycardia to 20% below baseline heart rate or oxygen desaturation below 80% of baseline.[4]

Apnea in Children and Adolescents

The apnea index (the number of apneas greater than 10 seconds duration/hour of sleep) can be used to quantify the amount of OA. In normal adults, this index ranges from 5-10.[7,8] In children and adolescents, in whom the episodes are much more frequent but shorter in duration, the apnea index range is 0.1 +/− 0.5.[9] Marcus et al.[9] consider that more than one obstructive event of any duration in the pediatric age group is abnormal. *Hypopnea,* or episodes of partial obstruction, are also more common in the pediatric population. Various definitions of hypopnea have been offered: (1) 50% reduction in airflow,[10] (2) 50% reduction in respiratory effort;[11] (3) reduction in airflow and a decrease in oxygen (O_2) desaturation;[12] and (4) reduction in both

Pediatric Otolaryngology, Edited by R.F. Wetmore, H.R. Muntz, and T.J. McGill. Thieme Medical Publishers, Inc., New York © 2000.

airflow and effort and a decrease in O_2 saturation.[13] Children tend to have more episodes of hypopnea than adults, in whom true apneas are more significant. For this reason, Rosen et al.[14] suggest that abnormalities of end tidal carbon dioxide (CO_2) and O_2 saturation during sleep are better indicators of upper airway obstruction. Abnormal end tidal CO_2 values are described by Marcus et al.[9] as peak end tidal CO_2 greater than 53 mmHg or as end tidal CO_2 greater than 45 mmHg for more than 60% of the total sleep time. Likewise, an O_2 saturation less than 92% should be considered abnormal in the pediatric age group.[9]

Episodes of CA greater than 10 seconds occur frequently in children and adolescents. Rarely is there an impairment of gas exchange during these episodes.[9] However, CA greater than 20 seconds are of uncertain clinical significance.[15] Marcus et al.[9] recommend that central events of any duration be considered abnormal if the O_2 saturation falls below 90%.

APNEA OF PREMATURITY AND INFANCY

Apnea in neonates before 37 weeks of gestational age is *apnea of prematurity. Apnea of infancy* is defined as apnea in neonates older than 37 weeks of gestational age. Preterm infants have more frequent episodes of apnea: 25% of infants weighing less than 2500 gm and 84% of infants weighing less than 1000 gm.[16] In fact, at 40 weeks of gestational age, preterm infants still show significantly more apnea than term infants. This difference in the amount of apnea persists until 64 weeks of gestational age.[17] Likewise, periodic breathing also decreases as the infant matures.[18]

Pathogenesis

Factors that predispose to infant apnea include those that affect the airway or neurologic control of respiration (Table 51-1). Anatomic and neurologic factors frequently result in MA. Small premature infants demonstrate MA (53-71%) more often than CA (10-25%) or OA (12-20%) alone.[19,20]

As in older children and adults, the most common site of anatomic obstruction in the apneic infant is in the pharynx.[21] Isolated lesions of the larynx that cause OA, such as subglottic stenosis, subglottic

TABLE 51–1:   Factors Predisposing to Infant Apnea

Airway anatomic abnormalities
Drugs
Electrolyte abnormalities
Gastroesophageal reflux (GER)
Metabolic errors
Poor thermoregulation
Prematurity
Seizure disorder

hemangioma, glottic web, or bilateral vocal cord paralysis (as seen with the Arnold-Chiari malformation), are rare.[22] Likewise, the occurrence of multiple lesions in the larynx and pharynx that cause apnea is uncommon. Collapse of the pharyngeal lumen, which is the result of a lack of activation of the genioglossus and other pharyngeal muscles that span the pharynx, is the major cause of airway obstruction.[23,24] The response of the pharyngeal musculature to hypercapnia tends to be delayed compared to the response of the diaphragmatic muscles, and this instability of the pharyngeal airway at a time when respiration is normal may explain why OA and MA events are more common after episodes of CA.[18]

Central control of groups of muscles that maintain the airway and provide respiratory effort suggests a common, neurologically-controlled pathway that results in either OA, CA, MA.[18] The respiratory center, located in the brainstem, may be susceptible to inhibition from a multitude of sources, including metabolic disorders, infection, gastroesophageal reflux (GER), thermal instability, or drugs.[25] Local reflexes that maintain the pharyngeal and laryngeal airway also may have inhibitory and excitatory influence from higher centers in the brain. For example, sensory receptors in the larynx serve as afferents for reflexes that may cause both CA and OA. These receptors may be stimulated by a variety of substances, including water and acid.[26,27] In preterm infants, even endogenous upper airway secretions may be a source of stimuli-inducing apneic spells.[28] Negative pressures within an isolated upper airway also have been shown to depress ventilation, and this is a finding that also may explain the coexistence of obstructive and central elements within MA.[29]

Other factors that predispose to the development of apnea include responses to CO_2 and O_2. Premature infants appear to exhibit a decreased response to CO_2, although the exact relationship of this finding to apnea is unclear.[30] Infants also demonstrate a biphasic response to a decrease in inspired O_2. Initially, there is an increase in ventilation that is followed by a return to baseline or a decrease in ventilation. This instability of respiration after exposure to O_2 may predispose the infant to apnea.[31]

As in children in general, the effects of apnea on the sleep patterns of infants remain unclear; however, apnea has been shown to be more common during rapid eye movement (REM) sleep when respiratory patterns are more irregular.[32] GER also may play a role in apnea in some infants, although usually after 6 weeks of age.[33] Some infants have been shown to have *pseudoreflux*—episodes of periodic breathing that mimic reflux-induced apnea but that are clinically benign.[34] Frequent swallowing is another finding that has been demonstrated both experimentally and clinically in infants with prolonged apnea.[35]

Adverse Effects of Apnea

Because apnea in infants tends to be of short duration, episodes of hypoxia and hypercarbia, which are seen in more prolonged apneas, may not be readily demonstrated. On the other hand, apnea frequently causes changes in heart rate; typically, bradycardia is thought to result from a complex reflex involving multiple sources.[18] Changes in blood pressure include increases in systolic blood pressure and an occasional fall in diastolic blood pressure.[36] With prolonged or repeated apneic episodes, the decrease in systolic blood flow may begin to compromise cerebral blood flow, causing a condition that may lead to cerebral anoxia in susceptible infants.[18]

Although the exact pathophysiology of SIDS remains elusive and is probably multi-factorial, apnea is implicated as a possible cause. Those who support this hypothesis believe that episodes of apnea are the final common pathway to SIDS.[37] Groups of infants who have been shown to be at high risk for SIDS have also been shown to have higher rates of apnea. These groups include premature infants, siblings of SIDS patients, and those who have undergone an apparent life-threatening event (ALTE), such as some combination of prolonged apnea, marked change in color (cyanosis) or muscle tone or choking or gagging spell.

Symptoms and Signs

Because of the high incidence of apnea in preterm infants, continuous monitoring of heart rate, respiratory patterns, and O_2 saturation are typically performed prior to discharge from the hospital.

SPECIAL CONSIDERATION:

Infants differ from their pediatric counterparts in that they may experience episodes of apnea even while they are awake.

Parents may be alerted to a problem because of their observation of an apneic event or an ALTE. Any infant with an ALTE should be hospitalized for observation and evaluation.

The frequency and duration of apparent apneic episodes are important to document in order to distinguish apnea from periodic breathing clinically. Sleep position has become an important etiologic factor for SIDS, and current American Academy of Pediatrics recommendations suggest that healthy newborn infants should be placed on their back or side to reduce their risk for SIDS. Careful questioning of the infant's sleep position should be included in any evaluation.

Other ominous symptoms include the appearance of cyanotic or gray spells or major changes in muscle tone. In infants with anatomic abnormalities that could cause apnea, the presence of stridor or snoring may help to localize the site of obstruction (e.g., to the larynx or pharynx). Staring or rigid posturing spells may suggest a seizure disorder or reflux-related apnea, especially if the episodes occur 1–2 hours after a feeding. Difficulty with feeding or frequent vomiting also suggests episodes of reflux that may have an effect on respiratory patterns.

Observation of an infant who is suspected of having apnea should be made while the infant is awake, asleep, and feeding. Although brief periods of central apnea may be difficult to detect from observation alone, even short episodes of OA may be apparent. Evaluation of infants suspected of apnea should include a careful cardiac, neurologic, and respiratory examination by physicians familiar with care of newborns (e.g., pediatricians, neonatologies, etc).

Diagnosis

Polysomnography is necessary to confirm the presence and type of apnea. This study is a continuous and simultaneous monitoring of respiratory and cardiac functions over a period of time that may range from 4–24 hours. A polygraphic record is compiled, and allows the observer to document the frequency, duration, and type of apnea, as well as associated events such as GER. Measured parameters are listed in Table 51–2.

Movement of the chest wall is determined by *impedance,* which is a technique that utilizes changes in current from electrocardiogram (EKG) electrodes that vary with changes in the amount of fluid and air within the chest cavity. When combined with a record of the electrical activity of the heart, this study is called a *pneumocardiogram.* Traditionally, this study is used to verify and monitor episodes of CA and it is still useful as a screening tool. Because the chest wall continues to move with obstructive events, the pneumogram may not detect episodes of OA. Newer monitoring units that have computer chips that can record pulse oximetry as well as oral and nasal airflow have replaced the pneumogram in many centers.

Changes in nasal and oral airflow are monitored by a *thermistor,* which is a device that detects differences in inspiratory and expiratory airflow temperature. O_2 saturation is monitored by pulse oximetry; very brief episodes of apnea demonstrate little change in O_2 saturation. A continuous tracing of the EKG may demonstrate bradycardia, which is a finding often seen in infants with significant apnea, or evidence of other arrhythmias. In infants in whom reflux is suspected, simultaneous recording with a pH probe may be correlated with episodes of OA or CA.

Once apnea is documented, an evaluation as to the possible cause should be undertaken. Structural cardiac defects or arrhythmias may be demonstrated on a 12-lead EKG. Although sleep stages are not typically monitored in infants, an electroencephalogram (EEG) may show evidence of a seizure focus. Radiographic studies that are helpful in the evaluation include a chest radiograph to exclude infection

or aspiration, lateral neck radiograph to visualize the upper airway, and a barium swallow to document reflux or a vascular anomaly of the mediastinum. Presence of infection, anemia, metabolic disorders, or electrolyte imbalance that would predispose to apnea may be demonstrated on blood studies, including a complete blood count (CBC), electrolytes, and glucose.

Treatment

Concerns about the adverse effects of apnea (i.e., failure to thrive, chronic hypoxia, and the risk of SIDS) necessitate aggressive treatment of this disorder. Because of the life-threatening nature of SIDS and the tendency of episodes to cluster, a history suggestive of apnea may warrant hospitalization for observation and evaluation.[38]

Although apnea is well recognized as a possible contributor to the pathophysiology of SIDS, not all experts agree that home monitoring is necessary.[39,40] Those in favor of home monitoring point to the monitor as a means of possibly averting a life-threatening event with the intervention of a caregiver trained in cardiopulmonary resuscitation (CPR). Families in whom an infant has died of SIDS or with an infant who has undergone an ALTE often feel more secure with monitoring. On the other hand, those opposed to home monitoring cite data that fails to demonstrate any decrease in the incidence of SIDS. Some families may suffer from the intrusion that a monitor may have on family life.

Early home monitoring systems surveyed for changes in both heart rate and respiration showed that heart rates that fell either above or below set limits activated the alarm. Likewise, respiratory rates outside of preset limits produced a signal. Unfortunately, these early monitors could not recognize the initial signs of distress associated with OA due to the continuation of respiratory attempts during these events. These monitoring systems only recognized obstruction that was severe enough to cause a change in heart rate, typically bradycardia. Recently, alarms have become more sophisticated, employing computer chips that not only monitor vital functions, including oxygen desaturation by way of pulse oximetry, but also store data that can be downloaded for analysis. These multichannel monitors also may have the ability to record nasal and oral airflow, permitting polysomnography to be performed in the home.

The treatment of CA, OA, or MA usually consists

TABLE 51–2: Infant Polysomnography: Recorded Parameters

Chest wall movements (impedance or strain gauges)
Electrocardiogram (EKG)
Nasal and oral airflow
Oxygen saturation
pH probe (if reflux suspected)

of treating the underlying disorders that affect either the upper airway or the centers within the brainstem that control respiratory effort. Methylxanthines, which are respiratory stimulants that act directly on brainstem neurons to stimulate the respiratory drive, are the mainstay of drug therapy for CA.[1] Although both theophylline and caffeine have been utilized as respiratory stimulants in infants, caffeine is preferred because it has a longer half-life and fewer major side effects. Doxapram is another potent respiratory stimulant that causes an increase in minute ventilation and tidal volume without a change in respiratory timing.[42] Other therapy that may lessen or abolish CA includes the discontinuation of medications that affect the respiratory drive, treatment of underlying electrolyte or metabolic abnormalities, and treatment of sepsis with antibiotics. Treatment of seizures may result in a decrease in both central and obstructive events.

Infants with evidence of obstruction of the upper airway require aggressive management, both surgical and nonsurgical. Swelling of the airway, causing acute events of apnea, may be relieved with corticosteroids. Obstruction as the result of upper airway infection may respond to antibiotic therapy. Infants with choanal atresia may be treated with the temporary use of a McGovern nipple or may undergo primary repair of the atresia. Infants with Robin sequence may respond to placement of a nasogastric tube that pushes the tongue forward, re-establishing the airway, or may require a tongue-lip adhesion (glossopexy) to advance the tongue.[43] Airway obstruction that is transient and may improve in a self-limited fashion may be treated temporarily with placement of a nasal or oral airway or endotracheal intubation. Nasal continuous positive airway pressure (CPAP), which is delivered by either nasal prongs, a mask, or a shortened endotracheal tube used as a nasal airway, may improve OA and MA by stenting the airway with positive pressure.[20] Although rare in the infant age group, enlarged adenoid or tonsil tissue may cause obstruction, and improvement may be seen following its removal.[44] In some cases, a tracheotomy may be required to maintain a stable airway.

Infants in whom both GER and apnea have been diagnosed require aggressive treatment of their reflux. Upright positioning and thickened feedings may suffice in some infants. The pharmacologic armamentarium for reflux includes use of H_2-receptor blockers, such as cimetidine or ranitidine, that in-hibit gastric acid secretion and prokinetic agents, such as cisapride, that improve gastric emptying and increase sphincteric pressure.[45] Cases of reflux unresponsive to medical therapy may warrant surgical intervention, typically a Nissen fundoplication.

Practice Pathway

Practice Pathway 51-1 illustrates the diagnosis and treatment of infant apnea. Polysomnography is crucial in the identification of infants with suspected apnea. Infants with a central component to their apnea should be evaluated and treated medically. Persistence of apnea following treatment necessitates monitoring until the apnea resolves. Those infants with an obstructive component to their apnea require radiologic and perhaps endoscopic evaluation prior to treatment.

AT A GLANCE. . .

Apnea of Prematurity and Infancy

Pathogenesis: airway anatomic abnormalities, drugs, electrolyte abnormalities, GER, metabolic errors, poor thermoregulation, prematurity, seizure disorder

Adverse Effects: changes in heart rate and blood pressure, possibly SIDS

Symptoms and Signs: cyanotic or gray spells, change in muscle tone, stridor or snoring, staring or rigid posturing spells, difficulty with feeding or frequent vomiting

Diagnosis: home monitoring, polysomnography, EKG, chest radiograph, lateral neck radiograph, barium swallow, blood studies

Treatment: treatment of underlying disorders with surgical or nonsurgical management

---

OBSTRUCTIVE APNEA IN THE CHILD AND ADOLESCENT

OSA spans the range of pediatric medicine through adolescence. Recognition of OSA as a relatively common problem has improved over the past two decades, and OSA's reported incidence in 4- to 5-

Practice Pathway 51–1   DIAGNOSIS AND TREATMENT OF APNEA IN INFANTS

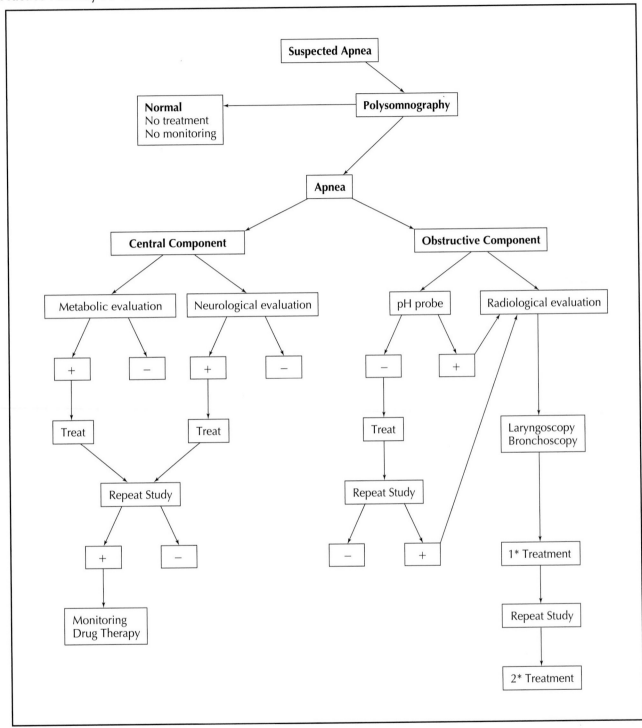

year-old children, in whom lymphoid tissue is most prolific, is reported to be as high as 2%.[46]

Pathogenesis

Many of the same conditions that predispose to OA in neonates and infants are also causative in children and adolescents. The occurrence of OSA seems di-

rectly related to some combination of abnormal craniofacial morphology, space occupying lesions, within the airway, and neuromuscular status[47] (Table 51–3). Obesity is widely recognized as an etiologic component in adult OSA and has been similarly cited in children.[48] As in adults, the exact manner by which obesity contributes to this condition remains unclear; however, magnetic resonance im-

TABLE 51–3: Factors Predisposing
to Pediatric Apnea

Adenotonsillar hypertrophy
Cleft palate (posterior pharyngeal flap)
Craniofacial disorders
  Apert syndrome
  Crouzon syndrome
  Down syndrome
  Hunter syndrome
  Hurler syndrome
  Klippel-Feil syndrome
  Pfeiffer syndrome
  Robin sequence
  Treacher Collins syndrome
Familial factors
Nasal obstruction
  Allergic rhinitis
  Chronic sinusitis
  Cystic fibrosis
  Nasal masses and tumors
  Nasopharyngeal stenosis
  Septal deviation
Laryngeal and tracheobronchial lesions
  Bilateral vocal cord paralysis
  Laryngeal masses
  Laryngomalacia
  Tracheobronchomalacia
Neurologic impairment
  Anoxic encephalopathy
  Cerebral palsy
  Myopathies
Obesity

aging (MRI) suggests that increased fat in the fascial planes surrounding the pharynx compromises the airway.[49]

As in infants, children with neurologic impairment suffer a higher incidence of OSA, and the severity of OSA is often directly proportional to the severity of the neurologic impairment. Examples include children with cerebral palsy, muscular dystrophy and other myopathies, and anoxic encephalopathy. Neurologic disorders are thought to affect respiration by two mechanisms. The bellows action of the diaphragm that powers respiration may be compromised. Accessory respiratory muscles in the pharynx such as the genioglossus and stylopharyngeus, which are responsible for maintaining the airway during sleep, may be less reactive. Drugs that have sedative side effects may compromise both the respiratory drive and pharyngeal muscle activity.

Familial apnea is a recognized entity, and affected members have been shown to have a decrease in genioglossus muscle activity on electromyography (EMG) during sleep.[50] Some teenagers who underwent a tonsillectomy and adenoidectomy for airway obstruction during their early childhood years may

have suffered morphometric facial changes during that period of obstruction that may predispose to sleep apnea during the teenage years.[51]

The pathophysiology of obstructive events in children mirrors that speculated in adults.[52] Inspiratory force collapses an airway that already may be narrowed by other anatomic factors. This intermittent closure of the pharyngeal airway may be either partial, producing hypopnea, or total, resulting in apnea. The muscles that span the pharynx (i.e., the genioglossus and stylopharyngeus) are thought to be most responsible for maintaining the airway during sleep and are implicated in the pathogenesis of OSA. Apneic events in children are briefer, more frequent, and more complex than those seen in adults.[53] Apneic events are punctuated by arousals that represent either a complete awakening or a lighter sleep stage. During these arousals, the pharyngeal dilators are activated. These arousals may be signaled by a gasping respiration as the airway opens. The child returns to a deeper sleep stage, only to have the whole cycle repeat itself again. Episodes of apnea and hypopneas may be bunched together depending on the level of sleep and factors that influence the airway, such as sleep position.

Physiologic effects on children suffering from OSA depend on the length and frequency of apneas and hypopneas. As in adults, O_2 desaturation, hypercarbia, and a decrease in pH may be demonstrated. Another factor that may interfere with efficient respiration includes aspiration of secretions, which is a finding reported in children with OSA but not in normal controls.[54]

In contrast to adults, in whom the effects of OSA on sleep have been well documented, children may show a variety of sleep patterns depending on the severity of apnea. Mildly affected children will have more normal amounts of sleep than adults and may also show less sleep fragmentation.[55,56] EEG arousals may not be as obvious as in adults, and when present may be of such short duration that they are termed mini or microarousals.[57] On the other hand, severely affected children may show a marked alteration in sleep architecture that includes changes in sleep cycles and a decrease in REM sleep.[58] Children so affected may suffer from chronic sleep deprivation. Because there are no good EEG guidelines to evaluate sleep quality, one must look for normal proportions of REM and delta sleep and review the overall sleep architecture.[46]

As in the adult population, the site of obstruction in most cases of pediatric OSA is in the pharynx.

TABLE 51–4:   Mechanisms of Pharyngeal Obstruction

Type 1: the obstruction consists of the posterior movement of the dorsum of the tongue to the posterior pharyngeal wall so that the majority of the airway constriction is anteroposterior.

Type 2: the tongue moves posteriorly, but instead of contracting the posterior pharyngeal wall, the tongue compresses the soft palate posteriorly against the posterior pharynx so that there is a junction of the tongue, velum, and pharyngeal wall in the upper portion of the oropharynx.

Type 3: the lateral pharyngeal walls move medially, causing them to appose one another.

Type 4: the pharynx constricts in a circular or sphincteric manner with movements occurring in all directions.

From reference 59, with permission.

Sher[59] has described four mechanisms of pharyngeal obstruction (Table 51–4). By far, the most common cause of pharyngeal obstruction in children is adenotonsillar hypertrophy. The highest incidence of OSA coincides with the time of greatest hypertrophy of the tonsils and adenoids, typically during the 4th to 6th years of life.[60] Symptoms may appear even earlier: in one study, 14 patients with OSA aged under 18 months were reported to have symptoms that first appeared at 2 to 6 months of age.[61] Whereas neither the size of the adenoid pad nor the size of the airway is predictive for the degree of airway obstruction, the size of the tonsils is weakly associated with the amount of obstruction.[60-63] Rarely, lingual tonsils may obstruct the pharynx of a child.[64] Other space occupying masses in the pharynx include tumors such as rhabdomyosarcoma and lymphoma.

A variety of craniofacial disorders have been reported to cause OSA, especially those with midface hypoplasia, such as Crouzon, Pfeiffer, Apert, and Treacher Collins.[65-67] Obstruction in Crouzon and Pfeiffer patients may be worse compared to those afflicted with Apert syndrome.[65] Although the mechanism of obstruction may be complex in these craniofacial patients, a narrow nasopharynx is frequently the site of obstruction. Glossoptosis as seen in Robin sequence affects infants; however, older children may suffer analogous obstruction with posterior displacement of the tongue (see Table 51–4, type 1). Children with Down syndrome have several abnormalities that predispose to OSA, including a small nasopharynx and oropharynx, relative macroglossia, and generalized hypotonia.[68] Cleft palate patients who undergo surgery to create a posterior pharyngeal flap due to residual velopharyngeal insufficiency may require removal or revision of the flap, if it causes airway obstruction at night.[69,70] Children with achondroplasia and other orthopedic syndromes, such as Klippel-Feil syndrome may suffer from OSA; a narrow nasopharynx and oropharynx have been implicated as the site of obstruction.[71] Children with mucopolysaccaridoses, specifically the Hurler and Hunter syndromes, are at high risk for OSA due to redundant pharyngeal tissue, generalized hypotonia, and macroglossia.[72,73]

Conditions that cause nasal obstruction may lead to OSA. These include anatomic disorders such as septal deviation or nasopharyngeal stenosis.[74] Allergic rhinitis, chronic sinusitis, and other chronic inflammatory and infectious conditions that compromise the nasal airway may contribute to OSA in susceptible patients, as do tumors or masses in the nasopharynx, such as a teratoma, encephalocele, or an antral choanal polyp.[75] A variety of laryngeal and tracheobronchial lesions, including laryngomalacia, tracheobronchomalacia, vocal cord paralysis, and space-occupying lesions of the larynx (i.e., papillomatosis) may rarely cause OSA.[22]

Adverse Effects of OSA

As opposed to the rare child with the pickwickian constellation of symptoms that includes OSA in association with obesity, the overwhelming majority of children with OSA have either a normal body habitus or a body weight below normal.[76] Some children develop frank failure to thrive.[44] Children affected by chronic airway obstruction are often slow eaters who are forced to chew and swallow between episodes of mouth breathing. Their dislike of food that requires a great deal of chewing, such as meat, limits their diet. Food may also lack appeal if nasal obstruction causes anosmia. Another factor responsible for less than projected growth is that growth hormone has been shown to be released during REM sleep, and a reduction in REM sleep in apneic patients may affect growth hormone secretion.[77,78] Schiffman et al.[44] showed improvement in affected patients following tonsillectomy and adenoidectomy. In OSA patients treated with tonsillectomy and adenoidectomy, Williams et al.[79] reported weight gain in 75% of 41 patients with increases in weight of 15% or more in 65% of patients.

Clinically evident effects of OSA on the cardiovascular system are rare. The development of frank cor pulmonale and other signs of right heart failure, such as cardiomegaly on chest radiograph and right ventricular strain on echocardiogram and EKG, are extremely uncommon, but suspicion of such cardiac compromise should be investigated before proceeding with any surgical intervention of OSA.[3,80,81] Sustained peripheral hypertension as a result of OSA has been documented in adults but not in children. The most frequent cardiac arrhythmia associated with OSA in children is heart rate changes, usually bradycardia.

A variety of daytime behavioral changes that result from OSA have been reported and range from irritability to severe hypersomnolence. The incidence of daytime hypersomnolence in children appears to be less than in adults, although the literature is confusing on this issue.[82] In any case, school performance may be affected adversely due to impairment of memory and concentration associated with chronic sleep deprivation. Likewise, there have been suggestions that OSA may cause developmental delays, although apparent delays may be due, in reality, to behavioral changes associated with OSA.[83]

Chronic nasal obstruction may result in an "adenoid facies," or a prolongation of the midface.[84] The development of this craniofacial anomaly is controversial and not shared universally.[85] Patients with chronic airway obstruction have been shown to have a higher incidence of malocclusion, an abnormality that corrects itself, although sometimes not completely, in patients who undergo surgical relief of their airway obstruction.[86]

Symptoms and Signs

Daytime symptoms of OSA may be nonexistent. In fact, many parents may assume that their child does not have a problem, because he/she may function well during the daytime. Other children have symptoms of chronic nasal obstruction, including a history of mouth-breathing, chronic rhinorrhea, changes in the quality of speech, and complaints of hyposmia. Parents may report that their child takes longer to eat than other family members. There may be episodes of choking or gagging on food, and affected children frequently avoid food that requires chewing such as meat, preferring soft foods instead. A decrease in appetite may be the result of hyposmia and problems eating and breathing at the same time. Children may complain of morning headaches that are the result of chronic hypoxia or CO_2 retention. Behavioral abnormalities during the daytime in children affected with OSA range from crankiness and

irritability to hypersomnolence, although the latter behavior appears not be as prevalent as in adults.[82]

In contrast, night-time symptoms frequently frighten parents, who express fears that their child may stop breathing during sleep. In some cases, parents actually sit at the bedside arousing their child to breath. Loud snoring may be "heard down the hall," "downstairs," or "shaking the entire house." There also may be associated symptoms of gasping, choking, or coughing. To parents, episodes of apnea may seem exceedingly long, when infact they last mere seconds. In questioning a parent, it is important to elicit a description of the breathing abnormality, because some parents will describe normal changes in respiratory patterns. Restless sleep is a frequent symptom, as is extending the head in an effort to maximize the airway. Sleepwalking, night terrors, and diaphoresis are not uncommon. The appearance of enuresis after the child has been previously toilet trained has been reported in OSA patients, although this association is somewhat controversial.[82,87]

Most children with OSA present with a slender body habitus suggestive of failure to thrive. Rarely, a child may present with an obese body habitus and OSA.[48] Simpser et al.[88] reported a case of an obese child with OSA and scant tonsil and adenoid tissue whose apnea disappeared following weight loss alone. Frequently, affected children have audible mouth-breathing, the result of enlarged tonsils and adenoids, that can be heard throughout the examination room. Hyponasal speech is seen in children with adenoid hypertrophy and muffled speech or a "hot potato" voice is the result of enlarged tonsils. Development of midface elongation into an "adenoid facies" remains controversial, although children with chronic upper airway obstruction will typically assume a classic appearance with the mouth gaped open due to nasal obstruction.[85] In children with a craniofacial disorder, there may be abnormalities of the nose or midface hypoplasia that result in a narrow nasopharynx. In cystic fibrosis patients, the nasal cavities may be occluded with polyps. Upon pharyngeal examination, the tonsils may be enlarged or pedicled on the tonsillar pillars, allowing them to rotate into the pharynx, causing obstruction during sleep. Other pharyngeal abnormalities include redundant pharyngeal mucosa, which is a finding seen frequently in mucopolysaccaridosis patients, and an elongated soft palate. In cleft palate patients, examination of the pharynx should include inspection for a posterior pharyngeal flap that may compromise the airway during sleep. Rarely, there may be clinical evidence of right heart failure that produces signs of hepatomegaly and polycythemia.

SPECIAL CONSIDERATION:

Neuromuscular disorders that predispose to OSA, such as cerebral palsy and anaxic encephalopathy, are usually obvious, although mild cases of hypotonia may not be readily apparent and should be sought by questioning.

Diagnosis

The initial evaluation of a child with suspected OSA begins with a careful sleep history and questions about symptoms that occur during the daytime that suggest chronic upper airway obstruction. Typically, this history is given by the parents or caregivers, but may also include information from others such as siblings who may sleep with the affected child. The physical examination should include a total assessment of the child with special attention to the nose and pharynx where conditions that adversely affect the airway may be found. The clinical evaluation of the child with suspected OSA is sensitive in a high proportion of patients, but may not be very specific. Goldstein et al.[89] and Suen et al.[90] have suggested that clinical assessment alone is not enough to identify children with OSA and that polysomnography should be performed in all suspected cases. Brouilette et al.[91] described the use of an OSA score that weighted the severity of three factors: difficulty breathing, snoring, and apnea. This score was useful in predicting those with significant obstruction on formal polysomnography. The need for polysomnography in children with suspected OSA due to adenotonsillar hypertrophy remains controversial and has enormous cost implications.

There are several methods by which a child may be monitored in the home setting. Not only is this less costly and easier for the parents, but home monitoring better simulates normal sleeping conditions. Audio monitoring of the child's breathing during sleep (sleep sonography) is accomplished by using a small tape recorder connected to a precordial stethoscope that overlies the trachea. Sleep sounds

are recorded and then subjected to computer-aided analysis to confirm irregularities of breathing, including loud and obstructed snoring, and potential periods of apnea.[92] Potsic[93] has shown a good correlation between sleep sonography and polysomnography in the evaluation of respiratory patterns and obstructive apnea.

By using a camcorder, parents can make video recordings of their child's sleep. This method of analyzing sleep in the home may uncover episodes of apnea that are not evident on audio recordings. This technique also allows the examiner to view positions and breathing patterns during sleep. Finally, newer home monitors permit overnight recording of O_2 saturation levels with pulse oximetry. The disadvantage of studying children with pulse oximetry is that many apneic episodes are of such short duration that they may not have any effect on O_2 saturation.

Polysomnography remains the gold standard for the evaluation of a child with suspected OSA. Although monitoring of physiologic parameters and sleep stages may be made, the major disadvantage of polysomnography performed in the hospital setting is that it does not reproduce conditions in the home. In children the study is performed in the same manner as in adults. Chest wall movements are monitored by either impedance or chest and abdominal strain gauges and recorded on a polygraph. Likewise, thermistors are used to measure changes in nasal and oral airflow. Polygraphic recording of the EKG and O_2 saturation complete the analysis of the cardio-respiratory system. The EEG, a record of sleep stages, is essential to complete a standard polysomnographic study. Electro-oculography (EOG), an accurate determinant of REM sleep, and suprahyoid electromyogram (EMG), a measure of the tone of the muscles that maintain the pharyngeal lumen, are two studies that are less commonly employed in children. Use of a pH probe during polysomnography can identify episodes of GER in suspected patients. As noted earlier in this chapter, analysis of polysomnographic data in children is difficult due to a lack of widely accepted standards.[82] Other factors that make analysis difficult include shorter and more frequent episodes of apnea, more episodes of hypopnea, and less severe gas exchange abnormalities.

The lateral neck film is the single most useful radiologic study in the evaluation of OSA. The nasal and oral airway can be visualized in addition to the larynx and trachea. This study allows for particular attention to the base of tongue region and the naso-pharynx, two common sites of pharyngeal obstruc-tion. No difference has been shown between the size of adenoid tissue on erect or supine lateral neck films.[94] The size of the adenoid pad is also not pre-dictive of the degree of upper airway obstruction. Tonsillar size is best determined by physical exami-nation, rather than by lateral or AP neck radio-graphs. Cephalometric analysis is not useful in ana-lyzing most children with OSA, although it may be of some benefit in patients with a craniofacial disor-der.[94] Whereas static films of the upper airway do not provide a dynamic analysis of the upper airway during sleep, videofluoroscopy in the supine posi-tion may reproduce those conditions more closely. Specific areas of interest include posterior displace-ment of the tongue and mandible, forward move-ment of retropharyngeal tissue, inferior and poste-rior displacement of the tonsils, and narrowing of the nasopharyngeal airway between the soft palate and the adenoid pad. Ultrafast or cine computed tomography (CT) has been used to evaluate adult patients with OSA to measure the cross-sectional area of the airway during sleep.[95]

Direct examination of the site of pharyngeal ob-struction can be performed using a fiberoptic naso-pharyngoscope or bronchoscope. This study may be performed under local anesthesia with sedation or general anesthesia in children who are uncooper-ative. These two methods of examination do not reproduce normal sleep, but closely approximate it.

Treatment

Nonsurgical

Nonsurgical treatments of OSA in children are listed in Table 51–5. Respiratory stimulants such as caf-feine and theophylline, which are useful in infants who have a more significant central component to their apneic episodes, may be helpful in correcting the central component of MA in children; however, they are rarely employed in this manner. Methyl-phenidate, a central nervous system (CNS) stimu-lant, is indicated for the treatment of narcolepsy, and has been utilized in some patients with daytime hypersomnolence.

Use of an artificial airway may be helpful in the acute management of selected children with OSA. Several types of oral or tongue retaining devices have been described but most are cumbersome and

TABLE 51–5: Treatment of Pediatric Apnea

Nonsurgical
 Artificial airway
 BiPAP/CPAP
 Drug therapy
 Treatment of allergies
 Treatment of GER
 Weight loss
Surgical
 Craniofacial surgery
 Nasal surgery
 Revision of posterior pharyngeal flap
 Tonsillecromy +/− adenoidectomy
 Tracheotomy
 Uvulopalatopharyngoplasty

poorly tolerated by children. Night-time insertion of a soft rubber nasal airway has greater acceptance in children and may be an alternative to a tracheotomy. Overall, long-term use of both nasal and oral devices has met with poor compliance.[76,96]

Use of CPAP delivered through the nose by way of a mask has been shown to overcome pharyngeal obstruction.[97] Problems with this form of therapy include poor compliance and difficulty with mask fit, although some centers report good results.[98] Bi-phasic positive airway pressure (BiPAP) has been used with increasing frequency as a nonsurgical al-ternative to a tracheotomy. As with nasal CPAP, BiPAP is plagued by problems with compliance and mask fit; however, some authors report better com-pliance than with nasal CPAP.[82]

Although it is unlikely that seasonal allergies alone will cause OSA, the nasal congestion that they pro-duce may be contributory. Treatment with decon-gestants, nasal steroids, or immunotherapy may cause improvement in symptoms of nasal obstruc-tion. Initial treatment of GER includes elevating the head of the bed at night, antacids, H_2 blockers, and prokinetic agents such as cisapride. In refractory cases, a Nissen fundoplication may become neces-sary. Finally, in those rare cases in which obesity is felt to play a role in the etiology of OSA, a nutritional program geared to weight loss may be very effec-tive.

Surgical

The surgical management of OSA in children is also listed in Table 51–5. Because adenotonsillar hyper-trophy is the most common cause of chronic airway obstruction and OSA in children, tonsillectomy and/or adenoidectomy relieves symptoms in almost all patients, some of whom may undergo a subsequent growth spurt.[99,100] Although symptoms of nasal obstruction may be relieved by adenoidectomy alone, removal of both tonsils and adenoid tissue should be considered when apnea has been documented. Even when the tonsils appear small on physical examination, they may rotate into the pharynx during sleep and obstruct the airway.

Careful postoperative management of children undergoing tonsillectomy and adenoidectomy for OSA is crucial to success of the procedure. Young patients, especially those under the age of 4 years who already have a small pharyngeal airway, are susceptible to airway obstruction in the immediate postoperative period due to increased edema and secretions. Whereas selected older patients may be sent home the day of surgery following a period of close observation for several hours, young children should be observed overnight in the hospital where their airway and vital signs can be monitored. Children 36 months of age and younger have been shown to have a higher incidence of postoperative complications, usually airway obstruction that results in O_2 desaturation. Tom et al.[101] reported an 8% incidence of observation in the intensive care setting in this age group.

SPECIAL CONSIDERATION:

Children most at risk for complications in this age category include those with severe apnea preoperatively or with significant medical conditions, such as asthma, cardiac disease, Down's syndrome, craniofacial disorders, or the mucopolysaccharidoses.

In addition to observation, hospitalization allows aggressive treatment with humidification and oxygen, if necessary. Use of corticosteroids has been shown to be helpful in reducing the incidence of postoperative vomiting and throat pain and improving oral intake in the first few hours following surgery.[102] The decision to observe a child overnight needs to be made on an individual basis, taking into consideration the following factors: age, severity of preoperative symptoms, respiratory status during

the immediate postoperative period, frequency of vomiting, family situation, and distance to home.

The goal of nasal surgery in OSA patients is to restore patency to the nasal airway. Usually the nasal septum is straight in children; however, it may be deviated as the result of trauma or growth patterns. Deviation is especially prominent in children with a cleft palate. Although septoplasty is usually avoided in children because of concern about violating cartilage growth centers in the septum, a conservative procedure can be performed to improve breathing. Enlargement of the inferior turbinates that fails to respond to allergic therapy, including decongestants and nasal steroid sprays, may be treated successfully with partial resection of the anterior portion of the turbinates. Cystic fibrosis patients with nasal polyposis unresponsive to medical therapy often show significant improvement following either nasal polypectomy or functional endoscopic sinus surgery.

Craniofacial surgery in which the midface is advanced may prove helpful in children with Apert's or Crouzon's syndromes.[65] Because of the potential blood loss during surgery, these procedures are typically not performed until the child approaches the teenage years. Cephalometric studies are important in the preoperative analysis of these patients.[103]

In cleft palate patients who have undergone placement of a posterior pharyngeal flap because of velopharyngeal insufficiency, revision may need to be performed if upper airway obstruction occurs at night. Examination of the nasopharynx with a fiberoptic nasopharyngoscope or bronchoscope allows appraisal of the lateral ports. A flap that is too wide may be thinned or taken down to relieve symptoms.

Uvulopalatopharyngoplasty (UPPP) as described by Fujita et al.[104] is most effective in patients with redundant pharyngeal mucosa, especially a large uvula and redundant tissue in the regions of the tonsillar pillars. A conservative UPPP in addition to or following tonsillectomy or adenoidectomy may improve symptoms of obstruction, even if the tonsil and adenoid tissue was not particularly enlarged prior to surgery.[105] The Müller maneuver is a method for identifying patients who will benefit from UPPP.[106] Performing this maneuver while observing with a fiberoptic nasopharyngoscope should show pharyngeal collapse in the region of the soft palate and tonsillar region for UPPP to be successful. The use of UPPP in children should be reserved for only those children with severe ob-

Practice Pathway 51–2 DIAGNOSIS AND TREATMENT OF APNEA IN CHILDREN AND ADOLESCENTS

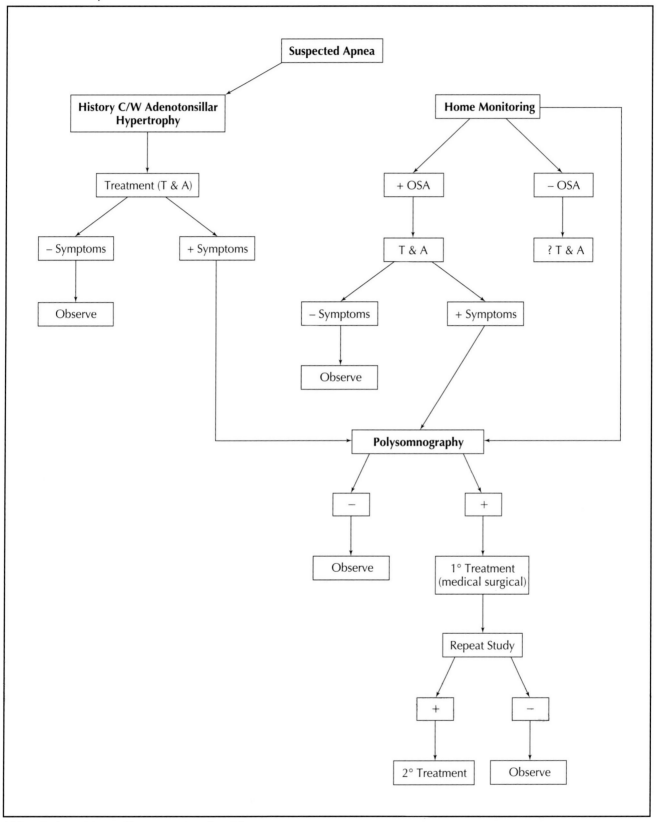

Abbreviations: T, tonsillectomy; A, adenoidectomy.

struction and anatomic evidence for improvement postoperatively because overly aggressive surgery may result in velopharyngeal insufficiency.

A variety of surgical procedures to open the hypopharynx in adults have been described. These include hyoid myotomy and suspension and advancement of the genioglossus.[107] There is little experience with these procedures in children.

Tracheotomy is frequently the treatment of last resort in children with OSA. In some children, a tracheotomy may be temporary until the child grows out of the condition that predisposed to apnea. In other children, especially those in whom neurologic impairment is felt to be permanent, the tracheotomy may need to remain for the child's entire life. A young child with a tracheotomy needs a great deal of care and support from the caregivers. Adolescents with a tracheotomy, on the other hand, may become very self sufficient. In an adolescent patient with a permanent tracheotomy, use of a plug or tracheotomy button during the daytime may restore speech and the ability to function in a normal fashion.

AT A GLANCE...

Obstructive Apnea in Childhood and Adolescence

Pathogenesis: adenotonsillar hypertrophy, cleft palate, craniofacial disorders, familial factors, nasal obstruction, laryngeal and tracheobronchial lesions, neurologic impairment, obesity

Adverse Effects: failure to thrive, frank cor pulmonale or other signs of right heart failure, sustained peripheral hypertension, behavioral changes, adenoid facies(?)

Symptoms and Signs: Daytime: mouth breathing, chronic rhinorrhea, change in quality of speech, hyposomia, choking or gagging while eating, morning headaches, behavioral abnormalities. Night-time: loud snoring; episodes of gasping, choking, or coughing; change in respiratory pattern; restless sleep; sleepwalking; night terrors; diaphoresis; enuresis(?)

Diagnosis: sleep history, physical examination, home monitoring, polysomnography, lateral neck film, nasopharyngoscopy or bronchoscopy

Treatment: *Nonsurgical:* respiratory stimulants, artificial airway, CPAP. *Surgical:* tonsillectomy and/or adenoidectomy, septoplasty, craniofacial surgery, UPPP, tracheotomy

---

Practice Pathway

Practice Pathway 51-2 illustrates the diagnosis and treatment of pediatric apnea. Cases with adenotonsillar hypertrophy as a clear-cut cause for OSA do not require polysomnography in most instances. Home audio or video monitoring are useful tools to identify those children with significant obstruction at night. A positive polysomnographic study for OSA warrants medical and/or surgical therapy and a follow-up study to ensure that treatment has been successful.

REFERENCES

1. Osler W. *The Principles and Practice of Medicine.* New York: Appleton, 1906, p. 431.
2. Cole VN, Alexander JK. Clinical effect of extreme obesity in cardiopulmonary function. South Med J 1959; 52:435.
3. Menashe VD, Farrehi C, Miller M. Hypoventilation and cor pulmonale due to chronic upper airway obstruction. J Pediatr 1965; 67:198-203.
4. Gibson E. Apnea. In: Spitzer AR, ed. *Intensive Care of the Fetus and Neonate.* New York: Mosby, 1996, p. 470-481.
5. Glotzbach SF, Baldwin RB, Lederer NE, et al. Periodic breathing in preterm infants: Incidence and characteristics. Pediatrics 1989; 84:785-792.
6. Miller MJ, Carlo WA, DiFiore JM, et al. Airway obstruction during periodic breathing in premature infants. J Appl Physiol 1988; 64:2496-2500.
7. Guilleminault C, van den Hoed J, Mitler MM. Clinical overview of the sleep apnea syndromes. In: Guilleminault C, Dement WC, eds. *Sleep Apnea Syndromes.* New York: Alan R. Liss, 1978, p. 1-12.
8. Schmidt-Nowara WW, Jennum P. Epidemiology of sleep apnea. In: Guilleminault C, Parrinen M, eds. *Obstructive Sleep Apnea Syndrome.* New York: Raven Press, 1990, p. 1-8.
9. Marcus CL, Omlin KJ, Basinki DJ, et al. Normal polysomnographic values for children and adolescents. Am Rev Respir Dis 1992; 146:1235-1239.
10. Catterall JR, Calverley PMA, Shapiro CM, et al. Breathing and oxygenation during sleep are similar in normal men and normal women. Am Rev Respir Dis 1985; 132:86-88.
11. Gould GA, Whyte KF, Rhind GB, et al. The sleep hypopnea syndrome. Am Rev Respir Dis 1988; 137:895-898.
12. Guilleminault C, Connolly S, Winkle R, et al. Cyclical variation of heart rate in sleep apnoea syndrome. Lancet 1984; 1:126-131.
13. Block AJ, Boysen PG, Wynne JW, et al. Sleep apnea, hypopnea and oxygen desaturation in normal sub-

jects. A strong male predominance. N Engl J Med 1979; 300:513-517.

14. Rosen CL, D'Andrea L, Haddad GG. Adult criteria for obstructive sleep apnea do not identify children with serious obstruction. Am Rev Respir Dis 1992; 146:1231-1234.

15. Weese-Mayer DE, Morrow AS, Conway LP, et al. Assessing clinical significance of apnea exceeding fifteen seconds with event recording. J Pediatr 1990; 117:568-574.

16. Alden ER, Mandelkorn T, Woodrum DE, et al. Morbidity and mortality of infants weighing less than 1000 grams in an intensive care nursery. Pediatrics 1972; 50:40-49.

17. Albani M, Bentele KHP, Budde C, et al. Infant sleep apnea profile: Preterm vs. term infants. Eur J Pediatr 1985; 143:261-268.

18. Miller MJ, Martin RJ. The pathophysiology of apnea of prematurity. In: Polin RA, Fox WW, eds. Fetal and Neonatal Physiology. Philadelphia: Saunders, 1992, p. 872-885.

19. Dransfield DA, Spitzer AR, Fox WW. Episodic airway obstruction in premature infants. Am J Dis Child 1983; 137:441-443.

20. Miller MJ, Carlo WA, Martin RJ. Continuous positive airway pressure selectively reduces obstructive apnea in preterm infants. J Pediatr 1985; 106: 91-94.

21. Mathew OP, Roberts JL, Thach BT. Pharyngeal airway obstruction in preterm infants during mixed and obstructive apnea. J Pediatr 1982; 100: 964-968.

22. Holinger PC, Holinger LD, Reichert TJ, et al. Respiratory obstruction and apnea in infants with bilateral abductor vocal cord paralysis, meningomyelocele, and Arnold-Chiari malformation. J Pediatr 1978; 92:368-373.

23. Remmers JE, de Groot WJ, Sauerland EK, et al. Pathogenesis of upper airway occlusion during sleep. J Appl Physiol 1978; 44:931-938.

24. Roberts JL, Reed WR, Mathew OP, et al. Control of respiratory activity of the genioglossus muscle in micrognathic infants. J Appl Physiol 1986; 61: 1523-1533.

25. Martin RJ, Miller MJ, Carlo WA. Pathogenesis of apnea in preterm infants. J Pediatr 1986; 109:733.

26. Menon AP, Schefft GL, Thach BT. Apnea associated with regurgitation in infants. J Pediatr 1985; 106: 625-629.

27. Wetmore RF. The effects of acid on the larynx of maturing rabbits and their possible significance to the sudden infant death syndrome. Laryngoscope 1993; 103:1242-1254.

28. Pickens DL, Schefft G, Thach BT. Prolonged apnea associated with upper airway protective reflexes in apnea of prematurity. Am Rev Respir Dis 1988; 137: 113-118.

29. Thach BT, Menon AP, Schefft G. Negative upper airway pressure decreases inspiratory airflow and tidal volume in tracheostomized sleeping human infants. Am Rev Resp Dis 1985; 131:A295.

30. Durand M, Cabal LA, Gonzalez F, et al. Ventilatory control and carbon dioxide response in preterm infants with idiopathic apnea. Am J Dis Child 1985; 139:717-720.

31. Cross KW, Oppe TE. The effect of inhalation of high and low concentrations of oxygen on the respiration of the premature infant. J Physiol 1952; 117: 38-55.

32. Hathorn MKS. The rate and depth of breathing in newborn infants in different sleep states. J Physiol 1974; 243:101.

33. Spitzer AR, Boyle T, Tuchman DN, et al. Awake apnea associated with gastroesophageal reflux: A specific clinical syndrome. J Pediatr 1984; 104: 200-205.

34. Spitzer AR, Newbold M, Alicea-Alvarex N, et al. Pseudoreflux syndrome—increased periodic breathing during the neonatal period presenting as feeding-related difficulties. Clin Pediatr 1991; 30: 531-537.

35. Menon AP, Schefft GL, Thach BT. Frequency and significance of swallowing during prolonged apnea in infants. Am Rev Respir Dis 1984; 130:969-973.

36. Girling DJ. Changes in heart rate, blood pressure, and pulse pressure during apnoeic attacks in newborn babies. Arch Dis Child 1972; 47:405-410.

37. Gibson E. Sudden infant death syndrome. In: Spitzer AR, ed. Intensive Care of the Fetus and Neonate. St. Louis: Mosby, 1996, p. 482-493.

38. Spitzer AR, Fox WW. Infant apnea. Clin Pediatr 1984; 23:374-380.

39. Hodgman JE, Hoppenbrouwers T. Home monitoring for sudden infant death syndrome: The case against. Ann NY Acad Sci 1988; 533:164-175.

40. Kelly DH. Home monitoring for the sudden infant death syndrome: The case for. Ann NY Acad Sci 1988; 533:158-163.

41. Eldridge FL, Millhorn DE, Waldrop TG, et al. Mechanism of respiratory effects of methylxanthines. Respir Physiol 1983; 53:239-261.

42. Barrington KJ, Finer NN, Peters KL, et al. Physiologic effects of doxapram in idiopathic apnea of prematurity. J Pediatr 1986; 108:124-129.

43. Freed G, Pearlman MA, Brown AS, et al. Polysomnographic indications for surgical intervention in Pierre-Robin sequence: Acute airway management and follow-up studies after repair and take-down of tongue-lip adhesion. Cleft Palate J 1988; 25: 151-155.

44. Schiffmann R, Faber J, Eidelman AI. Obstructive hypertrophic adenoids and tonsils as a cause of infantile failure to thrive: Reversed by tonsillectomy and

adenoidectomy. Int J Pediatr Otorhinolaryngol 1985; 9:183–187.

45. Orenstein SR. Disorders of esophageal motility. In: Rudolph AM, Hoffman JIE, Rudolph CD, eds. *Rudolph's Pediatrics,* 20th ed. Stamford: Appleton Lange, 1996, pp. 1057–1060.

46. Ali NJ, Pitson D, Stradling JR. The prevalence of snoring, sleep disturbance and sleep related breathing disorders and their relation to daytime sleepiness in 4–5 year old children. Am Rev Respir Dis 1991; 143:A381.

47. Sher AE. Obstructive sleep apnea syndrome: A complex disorder of the upper airway. Otolaryngol Clin North Am 1990; 23:593–608.

48. Mallory GB, Fiser DH, Jackson R. Sleep-associated breathing disorders in morbidly obese children and adolescents. J Pediatr 1989; 115:892–897.

49. Horner RL, Mohiaddin RH, Lowell DG, et al. Sites and sizes of fat deposits around the pharynx in obese patients with obstructive sleep apnea and weight matched controls. Eur Respir J 1989; 2: 613–622.

50. Strohl KP, Saunders NA, Feldman NT, et al. Obstructive sleep apnea in family members. N Engl J Med 1978; 299:969–973.

51. Guilleminault C, Partinen M, Praud JP, et al. Morphometric facial changes and obstructive sleep apnea in adolescents. J Pediatr 1989; 114:997–999.

52. Remmers JE, deGroot WJ, Sauerland EK, et al. Pathogenesis of upper airway occlusion during sleep. J Appl Physiol 1978; 44:931–938.

53. Brouillette RT, Fernbach SK, Hunt CE. Obstructive sleep apnea in infants and children. J Pediatr 1982; 100:31–40.

54. Konno A, Hoshino T, Togawa K. Influence of upper airway obstruction by enlarged tonsils and adenoids upon recurrent infection of the lower airway in childhood. Laryngoscope 1980; 90:1709–1716.

55. Frank Y, Kravath RE, Pollak CP, et al. Obstructive sleep apnea and its therapy: Clinical and polysomnography manifestations. Pediatrics 1983; 71: 737–742.

56. Guilleminault C, Winkle R, Korobkin R, et al. Children and nocturnal snoring: Evaluation of the effects of sleep related respiratory resistive load and daytime functioning. Eur J Pediatr 1982; 139: 165–171.

57. McGrath-Morrow SA, Carroll JL, McColley SA, et al. Termination of obstructive apnea in children is not associated with arousal. Am Rev Resp Dis 1990; 141:A195.

58. Mangat D, Orr WC, Smith RO. Sleep apnea, hypersomnolence, and upper airway obstruction secondary to adenotonsillar enlargement. Arch Otolaryngol 1977; 103:383–386.

59. Sher AE, Shprintzen RJ, Thorpy MJ. Endoscopic observations of obstructive sleep apnea in children

with anomalous upper airways: Predictive and therapeutic value. Int J Pediatr Otorhinolaryngol 1986; 11:135–146.

60. Crepeau J, Patriquin HB, Poliquin JF, et al. Radiographic evaluation of the symptom-producing adenoid. Otolaryngol Head Neck Surg 1982; 90: 548–554.

61. Leiberman A, Tal A, Brama I, et al. Obstructive sleep apnea in young infants. Int J Pediatr Otorhinolaryngol 1988; 16:39–44.

62. Laurikainen E, Erkinjuntti M, Alihanka J, et al. Radiological parameters of the bony nasopharynx and the adenotonsillar size compared with sleep apnea episodes in children. Int J Pediatr Otorhinolaryngol 1987; 12:303–310.

63. Brodsky L, Adler E, Stanievich JF. Naso- and oropharyngeal dimensions in children with obstructive sleep apnea. Int J Pediatr Otorhinolaryngol 1989; 17:1–11.

64. Guarisco JL, Littlewood SC, Butcher RB III. Severe upper airway obstruction in children secondary to lingual tonsil hypertrophy. Ann Otol Rhinol Laryngol 1990; 99:621–624.

65. Moore MH. Upper airway obstruction in the syndromal craniosynostoses. Br J Plast Surg 1993; 46: 355–362.

66. Mixter RC, David DJ, Perloff WH, et al. Obstructive sleep apnea in Apert's and Pfeiffer's syndromes: More than a craniofacial abnormality. Plast Reconstr Surg 1990; 86:457–463.

67. Johnson C, Taussig LM, Koopman C, et al. Obstructive sleep apnea in Treacher-Collins syndrome. Cleft Palate J 1981; 18:39–44.

68. Strome M. Obstructive sleep apnea in Down syndrome children: A surgical approach. Laryngoscope 1986: 96:1340–1342.

69. Kravath RE, Pollak CP, Borowiecki B, et al. Obstructive sleep apnea and death associated with surgical correction of velopharyngeal incompetence. J Pediatr 1980; 96:645–648.

70. Orr WC, Levine NS, Buchanan RT. Effect of cleft palate repair and pharyngeal flap surgery on upper airway obstruction during sleep. Plast Reconstr Surg 1987; 80:226–232.

71. Larsen P, Snyder EW, Matsuo F, et al. Achondroplasia associated with obstructive sleep apnea. Arch Neurol 1983; 40:769.

72. Malone BN, Whitley CB, Duvall AJ, et al. Resolution of obstructive sleep apnea in Hurler syndrome after bone marrow transplantation. Int J Pediatr Otorhinolaryngol 1988; 15:23–31.

73. Sasaki CT, Ruiz R, Gaito R, et al. Hunter's syndrome: A study in airway obstruction. Laryngoscope 1987; 97:280–285.

74. Mauer KW, Staats BA, Osen KD. Upper airway obstruction and disordered nocturnal breathing in children. Mayo Clin Proc 1983; 58:349–353.

75. Rodgers GK, Chan KH, Dahl RE. Antral choanal polyp presenting as obstructive sleep apnea syndrome. Arch Otolaryngol Head Neck Surg 1991; 117:914-916.

76. Kravath RE, Pollak CP, Borowiecki B. Hypoventilation during sleep in children who have lymphoid airway obstruction treated by nasopharyngeal tube and T and A. Pediatrics 1977; 59:865-871.

77. Underwood LE, Azumi K, Voina SJ, et al. Growth hormone levels during sleep in normal and growth hormone deficient children. Pediatrics 1971; 48: 946-954.

78. Sackner MA, Landa J, Forrest T, et al. Periodic sleep apnea: Chronic sleep deprivation related to intermittent upper airway obstruction and central nervous system disturbance. Chest 1975; 67:164-171.

79. Williams EF, Woo P, Miller R, et al. The effects of adenotonsillectomy on growth in young children. Otolaryngol Head Neck Surg 1991; 104:509-516.

80. Macartney FJ, Panday J, Scott O. Cor pulmonale as a result of chronic nasopharyngeal obstruction due to hypertrophied tonsils and adenoids. Arch Dis Child 1969; 44:585-592.

81. Luke MJ, Mehrizi A, Folger GM, et al. Chronic nasopharyngeal obstruction as a cause of cardiomegaly, cor pulmonale, and pulmonary edema. Pediatrics 1966; 37:762-768.

82. Carroll JL. Sleep-related upper-airway obstruction in children and adolescents. Child Adolesc Psychiatr Clin North Am 1996; 5:617.

83. Lind MG, Lundell BPW. Tonsillar hyperplasia in children: A cause of obstructive sleep apneas, CO_2 retention, and retarded growth. Arch Otolaryngol 1982; 108:650-654.

84. Linder-Aronson S, Woodside DG, Lundstrom A. Mandibular growth direction following adenoidectomy. Am J Orthod 1986; 89:273-284.

85. Klein JC. Nasal respiratory function and craniofacial growth. Arch Otolaryngol Head Neck Surg 1986; 112:843-849.

86. Hultcrantz E, Larson M, Hellquish R, et al. The influence of tonsillar obstruction and tonsillectomy on facial growth and dental arch morphology. Int J Pediatr Otorhinolaryngol 1991; 22:125-134.

87. Weider DJ, Hauri PJ. Nocturnal enuresis in children with upper airway obstruction. Int J Pediatr Otorhinolaryngol 1985; 9:173-182.

88. Simpser MD, Strieder DJ, Wohl ME, et al. Sleep apnea in a child with the Pickwickian syndrome. Pediatrics 1977; 60:290-293.

89. Goldstein NA, Sculerati N, Walsleben JA, et al. Clinical diagnosis of pediatric obstructive sleep apnea validated by polysomnography. Otolaryngol Head Neck Surg 1994; 111:611-617.

90. Suen JS, Arnold JE, Brooks LJ. Adenotonsillectomy for treatment of obstructive sleep apnea in children. Arch Otolaryngol Head Neck Surg 1995; 121: 525-530.

91. Brouillette R, Hanson D, David R, et al. A diagnostic approach to suspected obstructive sleep apnea in children. J Pediatr 1984; 105:10-14.

92. Marsh RR, Potsic WP, Pasquariello C. Recorder for assessment of upper airway disorders. Otolaryngol Head Neck Surg 1983; 91:584-585.

93. Potsic WP. Comparison of polysomnography and sonography for assessing regularity of respiration during sleep in adenotonsillar hypertrophy. Laryngoscope 1987; 97:1430-1437.

94. Mahboubi S, Marsh RR, Potsic WP, et al. The lateral neck radiograph in adenotonsillar hyperplasia. Int J Pediatr Otorhinolaryngol 1985; 10:67-73.

95. Stein MG, Gamsu G, de Geer G, et al. Cine CT in obstructive sleep apnea. AJR 1987; 148:1069-1074.

96. Eavey RD, Casagrande A, Blasberg G, et al. Relief of chronic upper airway obstruction using a dental prosthesis: A nonsurgical approach. Pediatrics 1977; 59:288-292.

97. Guilleminault C, Nino-Murcia G, Heldt G, et al. Alternative treatment to tracheostomy in obstructive sleep apnea syndrome: Nasal continuous positive airway pressure in young children. Pediatrics 1986; 78:797-802.

98. Brooks LJ, Crooks RL, Sleeper GP. Compliance with nasal CPAP by children with obstructive sleep apnea. Am Rev Resp Dis 1992; 145:A556.

99. Potsic WP, Pasquariello PS, Baranak CC, et al. Relief of upper airway obstruction by adenotonsillectomy. Otolaryngol Head Neck Surg 1986; 94: 476-480.

100. Stradling JR, Thomas G, Warley ARH, et al. Effect of adenotonsillectomy on nocturnal hypoxaemia, sleep disturbance, and symptoms in snoring children. Lancet 1990; 335:249-253.

101. Tom LWC, DeDio RM, Cohen DE, et al. Is outpatient tonsillectomy appropriate for young children? Laryngoscope 1992; 102:277-280.

102. Tom LWC, Templeton JJ, Thompson ME, et al. Dexamethasone in adenotonsillectomy. Int J Pediatr Otorhinolaryngol 1996; 37:115-120.

103. Borowiecki B, Kukwa A, Blanks RHI. Cephalometric analysis for diagnosis and treatment of obstructive sleep apnea. Laryngoscope 1988; 98:226-234.

104. Fujita S, Conway W, Zorick F, et al. Surgical correction of anatomic abnormalities in obstructive sleep apnea syndrome: Uvulopalatopharyngoplasty. Otolaryngol Head Neck Surg 1981; 89:923-934.

105. Hultcrantz E, Svanholm H, Ahlqvist-Rastad J. Sleep apnea in children without hypertrophy of the tonsils. Clin Pediatr 1988; 27:350-352.

106. Sher AE, Thorpy MJ, Shprintzen RJ, et al. Predictive value of Müller maneuver in selection of patients for uvulopalatopharyngoplasty. Laryngoscope 1985; 95:1483-1486.

52 Management of Acute Airway Obstruction

Ralph F. Wetmore

A young child who presents with acute respiratory distress represents one of the most critically ill patients in all of medicine. Because their physiology differs from their adult counterparts, children may look surprisingly well in spite of being on the verge of respiratory or circulatory collapse. For this reason, their decompensation may be swift and difficult to reverse. Children also have less respiratory reserve and smaller airways than adults, making them more easily compromised. They are also more susceptible to upper respiratory illnesses that cause edema of the airways and an increase in secretions, and both of these may affect ventilation.

SPECIAL CONSIDERATION:

Because of their diminished reserve, children suffer respiratory collapse relatively quickly.

Prior to the development of antibiotic therapy and the ability to control an airway with either endotracheal intubation or tracheostomy, many children succumbed to illnesses that resulted in acute upper airway obstruction. While the morbidity and mortality of such illnesses has decreased dramatically over the last 50 years, a logical and decisive approach to the child with acute airway obstruction (AAO) is necessary in order to prevent catastrophic results. The evaluation and management of children with this condition should be performed with a health care team that includes emergency room physicians, anesthesiologists, critical care specialists, and otolaryngologists familiar with the pediatric airway.

Pediatric Otolaryngology, Edited by R.F. Wetmore, H.R. Muntz, and T.J. McGill. Thieme Medical Publishers, Inc., New York © 2000.

SYMPTOMS AND SIGNS OF ACUTE AIRWAY OBSTRUCTION

Symptoms

Dyspnea

Dyspnea is the most obvious symptom in a child with AAO. The child or the child's caretakers may complain that he/she is breathing fast or cannot seem to catch his/her breath. This symptom may appear to worsen when the child assumes certain positions; conversely, other positions may serve to relieve the symptom of air hunger.

Vocal changes

Depending upon the severity and location of the disease process, changes in the voice may range from slight hoarseness or a change in vocal quality to complete aphonia. A muffled cry may result from an increase in mass within the pharynx (e.g., an enlargement of the tonsils). An infant with poor muscle tone may be able to produce a weak cry only. A child with croup (laryngotracheobronchitis [LTB]) may present with hoarseness and intermittent aphonia.

Cough

A stimulus anywhere throughout the airway may result in cough. Thus, infected tonsils or inflammation of the larynx during croup may cause cough. Mucopurulent secretions in the tracheobronchial tree or pneumonia involving the lung parenchyma may also produce this symptom. With the exception of the barking cough that is seen in patients with croup, it is often difficult to localize the site of inflammation from the cough alone.

Dysphagia

Depending upon the site of the airway obstruction, there may be dysphagia for both liquids and solids. Children with acutely enlarged tonsils may have difficulty swallowing solid food, yet may do well with liquids. A child with supraglottitis that involves the entire supraglottic larynx and hypopharynx may be unable to swallow either liquids or solids.

Sore throat

Complaints of throat pain are usually nonspecific and may be seen with a variety of conditions that cause AAO. Children who have ingested a foreign body typically will complain of odynophagia, whereas a child with an allergic reaction involving the pharynx may complain that the throat feels full or swollen. Acute infectious processes involving the pharynx and larynx usually produce a diffuse discomfort in the throat that may be difficult to localize.

Signs

General appearance

In evaluating the child with AAO, it is initially important to observe the child's overall appearance because this frequently will determine the speed and sequence of therapeutic actions. The level of consciousness should be assessed immediately because the child who is unconscious or obtunded may require immediate control of the airway. Restlessness, diaphoresis, and anxiety need to be recognized because they usually accompany air hunger. Because of their diminished respiratory reserve, children may undergo oxygen (O_2) desaturation relatively quickly, and cyanosis is an ominous sign in a child without underlying cyanotic cardiac disease. Although the respiratory rate in children varies depending on the age, children in distress appear to be breathing with difficulty, employing all of their accessory respiratory muscles. Substernal retractions and use of the intercostal muscles are all signs of respiratory distress. Initially, the child with AAO will have tachycardia; bradycardia is a late indication of severe hypoxia. Frequently, the child will position himself/herself in an attempt to improve his airway or reduce pain, which portends cardiopulmonary collapse. Thus, children with supraglottitis will sit erect with the head tilted forward in the "sniffing position," whereas a child with a retropharyngeal abscess will assume a head tilt or opisthotonic posture because of spasm of the muscles supporting the cervical spine.

Vocal changes

Changes in the voice may range from slight hoarseness to complete aphonia. These changes are the result of inflammation of the true vocal folds, which determine the quality of the voice and structures that control airflow in the trachea, larynx, and pharynx. Thus, edema of the cords and subglottis, seen in patients with croup, produces a barking quality to the cough and a low-pitched hoarse sound to the cry. Supraglottitis and adenotonsillar hypertrophy do not typically affect the quality of the sound as much as they muffle it due to a decrease in the airflow.

Stridor and other airway sounds

Depending upon the level of airway obstruction, the examiner can localize it by the character of the turbulent airflow that produces noise upon breathing. *Stertor* is a snoring or snorting sound that is produced by turbulence within the nasopharynx. In the oropharynx, turbulence produces a gurgling sound due to the mixture of air and secretions.

Stridor is sound produced by turbulent flow within the laryngeal or tracheal airway. With a stethoscope, the examiner can use these stridor sounds to localize the level of airway obstruction. Because the laryngeal airway is the most narrow, stridor that originates from this region is high-pitched and often the loudest due to the large gradient that the air must cross. On the other hand, low-pitched wheezing sounds are often produced by minor bronchi and bronchioles. Hirschberg has described four types of stridor: (1) *pharyngeal stridor* is noise-like, with frequent interruptions, and may occur during both inspiration and expiration; (2) *laryngeal stridor* is phonation-like with musical elements and an overtone that resembles crying; (3) *subglottic* and *tracheal stridor* has a hollow timbre and a continuous breathing noise that is mainly inspiratory; and (4) *bronchial stridor* is a noise-like acoustic phenomenon that appears in expiration and is often spastic.[1]

Inspiratory stridor is produced by an abnormality at or above the glottis, and is due to soft tissue that is pulled into the airway during an exaggerated inspiration used to try to overcome airway obstruction.[2,3] *Expiratory stridor* results from an abnormality in the distal trachea and bronchi. During expiration, contraction of the bronchus makes an obstructed airway even narrower, causing an increased noise. Stridor that is both inspiratory and expiratory is usually the result of a lesion in the mid-trachea.

The degree and loudness of stridor is not necessarily indicative of the degree of obstruction; for example, stridor may become less noisy just before complete obstruction due to diminishing airflow. The intensity and pitch of stridor is dependent upon the diameter of the airway, the velocity of airflow, and the pressure gradient across the site of obstruction. As the diameter of the airway narrows, the frequency of the sound takes on a higher pitch. The loudness of the stridor is a function of the velocity of airflow and the pressure gradient. Obstruction in the upper airway lengthens the inspiratory component of respiration, and lower-airway obstruction lengthens the expiratory component.

SPECIAL CONSIDERATION:

The intensity and pitch of stridor is dependent upon the diameter of the airway, the velocity of airflow, and the pressure gradient across the site of obstruction.

Drooling

Drooling is the result of an inability to swallow. This dysphagia may be due to either pain or swelling of affected tissues. Drooling, dysphagia for liquids and solids, and sore throat are typical symptoms of supraglottic pathology (e.g., supraglottitis).

Accessory respiratory muscles

Suprasternal and substernal retractions, nasal flaring, and use of the intercostal muscles are all due to the increased work of breathing. Use of these accessory respiratory muscles is nonspecific and may represent problems with ventilation anywhere within the airway and lungs.

Subcutaneous emphysema

Subcutaneous emphysema is the result of a rupture in the integrity of either the respiratory or digestive

tracts, with dissection of air into the surrounding planes of the neck.

AT A GLANCE. . .

Acute Airway Obstruction

Symptoms: dyspnea, vocal changes, cough dysphagia, sore throat

Signs: general appearance, vocal changes, airway sounds, drooling, use of accessory respiratory muscles, subcutaneous emphysema

Radiologic Evaluation: lateral and AP neck radiography, chest radiography, AP neck film barium swallow, airway fluoroscopy

Endoscopic Evaluation: flexible nasopharyngoscope and bronchoscope, rigid bronchoscopy

DIFFERENTIAL DIAGNOSIS OF ACUTE AIRWAY OBSTRUCTION

Infectious and noninfectious differential diagnoses of acute airway obstruction are listed in Table 52-1.

Infectious Problems

Laryngotracheobronchitis (LTB)

LTB or *croup* is usually the result of a viral infection, either parainfluenza virus 1 and 2, influenza A, or

TABLE 52-1: Differential Diagnoses of Acute Airway Obstruction

Infectious
  Laryngotracheobronchitis
  Acute supraglottitis
  Bacterial tracheitis
  Adenotonsillar hypertrophy
  Retropharyngeal/parapharyngeal abscess
Noninfectious
  Acute anaphylaxis
  Spasmodic croup
  Foreign body
  Laryngeal trauma
  Congenital laryngeal abnormalities
  Laryngeal neoplasms

respiratory syncytial virus (RSV). LTB strikes children from 3 months to 3 years of age, and males are more commonly affected.[4] Croup is seen most often during the fall and winter season (September to February), especially with a change in weather, and has a peak incidence during October.[5]

The onset of LTB is gradual with a low-grade fever and hoarseness that follows a viral upper respiratory infection (URI). The classic harsh cough or bark may progress to inspiratory stridor and frank dyspnea. LTB typically lasts from 3 to 7 days but may linger for as long as 14 days in severe cases. Assessment of the severity of LTB may be made by scoring the following five parameters: level of consciousness, cyanosis, stridor, air entry, and retractions.[6] Most children with LTB are managed conservatively with observation and humidity, although some may require treatment with corticosteroids or racemic epinephrine. Rarely, intubation or tracheostomy may be necessary.

Acute supraglottitis

Acute supraglottitis classically occurs in the 2 to 6 year age group, and is almost always the result of *Hemophilus influenzae*, Type B (HIB) infection. Since the development and widespread use of the conjugated HIB vaccine, there has been a decreasing incidence of this disease in children.[7] Acute supraglottitis begins with the abrupt onset of fever, sore throat, dysphagia, and drooling. Affected children assume a characteristic sniffing position in an attempt to maximize their airway. The voice tends to be muffled, rather than hoarse as in LTB.

Because the symptoms and signs are classic, the diagnosis of acute supraglottitis often is made clinically. Any attempt to visualize the epiglottis in order to confirm the diagnosis remains controversial. A lateral neck radiograph performed under closely supervised conditions shows thickening of the epiglottis and other supraglottic structures (Fig. 52-1).

Prior to the 1970s, airway management in cases of acute supraglottitis consisted of a tracheostomy. Since the mid-1970s, endotracheal intubation has replaced tracheostomy as the airway management of choice (Fig. 52-2). In early cases of supraglottitis, observation alone in the intensive care unit (ICU) may be considered, although conservative management is to secure the airway.[8]

If conditions permit, endotracheal intubation is best performed in the operating room under an inhalational anesthetic. With a surgeon familiar with

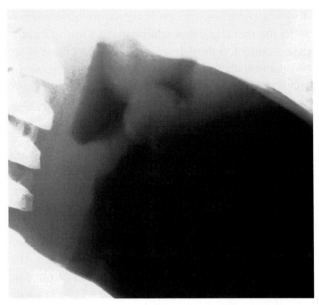

Figure 52–1: Lateral neck radiograph in a child with acute supraglottitis demonstrates classic thumbprint sign, thickening of the epiglottis, and other supraglottic structures.

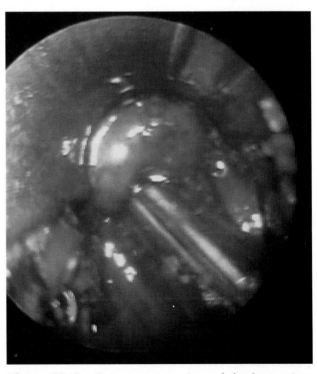

Figure 52–2: Laryngoscopic view of the larynx in a child with acute supraglottitis. An endotracheal tube maintains the airway. Note the poor definition of supraglottic structures due to marked edema and inflammation.

the pediatric airway in attendance, intravenous access is obtained and anesthesia typically is induced without the aid of muscle relaxants. The use of muscle relaxants during intubation of a patient with supraglottitis remains controversial.[9] After examination and culture of the larynx, the intubated child is returned to the ICU. Antibiotic therapy should include either ampicillin and chloramphenicol or a third-generation cephalosporin. The decision to extubate after 24 to 48 hours is usually made after direct inspection of the supraglottis at the bedside.

Bacterial tracheitis

This type of acute bacterial infection of the airway includes the tracheobronchial tree and larynx and is characterized by subglottic edema, narrowing of the airway, and copious purulent secretions. Most cases are caused by *Staphylococcus aureus* or *Hemophilus influenzae;* however, anaerobic bacteria have been recovered in 57% of tracheal aspirates.[10] Parainfluenza has been documented as a prodromal infection in many cases.[11]

Children with bacterial tracheitis quickly develop severe airway obstruction, although not as quickly as in supraglottitis. Affected children show signs of systemic toxicity, including high fever, and pneumonia was an associated condition in 60% of cases in one series.[11] Unlike LTB, symptoms of stridor and dyspnea are not relieved by treatment with corticosteroids or racemic epinephrine. The lateral neck radiograph confirms subglottic narrowing and may also demonstrate large crusts within the airway. The diagnosis is made by endoscopic examination of the airway, during which crusts should be debrided and cultures obtained.

After confirming the diagnosis, the airway should be secured with an endotracheal tube. Repeated endoscopies may be required because of recurrent plugging and crusting. Tracheostomy may be necessary in severe cases.[12] Antibiotic therapy should be guided by culture results, but should initially include coverage for *Staphylococcus aureus.*

Adenotonsillar hypertrophy

Adenotonsillar hypertrophy is usually the result of infection, either viral or bacterial.[13] The overwhelming majority of children with adenotonsillar hypertrophy present with symptoms of chronic airway obstruction, especially at nighttime; however, a small group may present suddenly during an acute URI that causes additional swelling. Epstein-Barr virus (i.e., infectious mononucleosis) typically causes enlargement of lymphoid tissue and may precipitate acute obstruction.[14] Lymphoid enlargement may affect not only the tonsils and adenoid tissue, but also the lymph nodes surrounding the pharynx.[15] Children with underlying craniofacial abnormalities such as Down, Apert, or Crouzon syndromes and children with hypotonia are more susceptible to acute episodes of obstruction that result from adenotonsillar swelling.

Careful questioning of caregivers will often elicit a history of preceding chronic airway obstruction, especially at nighttime with loud snoring, obstructed and irregular breathing, and even short periods of apnea. During an infection, these symptoms become more severe and may progress to cor pulmonale and right heart failure. Tonsillar size does not always correlate with the severity of symptoms (Fig. 52-3).[16] It is important to view the lower poles of the tonsils because there may be hypertrophy of the caudal portion of the tonsils that may not be evident when viewing the superior poles.[17] With acute infection, there is usually erythema of the pharynx and often exudative tonsillitis. There may also be signs of infection elsewhere, such as acute otitis media or mucopurulence in the nasal cavities. In most cases of acute obstruction secondary to adenotonsillar hypertrophy, the diagnosis is clinically obvious; in ambiguous cases, polysomnography can document the severity of obstruction.

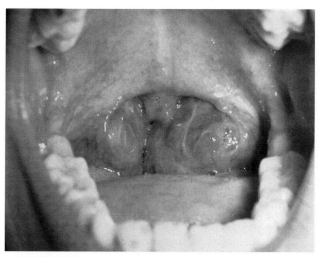

Figure 52-3: Significant tonsillar hypertrophy with almost complete obstruction of the oropharyngeal airway.

SPECIAL CONSIDERATION:

The size of the tonsils on examination does not always correlate with the degree of obstruction that they cause.

The initial treatment of acute obstruction as the result of adenotonsillar hypertrophy is to stabilize the airway. Use of a nasopharyngeal airway may suffice, although endotracheal intubation may be necessary, especially if right heart failure is present. Antibiotics and corticosteroids are helpful in reducing infection and the size of the lymphoid tissue.[16] Corticosteroids are particularly effective in the treatment of lymphoid hypertrophy as a result of infectious mononucleosis. Cases that fail to respond to medical therapy are candidates for an urgent tonsillectomy and adenoidectomy.[18]

Retropharyngeal/parapharyngeal abscess

An abscess in one of the deep spaces of the neck (e.g., the retropharyngeal or parapharyngeal spaces) may present with symptoms of upper airway obstruction. In one series of such infections, 7% of children presented with difficulty breathing.[19] Endotracheal intubation was required in 3%; a tracheostomy was not utilized in any case. *Staphylococcus aureus* is the most common organism in this type of infection, although streptococcal species and anaerobic bacteria such as Bacteroides and *Veillonella* have also been documented.[19,20]

Fever is the most common symptom in patients with a deep neck abscess and is usually associated with sore throat, dysphagia and limited neck motion, or torticollis. Airway symptoms include stridor or stertor and difficulty breathing. Physical findings in the pharynx may include diffuse erythema, tonsillar exudates, and swelling or bulging of the involved tonsillar region. Cervical adenopathy appears to be greatest on the side of the neck where the deep neck infection is most involved.

A lateral neck radiograph may show impingement upon the airway in cases where the abscess is in the retropharynx (Fig. 52-4). Computed tomography (CT) with contrast is the procedure of choice because it confirms the presence of an abscess, determines its extent, and identifies its relationship to the airway. In children with deep neck infections,

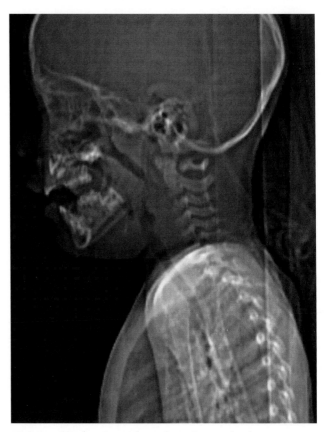

Figure 52–4: Lateral neck radiograph demonstrates widening of the retropharyngeal space in a child with a retropharyngeal abscess.

Ungkanont et al. demonstrated 91% sensitivity and 60% specificity with CT in determining the presence of an abscess, whereas Wetmore et al. showed a 92% correlation between findings of rim enhancement on contrast CT and evidence of an abscess at the time of surgical intervention (Fig. 52-5).[19,20]

Intravenous (IV) antibiotic therapy with broad spectrum coverage is the initial management of a deep space infection. Parapharyngeal infections may be therapeutically needled, and a specimen sent for culture. Depending upon the degree of the child's cooperation, retropharyngeal infections may be treated in a similar manner. Failure of an abscess to respond to antibiotics and aspiration is an indication for surgical drainage through either an intraoral or external neck approach. Surgical drainage has almost a 100% success rate; a small percentage of patients will require repeat drainage.[19]

Noninfectious Problems

Acute anaphylaxis

An anaphylactic reaction is the result of immunoglobulin E (IgE) activation of mast cells that cause

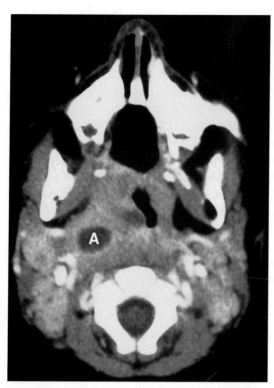

Figure 52–5: CT with contrast in a child with a parapharyngeal abscess (A). Note impingement on the pharyngeal airway by two hypolucent areas; one has rim enhancement suggestive of an abscess.

the release of histamine and other mediators.[21] Approximately 15 minutes after exposure to the antigen, anaphylaxis begins as a generalized reaction that may progress to respiratory and circulatory collapse.[22] Early symptoms include itching of the eyes, nose, and throat associated with facial flushing and a tightening sensation in the throat. Tachycardia, bronchospasm, urticaria, and a feeling of impending doom are other symptoms suggestive of anaphylaxis. Respiratory distress is the result of edema of the larynx, trachea, and even hypopharynx. Death may result from airway and cardiovascular collapse.

Establishing an airway and preventing circulatory collapse are the two major objectives in the treatment of anaphylaxis. Endotracheal intubation may be necessary to secure the airway. Starting IV fluids and giving epinephrine either subcutaneously or slowly by IV will help to maintain circulatory stability. Antihistamines and corticosteroids may be helpful in reversing the effects of the offending antigen.

Spasmodic croup

Spasmodic croup is thought to be an allergic condition that causes edema and inflammation of the upper airway. Like LTB, affected children are in the 1 to 3 year age group, although the symptoms of inspiratory stridor and a harsh barking cough are much milder than when seen with LTB. Spasmodic croup also differs from LTB in that there are few prodromal symptoms: there is rarely fever, onset is often at night, and attacks are frequently recurrent. Spasmodic croup usually responds to corticosteroid therapy and changes with environment, such as with the addition of cool mist.

Foreign bodies

Depending on their location, the ingestion or aspiration of foreign bodies may produce stridor. Objects, such as small pieces of plastic, that are caught in the glottic or subglottic airway often produce symptoms that mimic croup, such as the sudden onset of stridor and respiratory distress. Objects trapped in the distal trachea tend to produce coughing and wheezing. Large objects that are lodged in the proximal esophagus and apply pressure to the posterior larynx may also produce stridor and signs of airway obstruction. Coins are the most commonly ingested foreign bodies, which is fortunate since their presence is easy to diagnose and their extraction is frequently simple.[23] Boys are at greater risk of injury or death from the aspiration or ingestion of foreign bodies, and spherical objects are most likely to cause asphyxiation.[23]

Radiopaque foreign objects can be demonstrated on lateral neck or chest radiographs (Fig. 52-6). Radiolucent foreign bodies in the upper esophagus may be demonstrated with barium swallow; however, this study is often avoided because the barium may make the endoscopic extraction of the object more difficult. Radiolucent foreign objects within the proximal trachea may produce edema in the subglottis, mimicking croup. More distal tracheal or bronchial foreign objects can be demonstrated on inspiratory/expiratory films, on lateral decubitus views, or on fluoroscopy of the lung fields. Extraction of foreign bodies in the upper aerodigestive tract is by rigid endoscopy in almost all cases (Fig. 52-7).

Laryngeal trauma

In children the major causes of laryngeal trauma are blunt or sharp trauma to the neck, burns of the upper airway, or iatrogenic injury to the larynx or the nerves that innervate the larynx. Unilateral or

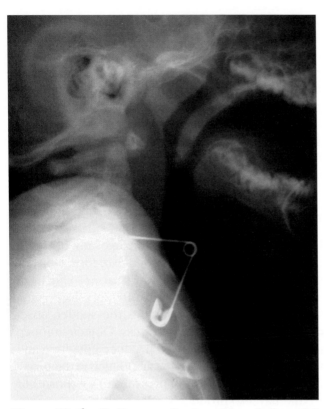

Figure 52–6: Radiopaque foreign object (safety pin) visible on lateral neck radiograph. The pointed end of the pin is impaled into the posterior pharyngeal wall and the keeper is through the larynx.

bilateral vocal cord paralysis may occur following repair of vascular or tracheoesophageal abnormalities in the chest. Although rare, endotracheal intubation may injure the larynx, producing symptoms of AAO after extubation.[24] The tip of the tube and cuff, if present, may press against the anterior tracheal wall, the shaft may press against the arytenoid cartilages, or the tube may injure the mucosa in the most narrow portion of the airway, which in children is the subglottis at the level of the cricoid cartilage.[25] Mucosal injury, if significant, may progress to necrosis and scarring and ultimately to subglottic or tracheal stenosis.

The best form of treatment for all of these conditions is prevention. Identification of the recurrent laryngeal nerves during chest or thyroid surgery may prevent iatrogenic injury. Use of an appropriately sized endotracheal tube and maintenance of a leak around it lower the incidence of mucosal injury. Careful securing of the tube prevents repeated rubbing against the laryngeal mucosa. Use of a nasotracheal tube rather than an orotracheal tube allows better securing and prevention of rubbing, but does increase the chances of mucosal injury in the posterior commissure region.

Congenital laryngeal abnormalities

Subglottic hemangioma rarely presents with AAO, but an affected child may decompensate acutely

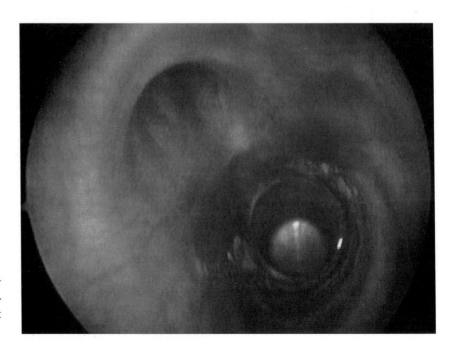

Figure 52–7: Telescopic view through a rigid bronchoscope of an aspirated pen cap lodged in the right mainstem bronchus.

during an URI. A majority of infants with a subglottic hemangioma present by 6 months of age with stridor and a "croupy" cough.[26] *Cutaneous hemangiomas* are often present, but their absence does not rule out the diagnosis. Although the diagnosis may be suspected from a lateral neck radiograph, endoscopic examination of the airway confirms the diagnosis. Treatment may be with local or systemic corticosteroids, laser excision, open surgical excision, or tracheostomy.[26]

Subglottic stenosis will occasionally present with AAO during a viral URI. A history of previous intubation dramatically increases the incidence of subglottic injury.[27] The diagnosis is suspected also on lateral neck film, but is confirmed by endoscopic examination. Depending upon the severity of stenosis, treatment ranges from observation to tracheostomy and laryngeal reconstruction.

Congenital bilateral vocal cord paralysis may be due to a variety of causes including Arnold-Chiari malformation or thoracic malformations, or may be inherited.[28,29] Presentation may be acute, and the diagnosis is made by endoscopy. Treatment varies from observation to tracheostomy, depending upon the severity of airway obstruction.

Laryngeal atresia is the rarest of all congenital laryngeal abnormalities and presents as AAO in the delivery suite.[30] Survival is dependent upon immediate tracheostomy.

Laryngeal neoplasms

With the exception of laryngeal papillomatosis, laryngeal tumors are rare in children. Typically, *laryngeal papillomatosis* presents with hoarseness or aphonia that progresses to stridor and retractions. Diagnosis may be suspected from a lateral neck radiograph, but both the diagnosis and treatment are endoscopic (Fig. 52–8).

DIAGNOSTIC EVALUATION

Ventilation Assessment

Depending on the severity of the upper airway obstruction, the clinical evaluation of an affected child should include an assessment of the ventilation status. The metabolic rate of children is much higher than adults, so both O_2 consumption and carbon dioxide (CO_2) production are greater. For this reason, the respiratory reserve depends on the age of the child, and infants have much less reserve due to their higher metabolic rate.

The use of pulse oximetry and transcutaneous monitoring of CO_2 can provide an ongoing record of ventilation.[31] Many children struggle and cry during the drawing of arterial blood gases, and gases drawn under such conditions may not be a true reflection

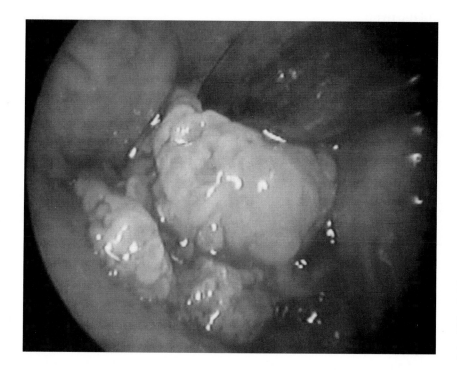

Figure 52–8: Endoscopic view of the larynx in a child with laryngeal papillomatosis. As is often the case in these patients, the true glottis is completely obscured.

of the instantaneous ventilation status unless an arterial line is already in place.

In occasional cases following the sudden relief of severe upper airway obstruction, postobstructive pulmonary edema may result. This condition is the result of alveolar hypoxia, an increased alveolar-capillary transmural pressure gradient, and a catechol-mediated shift of blood volume from systemic to pulmonary circulation.[32] Treatment of this form of noncardiac pulmonary edema with positive pressure ventilation and diuretics allows for swift resolution.

Radiologic Evaluation

Lateral neck radiograph

The lateral neck radiograph remains the single best initial study in the evaluation of the child who presents with acute upper airway obstruction and in whom emergent airway intervention is not warranted.[5] The film is best produced with a high kilovoltage source (150 to 250 kV) and a short exposure time (1/30 to 1/60 second). It is important to position the child well, with the head completely extended and the arms held posteriorly and inferiorly.[33] The tracheal lumen normally narrows on expiration and re-expands on inspiration due to changes in intrathoracic pressure.[33] It is a normal finding to see the trachea deviated somewhat anteriorly, simulating a mass that is posterior to the trachea. In an obstructed child, ballooning of the hypopharynx may be seen on the lateral neck radiograph. This ballooning disappears during expiration but is replaced by dilatation of the trachea distal to the obstruction (Fig. 52-9).

> ## SPECIAL CONSIDERATION:
>
> The lateral neck radiograph remains the single best initial study in the evaluation of the child with AAO.

AP neck film

An AP neck film is helpful in determining the caliber of the tracheal airway, and may identify pathology that narrows the airway in a coronal plane. A steeple

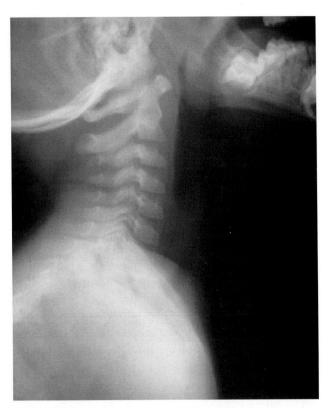

Figure 52–9: Lateral neck radiograph demonstrates haziness of the subglottic airway in a child with laryngotracheobronchitis. Note ballooning of the hypopharynx proximal to the level of acute obstruction.

sign may be seen with LTB and other conditions that cause subglottic edema (Fig. 52-10).

Chest radiograph

In a child who presents with acute upper airway obstruction, a chest radiograph may be invaluable. For example, a pathologic condition within the trachea may alter the tracheal air shadow. Radiopaque foreign bodies within the airway may be identified. Because obstruction of the upper airway may be associated with pulmonary infection, the chest radiograph is important for identifying such conditions.

Barium swallow/airway fluoroscopy

These two studies, which are frequently performed together, are most useful in the evaluation of chronic, not acute, airway obstruction. The barium swallow may be helpful in identifying vascular abnormalities in the chest by showing a posterior and lateral tracheoesophageal indentation.[34] Fluoroscopy is helpful in the evaluation of the infant airway

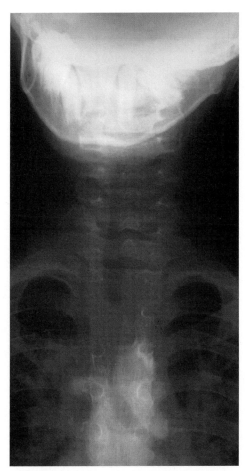

Figure 52–10: Neck radiograph (AP view) demonstrates classic steeple sign that is seen in patients with laryngotracheobronchitis.

because it allows image intensification of that portion of the airway that is movable.[33] Both unilateral and bilateral vocal cord paralysis may also be demonstrated on videofluoroscopy.[29]

Endoscopic Evaluation

In selected patients, judicious use of either a flexible nasopharyngoscope or bronchoscope in the emergency room or outpatient clinic may identify the cause of AAO. Prior to flexible endoscopy in these settings, the nose may be anesthetized with 2% lidocaine solution in combination with either oxymetazoline or phenylephrine spray or drops. In patients with suspected vocal fold paralysis, one should look for paradoxical movement of the vocal fold such as adduction on inspiration. This method of examination should be avoided in any patient with suspected supraglottitis because of the possibility of precipitating complete obstruction of the airway.

Whereas the airway from the nares to the true vocal folds can be inspected under local anesthesia, examination distal to the glottis is usually performed under general anesthesia in most children. With inhalation anesthesia and in the absence of neuromuscular blockade, the dynamics of the airway can be evaluated with a flexible bronchoscope.[35] Endoscopic examination in the operating room also should include use of the rigid bronchoscope, which has the advantages of superior optics and the ability to establish and maintain the airway.[35] In a review of the efficacy of rigid bronchoscopy for diagnosing both airway and pulmonary problems, upper airway obstruction was present in 30% of cases and lower airway disease in the remainder.[36] In other series, many patients undergoing endoscopy have been found to have multiple airway lesions.[27,37,38] The presence of cyanosis in addition to stridor suggests an increased incidence of multiple airway lesions.[27]

The risks of rigid endoscopy are small, in the range of 2 to 4% in five series.[39] These series include patients at higher risk of complication (i.e., children with a foreign body or other major tracheal pathology such as tracheal stenosis) so, the risks of diagnostic bronchoscopy in institutions that routinely care for children may be much lower.

MANAGEMENT OF ACUTE AIRWAY OBSTRUCTION

Impending loss of the airway requires immediate airway intervention. Depending upon the degree of obstruction and the etiology, the child may be observed or treated medically or surgically (Practice Pathway 52–1).

Nonsurgical Intervention

Observation

After assessing the patient and deciding that the airway is stable and that, in fact, intervening may make it unstable, the examiner may elect to just observe the patient in a setting where trained personnel can secure the airway if necessary. This setting is typically an ICU or other high-surveillance unit where constant observation and airway intervention can take place immediately.

Practice Pathway 52–1   ACUTE AIRWAY OBSTRUCTION

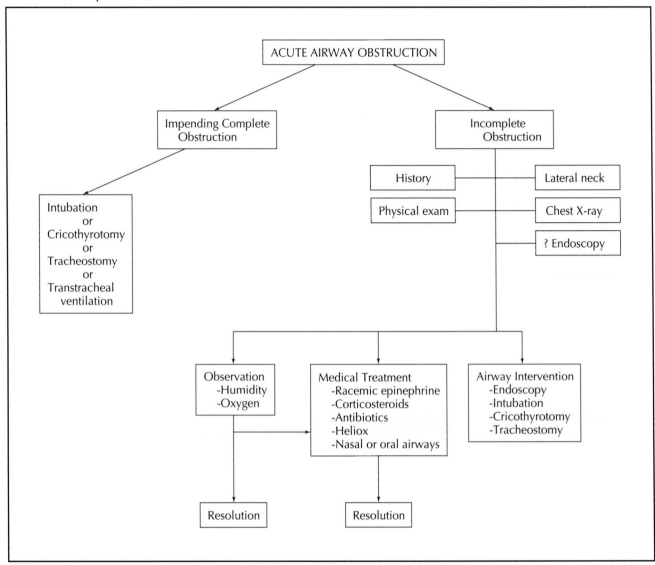

Oxygen and humidity

Humidified O_2 may be administered by face mask and may increase the actual inspired O_2 to approximately 50%. Humidification of inspired O_2 or air liquifies secretions and aids in their clearance. In patients with croup, there is no evidence that humidification actually improves symptoms, although it makes empirical sense that it may help.[40]

Racemic epinephrine

The administration of racemic epinephrine by nebulization acts by its alpha-agonist constrictor properties to decrease mucosal edema. Its effects last approximately 30 to 60 minutes. When used in patients with LTB, racemic epinephrine improves croup scores at 10 and 30 minutes, but not at 120 minutes.[6] Use of racemic epinephrine has also been shown to decrease the need for either intubation or tracheostomy in LTB.[31] When compared to nebulized saline alone, racemic epinephrine is more efficacious in the management of croup.[6,41] Rebound or worsening of airway obstruction after the drug effect wears off may occur with the use of racemic epinephrine. For this reason, treated patients should be observed for 4 to 6 hours after administration.

Corticosteroids

The rationale for using corticosteroids in the management of upper airway obstruction is their ability to suppress the progressive cycle of inflammation that results in edema of injured tissue.[42] Dexamethasone and methylprednisolone are two preparations of corticosteroids that are water-soluble with rapid absorption and high blood levels within a short period of time.[42] Dexamethasone is the most commonly used corticosteroid in the treatment of airway obstruction because of its long half-life, high antiinflammatory potency and low mineralocorticoid effect.[43] The usual dosage for dexamethasone for upper airway problems is 1.0 to 1.5 mg/kg/day, with the first dose one-half of the daily dose and the remainder given at 6 to 8 hour intervals. The maximum dosage of dexamethasone per day is unknown but is thought to be in the 10 to 30 mg range.[42] The dosage of methylprednisolone is approximately five times the dosage of dexamethasone: 5 to 7 mg/kg/day.[42]

The use of corticosteroids in children with LTB remains controversial. After reviewing the literature on their use, Hawkins et al. suggested that the effect of corticosteroids was local, directly proportional to their concentration, and helpful in the management of LTB when given in appropriate doses.[42] In two separate studies, Postma et al. and Tiballs et al. have shown the efficacy of corticosteroids in the treatment of croup.[44,45] Kairys et al. performed a meta-analysis of nine randomized trials of the efficacy of corticosteroids in LTB and showed an improvement at both 12 and 24 hours and an 80% reduction in the incidence of intubation.[46]

Corticosteroids have also been demonstrated to be of value in the treatment of other airway problems including postintubation edema, adenotonsillar hypertrophy as the result of Epstein-Barr viral infection, and allergic edema.[42,47-49] In patients who were intubated with acute supraglottis, corticosteriods have been shown to be of benefit prior to extubation.[5] Spasmodic croup, which has an allergic etiology (as opposed to LTB, which is infectious), appears to have a better response to corticosteroid therapy.[50] The use of corticosteroids in the management of subglottic hemangioma is controversial, although several studies support their value.[42]

Antibiotics

Although the etiology of many infections of the upper respiratory tract are viral, there may be bacterial superinfection or injury to the respiratory mucosal that may invite bacterial infection. LTB is a

viral illness and when uncomplicated should not be treated with antibiotics. In patients who fail to improve or who require active airway intervention with endotracheal intubation, antibiotic therapy should be considered because of the possibility of mucosal injury. Both acute supraglottitis and bacterial tracheitis require aggressive IV antibiotic treatment. Likewise, infections involving the pharynx that result in airway obstruction, such as a retropharyngeal or parapharyngeal abscess, require IV antibiotic therapy.

In the past, ampicillin, which is a broad-spectrum semisynthetic penicillin, was the drug of choice for the treatment of upper airway infections. The development of bacterial resistance to the penicillins has resulted in the need for additional antibiotic coverage. When *Hemophilus influenzae* was thought to be the offending organism, chloramphenicol was typically added to ampicillin to counter resistant organisms. The use of these two antibiotics has been supplanted by the higher generation cephalosporins (i.e., cefuroxime, cefotaxime, or ceftizoxime).[51] *Staphylococcus aureus* is the usual organism in bacterial tracheitis, and antibiotic coverage in these cases should include the penicillinase-resistant penicillins, such as methicillin or nafcillin, that have been shown to be effective against resistant staphylococci. Anaerobic organisms may infect the pharynx, and clindamycin, which is an antibiotic with both good gram-positive and anaerobic coverage, is efficacious in the management of serious pharyngeal infections.[52]

Heliox

The use of a helium-oxygen mixture in the management of airway obstruction was first described by Barach in 1935.[53] Helium has the lowest specific gravity of any gas with the exception of hydrogen, which is explosive and therefore not a clinical option. The density of any gas is related to its specific gravity; thus, when helium is used to replace nitrogen, it lowers the density of the oxygen-gas mixture. This lower gas density means less air turbulence and therefore less gas resistance. In fact, the resistance to flow with heliox is less than when breathing any concentration of O_2 including 100% oxygen.[54] In emergent airway obstruction, heliox can be used to maintain oxygenation until a more stable solution can be found.[55]

SPECIAL CONSIDERATION:

In emergent airway obstruction, heliox can be used to maintain oxygenation until a more stable solution can be found.

Nasal and oral airways

Nasal airways are made of red or latex rubber and can be inserted into either naris with ease after sufficient lubrication. The airway should be long enough so that the distal end reaches the end of the soft palate. A shorter length fails to correct obstruction caused by collapse of the palate against the posterior pharyngeal wall, and a longer airway may induce gagging. Nasal airways are much better tolerated than their oral counterparts that are typically made of hard plastic. Nasal and oral airways may be used to overcome airway obstruction in the nose and superior pharynx. Because of compliance problems, they are typically employed as only a temporary solution.

Endotracheal intubation

In children with progressive airway obstruction or ventilation compromise, endotracheal intubation has become the airway treatment of choice. In the last 25 years, use of polyvinyl chloride tubes to maintain the airway has revolutionized the airway management in cases of acute supraglottitis and severe croup that were formerly treated with tracheostomy.[8]

In children, the subglottis is the most narrow region of the airway and dictates the size of the endotracheal tube that will pass through it. The tube should have a leak around it of less than 30 cm of water and yet still allow adequate suctioning. Age appears to correlate better with endotracheal tube size than height or weight. A list of endotracheal tube sizes for children is listed in Table 52–2.[56,57]

TABLE 52–2: List of Expected Endotracheal Tube Sizes for Children

Age	Internal Diameter (mm)
0–3 months	3.5
3–9 months	4.0
9 months–2 years	4.5
after 2 years	18 + age in years/4

From references 56 and 57, with permission.

In a study by Mostafa, the need for an endotracheal tube two sizes smaller (1.0 mm) was indicative of mild congenital subglottic stenosis and was seen in 0.91% of cases, whereas a tube three sizes smaller (1.5 mm) was indicative of moderate stenosis and seen in 0.06% of children.[56]

Several contraindications to oral intubation exist, most of which are related to trauma. In a child with a cervical spine injury, the neck needs to remain immobile, and nasal intubation may only be accomplished by flexible laryngoscopy. Intubation should not be performed in cases where visualization of the larynx may be difficult, such as in a patient who has sustained oral trauma, or in cases where the laryngeal or tracheal integrity may have been violated by trauma; it also should not be done when there is a risk that the tube may pass out of the airway and into either the neck or chest. The airway in such cases may be better managed with a tracheostomy.

Appropriate equipment is essential to perform intubation, especially in a child whose airway is already compromised (Fig. 52–11). Either a standard Jackson laryngoscope or an intubating laryngoscope with several types of blades (e.g., Miller, MacIntosh) may be used. An appropriately sized endotracheal tube, one or two smaller and larger endotracheal tubes, and a stylet should be available. Suction and forceps (e.g., Magill) should be available if needed. After intubation, the tube should be carefully, but adequately, secured to the child to prevent kinking or dislodgement. In children with a difficult airway

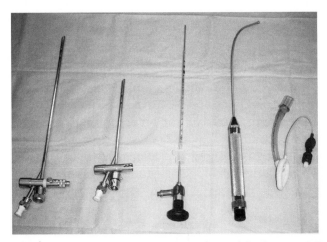

Figure 52–11: Instrumentation that might be crucial during the induction of a child with a difficult airway. These include from left to right: two rigid bronchoscopes, a telescope inserted through an endotracheal tube, a lighted stylet, and a laryngeal mask.

(i.e., Treacher Collins syndrome, Goldenhar's syndrome, etc.) a plan should be devised prior to attempts at intubation. These children may require an awake intubation, use of a flexible bronchoscope, a lighted stylet, or a laryngeal mask.

Nasal intubation may be performed safely using a standard laryngoscope. In children where the larynx is difficult to visualize, a flexible bronchoscope may be used to guide a nasally-placed endotracheal tube. Blind nasal intubation may be an option, especially if a cervical spine injury is present. This procedure, however, carries the risk that it will be unsuccessful and so other options should be made available. Nasal intubation has the advantages of being more comfortable for the patient and allowing the tube to be better secured than an oral tube.

The intubated child should remain in the ICU or equivalent high-surveillance unit where recognition of the problems of an artificial airway may be immediate. The child will require sedation, and the arms should be restrained to prevent accidental self-extubation. Immobilizing the child with neuromuscular paralyzing agents should be avoided because it requires mechanical ventilation and may allow problems with atelectasis to develop.

Transtracheal ventilation

This form of emergency ventilation has been described in adults as an alternative to an emergency tracheostomy or cricothyrotomy for complete airway obstruction; however, it should only be employed in children as last resort because of the difficulty in identifying the appropriate anatomic landmarks. Several canine studies have verified the success of this technique, although at least one author (Oppenheimer) has cautioned against its use in small children because of the softness of the cartilage and the extreme mobility of the trachea.[58-60]

After identifying the cricothyroid membrane, a 16 gauge needle is inserted through the membrane into the trachea, and O_2 may be delivered through an appropriate connecting tubing. This emergency type of ventilation should be performed only until a more stable airway can be obtained.

Surgical Intervention

Endoscopy

In the child with AAO, failure to secure the airway with endotracheal intubation necessitates endo-

scopic management or either a cricothyrotomy or tracheostomy. Endoscopic instrumentation, such as a standard Jackson laryngoscope and an appropriately sized pediatric bronchoscope, should be available immediately to secure the airway.

Endoscopic control of the airway in a child with AAO should be performed either while the child is awake or under inhalational anesthesia. Paralyzing the child with neuromuscular paralyzing agents may result in an inability to ventilate the child. The child who is still ventilating spontaneously maintains some tone of the pharyngeal musculature, and this may allow for better visualization of the larynx in difficult cases. In cases with difficult laryngeal visualization (e.g., the child with mandibular hypoplasia), use of an anterior commissure laryngoscope and bronchoscopic telescope may allow exposure of the glottis.[61]

Once the airway has been secured with a bronchoscope, a decision must be reached as to further airway management. If the pathologic condition can be treated, allowing the child to be successfully intubated, no additional therapy is required. Otherwise, a tracheostomy can be performed with the bronchoscope still controlling the airway.

Cricothyrotomy

Rarely in a child who presents with AAO will all attempts at obtaining an airway, including endoscopy, fail, necessitating immediate surgical intervention. *Cricothyrotomy* is a procedure that may be performed rapidly with a minimum of equipment, and it may avoid some of the risks of an emergency tracheostomy such as bleeding and pneumothorax. Unlike transtracheal ventilation, a small endotracheal or tracheostomy tube may be placed through the opening in the cricothyroid membrane and the airway secured for positive ventilation if necessary. Once performed, however, the airway should be converted to a more stable form by way of either endotracheal intubation or a tracheostomy. Leaving a tube through the cricothyroid membrane for a prolonged period of time may result in perichondritis of the cricoid cartilage with resultant subglottic stenosis.

When performed emergently, cricothyrotomy can be accomplished quickly. After identifying the cricoid and thyroid cartilages, the cricothyroid membrane can be palpated just superior to the cricoid cartilage. An incision is made in the overlying skin and a pointed instrument, such as a hemostat, can be used to enter the airway. Either a tracheostomy tube, endotracheal tube, or other large bore catheter can then be used to maintain the airway until a more secure airway can be established.

Tracheostomy

If the airway is stable or can be secured temporarily by some other means, a tracheostomy is preferable to either transtracheal ventilation or a cricothyrotomy. Although endotracheal intubation has replaced tracheostomy for many diseases, such as croup and supraglottitis, tracheostomy is still an option in cases where a translaryngeal airway has to be avoided.

The incidence of tracheostomy for the relief of upper airway obstruction, either acute or chronic, has remained relatively constant over the past 25 years as reported in two series from a major children's hospital.[62] In the first series that spanned a decade from 1971 to 1980, 39% of tracheostomies were performed for upper airway obstruction.[63] In a later series from 1981 to 1992, 38% of tracheostomies were performed for the same reason. Of note is that the use of tracheostomy in the management of LTB decreased from 7.6 to 1.1% during the second decade compared to the first.

Tracheostomies performed emergently are fraught with a higher incidence of complications. Bleeding may result from inadequate ligation of vessels or diffuse ooze from trauma to the thyroid gland. Subcutaneous emphysema, pneumomediastinum, and pneumothorax may all result from leakage of air into surrounding tissues or inadvertent violation of the pleura. Injury to adjacent structures in the neck, such as the esophagus or recurrent laryngeal nerves, are all possible. Lack of proper sterile technique may result in postoperative infection. Prompt recognition of these complications is necessary to prevent further morbidity.

AT A GLANCE...

Management of Acute Airway Obstruction

Nonsurgical intervention: observation, oxygen, humidity, racemic epinephrine, corticosteroids, antibiotics, heliox, nasal and oral airways, endotracheal intubation, transtracheal ventilation

Surgical intervention: endoscopy, cricothyrotomy, tracheostomy

---

REFERENCES

1. Hirschberg J. Acoustic analysis of pathological cries, stridors, and coughing sounds in infancy. Int J Pediatr Otorhinolaryngol 1980; 2:287–300.
2. Holinger LD. Etiology of stridor in the neonate, infant, and child. Ann Otol Rhinol Laryngol 1980; 89:397–400.
3. Snow JB. Clinical evaluation of noisy respiration in infancy. Lancet 1965; 85:504–509.
4. Denny FW, Murphy TF, Clyde WA, et al. Croup: An 11-year study in a pediatric practice. Pediatrics 1983; 71:871–876.
5. Hodge KM, Ganzel TM. Diagnostic and therapeutic efficiency in croup and epiglottitis. Laryngoscope 1987; 97:621–625.
6. Westley CR, Cotton EK, Brooks JG. Nebulized racemic epinephrine by IPPB for the treatment of croup. Am J Dis Child 1978; 132:484–487.
7. Kessler A, Wetmore RF, Marsh RR. Childhood epiglottitis in recent years. Int J Pediatr Otorhinolaryngol 1993; 25:155–162.
8. Wetmore RF, Handler SD. Epiglottitis: Evolution in management during the last decade. Ann Otol Rhinol Laryngol 1979; 88:822–826.
9. Schuller DE, Birsk HG. The safety of intubation in croup and epiglottitis: An eight-year follow-up. Laryngoscope 1975; 85:33–46.
10. Tobias JD. Heliox in children with airway obstruction. Pediatr Emerg Care 1997; 13:29–32.
11. Donnelly BW, McMillan JA, Weiner LB. Bacterial tracheitis: Report of eight new cases and review. Rev Infect Dis 1990; 12:729–735.
12. Denneny JC, Handler SD. Membranous laryngotracheobronchitis. Pediatrics 1982; 70:705–707.
13. Potsic WP. Assessment and treatment of adenotonsillar hypertrophy in children. Am J Otolaryngol 1992; 13:259–264.
14. Alpert G, Fleisher GR. Complications of infection with Epstein-Barr virus during childhood: A study of children admitted to the hospital. Pediatr Infect Dis 1984; 3:304–307.
15. Handler SD, Potsic WP. Neck masses and the airway. Int Anesthesiol Clin 1992; 30:45–48.
16. Potsic WP. Sleep apnea in children. Otolaryngol Clin North Am 1989; 22:537–544.
17. Grundfast KM, Wittich DJ. Adenotonsillar hypertrophy and upper airway obstruction in evolutionary perspective. Laryngoscope 1982; 92:650–656.
18. Potsic WP, Pasquariello PS, Baranak CC, et al. Relief of upper airway obstruction by adenotonsillectomy. Otolaryngol Head Neck Surg 1986; 94:476–480.
19. Ungkanont K, Yellon RF, Weissman JL, et al. Head and neck space infections in infants and children. Otolaryngol Head Neck Surg 1995; 112:375–382.

20. Wetmore RF, Mahboubi S, Soyupak SK. Computed tomography in the evaluation of pediatric neck infections. Otolaryngol Head Neck Surg 1998; 119: 624-627.

21. Dixon HS. Allergy and laryngeal disease. Otolaryngol Clin North Am 1992; 25:239-250.

22. Gordon BR. Prevention and management of office allergy emergencies. Otolaryngol Clin North Am 1992; 25:119-134.

23. Reilly JS, Walter MA. Consumer product aspiration and ingestion in children: Analysis of emergency room reports to the National Electronic Injury Surveillance System. Ann Otol Rhinol Laryngol 1992; 101:739-741.

24. Whited RE. A study of endotracheal tube injury to the subglottis. Laryngoscope 1985; 95:1216-1219.

25. Othersen HB. Intubation injuries of the trachea in children. Ann Surg 1979; 189:601-606.

26. Sie KCY, McGill T, Healy GB. Subglottic hemangioma: Ten years experience with the carbon dioxide laser. Ann Otol Rhinol Laryngol 1994; 103:167-172.

27. Gonzalez C, Reilly JS, Bluestone CD. Synchronous airway lesions in infancy. Ann Otol Rhinol Laryngol 1987; 96:77-80.

28. Isaacson G, Moya F. Hereditary congenital laryngeal abductor paralysis. Ann Otol Rhinol Laryngol 1987; 96:701-704.

29. Grundfast KM, Harley E. Vocal cord paralysis. Otolaryngol Clin North Am 1989; 22:569-597.

30. Gatti WM, MacDonald EM, Orfei E. Congenital laryngeal atresia. Laryngoscope 1987; 97:966-969.

31. Fanconi S, Burger R, Maurer H, et al. Transcutaneous carbon dioxide pressure for monitoring patients with severe croup. J Pediatr 1990; 117:701-705.

32. Travis KW, Todres ID, Shannon DC. Pulmonary edema associated with croup and epiglottitis. Pediatrics 1977; 59:695-698.

33. Jasin ME, Osguthorpe JD. The radiographic evaluation of infants with stridor. Otolaryngol Head Neck Surg 1982; 90:736-739.

34. Lima JA, Rosenblum BN, Reilly JS, et al. Airway obstruction in aortic arch anomalies. Otolaryngol Head Neck Surg 1983; 91:605-609.

35. Handler SD. Direct laryngoscopy in children: Rigid and flexible fiberoptic. Ear Nose Throat J 1995; 74: 100-106.

36. Wiseman NE, Sanchez I, Powell RE. Rigid bronchoscopy in the pediatric age group: Diagnostic effectiveness. J Pediatr Surg 1992; 27:1294-1297.

37. Friedman EM, Williams M, Healy GB, et al. Pediatric endoscopy: A review of 616 cases. Ann Otol Rhinol Laryngol 1984; 93:517-519.

38. Altman KW, Wetmore RF, Marsh RR. Congenital airway abnormalities requiring tracheostomy: A profile of 56 patients and their diagnoses over a 9 year period. Int J Pediatr Otorhinolaryngol 1997; 41: 199-206.

39. Hoeve LJ, Rombout J, Meursing AEE. Complications of rigid laryngobronchoscopy in children. Int J Pediatr Otorhinolaryngol 1993; 26:47-56.

40. Henry R. Moist air in the treatment of laryngotracheitis. Arch Dis Child 1983; 58:577.

41. Lenny W, Milner AD. Treatment of acute viral croup. Arch Dis Child 1978; 53:704-706.

42. Hawkins DB, Crockett DM, Shum TK. Corticosteroids in airway management. Otolaryngol Head Neck Surg 1983; 91:593-596.

43. Schimmer BP, Parker KL. Adrenocorticotropic hormone; Adrenocortical steroids and their synthetic analogs; Inhibitors of the synthesis and actions of adrenocortical hormones. In: Hardman JG, Limbird LE, eds. *Goodman & Gilman's The Pharmacological Basis of Therapeutics, 9th ed.* New York: McGraw-Hill, 1996, p. 1466.

44. Postma DS, Jones RO, Pillsbury HC. Severe hospitalized croup: Treatment trends and prognosis. Laryngoscope 1984; 94:1170-1175.

45. Tibballs J, Shann FA, Landau LI. Placebo-controlled trial of prednisolone in children intubated for croup. Lancet 1992; 340:745-748.

46. Kairys SW, Olmstead EM, O'Connor GT. Steroid treatment of laryngotracheitis: A meta-analysis of the evidence from randomized trials. Pediatrics 1989; 83:683-693.

47. Biller HF, Bone RC, Harvey JE, et al. Laryngeal edema. An experimental study. Ann Otol Rhinol Laryngol 1970; 79:1084-1087.

48. Mandel W, Marilley RJ, Gaines LM. Corticotropin in severe anginose infectious mononucleosis. JAMA 1955; 158:1021-1022.

49. Relkin R. The use of steroids in infectious mononucleosis. NY State J Med 1960; 60:168.

50. Koren G, Frand M, Barzilay Z, et al. Corticosteroid treatment of laryngotracheitis V. spasmodic croup in children. Am J Dis Child 1983; 137:941-944.

51. Neu HC. Contemporary antibiotic therapy in otolaryngology. Otolaryngol Clin North Am 1984; 17: 745-760.

52. Kapusnik-Uner JE, Sande MA, Chambers HF. Antimicrobial Agents. In: Hardman JG, Limbird LE, eds. *Goodman & Gilman's The Pharmacological Basis of Therapeutics, 9th ed.* New York: McGraw-Hill, 1996; p. 1141.

53. Barach AL. The use of helium in the treatment of asthma and obstructive lesions in the larynx and trachea. Ann Intern Med 1935; 9:739-765.

54. Brook I. Aerobic and anaerobic microbiology of bacterial tracheitis in children. Pediatr Emerg Care 1997; 13:16-18.

55. Mizrahi S, Yaari Y, Lugassy G, et al. Major airway

obstruction relieved by helium/oxygen breathing. Crit Care Med 1986; 14:986–987.

56. Mostafa SM. Variation in subglottic size in children. Proc R Soc Med 1976; 69:793–795.

57. Lee KW, Templeton JJ, Dougal RM. Tracheal tube size and post-intubation croup in children. Anesthesiology 1980; 53:S325.

58. Hughes RK. Needle tracheostomy. Arch Surg 1966; 93:834–837.

59. Oppenheimer P. Needle tracheotomy. Otorhinolaryngol Digest 1977; 39:9.

60. Cote C, Eavey R, Jones RD, et al. Cricothyroid membrane puncture: Oxygenation and ventilation in a dog model using an intravenous catheter. Crit Care Med 1988; 16:615–619.

61. Handler SD, Keon TP. Difficult laryngoscopy/intubation: The child with mandibular hypoplasia. Ann Otol Rhinol Laryngol 1983; 92:401–404.

62. Wetmore RF, Marsh RR, Thompson ME, et al. Pediatric tracheostomy: A changing procedure? Arch Otol Rhinolaryngol (in press).

63. Wetmore RF, Handler SD, Potsic WP. Pediatric Tracheostomy: Experience during the past decade. Ann Otol Rhinol Laryngol 1982; 91:628.

53 Management of Chronic Airway Obstruction

J. Scott McMurray and Charles M. Myer III

The treatment of pediatric chronic airway obstruction (CAO) is complex and controversial. This chapter discusses issues concerning the evaluation and management of CAO, specifically those related to laryngotracheal stenosis at the level of the subglottis and cervical trachea. CAO from other regions of the upper airway or tracheobronchial tree is not discussed. The chapter concludes with an overview of pediatric tracheostomy.

HISTORY OF MANAGEMENT

One of the most challenging problems confronting the otolaryngologist today remains the management of subglottic stenosis in infants and children. Although Caron performed the first successful tracheotomy in a child in 1808, airway reconstruction was not defined until the 20th century. This is due in part to refinements in the surgical management of children but also to changes in the prevalence of iatrogenic airway obstruction in children.

Previously, acquired subglottic stenosis was caused by trauma or infection and was seen in older children and adults. The most common inflammatory processes affecting the airway included syphilis, tuberculosis, typhoid, diphtheria, and croup. In children, the stenosis was frequently a complication of a high tracheotomy as treatment for these inflammatory conditions.

Since 1965, however, there has been a shift in the age group developing laryngotracheal stenosis. In 1965, McDonald and Stocks introduced long-term intubation as a method of airway management for prolonged ventilatory support in neonates.[1] As a re-

sult, the majority of patients who develop laryngotracheal stenosis today are infants and neonates. With improvements in medical management, more premature infants are surviving the neonatal period, occasionally at the cost of subglottic stenosis from long-term intubation and ventilation.

Improved medical treatment and antimicrobial therapy also have decreased the incidence of tracheotomy in those inflammatory processes that affect the airway. This has decreased the amount of stenosis seen in this group of patients.

The incidence of congenital subglottic stenosis from malformation of the cricoid cartilage or laryngotracheal web has not changed. Today, the incidence of acquired subglottic stenosis exceeds that of congenital origin. Congenital stenosis is often easier to manage surgically because the cases generally are not as severe. Acquired subglottic stenosis is usually more severe and may require more complex surgical intervention for correction.

> ### SPECIAL CONSIDERATION:
>
> Acquired subglottic stenosis is usually more severe and may require more complex surgical intervention for correction.

As early as 1932, Chevalier Jackson realized that many children with chronic laryngeal stenosis did not outgrow their obstruction. He also thought that surgical intervention, however, might inhibit future growth of the larynx. Reliable methods for surgical therapy were not available in the early part of this century and many patients were forced to live with a permanent tracheotomy.[2]

Pediatric Otolaryngology, Edited by R.F. Wetmore, H.R. Muntz, and T.J. McGill. Thieme Medical Publishers, Inc., New York © 2000.

As the etiology and severity of subglottic stenosis shifted over the next 30 years, there was a subsequent mortality increase in patients with a tracheotomy that was as high as 24% in some series.[3] Obviously, children with a severely stenotic airway and poor pulmonary reserve from serious lung disease were at greater risk of death if accidental decannulation occurred. The need to improve the airway of children with severe subglottic stenosis in the hope of decannulation or preventing disaster from accidental decannulation was then realized.

The treatment of subglottic stenosis in the early part of this century was relatively standard and often unsuccessful. Repeated dilatation using a variety of metal obturators or hollow tubes of rubber has been well documented with scattered success. The Réthi procedure, developed in 1956, was unique in that expansion of the airway through incisions of the anterior and posterior cricoid, prolonged stenting, and closure of the anterior cricoid were utilized rather than dilatation.[4] In 1971, Grahne modified the procedure by incorporating division of the anterior and posterior cricoid plate with an Aboulker stent wired to a metal tracheotomy tube, leaving the posterior and anterior cricoid distracted.[5] The limiting factor for stent size was the tracheal lumen below the stoma rather than the glottis or subglottis. Grahne left the airway stented for 4 months and published good long-term results from the technique.[6]

Evans and Todd developed another method for cricoid framework expansion without grafting at the Hospital for Sick Children, Great Ormond Street, London.[7] A castellated incision of the anterior cricoid cartilage and cervical trachea was performed, the airway was stented with a rolled Silastic™ sheet, and was left in position for 6 weeks. The effectiveness of this technique was confirmed by Cotton and Evans,[8] and MacRae and Barrie.[9]

To provide stabilization of the expanded cricoid framework and decrease the time that stenting is required, grafting material was introduced. Grafting techniques were described as early as 1938 in adults by Looper who used the hyoid bone.[10] Other successful materials included rib cartilage, iliac crest, septal cartilage, auricular cartilage, and composite clavicular bone-muscle flaps. None of these methods had been utilized in children or growing animals, however.[11] Lapido et al., in 1968, reported the successful use of a pedicled thyroid cartilage flap in piglets.[12] This study was important as it demonstrated the viability of a pedicled cartilage graft

and significant growth of the subglottis over a 6-month period. This finding placed in question Jackson's theory that surgical intervention of the pediatric larynx may result in impaired growth.

Further published series have demonstrated that surgery on the pediatric laryngeal framework is not contraindicated. Fearon and Cotton reported their experience using free and pedicled thyroid cartilage grafts in 2-year-old African green monkeys weighing 2.5 kg,[3] and then later Fearon and Cinnamond used this method in six children.[13] Calcaterra et al. showed the efficacy and safety of vertical median thyrotomy in the developing larynx in a canine model without impairment of development and function.[14] Using rigid grafting material, it became possible to expand the airway without the need for stenting in selected patients.[15]

The use of a composite hyoid-muscle flap was first demonstrated in children by Ward et al.[16] This technique was documented by many other investigators between 1978 and 1986.[17-21] Unfortunately, the utility of this technique is limited because the graft can be placed anteriorly only and cannot be used for severe posterior glottic and posterior subglottic stenosis.[11]

The use of autogenous costal cartilage has been shown in several studies to be efficacious. Histopathologic studies have demonstrated viability of grafts placed both in the anterior and posterior cricoid plate.[8,15,22,23] To reduce donor site morbidity, attempts were made to use irradiated costal cartilage and alcohol-stored homograft auricular cartilage for laryngotracheal reconstruction in rabbits. Unfortunately, there was a significantly higher rate of resorption in both instances, and autogenous fresh cartilage has become the preferred material.[24] Following the initial reports of success using costal cartilage anteriorly, there have been many reports documenting the use of this grafting material in the posterior cricoid lamina in combination with stenting. The largest series to date was presented by Cotton in 1991 when he reported that 59 of 61 patients were decannulated following laryngotracheal reconstruction utilizing autogenous cartilage grafts placed between the divided posterior lamina of the cricoid cartilage.[11]

Posterior cartilage grafting has become more common since 1979. Prior to that time, stenosis was generally anterior and could be corrected surgically with an anterior costal cartilage graft. More recently, it appears that stenosis is of a higher grade and requires a different operative approach, often incorporating posterior costal cartilage grafting. Although no studies exist to confirm this, the change in the severity of stenosis seems to correlate with an increase in the length of time of intubation of infants and children and a change in the etiology of stenosis.

Finally, some severe subglottic stenosis is not readily amenable to expansion surgery. Resection of the stenotic area has been employed successfully in adults and, more recently, in children. If the stenotic area is short and complete or if the supporting cartilaginous framework is poor and unable to support grafting, resecting the area and performing a thyrotracheal anastomosis has been shown to be successful.[25-27] Subglottic growth in the resected area has been shown to be no different from littermate controls in the canine model.[28] This model utilized primary thyrotracheal reanastomsis after the resection of normal cricoid cartilage. Partial cricotracheal resection has been used in adults with good results,[26,27,29] and recently, cricotracheal resection has been attempted in the pediatric population with initial good results.[25,30]

SPECIAL CONSIDERATION:

Some cases of severe subglottic stenosis that are not amenable to expansion surgery may be treated with cricotracheal resection.

It appears that the best results for cricotracheal resection occur in patients with discrete, short, complete stenosis that is distinct from the vocal cords. Although there are no contraindications for cricotracheal resection in patients that have a transglottic stenosis, it is intuitively obvious that these patients may have poor voice and swallowing outcomes. More experience is needed with partial cricotracheal resection before its utility is determined completely but it remains a powerful tool for the treatment of subglottic stenosis.

Treatment pathways for subglottic stenosis include expansion surgery with or without stenting or resection surgery with or without prolonged airway management. Historically, each has shown utility. The decision making process is important in determining the correct initial path to take, and this is outlined in the next sections.

EVALUATION

Many patients with CAO have multisystem disease processes. A multidisciplinary approach is often required, involving the pediatric otolaryngologist, pediatric swallowing specialist, pediatric pulmonologist and pediatric gastroenterologist. Table 53-1 outlines the preoperative evaluation.

TABLE 53–1: Preoperative Evaluation for Laryngotracheal Reconstruction

History
Progression of symptoms
Feeding difficulty
Voice change
Gestational age at birth
Intubation history
Physical Exam
Stridor
Retractions
Nasal airway
Cutaneous hemangioma
Neck mass
Awake Flexible Nasopharyngoscopy
Nasopharynx
Hypopharynx
Supraglottis and glottis
Vocal cord motion
Airway Radiographs
AP and lateral neck
PA and lateral chest
Airway fluoroscopy
MRI
CT scan
Rigid Endoscopy
Laryngoscopy
Tracheoscopy
Bronchoscopy
Esophagoscopy
Gastroenterology Consultation
(dual) pH probe
Mucosal biopsy
Barium esophogram
Pulmonary Consultation
Pulmonary assessment
Pulmonary Function Tests
Swallowing Assessment
Flexible endoscopic evaluation of swallowing
Modified barium swallow
Swallowing specialist evaluation

Abbreviations: AP, anteroposterior; PA, Posteroanterior; MRI, Magnetic Resonance imaging; CT, Computed Tomography.

History

The clinical presentation of patients with subglottic stenosis is variable, and is dependent on age, the overall medical condition, and the extent of the stenosis. The major signs and symptoms related to subglottic stenosis concern issues with feeding, voice, and the airway. Feeding disorders commonly are due to the stress placed upon the airway during feeding. Reference growth charts often show a child who is underweight or has fallen off the growth curve for age. Voice may or may not be affected depending on the extent of stenosis and the proximity and involvement of the vocal folds. The most common presentation of subglottic stenosis, however, is progressive respiratory difficulty with biphasic stridor. The stridor may present only during agitation or feeding, when the airway is stressed. Airway compromise also may present only during respiratory tract infections such as recurrent croup. Asthma refractory to medical therapy may be a sign of a fixed structural stenosis. The degree of dyspnea varies depending on the rapidity with which the stenosis develops. Severe stenosis that has developed gradually is occasionally better tolerated than the acutely-occluded airway. Retractions commonly are seen in the suprasternal, intercostal, and diaphragmatic areas.

The true incidence of subglottic stenosis is unknown. An incidence of 1.5 cases/1,000,000 population in adults in the United Kingdom has been estimated.[31] Neonates requiring endotracheal intubation for any reason have an incidence of subglottic stenosis ranging from 1 to 8%.[32-34] A history of endotracheal intubation should alert the clinician to the possibility of subglottic stenosis resulting from either scar formation or subglottic cysts. Generally, the time from intubation to presentation is from 1 to 4 weeks, although infrequently, a longer latency period is possible from the time of laryngeal injury to the development of symptoms.[35] Significant congenital subglottic stenosis generally presents within the first few weeks of life. Children with a mild or moderate subglottic stenosis may not present with symptoms until an upper respiratory infection (URI) further narrows the subglottis with edema. These patients generally present with recurrent croup that has a protracted course despite the advancing age of the patient.

> ### Special Consideration:
> A history of endotracheal intubation should alert the clinician to the possibility of subglottic stenosis resulting from either scar formation or subglottic cysts.

Physical

A complete physical examination should be performed to identify any associated abnormalities. The supraglottic and glottic larynx should be evaluated as a routine part of the examination, utilizing flexible fiberoptic nasopharyngoscopy to evaluate laryngeal function. Vocal cord motion and hypopharyngeal pooling of secretions should be documented, as well as any other abnormalities of the supraglottis. If vocal cord motion impairment or hypopharyngeal pooling of secretions is identified, the child also should be evaluated for potential swallowing disorders.

Due to the risk of reflex laryngospasm and severe vasovagal reflexes, passing the flexible telescope through the glottis is not recommended in the office setting. Infrequently, the diagnosis of subglottic stenosis is made during flexible office endoscopy by visualizing the subglottis between open vocal cords. Flexible fiberoptic nasopharyngoscopy confirms a normal glottis and supraglottis before proceeding with an evaluation of the subglottis and trachea utilizing general anesthesia and rigid endoscopy.

Radiographic Exam

Radiographic studies are useful in determining the site and extent of subglottic stenosis (Table 53–2).[36] High-kilovoltage anteroposterior (AP) and lateral neck radiographs and posteroanterior (PA) and lateral chest radiographs are essential in every child under evaluation for CAO. The lateral neck radio-

Table 53–2: Airway Radiographs for Evaluation of Chronic Laryngotracheal Stenosis

AP and lateral neck
PA and lateral chest
Airway fluoroscopy (level of airway collapse)
MRI or CT (vascular compression)

graph is likely the most useful view, although asymmetry in the subglottic region in the AP view may suggest a subglottic hemangioma or cyst. Videofluroscopy occasionally may be useful in evaluating respiratory dynamics, as subglottic stenosis can worsen the effects of tracheomalacia. Cardiac enlargement may be a late sign of CAO.

Computed tomography (CT) and magnetic resonance imaging (MRI) may be useful in determining the length and severity of subglottic stenosis. These scans are not used routinely unless specific information is required after diagnostic endoscopy. These evaluations never replace rigid endoscopy and often add little information as to the management of the patient with routine subglottic stenosis. The role of CT and MRI is important when tracheal compression by a vascular anomaly is considered.

Endoscopy

The mainstay for diagnosis of subglottic stenosis is rigid endoscopy under general anesthesia. The entire aerodigestive tract (ADT) may be evaluated by telescopic laryngoscopy, tracheoscopy, bronchoscopy, and esophagoscopy. Close attention to each anatomic subunit of the larynx, supraglottis, glottis, and subglottis, as well as the immediate cervical trachea, should be given so that an accurate identification of the stenotic area and its related parts may be determined. The size, length, thickness, and character of the stenotic region and adjacent affected regions should be documented. Photo-

graphic documentation should be obtained for the permanent record.

> ## SPECIAL CONSIDERATION:
>
> The mainstay for diagnosis of subglottic stenosis is rigid endoscopy under general anesthesia.

The accurate sizing of subglottic stenosis can be difficult due to eccentric shapes and varying lengths of stenosis. One staging system for subglottic stenosis was developed at Children's Hospital Medical Center in Cincinnati and was based on the degree of stenosis of the subglottis.[37] This method originally relied on subjective estimates of the percentage of stenosis observed. A modification was developed in an attempt to determine the degree of the subglottic stenosis objectively.[38] After visualizing the airway and estimating the appropriate-sized endotracheal tube, the surgeon intubates the child and performs a leak test. The endotracheal tube size is then increased until a leak is permitted at just <25 cm of water. This gives the appropriate-sized endotracheal tube for the patient's larynx. The endotracheal tube size is then compared to a chart listing the average endotracheal tube size that is appropriate for that and this allows the surgeon to determine the percentage of stenosis (Fig. 53-1). This technique

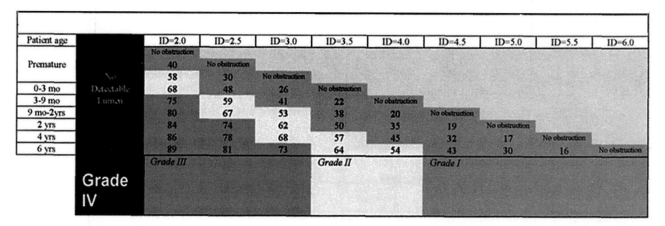

Patient age		ID=2.0	ID=2.5	ID=3.0	ID=3.5	ID=4.0	ID=4.5	ID=5.0	ID=5.5	ID=6.0
Premature		No obstruction								
	No Detectable Lumen	40	No obstruction							
		58	30	No obstruction						
0-3 mo		68	48	26	No obstruction					
3-9 mo		75	59	41	22	No obstruction				
9 mo-2yrs		80	67	53	38	20	No obstruction			
2 yrs		84	74	62	50	35	19	No obstruction		
4 yrs		86	78	68	57	45	32	17	No obstruction	
6 yrs		89	81	73	64	54	43	30	16	No obstruction
Grade IV		Grade III			Grade II		Grade I			

Figure 53–1: Classification of stenosis with actual endotracheal tube size. The numbers in the columns represent the estimated percent stenosis. The grade can be determined by sizing the airway with an endotracheal tube and comparing the estimated size with the age of the patient on the chart. The appropriate endotracheal tube leaks with 10-25 cm H_2O positive pressure applied. (Adapted from reference 38, with permission.)

shows for easy, objective documentation and comparisons after reconstruction. It is best used in circular and firm stenotic segments. It is not as useful for evaluating subglottic stenosis from functional collapse secondary to poor cartilage support. In those cases, the endotracheal tube acts to stent the collapsing segment open during sizing. Using this endotracheal tube system, a grading system was developed such that grade I is 0 to 50% stenosis, grade II is 51 to 70% stenosis, grade III is 71 to 99% stenosis, and grade IV is no detectable lumen (Fig. 53-2).[38]

It is important to minimize trauma to the larynx during endoscopy. Skilled endoscopy, with an appropriately-sized endoscope and a minimum number of endotracheal intubations during the sizing procedure, minimizes the amount of postoperative edema. Patients who are symptomatic preoperatively and without tracheotomy may benefit from a single perioperative dose of systemic steroids (dexamethasone sodium phosphate 0.6-1.0 mg/kg up to a maximum of 20 mg). Although not performed routinely diagnostic biopsies may be taken of the stenosis during endoscopy.

Along with the extent of stenosis encountered, the maturity of the stenosis may be judged. Active granulation tissue and acute inflammatory changes indicate immature and evolving lesions that are termed "active larynx" unless no other causes for the inflammation can be determined. Surgical reconstruction performed on evolving, immature lesions may result in an inadequate or too aggressive surgical repair. If inflammation is seen in the larynx, an evaluation for gastroesophageal reflux (GER) should be performed also. Although still controversial, GER has been implicated as a causative agent in subglottic stenosis.

Swallowing

Preoperative evaluation of swallowing function is important in children undergoing laryngotracheal reconstruction. Some children who have a complete stenosis may develop chronic aspiration following surgical relief of their airway obstruction. Several techniques are available for the preoperative evaluation of swallowing to predict the postoperative ability of swallowing.

Modified barium swallows in conjunction with an evaluation by a swallowing specialist, usually a speech language pathologist or an occupational therapist, may be helpful in the preoperative period. Hypopharyngeal pooling of secretions and delayed transit time of the contrast medium may be identified with this technique. Penetration and aspiration may be missed in patients with complete stenosis.

Flexible endoscopic evaluation of swallowing (FEES) (Table 53-3) gives a more dynamic assessment of laryngeal mobility, laryngeal function, hypopharyngeal pooling, and clearing of the bolus during the swallow. Penetration of food material into the endolarynx above a complete stenosis also can be identified. Performed in conjunction with an examination by the otolaryngologist and the swallowing specialist, different food textures and consistencies may be tried to identify those that are swallowed

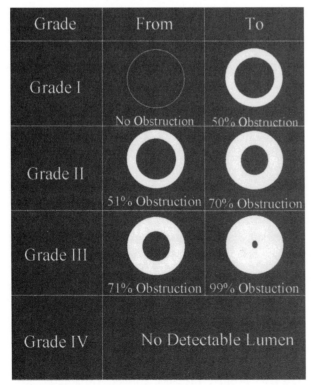

Grade	From	To
Grade I	No Obstruction	50% Obstruction
Grade II	51% Obstruction	70% Obstruction
Grade III	71% Obstruction	99% Obstuction
Grade IV	No Detectable Lumen	

Figure 53-2: Grading scale for subglottis stenosis. (Adapted from reference 38, with permission.)

TABLE 53-3:   Flexible Endoscopic Evaluation of Swallowing

Nasopharynx	Pharyngeal transit
Velopharyngeal closure	Laryngeal penetration
Oropharynx	Premature spillage
Tongue base	Aspiration
Hypopharynx	Hypopharyngeal clearance
Laryngeal movement	Hypopharyngeal pooling
vocal cord motion	Laryngeal and hypopharyngeal
laryngeal elevation	sensation

more efficiently. Immediate feedback also is given when different positions are attempted during the swallow. No radiation is used during the procedure and so it may be repeated in the postoperative period without worry of additional radiation exposure.

Children who have decreased sensation, hypopharyngeal pooling, and decreased pharyngoesophageal transit times are at risk of postoperative aspiration. The baseline FEES gives an excellent assessment of the swallowing skills and allows for a preoperative discussion with the family regarding the risk of the surgery in terms of postoperative swallowing disorders.

It is also useful when postoperative aspiration persists. During the examination, changes in laryngeal dynamics may be assessed. Disorders, such as a persistent posterior glottic opening due to redundant mucosa in the interarytenoid area, may be identified for subsequent laser ablation.

Pulmonary

The patient's pulmonary status determines many aspects of the reconstruction. Choosing between single-stage and prolonged stenting with a tracheotomy tube or a T tube is often determined by the patient's pulmonary reserve. During the perioperative period, secretions are often increased. A good pulmonary reserve is required to perform a single-stage procedure with brief endotracheal tube stenting successfully.

If questions about pulmonary status arise, consultation with a pediatric pulmonologist is important. An accurate assessment of pulmonary reserve as well as optimization of the current pulmonary status may be obtained. In general, patients who have good pulse oximetry on room air and no recent oxygen or artificial ventilatory requirements are good candidates for single-stage procedures. Patients with a history of bronchopulmonary dysplasia, oxygen requirements, or recurrent pulmonary infections may best be served with prolonged airway management with a tracheotomy tube or a T tube. The surgical airway provides an excellent route for perioperative pulmonary toilet.

Although an oxygen requirement may determine single-stage versus multiple-stage surgical airway management, it does not preclude laryngotracheal reconstruction. Oxygen may be delivered by nasal cannula in patients who continue to have a postoperative oxygen requirement.

Gastropharyngeal Reflux

Although controversial gastropharyngeal reflux (GPR) has been implicated as an inciting factor in the development of laryngotracheal disorders.[39] Animal models have shown that periodic, but infrequent, soiling of the subglottis with gastric secretions can induce a stenosis through scar formation.[40] Other components of gastric secretions, such as pepsin, have been implicated in cases where laryngeal mucosal damage occurred in the presence of nonacidic gastric contents.[39] A less controlled study, however, suggested that testing and treating gastroesophageal reflux disease (GERD) does not affect the outcome of laryngotracheal reconstruction.[41] No definitive prospective studies are available.

> **SPECIAL CONSIDERATION:**
> Although controversial, GER has been implicated as an inciting factor in the development of laryngotracheal disorders.

Consultation with a pediatric gastroenterologist is helpful in children who are candidates for laryngotracheal reconstruction if significant GER is suspected. This is especially true in infants in whom reflux and regurgitation are common. Because no definitive studies exist regarding the amount of GPR required to induce subglottic stenosis, standards for the detection of the minimum harmful refluxate have not been established. Unpublished data from Children's Hospital Medical Center in Cincinnati has revealed little correlation between laryngoscopic exam, dual pH-probe data, and histologic examination of the lower and upper esophagus and the postcricoid and interarytenoid regions of the larynx for the determination of significant GPR.

Dual pH-probe and mucosal biopsies, however, are the best tools presently available for the determination of significant reflux of gastric contents to the level of the esophagus and pharynx. Reflux is significant if the time with pH <4 is >5 to 10% at the lower probe and >4% at the upper probe. Patients with significant GPR should be treated with aggressive medical management including a proton pump inhibitor and a prokinetic agent. These patients are then reexamined for significant reflux by rigid endoscopy and repeat pH-probe. If medical therapy has not been sufficient, surgical antireflux treatment is recommended prior to laryngotracheal reconstruction. Since medical therapy for reflux has few side effects, all other patients should be placed on reflux medications during the perioperative period of laryngotracheal reconstruction.

AT A GLANCE . . .

Evaluation of Chronic Airway Obstruction

Physical Exam: examination of the supraglottic and glottic larynx using flexible fiberoptic nasopharyngoscopy.

Radiographic Exam: high-kv AP and lateral neck radiographs and PA and lateral chest radiographs; CT and MRI to determine the length and severity of stenosis.

Endoscopy: rigid endoscopy under general anesthesia to identify the stenoic area accurately.

Swallowing Studies: modified barium swallow to identify hypopharyngeal pooling of secretions and delayed transit time of the contrast; flexible endoscopic evaluation of swallowing to assess laryngeal mobility, laryngeal function, hypopharyngeal pooling, and clearing of the bolus during swallow.

Pulmonary Evaluation: used to determine type of reconstruction that the patient can undergo.

Gastropharyngeal Reflux Evaluation: dual pH-probe and mucosal biopsies to determine if there is significant reflux to the level of the esophagus and pharynx.

PATIENT SELECTION:

Although some authors have reported a higher incidence of revision laryngotracheal reconstruction in patients who were first treated when they weighed <10 Km,[42] there is no absolute minimum age or weight requirement before attempts at surgical reconstruction for CAO. The most important factors for determining the timing of laryngotracheal reconstruction are the patient's overall health and pulmonary reserve. With these factors in mind, some mini-

mum criteria have been set for anterior cricoid split in the neonate (see **AT A GLANCE . . . Criteria for Performing Anterior Cricoid Split**).

SPECIAL CONSIDERATION:

The most important factors for determining the timing of laryngotracheal reconstruction are the patient's overall health and pulmonary reserve.

The main reasons for performing reconstructive surgery for CAO are to reduce the morbidity associated with tracheotomy in young infants and children with severe stenosis, to permit air escape through the glottis for phonation and the development of verbal communicative skills, and to permit decannulation. Nearly all infants and children with chronic laryngotracheal stenosis meet these criteria for surgical intervention.

AT A GLANCE . . .

Criteria for Performing Anterior Cricoid Split

1. Extubation failure on at least two occasions secondary to laryngeal pathology
2. Weight >1500 gms
3. No assisted ventilation for 10 days prior to evaluation
4. Supplemental oxygen requirement of <35%
5. No congestive heart failure for 1 month prior to evaluation
6. No acute upper or lower respiratory tract infection at the time of the evaluation
7. No antihypertensive medications for 10 days prior to the evaluation

---

Children with contraindications for laryngotracheal reconstruction include those with absolute contraindications for general anesthesia and those with severe incompetence of the gastroesophageal sphincter and reflux. Children with severe reflux must be treated medically or surgically to correct this disorder prior to laryngotracheal reconstruction. A relative contraindication would be in those children who would require tracheotomy after laryngotracheal reconstruction. A reconstructive procedure still may be beneficial, however, if performed to provide a conduit for phonation and the development of communicative skills.

TREATMENT

The current open surgical treatment options that are available for laryngotracheal reconstruction include expansion surgery with or without prolonged stenting and resection surgery with or without prolonged airway management Practice Pathway 53-1). Expansion surgery may be performed with or without stabilization with grafting material. Generally, costal cartilage is employed as the grafting material. Some authors also have had success with auricular cartilage in mild to moderate anterior stenoses. Auricular cartilage is very useful when no

rigid support is needed; the curve of the cartilage also adds to the anteroposterior dimension when used as an overlay cap.

The airway may be managed with either an endotracheal tube, as in single-stage procedures, a tracheotomy tube, or a T tube. Tracheotomy may be used with or without prolonged stenting. Such prolonged stenting might include a Teflon stent placed in the trachea above the tracheostomy stoma. A T tube serves to manage the airway and provide prolonged stenting, but requires meticulous care to prevent obstruction. T tubes have been used safely and successfully in the pediatric population, as described by Stern, Willging, and Cotton.[43]

Determining the procedure of choice, either resection or expansion surgery, requires a complete understanding of the underlying pathology of laryngotracheal stenosis, facility with both expansion and resection techniques, and multidisciplinary resources to care for the patient in the perioperative period adequately.

Laryngotracheal reconstruction is presented in Practice Pathway 53-2. As with any strict flow dia-

Practice Pathway 53-1: OPTIONS IN LARYNGOTRACHEAL RECONSTRUCTION

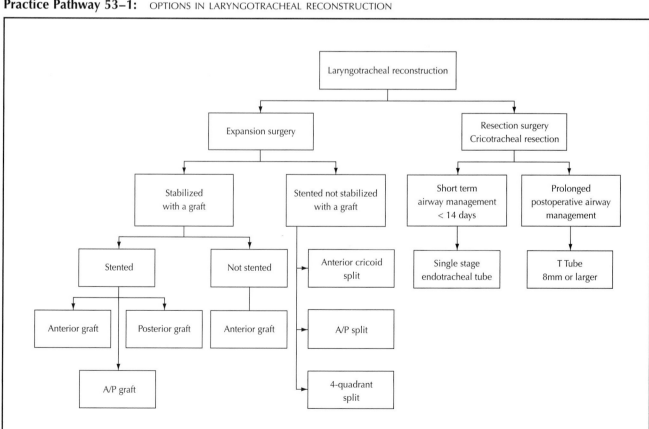

Abbreviations: A/P, Anterior and Posterior.

Practice Pathway 53–2: SURGICAL MANAGEMENT OF LARYNGOTRACHEAL STENOSIS

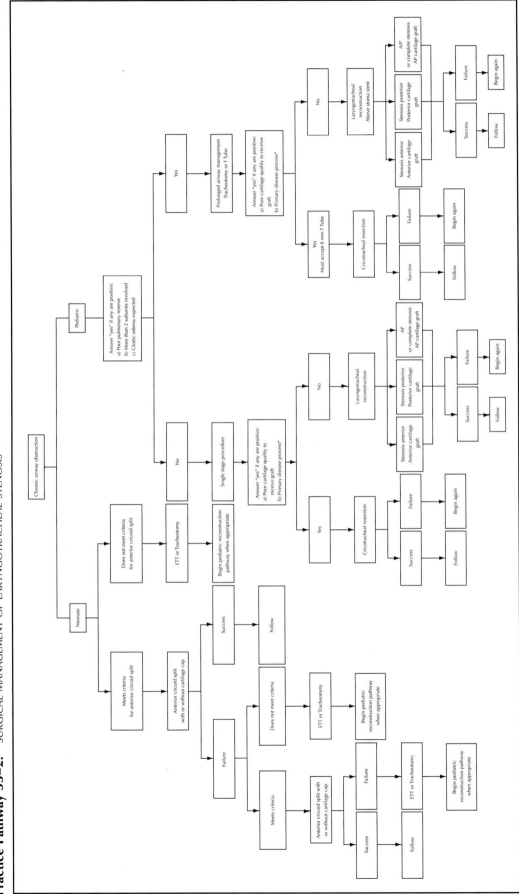

Abbreviations: ETT, Endotracheal Tube: A/P, Anterior and Posterior. *Primary disease process means subglottic stenosis from primary disease processes such as Wegener's granulomatosis, Sarcoidosis, or relapsing polychondritis. Resection surgery with medical management of the systemic disease process is the procedure of choice in this population.

gram describing the management of complex laryngotracheal disorders, there may arise a rare case that does not fit the chart. Also, this pathway is designed specifically for the treatment of subglottic stenosis. Glottic and supraglottic components must be assessed and managed separately. If more than two laryngotracheal subunits are involved, however, prolonged airway management is best used. Expansion or resection surgery may be used in conjunction with open or laser arytenoidectomy if a glottic component is identified. Supraglottic stenosis also may be addressed with endoscopic mucosal flap elevation and excision of the underlying scar.

Neonate

The neonate with CAO generally has been intubated since birth and has failed extubation repeatedly. Once all other forms of airway obstruction in this group have been ruled out by physical examination, flexible fiberoptic endoscopy (FFE) airway radiography, and rigid endoscopy, surgical management may be contemplated to avoid tracheotomy. The child must be evaluated for nasal stenosis, nasolacrimal duct cysts, retrognathia, glossoptosis, laryngomalacia, vocal fold motion impairment, and subglottic cysts. If found, these conditions should be corrected prior to any surgery for subglottic stenosis. If the evaluation reveals subglottic stenosis, the child's general medical health is assessed. If the child meets the minimum criteria described in AT A GLANCE . . . Criteria for Performing Anterior Cricoid Split, an anterior cricoid split may be performed to avoid a tracheotomy.[44,45]

A neonate who fails extubation may (1) meet the criteria for anterior cricoid split; (2) fail to meet the criteria but show signs of improvement; or (3) may not meet the criteria and may not show signs of improvement. Infants meeting the criteria for anterior cricoid split may undergo this procedure. If the child shows signs of improvement, a trial of continued intubation with supportive care followed by reevaluation and extubation may be warranted. Some neonates may never reach the minimum criteria for anterior cricoid split due to poor pulmonary reserve, and they are served better by a tracheotomy. These children should be followed with periodic endoscopy and reentered into the airway management decision tree as their condition improves.

Pediatric

There are many approaches to the surgical correction of CAO in the pediatric group. Familiarity and expertise in all the available surgical techniques is important for appropriate management. The key decision making points are between patients who need short-term airway management with an endotracheal tube and those who require long-term surgical airway support. The decision between resection surgery and expansion surgery should be considered next. If expansion surgery is considered, the final decision should be where to perform the expansion cuts and if to place stabilizing grafting material.

Single–stage versus long-term airway management

If a child undergoing airway reconstruction has good pulmonary reserve, two or fewer laryngotracheal subunits involved, and no glottic edema expected after the procedure, she is a candidate for a single-stage procedure. The airway reconstruction is performed with an endotracheal tube for short-term airway management and to act as a stent. The amount of postoperative sedation is tailored to the child. Rarely is it necessary to sedate and paralyze a child (Fig. 53–3). This policy relies on close and careful observation in the intensive care unit (ICU).

The duration of endotracheal intubated for 7

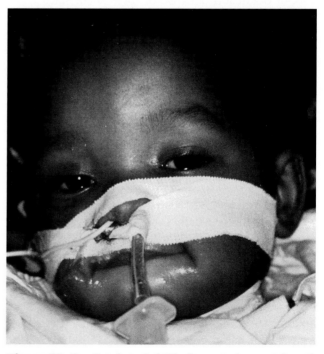

Figure 53–3: Intubated child after anterior costal cartilage laryngotracheal reconstruction. She received minimal sedation during her single-stage reconstruction.

days, posterior grafts for 14 days, and cricotracheal resection for 7 days. Operative laryngoscopy is performed and the endotracheal tube can be downsized at that point. The child is returned to the ICU and extubated once the anesthetic or required sedation has been metabolized. The child is observed in the ICU for 24 hours and transferred to a monitored setting once stable. Reevaluation by rigid endoscopy at appropriate intervals is helpful in the management of these children.

A child who has poor pulmonary reserve and more than two laryngotracheal subunits or who is predicted to have glottic edema in the perioperative period should be managed with long-term airway support. The airway may be managed with a tracheotomy or a T tube while the operative site heals. This gives the caregivers an easy route for pulmonary toilet.

The choice between a T tube and a tracheotomy depends on the child and the procedure. If the stoma is not involved in the airway obstruction and the repair does not require opening the stoma, a well-established tracheotomy tract may be left and utilized. If necessary, the tracheotomy tube may be increased 0.5 to 1.0 mm in inner diameter to allow for the management of increased secretions. If the child's larynx will not accept a T tube with a minimum diameter of 8 mm, a tracheotomy should be used. T tubes <8 mm in diameter have an increased risk of occlusion because of their small size.

Stent or no stent

The decision between a T tube and a tracheotomy with an above-stoma stent is more arbitrary. Both serve to manage the airway and provide support for the healing reconstruction. Unless an uncomplicated anterior graft is performed, at least some period of stenting is required. Single stage procedures are stented by an endotracheal tube for 7 to 14 days. When no stabilizing grafts are used, the stent serves to keep the cut cricoid cartilage distracted. Laryngotracheal reconstruction with stabilizing cartilage grafts is stented usually for 6 to 8 weeks. The stent serves to stabilize the cartilaginous framework and the grafted cartilage. Additionally, the grafts speed stabilization of the reconstruction.

A T tube and an above-stoma stent are similar in their ability to stent. Both are hollow and may lead to aspiration, but an Aboulker stent may be capped to prevent aspiration if necessary.[46] If the T tube causes aspiration that cannot be corrected by the suspension of oral feedings, the T tube should be removed. Fortunately, this occurs infrequently.

The T tube gives a smooth continuous stent through the reconstructed area to the cervical trachea. The Aboulker stent sired to the tracheotomy tube also performs the same type of stenting. Wired in stents are used less frequently and are being replaced with the Silastic™ T tube. Difficulties with proper fit, material failure, and the rigid nature of the wired-in stent makes it less desirable than the T tube.

The above-stoma stent ends superior to the tracheotomy tube. Problematic granulation may develop between the tracheotomy and the stent. This usually resolves once the stent is removed. Residual granulation may be removed with optical forceps during interval laryngoscopy.

Expansion surgery versus resection surgery

The decision between expansion and resection surgery can be difficult. Although expansion surgery has been used for years and its utility has been well documented, pediatric resection surgery is still in its infancy. There will always be cases when the choice between expansion and resection will not be clear. The experience of the surgeon must then guide the decision making process. As more experience with these two surgical modalities for correction of the obstructed airway is gained, the decision making process will become clearer.

Some types of stenosis, however, lend themselves to definitive decisions regarding technique (Fig. 53–4). Short, discreet, complete stenosis, at least 5 mm from the vocal cords, are prime candidates for cricotracheal resection. Stenotic segments that are associated with poor-quality surrounding cartilage also may be suited better for resection. If grafted, the airway may be patent but could collapse functionally during respiration. Resecting the floppy, stenotic area has worked well in these situations.[47] Finally, some primary disease processes such as Wegener's granulomatosis (WG) or relapsing polychondritis may benefit from resection of the affected area with reanastomosis, rather than grafting in an area with active disease.

SPECIAL CONSIDERATION:

Short, discreet complete stenosis at least 5 mm from the vocal cords are prime candidates for cricotracheal resection.

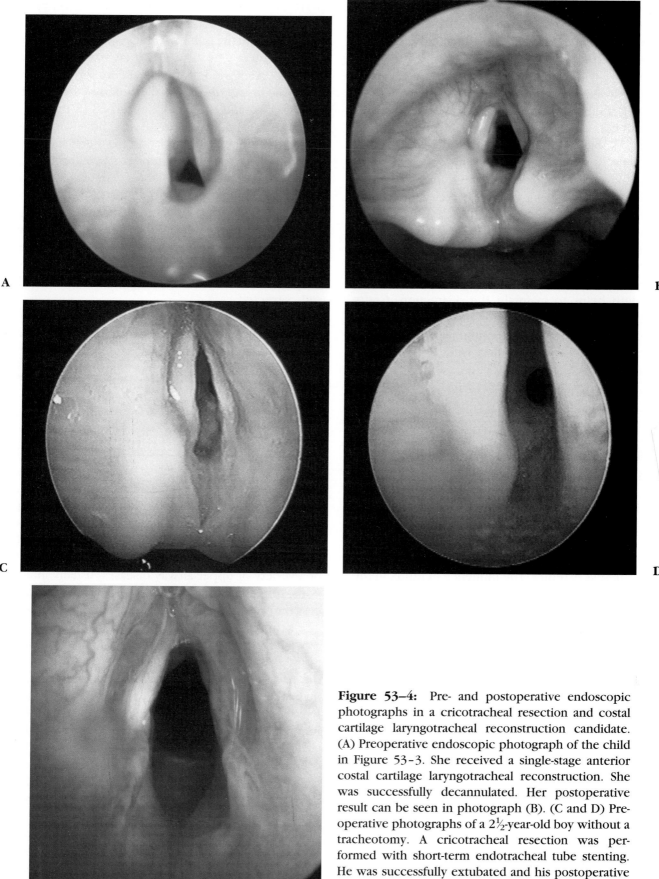

Figure 53–4: Pre- and postoperative endoscopic photographs in a cricotracheal resection and costal cartilage laryngotracheal reconstruction candidate. (A) Preoperative endoscopic photograph of the child in Figure 53–3. She received a single-stage anterior costal cartilage laryngotracheal reconstruction. She was successfully decannulated. Her postoperative result can be seen in photograph (B). (C and D) Preoperative photographs of a 2½-year-old boy without a tracheotomy. A cricotracheal resection was performed with short-term endotracheal tube stenting. He was successfully extubated and his postoperative result can be seen in plate (E).

Expansion surgery has been used more commonly and currently is the workhorse for airway reconstruction. Stenosis that is long, close to or involving the vocal cords, or grade III or less may be expanded with or without cartilage grafts. The type of expansion surgery (i.e., anterior, posterior, or both) depends on the site of the stenosis. The cartilage cuts in the cricoid are made at the site where the stenosis is found. If this site is anterior, an anterior split can be performed. If the stenosis is posterior, the posterior plate of the cricoid should be distracted. If the stenosis is either circumferential or severe, both the anterior and posterior cricoid plates are distracted. Additionally, lateral cricoid cuts may be utilized. Grafting material is used to stabilize the distraction and speed the healing process. Usually costal cartilage is used because its strength helps to maintain the distraction. Grafts may be placed in the anterior and/or posterior cricoid plates. Temporary stenting with an endotracheal tube, T tube, or Teflon stent has been discussed above.

Perioperative Management

No definitive studies are available investigating the perioperative management of laryngotracheal reconstruction patients. Generally, antibiotics are giving during the initial healing phase to avoid chondritis during reepithelialization. Empiric antireflux measures are given with either H_2-receptor blockers or proton pump inhibitors as well as prokinetic agents, even if the preoperative evaluation did not indicate severe reflux. The influence of reflux in the postoperative period is controversial and not well studied. It has been stated that the success rate of laryngotracheal reconstruction has not changed since the recognition and treatment of reflux has come into fashion.[41] It may be that the stenosis seen today is more severe because neonatal management has improved. As a result, the lack of change in the success rate may be misleading. Steroids (dexamethasone sodium phosphate 0.6 mg/kg up to 20 mg) are given if edema and granulation tissue become problematic.

Extubation or Decannulation

After the initial healing phase has been completed, both the single-stage and the prolonged stented patients are returned to the operating room to evaluate the status of the reconstruction. Laryngoscopy is performed after the endotracheal tube, T tube, or Teflon stent has been removed. Reepithelialization is assessed and the stability of the reconstructed area is determined. The airway is then sized as in the preoperative period. If the procedure was a single-stage reconstruction, a smaller endotracheal tube is reinserted and the child is returned to the ICU. Extubation is performed in the ICU once the anesthetic and any residual sedation has been metabolized. If a Teflon stent or T tube has been removed, an appropriately-sized tracheotomy tube is inserted through the stoma.

Systemic steroids and nebulized racemic epinephrine are given to the newly-extubated child if stridor or mild airway obstruction is encountered. If the child does not tolerate extubation, reintubation is performed and the cause of the failure is determined and corrected.

Single-stage and prolonged stented patients may be reevaluated by rigid endoscopy at 1 week for removal of granulation tissue and to inspect the progress of healing. All patients are evaluated again at about 4 weeks with rigid endoscopy.

PEDIATRIC TRACHEOTOMY

Indications and Incidence

The mainstay of pediatric airway management for both acute and chronic airway problems remains a tracheotomy (Table 53–4). Whereas the original indication for a tracheotomy in a child was for relief of a variety of upper airway diseases, usually infectious, the indications have expanded to include access for prolonged ventilation and pulmonary toilet. The proportion of tracheotomies done for relief of airway obstruction (~40%) and prolonged ventilation (~50%) has remained relatively constant over the past 25 years in two sequential reports from a major children's hospital.[48,49] Other recent series have reported either an increase or decrease in the number of procedures for the relief of airway obstruction.[50,51] The decrease in the number of tracheotomies for both croup and epiglottitis has been the result of careful airway management and the development of the *Hemophilus influenzae B* vaccine.[48,49,52] A decrease in tracheotomies required to maintain the airway during craniofacial procedures has resulted from improvements in airway management by pediatric anesthesiologists.[48] Prolonged ventilation as an indication for tracheotomy has

TABLE 53–4: Size Comparison of Endotracheal Tubes, Tracheostomy Tubes, and Pediatric Bronchoscopes

Cannula	Inner Diameter	Outer Diameter	Overall Length
Endotracheal Tubes			
2.5	2.5 mm	3.6 mm	12 cm
3.0	3.0 mm	4.3 mm	14 cm
3.5	3.5 mm	4.9 mm	16 cm
4.0	4.0 mm	5.6 mm	18 cm
4.5	4.5 mm	6.2 mm	20 cm
5.0	5.0 mm	6.9 mm	22 cm
5.5	5.5 mm	7.5 mm	25 cm
6.0	6.0 mm	8.2 mm	26 cm
Shiley			
3.0 Neonatal (00NT)	3.0 mm	4.5 mm	30 mm
3.5 Neonatal (0NT)	3.5 mm	5.2 mm	32 mm
4.0 Neonatal (1NT)	4.0 mm	5.9 mm	34 mm
3.0 Pediatric (00PT)	3.0 mm	4.5 mm	39 mm
3.5 Pediatric (0PT)	3.5 mm	5.2 mm	40 mm
4.0 Pediatric (1PT)	4.0 mm	5.9 mm	41 mm
4.5 Pediatric (2PT)	4.5 mm	6.0 mm	42 mm
5.0 Pediatric (3PT)	5.0 mm	7.1 mm	44 mm
5.5 Pediatric (4PT)	5.5 mm	7.7 mm	46 mm
Shiley Long Pediatric			
5.0 PDL	5.0 mm	7.1 mm	50 mm
5.5 PDL	5.5 mm	7.7 mm	52 mm
6.0 PDL	6.0 mm	8.3 mm	54 mm
6.5 PDL	6.5 mm	9.0 mm	56 mm
Portex			
3.0	3.0 mm	5.0 mm	36 mm
3.5	3.5 mm	5.8 mm	40 mm
4.0	4.0 mm	6.5 mm	44 mm
4.5	4.5 mm	7.1 mm	48 mm
5.0	5.0 mm	7.7 mm	50 mm
5.5	5.5 mm	8.3 mm	52 mm
Bivona Neonatal			
2.5	2.5 mm	4.0 mm	30 mm
3.0	3.0 mm	4.7 mm	32 mm
3.5	3.5 mm	5.3 mm	34 mm
4.0	4.0 mm	6.0 mm	36 mm
Bivona Pediatric			
2.5	2.5 mm	4.0 mm	38 mm
3.0	3.0 mm	4.7 mm	39 mm
3.5	3.5 mm	5.3 mm	40 mm
4.0	4.0 mm	6.0 mm	41 mm
4.5	4.5 mm	6.7 mm	42 mm
5.0	5.0 mm	7.3 mm	44 mm
5.5	5.5 mm	8.0 mm	46 mm
Bivona Phillyflex			
3.5	3.5 mm	5.3 mm	40 mm
4.0	4.0 mm	6.0 mm	44 mm
4.5	4.5 mm	6.7 mm	48 mm
5.0	5.0 mm	7.3 mm	50 mm
5.5	5.5 mm	8.0 mm	52 mm
Bronchoscopes			*Working Length*
2.5 short	2.8 mm	4.0 mm	14 cm
3.0 short	3.5 mm	5.0 mm	14 cm
3.5 short	4.3 mm	5.9 mm	13 cm
3.5 long	4.3 mm	5.9 mm	24.5 cm
4.0 long	5.1 mm	7.5 mm	25 cm
5.0 long	6.0 mm	7.7 mm	25 cm

Abbreviations: NT, neonatal; PT, pediatric; PDL, pediatric lung

Source: Shiley—Shiley Laboratories, Irvine, CA USA. Portex—Simms-Portex Division of Smith Industries, Keene, NH. Bivona—Bivona Corporation, Gary, IN.

shown a recent increase according to one study.[51] In a study spanning the 1970s, upper airway obstruction and neurologic disorders were the most common diagnoses in pediatric tracheotomy patients.[48] A similar study from the 1980s listed bronchopulmonary dysplasia and neurologic disorders as the most common diagnoses.[49]

A slight decrease in the incidence of pediatric tracheotomies has been demonstrated by several series.[53,54] A trend towards the procedure being performed in younger children also has been shown.[48,49] The male:female ratio for pediatric tracheotomy ranges from 1:1 to 2:1 in the literature.[49]

Operative Timing

The decision to perform an elective tracheotomy is complex, and depends up the child's condition, the status of the child's airway, and the length of intubation. The decision-making process should include the family, the pediatricians, and the critical care physicians who are caring for the child. Older children and adolescents should be managed like adults and considered candidates for tracheotomy after 2 weeks of intubation. On the other hand, because they have a more pliable airway, neonates may remain intubated for several months before tracheotomy is considered. Additional factors that may influence the timing of a tracheotomy include: (1) difficulty with intubation due to abnormal anatomy; (2) difficulty with intubation due to laryngeal or tracheal swelling; and (3) difficulty maintaining a translaryngeal airway due to secretions.

SPECIAL CONSIDERATION:

Cricothyrotomy remains the procedure of choice if an emergency tracheotomy needs to be performed.

In the emergency situation, tracheotomy should be reserved as the airway management of last resort. Other forms of airway management such as intubation or rigid bronchoscopy should be attempted first. Devices have been developed that assist the surgeon in performing an emergency tracheotomy in an adult; these devices should be avoided in infants and children because they present a higher risk

of complications due to poor anatomic definition. In infants and children, the cricothyroid membrane usually can be identified, and cricothyrotomy remains the procedure of choice for an emergent procedure because it lessens the risk of injury to the esophagus or major vascular structures of the neck. The use of transtracheal needles to establish an airway emergently in children remains controversial.[55-56]

Operative Complications

Excessive bleeding during a tracheotomy procedure may be due to a coagulation defect. Many patients undergoing a tracheotomy have complex medical problems such as liver disease and thrombocytopenia that may affect clotting. These clotting defects should be corrected prior to surgery. Injury to vascular structures in the neck or bleeding from thyroid tissue may be prevented by meticulous surgical technique.

The incidence of pneumothorax, pneumomediastinum, or subcutaneous emphysema range from 3 to 9% in the literature.[48,53,54] These complications are due to violation of the pleura, especially where it approaches the trachea low in the neck in children, or to closing the wound too tightly. The treatment of pneumomediastinum and subcutaneous emphysema usually is expectant. Depending on the size of the pneumothorax, treatment may include placement of a chest tube. A chest radiograph is warranted after every tracheotomy to check for these complications and to assess the position of the tube.

Injury to both the esophagus and the recurrent laryngeal nerves has been reported and can be prevented by careful surgical technique.[57] Respiratory arrest following a tracheotomy may occur due to a rapid washout of retained CO_2.[58] Pulmonary edema has been reported after the sudden relief of acute airway obstruction.[68] Both of these complications may be managed by ventilatory support.

Postoperative Complications

Episodes of hemorrhage from the trachea may be due to tracheitis or granulation tissue within the trachea. Tracheal infection may be treated with systemic antibiotics, and granulation tissue may be excised surgically. Rarely, the tip of the tracheotomy tube may erode into the innominate artery causing massive bleeding. This catastrophic event was more common when metal tracheotomy tubes were used. Bleeding that is suggestive of innominate trauma should be treated initially with either digital pressure or placement of a cuffed endotracheal tube to tamponade the bleeding. Then, the traumatized artery may be repaired surgically.

Pneumothorax, pneumomediastinum, or subcutaneous emphysema may all result from too vigorous ventilation and may occur in a child with either a tracheotomy or an endotracheal tube. Pneumomediastinum and subcutaneous emphysema may be treated expectantly, whereas a pneumothorax may require placement of a chest tube.

Subglottic stenosis does not result from placement of a tracheotomy tube, but rather is either congenital or due to injury of the subglottic mucosa. Tom et al. noted tracheal lesions in 44% of patients 1 week after a tracheotomy was performed.[60] These tracheal lesions were thought to be the result of prior injury from the endotracheal tube that was not evident at the time of tracheotomy. Tracheal stenosis and tracheomalacia may develop in the distal trachea due to chronic trauma and infection from the tracheotomy tube. The treatment of subglottic and tracheal stenosis is dependent on the severity of the lesion, but laryngotracheal reconstruction may be required. Tracheomalacia is managed expectantly either with tracheal resection or tracheopexy.

Both accidental decannulation and plugging of the tracheotomy tube occur commonly and if not recognized properly, may result in hypoxic brain injury or death.

Tracheitis, which is bacterial infection of the trachea, typically presents with symptoms of fever and cough. Examination of mucopurulent secretions reveals numerous white blood cells, and cultures are usually positive for a predominant organism. On the contrary, tracheal secretions in otherwise healthy tracheotomy patients are colonized by mixed flora and do not have large numbers of white blood cells usually. Tracheitis may be treated with either systemic or aerosolized antibiotics.

A persistant tracheocutaneous fistula has been reported to occur in more than 50% of children who have a tracheotomy for more than 1 year.[48] Treatment is by excision of the tract and a cosmetic closure.

Mortality

Tracheotomy-related mortality ranges from 0.5 to 5% in recent series.[48,49] Reviewing two series from the same institution over a 20-year period shows a decrease in mortality from 2 to 0.5%.[48,49] This decrease may be attributed to better caregiver education and the widespread use of pulse oximetry.

Tracheotomy Care

Because a tracheotomy bypasses the upper airway that is responsible for warming and humidifying the air, children with a tracheotomy require additional humidity to prevent the tracheal mucosa from suffering drying effects that may result in either infection or a plugged tube. Humidification may be supplied in several forms. Either a T-piece adapter or a tracheotomy collar may provide humidified air from an external source. Humidivents, artificial noses, or other such devices also may humidify inspired air. All of these devices should be cleaned thoroughly on a regular basis to prevent infection.

Suctioning of the trachea should be performed by skilled caregivers who are familiar with accepted clean technique. Sterile technique is not required. Instillation of physiologic saline often helps to mobilize secretions. Suctioning does not need to follow a set interval but rather should be performed when secretions accumulate. Care must be taken to avoid vigorous suctioning that may cause hypoxia or injury to the distal tracheal mucosa. Either stationary or portable suctions always should be available to keep the airway clear.

A variety of monitors including apnea and cardiorespiratory (CR) monitors and pulse oximetry have been employed in the care of children with a tracheotomy. Apnea and CR monitors alarm when the child stops breathing or becomes bradycardic and signal airway problems at a late stage. Pulse oximetry is more sensitive to airway problems but is fraught with false alarms.

Infections involving the tracheal stoma are common because of the presence of a foreign body, the tracheotomy tube. It is not uncommon for granulation tissue to form around the stoma. Granulation tissue may be treated with cautery, and infection may be managed with either systemic antibiotics or locally-applied antibiotic ointment. Keloids that form in this area of chronic irritation may require surgical excision if they are traumatized easily or interfere with changing of the tracheotomy tube.

All caregivers need to undergo teaching to handle all aspects of tracheotomy care. This includes suctioning, changing of the tube during an emergency, and cardiopulmonary resuscitation. A caregiver always should be in attendance or nearby in case an emergency such as plugging or accidental decannulation occurs.

Decannulation

Decannulation should not be considered until the underlying disease process that necessitated the tracheotomy has resolved. The patient should no longer be on a ventilator and should be breathing room air. Subglottic or tracheal stenosis should be corrected. Children with poor pulmonary toilet should not be decannulated until they can handle their secretions.

SPECIAL CONSIDERATION:

Decannulation should not be considered until the underlying disease process that necessitated the procedure has resolved.

Unless the tracheotomy tube has been present for only a few days, the airway should be examined endoscopically to search for any conditions that would prevent successful decannulation. Stenotic areas should be repaired and granulomas within the tracheal lumen should be excised.

Decannulation of an adolescent can be treated as that of an adult. The tube may be downsized and then capped. If capping is tolerated, decannulation can be performed. Decannulation of children is treated in a variety of ways. Some physicians downsize the tracheotomy tube and then cap it as in adults. Young children may have problems breathing around a smaller tube because of their narrow smaller airway; small tracheotomy tubes are also more prone to plugging. For this reason, other physicians do not downsize the tube, but instead just remove it in a setting where the child can be monitored adequately such as in the ICU or recovery room. All decannulated patients should be observed for a period of time in the hospital for signs of respiratory distress or difficulty with secretions. Use of sedation for decannulation is controversial.[61]

AT A GLANCE . . .

Pediatric Tracheotomy

Indications: relief of upper airway disease, prolonged ventilation, and pulmonary toilet.

Complications: excessive bleeding, hemorrhage, tracheal infection, pneumothorax, pneumomediastinum, subcutaneous emphysema, subglottic stenosis, injury to the esophagus and recurrent laryngeal nerves, respiratory arrest, and pulmonary edema.

Tracheotomy Care: T-piece adapter or a tracheotomy collar for humidification, suctioning of the trachea, and removal of granulation tissue and keloids.

CONCLUSION

The management of the child with CAO is highly rewarding. Creating a safe airway for the tracheotomy-dependent child with the ultimate goal of decannulation requires a thorough understanding of the available reconstruction techniques and a multidisciplinary evaluation of the child.

Resection or expansion surgery may be used to increase the caliber of the obstructed airway. Depending on the cause and location of the stenosis, the appropriate technique is chosen. Although controversial, evaluation and management of GER is recommended. A methodical and logical approach to the child with the obstructed airway is one of the keys to success.

REFERENCES

1. McDonald IH, Stocks JG. Prolonged nasotracheal intubation: A review of its development in a pediatric hospital. Br J Anaesth 1965; 37:161-173.
2. Jackson C. Laryngeal stenosis—Growth of the larynx as a factor in treatment. Laryngoscope 1932; 2: 887-889.
3. Fearon B, Cotton RT. Subglottic stenosis in infants and children: The clinical problem and experimental surgical correction. Can J Otolaryngol 1972; 1: 281-289.
4. Rethi A. An operation for cicatrical stenosis of the larynx. J Laryngol Otol 1956; 70:283-293.

5. Grahne B. Operative treatment of severe chronic traumatic laryngeal stenosis in infants up to three years old. Acta Otolaryngol (Stockh) 1971; 72: 134–137.

6. Rinne J, Grahne B, Sovijarvi AR. Long-term results after surgical treatment of laryngeal stenosis in small children. Int J Pediatr Otorhinolaryngol 1985; 10: 213–220.

7. Evans JNH, Todd GB. Laryngo-tracheoplasty. J Laryngol Otol 1974; 88:589–597.

8. Cotton RT, Evans JN. Laryngotracheal reconstruction in children. Five-year follow-up. Ann Otol Rhinol Laryngol 1981; 90:516–520.

9. MacRae D, Barrie P. "Swiss Roll" laryngotracheoplasty in young children. J Otolaryngol 1986; 15:115–118.

10. Looper EA. Use of the hyoid bone as a graft in laryngotracheal stenosis. Arch Otolaryngol 1938; 28: 106–111.

11. Cotton RT. The problem of pediatric laryngotracheal stenosis: A clinical and experimental study on the efficacy of autogenous cartilaginous grafts placed between the vertically divided halves of the posterior lamina of the cricoid cartilage. Laryngoscope 1991; 101:1–34.

12. Lapidot A, Sodagar R, Ratanaprashtporn S. Experimental repair of subglottic stenosis in piglets. "Trapdoor" thyrochondroplasty flap. Arch Otolaryngol 1968; 88:529–535.

13. Fearon B, Cinnamond M. Surgical correction of subglottic stenosis of the larynx. J Otolaryngol 1976; 5: 475–478.

14. Calcaterra TC, McClure R, Ward PH. Effect of laryngofissure on the developing canine larynx. Ann Otol Rhinol Laryngol 1974; 83: 810–813.

15. Cotton RT. Management of subglottic stenosis in infancy and childhood. Ann Otol Rhinol Laryngol 1978; 87:649–657.

16. Ward P, Canalis R, Fee W, et al. Composite hyoid sternohyoid muscle grafts in human. Arch Otolaryngol 1977; 103:531–534.

17. Wong ML, Finnegan DA, Kashima HK, et al. Vascularized hyoid interposition for subglottic and upper tracheal stenosis. Ann Otol Rhinol Laryngol 1978; 87: 491–497.

18. Freeland AP. Composite hyoid-sternohyoid graft in the correction of established subglottic stenosis in children. J R Soc Med 1981; 74:729–735.

19. Freeland AP. The long-term results of hyoid-sternohyoid grafts in the correction of subglottic stenosis. J Laryngol Otol 1986; 100:665–657.

20. Close LG, Lozano AJ, Schaefer SD. Sternohyoid myoosseus flap for acquired subglottic stenosis. Laryngoscope 1983; 93:433–439.

21. Burstein FD, Canalis R, Ward PH. Composite hyoid-sternohyoid interposition graft revisited: UCLA experience 1974–1984. Laryngoscope 1986; 96: 516–520.

22. Zalzal GH, Cotton RT, McAdams AJ. The survival of costal cartilage graft in laryngotracheal reconstruction. Otolaryngol Head Neck Surg 1986; 94:204–211.

23. Pashley RN, Jaskunas JM, Waldstein G. Laryngotracheoplasty with costochondral grafts—A clinical correlate of graft survival. Laryngoscope 1984; 94: 1493–1496.

24. Hubbell RN, Zalzal G, Cotton RT, et al. Irradiated costal cartilage graft in experimental laryngotracheal reconstruction. Int J Pediatr Otorhinolaryngol 1988; 15:67–72.

25. Monnier P, Savary M, Chapuis G. Cricotracheal resection for pediatric subglottic stenosis: Update of the Lausanne experience. Acta Otorhinolaryngol Belg 1995; 49:373–382.

26. Pearson FG, Cooper JD, Nelems JM, et al. Primary tracheal anastomosis after resection of the cricoid cartilage with preservation of recurrent laryngeal nerves. J Thorac Cardiovasc Surg 1975; 70:806–816.

27. Pearson FG, Brito-Filomeno L, Cooper JD. Experience with partial cricoid resection and thyrotracheal anastomosis. Ann Otol Rhinol Laryngol 1986; 95: 582–558.

28. Sullivan MJ, McClatchey KD, Passamani PP. Airway growth following cricotracheal resection in puppies. Arch Otolaryngol Head Neck Surg 1987; 113: 606–611.

29. Laccourreye H, Beutter P, Brasnu D. Laryngeal and laryngotracheal stenoses. Classification and treatment (author's transl). Annales d Oto-Laryngologie et de Chirurgie Cervico-Faciale 1981; 98:571–579.

30. Triglia JM, Belus JF, Portaspana T, et al. Laryngeal stenosis in children. Evaluation of 10 years of treatment. Ann Otolaryngol Chir Cervicofac 1995; 12: 279–284.

31. Stell PM, Maran AGD, Stanley RE, et al. Chronic laryngeal stenosis. Ann Otol Rhinol Laryngol 1985; 94: 108–113.

32. Ratner I, Whitfield J. Acquired subglottic stenosis in the very-low-birth-weight infant. Am J Dis Child 1983; 137:40–43.

33. Papsidero MJ, Pashley NRT. Acquired stenosis of the upper airway in neonates: An increasing problem. Ann Otol Rhinol Laryngol 1980; 89:512–514.

34. Marshak G, Grundfast KM. Subglottic stenosis. Pediatr Clin North Am 1981; 28:941–948.

35. Cotton RT. Prevention and management of longitudinal stenosis in infants and children. J Ped Surg; 1985; 20(6):845–851.

36. Dunbar JS. Upper respiratory tract obstruction in infants and children. Am J Roentgenol 1970; 109: 227–246.

37. Cotton RT, Gray SD, Miller RP. Update of the Cincin-

nati experience in pediatric laryngotracheal reconstruction. Laryngoscope 1989; 99:1111–1116.

38. Myer CM III, O'Connor DM, Cotton RT. Proposed grading system for subglottic stenosis based on endotracheal tube sizes. Ann Otol Rhinol Laryngol 1994; 103:319–323.

39. Koufman JA. The otolaryngologic manifestations of gastroesophageal reflux disease (GERD): A clinical investigation of 225 patients using ambulatory 24-hour pH monitoring and an experimental investigation of the role of acid and pepsin in the development of laryngeal injury. Laryngoscope 1991; 101: 1–78.

40. Little FB, Koufman JA, Kohut RI, et al. Effect of gastric acid on the pathogenesis of subglottic stenosis. Ann Otol Rhinol Laryngol 1985; 94:516–519.

41. Zalzal GH, Choi SS, Patel KM. The effect of gastroesophageal reflux on laryngotracheal reconstruction. Arch Otolaryngol Head Neck Surg 1996; 122: 297–300.

42. Zalzal GH, Choi SS, Patel KM. Ideal timing of pediatric laryngotracheal reconstruction. Arch Otolaryngol Head Neck Surg 1997; 123:206–208.

43. Stern Y, Willging JP, Cotton RT. Use of the Montgomery T-tube in Laryngotracheal reconstruction in children: Is it safe? Anals of Otolaryngology Rhinology & Laryngology 1998; 107(12):1006–1009.

44. Cotton RT, Seid AB. Management of the extubation problem in the premature child. Anterior cricoid split as an alternative to tracheotomy. Ann Otol Rhinol Laryngol 1980; 89:508–511.

45. Cotton RT, Myer CMD, Bratcher GO, et al. Anterior cricoid split, 1977–1987. Evolution of a technique. Arch Otolaryngol Head Neck Surg 1988; 114: 1300–1302.

46. Stern Y, Willging JP, Cotton RT. Treatment of chronic aspiration secondary to laryngeal stent by endoscopic capping. Arch Otolaryngol Head Neck Surg 1998; 124:93–94.

47. Stern Y, Gerber ME, Walner DL, et al. Partial cricotracheal resection with primary anastomosis in the pediatric age group. Ann Otol Rhinol Laryngol 1997; 106:891–896.

48. Wetmore RF, Handler SD, Potsic WP. Pediatric tracheostomy: Experience during the past decade. Ann Otol Rhinol Laryngol 1982; 91:628–632.

49. Wetmore RF, Marsh RR, Thompson ME, Tom LWC. Pediatric tracheostomy: A changing procedure? Ann Otol Rhinol Laryngol *(in press)*.

50. Waki EY, Madgy DN, Zablocki H, et al. An analysis of the inferior based tracheal flap for pediatric tracheotomy. Int J Pediatr Otorhinolaryngol 1993; 27: 47–54.

51. Ward RF, Jones J, Carew JF. Current trends in pediatric tracheotomy. Int J Pediatr Otorhinolaryngol 1995; 32:233–239.

52. Wetmore RF, Handler SD. Epiglottitis: Evolution in management during the last decade. Ann Otol Rhinol Laryngol 1979; 88:822–826.

53. Arcand P, Granger J. Pediatric tracheostomies: Changing trends. J Otolaryngol 1988; 17:2.

54. Line WS, Hawkins DB, Kohlstrom EJ, et al. Tracheotomy in infants and young children: The changing perspective 1970–1985. Laryngoscope 1986; 96: 510–515.

55. Cote C, Eavey R, Jones RD, et al. Cricothyroid membrane puncture: Oxygenation and ventilation in a dog model using an intravenous catheter. Crit Care Med 1988; 16:615–619.

56. Hughes RK. Needle tracheostomy–further evaluation. Arch Surg 1966; 93(5):843–847.

57. Hawkins DB, Williams EH. Tracheostomy in infants and young children. Laryngoscope 1976; 86: 331–340.

58. Greene NM. Fatal cardiovascular and respiratory failure associated with tracheotomy. N Engl J Med 1959; 261:846–848.

59. Kanter RK, Watchko JF. Pulmonary edema associated with upper airway obstruction. Am J Dis Child 1984; 138:356–358.

60. Tom LWC, Miller L, Wetmore RF, et al. Endoscopic assessment in children with tracheotomies. Arch Otolaryngol Head Neck Surg 1993; 119:321–324.

61. Handler SD. The difficult decannulation. In: Gates G, ed. *Current Therapy in Otolaryngology—Head and Neck Surgery.* Philadelphia: Decker, 1986, pp. 327–329.

54 Traumatic Injury to the Larynx, Trachea, Esophagus, and Neck

Joseph Haddad Jr, and Thomas G. Takoudes

The major structures of the neck, including the laryngotracheal complex, the esophagus, and the great vessels, may be injured extensively during trauma. Often, these neck injuries are associated with trauma to other major organs, and basic principles of pediatric trauma management should be followed in all patients. In one series, 50% of tracheobronchial disruptions had associated severe injuries with a mortality rate of 30%, and other authors have reported greater than 50% associated injuries.[1] Of immediate concern is maintenance of the airway and respiratory support. The airway may be secured at the scene of the injury, but occasionally a child may present to a hospital or trauma center with an unrecognized severe injury such as laryngotracheal separation. In addition to securing the airway, control of hemorrhage and maintenance of the cardiovascular system is paramount for the child's survival.

Neck trauma may be categorized as either blunt or penetrating, depending upon the force that causes the injury. Both blunt and penetrating injuries may involve the airway, the esophagus, and the great vessels either singly or in any combination. For this reason, a systematic and comprehensive approach to neck trauma optimizes care and prevents overlooking an occult and potentially life-threatening injury.

ANATOMY

The pediatric larynx differs from the adult in position, size, shape, and consistency. The higher position of the larynx in the neck of children is protective, and along with a relatively larger head and jaw, may help to explain the infrequency of laryngeal trauma in children. The laryngeal framework consists of soft and pliable cartilage that make laryngeal fractures rare. Alternatively, the intercartilaginous connecting membranes and ligaments are immature, making laryngotracheal disruption more likely.

> **SPECIAL CONSIDERATION:**
>
> The pediatric larynx differs from the adult in that it is higher in the neck, narrow at the cricoid cartilage, and less likely to fracture because it is soft and pliable.

The relative dimensions of the pediatric larynx differ from those of its adult counterpart; the pediatric larynx contains relatively larger arytenoid cartilages, an omega-shaped epiglottis, and a funnel-shaped larynx that is narrowest in the subglottis. In children, the narrowest region of the trachea is at C3, at the level of the cricoid cartilage, whereas the narrowest area in adults is significantly lower at C7. The effects of narrowing also differ by age; whereas an adolescent or adult may tolerate a 50% narrowing of the airway without distress, the child with similar compromise may demonstrate significant respiratory distress.

LARYNGEAL INJURIES

Blunt Laryngotracheal Injuries

Blunt injury to the laryngotracheal complex is less common than penetrating injury but may be life-

Pediatric Otolaryngology, Edited by R.F. Wetmore, H.R. Muntz, and T.J. McGill. Thieme Medical Publishers, Inc., New York © 2000.

threatening. In a series of 30,000 trauma cases from a level-1 trauma center, 12 patients had cervical laryngotracheal trauma and only one was a pediatric patient.[2] The incidence of blunt laryngotracheal trauma may indeed be higher because many children with these severe injuries may die before ever reaching a hospital.

Adult laryngeal trauma may arise when the anterior neck strikes the steering wheel during the sudden deceleration forces of a motor vehicle accident (MVA). Unless properly restrained, children may suffer similar laryngeal injuries; however, the frequency of these injuries is recognized much less in children than in adults because children typically sustain severe or mortal brain injury when subjected to severe forces during a MVA. Children also may be the object of direct blows to the neck during sporting events, especially football, karate, hockey, and others. In addition, strangulation attempts during physical abuse or attempted suicide may result in laryngeal injury. Older children may suffer "clothes line" injuries either while driving or as a passenger on all-terrain vehicles, motorcycles, bicycles, or snowmobiles. Seat belt injuries to the neck also have been reported in children.[3]

Blunt trauma to the larynx may include soft tissue edema, ecchymosis, mucosal laceration, submucosal hematoma, avulsion of a true or false cord, disruption of the thyroepiglottic ligament, and fracture of the thyroid or cricoid cartilage. Additional injuries may include recurrent laryngeal nerve injury, arytenoid joint subluxation, or complete laryngotracheal separation. The latter condition makes airway management difficult if the trachea retracts into the mediastinum. The care of these children also may be complicated by associated trauma, including cervical spine and great vessel injury. In one series, 50% of patients with tracheal transection had an associated cervical spine fracture.[4]

SPECIAL CONSIDERATION:

Many children who suffer laryngotracheal trauma also have sustained cervical spine injuries.

Assessment

Depending on the condition of the child and the availability of observers to the injury, the initial eval-uation should begin with an inquiry as to the mechanism of injury. Important symptoms include change in voice, pain on swallowing or speaking, dysphagia, stridor, dyspnea, and hemoptysis.

In contrast to penetrating trauma, the child with blunt trauma to the laryngotracheal complex may present with minimal external evidence of injury. There may be ecchymosis or abrasions on the neck with both major and minor injuries (Fig. 54–1), but some children may present only with symptoms of airway distress such as stridor and retractions.[5] If the child's airway has been controlled "in the field" with an endotracheal tube, a blunt laryngeal injury may go unrecognized until an attempt is made at extubation. Other significant signs include hoarseness, dysphonia, and aphonia. The inability to tolerate the supine position may be a another clue to a laryngeal injury.

The neck examination should include a search for evidence of subcutaneous emphysema and palpation of the laryngeal framework for pain or crepitus. In one review, three of four pediatric patients with tracheal and bronchial disruptions from blunt chest trauma had subcutaneous air on examination, chest radiography, or both; all were intubated successfully.[6] Numerous case reports have demonstrated the association of subcutaneous air, either on clinical or radiographic examination, with a tracheal tear. Not all children had respiratory distress, but some had tenderness over the larynx or trachea. Dyspnea, hoarseness, or dysphagia were uncommon findings in these patients, and the endoscopic evaluation was crucial to the diagnosis.[6-10]

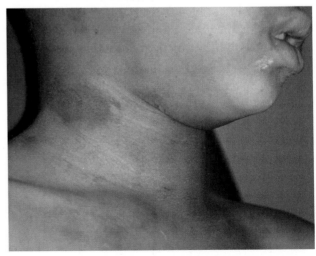

Figure 54–1:   Children who have suffered blunt laryngeal trauma may have minimal evidence of injury, that is only ecchymosis or abrasions of the neck.

In the stable patient, radiographic studies of the neck and chest should be performed to identify pneumothorax, pneumomediastinum, an abnormal tracheal outline, and subcutaneous emphysema. Cervical spine films should be obtained as soon as possible to exclude a cervical spine injury. In an unstable patient, the neck should be immobilized with a cervical collar or sandbags until the clinical and radiographic evaluation of the neck is complete.

Evaluation of the stable patient usually requires flexible fiberoptic laryngoscopy (FFL) to examine the mobility of the cords and evidence of avulsion, edema, laceration, or hematoma of the cords. Until the examination is completed, topical anesthesia should be avoided.

Computed tomography (CT) of the larynx may be performed electively when the patient's condition has stabilized, and it may be helpful in identifying the location and extent of laryngeal fractures (Figs. 54-2, 54-3, and 54-4). Delayed ossification of the thyroid cartilage in children may complicate the interpretation of findings on CT scan. CT is not necessary if an open exploration of the larynx is to be performed.

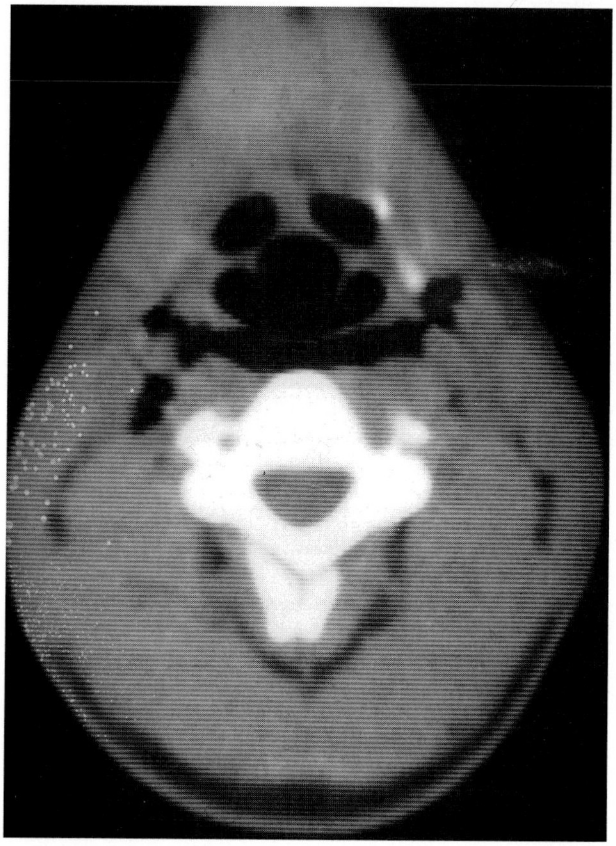

Figure 54–2: CT demonstrates a fracture of the larynx with disruption of the thyroid cartilage and dissection of air throughout the soft tissues of the neck.

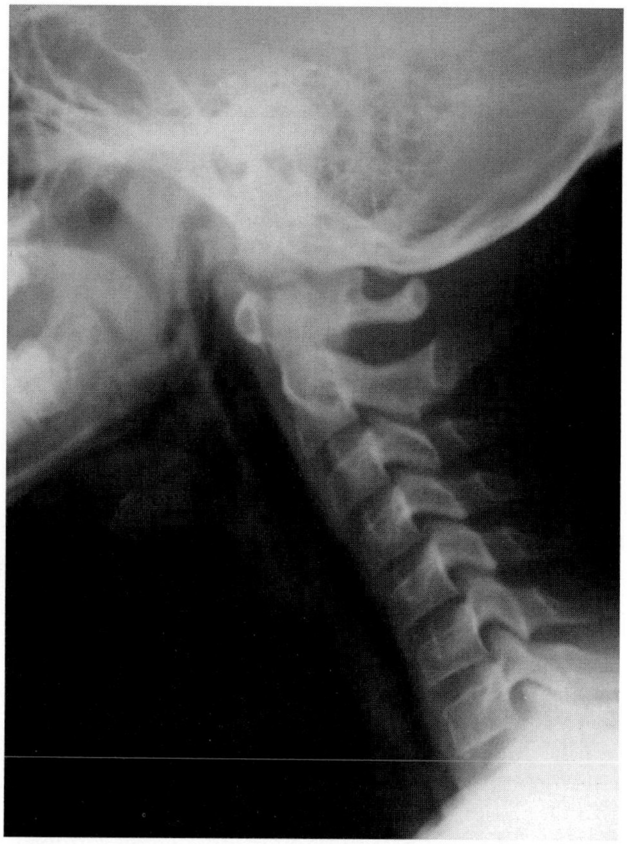

Figure 54–3: Lateral neck radiograph in a child with disruption of the trachea demonstrates dissection of air throughout the neck.

Management of laryngeal injuries

Practice Pathway 54-1 outlines the diagnosis and management of pediatric laryngeal injuries. Supplemental oxygen, continuous pulse oximetry, and close observation should be carried out during evaluation and management of the injured child. The use of corticosteroids is controversial; they must be started within hours of the initial injury to be effective. In selected cases, they may be helpful to reduce soft-tissue edema.

Some controversy exists as to the best way to manage the airway with laryngotracheal trauma initially. Tracheostomy (or cricothyroidotomy) has long been advocated to treat the potentially unstable airway in adults. Endotracheal intubation has been recommended by some because it is faster and avoids iatrogenic tracheal injury, which might occur from an emergency tracheostomy. Gussack reserves tracheostomy for patients with significant laryngo-

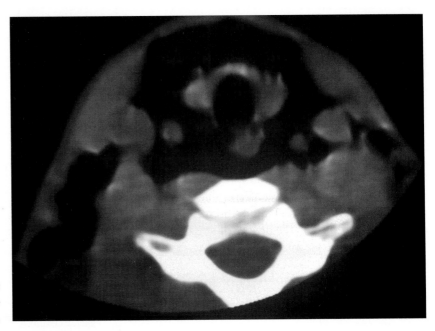

Figure 54–4: CT of the neck in the same patient illustrates massive dissection of air in the surrounding soft tissue.

tracheal disruption or if intubation cannot be performed easily.[11]

The proponents of tracheostomy recommend it for the patient with an unstable airway and point to the risk of intubation converting a small mucosal laceration of the airway into a complicated airway problem.[7] There is also potential for the endotracheal tube to create a false passage. A tenuous airway may be converted quickly into a completely-obstructed airway in these situations. In cases of laryngotracheal separation, the transected ends of the trachea may be separated by as much as 8 cm, making passage of an endotracheal tube not only difficult, but also dangerous.[12]

Most children will not cooperate for an elective tracheostomy under local anesthesia. Emergent tracheostomy is extremely difficult in the awake child, especially if anatomic landmarks are obscured by soft-tissue edema or hematoma. In children, some physicians recommend careful oral intubation, reserving tracheostomy only if there is poor airway visualization due to blood or edema.[5]

Perhaps the best approach in children is to induce general anesthesia with an inhalational agent in the operating room, maintaining spontaneous respiration. In cases of suspected laryngeal or tracheal injury, a rigid bronchoscope may then be used to obtain an airway under direct visualization. Tracheostomy can be performed over the bronchoscope once the airway is secured,[13] or the patient can be intubated if tracheostomy is unnecessary. Care should be taken to place the tracheostomy

tube low enough to avoid compromising the cricoid ring. Those patients undergoing cricothyrotomy as a life-saving measure should have the tracheostomy revised and placed more inferior once other medical problems have been stabilized.

Once the airway is secured, laryngoscopy and bronchoscopy should be performed to identify airway injuries that may be amenable to repair. Surgical repair of problems identified by endoscopy is best done early; an immediate open approach is advocated in patients with hematemesis, hemoptysis, exposed cartilage, cord paralysis, displaced fractures, or significant mucosal injury.

The importance of direct laryngoscopy and bronchoscopy in evaluating children with blunt cervical trauma has been highlighted in one series that included nine patients with blunt injury identified in a 5-year period. All underwent endoscopy and eight of the procedures identified injuries. Seven patients underwent neck exploration and successful repair of the laryngotracheal injuries.[14]

> **SPECIAL CONSIDERATION:**
>
> Delays in the evaluation and treatment of laryngeal trauma lead to the development of infection, granulation tissue, and scarring.

Minor laryngeal injuries with intact mucosa and no displacement of the cartilaginous framework can

Practice Pathway 54–1   DIAGNOSIS AND MANAGEMENT OF PEDIATRIC LARYNGEAL INJURY

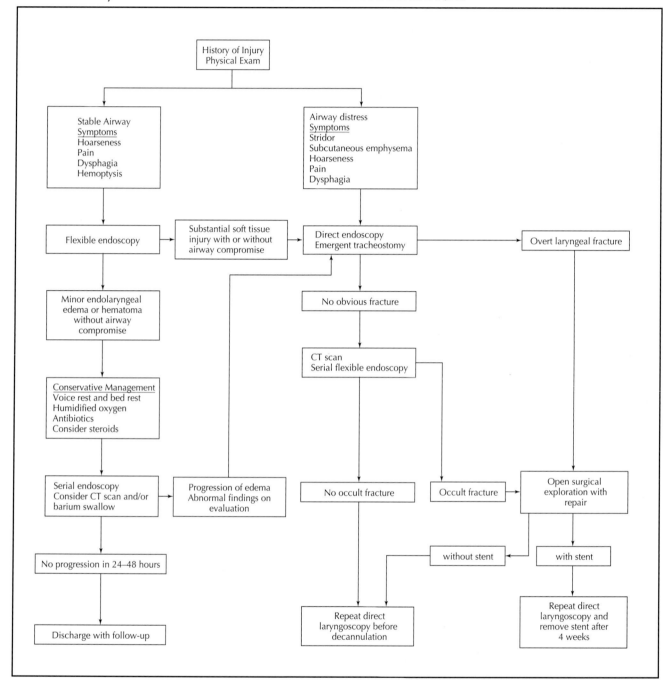

be managed conservatively. A hematoma of the vocal cord with normal function can likewise be observed. Conservative management includes voice rest, soft diet, humidified oxygen, and possibly antibiotics and corticosteroids.

Delays in the evaluation and treatment of laryngeal trauma lead to the development of infection, granulation tissue, and scarring. In this setting, it becomes difficult to identify landmarks and restore

function. The CO_2 laser can be useful in late repairs or in treating complications of scarring or granulation tissue after early surgical repair.

Major injuries to the larynx necessitate a midline thyrotomy in order to make repairs. A tracheostomy should be performed prior to surgical exploration of the larynx so that the larynx can be examined closely without the encumbrance of a translaryngeal airway. Mucosal integrity should be restored by early repair of any lacerations using absorbable sutures. An operating microscope may be utilized in small children to facilitate mucosal repair. Soft-tissue loss can be replaced using local sliding advancement flaps, split-thickness skin grafts, or free mucosal grafts.[15] Fractures of the thyroid and cricoid cartilages should be repaired with either nonabsorbable sutures or stainless steel wire if necessary. Care must be taken to maintain laryngeal landmarks, especially the location of the vocal cords, in performing the laryngeal reconstruction. A variety of laryngeal stents are available to aid in the restoration of a normal lumen.

Following the repair of a major laryngeal injury, careful follow-up is necessary to determine laryngeal function. Impairment of vocal cord mobility may be temporary or permanent; FFL can be used to monitor any improvement. In selected cases, electromyography (EMG) of the larynx may be necessary to document paresis or paralysis. Injuries to the laryngeal framework may affect cartilage growth centers, and long-term follow-up should be performed to monitor laryngeal function.

Although airway stability is a primary concern in these children, voice problems cannot be ignored and may be of great significance for the child in school and at home. Speech therapy may play a role in this regard, and further surgery aimed at voice improvement should be individualized to the child's particular problems.

Penetrating Neck Injuries in Children

Penetrating injuries of the neck in children can be caused by gun shots, knives, or other sharp objects during play, assault, or MVAs. These injuries are difficult to assess and treat because the complex anatomy of the neck includes vital blood vessels and important structures of the aerodigestive tract (ADT) and nervous system. Vascular injuries are particularly dangerous and can lead to severe hemorrhage, shock, and death. One series attributed 50% of deaths in penetrating neck trauma to exsanguinating hemorrhage from lacerated arteries or veins.[16]

Upper ADT injuries are also potentially life-threatening, as approximately 10% of patients with penetrating neck trauma present with airway compromise.[17] Esophageal tears, if not recognized and repaired early, can be fatal.

The nervous system may be damaged by hypoperfusion secondary to vascular injuries. Specifically, carotid artery injury causes a neurologic deficit in 20 to 30% of patients.[18,19] Cervical spinal cord injuries are uncommon but may lead to disabling paresis or paralysis. Cranial nerve injuries are rare, occurring in < 1% of patients.[20]

Although predictors of patient mortality are well described in the adult literature, there are no large studies involving exclusively pediatric patients. An analysis of 2495 patients of all ages with penetrating neck trauma estimated a 4.2% mortality rate.[20] Deaths were more likely to occur in those patients with gunshot wounds, Zone-1 injuries (See, Injuries to the Great Vessels of the Neck, later), spinal cord injuries, and shock on admission to the hospital. Vascular trauma may be an ominous sign because the leading cause of death in penetrating neck trauma is hemorrhage from vascular injury.[20]

Management

Initial care of penetrating neck trauma should be directed towards stabilizing the patient and considering the potential sources of morbidity and mortality. Patients with vascular injuries should receive aggressive fluid resuscitation and direct pressure over the wound. Airway injuries should be treated with fiberoptic intubation if the patient is stable and direct oropharyngeal intubation in an urgent situation.[21] A thorough neurologic examination should be performed if the situation allows.

The management of penetrating neck wounds remains controversial. The debate centers around the use of exploratory surgery as "mandatory" for all neck wounds versus selective operation for wounds that meet specific criteria during the initial evaluation. Typically, with the selective option, patient care is based on the results of the physical examination and various diagnostic modalities.

The medical team treating penetrating injuries of the neck should consider two important factors during the decision-making process. These are: (1) the nature of the injury and (2) the resources available at the medical center. There is little debate that a patient with signs and symptoms of major vascular or ADT injury needs emergent surgery. However, patients without clinical signs or with soft signs of significant injury may be treated with either surgical exploration or conservative management.

Those who favor surgical exploration, regardless of clinical signs, argue that the physical examination is unreliable, and that serious injuries may be missed by observation alone. One study of 393 patients with stab wounds penetrating the platysma found no clinical signs in 30% of patients with positive neck explorations and in 58% of patients with negative neck explorations.[22] They concluded that the five minor complications in patients with negative neck explorations outweighed the potential for missed injuries in patients with positive explorations. Additionally, those patients with negative explorations were hospitalized for an average of only 1.5 days.

Proponents of selective management argue that conservative treatment that utilizes surgery in only selected cases is safer. They claim that data from the physical examination coupled with investigative modalities, such as angiography, color flow Doppler, endoscopy, and fluoroscopy, can reliably diagnose significant injuries (Fig. 54–5). The benefit is that patients are less likely to receive unnecessary surgical exploration while still being diagnosed for major injuries. Although the practice of selective management is employed more commonly, its success depends on both access to the proper diagnostic modalities and on appropriate staffing to perform routine examinations properly.

AT A GLANCE . . .

Laryngeal Injury

Pathogenesis: penetrating wounds and blunt trauma from sports-related injuries, seat belts, and child abuse

Assessment: voice change, pain on swallowing or speaking, dysphagia, stridor, dyspnea, or hemoptysis

Diagnosis: flexible fiberoptic laryngoscopy, radiography, computed tomography

Management: observation with supplemental oxygen and monitoring *or* endotracheal intubation *or* tracheostomy followed by surgical repair of laryngeal fracture

---

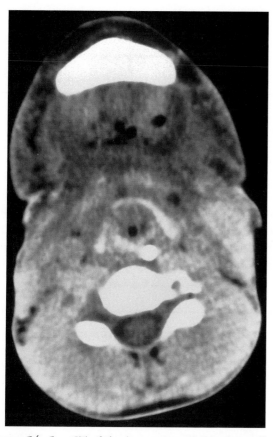

Figure 54–5: CT of the larynx in a child who suffered a gunshot wound to the neck. Extensive subcutaneous emphysema and fracture of the thyroid cartilage are evident.

ESOPHAGEAL TRAUMA

Practice Pathway 54-2 outlines the diagnosis and management of pediatric esophageal injury.

The esophagus in the neck is susceptible to injury from a variety of mechanisms, including blunt and penetrating trauma and ingestion of caustic agents and foreign bodies. Blunt force to the neck can damage the esophagus if it is compressed against the vertebra. Serious injury may occur even with minimal evidence of external trauma, as in an MVA when the neck hits the dashboard or in a motorcycle or snowmobile accident when a "clothes-line" injury occurs from riding across an unexpected wire.

Penetrating neck trauma is often secondary to gunshot or stab wounds. Despite the deep location of the esophagus in the neck, esophageal perforation must be suspected with these types of injury. McConnell combined data from 16 papers with 2495 patients to estimate that injury to the pharynx and esophagus together occurred 9.6% of the time with penetrating neck trauma, and injury to the esophagus alone occurred 6.6% of the time.[20] In addition to external sources of trauma, perforation of the esophagus may be iatrogenic in origin as it can occur during instrumentation procedures such as endoscopy or dilation of a stricture.[23]

Esophageal injury may result from the ingestion

Practice Pathway 54–2   DIAGNOSIS AND MANAGEMENT OF PEDIATRIC ESOPHAGEAL INJURY

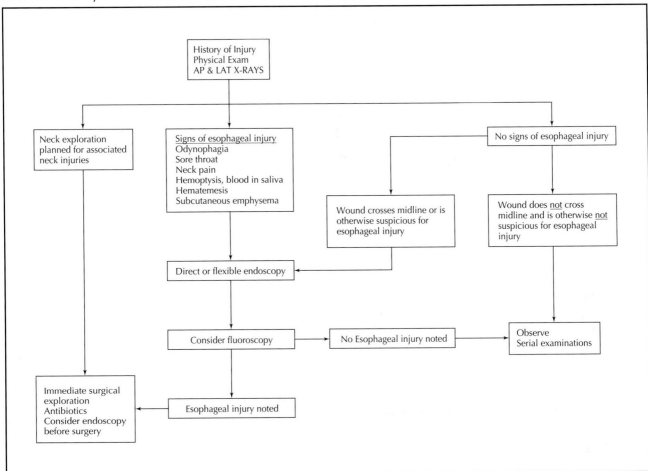

of caustic substances that are found in common household products that are accessible to children (See Chap. 38). Additionally, foreign bodies may become lodged in the esophagus and cause damage (See Chap. 49).

Assessment

Neck trauma should always lead the clinician to consider esophageal injury. Blunt force can cause esophageal perforation without skin laceration, and perforation resulting from penetrating neck trauma is not always obvious on presentation.[23] As few as 70% of patients with esophageal laceration from penetrating neck injury have signs and symptoms consistent with perforation on arrival to the emergency department.[24]

In the immediate evaluation of the patient, signs and symptoms consistent with esophageal perfora-

tion include a sore throat, neck pain, fever, tachycardia, subcutaneous emphysema, blood in the saliva, and hematemesis.[21] Later, the patient may complain of increasing neck pain, odynophagia, and chest pain as a result of sequelae of untreated perforations, including abscess formation, fistula formation, pleural effusion, and mediastinitis.[25,26]

SPECIAL CONSIDERATION:

Esophageal injury should always be suspected in patients with neck trauma because as few as 70% of patients with esophageal lacerations that result from penetrating neck injury have signs and symptoms consistent with a perforation upon arrival to the emergency room.

Iatrogenic perforation occurs most often during endoscopy. The typical clinical picture is similar to penetrating neck trauma and includes the presence of a sore throat immediately following the procedure, tachycardia, and subcutaneous emphysema.[27]

Diagnosis of esophageal injury is difficult, causing it to be the most commonly missed lesion in neck trauma.[28] Delay in the diagnosis may result in severe complications and death. Perforation should be suspected with any penetrating injury that is either in the midline or that crosses the midline.[25]

Although both rigid and flexible endoscopy are safe and effective means of evaluating the esophagus for the location and extent of any laceration, endoscopy does carry a risk of perforation.[29] Additional information may be obtained from fluoroscopic studies; however, this method is less accurate and identifies transmural perforation only 62 to 80% of the time. Endoscopy has been shown to have a sensitivity of 89 to 100% in diagnosing cervical esophageal injuries.[24,25,30-32] If a torn viscus is suspected prior to fluoroscopy, an isosmolar nonionic contrast material should be used. Finally, surgical exploration to rule out esophageal injury may be performed, although a tear can be overlooked during exploration.[29]

Management

Esophageal tears should be treated with broad-spectrum antibiotics and repaired promptly in one or two layers. In two separate series, Bladergroen[33] and Attar[34] studied consecutive patients with esophageal perforation from neck trauma. Repair of the lesion within 24 hours resulted in 92% and 91% survival, respectively. When repair was delayed more than 24 hours, survival dropped to 67% and 75%, respectively. There has been some interest in nonoperative treatment of esophageal perforation.[35] If repair is delayed, treatment may consist of drainage alone, T tube insertion, or esophagectomy.

Complications from esophageal repair are problematic. Stanley[36] noted that 39% of 23 patients treated for cervical esophageal wounds eventually developed a fistula or a deep neck infection requiring drainage, and Winter[37] noted that 9% of 46 patients with such wounds developed esophageal fistulas. Management of complications includes appropriate local wound care and drainage.

AT A GLANCE . . .

Esophageal Injury

Pathogenesis: gunshot and stab wounds, "clothesline" injuries, and blunt force injuries (e.g., hitting dashboard, sports, etc.) may cause serious esophageal trauma with minimal external evidence of trauma

Assessment: signs and symptoms include sore throat, neck pain, subcutaneous emphysema, bloody saliva, or hematemesis

Diagnosis: endoscopy, radiography, surgical exploration

Management: broad-spectrum antibiotics and surgical repair within 24 hours

---

INJURIES TO THE GREAT VESSELS OF THE NECK

Practice Pathway 54-3 outlines the diagnosis and management of vascular injury of the neck.

Vascular injuries can be caused by penetrating and blunt neck trauma and are the most common cause of death in penetrating wounds.[38] The most frequently injured arteries in penetrating neck trauma are the common carotid (6.7% of the time), the subclavian (2.2%), the external carotid (2.0%), and the vertebral (1.3%); the internal jugular vein is injured 9% of the time, followed by the subclavian vein (1.7%).[20] In children, blunt trauma is typically secondary to MVAs and sports-related accidents and accounts for 3 to 10% of total cervical vascular injuries.[39]

SPECIAL CONSIDERATION:

Vascular injuries are the most common cause of death in patients with penetrating neck wounds.

The neck may be divided into anatomic zones in order to facilitate decision making about diagnostic

Practice Pathway 54–3   DIAGNOSIS AND MANAGEMENT OF VASCULAR INJURY OF THE NECK IN CHILDREN

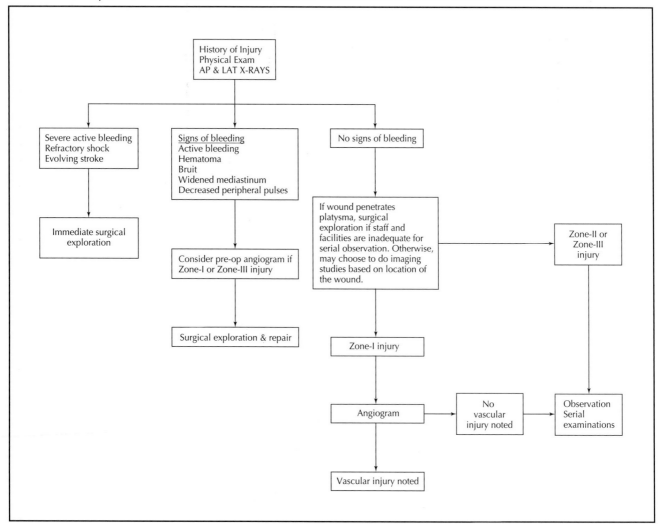

and therapeutic interventions. *Zone I* includes the area between the clavicles and the inferior margin of the cricoid cartilage. The major anatomic structures in this region include the great vessels of the superior mediastinum, the trachea, and the esophagus. *Zone II* extends from the inferior margin of the cricoid cartilage to the angle of the mandible. This region contains the carotid arteries, jugular veins, esophagus, pharynx, larynx, and trachea. *Zone III* is the area superior to the angle of the mandible and extends to the base of the skull. It contains the distal extracranial carotid arteries, vertebral arteries, and jugular veins.

Assessment

Signs of vascular injury in the neck include persistent bleeding from the neck wound, hematoma formation, and the presence of a bruit. A large hema-

toma may compress the airway and cause stridor and respiratory distress. Neurologic deficits may be global, caused by brain hypoperfusion that is secondary to significant blood loss, or specific, caused by a lesion of a major artery that supplies the brain. For example, injury to the carotid artery leads to neurologic changes 20 to 30% of the time, depending upon the carotid anatomy and the severity and location of the wound. Vertebral artery lesions rarely cause neurologic deficits.[18,19]

Physical examination is the earliest and most accessible diagnostic tool available, and findings consistent with vascular injury have already been discussed. Although some physicians believe that a physical examination is an unreliable method of identifying significant vascular lesions, others consider it to be a safe method to triage patients. One investigator[40] studied 335 consecutive patients with penetrating neck injuries who underwent an extensive screening physical examination. Based on these physical findings, patients were either observed, evaluated by angiography, or surgically explored. There were no significant findings on physical examination for 269 patients (80%) treated nonoperatively with observation. Of these, only two patients subsequently required neck exploration. Both of these surgeries occurred during the time they were being hospitalized for observation. Only seven of the 335 patients in the study (2%) underwent angiography.

Angiography has been advocated by others as an important tool that adds pertinent information to the physical examination. It has been used by various physicians as both a routine and an elective procedure to evaluate neck trauma. Its major benefit is its high sensitivity for detecting vascular injury and, therefore, its potential to avoid unnecessary exploratory surgery; negative considerations include its invasiveness and cost. In one study of 176 consecutive hemodynamically-stable neck trauma patients who were evaluated with routine angiography, none went on to have an unnecessary operation.[40] In an attempt to reduce unnecessary surgery, angiography also has been used to evaluate selected patients, such as those with Zone-I or Zone-III injuries (which are more difficult to assess on physical examination and to repair surgically without angiographic images).[41]

The role of color flow Doppler imaging as a screening test for vascular injury is uncertain. In a small series, one investigator demonstrated that Doppler may be useful as a less expensive alternative to angiography in Zone-II and Zone-III injuries.[42]

Management

Patients with penetrating neck injury and suspected vascular trauma require aggressive resuscitation if they are actively bleeding on arrival to the emergency room. In that setting, bleeding wounds should be compressed and not probed or blindly clamped. Direct pressure helps control the bleeding and reduces the risk of an air embolus.

Once the initial assessment and attempts at stabilizing the patient have been made, the treatment plan may follow one of three options: (1) surgical exploration; (2) diagnostic study, such as angiography; or (3) observation. Although there is general agreement that patients who have severe bleeding or who are in shock should undergo immediate exploratory surgery, the management of other patients is controversial. Some surgeons advocate mandatory exploration of any wound that penetrates the platysma, citing data that up to 30% of positive neck explorations had no clinical signs of vascular injury on physical examination.[22] Others advocate the use of selective exploration. With this method, patients with low-risk injuries and negative physical exams are admitted and observed. Patients with intermediate or high-risk injuries are selected for angiography, exploration, or both.[43,44]

Most surgeons practice selective exploratory surgery when managing penetrating neck trauma. Wounds that do not penetrate the platysma are often treated with observation, with or without angiography, if there are no signs or symptoms of vascular injury. Mansour et al. recommend performing angiography on even asymptomatic Zone-I injuries, because unrecognized bleeding in this region may result in complications.[44] Most surgeons surgically explore wounds that penetrate the platysma. Preoperative angiography can be helpful in Zone-I and Zone-III injuries to help define the anatomy.

Repair should be attempted when the injury involves the internal, common carotid, or subclavian artery. If simple closure is not possible, then a vein patch or interposition graft may be necessary. Jugular vein tears should be repaired, although ligation may be necessary if the injury is extensive. The role of interventional radiology remains to be defined. Although embolization of the vertebral artery in trauma is convenient, the advantages of embolization, including the use of local anesthesia and radiographic guidance, need to be weighed against the potential pitfalls such as pseudoaneurysm formation and loss of access to the proximal portion of the artery.[45,46]

AT A GLANCE . . .
Cervical Vascular Injury

Pathogenesis: penetrating wounds, more so than blunt trauma, more commonly injure the great vessels of the neck

Assessment: continuous bleeding from wound, hematoma formation, bruit, neurologic deficits, shock

Diagnosis: indications for angiography and surgical exploration remain controversial

Management: selective surgical exploration with or without preoperative angiography is commonly used for wounds that penetrate the platysma

REFERENCES

1. Kirsh M, Orringer M, Behrendt D. Management of tracheobronchial disruption secondary to nonpenetrating trauma. Ann Thorac Surg 1976; 22:93–101.

2. Jurkovich G, Luterman A. Laryngotracheal trauma: A protocol approach to a rare injury. Laryngoscope 1986; 96:660–665.

3. Hoy GA, Cole WG. The paediatric cervical seat belt syndrome. Injury 1993; 24:297–299.

4. Fitz-Hugh G, Wallenborn W, McGovern F. Injuries of the larynx and cervical trauma. Ann Otol Rhino Laryngol 1962; 71:419.

5. Gold SM, Gerber ME, Shott SR, et al. Blunt laryngotracheal trauma in children. Arch Otolaryngol Head Neck Surg 1997; 123:83–87.

6. Baumgartner F, Sheppard B, Virgilio C. Tracheal and main bronchial disruptions after blunt chest trauma: Presentation and management. Ann Thorac Surg 1990; 50:569–574.

7. Kadish H, Schunk J, Woodward G. Blunt pediatric laryngotracheal trauma: Case reports and review of the literature. Am J Emerg Med 1994; 12:207–211.

8. Humar A, Pittes C. Emergency department management of blunt cervical tracheal trauma in children. Pediatr Emerg Care 1991; 7(5):291–293.

9. Lusk R. The evaluation of minor cervical blunt trauma in the pediatric patient. Clin Pediatr 1986; 25:445–447.

10. Kielmovitch I, Friedman W. Lacerations of the cervical trachea in children. Int J Pediatr Otorhinolaryngol 1988; 15:73–78.

11. Gussack G, Jurkovich G. Treatment dilemmas in laryngotracheal trauma. J Trauma 1988; 28: 1439–1444.

12. Fuhrman G, Stieg F, Buerk C. Blunt laryngeal trauma: Classification and management protocol. J Trauma 1990; 30:87–92.

13. Myer CM III, Orobello P, Cotton RT, et al. Blunt laryngeal trauma in children. Laryngoscope. 1987; 97: 1043–1048.

14. Ford HR, Gardner MJ, Lynch JM. Laryngotracheal disruption from blunt pediatric neck injuries: Impact of early recognition and intervention on outcome. J Pediatr Surg 1995; 30:331–334.

15. Thompson JN, Strausbaugh PL, Koufman JA, et al. Penetrating injuries of the larynx. South Med J 1984; 77:41–45.

16. Stone HH, Callahan GS. Soft tissue injuries of the neck. Surg Gynecol Obstet 1963; 117:745–752.

17. Pate JW. Tracheobronchial and esophageal injuries. Surg Clin North Am 1989; 69:111–123.

18. Pearce WH, Whitehill TA. Carotid and vertebral arterial artery injuries. Surg Clin North Am 1988; 68: 705–722.

19. Unger SW, Tucker WS Jr, Mideza MA. Carotid artery trauma. Surg 1980; 87:477–487.

20. McConnell DB, Trunkey DD. Management of penetrating trauma to the neck. Adv Surg 1994; 27: 97–127.

21. Demetriades D, Asensio JA, Velmahos G, et al. Complex problems in penetrating neck trauma. Surg Clin North Am 1996; 76(4):661–683.

22. Apffelstaedt JP, Muller R. Results of mandatory exploration for penetrating neck trauma. World J Surg 1994; 18:917–919.

23. Offerson HB Jr. Cardiothoracic injuries. In: Touloukian RJ, ed. Pediatric Trauma, St. Louis: Mosby-Year Book, 1990 pp. 266–311.

24. Weigelt JA, Thal ER, Snyder WH III, et al. Diagnosis of penetrating cervical esophageal injuries. Am J Surg 1987; 154:619–622.

25. Donat TL, Maisel RH, Mathog RH. Injuries of the mouth, pharynx, and esophagus. In: Bluestone CD, Stool SE, Kenna MA, eds. Pediatric Otolaryngology. Philadelphia: Saunders, 1996, pp. 1181–1191.

26. Kerr HH, Sloan H, O'Brien CE. Rupture of the esophagus by compressed air. Surgery 1953; 33:417–420.

27. Jones KR. The esophagus. In: Lee KJ, ed. Essential Otolaryngology Head & Neck Surgery. Norwalk, CT: Appleton & Lange, 1995, pp. 481–497.

28. Shama DM, Odell J. Penetrating neck trauma with tracheal and esophagus injuries. Br J Surg 1984; 71: 534–536.

29. Asensio JA, Valenziano CP, Falcone RE, et al. Management of penetrating neck injuries. The controversy surrounding Zone II injuries. Surg Clin North Am 1991; 71(2):267–296.

30. Flowers JL, Graham SM, Ugarte MA, et al. Flexible endoscopy for the diagnosis of esophageal trauma. J Trauma 1996; 40(2):261–265.

31. Armstrong WB, Detar TR, Stanley RB. Diagnosis and management of external penetrating cervical esophageal injuries. Ann Otol Rhinol Laryngol 1994; 103(11):863–871.

32. Ghahremani GG. Esophageal trauma. Semin Roentgenol. 1994; 29(4):387–400.

33. Bladergroen MR, Lowe JE, Postlethwalt MD. Diagnosis and recommended management of esophageal perforation and rupture. Ann Thor Surg 1986; 42: 235–239.

34. Attar S, Hankins JR, Suter, et al. Esophageal perforation: A therapeutic challenge. Ann Thorac Surg 1990; 50(1):45–49.

35. Hatzitheofilou C, Strahlendorf C, Kakoyiannis S, et al. Penetrating external injuries of the oesophagus and pharynx. Br J Surg 1993; 80:1147–1149.

36. Stanley Jr RB, Armstrong WB, Fetterman BL, et al.

Management of external penetrating injuries into the hypopharyngeal-cervical esophageal funnel. J Trauma 1997; 42(4):675-679.

37. Winter RP, Weigelt JA. Cervical esophageal trauma. Incidence and cause of esophageal fistulas. Arch Surg 1990; 125(7):849-851.

38. Miller RH, Duplechain JK. Penetrating wounds of the neck. Otolaryngol Clin North Am 1991; 24(1):15-29.

39. Fakhry SM, Jaques PF, Proctor HJ. Cervical vessel injury in infants and young children. F Vasc Surg 1988; 8(4):501-508.

40. Demetriades D, Charalambides D, Lakhoo M. Physical examination and selective conservative management in patients with penetrating injuries of the neck. Br J Surg 1993; 80:1534-1536.

41. Rao PM, Ivatury RR, Sharma P, et al. Cervical vascular injury: A trauma center experience. Surg 1993; 114: 527-531.

42. Montalvo BM, LeBlang SD, Nunez DB Jr, et al. Color Doppler sonography in penetrating injuries of the neck. Am J Neuroradiol 1996; 17(5):943-951.

43. Roon AJ, Christensen N. Evaluation and treatment of penetrating cervical injuries. J Trauma 1979; 19: 391-397.

44. Mansour MA, Moore EE, Moore FA, et al. Validating the selective management of penetrating neck wounds. Am J Surg 1991; 162:517-520.

45. Golueke P, Sclafani S, Phillips T, et al. Vertebral artery injury, diagnosis and management. J Trauma 1987; 27:856-865.

46. Reid JDS, Weigelt JA. Forty-three cases of vertebral artery trauma. J Trauma 1988; 28:1007-1012.

55 Neoplasms of the Larynx and Trachea

Craig S. Derkay and David H. Darrow

Neoplasms in the airway usually present with signs and symptoms of airway obstruction and may initially be confused with inflammatory and infectious diseases such as asthma and croup. Left untreated, these tumors lead to a significant degree of airway compromise and may result in respiratory distress or death.

This chapter aims to acquaint the reader with the presentation and management of neoplasms affecting the larynx and trachea in children (Table 55-1). The commonly encountered benign lesions, recurrent respiratory papillomatosis (RRP) and subglottic hemangioma, are covered comprehensively. The less common benign and malignant tumors of the pediatric airway also are discussed.

ASSESSMENT OF PATIENT

History

Patients with lesions of the airway typically present with a history of hoarseness and/or stridor. *Hoarseness* suggests a lesion of the glottis, especially when the anterior larynx is affected. *Stridor* may develop in the presence of glottic lesions that involve the posterior larynx, or may suggest a supraglottic or subglottic lesion. Not uncommonly, a mistaken diagnosis of asthma, croup, allergy, vocal nodules, or bronchitis is entertained before the true diagnosis is made. Acute respiratory distress or arrest may occasionally be the initial presentation. Additional clinical features include chronic cough, recurrent pneumonia, failure to thrive, dysphagia, and dyspnea.

In the absence of severe respiratory distress, a careful history should be obtained. The age of the patient may suggest an etiology: hemangiomas and congenital lesions are more common in infants, whereas papillomas and acquired lesions are more common in toddlers. There is, however, considerable overlap between these two groups. Other useful information such as the time of onset of symptoms, airway trauma including a history of previous intubation, characteristics of the cry, and history of maternal condylomata may be useful in determining the responsible etiology.

Physical Examination

Children presenting with symptoms of airway lesions must undergo a thorough and methodical physical examination. The child's respiratory rate and degree of distress must be assessed first. Pulse oximetry may be helpful in determining the need for urgent intervention. If a child is gravely ill, additional examination should not be undertaken outside of the operating room (OR), the emergency room (ER), or the intensive care unit (ICU) where equipment for intubation of the airway, endoscopic evaluation, and possible tracheotomy is available. In the stable, well-oxygenated child, additional examination can proceed.

The most important part of the examination is auscultation with the aid of a stethoscope. The physician should listen over the nose, open mouth, neck, and chest to help localize the probable site of the respiratory obstruction. Stridor of a supraglottic origin is most often inspiratory, whereas biphasic stridor suggests involvement of the glottic or subglottic larynx. Tracheal lesions most often present with wheezing or expiratory stridor. Stridor due to fixed intrinsic lesions of the airway does not change with position.

Imaging

In patients without acute airway distress, radiologic evaluation of the upper aerodigestive tract (UADT)

Pediatric Otolaryngology, Edited by R.F. Wetmore, H.R. Muntz, and T.J. McGill. Thieme Medical Publishers, Inc., New York © 2000.

TABLE 55–1: Benign and Malignant Neoplams of the Larynx in Children

Cell of Origin	
Epithelial	*Neurogenic*
Benign	Benign
Papilloma	Neurofibroma
Malignant	Neurilemoma
Squamous cell carcinoma	Chemodectoma
Verrucous carcinoma	Granular cell tumor
Spindle cell carcinoma	Carcinoid tumor
Malignant melanoma	*Hematopoietic*
Adenoid cystic carcinoma	Benign
Adenocarcinoma	Plasmacytoma
Rhabdomyosarcoma	Hemangioendothelioma
Mucoepidermoid carcinoma	Malignant
Connective Tissue	Reticulosarcoma
Benign	Acute leukemia
Fibroma	*Miscellaneous*
Chondroma	Benign
Hemangioma	Hamartoma
Leiomyoma	Adenolipoma
Lipoma	Plascacytoma
Lymphangioma	Fibrous Histiocytoma
Malignant	Malignant
Rhabdomyosarcoma	Metastatic carcinoma
Chondrosarcoma	Lymphoma
Liposarcoma	
Spindle cell sarcoma	
Leiomysarcoma	

may be indicated. Fluoroscopy with the use of barium contrast medium is the radiographic study of choice in the child with stridor of uncertain etiology. This allows evaluation of both the inspiratory and expiratory phases of respiration as well as the contribution of gastroesophageal reflux (GER) to the child's symptoms. Foreign bodies and airway neoplasms also may be evident occasionally. Computed tomography (CT) and magnetic resonance imaging (MRI) are rarely necessary, although they may be helpful in evaluating the mediastinum for masses or compression of the airway by aberrant vessels.

Flexible Airway Endoscopy

Flexible fiberoptic laryngoscopy (FFL) alone may be sufficient to diagnose lesions of the supraglottic and glottic larynx. Patients should be in no acute respiratory distress and the examination should be kept as brief as possible. Patients who will not tolerate passage of an FFL in the outpatient setting should proceed directly to operative direct laryngoscopy and bronchoscopy.

Advances in instrumentation have produced flexible nasopharyngoscopes as small as 1.9 mm in diam-

eter, allowing passage in even the smallest newborns. Topical decongestion and local anesthesia can be applied by spray, dropper, or pledget. Oxymetazoline is the decongestant of choice because of its lack of cardiac side-effects. Either topical tetracaine or lidocaine may be used in addition to the oxymetazoline to enhance patient cooperation, but overdosage may result in cardiotoxicity, and aspiration may occur in infants who feed postlaryngoscopy.

Infants can be restrained easily for FFL, sitting up in the parent's or nurse's lap. Most children over the age of 7 years can be reassured through the examination. Children between 1 and 6 years of age may be the most difficult to examine, requiring the greatest patience and skill on the part of the clinician. Although dynamic evaluation is best appreciated when children are breathing spontaneously, endoscopy in the OR under general anesthesia is warranted in any child suspected of having an airway lesion who cannot be examined fully in the outpatient setting.

Rigid Airway Endoscopy

Definite diagnosis of airway lesions is established by direct laryngoscopy and biopsy. The procedures are performed ideally in the operating room where resuscitation equipment, small endotracheal tubes, and a tracheotomy set are readily available. Cooperation between the surgeon, anesthesiologist, and the OR staff is imperative in the examination of the upper airway in children.

Before the child enters the operating suite, the surgeon, anesthesiologist, and OR team must select the proper-sized endotracheal tubes, laryngoscopes, and bronchoscopes. All ancillary equipment including telescopes, light cords, suction tips, and forceps should be available and checked for proper functioning. All OR personnel are required to wear eye protection whenever working around the laser. Specially-designed laser masks are worn by OR personnel during the surgery to prevent the inhalation of plume containing viral particles liberated during laser procedures.

Before the institution of any anesthesia, the surgeon should discuss the possible pathology with the anesthesiologist. Additionally, the operative staff should be informed of the surgeon's concerns so that appropriate instrumentation is available. Intraoperative teamwork is enhanced by the presence of video monitors during the procedure because this allows the entire OR staff to follow the operation as it progresses. A dialogue between the surgeon and the anesthesiologist continues throughout the surgical procedure regarding the current status of ventilation, the amount of bleeding encountered, the motion of the vocal cords, the timing of laser use in conjunction with respiration, and the concentration of inspired oxygen.

The ultimate decision about the technique of anesthesia should be shared between the anesthesiologist and the surgeon. A variety of alternatives may be used, including endotracheal intubation with a laser-safe tube; insufflation through nasal cannulae; or laryngoscope, supraglottic, or subglottic jet ventilation and apneic technique. When the laser is used, the smallest possible laser-safe endotracheal tube should be used that allows for adequate ventilation. If a cuffed tube must be used in laser surgery, then the cuff should be filled with saline so that if it is inadvertently struck by laser energy, the saline acts as a heat sink to prevent combustion.

Careful sequential inspection of the pharynx, hypopharynx, larynx, and trachea provides the critical information necessary to make a presumptive diagnosis and determines the adequacy of the airway, vocal cord mobility, and the options for operative intervention. The surgical sequence begins with a mask induction and establishment of intravenous (IV) access. Spontaneous ventilation is used whenever possible to assess airway dynamics and to permit some ventilation in the event of a lesion that causes nearly complete obstruction. After exposure by the surgeon, the vocal folds are sprayed with topical lidocaine. Whenever possible, operative laryngoscopy and tracheobronchoscopy are performed with the telescope alone to assess the site and degree of airway obstruction while minimizing airway trauma. The airway is then secured with a ventilating bronchoscope or endotracheal tube while appropriate operative intervention is planned.

RECURRENT RESPIRATORY PAPILLOMATOSIS

The squamous papilloma is the most common benign neoplasm of the larynx among children.[1] The lesion typically is associated with *recurrent respiratory papillomatosis* (RRP), a disease of viral etiology that is associated with exophytic lesions of the air-

way. Despite its benign histology, RRP has potentially morbid consequences due to the severity of its involvement in the airway and to the risk of malignant degeneration. It is often difficult to treat because of its tendency to recur and spread throughout the respiratory tract.

Epidemiology and Pathogenesis

RRP may affect humans of any age; reports have documented affected patients as young as 1 day of age and as old as 84 years of age.[2] However, two distinct clinical forms are generally recognized: a juvenile or aggressive form (previously referred to as *juvenile laryngeal papillomatosis*) and an adult or less aggressive form. This distinction is somewhat artificial because the aggressive form also can occur in adults and the less aggressive form may be seen in children. Childhood-onset RRP is most often diagnosed between 2 and 3 years of age, with distribution among boys and girls approximately equal.[3] It is considered the second most common cause of hoarseness in children,[4] and 75% of affected children are diagnosed by 5 years of age[5,6] In contrast, adult RRP peaks between the ages of 20 and 40 and has a slight male predilection.[7] The incidence of RRP in children is estimated at 0.6 to 4.3/100,000 with approximately 2350 new cases occurring in the United States per year. The incidence of RRP in adults may be as high as 1.6 to 3.8/100,000 with 3600 new cases appearing in the United States yearly.[2] The true incidence and prevalence of RRP is uncertain. In a Danish subpopulation incorporating 50% of the population of that country, the incidence of laryngeal papillomatosis was 3.84 cases/100,000. The rate among children was 3.62/100,000, whereas adult onset cases occurred at a rate of 3.94/100,000.[8] Anecdotal observations suggest that most children with RRP are first-born, have young primigravid mothers, and come from families of lower socioeconomic status.[2,9] (Table 55-2)

Before the 1990s, the *human papilloma virus*

TABLE 55-2: Possible Risk Factors Predisposing Children to Develop RRP

Maternal or paternal newly acquired human papilloma virus (HPV) lesion

Primigravid young mother with prolonged second stage of labor

Low socioeconomic status

Bronchopulmonary dysplasia with history of endotracheal intubation

(HPV) had been suspected but not confirmed as the causative agent in RRP. This uncertainty had arisen from an inability to culture the virus in vitro and from the failure to demonstrate consistently viral particles in papilloma lesions using electron microscopy or HPV antibodies. Through the use of viral probes, HPV deoxyribonucleic acid (DNA) has now been identified in virtually every papilloma lesion studied.[10] HPV is a nonenveloped icosahedral capsid virus with a double-stranded circular DNA that is 7900 base pairs long. A member of the papovavirdae family, HPV has an outer surface protein coat without a membrane. It is approximately 55 nm in diameter with 72 capsomers. As a result of molecular biological techniques, including polymerase chain reaction (PCR), filter hybridization, and southern blot hybridization, 77 HPV types have been differentiated.

HPV subtypes 6 and 11 are those most commonly identified with RRP, though subtype 16 and 18 also have been isolated from the respiratory tract of humans.[11] HPV subtypes 6 and 11 are responsible for approximately 90% of genital warts, whereas HPV subtypes 16 and 18 have been associated with cervical and laryngeal cancers. The two most common HPV subtypes are subtype 1, which is associated with plantar warts, and subtype 2 which is associated with common cutaneous warts.

Viral DNA has been detected in areas of "normal appearing mucosa" adjacent to papilloma lesions, suggesting a possible explanation for the recurrence of the disease following thorough surgical removal.[12,13] The present understanding is that HPV establishes itself in the basal layer, where viral DNA enters the cell, and elaborates RNA to produce viral proteins. In the aerodigestive tract (ADT), HPV frequently causes latent infection (viral DNA is present in tissue but without evidence of clinical or histologic disease). Brandsma reported finding HPV DNA in 4% of random, clinically-normal biopsies of the airway.[14] Adult onset respiratory papillomas thus could reflect either activation of virus present since birth or an infection acquired in adolescence or adult life.

Although any site along the UADT can be affected, HPV shows a predilection to infect sites where ciliated columnar and squamous epithelia are juxtaposed.[15] This explains the frequent involvement of the false vocal folds, the upper and lower margins of the ventricle, and the undersurface of the true vocal folds. Less frequently, lesions are found on the nasopharyngeal surface of the soft pal-

ate, the mid-zone of the laryngeal surface of the epiglottis, and mucosa of the carina. In tracheotomized patients, papillomas often are encountered at the stoma and in the midthoracic trachea, which are areas where iatrogenic trauma to ciliated epithilum often induces squamous metaplasia. It is postulated that an eddying flow of the mucous blanket at squamociliary junctions may concentrate infectious viral particles at these sites. Children with bronchopulmonary dysplasia (BPD) who require prolonged endotracheal intubation also may be at increased risk for development of RRP. An endotracheal tube may play the same role in the mechanical dissemination or implantation of papilloma virus as a tracheotomy in this setting, through the interruption of the continuous respiratory mucosal surface.

Transmission

An association between cervical HPV infection of the mother and the development of RRP has been well established.[16] Clinically-apparent genital condylomata acuminata has been reported in greater than 60% of mothers of affected children either during pregnancy or at parturition.[2] However, since only 1:400 at-risk infants seems to develop RRP, the presence of HPV alone is not sufficient to cause disease.[17] Other factors postulated to influence disease expression include host human leukocyte antigen (HLA) type, hormones, trauma, malnutrition, and viral coinfection.

The universality of HPV in the lower genital tract rivals that of any other sexually-transmitted disease. It is estimated that at least 1,000,000 cases of genital papillomatosis occur per year in the United States.[18] These most often manifest as condylomata acuminata involving the cervix, vulva, and anogenital sites in women or involving the penis of male sexual partners of affected women. HPV is present in the genital tracts of 25% of all women of child-bearing age worldwide.[19] Clinically-apparent HPV infection has been noted in 1.5 to 5% of pregnant women in the United States.[20] Ten percent of sexually active men and women with no evidence of disease have been shown to have HPV identified on the penis or cervix by southern blot hybridization analysis.[18]

The precise mode of HPV transmission remains unclear. Several retrospective studies suggest that 50 to 67% of children with RRP are born to mothers with a history of genital warts.[21,22] Circumstantial evidence suggests that adult disease also may be acquired by oral-genital contact. Nosocomial acquisition of virus by patients in the OR also may result theoretically from improper equipment sterilization or room preparation; however, current Occupational Safety and Health Administration (OSHA) recommendations have eliminated this risk virtually.

Several theories have been proposed to explain the possibility of transmission of HPV from mother to child. The first, *infection in utero,* implicates ascending transplacental spread.[16] A second mechanism by which HPV may spread from mother to child is by perinatal infection as the fetus passes through the birth canal (*vertical transmission*). HPV also may be transmitted by direct sexual contact or by social or sexual contact of a digital-genital or urogenital nature. In the pediatric population, such transmission may involve child abuse, and the history must be elucidated delicately to evaluate this possibility.

Despite the aforementioned theories, there is presently no concrete evidence that RRP in children results directly from maternal HPV infection. No studies have unequivocally shown that children born to mothers with HPV are more likely to develop laryngeal papillomas. Only four sibling sets with RRP have ever been identified; and of the two reported cases of RRP with twin siblings, in only one was the twin affected.[2] Furthermore, neither cesarean delivery nor predelivery removal of condylomata has been demonstrated to reduce the risk of HPV transmission in the presence of these lesions. Retrospective studies and a recent prospective study confirm that HPV may be passed by vertical transmission from mother to child.[20,23] In a report by Kashima that has been corroborated by the anecdotal observations in a U.S. survey of otolaryngologists,[2,9] it was found that childhood onset RRP patients were most likely to be firstborn and vaginally delivered. Kashima hypothesized that primigravid mothers are more likely to have a long second stage of labor, and that the prolonged exposure to the virus leads to a higher risk of infection in the firstborn child. He also suggests that newly-acquired genital HPV lesions are more likely to shed virus than long-standing lesions.[9] This may explain the higher incidence of papilloma disease observed among the offspring of young mothers of low socio-economic status (the same group that is more likely to acquire sexually-transmitted diseases such as HPV). Despite the apparent close association between maternal condylomata and the development of RRP, few children exposed to genital warts at birth actually develop clinical symptoms.[17] It is not well understood why RRP develops in so few children whose mothers have condylomata.

The most likely method of maternal-fetal HPV transmission is through direct contact in the birth canal. This would explain the clinical observation that most children in whom papillomas develop are delivered vaginally to mothers with a history of genital condylomatas. However, other factors such as patient immunity, timing, length and volume of exposure, and local trauma must also be important in the of development of RRP. Shah reported that only 1% of 109 childhood-onset RRP cases reviewed gave a history of birth by cesarean section before rupture of uterine membranes.[17] However, there are at least five reported cases in the literature and six self-reported cases of cesarean section birth in children with RRP.[2] Even though cesarean section would seem to reduce the risk of transmission of the disease, this procedure is associated with a higher morbidity and mortality for the mother at a much higher economic cost than elective vaginal delivery. Shah estimates that the risk of a child contracting the disease from a mother who has an active condylomatous lesion and delivers vaginally to be only about 1:400.[17] The characteristics that differentiate this one child from the other 399 are elusive. As a result, the use of cesarean section in HPV infected mothers remains controversial. In light of the uncertainty surrounding intrapartum exposure, there is presently insufficient evidence to support delivery by cesarean section in all pregnant women with condylomata.[16] A better understanding of the risk factors associated with RRP is needed before the efficacy of cesarean delivery in preventing papilloma disease can be fully assessed. In a more definitive statement, the American College of Obstetricians and Gynecologists advises, Because the risk of respiratory papillomatosis is low, it (cesarean section) is *not* recommended solely to protect the neonate from HPV infection.[24] The issue as to whether or not aggressive treatment of genital condylomata acuminata during the third trimester of pregnancy would alter the transmission of HPV to the neonate still has to be studied.

Histopathology

Papilloma lesions may be either sessile or pedunculated and often occur in irregular exophytic clusters (Fig. 55-1). Typical lesions are pinkish to white in color.

Histologically, papillomas demonstrate finger-like

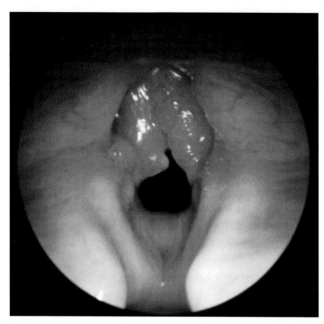

Figure 55–1:   Papilloma lesions often occur in irregular clusters.

projections of nonkeratinized stratified squamous epithelium supported by a core of highly-vascularized connective tissue stroma (Fig. 55–2). The basal layer may be either normal or hyperplastic and mitotic figures generally are limited to this layer. Cellular differentiation appears to be abnormal with altered expression and production of keratins. Though subtypes do not correlate strongly with clinical outcomes, the degree of atypia may be a sign of premalignant tendency.[25] Atypia may be re-

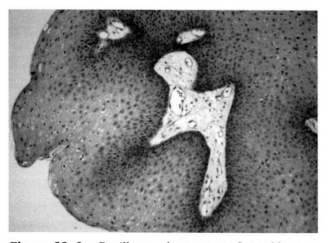

Figure 55–2:   Papillomas demonstrate finger-like projections of nonkeratinized stratified squamous epithelium supported by a core of highly-vascularized connective tissue stroma.

lated to the high levels of epidermal growth factor receptors present in affected cells.

Clinical Course

Patients with RRP typically present with hoarseness, but may have significant stridor as well if the disease is advanced. The duration of symptoms until diagnosis ranges from 1 to 8 years with a mean of 2 years.[3,8] RRP presenting in the neonatal period is thought to be a negative prognostic factor with a greater likelihood for mortality and need for tracheotomy.[26,27]

SPECIAL CONSIDERATION:

A triad of relentlessly-progressive hoarseness, stridor, and respiratory distress strongly suggests a diagnosis of RRP in children under 5 years.

A surgical scoring system to assess the severity and clinical course of RRP disease is helpful in tracking the course of a child's disease and in communicating to other surgeons when treating patients in a protocol format. Though several staging and scoring systems have been proposed, clinicians and researchers have not yet adopted a uniformally-acceptable nomenclature for describing RRP lesions that is simple yet comprehensive. A format that incorporates the best qualities of the existing systems, including numerically grading the extent of papillomatosis at defined aerodigestive subsites, assessing functional parameters, diagrammatically cataloging subsite involvement, and assigning a final numeric score to the patient's current extent of disease, has been adopted by the Centers for Disease Control (CDC) sponsored multiinstituional task force on RRP.[28]

In a survey of practicing otolaryngologists in the United States, half of the adults with RRP had required fewer than five procedures over their lifetime compared with < 25% of the children. Approximately equal percentages of children and adults (17% of children versus 19% of adults) had very aggressive RRPs (defined as requiring more than 40 lifetime operations), although adults had more years to accumulate these operations.[2] Tracheotomy was necessary at some point in the management of 14% of children in two independent series. The frequency of tracheotomy in adults with RRP was estimated at 6%.[2,8]

The clinical course of RRP is highly variable. Childhood-onset disease commonly persists until puberty but can extend into adulthood. Endocrine and/or hormonal influences on RRP have been implicated by the proliferation of uterine, cervical, and laryngeal HPV lesions observed during pregnancy.

Extralaryngeal spread of respiratory papillomas has been identified in approximately 30% of children and 16% of adults with RRP.[2] The most frequent sites of extralaryngeal spread were, in order of frequency, the oral cavity, trachea, and bronchi. A possible link between RRP and immunodeficiency states also has been observed. Children and adults with acquired immune deficiency syndrome (AIDS) or congenital immune deficiencies and those on immune-suppression after organ transplantation all have been identified with RRP.[2]

Malignant transformation of RRP into squamous cell carcinoma has been documented in several case reports. A total of 26 patients were identified as having progressed to squamous cell carcinoma in the Task Force Survey.[2] Lindeberg recorded three adult RRP patients with neoplastic progression.[29] Interestingly, all three had received prior radiation therapy and two were heavy smokers, suggesting that these may be important cofactors for malignant transformation.

Surgical Management

No single modality has been effective consistently in eradicating RRP. The current standard is surgical therapy with a goal of maintaining an airway and doing no harm. For patients with anterior commissure disease or highly-aggressive papilloma, the goal may be subtotal removal to avoid excessive scarring. Overzealous laser use, however, can lead to significant scar injury that can leave the patient with continued airway or vocal dysfunction once the disease goes into remission. When in doubt, it is best to leave disease behind in the anterior commissure and interarytenoid areas because the majority of complications following disease remission are related to damage in these areas. The majority of patients require repeated laser surgery with a median of 7 surgeries in Lindenberg and Elbrond's[8] series and 13 surgeries in that of Morgan and Zitscho.[4]

The CO_2 laser has been favored over cold instru-

ments in the treatment of RRP involving the larynx, pharynx, upper trachea, and nasal and oral cavities.[2] When coupled to an operating microscope, the laser vaporizes the lesion with precision causing minimal bleeding. When used with a no touch technique, it minimizes damage to the vocal folds and limits scarring. The CO_2 laser has an emission wavelength of 10,600 nm, and converts light to thermal energy. It provides a controlled destruction of tissues with vaporization of water and also cauterizes tissue surfaces. Three other common surgical lasers that have been used for papilloma are the argon, neodynium yag (Nd-Yag), and potassium titanyl phosphate (KTP lasers). These lasers offer no significant advantage in terms of achieving disease remission; however, they can be transmitted fiberoptically through flexible or rigid bronchoscopes, which can be an advantage when dealing with distal airway disease.

After intubation of the patient by the operating surgeon with a laser-safe tube, the larynx is visualized by laryngoscopy and suspended for operative microsurgery. Alternatives to this approach include apneic technique without intubation and the use of jet ventilation for microsurgery of the larynx. Cup forceps may be used for biopsy and debulking of the lesions. The CO_2 laser is then used for smaller lesions in critical areas. The supraglottis is usually debrided first followed by the anterior larynx. An apneic or spontaneous ventilation technique is then used so that the endotracheal tube can be removed and any posterior glottic or subglottic disease can be ablated. At the end of the procedure, the child is reintubated with a standard endotracheal tube and extubated only when fully awake. High humidity is provided and occasionally racemic epinephrine or steroids are administered postoperatively. The patient is monitored closely for several hours prior to discharge; often an overnight stay in a monitored bed is necessary if the patient's condition or social circumstances are not conducive to outpatient surgery.

Potential complications of laser surgery include the development of anterior commissure webs, laryngeal and subglottic stenosis, and the possibility of a laser-induced endotracheal tube fire. A laser fire is more likely to occur in the setting of high oxygen concentrations and in the presence of a polyvinyl chloride endotracheal tube. Direct thermal injury to local tissues or chemical burn may result from such a mishap. Prevention is the best treatment and consists of limiting the oxygen concentration to < 40%

or ventilating with room air. Commercially-available laser-safe tubes are generally preferable to aluminum-wrapped red rubber tubes. In the event of a laser fire, emergency care consists of immediate extubation of the patient and disconnection of the tube from its oxygen source. The child is then reintubated and examined through a ventilating bronchoscope. Antibiotics are given and a tracheotomy may be necessary based on the degree of damage. Tertiary care consists of positive end expiratory pressure (PEEP) and reverse isolation.

> ## SPECIAL CONSIDERATION:
>
> Surgical management of RRP is challenging. Whenever possible, utilize the most-experienced pediatric-trained anesthesiologist and OR staff available.

Tracheotomy is occasionally used as an alternative or an adjuvant to repeated laser surgery. However, it has been suggested that tracheotomy may activate or spread disease lower in the respiratory tract. Cole reported on the Cincinnati Children's Hospital experience in which tracheal papillomas developed in half of their tracheotomy patients. Despite attempts to avoid this procedure, 21% of their patients still required a long-term tracheotomy.[27] Shapiro, on the other hand, reported on the favorable experience with the placement of tracheotomies in children with papilloma disease at the Children's Hospital of Pittsburgh.[30] Thirty-seven percent of the RRP patients studied required a tracheotomy, though this did not seem to change the incidence of extralaryngeal spread of the disease. When a tracheotomy is unavoidable, decannulation should be considered as soon as the disease is managed effectively with endoscopic techniques.

Medical Management

Though surgical management remains the mainstay of therapy for RRP, ultimately more than 10% of patients with the disease require some form of adjuvant therapy.[2] The most widely adopted criteria for initiating adjuvant therapy are a requirement of more than four surgical procedures per year, distal or metastatic disease, and/or rapid regrowth of pap-

illoma disease with airway compromise.[31] The most commonly recommended adjuvant therapy is alpha-interferon.[2] The exact mechanism by which interferon elicits its response is unknown. It appears to modulate host immune response by increasing production of a protein kinase and endonuclease, which inhibits viral protein synthesis. Interferon produced by recombinant DNA techniques appears to have fewer side effects and better efficacy then blood bank harvested interferon.[32] Common side effects of interferon include headache, fever, and a flu-like state. Use of interferon in infants prior to the development of gross motor skills potentially could predispose these children to spastic diplegia, a form of cerebral palsy, due to a theoretical delay in the development of the pyramidal tracts. Though a rare complication, this has prompted the recommendation of a neurologic and developmental assessment prior to treatment initiation in infants.

Several large, multiinstitutional studies regarding interferon have arrived at seemingly conflicting conclusions regarding its efficacy. Healy reported on 118 patients randomly assigned to surgery plus interferon or interferon alone.[33] Those in the interferon group received human alpha-interferon at 2 $\times$ 10^6 IU/m^2 daily for 1 month and then 3 times a week for 11 months. This study had a distinct and separate control group that never received therapy. Findings revealed a significant decrease in the growth rate of papillomas in the interferon group in the first 6 months of therapy, but the difference was not significant in the second 6 months of the study. One of the reasons that there is no statistical significance between the control group and the interferon group is that the control group in this study had a high rate of spontaneous remission during the 12-month study. This high rate of improvement of untreated patients must be considered when reviewing articles on experimental drug therapies given to few patients with no control group used as a comparison. Critics of the Healy study have cited the type of interferon used and the low-dosing strategy.

Leventhal and Kashima reported on 66 children who were randomized to treatment plus surgery for 6 months followed by surgery alone or surgery alone for 6 months followed by treatment plus surgery for 6 months.[31] They were administered alpha-N1-interferon at 5 $\times$ 10^6 IU/m^2 daily for 28 days followed by the same dose 3 times weekly for 5 months. Patients in the interferon treatment arms showed a significant decrease in the amount of disease present. One-third of patients had a complete remission and 25/26 experienced a partial remission with a median duration of 550 days. They also found that a response could be reintroduced after a period of nontreatment with interferon. A 1997 Cuban study regarding that country's 8-year experience with alpha-interferon also showed significant efficacy; however, this study was designed poorly and lacked controls, which make the data somewhat suspect.[34] In this report, 125 patients (92 children) received interferon 3 times per week for 5 weeks and then weekly for 1 year. Seventy-one percent achieved a complete response, 18% a partial response, and 11% had persistent disease. The researchers found that interferon was most efficacious if started within the first 3 months of diagnosis. Intralesional injection of interferon also has been tried for RRP but has been reported only in uncontrolled reports of patients with limited laryngeal involvement. Heberhold reported on 11 patients who underwent intralesional injection with alpha-2A-interferon following laser surgery with excellent results.[35]

Based on these data, it seems reasonable to recommend the initiation of interferon therapy for patients who are being operated on at least every 2 months or less for a 6-month trial at a dose of 4 to 5×10^6 IU/m² every day for 30 days and then 3 times weekly. If there is no response, then treatment should be discontinued.

SPECIAL CONSIDERATION:

Children requiring laser therapy more frequently than 6 times in 12 months or who have evidence of distal spread of RRP should be considered for adjuvant medical therapy.

Photodynamic therapy (PDT) in the treatment of RRP has been studied extensively by Abramson, Shikowitz, and Steinberg.[36] PDT is based upon the transfer of energy to a photosensitive drug. The most commonly utilized drug has been dihematoporphyrin ether (DHE), which has a tendency to concentrate within papillomas more so that in surrounding normal tissue. A new drug, M-tetra (Hydrozyphenyl) chlorine also has shown efficacy in HPV tumors in rabbits with minimal tissue damage, and a clinical trial utilizing this drug is now ongoing. The use of PDT and DHE show a small but statistically significant decrease in RRP growth, especially in those patients with the worst disease. Unfortunately, many patients became markedly photosensitive for periods of time lasting from 2 to 8 weeks.

Recent interest has focused on chemically-pure indole-3-carbinol (I3C), which has been shown to inhibit papilloma formation in mice.[37] This compound is found in high concentration in cruciferous vegetables such as cabbage, broccoli, and cauliflower. Initial reports of this vitamin supplement given in an uncontrolled fashion showed a marked reduction in the visible growth of lesions. Multiinstitutional, controlled studies currently are being carried out in Pittsburgh, PA and Memphis, TN. I3C appears to influence estrogen metabolism and induces 2-hydroxylation of extradiol resulting in 2-methoxy-estrone. The recommended dosage for adults is 200 to 400 mg/day and 100 to 200 mg/day for children under 20 kg. Although the product is probably safe at these dosages, its distribution is not controlled by the Food and Drug Administration (FDA) because it is listed as a dietary supplement.

Small series reports of RRP patients treated with acyclovir, isotretinoin, ribavirin, and methotrexate all suffer from poor scientific design and small patient numbers. A larger ribavirin study conducted at the University of Minnesota has been completed recently, though the results are not very encouraging. An FDA-sponsored study of Cidofivir has recently been launched through the University of Alabama at Birmingham. It should be stressed that participation in national or regional treatment protocols is essential for the scientific community to learn more about RRP. A national registry of pediatric patients with RRP is being formed through the cooperation of the CDC and the American Society of Pediatric Otolaryngology. This will aid in the identification of patients suitable for enrollment in multiinstitutional studies of adjuvant therapies and will better define the risk factors for transmission of HPV and the cofactors that may determine the aggressiveness of RRP.

Practice Pathway

Practice Pathway 55-1 illustrates the diagnosis and treatment of children with RRP. FFL and rigid laryngoscopy with biopsy are essential for making the initial diagnosis. Outpatient observation and FFL will determine the appropriate interval for repeat rigid endoscopy and laser surgery. Those children requiring surgery more than six times per year or

Practice Pathway 55-1   RECURRENT RESPIRATORY PAPILLOMATOSIS

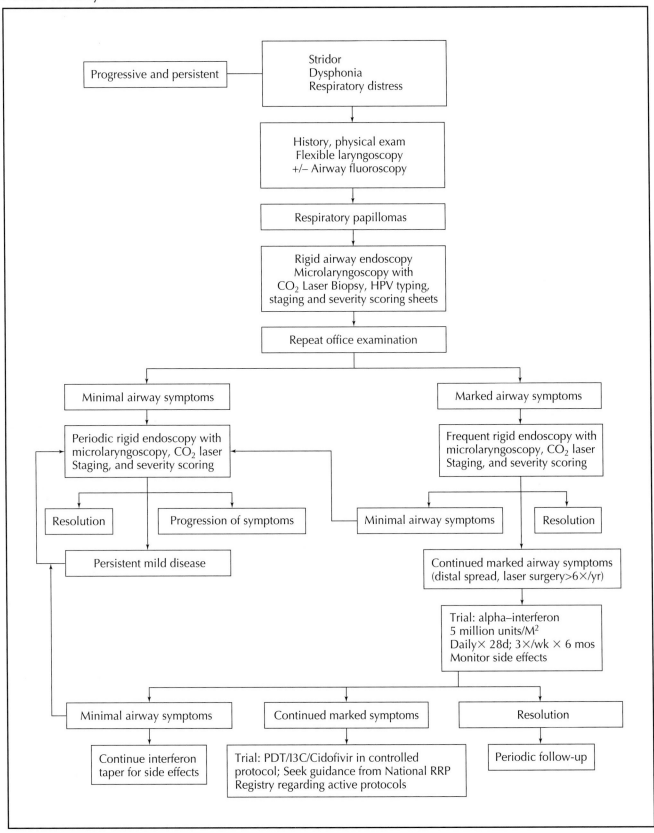

with distal spread of disease may benefit from adjuvant therapy. The best studied adjuvant therapy is alpha-interferon; alternatives include I3C, PDT, cidofivir, and ribavirin utilized in a protocol fashion.

Children who are newly diagnosed with RRP warrant a substantial time commitment on the part of the otolaryngologist in order to provide the family with a frank and open discussion of the disease and its management. We find that support groups such as the Recurrent Respiratory Papilloma Foundation (U.S. telephone number, 609-530-1443) can be a tremendous resource to the families for information and support. Most RRP patients require frequent office visits and endoscopic procedures after the initial diagnosis is made in order to establish the aggressiveness of their disease.

AT A GLANCE . . .

Recurrent Respiratory Papillomatosis

Pathogenesis: viral etiology, HPV types 6 and 11, maternal-fetal transmission or STD, occur at sites in which ciliated and squamous epithelium are juxtaposed

Adverse Effects: life-threatening airway obstruction, acute and chronic respiratory obstruction, voice changes, malignant transformation, psycho-social stress of repeated need for surgery

Symptoms and Signs: hoarseness, stridor, acute respiratory distress, cough, recurrent pneumonia, failure to thrive, dysphagia, or dyspnea

Diagnosis: direct visualization of lesions using FFL or rigid laryngoscopy and bronchoscopy along with biopsy of lesions

Treatment: CO_2 laser vaporization of laryngeal lesions, KTP laser vaporization of tracheobronchal lesions, adjuvant medical therapies (e.g., alpha-interferon, I3C) for recalcitrant cases and distal spread of disease

---

Children with stable papilloma disease requiring fewer than four laser procedures per year and whose parents reliably bring them in before showing signs of respiratory distress can be monitored at home with commercially available infant home intercom-type monitors (e.g., Fisher-Price®). Those with rapidly-recurring papillomas and those whose parents wait until the child is in distress before seeking medical attention may warrant home pulse oximetry with frequent home health nurse visits. Speech and language therapy is offered early in the course of the disease to RRP families.

SUBGLOTTIC HEMANGIOMA

The exact incidence of airway hemangioma is not documented, though cutaneous hemangioma is considered the most common benign tumor of infancy, occurring in as many as 10% of white children.[38,39] The airway may be involved at any level, although the subglottis is the most common site. Reasons for this predilection remain unknown. Considered a congenital lesion, symptoms do not usually occur until a period of increased growth in the first few months of life. It is estimated that 80 to 90% will present within the first 6 months of life with the mean age 3.6 months at diagnosis.[40] About half of the infants with subglottic hemangioma also will have a cutaneous hemangioma. Yet only 1 to 2% of children with cutaneous hemangiomas also have subglottic hemangiomas.[41] Subglottic hemangiomas occur more frequently in females with a 2:1 female to male preponderance.

SPECIAL CONSIDERATION:

Whereas roughly 50% of children with a subglottic hemangioma will also have a cutaneous hemangioma, only about 1 to 2% of children with a cutaneous hemangioma will also have a subglottic hemangioma.

Pathogenesis

Histologically, subglottic hemangiomas are benign. Classic histologic features of proliferating hemangiomas include tubules of plump, proliferating endothelial cells surrounding narrow vessels and an abundance of mast cells.[42] During the involution phase, the color may change from a bright red to a more dusky purple. There is also a progressive flattening of the endothelial cells until an end point of flat, inactive cells surrounding ectatic thin-walled vessels. As the lesions shrink, the number of vessels diminish and are replaced by fibro-fatty tissue.

The widely held notion that the majority of cutaneous cervicofacial hemangiomas disappear completely should be dispelled. In general, the more rapid the rate of involution the more complete the process. Early involuters, in whom the process lasts less than 2 years, can be expected to have an excellent cosmetic result in about 60% of patients. Late involuters, those in which the process lasts more than 4 years, are far less likely to have complete involution with only about 20% achieving an overall favorable outcome.[42] These general principles appear to apply to subglottic hemangiomas as well.

Clinical Course

Subglottic hemangiomas typically present with biphasic stridor and a normal cry. Occasionally, symptoms include cough, cyanosis, and hoarseness. Swallowing is also usually normal. Respiratory symptoms usually are increased when the child becomes agitated. Upper respiratory infections (URI) frequently worsen the symptoms. A diagnosis of recurrent croup may be entertained before the definitive diagnosis is confirmed. As airway obstruction progresses, the child may begin to exhibit feeding problems, cyanotic episodes, dyspnea, and failure to thrive. Preoperative fluoroscopy or anterior-posterior radiographs of the neck may demonstrate an asymmetric subglottic narrowing.

Diagnosis of subglottic hemangioma is based upon characteristic findings at bronchoscopy. The classic appearance is one of an asymmetric, smooth, submucosal, compressible, pink or blue subglottic mass (Fig. 55–3). A left-sided predominance has been reported, but hemangiomas may be bilateral, circumferential, or multiple. The typical lesion is unilateral and sessile. Biopsy usually is not necessary to establish the diagnosis and theoretically may result in significant hemorrhage. The natural history of hemangioma is one of rapid growth for 8 to 18 months (i.e., the *proliferative phase*) followed by a slow regression (i.e., the *involutive phase*) over the next 5 to 8 years. Though it is extremely unusual for hemangiomas to involute spontaneously during the first year of life, about 50% do show a complete regression by age 5 years and 70% by age 7 years.[43]

Adverse Affects

Certainly, the most dreaded complication of subglottic hemangiomas is airway obstruction. Given

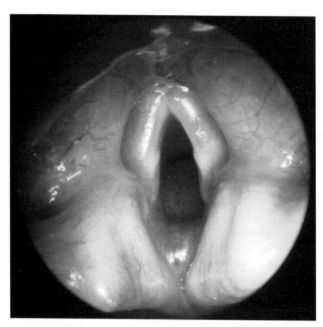

Figure 55–3: A subglottic hemangioma typically appears as an asymmetric, smooth, submucosal subglottic mass with a left-sided predominance.

the relative size of the infant larynx, hemangiomas in this area may sometimes present with life-threatening obstruction requiring a tracheotomy. Depending on the location of the hemangioma, there is also the possibility of voice changes. When subglottic hemangioma is associated with a large, cervicofacial, compound hemangioma, the patient may experience high output cardiac failure. This is usually incipient and more often is associated with a single large hemangioma or multiple large lesions. The *Kasabach-Merritt syndrome* is a phenomenon resulting from platelet sequestration and destruction within the hemangioma as well as a consumptive coagulopathy. This, too, is associated mostly with massive, cervicofacial, compound hemangiomas. Left untreated, a profound thrombocytopenia results and a generalized bleeding disorder occurs. The Kasabach-Merritt syndrome is usually clinically evident within the first few weeks of life, and the patient usually presents with edema and ecchymosis surrounding a rapidly-proliferating hemangioma. This syndrome may be fatal in up to 60% of children.[42]

Treatment

Many different therapies have been advocated to treat subglottic hemangiomas. Because the natural history of these lesions can be unpredictable, the question remains how to best deal with a potential life-threatening airway compromise until involution occurs. In patients with mild symptoms, spontaneous involution is anticipated and "watchful waiting" is reasonable. Symptomatic obstruction demands more aggressive intervention. Tracheotomy can "buy time" allowing the tracheal lumen to enlarge with the growth of the child and, more importantly, giving the hemangioma an opportunity to involute spontaneously. However, tracheotomy requires considerable home care and may be associated with language delay and complications such as tube obstruction. Alternatives include systemic corticosteroids, laser surgery, open surgical excision, and alpha-interferon therapy.

The first line of treatment for a hemangioma that affects a vital function such as breathing is oral corticosteroids. These medications inhibit growth of the lesion during the proliferative phase of hemangioma growth.[42] Once the lesion has begun to involute, they are no longer effective. High starting doses of prednisone at 4 mg/kg/day or 8 mg/kg every other day for a period of 4 weeks are appropriate. The medication is then tapered over a 2-week period. At this high dosage, a significant response is seen in about 75% of patients,[42] although regrowth resumes within a few days of completion of this course in about 40% of patients. A second 6-week course after a rest of several weeks may be tried if the initial response was good. Unfortunately, proliferation often recurs anew after the second course has been completed. Daily maintenance doses of approximately 1 mg/kg body weight may then be considered. The child should be followed closely by a pediatrician and monitored for any significant steroid side effects. It is important to remember that the immunization schedule should be discontinued while the child is on high-dose steroids.

SPECIAL CONSIDERATION:

High-dose steroid therapy can be expected to reduce markedly the size of a subglottic hemangioma in about 70% of cases, though short-lived steroid side effects should be anticipated and immunizations need to be discontinued.

Surgical excision using the CO_2 laser has been used widely for treatment of this lesion.[41] The pro-

cedure begins with biopsy as necessary, followed by simple vaporization of remaining abnormal tissue. If a tracheotomy for airway maintenance has not been required before the surgery, it is usually unnecessary for the procedure itself. However, the physician must provide intense humidification in the immediate postoperative period to prevent airway obstruction from eschar formation. Cotton and Tewfik advocate caution in the use of the CO_2 laser because of the risk of developing subglottic stenosis.[44] They reported three such cases after laser therapy. Mizono and Dedo suggest that the following guidelines be kept in mind when utilizing laser therapy for treatment of subglottic hemangioma[45]:

(1) Use of laser therapy only on capillary-type lesions.
(2) Use of laser therapy only in patients with subglottic lesions and not in those with diffuse hemangioma extending to the trachea.
(3) The staged resection of large subglottic lesions to prevent the apposition of raw mucosal surfaces.

Open surgical excision is another option that had received less attention previously, but that now appears to have several advantages in selected patients. Froehlich,[46] Seid,[47] and Phipps[48] advocate this as their treatment of choice when airway obstruction is significant enough to require a tracheotomy. The lesion may be approached through a laryngofissure and removed through submucosal dissection. However, the long-term sequelae of laryngofissure in this age group are not established. Advocates also caution against open surgical excision when there is the suggestion of a significant extra-laryngeal extent of the disease, such as a supraglottic or tracheal blush. Skilled pediatric intensive care capabilities and pediatric anesthesia are necessary to make this a more appealing option.

SPECIAL CONSIDERATION:

Caution needs to be exercised in use of the CO_2 laser for treatment of subglottic hemangioma, especially if more extensive than a unilateral lesion, to prevent the development of a subglottic stenosis.

Alpha-interferon has been utilized to treat hemangiomas with good success and can be considered when traditional modalities fail.[43,49-51] Ohlms[49] et al. reported on their experience with the use of alpha-interferon in 15 patients with airway-obstructing hemangiomas that had not responded to laser or corticosteroid therapy. An interferon dose of 3×10^6 IU/m^2 body surface given subcutaneously was administered daily until a 50% or greater regression in tumor size and a stable airway was achieved. All previously nontracheotomized patients (8/15) responded and did not require a tracheotomy after starting interferon therapy, and six of the seven patients who were tracheotomized before interferon were able to be decannulated after completion of therapy. No long-term morbidity of interferon therapy was encountered. Ohlms et al. suggest the use of interferon when traditional therapeutic modalities such as steroid and laser therapy fail, and especially when subglottic hemangioma presents as part of a massive life-threatening cervicofacial hemangioma.

AT A GLANCE . . .

Subglottic Hemangioma

Pathogenesis: Congenital lesion consisting of abnormal proliferating endothelial cells, airway predilection for subglottis with rapid growth followed by slow regression

Adverse Effects: airway obstruction, voice changes, Kasabach-Merritt Syndrome, congestive heart failure

Symptoms and Signs: biphasic stridor that increases with agitation or respiratory infection, coinciding cervicofacial cutaneous hemangioma, cough, cyanosis, hoarseness, platelet dysfunction

Diagnosis: based on history and direct observation during laryngoscopy and bronchoscopy of a typically unilateral, sessile, compressible, submucosal, reddish-blue mass in the subglottis

Treatment: controversial depending on severity of airway compromise; may choose observation, CO_2 laser, tracheotomy, interferon, steroids and/or surgical excision

---

Practice Pathway

Practice Pathway 55-2 illustrates the diagnosis and treatment of children with subglottic hemangioma.

Either FFL or rigid laryngoscopy and bronchoscopy are essential for making the initial diagnosis. The first modality chosen for treatment depends greatly on the degree of airway compromise, ranging from watchful waiting to tracheotomy. Options include high-dose corticosteroids, use of the CO_2 laser, open surgical excision, and systemic alpha-interferon therapy.

OTHER BENIGN AND MALIGNANT NEOPLASMS OF THE PEDIATRIC AIRWAY

Other benign and malignant neoplasms affecting the pediatric airway are extremely rare. Table 55-1 lists the most common benign and malignant neoplasms of the larynx in children by their cell of origin.

Malignant tumors of the larynx are extremely uncommon in children. Previous, radiation therapy RRP as well as malignant degeneration of invasive papillomas has been implicated in the development of squamous cell carcinoma. Other risks factors include, smoking, chemical carcinogens, and intrauterine exposure to ionizing radiation. RRP caused by HPV subtypes 16 and 18 appear to be more likely to develop malignant degeneration.

Histopathologically, grossly, and clinically, squamous cell carcinoma in the child is similar to that in the adult. However, pediatric laryngeal carcinomas tend to have been present for a longer period of time before diagnosis, likely because of a lower index of suspicion, and the disease tends to present at a more advanced state. Treatment modalities are the same for childhood laryngeal carcinoma as for adult disease. Prompt recognition and treatment of any abnormal laryngeal mass in a young child with hoarseness is critical.

The most common malignant tumor of connective tissue origin is the *rhabdomyosarcoma*. The embryonal cell type has been found to be the predominant variety of rhabdomyosarcoma affecting the larynx.[52] As with other rhabdomyosarcomas, nonmutilating surgical excision, radiation therapy, and chemotherapy are the recommended treatment modalities.

Neurogenic tumors of the larynx are also extremely rare in children. They may be more common in female patients and tend to occur in the

Practice Pathway 55–2   SUBGLOTTIC HEMANGIOMA

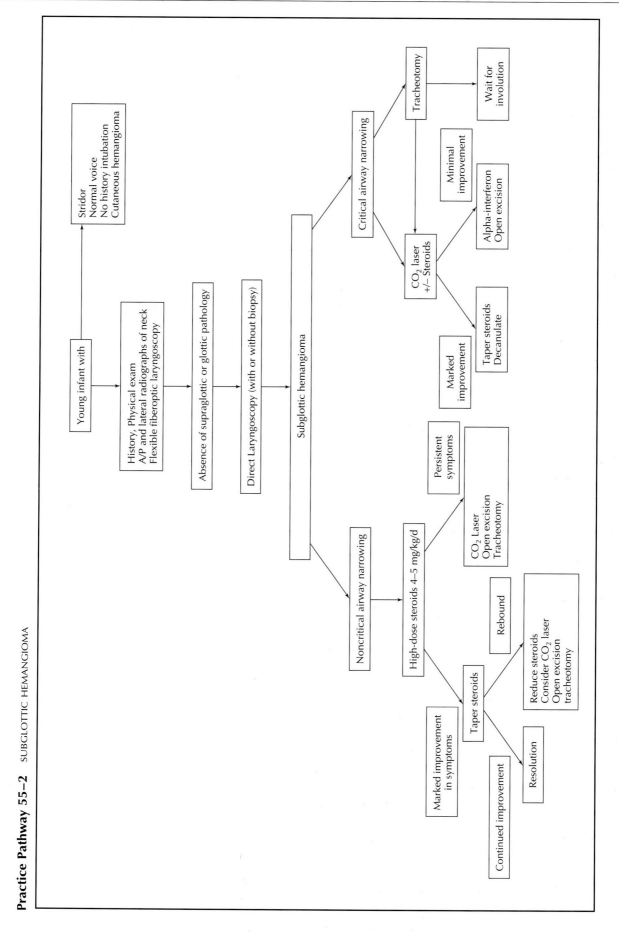

supraglottic region. The most common neurogenic tumors of the larynx included *neurofibroma, neurilemmoma, granular cell tumor,* and *carcinoid tumor.* Neurofibroma and neurilemmoma are of Schwann cell origin. Neurilemmomas are typically solitary and encapsulated and may occur in association with neurofibromatosis (i.e., *Von Recklinghausen's disease*), especially in children. In such cases, the presence of six or more "cafe-au-lait" spots greater than 1.5 cm in diameter establishes the diagnosis. Nearly all the tumors described involve the arytenoid or aryepiglottic folds. A biopsy specimen should be obtained for diagnosis if a submucosal mass is discovered in the larynx, especially in a patient with other manifestations of neurofibromatosis. Complete surgical excision of the lesion is recommended, and this often requires a supraglottic laryngectomy.[53] It is important to remember that this is a benign lesion and that judicious subtotal removal is indicated when vital structures are involved.

Granular cell tumors are also extremely rare in children. Clinically, the lesions appear as a polypoid or sessile mass that may be solitary or multiple. The tumor generally takes a benign course and most pediatric patients respond well to local excision performed endoscopically.

Cartilaginous and bony tumors also can occur in the trachea and larynx of children. They may appear as enlargements of existing tracheal or bronchial cartilage, are firm, and may be as hard as glass when ossified. These tumors grow slowly and may cause extensive bronchopulmonary destruction. Most cartilaginous tumors arise in the cricoid cartilage, primarily from the posterior plate. Their growth is mostly intraluminal and even chondrosarcomas are usually indolent and rarely metastasize, making local resection adequate treatment if it is technically feasible.

In summary, the basic principles for treatment of these rare benign and malignant tumors of the larynx and trachea are similar regardless of the cell of origin. Removal should be as complete as possible, but conservative to spare voice, with the surgical approach determined primarily by the tumor size and location. With more systemic diseases such as leukemia or rhabdomyosarcoma, the addition of radiation and chemotherapy may be indicated.

REFERENCES

1. Jones S, Myers GN. Benign neoplasm's of the larynx. Otolaryngol Clin North Am. 1985; 17(1):151–178.

2. Derkay CS. Task force on recurrent respiratory papillomas. Arch Otolaryngol Head Neck Surg. 1995; 121: 1386–1391.

3. Mounts P, Shah KV, Kashima H. Viral etiology of juvenile and adult onset squamous papilloma of the larynx. Proc Natl Acad Sci USA 1982; 79:5425–5429.

4. Morgan AH, Zitsch RP. Recurrent respiratory papillomatosis in children: A retrospective study of management and complications. Ear Nose Throat J, 1986; 65:19–28.

5. Cohn AM, Kos JT, Taber LH, et al. Recurring laryngeal papilloma. Am J Otolaryngol 1981; 2:129–5429.

6. Strong MS, Jako GJ. Recurrent respiratory papillomatosis: Management with the CO_2 laser. Ann Otol Rhinol Laryngol 1976; 8:508–516.

7. Fox CF, Kashima HK, Kurman RJ, et al. Papillomaviruses: Biological and clinical implications. Clinical Courier (Gardner-Caldwell SynerMed/CICLA Continuing Education) 1985; 3(6):1–8.

8. Lindeberg H, Elbrond O. Laryngeal papillomas: The epidemiology in a Danish subpopulation 1965–1984. Clin Otolaryngol 1991; 15:125–131.

9. Kashima HK, Shah F, Lyles A, et al. Factors in juvenile-onset and adult recurrent respiratory papillomas. Laryngoscope 1992; 102:9–13.

10. Steinberg BM, Auborn KJ. Papillomaviruses in head and neck disease: Pathophysiology and possible regulation. J Cell Biochem, 1993; 17F(Supplement): 155–164.

11. Kashima HK, Kessis T, Mounts P, et al. Polymerase chain reaction identification of human papilloma virus DNA in CO_2 laser plume from recurrent respiratory papillomatosis. Otolaryngol Head Neck Surg 1991; 104:191–195.

12. Steinberg BM, Topp WC, Schneider PS, et al. Laryngeal papillomavirus infection during clinical remission N Engl J Med 1983; 308:1261–1264.

13. Rihkaren H, Aaltonen LM, Syranen SM. Human papillomavirus in laryngeal papillomas and in adjacent normal epithelium. Clin Otolaryngol 1993; 18: 470–474.

14. Brandsma JL, Abramson AL. Association of papillomavirus with cancers of the head and neck. Arch Otolaryngol Head Neck Surg 1989; 115:621–625.

15. Kashima HK, Mounts P, Leventhal B, et al. Sites of predilection in recurrent respiratory papillomatosis. Ann Otol Rhinol Laryngeal 1993; 102:580–583.

16. Kosko J, Derkay CS. Role of cesarean section in the prevention of recurrent respiratory papillomas: Is there one? Int J Pediatr Otorhinolaryngol 1996; 1:31–38.

17. Shah K, Kashima H, Polk BF, et al. Rarity of caesarean delivery in cases of juvenile onset respiratory papillomatosis. Obstet Gynecol 1986; 68:795–799.

18. Koutsky LA, Wolner-Hanssen P. Genital papillomavi-

rus infection: Current knowledge and future prospects. Obstet Gynecol Clin North Am 1989; 16: 541–561.

19. Reid R, Laverty CR, Copplesen M, et al. Non-condylomotous cervical wart virus infection. Obst Gyn J 1982; SS:476–482.

20. Bennett RS, Powell KR. Human papillomavirus: Association between laryngeal papillomas and genital warts. Pediatr Infect Dis J 1987; C:229–232.

21. Cook TA, Brunchswig JP, Butel JS, et al. Laryngeal Papilloma: Etiologic and therapeutic considerations. Ann Otol Rhinol Laryngol 1973; 82:649–655.

22. Hallen C, Majmudar B. The relationship between juvenile laryngeal papillomatosis and maternal condylomata acuminata. J Reprod Med 1986; 31:804–807.

23. Smith EM, Johnson SR, Pignatari S, et al. Perinatal vertical transmission of human papilloma virus and subsequent development of respiratory tract papillomatosis. Ann Otol Rhinol Laryngol 1991; 100: 479–483.

24. *Guidelines for Perinatal Care, 3rd ed.* American Academy of Pediatrics American College of Obstetrics and Gynecology. 1990, pp 127–128.

25. Mounts P, Kashima H. Association of human papillomavirus subtype and clinical course in respiratory papillomatosis. Laryngoscope 1984; 94: 28–33.

26. Chipps BE, DonMcClug FL, Freidman EM, et al. Respiratory papillomas: Presentation before six months Pediatr Pulmonol 1990; 9:125–130.

27. Cole RR, Myer CM, Cotton RT. Tracheotomy in children with recurrent respiratory papillomatosis. Head Neck 1989; 11:226–230.

28. Derkay CS, Malis D, Zalzel G, et al. Uniform staging/scoring system for RRP. Laryngoscope 108: 935–937.

29. Lindeberg H, Elbrond O. Laryngeal papillomas: Clinical aspects in a series of 231 patients. Clin Otolaryngol 1989; 14:333–342.

30. Shapiro AM, Rimell FL, Pou A, et al. Tracheotomy in children with juvenile-onset recurrent respiratory papillomatosis: The Children's Hospital of Pittsburg experience. Ann Otol Rhinol Laryngol 1996; 105: 1–5.

31. Leventhal BG, Kashima HK, Mounts P, et al. Long-term response of recurrent respiratory papillomatosis to treatment with lymphoblasoid interferon alfa-nl. N Engl J Med 1991; 325:613–617.

32. Zemer HP, Dley W, Claros A, et al. Recombinant Interferson-alpha-2C in laryngeal papillomatosis: Preliminary results of a prospective mulicenter trial. Oncology 1985; 42(Supplement 1):15–18.

33. Healy GB, Gelber RD, Trowbridge AL, et al. Treatment of recurrent respiratory papillomatosis with human leukocyte interferon: Results of a multicenter

randomized clinical trial. N Engl J Med 1988; 319: 401–407.

34. Deunes L, et al. Use of interferon-alpha in laryngeal papillomatosis: 8 years of the Cuban National Programme. J Laryngol Otol 1997; 111:(2)134–140.

35. Heberhold C, Walther EK. Combined laser surgery and adjuvant intra-lesional interferon injections in patients with laryngotracheal papillomatosis. In: *Laser in Otolaryngology Head and Neck Surgery. Adv Otorhinolaryngol.* Basel, Karger, 1995; 49:166–169.

36. Abramson AL, Shikowitz MJ, Mullooly VM, et al. Clinical effects of photodynamic therapy on recurrent laryngeal papillomas. Arch Otolaryngol Head Neck Surg 1992; 118:25–29.

37. Newfield L, Goldsmith A, Bradlow HL, et al. Estrogen metabolism and human papillomavirus-induced tumors of the larynx: Chemo-prophylaxis with Indole-3-Carbinol. Anticancer Res 1993; 13:337–341.

38. Finn MC, Glowacki J, Mulliken JB. Congenital vascular lesions: Clinical application of a new classification. J Pediatr Surg 1983; 18:894–900.

39. Mulliken JB, Glowacki J. Hemangiomas and vascular malformations in infants and children: A classification based on endothelial characteristics. Plast Reconstr Surg 1982; 69:412–422.

40. Shikhani AH, Marsh BR, Jones MM, et al. Infantile subglottic hemangiomas: An update. Ann Otol Rhinol Laryngol 1986; 95:336–347.

41. Sie KC, McGill T, Healy GB. Subglottic hemangiomas: 10 years experience with the carbon dioxide laser. Ann Otol Rhino Laryngol 1994; 103:167–172.

42. Waner M, Suen JY. Advances in the management of congenital vascular lesions of the head and neck. Adv Otorhinolaryngol 1996; 10:31–54.

43. Ezekowtiz RAB, Mulliken JB, Folkman J. Interferon alfa-2A therapy for life-threatening hemangiomas of infancy. N Engl J Med 1992; 326:1456–1463.

44. Cotton RT, Tewfik TL. Laryngeal stenosis following carbon dioxide laser in subglottic hemangioma: Report of three cases. Ann Otol Rhinol Laryngol 1985; 94:494–497.

45. Mizono G, Dedo HH. Subglottic hemangiomas in infants: Treatment with CO_2 laser. Laryngoscope 1984; 94:638–41.

46. Froehlich P, Stamm D, Floret D, et al. Management of Subglottic hemangioma. Clin Otolaryngol 1995; 4: 336–339.

47. Seid AB, Pransky SM, Kearns DB. The open surgical approach to subglottic hemangioma. Int J Pediatr Otorhinolaryngol 1993; 22:85–90.

48. Phipps CD, Gibson WS, Wood WE. Infantile subglottic hemangioma: A review and presentation of two cases of surgical excision. Int J Ped Otorhinolaryngol 1997; 41:71–79.

49. Ohlms LA, Jones DT, McGill TJ, et al. Interferon alfa-

2A therapy for airway hemangiomas. Ann Otol Rhinol Laryngol 1994; 103:1–8.

50. Bauman MN, Burke DK, Smith RJH. Treatment of massive or life-threatening hemangiomas with recombinant α 2a-interferon. Otolaryngol Head Neck Surg 1997; 117:99–110.

51. MacArthur CJ, Senders CW, Katz J. The use of interferon Alfa-2A for life-threatening hemangiomas. Arch Otolaryngol Head Neck Surg 1995; 121:690–693.

52. Dodd-o JM, Wieneke, KF, Rosman PM. Laryngeal Rhabdomyosarcoma. Cancer 1987; 59:1012.

53. Greinwald J, Derkay CS, Schechter GL. Management of massive had and neck neurofibromas in children. Am J Otolaryngol 1996; 17:136–142.

VI

THE NECK

56 Embryology and Anatomy of the Neck

Carol J. MacArthur

EMBRYOLOGY OF THE NECK

Early in development, the primitive foregut differentiates into the pharynx, esophagus, stomach, and proximal duodenum. The *pharynx* occupies most of the foregut during the first few weeks of development.[1] The *foregut* sits below the developing brain and above the primitive heart. Initially, the mouth is separated from the pharynx by the *buccopharyngeal membrane.* The buccopharyngeal membrane disappears by the end of the third week. At this time, *mesodermal bars* appear in the walls of the pharynx. These become the *pharyngeal* (or *branchial*) *arches,* which fuse ventrally to form U-shaped structures that support the pharynx.[2] At 5 weeks of age, there are six pairs of *mesodermal arches* lying in the transverse plane of the neck or lateral wall of the foregut. The arches are numbered in a cranial to caudal direction. The fifth arch is small, does not appear on the surface, and disappears early. Therefore, only arches I, II, III, IV, and VI are important in terms of anatomic derivatives in the human infant. The arches are separated externally by ectodermal-lined clefts and internally by endodermal-lined pouches (Fig. 56-1). Each arch contains a core cartilaginous skeleton, muscle rudiment, a cranial nerve, and an artery. Derivatives of the arches are therefore cartilage, bone, muscle, and connective tissue. Derivatives of the pouches are glandular or associated with the digestive tract. Each arch is innervated by a cranial nerve, which follows the muscle wherever it may eventually migrate; therefore, the origin of the muscles associated with each arch can always

be traced by their innervation. From the primitive heart tube, a ventral aorta divides right and left into two branches that curve caudally as the two dorsal aortae. As the pharyngeal arches develop, a vessel in each arch joins the ventral and dorsal aorta. The transitory branchial pattern is gone by the seventh week of development; however, much attention has been devoted to the pharyngeal arches in the embryo because of their complexity and phylogenetic significance.[1] The term *branchial* rather than *pharyngeal* is used here because of its wide usage and acceptance; however, pharyngeal is more accurate because the development of the pharynx and its derivatives does not proceed in the same fashion as the gills of nonmammalian aquatic vertebrates.

The structures formed from the primitive pharynx consist not only of the lateral branchial appartus, but also the unpaired ventral endodermal floor. The *endodermal floor* produces the tongue, thyroid gland, larynx, and trachea.

Most of the musculature of the neck is formed by differentiation of branchial arch mesoderm and mesenchyme with contribution from cervical somites. For instance, the sternocleidomastoid and trapezius muscles are derived from branchiomeric tissue with contribution from the occipital somite muscle cell migration. These two muscles are innervated by the spinal accessory nerve. The infrahyoid strap muscles are completely of somitic origin, with innervation from branches of the hypoglossal nerve, C1, and C2.

The fate of the branchial arches cranially is known in greater detail than it is caudally. Table 56-1 shows the derivatives of the branchial arches. As the branchial apparatus develops, the first and second arches grow in a caudal direction, creating the epipericardial ridge and the cervical sinus of His. The *epipericardial ridge* grows from development

Pediatric Otolaryngology, Edited by R.F. Wetmore, H.R. Muntz, and T.J. McGill. Thieme Medical Publishers, Inc., New York © 2000.

TABLE 56–1:   Derivatives of Branchial Arches, Clefts, and Pouches

First Cleft	First Arch	First Pouch
External auditory canal Tympanic membrane	Incus Malleus Meckel's cartilage Muscles of mestication Tensor tympani muscle Tensor veli palatini muscle Mylohyold muscle Digastric muscle (anterior belly) Pinna Fifth cranial nerve External maxillary artery	Eustachian tube Middle ear Mastoid air cells

Second Cleft	Second Arch	Second Pouch
Cervical sinus of His	Stapes suprastructure Hyoid (lesser cornu, body) Styloid process Stylohyoid ligament Muscles of facial expression Buccinator muscle Platysma muscle Digastric muscle (posterior belly) Stylohyoid muscle Stapedius muscle Seventh and eighth cranial nerves Stapedial artery	Middle ear Palatine tonsil

Third Cleft	Third Arch	Third Pouch
Cervical sinus of His	Hyoid (greater cornu, body) Stylopharyngeus muscle Constrictor muscle (superior middle) Ninth cranial nerve Internal carotid artery	Inferior parathyroids Thymus, thymic duct

Fourth Cleft	Fourth Arch	Fourth Pouch
Cervical sinus of His	Thyroid cartilage Cuneiform cartilage Cricothyroid muscle Constrictor muscle (inferior) Tenth cranial nerve Aortic arch (left) Subclavian Artery (right)	Superior parathyroids

Sixth Cleft	Sixth Arch	Sixth Pouch
	Cricoid cartilage Arytenoid cartilage Corniculate cartilage Intrinsic muscles of larynx Recurrent laryngeal nerve Ductus arteriosus (left) Pulmonary artery (right)	

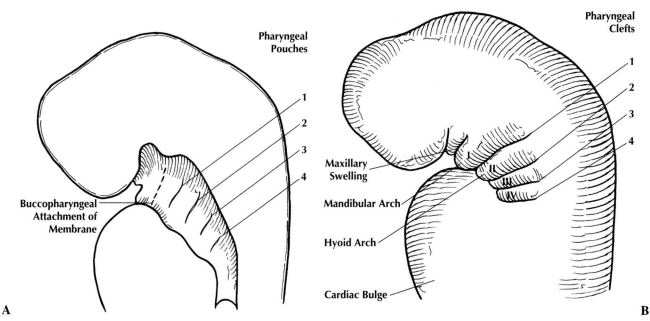

Figure 56–1: (A) Sagittal section through the cephalic end of a 5-week embryo (approximately 6 mm), showing the openings of the pharyngeal pouches along the lateral wall of the gut. Broken line represents the approximate site of attachment of the buccopharyngeal membrane. (B) The pharyngeal arches and clefts in a 5-week embryo. (From Langman J, ed. *Medical Embryology: Human Development—Normal and Abnormal, 3rd ed.* Baltimore: Williams & Wilkins, 1975, p. 262, with permission.)

of mesoderm in this area and contains rudiments of the future sternocleidomastoid, trapezius, infrahyoid, and lingual musculature. The nerves of the epipericardial ridge are spinal (spinal accessory and hypoglossal), not cranial. As the epipericardial ridge grows, the third, fourth and sixth arches become recessed, creating a deep ectodermal pit, known as the *cervical sinus of His* (Fig. 56-2). This sinus is eventually obliterated. If the sinus fails to be obliterated or is incompletely obliterated, a branchial cleft cyst, sinus, or fistula can occur of types II, III, or IV.

Branchial Arches

Early in the development of each arch, a cartilage bar is present that remodels into cartilage, bone, or connective tissue. Figure 56-3 shows the skeletal derivatives of each branchial arch schematically.

First branchial arch

The cartilage of the *first branchial arch* contains a dorsal portion, the maxillary process, and a ventral portion known as *Meckel's cartilage* or the *mandibular process.* Both the maxillary and mandibular processes eventually regress. The incus and malleus

are the only bony structures that persist from Meckel's cartilage. The *mandible* subsequently is formed by intramembranous ossification of mesodermal tissue around Meckel's cartilage. The sphenomandibular ligament and anterior ligament of the malleus are also remnants of Meckel's cartilage.

The muscles derived from the first arch are the muscles of mastication (i.e., temporalis, masseter, and pterygoids), the anterior belly of the digastric, the mylohyoid, the tensor tympani, and the tensor veli palatini. The nerve supplying the first arch muscles is the *trigeminal nerve.* As well, the mandibular branch of the trigeminal nerve also provides sensation to the skin over the mandible and the anterior two-thirds of the mucosa of the tongue. The glands and mucous membrane of the anterior two-thirds of the tongue are also derived from the first arch. The first arch artery degenerates before the other arch arteries are formed. However, ventral portions of the first arch artery may persist and contribute to the development of the *maxillary artery.*[2] The *pinna* is formed from six tubercles at the dorsal end of the first and second arches. These tubercles surround the dorsal end of the first branchial groove, which becomes the external ear canal (Fig. 56-4).

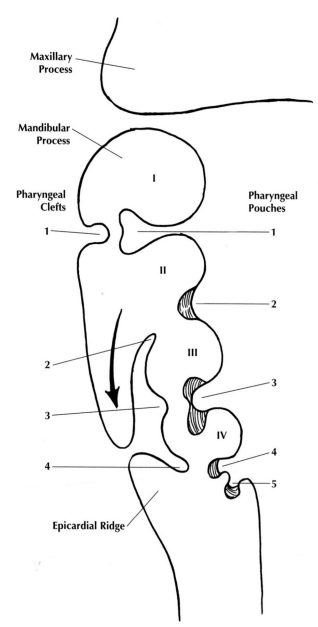

Figure 56–2: Schematic representation of the development of the pharyngeal clefts and pouches. Note how the second arch grows over the third and fourth arches, thereby burying the second, third, and fourth pharyngeal clefts. (From Langman J, ed. *Medical Embryology: Human Development—Normal and Abnormal, 3rd ed.* Baltimore: Williams & Wilkins, 1975, p. 266, with permission.)

Second branchial arch

The cartilage of the *second branchial arch* is known as *Reichert's cartilage.* Derivatives of this arch cartilage are the upper body and lesser cornu of the hyoid bone, styloid process, stylohoid ligament,

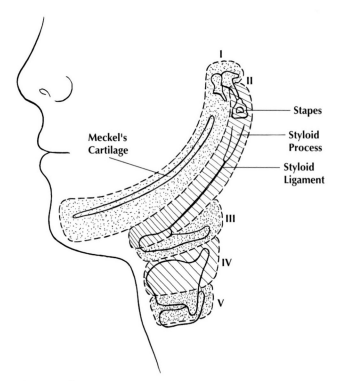

Figure 56–3: Skeletal derivatives of branchial arches. (From Graney DO. Anatomy. In: Cummings CW, Fredrickson JM, Harker LA, et al., eds. *Otolaryngology—Head and Neck Surgery, 2nd ed.* St. Louis: Mosby-Year Book, 1993; p. 1562, with permission.)

and stapes suprastructure (the stapes footplate is derived from the otic capsule).

Second arch muscles include the muscles of facial expression, buccinator, platysma, posterior belly of the digastric, stylohoid, and stapedius. The second arch nerve is the *seventh cranial nerve,* supplying motor innervation to the muscles of facial expression and sensation to a portion of the external auditory canal (EAC). The second arch artery may persist as the *stapedial artery,* which is an abnormal variant coursing through the crura of the stapes. Ventral portions of the second arch artery may also contribute to the maxillary artery.

Third branchial arch

The derivatives of the *third branchial arch* cartilage are the greater cornu and inferior body of the hyoid bone. The third arch muscles are the stylopharyngeus and possibly the superior and middle pharyngeal constrictors.[3] The mucous membrane and

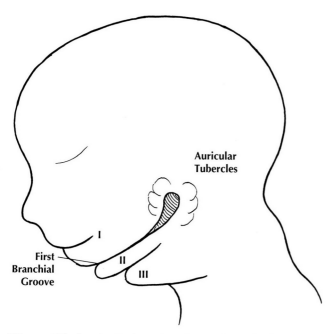

Figure 56–4: Auricular tubercles at the end of the first branchial cleft. (From Ellis P.DM. Branchial cleft anomalies, thyroglossal cysts, and fistulae. In: Evans JNG, ed. *Scott-Brown's Otolaryngology: Vol. 6, Pediatric Otolaryngology, 5th ed.* London: Butter North—Heinemann, 1987, p. 298, with permission. Originally modified from Frazer JE. Journal of Anatomy 1926; 61.)

glands of the posterior third of the tongue, valleculae, and anterior surface of the epiglottis also derive form the third arch.[2] The nerve of the third arch is the *glossopharyngeal* or *ninth cranial nerve.* The third arch artery contributes to the proximal internal carotid artery, external carotid artery, and common carotid artery.

Fourth and sixth branchial arches

The cartilaginous derivatives from the *fourth and sixth branchial arches* fuse to form the laryngeal cartilages: the thyroid, cricoid, arytenoid, corniculate, and cuneiform. The muscles arising from the fourth arch are the cricothyroid and the inferior pharyngeal constrictor. The nerve of the fourth arch is the superior laryngeal branch of the vagus nerve. The fourth arch artery gives rise to the arch of the aorta on the left side and the proximal subclavian on the right. An aortic ring surrounding the trachea and esophagus can occur as a result of persistence of the right and left fourth arch arteries and dorsal aortic root. An aberrant subclavian artery can arise

if the subclavian artery on the right passes from the dorsal aortic root behind the esophagus.

The muscles arising form the sixth arch are the intrinsic muscles of the larynx. The recurrent laryngeal branch of the vagus is the nerve of the sixth arch. The sixth arch artery becomes the *ductus arteriosus* on the left (connecting the left pulmonary artery to the arch of the aorta), and the *pulmonary artery* on the right (Fig. 56-5).

Branchial Pouches

The *first pouch* gives rise to the eustachian tube (ET), middle ear, and mastoid antrum. This occurs by lateral extension of the first pouch to meet the first cleft at the tympanic membrane (TM). The second, third, and fourth pouches have at their distal extremity a dorsal and ventral wing. The *second pouch* dorsally contributes to the middle ear and ventrally to the palatine tonsil. The *third pouch* dorsally contributes to the inferior parathyroids and ventrally to the thymus and thymic duct. The *inferior parathyroids* are drawn inferiorly with the thymus toward the chest as the thymus descends. As the thymus descends, it has a connection with the third pouch, the *thymopharyngeal duct.* This duct disappears by the eighth to ninth week of life. If the thymic duct persists, a cervical thymic cyst may occur. The dorsal part of the *fourth pouch* contributes to the superior parathyroids. The ventral part of the fourth pouch may contribute to the thymus gland and to the thyroid gland, but solid evidence is lacking as to the derivatives of the ventral part of the fourth branchial pouch.[3]

The dorsal portion of the fourth pouch and the *fifth pouch* (termed the *caudal pharyngeal pouch complex* or *ultimobranchial body*[1]) probably fuse with the superior parathyroids and become lost in the developing thyroid gland. However, much debate still exists as to the fate of these structures. The term "lateral thyroid primordia" also has been used for the products of pouches four and five. It is thought by some that the ultimobranchial body contributes to thyroid follicles, thymic tissue, or the parafollicular C cells of the thyroid (i.e., the cells that produce calcitonin, which is the calcium regulating hormone).[3] Also, neural crest cells contribute to the development of the *ultimobranchial gland.*[1] The lateral thyroid primordia may contribute to the development of the thyroid gland, along with the median thyroid anlage.[1]

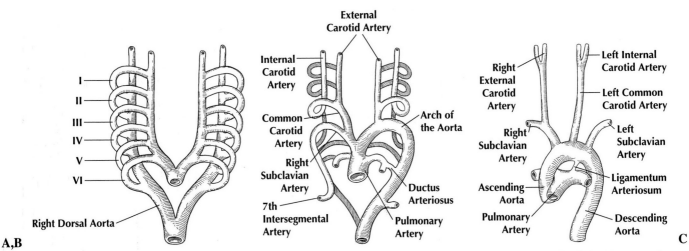

A,B   C

Figure 56–5: (A) Diagram of the aortic arches and dorsal aortae before transformation into the definitive vascular pattern. (B) Diagram of the aortic arches and dorsal aortae after the transformation. The obliterated components are indicated by broken lines. (C) The great arteries in the adult. (From Langman J, ed. *Medical Embryology: Human development—Normal and Abnormal, 3rd ed.* Baltimore: Williams & Wilkins, 1975, p. 235, with permission.)

SPECIAL CONSIDERATION:

There is still much debate about what happens to the dorsal portions of the fourth and fifth branchial pouches. Some think that they contribute to thyroid follicles, thymic tissue, or the parafollicular C cells of the thyroid.

Branchial Clefts

Although there are four branchial clefts present in the 5-week-old embryo, only the first one contributes to any definitive structure. The *first branchial cleft* gives rise to the EAC, and the epithelial lining at the bottom of the canal contributes to the formation of the eardrum. Duplication anomalies give rise to first branchial cleft cysts, sinuses, or fistulae. The *second, third,* and *fourth branchial clefts* temporarily give rise to the cervical sinus of His, but this sinus is obliterated in the embryo by 6 to 7 weeks of age in the normal situation.

Thyroid Gland

The *thyroid gland* appears in the fourth week of development as a midline thickening of the endoderm of the floor of the pharynx between the first and second branchial pouches, between the tuberculum impar and the copula. This point of origin is visible later as the *foramen cecum* (Fig. 56–6). The *bilobed thyroid primordium* descends into the neck, remaining attached to the *thyroglossal duct.* The thyroid gland reaches the level of the laryngeal primordium by the age of 7-weeks gestation. The thyroglossal duct is obliterated, but if it persists, a thyroglossal duct cyst can occur. Because the thyroglossal duct with the thyroid primordium passes between the first and second branchial arches, it descends between the mandible cranially (first arch) and the hyoid bone caudally (second and third arches). Therefore, the duct is associated intimately with the hyoid bone and lies anterior to it. It also hooks around the inferior border of the hyoid bone, and occasionally may pass behind or, more rarely, through the hyoid bone.[2] If the thyroid gland does not descend, a *lingual thyroid* can occur. Accessory thyroid tissue may be found in the neck, along the path it descends from the foramen cecum to the lower neck. Whether or not a part of the thyroid

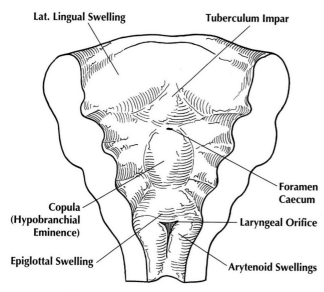

Lat. Lingual Swelling

Tuberculum Impar

Foramen Caecum

Copula (Hypobranchial Eminence)

Laryngeal Orifice

Epiglottal Swelling

Arytenoid Swellings

Figure 56–6: The ventral portions of the pharyngeal arches seen from above at approximately 5 weeks (6 mm). Note the foramen cecum, the site of origin of the thyroid primordium. (From Langman J, ed. *Medical Embryology: Human development—Normal and Abnormal, 3rd ed.* Baltimore: Williams & Wilkins, 1975, p. 270, with permission.)

gland is formed by epithelial proliferation of the fourth branchial pouch is still under debate.

ANATOMY OF THE NECK

Surface Anatomy

The neck is divided into two regions, the anterior neck (i.e., the *cervix*) and the porterior aspect (i.e., the *nucha*). The nuchal region belongs more properly to the back and spine. The cervical area is of the most interest to the otolaryngologist. Its boundaries are the mandible, the mastoid tip, the anterior border of the trapezius muscle, the clavicle, and the midline of the neck.

Triangles of the Neck

Posterior triangle

The sternocleidomastoid muscle divides the neck into the anterior and posterior triangles (Fig. 56-7). The boundaries of the *posterior triangle* are the trapezius muscle, the clavicle, and the sternocleido-

mastoid muscle. The floor is the deep layer of the deep cervical fascia. The roof is the superficial layer of the deep cervical fascia. The contents are the subclavian artery, brachial plexus, the spinal accessory nerve, two branches of the thyrocervical trunk artery, and posterior cervical nodes. The omohyoid muscle further divides the posterior triangle into the *occipital triangle* superiorly and the *subclavian,* or *supraclavicular, triangle* inferiorly.

Anterior triangle

The boundaries of the *anterior cervical triangle* are the sternocleidomastoid muscle, the midline of the neck, and the mandible. The floor is the mylohyoid, hyoglossus, thyrohyoid, and constrictor muscles (deep). The roof is the superficial layer of the deep cervical fascia and platysma. The anterior triangle is further divided into four triangles by the digastric, stylohyoid, and omohyoid muscles. The four subdivisions of the anterior triangle are the *submandibular, submental, carotid,* and *muscular* (inferior carotid) *triangles.* The primary contents of the anterior triangle are the common carotid, internal carotid, and external carotid arteries; the internal jugular vein; the laryngeal, pharyngeal, vagal, and recurrent laryngeal nerves; the submandibular gland; and lymphatic tissue. Subdividing the neck into compartments, or triangles, helps the surgeon simplify the organization of the complex anatomy of the neck.

Lymph Nodes of the Neck

Superficial lymph nodes

Superficial cervical lymph nodes are present as far superior as the face and extend posteriorly to the occipital area of the scalp. These nodes drain from the auricular and parotid areas. They lie adjacent to the external jugular vein and are superficial to the sternocleidomastoid muscle. These nodes drain into the submandibular triangle and the submandibular nodes.

Submandibular lymph nodes

The *submandibular lymph nodes* lie in the submandibular triangle. These nodes drain the cheek, medial canthus, lateral nose, upper lip, gingiva, and

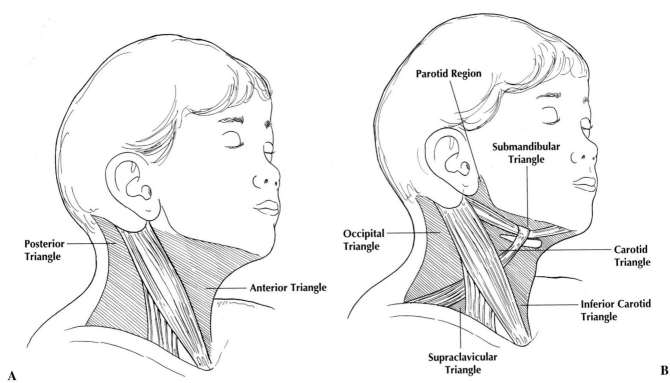

Figure 56–7: Triangles of the neck. (From Richardson MAT. The neck: Embryology and anatomy. In: Bluestone CD, Stool SE, Schetz MD, ed. *Pediatric Otolaryngology, 2nd ed.* Philadelphia: Saunders; 1990, p. 1273, with permission.)

the anterolateral tongue. The submandibular nodes subsequently drain to the superior deep cervical nodes.

Submental lymph nodes

The *submental lymph nodes* are found in the submental triangle. They drain the central lower lip, the floor of the mouth, and mobile tongue. They then drain to the submandibular lymph nodes and deep cervical nodes at the cricoid level.

Anterior cervical lymph nodes

The *anterior cervical nodes* lie ventral to the larynx and trachea. They drain the lower larynx, thyroid, and cervical trachea. These nodes drain to the deep cervical nodes.

Deep cervical lymph nodes

The *deep cervical lymph nodes* lie deep to the sternocleidomastoid muscle, intimately associated with

the great vessels (i.e., the internal jugular vein and carotid artery). Two distinct groups of nodes that are clinically important are the *jugulodigastric nodes* and the *juguloomohyoid nodes.* The jugulodigastric nodes lie at the point where the posterior belly of the digastric crosses the jugular vein. The juguloomohyoid nodes lie at the junction of the superior belly of the omohyoid and sternocleidomastoid muscle. These two groups of nodes often are easily palpable when enlarged in response to infection, inflammation, or neoplasm. The deep cervical nodes are divided into the superior and inferior group. The *superior deep cervical nodes* lie deep to the sternocleidomastoid muscle intimately associated with the internal jugular vein and eleventh cranial nerve. They drain the occipital region, the back of the neck, auricle, tongue, larynx, thyroid, trachea, nasopharynx, nose, palate, and esophagus. The *inferior deep cervical nodes* lie deep to the sternocleidomastoid muscle in the supraclavicular area. They drain the back of the scalp and neck and the pectoral region (Fig. 56-8).

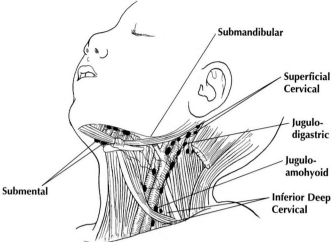

Figure 56–8: Superficial and deep lymph nodes of the neck. (From Rosse C, Gaddinn-Rosse P, eds. *Hollinshead's Textbook of Anatomy, 5th ed.* Philadelphia: Lippincott-Raven, 1997, with permission.)

SPECIAL CONSIDERATION:

The juguloomohyoid and jugulodigastric nodes are easily palpable when enlarged in response to infection, inflammation, or neoplasm.

Retropharyngeal lymph nodes

The *retropharyngeal nodes* lie in the buccopharyngeal fascia, behind the pharynx but anterior to the cervical vertebrae. They drain the nose and nasopharynx. These nodes subsequently drain to the superior deep cervical nodes. The retropharyngeal nodes are active in the pediatric patient, but not so much in the adult. When these nodes suppurate, a retropharyngeal abscess forms.

SPECIAL CONSIDERATION:

The retropharyngeal lymph nodes are not as active in the adult as they are in the child, and when these nodes suppurate, a retropharyngeal abscess forms.

Veins of the Neck

Superficial and subcutaneous veins of the neck

The *superficial veins of the neck* are tributaries of the external jugular vein (Fig. 56–9). The external jugular and anterior jugular veins are the two main subcutaneous veins of the neck, and they run a variable course. The *external jugular vein* begins on the surface of the sternocleidomastoid muscle at about the level of the angle of the mandible, where it is formed by the union of the posterior auricular vein and the retromandibular vein. The external jugular vein is closely paralled by the greater auricular nerve. The external jugular vein ends in the subclavian vein or the internal jugular vein. Before it terminates, it receives the transverse cervical, suprascapular, and anterior jugular veins. The *anterior jugular vein* begins in the suprahyoid region and descends on the infrahyoid muscles. In the lower neck, the right and left anterior jugular veins usually are joined by a venous arch horizontally. The anterior jugular vein empties into the external jugular vein or the subclavian vein.

Deep veins of the neck

The two *internal jugular veins* are the deep veins of the neck. The right vein is the larger. It starts at

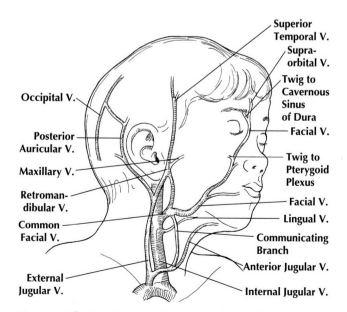

Figure 56–9: Superficial veins of the face. (From Becker RF, Wilson JW, Gehweiler JA, eds. *The Anatomical Basis of Medical Practice*. Baltimore: Williams & Wilkins, 1971, p. 361, with permission.)

the jugular foramen as a continuation of the sigmoid sinus. As it passes medial to the tympanic cavity, it forms the jugular bulb, often leaving an impression on the floor of the middle ear. At the level of the jugular bulb, the internal jugular vein has a minute amount of chemoreceptor tissue, which can give rise to glomus jugulare tumors. At the level of the jugular foramen, the internal jugular vein lies posterior to the internal carotid artery and is separated from it by the ninth, tenth, and eleventh cranial nerves. As the vein descends into the neck, it lies lateral to the internal and common carotid arteries. The internal jugular vein is associated intimately with the deep cervical nodes imbedded in the carotid sheath. The internal jugular vein receives blood from the inferior petrosal sinus, the middle meningeal vein, facial vein, posterior facial vein, superior thyroid vein, pharyngeal vein, and lingual vein. The internal jugular vein joins the subclavian vein to form the *innominate vein* (Fig. 56–10).

The thoracic and right lymphatic ducts

The *thoracic duct* on the left side of the neck drains lymphatic material from the lower extremities, the abdomen, the left side of the head and neck, and the left thorax. The thoracic duct terminates in the internal jugular vein, the subclavian vein, or where the two veins join in the supraclavicular area (see Fig. 56–10). The *right lymphatic duct,* which is a much smaller structure, may be difficult to identify or may exist as several channels. It drains the right side of the head and neck, right arm, and right thorax. It terminates in the same location as the thoracic duct, into either the internal jugular vein, the subclavian vein, or into the area of the junction of the two veins (see Fig. 56–10). Disorders of the lymphatic system can lead to lymphatic malformations (widely known as *cystic hygromas*). The neck is one of the most common areas for lymphatic malformations to occur.

> ## SPECIAL CONSIDERATION:
> Disorders of the lymphatic system can lead to lymphatic malformations that are known as cystic hygromas, and the neck is one of the most common areas for lymphatic malformations to occur.

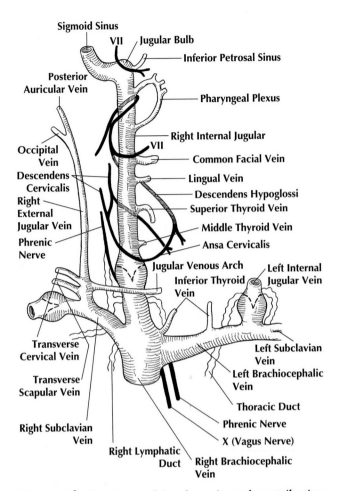

Figure 56–10: Internal jugular vein and contributing veins. (From Becker RF, Wilson JW, Gehweiler JA, eds. *The Anatomical Basis of Medical Practice.* Baltimore: Williams & Wilkins, 1971, p. 380, with permission.)

Arteries of the Neck

Along with the jugular vein, the carotid artery and its branches comprise the great vessels of the neck. The *common carotid artery* enters the neck as a branch of the innominate artery on the right, and as a branch of the arch of the aorta on the left. It appears from under cover of the omohyoid muscle in the carotid triangle and runs superiorly towards the thyroid cartilage before branching into the internal carotid and external carotid arteries. The common carotid artery and the internal carotid artery do not have any branches in the neck; only the external carotid artery gives arterial branches in the neck (Fig. 56–11). The *internal carotid* distributes inside the skull; the *external carotid* outside the skull. The internal carotid artery passes deep to the parotid gland; the external carotid artery enters into the parotid gland. The carotid bifurcation lies at about the level of the upper border of the thyroid cartilage. After the bifurcation, the internal carotid artery lies

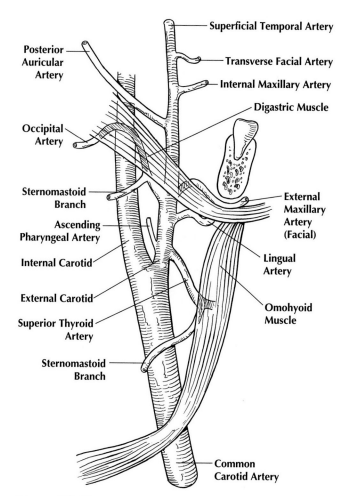

Figure 56–11: Common carotid, internal carotid, and external carotid arteries. (From Becker RF, Wilson JW, Gehweiler JA, eds. *The Anatomical Basis of Medical Practice.* Baltimore: Williams & Wilkins, 1971, p. 380, with permission.)

geal, occipital, facial, posterior auricular, maxillary, and superficial temporal (see Fig. 56–11).

The *thyrocervical trunk,* a branch of the subclavian artery, gives off three branches low in the neck: the transverse cervical, the transverse scapular, and the inferior thyroid artery. The *inferior thyroid artery* supplies branches to the thyroid gland, pharynx, larynx, and esophagus.

Fascial Layers of the Neck

The *cervical fascia* is rather complicated and opinions differ among investigators as to how the layers are arranged and as to which fascial spaces communicate with each other and which do not. However, there is consensus that there is a superficial and a deep component to the cervical fascia. The *deep cervical fascia* is further subdivided into three parts: the superficial (investing) layer, the middle (pretracheal or visceral) layer, and the deep (prevertebral) layer (Fig. 56–12).

Superficial cervical fascia

The *superficial cervical fascia* surrounds the neck, and is continuous with the superficial fascia of the pectoral, deltoid, and back regions (inferiorly) and the fascia of the facial muscles of expression (superiorly). It contains the platysma, external jugular vein, and superficial lymph nodes.

medial to the external branch as it runs upward to the skullbase. At the carotid bifurcation lies the *carotid sinus,* an area sensitive to changes in blood pressure. The carotid body is located behind the upper end of the common carotid artery. The *carotid body* responds to changes in oxygenation of the blood.

After branching off from the common carotid artery, the internal carotid artery lies deep to the stylohyoid and posterior belly of the digastric muscles. It runs upward, deep to the mandible to enter the skull. Again, it gives off no branches before entering the skull. The external carotid artery supplies most of the structures of the neck and head (except for the brain and orbit). It gives off eight named branches and most of the branches rebranch extensively. The branches of the external carotid artery are the superior thyroid, lingual, ascending pharyn-

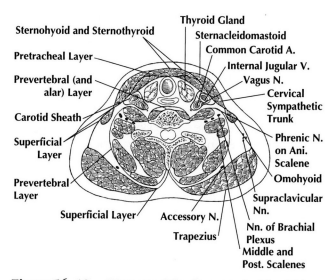

Figure 56–12: Diagram of the deep cervical fascial layers of the neck, in a cross-section below the level of the larynx. (From Rosse C, Gaddinn-Rosse P, eds. *Hollingshead's Textbook of Anatomy, 5th ed.* Philadelphia: Lippincott-Raven, 1997, with permission.)

Deep cervical fascia

The three layers of the *deep cervical fascia* divide the neck into spaces that communicate at different levels of the neck. An understanding of the relationships between the spaces of the neck becomes especially important in the diagnosis and treatment of deep space neck infections.

The *superficial (investing) layer* of the deep cervical fascia surrounds the neck like a collar surrounding the trapezius muscle, and splits to surround the sternocleidomastoid muscle. Above its attachment to the hyoid bone, it splits to surround the parotid and submandibular glands. It thickens in the area between the styloid process and the angle of the mandible to become the *stylohyoid ligament*. Below the hyoid, it attaches to the anterior and posterior aspects of the manubrium, forming the *suprasternal space of Burns.* This space contains the anterior jugular vein and a few lymph nodes. The superficial layer of the deep cervical fascia contributes to the carotid sheath.

The *middle (pretracheal or visceral) layer* of the deep cervical fascia surrounds the strap muscles, the sternohyoid, thyrohyoid, and omohyoid muscles. It also surrounds the trachea, thyroid, and esophagus. This layer contributes to the carotid sheath. It also envelopes the constrictor muscles and attaches to the base of the skull, forming the anterior aspect of the retropharyngeal space. The posterior-superior portion of the middle layer is also known as the *buccopharyngeal fascia* (Fig. 56–13).

The *deep (prevertebral) layer* of the deep cervical fascia begins in the posterior midline of the neck and surrounds the neck. It covers the prevertebral muscles, the brachial plexus, and the subclavian artery. It attaches to the transverse processes of the cervical vertebrae then splits into two layers in front of the vertebrae, forming a potential space known as the *danger space* (see Fig. 56–13). The deep layer originates at the base of the skull and fuses with the fascia of the esophagus in the superior mediastinum, forming the posterior wall of the retropharyngeal space. The deep layer also contributes to the carotid sheath. One of the important functions of the deep layer of the deep cervical fascia is to provide a free-moving surface for the mobile viscera of the neck.

The *carotid sheath* is a condensation of the fascia surrounding the internal carotid artery, internal jugular vein, and the vagus nerve. It has contributions from all three layers of the deep cervical fascia. The carotid sheath extends from the skullbase to the

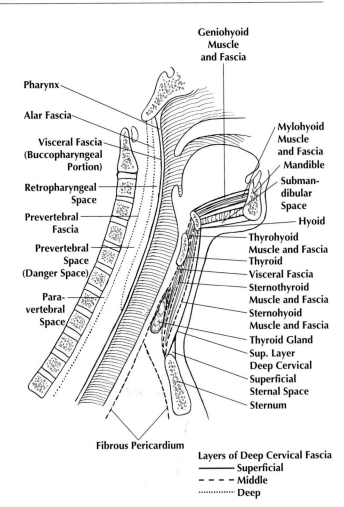

Figure 56–13: Midsaggital section showing pertinent spaces and fascial layers. Note the division of the space posterior to the visceral layer into the retropharyngeal and prevertebral spaces by the alar fascia. (From Shumrick KA, Sheft SA. Deep neck infections. In: Paparella MM, Shumrick DA, Gluckman JL, et al., eds. *Otolaryngology: Vol. 3, Head and Neck, 3rd ed.* Philadelphia: Saunders, 1991, p. 2547, with permission.)

superior mediastinum, passing through the parapharyngeal space and superficial layer to the deep layer of the deep cervical fascia.

Potential Neck Spaces

As there is dissent among investigators as to the exact description of the layers of the cervical fascia, there is also conflict of opinion over the communication and naming of the potential spaces of the neck. The potential spaces of the neck are important, however, because of the propensity of certain deep neck space infections to spread to contiguous areas or to other areas of the body such as the mediastinum. The four main potential spaces to appreciate are the parapharyngeal (or pharyngomaxillary), the retropharyngeal, the pretracheal, and the vascular. Also mentioned briefly are the submandibular, masticator, parotid, and peritonsillar spaces.

Parapharyngeal (pharyngomaxillary) space

The *parapharyngeal space* is a cone-shaped potential space in the neck. The base of the cone is the skullbase along the sphenoid bone, the apex is the hyoid bone, and the medial boundary is the buccopharyngeal fascia covering the superior constrictor muscle. The lateral border is the superficial layer of the deep cervical fascia covering the mandible, medial pterygoid muscle, and deep lobe of the parotid gland. Anteriorly, the space is limited by the pterygomandibular raphe: and posteriorly, the space is limited by the prevertebral fascia. The styloid process divides the space into an anterior muscular compartment and the posterior neurovascular compartment. The neurovascular compartment contains the carotid sheath and cranial nerves nine through twelve. Infections in the nasopharynx, pharynx, nasal cavity, sinuses, and mastoid tip drain to this area.

Retropharyngeal space

The *retropharyngeal space* is comprised of three parts: the retroesophageal, the prevertebral, and the danger space (see Fig. 56–13). The *retroesophageal space* is situated between the prevertebral fascia (i.e., the deep layer of the deep cervical fascia, or in this area of the neck, an ancillary portion of the deep cervical fascia called the *alar fascia*) and the middle layer of the deep cervical fascia. This potential space extends from the base of the skull to the posterior mediastinum, where the middle and deep layers of the deep cervical fascia fuse at approximately T2. This space contains retropharyngeal nodes. It drains infections from the nasopharynx, the nasal cavity, and the posterior ethmoid sinus.

The *prevertebral space* is limited anteriorly by the prevertebral of the deep cervical fascia and posteriorly by the bodies of the cervical vetebrae. It extends from the base of the skull to the coccyx. The *danger space* is a potential space formed by the two layers of the prevertebral fascia (or between the deep layer of the deep cervical fascia and the alar fascia) in front of the vertebral column. This space starts at the base of the skull and extends through the mediastinum. This space potentially allows abscesses in the prevertebral, retroesophageal, and parapharyngeal spaces to spread to the mediastinum.

Pretracheal space

The *pretracheal space* is a potential space in the front of the trachea and behind the infrahyoid muscles and pretracheal fascia. It is limited above by the attachment of fascia to the thyroid cartilage and below by the union of the pretracheal fascia with connective tissue in the anterior mediastinum.

Vascular space

The potential space within the carotid sheath is termed the *vascular space*. It extends from the base of the skull into the superior mediastinum. Because all three layers of the deep cervical fascia contribute to the carotid sheath, infection in any compartment of the deep cervical fascia may contribute to infection in the vascular space.

SPECIAL CONSIDERATION:

Because all three layers of the deep cervical fascia contribute to the carotid sheath, infection in any compartment of the deep cervical fascia may contribute to infection in the vascular space.

Submandibular space

This space is limited superiorly by the mucosa of the floor of the mouth. It is limited anteriorly and laterally by the mandible, posteriorly by the intrinsic muscles of the base of the tongue, and inferiorly by the hyoid and the superficial layer of the deep cervical fascia. Within this space are connections with the sublingual, submaxillary, and submental spaces. Multicompartment infection within these spaces is seen in Ludwig's angina.

Masticator space

Dental infections, usually from molar teeth, can cause abscess formation in this space. It is limited

AT A GLANCE . . .

Anatomy of the Neck

Triangles: the *posterior triangle* contains the subclavian artery, brachial plexus, spinal accessory nerve, two branches of the thyrocervical trunk artery, and posterior cervical nodes. The *anterior triangle* contains the common carotid, the internal carotid, and external carotid arteries; the internal jugular vein; the laryngeal, pharyngeal, vagal, and recurrent laryngeal nerves; the submandibular gland; and lymphatic tissue

Lymph Nodes: *superficial* (drain into the submandibular triangle and the submandibular nodes), *submandibular* (drain the cheek, medial canthus, lateral nose, upper lip, gingiva, and anterolateral tongue), *submental* (drain the central lower lip, the floor of the mouth, and mobile tongue), *anterior cervical* (drain the lower larynx, thyroid, and cervical trachea), *deep cervical* (divided into the superior deep nodes, which drain the occipital region, the back of the neck, auricle, tongue, larynx, thyroid, trachea, nasopharynx, nose, palate, and esophagus, and the inferior deep nodes, which drain the back of the scalp and neck and the pectoral region), *retropharyngeal* (drain the nose and nasopharynx)

Veins: external jugular vein, anterior jugular vein, internal jugular veins

Arteries: common carotid, internal carotid (distributes inside the skull), and external carotid (distributes outside the skull)

Fascial Layers: the *superficial cervical fascia* contains the platysma, external jugular vein, and the superficial lymph nodes. The *deep cervical fascia* is divided into three layers: the superficial layer, which contains the anterior jugular vein and a few lymph nodes; the middle layer, which surrounds the trachea, thyroid, and esophagus; and the deep layer, which covers the prevertebral muscles, the brachial plexus, and the subclavian artery

Potential Spaces: parapharyngeal, retropharyngeal, pretracheal, vascular submandibular, masticator, parotid, peritonsillar

medially by the pterygoid muscles and laterally by the superficial layer of the deep cervical fascia. The space contains the masseter muscle, the pterygoid muscles; the ramus of the mandible, and the inferior alveolar neurovascular bundle.

Parotid space

This potential space is formed by the splitting of the superficial layer of the deep cervical fascia as it surrounds the parotid gland. It is separated from the submandibular space by the stylomandibular ligament. The medial aspect of the capsule of the parotid gland is incomplete, therefore deep infections in the parotid gland can spread to the parapharyngeal space from the parotid space.

Peritonsillar space

The *peritonsillar space* lies between the capsule of the palatine tonsil medially, the superior constrictor muscle laterally, and the anterior and posterior tonsillar pillars. Infection in this space can spread to the parapharyngeal space and the vascular space.

REFERENCES

1. Skandalakis JE, Gray SW, Todd NW. The pharynx and its derivatives. In: Skandalakis JE, Gray SW, eds. *Embryology for Surgeons: The Embryological Basis for the Treatment of Congenital Anomalies.* Baltimore: Williams & Wilkins, 1994; pp. 17–64.
2. Last RJ, ed. *Anatomy: Regional and Applied, 6th ed.* Edinburgh; Churchill Livingstone, 1978, pp. 40–46.
3. Langman J, ed. *Medical Embryology: Human development-Normal and Abnormal, 3rd ed.* Baltimore: Williams & Wilkins, 1975, pp. 258–281.
4. Hollinshead WH, Rosse C, eds. *Textbook of Anatomy.* Philadelphia: Harper & Row, 1985, pp. 817–851.

57 Clinical Evaluation of the Neck

Brian J. Wiatrak

A child presenting with a neck mass is a clinical scenario that is encountered commonly by both otolaryngologists and primary care physicians (PCP) who routinely see children in their medical practices. Unlike adults in whom a neck mass is considered malignant until proven otherwise, the vast majority of neck masses presenting in children are benign lesions.[1,2] Disorders, such as congenital masses, chronic inflammatory lesions, noninflammatory benign masses, and malignant and benign neoplasms also may be encountered. Malignant neck lesions in children are rare; however, some conditions such as lymphoma frequently present as a neck mass initially.[1,3] It is extremely important that the practitioner have an organized and focused approach in evaluating a child with a neck mass so that an appropriate differential diagnosis can be made and those children at risk for malignancy are expeditiously evaluated, diagnosed, and treated. A thorough history and physical examination allows the physician to arrive at an accurate differential diagnosis. Appropriate radiologic and laboratory testing also may be beneficial. The vast majority of neck masses requiring surgical therapy in children are of congenital origin.

INITIAL EVALUATION

History and Physical Examination

A thorough systematic history and physical examination are important first steps towards the appropriate diagnosis and management of a child presenting with a neck mass. Important aspects of the history include: (1) age at onset of the mass; (2) duration; (3) symptoms related specifically to the mass; and (4) symptoms suggestive of a systemic process, such as fever, night sweats, fatigue, or weight loss.

AT A GLANCE . . .

Important Historical Aspects of a Neck Mass

- Age at onset of mass
- Duration of the mass
- Specific symptoms related to the mass
- Symptoms suggestive of a systemic process

A maternal history of infectious disease is important in cases of neck masses in neonates, which may be caused by adenopathy secondary to congenital syphilis or possibly human immunodeficiency virus (HIV). A mass presenting in the perinatal period or in early infancy may suggest a congenital lesion, such as a brachial cleft cyst, thyroglossal duct cyst, or lymphatic malformation. A mass presenting in later childhood may be more suggestive of reactive lymphadenopathy or possibly a malignancy. Lesions that have been present for many months or years are more consistent with congenital lesions or benign inflammatory processes.

Lesions that are rapidly growing over a period of 4 to 8 weeks are more likely to be malignant. Rapid enlargement associated with fever may suggest an acute inflammatory process, such as a neck abscess. However, this presentation also can be seen in cases of congenital masses such as lymphatic malformations or brachial cleft cysts, which either become acutely infected or undergo hemorrhage and sudden rapid enlargement. Systemic signs and symptoms such as fever, malaise, and night sweats that are associated with an enlarging neck mass should be considered a malignant process until proven otherwise. Lesions that fluctuate in size are more

Pediatric Otolaryngology, Edited by R.F. Wetmore, H.R. Muntz, and T.J. McGill. Thieme Medical Publishers, Inc., New York © 2000.

commonly associated with congenital or inflammatory processes. A history of trauma to the area may suggest a lesion, such as a hematoma that may become infected secondarily causing enlargement. A salivary gland duct obstruction should be considered in cases when pain accompanies a mass of the salivary gland.

A history of exposure to various inciting agents should be elicited. A prior history of radiation therapy to the head and neck region may predispose patients to secondary malignancies, such as thyroid and salivary gland cancer.[4] Unusual chronic cervical infections should be considered in patients exposed to cats, nondomestic animals, and ticks.

A family history may be important in cases of genetic syndromes that are associated with cervical masses or malignancies, such as branchial-oto-renal syndrome (otologic malformations, hearing loss, and renal malformations), which is an autosomal dominant condition associated with branchial cleft abnormalities. Multiple endocrine neoplasia (MEN) syndromes may be associated with neuroblastoma or possibly thyroid cancer.

The physical examination is a crucial part of evaluating a child with a neck mass, and it may give valuable information regarding the quality of the mass and the likelihood that the lesion is malignant. Some points to assess include whether the mass is solid, cystic, associated with overlying cutaneous skin changes or a draining fistula, tender, warm, fluctuating, colored, and mobile. In addition, the laterality of the mass as well as the presence of other associated mass lesions in the neck are important.

AT A GLANCE . . .

Important Signs in Evaluating a Neck Mass

- Consistency (solid, cystic, fluctuating, etc)
- Overlying skin changes/fistula
- Tenderness
- Erythema
- Mobility
- Location in the neck

A cystic lesion in the anterior midline is most consistent with a thyroglossal duct cyst; one at the ante-rior border of the sternocleidomastoid muscle is usually a branchial cleft cyst; and one in the posterior triangle is most likely a lymphatic malformation. A solid mass in the posterior triangle or supraclavicular area often heralds a malignancy. Torsiglieri et al. reported that 35% of their patients with a solid supraclavicular mass were diagnosed with lymphoma.[1] Flexible fiberoptic laryngoscopy (FFL) should be considered in selected cases because it has been reported that one of every six children with a malignant neck mass has an associated oral cavity or pharyngeal lesion.[5]

SPECIAL CONSIDERATION:

A solid mass in the posterior cervical triangle or supraclavicular triangle often heralds a malignancy.

Patients also should have a focused systemic examination because many inflammatory or malignant lesions may present with other systemic findings. Examples include a heart murmur in a child with Kawasaki disease, spleen tenderness in a patient with mononucleosis, or possibly an abdominal mass in a child presenting with a metastatic mass to the neck. A complete lymph node examination should be performed including the inguinal and axillary nodes. A general review of the skin may give diagnostic clues, such as "café-au-lait" spots on a child with neurofibromatosis or hemangiomas on a child with a vascular lesion of the neck.

DIAGNOSTIC TESTING

Imaging Studies

Imaging studies that may be useful in appropriate cases include plain radiography, ultrasonography (US), computed tomography (CT), magnetic resonance imaging (MRI) scans, or nuclear radioisotope studies. Imaging studies should be obtained only when the additional information provided affects the management of the patient and expedites the correct diagnosis.

Plain radiographs are not always accurate at providing useful diagnostic information about specific neck masses. However, useful information may be obtained in certain situations. Retropharyngeal widening or air-fluid levels may be visualized in cases of retropharyngeal cellulitis or abscess. In cases of possible tuberculous cervical infections, the chest radiograph may give information regarding pulmonary involvement. Chest radiography also should be obtained whenever a malignant neck mass is suspected in order to detect any pulmonary or hilar nodal involvement as seen in cases of lymphoma, which is the most common malignancy diagnosed by cervical node biopsy.

SPECIAL CONSIDERATION:

Chest radiography should be obtained to detect any pulmonary or hilar nodal involvement whenever a malignant neck mass is suspected.

Ultrasonography (US) may be extremely valuable in the evaluation of neck masses. The most important features of US are its ability to determine whether a mass is cystic or solid. The anatomic relationship of a mass also can be determined, as well as whether one mass is involved or whether there is multicentricity, such as in the case of a group of inflamed lymph nodes. In cases of thyroglossal duct cysts, US can be utilized to determine the cystic nature of the mass, as well as the presence or absence of a normal thyroid gland. In an infant with fibromatosis coli (i.e., congenital muscular torticollis), the solid nature of the mass and its intrinsic nature to the sternocleidomastoid muscle can be determined. With an acutely-inflamed neck mass, US can determine the fluid nature of an abscess and whether it is multilocular. In such cases, US also may assist in needle aspiration. US is well tolerated by patients, is relatively inexpensive, and does not expose a patient to ionizing radiation.

Computed tomography (CT) can provide much more detail with regards to a neck mass and its relationship to surrounding anatomic structures. In cases of deep neck abscesses that require surgical drainage, the anatomic information provided by CT is superior to US and should be obtained before surgery is attempted. When contrast is utilized, ring enhancement around a low-attenuation area within a soft-tissue inflammatory mass is suggestive of an

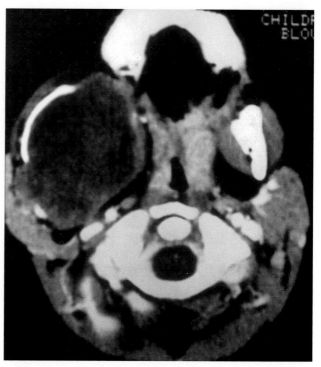

Figure 57–1: Destructive lesion of the right mandible presenting as a right mandibular and submandibular neck mass and diagnosed as aggressive fibromatosis.

abscess (Fig. 57-1). However, this appearance also may be demonstrated in a necrotic, metastatic node. CT is the best modality to evaluate bony structures, and may be necessary if a malignant or locally-aggressive process is suspected (Fig. 57-2).

Magnetic resonance imaging (MRI) may provide more extensive soft-tissue anatomic information that may be useful particularly in cases of extensive lesions requiring aggressive surgical resection. Bone anatomy is not demonstrated nearly as well on MRI as it is with CT. Vascular lesions are better assessed utilizing MRI, and in most cases, the diagnosis may be made with confidence avoiding open surgical biopsy. The cost of MRI is higher than other modalities and may require a longer period of immobility for the patient.

Nuclear medicine studies are indicated rarely for the evaluation of neck masses in children. In the past, thyroid scans were obtained routinely in the evaluation of suspected thyroglossal duct cysts; however, the cost of testing, the potential risks of sedation, and a lower positive yield make this test less than ideal for the initial evaluation of thyroglossal duct cysts. Currently, ultrasound is more commonly utilized. In cases of suspected ectopic thyroid tissue presenting as a neck mass, a thyroid scan may be beneficial (Fig. 57-3).

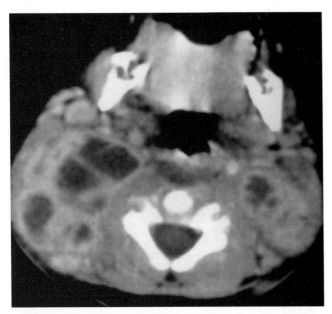

Figure 57–2: A contrast-enhanced CT scan of child with bilateral neck abscesses demonstrates a multilocular abscess with ring enhancement.

Laboratory Studies

The laboratory testing for all patients undergoing evaluation of a neck mass should be individualized. A complete blood count (CBC) with differential is frequently beneficial. In cases of acute inflammation, such as a neck abscess, a high white blood cell count with a leukocytosis helps confirm the diagnosis and also assists in monitoring response to therapy. Atypical lymphocytes may suggest infectious mononucleosis; heterophile antibody titers may help to confirm the diagnosis. Evidence of neoplastic activity also may be revealed in the CBC.

Suspected cases of cervical adenitis caused by mycobacterial infection, both tuberculous and atypical, should undergo skin testing with a purified protein derivative (PPD). Chest radiography also should be obtained in these cases, although most children with atypical mycobacteria cervical adenitis do not have pulmonary disease unless there is an associated immunologic disorder. Serologic testing for various viral and protozoan agents also may be required in selected situations. Serologic testing in cases of cat-scratch disease for the inciting agent *Bartonella henselae* may assist greatly in making the diagnosis.[6] However, the cat-scratch *Bacillus* may be identified

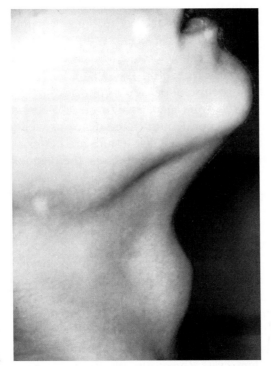

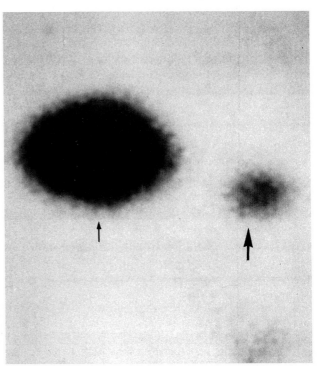

A   B

Figure 57–3: (A) An adolescent patient who presented with an anterior midline neck mass that was diagnosed as ectopic thyroid tissue. (B) Thyroid scan demonstrating ectopic thyroid tissue (small arrow demonstrates thyroid gland, large arrow is ectopic thyroid tissue).

on histologic section utilizing the Warthin-Starry silver stain. Serologic testing also may assist in the diagnosis of toxoplasmosis, cytomegalovirus (CMV), tularemia, brucellosis, histoplasmosis, and coccidioidomycosis. A focused history with special attention to recent travel or exposure to some of these more unusual infections aids in deciding which serologic testing is warranted, if any.

There is also a role for fine needle aspiration (FNA) of neck masses in children. Although the utilization of this technique is described well in adults, it is less consistent in the pediatric population. This technique is very limited to the experience and comfort level of the cytologists, with the most reported success occurring in institutions that utilize FNA frequently. The ability to determine malignancy utilizing FNA, without the utilization of general anesthesia has been reported.[7,8] Limitation in sample size may necessitate biopsy for electron microscopy and cytologic testing.

After a complete evaluation of the neck mass, open surgical biopsy may be required if a diagnosis has not been determined yet. If a mass is suspicious for malignancy based on location, physical examination, history, or an unsatisfactory resolution with medical therapy for a clinically-suspicious mass, open surgical biopsy is then warranted. It is wise to consult the hematology/oncology service preoperatively in cases suspicious for malignancy. If the biopsy is confirmed to be malignant by frozen section intraoperatively, further appropriate testing can be performed, such as bone marrow biopsy. It is important that enough tissue be obtained during the biopsy to arrive at an appropriate diagnosis, and the surgical case should not be terminated until the pathologist has confirmed that there is enough tissue for all appropriate testing. Definitive surgical excision should not be performed until a final tissue diagnosis has been determined. Practice Pathways 57-1 and 57-2 demonstrate the management of in-

Practice Pathway 57–1   EVALUATION AND MANAGEMENT OF AN INFANT WITH A NECK MASS

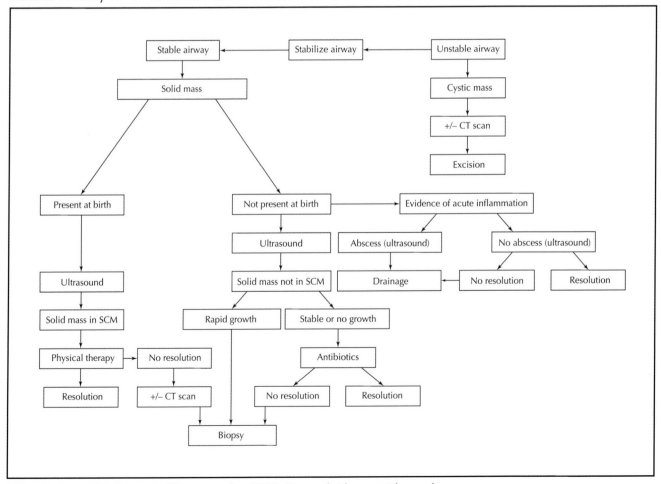

Abbreviations: CT, Computed Tomography; SCM, Sternocleidomastoid muscle.

Practice Pathway 57–2   EVALUATION AND MANAGEMENT OF A CHILD WITH A NECK MASS

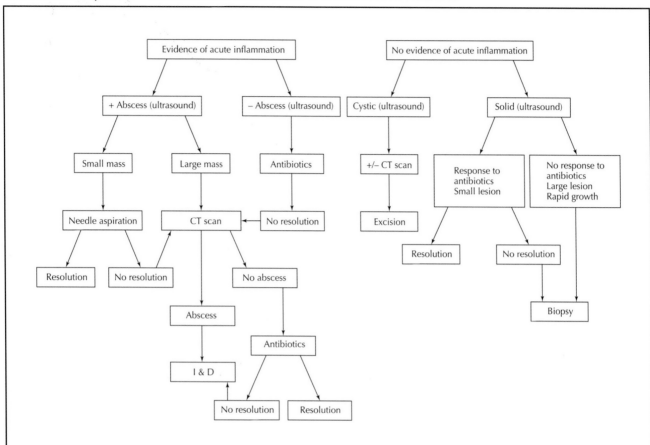

Abbreviations: CT, Computed Tomography; I = incision; & D = drainage.

fants and older children presenting with a neck mass.

AT A GLANCE . . .

Indications for Cervical Lymph Node Biopsy

1. Palpable node in a neonate that does not respond to medical therapy
2. Lymph node enlargement despite medical therapy
3. Supraclavicular or lower neck adenopathy that does not respond to medical therapy
4. Adenopathy associated with prolonged systemic symptoms (e.g., fever, weight loss, night sweats)
5. Hard or fixed node, posterior cervical triangle node greater than 1 cm in diameter that does not respond to medical therapy

---

SPECIAL CONSIDERATION:

After a complete evaluation of the neck mass, open surgical biopsy may be required if a diagnosis has not been determined.

DIFFERENTIAL DIAGNOSIS OF A PEDIATRIC NECK MASS

The vast majority of pediatric neck masses are benign, although the risk of a malignant lesion cannot be excluded. Torsiglieri et al. reviewed the charts of 445 patients at the Children's Hospital of Philadelphia who underwent biopsy of a neck mass.[1] Fifty-five percent of these lesions were congenital, 27% inflammatory, 5% noninflammatory benign masses, and 3% benign neoplasms. Eleven percent of the biopsies identified a malignancy.

TABLE 57–1: Diagnosis of Pediatric Neck Masses by Cervical Location

Preauricular and Parotid Region
Congenital
  Lymphatic malformation
  Cystic hygroma
  Hemangioma
  Vascular malformation
  First branchial cleft cyst
Inflammatory
  Parotitis
  Lymphadenitis
  Atypical mycobacterial infection
  Tuberculosis
Neoplastic
  Pleomorphic adenoma
  Mucoepidermoid carcinoma
  Lymphoma
  Other
Traumatic
  Sialocele
Idiopathic
  Sjögren's syndrome
  Sarcoidosis (Uveo-parotid fever)
Postauricular Region
Congenital
  First branchial cleft cyst
Inflammatory
  Lymphadenitis
Submental Region
Congenital
  Thyroglossal duct cyst
  Lymphatic malformation
  Dermoid cyst
  Vascular malformation
Inflammatory
  Lymphadenitis
Neoplastic
  Thyroglossal duct adenocarcinoma
Submandibular Region
Congenital
  Lymphatic malformation
  Vascular malformation
Inflammatory
  Lymphadenitis
  Submandibular sialoadenitis
Neoplastic
  Pleomorphic adenoma
  Mucoepidermoid carcinoma
  Adenoid cystic carcinoma
Other
  Cervical or plunging ranula
Jugulodigastric Region
Congenital
  First or second branchial cleft cyst
  Hemangioma
  Lymphatic malformation

Inflammatory
  Lymphadenitis
Neoplastic
  Lymphoma
  Parotid neoplasm (tail of parotid)
Anterior Midline Region
Congenital
  Thyroglossal duct cyst
  Dermoid cyst
  Ectopic thyroid gland
Inflammatory
  Lymphadenitis
Anterior Border Sternocleidomastoid Muscle
Congenital
  First, second, or third branchial cleft cyst
  Hemangioma
  Laryngocele
  Lymphatic malformation
  Fibromatosis coli (sternocleidomastoid tumor of infancy)
Neoplastic
  Lymphoma
  Sarcoma
  Carotid body tumor
Posterior Triangle (Spinal Accessory Region)
Congenital
  Lymphatic malformation
  Vascular malformation
Inflammatory
  Inflammatory lymphadenitis
Neoplastic
  Lymphoma
  Metastatic lesion from nasopharynx
Peritracheal Anterior Region
Congenital
  Thyroglossal duct cyst
Inflammatory
  Lymphadenitis
  Thyroiditis
Neoplastic
  Thyroid neoplasm
Supraclavicular
Congenital
  Lymphatic malformation
  Vascular malformation
  Hemangioma
Neoplastic
  Lipoma
  Lymphoma
  Metastatic lesion
Suprasternal
Congenital
  Dermoid cyst
  Thymic cyst
Neoplastic
  Lipoma
  Metastatic lesion

TABLE 57–2: Pediatric Neck Masses Categorized by Histology

Skeletal Muscle	Benign tumors
Rhabdomyosarcoma	Malignant tumors
Fat	*Vascular*
Lipoma	Aneurysm
Liposarcoma	Hemangioma
Fibrous Tissue	Arteriovenous malformation
Fibroma	Angiocarcinoma
Fibrosarcoma	*Endocrine*
Embryonic	Neuroblastoma
Thyroglossal duct cyst	Neurofibroma
Branchial cleft cyst	Schwannoma
Dermoid cyst	*Bone*
Teratoma	Osteogenic tumors
Cervical thymic cyst	Chondrogenic tumors
Mucosal Defect	*Miscellaneous*
Laryngocele	Amyloidosis
Thyroid/Parathyroid	Foreign body
Cyst	Hematoma
Adenoma	*Lymphatic*
Carcinoma	Lymphatic malformation
Other malignancies	*Lymph Node*
Salivary Glands	Metastatic Lesion
Ductal obstruction	Hyperplasia
Inflammation	Leukemia
Stones	Lymphoma
Cysts or sialoceles	Sarcoidosis
Ranula	

The differential diagnosis of children with a neck mass is extensive and can be organized by anatomic site and etiology (Table 57–1) or by the histology of the tissue from which the mass arises (Table 57–2). The best way to organize the discussion of the more commonly-encountered lesions, is to present them based on their etiologies. Although most neck masses presenting in children are the result of a pathologic process, it should be noted that the normal structures in the neck (e.g., the thyroid gland, hyoid bone, thyroid cartilage, carotid bulb, transverse process of the second cervical vertebra, and the styloid process) may be palpated and interpreted as a pathologic structure.

Congenital Neck Masses

Thyroglossal duct cyst

Thyroglossal duct cysts, along with branchial cleft cysts, are the most common congenital neck masses in children. They result from the persistence of the portion of the embryonic thyroglossal duct that is involved with the migration of the thyroid gland from the foramen cecum at the base of the tongue. This portion of the embryonic thyroglossal duct is obliterated during embryogenesis after the thyroid gland descends to its normal resting position in the neck. During the embryogenesis, the thyroglossal duct is involved closely with the development of the midportion of the hyoid bone. Although a sinus tract may be associated with a thyroglossal duct cyst, this more commonly occurs as the result of recurrence after surgical resection. The majority of thyroglossal duct cysts present in childhood, but they may remain asymptomatic until adolescence or adulthood. Up to one-third of thyroglossal duct cysts may not become apparent until after age 20.[9,10] As with other congenital cysts, thyroglossal duct cysts may become enlarged during the occurrence of an upper respiratory tract infection (URI).

> ## SPECIAL CONSIDERATION:
> Up to one-third of thyroglossal duct cysts may not become apparent until after age 20.

Classically, the thyroglossal duct cyst arises in the midline of the neck at or below the level of the hyoid bone (Fig. 57–4). However, a small number of these lesions may occur lateral to the midline. During physical examination, the mass may elevate with protrusion of the tongue due to its attachment to the hyoid bone. Other lesions that may have a similar presentation include a dermoid cyst and an enlarged lymph node. Lymph nodes and dermoid cysts typically do not move with tongue protrusion.

The treatment of choice is surgical resection utilizing the *Sistrunk procedure,* which consists of resection of the mass, including its attachment to the central portion of the hyoid bone and the suprahyoid musculature, leading up to the base of the tongue. It has been noted that numerous small epithelially-lined tracts may be present in the suprahyoid musculature; a generous resection of this area is required to decrease the recurrence rate.[11] It is important to determine preoperatively if normal thyroid tissue is present. If there is the possibility that ectopic thyroid tissue within the thyroglossal duct cyst may be the patient's only functioning thyroid tissue, resection will result in a hypothyroid state. In the past, radioisotope scans were frequently utilized. However, studies have shown the detection rate for ectopic thyroid is extremely

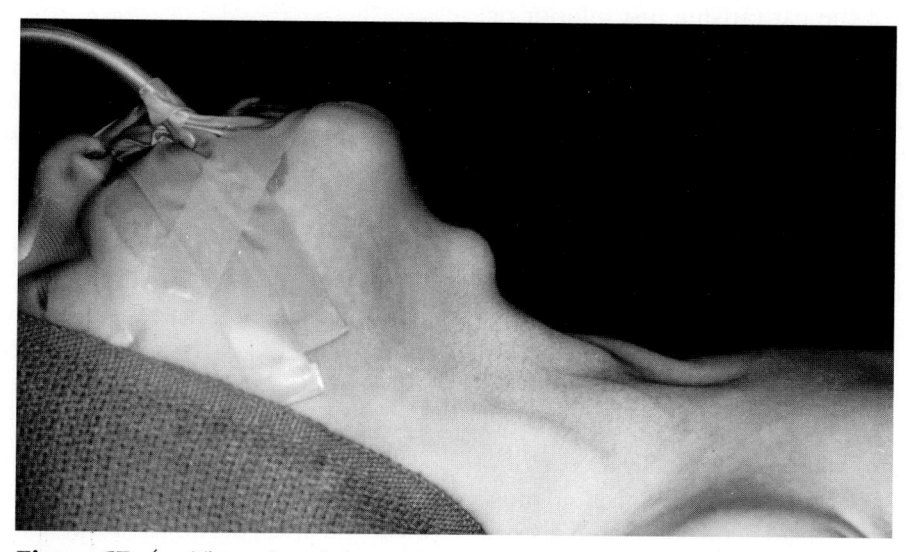

Figure 57–4: Thyroglossal duct cyst presenting in the interior midline of the neck, just prior to surgical resection.

low.[12] US is a noninvasive technique that may evaluate a thyroid gland, and it requires no exposure to ionizing radiation and costs less.

Branchial cleft cyst

Branchial cleft cysts arise from remnants of the branchial system when abnormalities arise within the normal persistence of fetal tissue or from the failure of dissolution of the embryologic branchial tissue. During embryogenesis, the branchial arch is associated with an external cleft of ectodermal origin and an internal pouch that is of endodermal origin. Anomalies arising from the branchial system include branchial cleft cysts, sinuses, or fistulae. A sinus tract usually has an external opening to the neck, typically along the anterior border of the sternocleidomastoid muscle, and a fistula has both an internal and external opening. A branchial cyst may arise anywhere along the course of a sinus or fistula tract. Abnomalities have been noted from the first through the fourth branchial clefts.

As with thyroglossal duct cysts, branchial cleft cysts may not be recognizable until later in childhood or possibly adulthood, whereas congenital sinus tracts and fistulae are usually apparent at birth. Branchial cleft cysts often become apparent at times of acute infection or possibly abscess formation. It may be necessary to aspirate the mass or perform an open incision before a definitive resection can take place.

Approximately 8% are first branchial cleft cysts, and these are separated anatomically into type-1 or type-2 anomalies.[2] *Type-1 first branchial cleft cysts* (Fig. 57-5) usually are closely associated with the

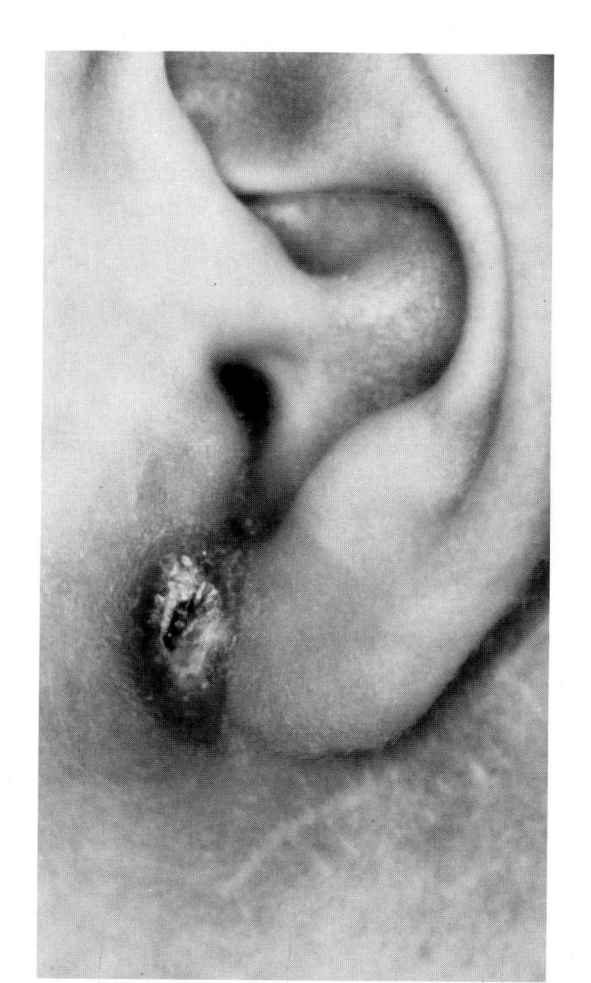

Figure 57–5: Type-1 first branchial cleft cyst presenting as recurrent infection of preauricular mass.

conchal cartilage of the ear (arising just inferior or posterior to the ear) and are occasionally associated with a sinus tract that parallels the direction of the external auditory canal (EAC) and ends blindly.[13] *Type-2 first branchial cleft cysts* usually arise in the upper neck, above the level of the hyoid bone. They have a sinus tract that typically courses through the parotid gland, that is closely associated with the facial nerve, and that ends at the bony-cartilaginous junction of the EAC. Great care must be taken to identify and preserve the facial nerve with surgical resection of first branchial cleft cysts and sinus tracts.

Second branchial cleft cysts typically arise along the anterior border of the sternocleidomastoid muscle with a sinus tract that, if present, courses between the internal and external carotid vessels and over the hypoglossal and glossopharyngeal nerves

to terminate in the tonsillar fossa if a complete fistula is present (Fig. 57-6). Branchial cleft cysts may occur anywhere along the course of the sinus tract; however, they most commonly arise in the anterior triangle of the neck, below the level of the hyoid bone.

Third and fourth branchial cleft cysts and sinus tracts are very rare. The external opening for a third branchial cleft anomaly is similar to that of a second branchial cleft, with the internal opening located in the region of the pyriform sinus. Theoretically, the external opening for a fourth branchial cleft is the same as the second and third branchial clefts sinus tracts, with the internal sinus opening terminating near the apex of the pyriform sinus. In these situations, a barium swallow may detect an internal sinus tract opening that may be associated with a third

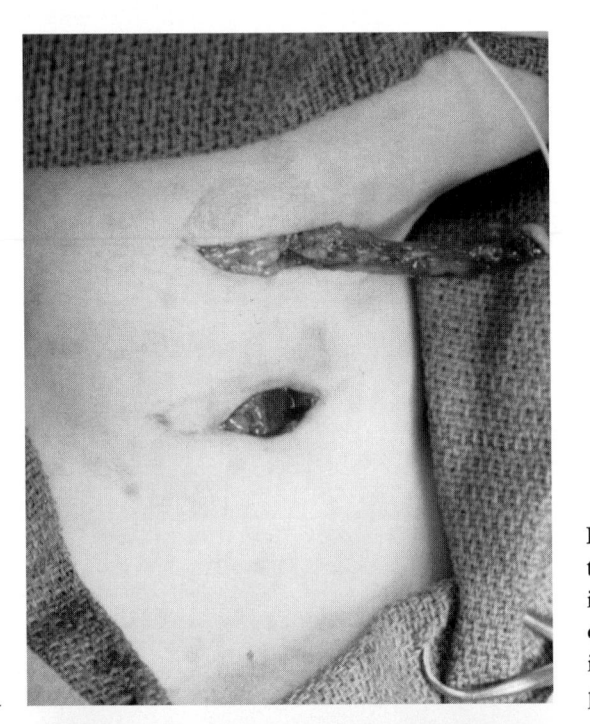

A

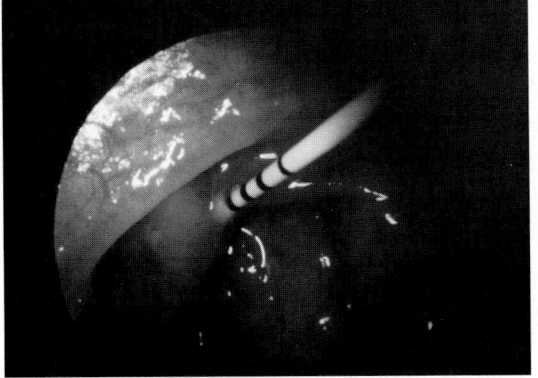

B

Figure 57–6: (A) Second branchial cleft fistula tract resected through a step-ladder incision. Note the Fogerty catheter entering the fistula tract. (B) Internal opening of the second branchial cleft fistula tract. Note the Fogerty catheter exiting through the internal opening in the region of the tonsillar fossa. (C) Completely resected second branchial cleft fistula tract.

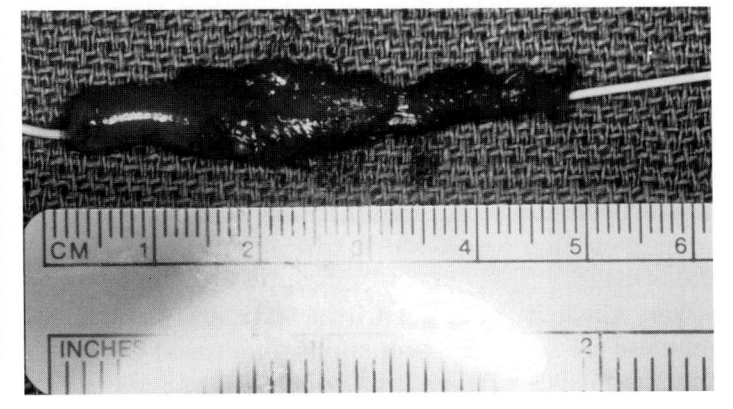

C

or fourth branchial cyst. Rigid endoscopy in the operating room may be necessary in these situations to detect an internal sinus opening.

Greater than 90% of branchial cleft anomalies arise from the second branchial cleft type, and approximately 8% are associated with the first branchial cleft. If an internal opening is apparent in the tonsillar fossa, then tonsillectomy should be performed and the intraoral component resected with closure of the mucosal defect.

Infected thyroglossal duct cysts and third branchial cleft cysts may be a cause of suppurative thyroiditis in children.[14,15] In cases of recurrent neck abscesses in a child, the diagnosis of a branchial cleft cyst should be considered. Postsurgical recurrence rates for branchial cleft cysts are approximately 3%; however, this rises to 20% in cases where prior surgical resection was attempted.[16]

> ### SPECIAL CONSIDERATION:
>
> Infected thyroglossal duct cysts and third branchial cleft cysts may be a cause of suppurative thyroiditis in children.

Lymphatic malformations

Lymphatic malformations (lymphangiomas) most likely arise from abnormal development of primordial lymphatic channels. Histologically, these lesions have been described as simple, cavernous, and cystic; the latter is the source of the frequently used term *cystic hygroma*. Histologic variability may occur within specific lesions. CT with contrast and MRI delineate the cystic or multilocular appearance of the lesion and its relative avascularity. Lymphatic malformations typically present within the first year of life as a compressible cystic mass, usually located in the posterior triangle of the neck. Other sites may be involved, including the floor of the mouth, tongue, larynx, or parotid region. Approximately 65% of lymphatic malformations are present at birth, and 90% are clinically detectable by the end of the second year of life.[17] Large lymphatic malformations of the neck may cause significant airway compromise at birth, requiring emergent airway intervention such as intubation or tracheotomy (Fig. 57-7). Although most lesions present early in in-

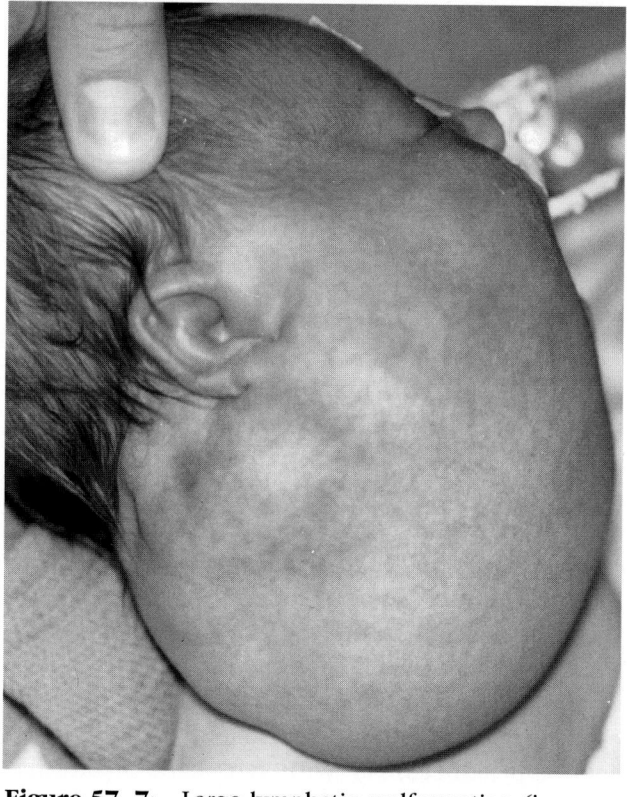

Figure 57–7: Large lymphatic malformation (i.e., cystic hygroma) presenting at birth with severe airway obstruction requiring urgent tracheotomy.

fancy, lymphatic malformations may arise with sudden enlargement later in childhood or even in adulthood. Sudden enlargement may result from inflammation secondary to an URI or possibly from hemorrhage into the cystic lesion. Unlike hemangiomas, which tend to involute within the first few years of life, lymphatic malformations do not involute over time.

> ### SPECIAL CONSIDERATION:
>
> Unlike hemangiomas, which tend to involute within the first few years of life, lymphatic malformations do not involute over time.

Surgical resection is the treatment of choice for lymphatic malformations, although other treatment modalities have been attempted in the past. Cyst aspiration and injection of sclerosing agents have been used successfully in malformations with a few large cysts. Surgical resection of large lesions may be fraught with much difficulty due to their proximity to important anatomic structures of the neck. Multiple stage resections may be required for extensive lesions.

Vascular lesions

Vascular lesions arising within the neck in children may be classified as hemangiomas or vascular malformations.[18,19] Hemangiomas typically present within the first few months of life. They demonstrate rapid growth and then a period of quiescence followed by a period of involution between the age of 3 to 5 years of age (Fig. 57–8). Although the majority of hemangiomas involute with time, a significant number of them do not involute completely and may result in cosmetic deformity for the child.[18] Vascular malformations typically are present at birth, do not go through a rapid growth phase, and do not undergo involution with time. Histologically, vascular malformations and hemangiomas have distinct appearances. As with lymphatic malformations, large hemangiomas may cause airway com-

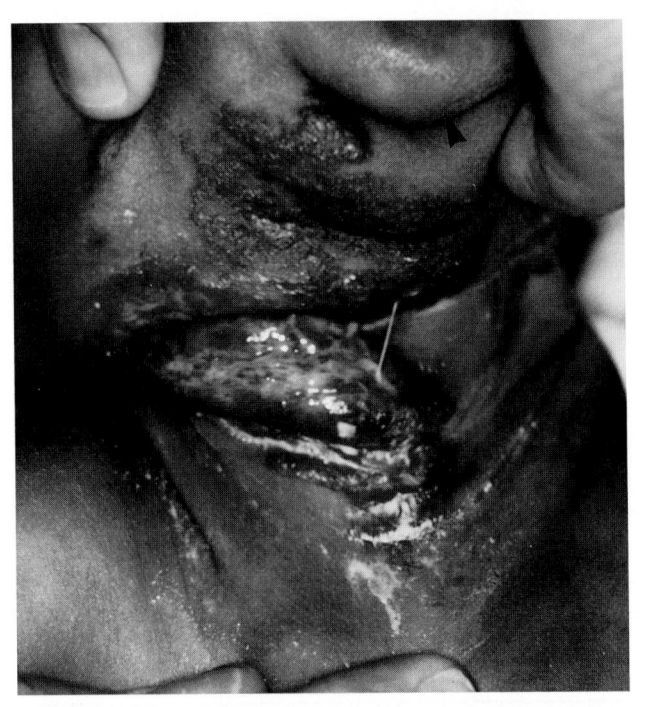

Figure 57–9: Large cervical hemangioma in a newborn presenting with extensive skin ulceration (arrow points to chin).

promise, requiring airway intervention. Most hemangiomas are soft, compressible lesions that may have a bluish discoloration. Extensive lesions may result in overlying skin ulcerations (Fig. 57–9).

Treatment for hemangiomas and vascular malformations is different. Diagnostic evaluation should include a CT with contrast or MRI with gadolinium, which will demonstrate the soft-tissue anatomy and vascularity of the lesion (Fig. 57–10). Hemangiomas undergoing rapid growth may benefit from high-dose corticosteroid therapy to control the growth rate and possibly reverse it. In lesions with significant cosmetic or functional deformities, surgical resection and possibly laser therapy with tunable dye lasers may be beneficial.[20] Vascular malformations typically do not involute and, therefore, may be treated by surgical resection in appropriate cases. Subglottic hemangiomas may be associated with cutaneous hemangiomas. It is imperative to perform airway endoscopy in patients with cutaneous vascular lesions associated with stridor.

Sternomastoid tumor of infancy

Sternomastoid tumor of infancy (SMTI) also is known by numerous other names, including fibromatosis coli, nodular fasciitis, or congenital muscular torticollis. SMTI is a fibrotic lesion that arises

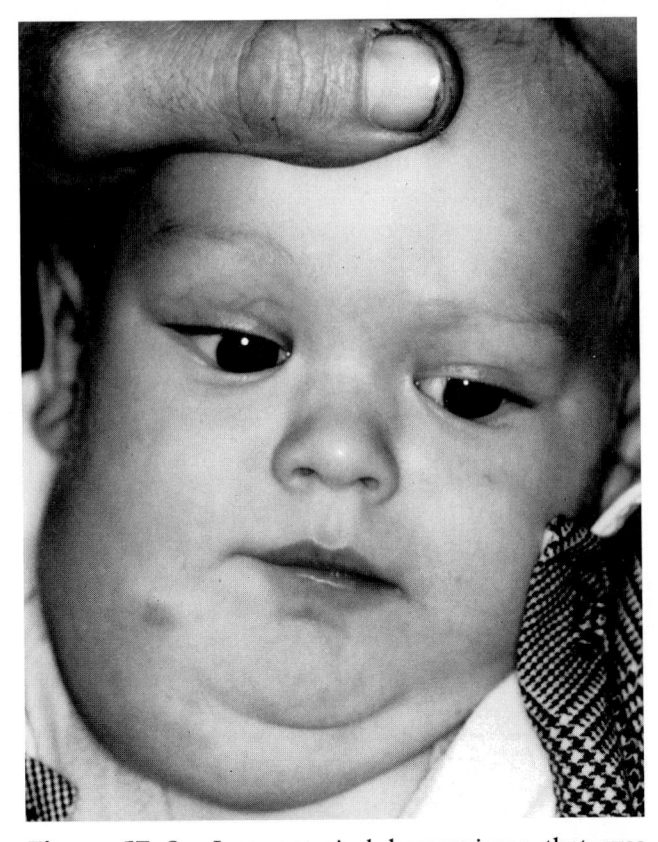

Figure 57–8: Large cervical hemangioma that was treated with corticosteroids and observation. No airway intervention was necessary.

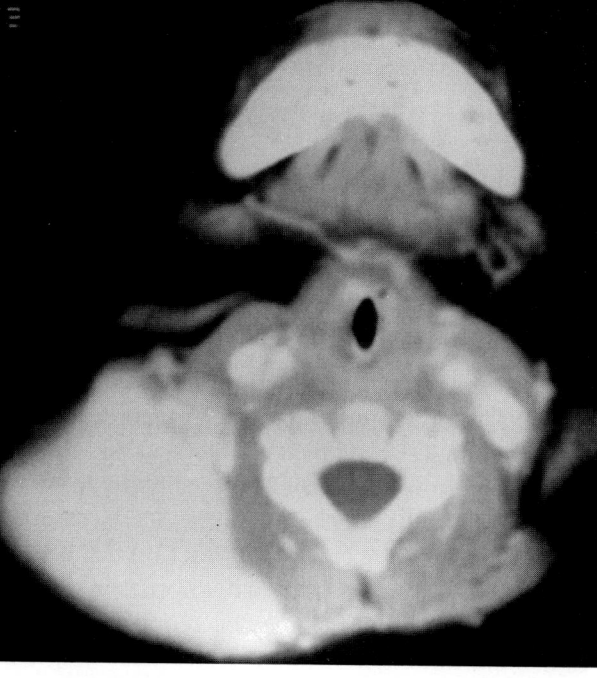
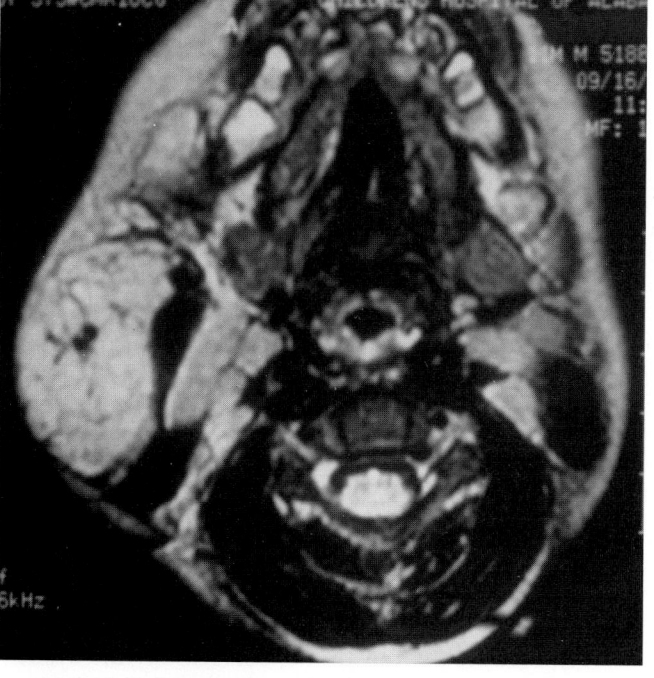

A

B

Figure 57–10: (A) CT with contrast demonstrates a cervical and supraclavicular hemangioma. (B) MRI with contrast demonstrates a hemangioma of the right parotid region.

within the substance of the sternocleidomastoid muscle. It typically presents as a firm, nontender mass in the distal third of the sternocleidomastoid muscle in the neonatal period. The lesion unusually presents within 7 to 28 days of birth.[21] Bilateral lesions have been reported rarely. The etiology of SMTI is unclear. An association with breach and forcep deliveries has been reported, leading to the conclusion that a difficult delivery may predispose an infant to the development of this lesion. The theory that hematoma formation within the sternocleidomastoid muscle during traumatic birth may result in the subsequent fibrosis is a commonly-accepted explanation.[22] However, SMTI following birth by cesarean section also has been reported.[23] Speculation also exists that a prenatal fibrotic process may be the lesion that subsequently leads to a difficult delivery.[21,24,25]

In untreated cases of SMTI, long term torticollis leads to subsequent plagiocephaly and facial asymmetry. Early surgical management is not recommended for treatment. Usually, aggressive physical therapy with cervical range of motion exercises leads to successful resolution within 6 months. Pretreatment evaluation should include an ultrasound to confirm that the mass is solid and intrinsic to the sternocleidomastoid muscle. Cervical spine films may be beneficial to rule out abnormalities that may preclude aggressive cervical range of motion exer-

cises. If physical therapy does not result in successful resolution and torticollis persists, then surgical division of the sternocleidomastoid muscle is indicated.

Other congenital neck masses

Dermoid or *epidermoid cysts* may arise within the neck, usually in the anterior midline region, and may be confused with thyroglossal duct cysts. Histologically, these lesions may be lined by epidermis and contain epidermal appendages, such as hair follicles, hair, and sebaceous glands within the cyst wall.[2] Although dermoid cysts are a distinct entity from thyroglossal duct cysts, they may have attachments to the hyoid bone, similar to thyroglossal duct cysts. It is recommended that the Sistrunk procedure be performed on all midline cystic lesions regardless of histologic type to prevent recurrence of these lesions.[2]

SPECIAL CONSIDERATION:

It is recommended that the Sistrunk procedure be performed on all midline cystic lesions regardless of histologic type to prevent recurrence of these lesions.

Other congenital cystic lesions that may be encountered include teratoid cysts and teratomas. These are usually present at birth, and 20% are associated with maternal polyhydramnois. Evidence of the lesion may be apparent on prenatal ultrasound.[26]

Extensive neck lesions that may produce significant airway compromise can be anticipated before birth when detected by prenatal ultrasound, thereby allowing time to plan for potential airway intervention and surgical resection at the time of birth. CT typically shows a cystic lesion with calcifications that distinguishes it from other congenital lesions. Although endotracheal intubation or tracheotomy may be required, there is a role for extracorporeal membrane oxygenation (ECMO) in newborn infants when airway compromise is severe.[27]

Other, more unusual congenital lesions, that may be included are ectopic thyroid tissue (see Fig. 57–3), ectopic thymus tissue, cervical thymic cysts, laryngoceles, or cervical (plunging) ranulas (Fig. 57–11). A *plunging ranula* results from abnormal cystic dilatation of a sublingual salivary gland that descends beyond the mylohyoid muscle, out of the submandibular space, and into the lower neck.

Inflammatory Neck Masses

Cervical adenitis

Benign cervical adenopathy is the most common cause of neck masses in the pediatric age group. Palpable cervical lymph nodes are present in 40% of infants, and approximately 55% of children in all pediatric age groups have lymph nodes that are palpable but not necessarily associated with an underlying systemic infection or illness.[28,29] Cervical nodes that are asymptomatic and < 1 cm in diameter may be considered normal in children under 12 years of age.

SPECIAL CONSIDERATION:

Cervical nodes that are asymptomatic and < 1 cm in diameter may be considered normal in children under 12 years of age.

Lymphadenitis in children may have a viral, bacterial, fungal, parasitic, or noninfectious etiology. The anatomy of facial and cervical lymph nodes is shown in Figure 57–12. The most common site of involvement for cervical adenitis in children is the submandibular or deep cervical nodes because the majority of head and neck lymphatics drain to these areas.[30]

Infection of the upper respiratory tract in children probably accounts for the majority of the cases of cervical lymphadenopathy. Most episodes of adenitis are fairly self-limited and do not require biopsy or drainage. Infectious mononucleosis, which is an Epstein-Barr viral (EBV) infection, may cause a particularly-severe viral adenopathy, as well as inflammation and enlargement of the remainder of Waldeyer's ring. Exudative tonsillitis also may be present and the diagnosis is typically made by heterophil and EBV antibody titers. Corticosteroids may help to reduce airway obstruction from adenotonsillar hypertrophy and discomfort from cervical adenopathy. Antibiotics may be required for bacterial superinfection. Amoxicillin and ampicillin should be avoided because approximately 90% of patients with EBV infection develop significant hypersensitivity reactions to these antibiotics.[31] Other viral infections that may cause adenopathy in children include HIV, human herpesvirus type 6, CMV, and varicella zoster.

The most common bacterial cause of cervical adenitis in children is *Staphylococcus aureus* and group A streptococci.[32,33] Anaerobic bacteria also may be involved. In suspected cases of bacterial adenitis, a 10-day course of oral antibiotics utilizing a beta-lactamase-resistant agent usually will result in complete regression of the adenitis within 4 to 6 weeks. However, in cases of progressive symptomatology, enlargement of nodes, or the development of fluctuation, a neck abscess should be suspected and aspiration under ultrasound guidance or open incision and drainage procedures should be performed. CT with contrast helps delineate the abscess by the demonstration of a ring-enhancing region around the abscess cavity (Fig. 57–2).

Mycobacterial cervical adenitis is another common cause of infectious cervical adenitis in children. Etiologic agents include tuberculous and nontuberculous mycobacteria. Nontuberculous mycobacterial or atypical nontuberculous mycobacteria are the most common causes arising from *Mycobacterium avium-intracellulare* or *Mycobacterium scrofulaceum*. Other mycobacterial agents also may be causative.[34,35] Typically, skin overlying the involved area undergoes a violaceous color change, with skin breakdown and drainage

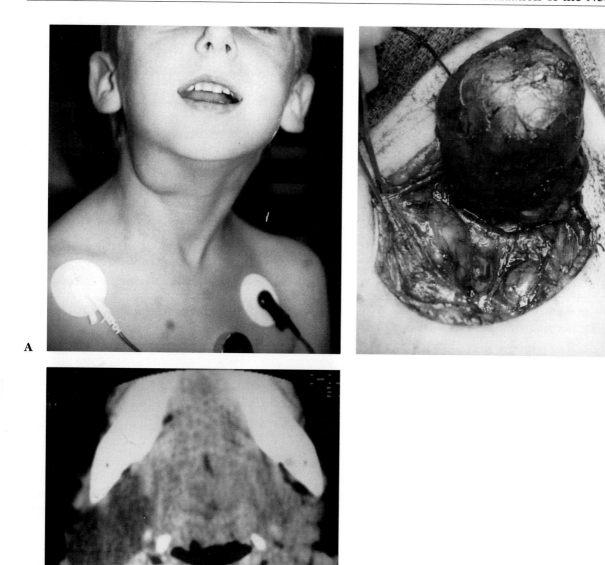

Figure 57–11: (A) 8-year-old boy presenting with a right neck mass that was identified as a plunging cervical ranula. (B) CT demonstrating the cervical ranula. (C) Intraoperative photograph demonstrating the resection of the cervical ranula.

frequently observed also (Fig. 57-13). Calcifications may be noted within the mass on CT. PPD tests are available for nontuberculous and tuberculous agents, and testing is indicated to help confirm the diagnosis. In cases of tuberculous cervical adenitis, chest radiography is warranted and antituberculous chemotherapy should be initiated. In cases of nontuberculous mycobacterial infection, pulmonary involvement is very unusual unless the patient is immunocompromised. Antituberculous chemotherapy, in general, is not helpful in these cases. The treatment of choice for nontuberculous mycobacterial adenitis is open surgical excision, although some have advocated curetage.[36] Histopathologic findings typically reveal granulomas with caseating necrosis. Acid-fast staining may reveal the mycobacterial organisms. Cultures also should be obtained for definitive diagnosis.

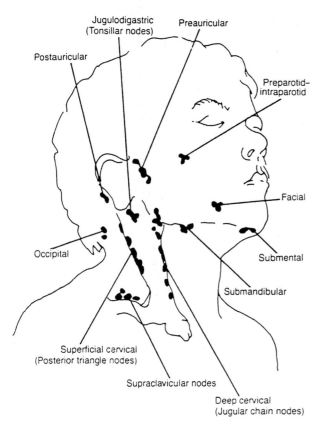

Figure 57–12: Regional lymph node drainage patterns in a child.

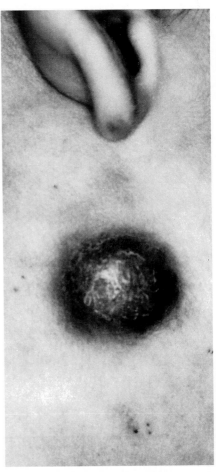

Figure 57–13: Atypical mycobacterial infection of the neck presenting with overlying violaceous skin changes.

Other Causes of Infectious Cervical Adenitis

Cat-Scratch Disease. *Cat-scratch disease* is a relatively unusual cause of cervical adenitis in children, accounting for < 3% of open lymph node procedures performed on pediatric patients.[30] Cervical adenopathy usually develops several weeks after the initial inoculation by a cat scratch. Systemic symptoms such as fever may accompany the infection. More severe systemic findings may occur in 10% of the cases, and these include encephalitis, pneumonia, hepatitis, osteomyelitis, and oculoglandular syndrome of Parinaud (which includes unilateral conjunctivitis and preauricular adenitis). Suspected etiologic bacterial agents include *Bartonella henselae* and *Afipia felis.*[37] Serologic testing for the *Bartonella* may be positive in 90% of cases and may help confirm the diagnosis. Histologically, after lymph node excision, the cat-scratch *Bacillus* may be identified by the Warthin-Starry silver stain. The use of antibiotics is somewhat controversial. Antibiotics that have been used in the treatment of cat-scratch disease include aminoglycosides, ciprofloxacin, rifampin, or trimethoprim-sulfamethoxazole; however, there is no convincing evidence that anti-microbial therapy is efficacious, as the process may resolve spontaneously.[38] Complete resolution of cat-scratch cervical adenitis may require several months.

Other unusual infectious agents that may cause cervical adenitis in children include tularemia, *Mycoplasma pneumoniae,* and actinomycosis. Fungal infections and parasitic infections such as toxoplasmosis also may be involved.

Noninfectious inflammatory cervical adenitis

Numerous noninfectious entities may result in cervical adenitis in children and should be considered in the differential diagnosis. These include *Kawasaki disease,* which is an acute multisystem vasculitis of unknown etiology that is most commonly seen in children < 5 years of age. These patients present with the abrupt onset of fever and may have nonexudative conjunctivitis, oral cavity mucosal changes, polymorphous exanthem, and changes in the ex-

tremities, including erythema of the palms and
soles, pitting edema of the hands and feet, and desquamation of the fingers and toes. Nonsuppurative
cervical adenopathy > 1.5 cm is not uncommon in
this disease.[39] Treatment includes immunoglobulin
replacement therapy. In severe cases, coronary artery aneurysms may develop. Up to 0.5% of the children with this disease may suffer myocardial infarction.

Other conditions that should be considered include sarcoidosis, sinus histiocytosis with massive
lymphadenopathy, focal myositis, and FAPA syndrome (which includes periodic *fever*, *a*phthous
stomatitis, *p*haryngitis, and cervical *a*denitis).[40]

Neoplastic Causes of a Cervical Neck Mass

The vast majority of neoplastic lesions that cause
neck masses in children are malignant lesions. Most
malignancies of the head and neck in children occur
within the lymph nodes themselves. Malignant lesions account for 15% of pediatric cervical neck
mass biopsies.[41,42] A common malignant neoplasm
arising in the neck of children is lymphoma.[3] Although nonHodgkin's lymphoma is more common
than Hodgkin's lymphoma in children, Hodgkin's
lymphoma presents more commonly with a neck
mass.[3] Hodgkin's lymphoma presents in 80 to 90%
of cases as an asymptomatic cervical or supraclavicular neck mass, whereas nonHodgkin's lymphoma
is more likely to be associated with disseminated
systemic disease.[43] Soft-tissue sarcomas are the next
most common cervical malignancy noted in children. Of these, rhabdomyosarcoma is the most commonly encountered and accounts for 15% of malignant lesions arising within the neck, followed by
thyroid tumors, neuroblastoma, and nasopharyngeal carcinoma.[3] Clinically, malignant lymph nodes
are extremely firm on physical examination and
demonstrate rapid enlargement and resistance to antimicrobial therapy. Malignant adenopathy most frequently arises in the supraclavicular and posterior
cervical regions. Although there may be a role for
FNA to determine the presence of malignant cells
in a suspected malignant neck mass, the definitive
diagnosis should be made by open surgical biopsy.
When there is a high suspicion for a malignant lesion, the hematology service should be consulted
preoperatively so that on confirmation of malignancy by frozen section other testing, such as bone
marrow biopsy, may be performed intraoperatively.
Benign neoplasms that may present as a neck mass
include lipoma, pleomorphic adenoma, and neurofibroma.

REFERENCES

1. Torsiglieri AJ Jr, Tom LW, Ross AJ 3rd, et al. Pediatric neck masses: Guidelines for evaluation. Int J Pediatr Otorhinolaryngol 1988; 16:199-210.
2. Cunningham MJ. The management of congenital neck masses. Am J Otolaryngol 1992; 13:78-92.
3. Cunningham MJ, McGuirt WF, Myers EN. Malignant tumors of the head and neck. In: Bluestone CD, Stool SE, Kenna MA, eds. *Pediatric Otolaryngology, 3rd ed.* Philadelphia: Saunders, 1996, pp. 1557-1583.
4. Favus MJ, Schneider AB, Stachura ME, et al. Thyroid cancer occuring as a late consequence of head and neck irradiation. N Engl J Med 1976; 294:1019-1025
5. Jaffe B. Pediatric head and neck tumors: A study of 178 cases. Laryngoscope 1973; 83:1644-1651.
6. Dalton MJ, Robinson LE, Cooper J, et al. Use of *Bartonella* antigens for serologic diagnosis of cat-scratch disease at a national referral center. Arch Int Med 1995; 155:670-676.
7. Layfield LJ, Glasgow B, Ostrega N, et al. Fine needle aspiration cytology and the diagnosis of neoplasms in the pediatric age group. Diagn Cytopathol 1991; 7:451-461.
8. Wakely PE, Kardos TF, Frable WJ. Application of fine needle aspiration biopsy to pediatrics. Human Pathol 1988; 19:1383-1386.
9. Guarisco JL. Congenital head and neck masses in infants and children. Part I. Ear Nose Throat J 1991; 70:40-47.
10. Guarisco JL. Congenital head and neck masses in infants and children. Part II. Ear Nose Throat J 1991; 70:75-82.
11. Mickel RA, Calcaterra TC. Management of recurrent thyroglossal duct cysts. Arch Otolaryngol 1983; 109:34-36.
12. Lim-Dunham JE, Feinstein KA, Yousefzadeh DK, et al. Sonographic demonstration of a normal thyroid gland excludes ectopic thyroid in patients with thyroglossal duct cyst. Am J Roentgenol 1995; 1489-1491.
13. Myers EN, Cunningham MJ. Inflammatory presentations of congenital head and neck masses. Pediatr Infect Dis J 1988; 7(Supplement):162-168.
14. Takai S, Miyauchi A, Matsuzuka F, et al. Internal fistula as a route of infection in acute suppurative thyroiditis. Lancet 1979; 1:751-752.
15. Montgomery GL, Ballantine TV, Kleinman MB, et al. Ruptured branchial cleft cyst presenting as acute thyroid infection. Clin Pediatr 1982; 21:380-383.
16. Rood SR, Johnson JT, Lipman SP, et al. Diagnosis and management of congenital head and neck masses.

American Academy of Otolaryngology—Head and Neck Surgery SIPAC 76481. Washington, DC: US Government Printing Office 1981, pp. 12-24.

17. Radkowski D, Arnold J, Healy GB, et al. Thyroglossal duct remnants. Preoperative evaluation and management. Arch Otolaryngol Head Neck Surg 1991; 117: 1378-1381.

18. Waner M, Suen JY. Management of congenital vascular lesions of the head and neck. [Review]. Oncology 1999; 9:989-994.

19. Schwager K, Waner M, Hohmann D. Hemangioma: Differential diagnosis and necessary early laser treatment. Adv Otorhinolaryngol 1995; 49:70-74.

20. Waner M, Suen JY, Dinehart S. Treatment of hemangiomas of the head and neck. Laryngoscope 1992; 102:1123-1132.

21. Thomsen JR, Koltai PJ. Sternomastoid tumor of infancy. Ann Otol Rhinol Laryngol 1989; 98:955-959.

22. McDaniel A, Hirsch BE, Kornblutt AD, et al. Torticollis in infancy and adolescence. Ear Nose Throat J 1984; 63:478-487.

23. MacDonald D. Sternomastoid tumor and muscular torticollis. J Bone Joint Surg 1969; 51:432-443.

24. Coventry MB, Haris LE. Congenital muscular torticollis in infancy. J Bone Joint Surg 1959; 41:815-822.

25. Jones PG, Mustard WT, eds. *Pediatric Surgery.* Yearbook Medical Publishers, Mosby, St. Louis MO, 1969, pp. 293-298.

26. Rosenfeld CR, Coln CD, Duenhoelter JH. Fetal cervical teratomas as a cause of polyhydramnios. Pediatrics 1979; 64:176-179.

27. Stocks RM, Egerman RS, Woodson GE, et al. Airway management of neonates with antenatally detected head and neck anomalies. Arch Otolaryngol Head Neck Surg 1997; 123:641-645.

28. Bamji M, Stone RK, Kaul A, et al. Palpable lymph nodes in healthy newborns and infants. Pediatrics 1986; 78:573-575.

29. Park YW. Evaluation of neck masses in children. [Review]. Am Fam Physician 1995; 51:1904-1912.

30. Rosenfeld RM. Cervical adenopathy. In: Bluestone CD, Stool SE, Kenna MA, eds. *Pediatric Otolaryngology.* Philadelphia: Saunders, 1996, pp. 1512-1524.

31. Haverkos HW, Amsel Z, Drotman DP. Adverse virus-drug interactions. Rev Infect Dis 1991; 13:697-704.

32. Baker CJ. Group B streptococcal cellulitis-adenitis in infants. Am J Dis Child 1982; 136:631-633.

33. Dajani AS, Garcia RE, Wolinski E. Etiology of cervical lymphadenitis in children. N Engl J Med 1963; 268:1329.

34. Armstrong KL, James RW, Dawson DJ. Mycobacterium haemophilum causing perihilar or cervical lymphadenitis in healthy children. J Pediatr 1992; 121:202-205.

35. Spark RP, Fried ML, Bean CK, et al. Nontuberculous mycobacterial adenitis of childhood: The ten year experience at a community hospital. Am J Dis Child 1988; 142:106-108.

36. Olson NR. Nontuberculous mycobacterial infections of the face and neck—Practical considerations. Laryngoscope 1981; 91:1714-1726.

37. Margileth AM, Hayden GF. Cat scratch disease: From feline affection to human infection. N Engl J Med 1993; 329:53-54.

38. Jackson LA, Perkins BA, Wenger JD. Cat scratch disease in the United States: An analysis of three national databases. Am J Public Health 1993; 83:1707-1711.

39. Gersony WM. Diagnosis and management of Kawasaki Disease. JAMA 1991; 265:2699-2703.

40. Marshall GS, Edwards KM, Butler J, et al. Syndrome of periodic fever, pharyngitis, and aphthous stomatitis. J Pediatr 1987; 110:43-46.

41. Knight PJ, Hamoudi AB, Vassy LE. The diagnosis and treatment of midline neck masses in children. Surgery 1983; 93:603-611.

42. Moussatos GH, Baffes TG. Cervical masses in infants and children. Pediatrics 1963; 32:251-256.

43. Clary RA, Lusk RP. Neck masses. In: Bluestone CD, Stool SE, Kenna MA, eds. *Pediatric Otolaryngology.* Philadelphia: Saunders, 1996, pp. 1488-1496.

58 Congenital Masses in the Neck

Blake C. Papsin
and Jacob Friedberg

The neck is an active area during embryogenesis and therefore, not unexpectedly, a site of a considerable number of congenital anomalies that present to the otolaryngologist attending infants and children. Congenital neck masses in children are the second most common in frequency only to benign lymphadenopathy,[1] and consist of developmental anomalies of the muscle, skin, blood vessels, lymphatics, and the branchial apparatus. This chapter is designed to provide the clinician with an organized and logical approach to congenital neck masses based primarily on the age at which the child presents. It is intended to be complete but not encyclopedic.

PRENATAL NECK MASSES

Improved quality of prenatal ultrasound imaging and its widespread use have resulted in an increased number of neck masses being diagnosed prior to delivery.[2] Oropharyngeal masses, neck masses, teratomas,[3] and lymphatic malformations[4] can present with a constellation of symptoms, including oligohydramnios, flattened diaphragms, and masses that are identified with high-resolution ultrasonography (Fig. 58–1). The acronym *CHAOS* has been used to describe children with congenital high-airway obstruction syndrome, although the collection of symptoms is not truly syndromic.[5] Emergent airway management at delivery is the key for survival in these infants.[6]

At the Hospital for Sick Children, Toronto, a multidisciplinary team, which includes a high-risk obstetrician, a neonatologist, a pediatric otolaryngologist, anesthesiologists (both a maternal and pediatric team), and three nursing teams (labor and delivery,

AT A GLANCE . . .
Congenital High-Airway Obstruction Syndrome (CHAOS)

Pathogenesis: congenital lesions either obstructing the airway intrinsically or by externally compressing the airway, including teratomas, epignathus, lymphangiomas, or laryngeal lesions

Adverse Effects: oligohydramnios during pregnancy and potentially lethal airway compromise at delivery

Symptoms and Signs: may be absent—can occur in a completely asymptomatic pregnancy

Diagnosis: oligohydramnios, flattened diaphragms, and identification of a mass with high-resolution ultrasonography

Treatment: planned Caesarean section delivery with prepared team ready to establish the airway while the child is oxygenated via the placental vessels

Pediatric Otolaryngology, Edited by R.F. Wetmore, H.R. Muntz, and T.J. McGill. Thieme Medical Publishers, Inc., New York © 2000.

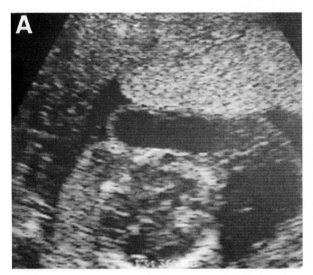

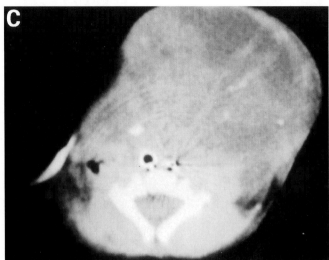

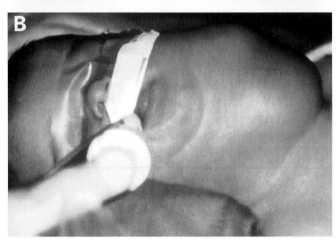

Figure 58–1: (A) An ultrasonographic image of a cystic hygroma that was detected prenatally with high-resolution ultrasound. (B) The mass shown at the time of surgical resection. (C) The corresponding CT scan shows the extent of the tumor and the degree of airway compression resulting from the mass.

neonatal, and pediatric surgical), attends all births of children with anticipated high-airway obstruction. Ideally, the child is delivered electively via Caesarean section, removed from the uterus, and oxygenated via the uterine vessels until the airway is secured.[3] With the infant placed at the same height as the mother's heart to minimize inappropriate transfusion of blood, the airway can be established via intubation or tracheostomy if necessary.

Practice Pathway

Practice Pathway 58-1 begins with high-resolution ultrasound, which identifies the problem and initiates referral to an institution in which the delivery and airway can be managed simultaneously. The critical aspect of management after diagnosis is the careful evaluation of the fetus for other potentially lethal anomalies that might preclude aggressive intervention. Time spent in discussion with the family prior to assembling team members and delivering

the infant is critical. The delivery via Caesarean section and establishment of an airway while on placental oxygenation are followed by another careful evaluation of the child for concomitant anomalies. If the child is otherwise well, surgical resection of the obstructing lesion or airway reconstruction follows.

NEONATAL NECK MASSES

Lymphangiomas

Forty percent of lymphatic malformations present in the neonatal period and often with some airway compromise due to the involvement of the tongue and the floor of the mouth or of the larynx, or as a result of external compression from a cervical mass.[7-9] Since the lesion was first described, there has been a considerable amount of debate about the development of the lymphatic system and the developmental error that leads to the formation of

Practice Pathway 58–1   FETUS AT RISK FOR CHAOS

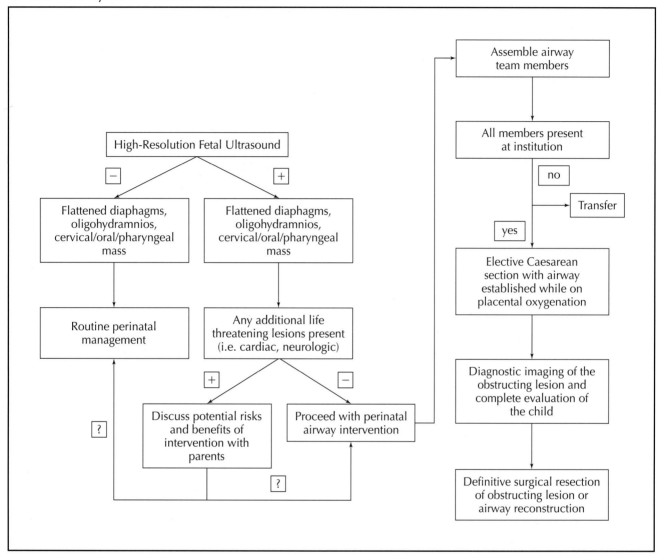

lymphangiomas. Some theorists have suggested that the lymphatic primordia grow outward (*centrifugal theory*) from venous channels,[10] whereas others believe the lymphatic system develops independently of the veins (centripetal theory) and establishes connection with the venous system later.[11] In either case, prominent lymph sacs, including the bilateral cervical jugular sacs, are detectable during the seventh week of embyonic life.[12] Whether these sacs fail to make contact with the venous system or fail to maintain their previously-developed connections is a point best left disputed by the embryologists. It is clear that, no matter which developmental theory is held, the pathologic lesion results from lymphatic cysts isolated from their normal route of drainage into the venous system. They cause their effect by expansion following this sequestration.

This drainage defect is likely incomplete in many instances, which accounts for the late presentation in some patients or apparent spontaneous resolution in others. Expansion may result from the sequestered tissue's proliferative growth potential[11] or may follow infection, trauma, or hemorrhage into a previously quiescent cyst (Fig. 58-2).[13]

Histologically, these lesions are comprised of normal mature lymphatic tissue, which can be subdivided into capillary, cavernous, and cystic types by the size of the lymphatic spaces. Commonly, all three subtypes coexist within a single lesion.[14] *Cystic hygroma* is a clinical term used to describe those large cystic neck masses that occur in areas where expansion can occur and large multiloculated cystic spaces can develop; these areas are typically deep to the sternocleidomastoid muscle, below the level

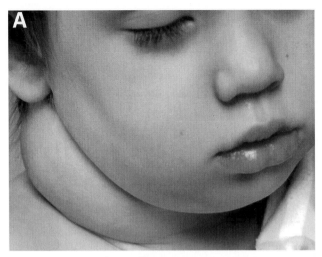
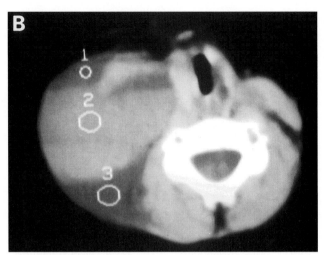

Figure 58–2: This 4-year-old girl presented with a rapidly-expanding neck mass resulting from hemorrhage into a cystic hygroma that is shown here clinically (A) and on a CT scan (B). The CT scan shows a cystic mass of the right neck with an obvious blood-fluid level present. This is not an uncommon presentation of cystic hygroma.

of the hyoid bone and intimately related to the neurovascular bundle.[8] Lymphangiomas, which occur more cephalad, are predominantly of the more infiltrative type and are not of great significance lower in the neck.

Cystic hygromas present as soft, painless, and easily-compressible masses. Although most commonly seen shortly after birth, increasingly, these lesions are being recognized prenatally with ultrasound imaging, allowing for airway management preparation in advance of delivery. Sixty percent of the lesions occur in the first year of life, and 90% will have presented by age 3 years.[15] Neonatal cystic hygromas often exhibit signs of hemorrhage into them, which makes them appear much more like hemangiomas. Cystic hygromas most commonly present in the posterior triangle and are initially only of cosmetic concern, but anterior triangle lesions and those involving the oral cavity and floor of the mouth may present with potential airway obstruction (Fig. 58–3).

Differential diagnoses include branchial cysts, thyroglossal duct cysts, lymphomas, and true neoplasms. Although they may be transilluminated readily, radiologic investigation is the best way to establish the diagnosis. Williams and Cole outline the diagnostic imaging currently used in the assessment of lymphangiomas and advocate the use of plain radiographs of the neck and chest to evaluate the extent of esophageal and laryngeal obstruction.[16] Ultrasound can be valuable in pre- and postnatal diagnosis and in monitoring the extent of the lesion.

Magnetic resonance imaging (MRI) delineates clearly the cystic mass from the surrounding normal tissue (Fig. 58–4), but computed tomography (CT) remains the modality of greatest value to differentiate the cystic lesion from vascular tumors and mucus retention cysts. CT remains the standard radiographic investigation especially if there is considerable mediastinal involvement (approximately 5% of the time) or if surgical excision is planned. Lymphangiography is no longer utilized.

Surgical excision remains the treatment of choice, although a rate of spontaneous regression between 8 and 15% has been reported.[8,17] The reported recurrence rate from residual lesions ranges from 10 to 52%.[8,15] The role of OK-432 sclerosis of macrocystic lymphangiomas is currently being evaluated, but initial reports suggest this modality may be of benefit only in the subset of lymphangiomas (the larger single cyst variety) that are resected most easily surgically.[18] When the larynx is involved directly, tracheostomy almost always is required.[8,19,20] Occasionally, more extensive resections are required, and modified radical neck dissections[9,17] and partial laryngectomy[21] have been used to control lesions in the neck with laryngeal involvement. Those lesions lower in the neck that are related closely to the carotid sheath and those in the anterior mediastinum[22] may be resected cleanly even if of significant size, whereas lesions in the submandibular region that involve the mandible, floor of the mouth, base of the tongue, or supraglottis seldom allow for complete removal. The benign

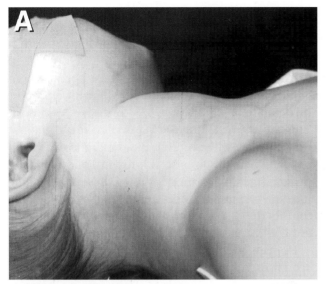

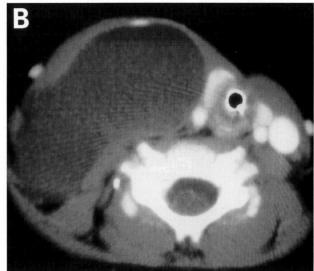

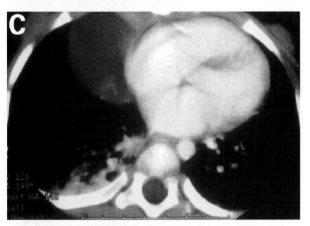

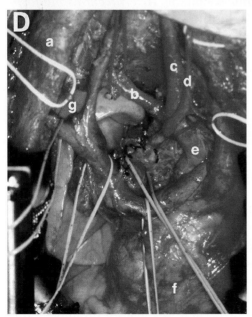

Figure 58–3: (A) A 20-month-old girl with an extensive lymphangioma presenting in the right neck. The lesion extends as shown in the CT scan from (B) the neck into the mediastinum almost to the level of (C) the diaphragm and compresses the airway. Resection of these extensive lesions often requires division of the manubrium to allow dissection of the mass from the pericardium and great vessels. (D) The dissection of the mediastinum is shown after the mass has been resected out of the right hilum. (a) right sternocleidomastoid muscle; (b) right subclavian artery; (c) right common carotid artery; (d) vagus nerve; (e) arch of the aorta; (f) the heart; (g) the phrenic nerve.

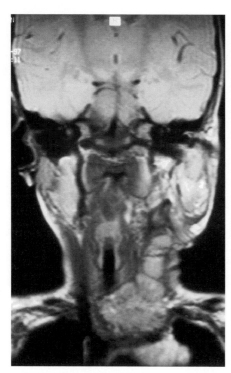

Figure 58–4: MRI of a cystic hygroma in a 6-year-old girl extending from the base of the skull into the mediastinum.

nature of lymphangiomas should be considered in treatment planning, and preservation of neurovascular structures accomplished whenever possible.[8,9,21] Undue risk to the facial, accessory, laryngeal, or hypoglossal nerves or to the brachial plexus cannot be justified.

AT A GLANCE . . .

Lymphangioma

Pathogenesis: developmental lesion that results from the failure of the distal lymphatic system to connect with the proximal system, leaving cystic lesions in the neck

Adverse Effects: potential airway compression; cosmetic and functional defects

Symptoms and Signs: large easily-compressible mass in head and/or neck; may enlarge after trauma or upper respiratory tract infection

Diagnosis: clinical suspicion with CT confirmation

Treatment: surgical resection with preservation of vital structures

---

Vascular Lesions

Hemangiomas are the most common vascular head and neck lesion in children. Although located primarily on mucosal or skin surfaces, hemangiomas can occur in deeper tissues and present as masses in neonates. Fewer than 33% of these lesions are present at birth, but the natural history of subsequent progressive, often rapid, enlargement within the first year of life is well known. Following their progressive enlargement, 90% of these lesions involute and require no additional therapy. The invasive tumors that involve muscles and deep fascial layers are less likely to involute spontaneously.[23]

Hemangiomas are benign lesions in which there are an increased number of normal and abnormal appearing blood vessels.[24] They can be hemodynamically-significant to the point of high-output cardiac failure due to the presence of arteriovenous shunting, and they may require treatment for this reason rather than because of expansion into soft tissue. Cutaneous *nevus flammeus lesions* and *strawberry nevi* are dermal capillary lesions that rarely present as neck masses. *Cavernous hemangiomas,* in contradistinction, are composed of much larger tortuous vascular channels with endothelial lining. These are far more likely to be associated with deeper tissue involvement, hemodynamic significance, and unfortunately, a much lower rate of spontaneous resolution. *Arteriovenous malformations* share histologic features with the cavernous hemangiomas, and in addition, have intimal thickening of the veins and multiple discrete arteriovenous connections. They are distinguishable clinically from other head and neck masses because they are pulsatile on palpation[25] and may be associated with an audible bruit (Fig. 58–5).

The diagnosis of a hemangioma is best done with CT, MRI, and angiography. With CT, the lesion enhances with intravenous contrast, allowing for evaluation of the extent of the mass and delineation of the relationship between the mass and the surrounding tissue. MRI is superior to CT in providing soft-tissue contrast resolution and can delineate clearly the extent of the lesion and its feeding vessels. On angiography, hemangiomas have a dense tissue stain and show association with several enlarged arteries. There is usually a prominent artery with several smaller communications between this larger feeding vessel and the mass.[26]

Soft-tissue hemangiomas, although benign, are difficult to remove surgically if there is extensive

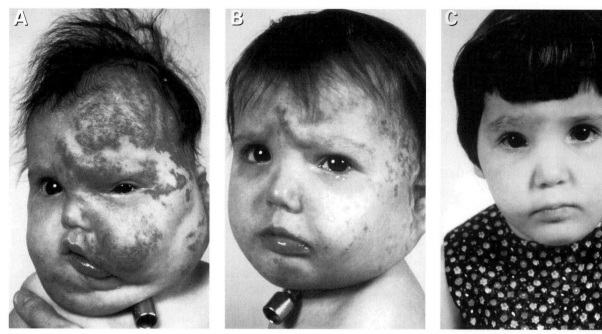

Figure 58–5: (A) An extensive cervicofacial hemangioma (note also the tracheostomy required because of a considerable subglottic stenosis). (B and C) The lesion's almost complete resolution with the passage of time. No surgical therapy except for the tracheostomy was required.

infiltration of the deep tissues of the neck. The mass is usually a well-circumscribed, rubbery, painless, and mobile lesion. A bruit is not present usually. There may or may not be cutaneous involvement over the mass. These masses most commonly present in the muscles of the neck and are associated with high recurrence rates after attempted exci-

---

AT A GLANCE . . .

Hemangioma

Pathogenesis: benign tumors with increased numbers of normal and abnormal appearing blood vessels

Adverse Effects: cosmetic and functional defects, potentially hemodynamic significance

Natural Course: progressive enlargement (often rapid in the first year of life) then spontaneous involution

Diagnosis: CT scan with contrast, angiography, MRI, and MRA (magnetic resonance angiography) show extent of the lesion and identification of dominant arterial feeding vessel

Treatment: surgery reserved for lesions in which there is cosmetic deformity or functional defects (e.g., oral commissure)

---

sion.[14] Conservative treatment is carried out whenever possible because these lesions are benign like lymphangiomas, and risk to underlying vital tissue must be minimized during treatment. Adjuvant therapy with interpheron alpha-2B may reduce the size of the lesion dramatically[27] and diminish proliferation of the hemangioma. Sclerosing agents and radiotherapy are no longer used.[23] Surgical excision of these masses should be reserved for cases in which there is serious cosmetic deformity or in which function is disturbed by the mass (i.e., laryngeal or subglottic involvement).

Teratoma, Hamartoma, and Choristoma

Teratomas are comprised of tissue that is foreign to the site of origin and are composed of all three germ layers.[28] They can be described as either mature or immature depending on the degree of differentiation in the cells contained. Often these tumors have poorly-differentiated tissue within them, which gives the histologic impression of malignancy. Unlike similar-appearing lesions in the sacrococcygeal region, these cervical teratomas are rarely malignant.[29,30] Cervical teratomas often present as neck masses in the neonatal period, and are diagnosed frequently in utero.[31] They rarely present after the first year of life.

Teratomas are evaluated best radiologically, and 50% show a soft-tissue mass on plain radiographs.[32] Ultrasonography shows mixed echogenicity that usually can be differentiated from a cystic hygroma. CT delineates the extent of the lesion and usually demonstrates a heterogeneous, partially-cystic, and well-encapsulated mass with speckled calcification. These masses often present with neonatal airway obstruction, but can present with less severe airway distress or esophageal compression. If possible, excision is the preferred method of management, and outcome is related largely to the extent of the tumor and associated anomalies.

Hamartomas contain tissue that is indigenous to the area of growth (e.g., ectopic tongue tissue in the floor of the mouth), and *choristomas* (Fig. 58–6) are similar to hamartomas but are composed of tissue from a foreign location (e.g., gastric tissue in the floor of the mouth). Choristomas display cellular differentiation that often allows recognition of organ structure; they usually present with symptoms that are related to their compression of normal tissue and distortion of anatomic architecture.

Midline Cervical Clefts

Midline cervical clefts are rare and manifest as linear erythematous vertical bands extending from the mandibular symphysis to the manubrium.[33,34] Their etiology is unknown, and they present with an absence of normal tissue in the midline vertical neck, which is replaced by a fibrous band up to 10 mm in width. They are more commonly found in females,[35] and are comprised of a characteristic cephalad skin tag, a mucosal surface, and a caudal sinus.[36] If untreated, these lesions deform and tether the mandible to the sternum. Treatment consists of early excision of the cleft and closure with multiple Z-plasties (Fig. 58–7).

Musculoskeletal Anomalies

Congenital muscular torticollis or *fibromatosis colli* is often noted at birth or may develop within

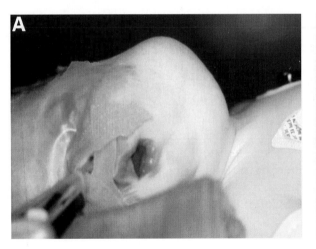

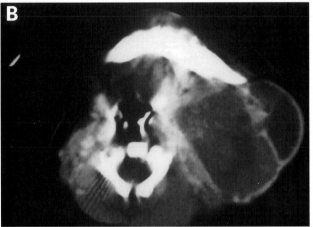

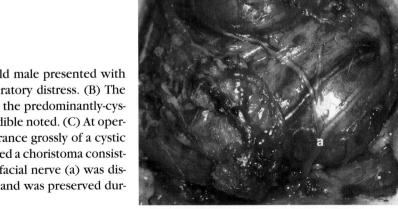

Figure 58–6: This 1-week-old male presented with the mass shown (A) and respiratory distress. (B) The corresponding CT scan shows the predominantly-cystic mass with flaring of the madible noted. (C) At operation, the mass had the appearance grossly of a cystic hygroma, but pathology revealed a choristoma consisting of neurogenic tissue. The facial nerve (a) was displaced laterally over the mass and was preserved during the dissection.

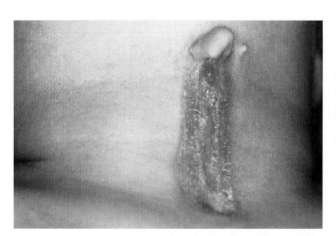

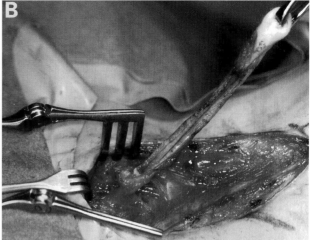

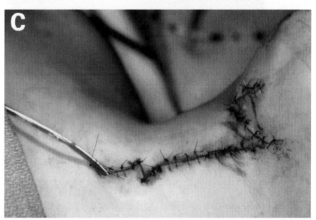

Figure 58–7: (A) A midline cervical cleft in an 8-month-old boy. (B) At surgery, a thick band was resected and (C) closure was carried out using multiple Z-plasties.

the first few postnatal weeks.[37–39] There is usually unilateral contracture of the sternocleidomastoid muscle with rotation of the chin away from the lesion and tilting of the head towards the lesion. A palpable, nontender "fibrous tumor" may be felt within the body of the sternocleidomastoid muscle (Fig. 58–8). The mass is an inflammatory lesion of unknown etiology wherein the muscle tissue becomes replaced by fibrosis. The mass grows to its maximum size within the first month and then usu-

ally regresses leaving little or no residual deformity. Treatment requires only range of motion exercises to prevent shortening of the sternocleidomastoid muscle. Follow-up is critical as those few patients in whom resolution does not occur may be left with an unsightly, difficult-to-manage, fixed cervical deformity that may require a myoplasty.[40]

Practice Pathway

Practice Pathway 58–2 begins by determining the amount of time over which evaluation and management can be performed. Airway symptoms of expansion of the mass obviously necessitate emergent evaluation and airway management. Next, the two, relatively-clear, nonmass lesions are identified. Midline cervical cleft is resected electively and hemangioma is observed unless there is a significant functional or cosmetic defect present. Then, the mass is evaluated for consistency. Cystic masses in this age group are imaged to confirm lymphangioma and its extent, and then they are resected electively. Solid lateral neck masses within the sternocleido-

SPECIAL CONSIDERATION:

A child with congenital muscular torticollis presents usually accompanied by alarmed parents and referring physicians. The urge to perform biopsy to rule out malignancy must be resisted for cases in which diagnostic imaging demonstrates the mass to be within the body of the sternocleidomastoid muscle.

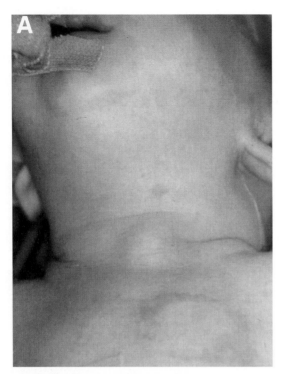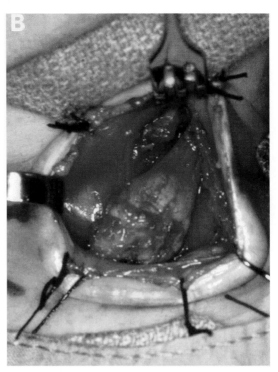

Figure 58–8: (A) Clinical presentation of a sternocleidomastoid tumor of infancy, and (B) the mass at operation at the time of myoplasty.

mastoid muscle confirmed by ultrasound are fibromatosis colli and are treated best with physiotherapy. Other solid lateral neck masses are imaged, and resection usually planned electively once a provisional diagnosis is determined.

NECK MASSES PRESENTING IN THE INFANTS

Branchial Anomalies

Neck embryology is covered in greater detail in Chapter 56, which includes a detailed discussion of the branchial apparatus. By the fifth week of embryogenesis, four visible and two rudimentary arches are present in the embryo. The branchial apparatus (arches, pouches, and grooves) develops into definitive structures of the head and neck,[41] and nondevelopment, maldevelopment, or duplication of any structure results in a branchial anomaly that can present as a mass in the neck.

First branchial cleft anomalies can be divided into four broad categories: aplasia, atresia, stenosis, and duplication.[42] Apart from easily-identifiable auricular tags, only duplication anomalies of the first arch can present as neck masses. These lesions

occur when there is duplication of the first branchial groove, usually in the presence of a normal external auditory canal (EAC). Two specific subtypes of this lesion have been described.[43] *Type I branchial cysts* exist as fistulous tracts near the lower portion of the parotid gland, and often present as sinus tracts or localized areas of swelling near the postauricular sulcus or anterior to the tragus. These lesions track parallel to the EAC and can end in continuity with the EAC or the middle ear, although a discrete opening is found uncommonly.[44] The cyst is lined by squamous epithelium without skin appendages. The less-commonly encountered *type II branchial lesion* (Fig. 58–9) presents as a superficial cyst or sinus tract in the neck below the angle of the mandible. This lesion represents an anomalous EAC and rudimentary pinna. For this reason, it is composed of both squamous epithelium plus skin appendages (epithelium) and may also contain cartilaginous elements (mesoderm). Both types of first branchial cleft anomalies may track in close approximation to the facial nerve, but type II lesions do this more consistently; commonly, the track runs from the neck to the EAC or middle ear by passing underneath the facial nerve in the posterior parotid and displacing the nerve laterally and inferiorly.[45] Both types of lesions are treated ideally by

Practice Pathway 58–2   NEONATAL NECK MASS

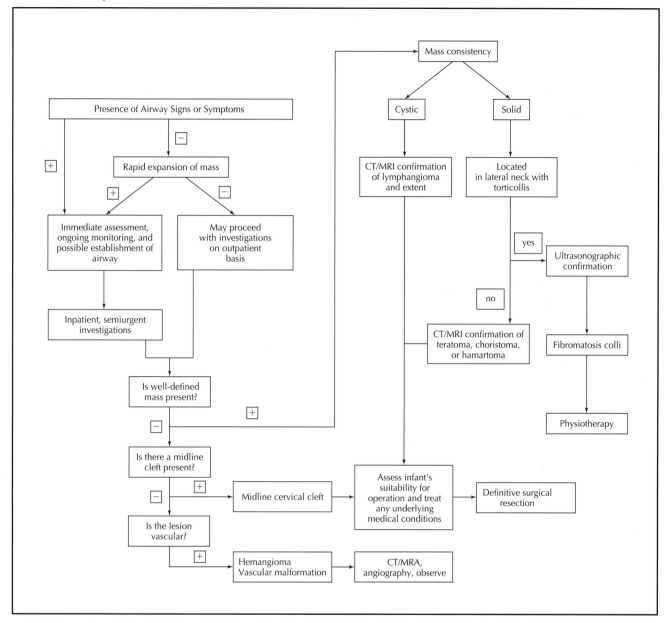

complete surgical excision, which usually is best attempted when the lesion is noninfected. CT or MRI of the lesion is helpful in planning the excision and may indicate the presence of a tract in continuity with the EAC.

The most common branchial cleft lesions encountered in the young child are derivatives of the second branchial groove.[46] Failure of obliteration of the cervical sinus of His results in an epithelial-lined space trapped in the neck. If the lesion is an isolated cyst, it is usually found high in the lateral neck, deep to the sternocleidomastoid muscle at its anterior aspect. It also can occur at the level of the carotid

bifurcation or even in the parapharyngeal space. Commonly, cysts enlarge and become clinically-apparent following an upper respiratory tract infection (URI) CT or MRI delineates the cyst well (Fig. 58-10) and distinguishes it from other lesions (e.g., carotid aneuryam, tumors of the parotid tail, etc.). Incision and drainage or aspiration of the cyst contents is not recommended. A fluid aspirate can demonstrate the presence of epithelial cells, which confirms the diagnosis. Infections within the cysts should be eliminated prior to any planned excision. Definitive treatment is surgical, and the mass usually is found lateral to the carotid bifurcation. A tract

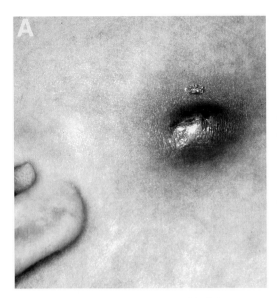

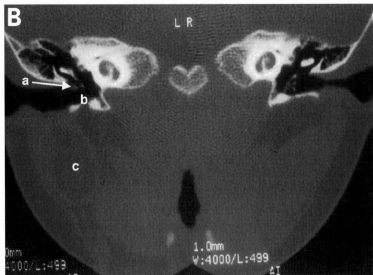

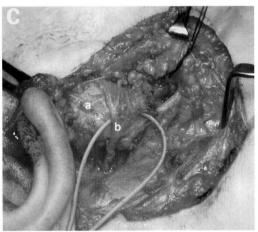

Figure 58–9: (A) This 2-year-old girl had a recurrent swelling in the right neck just anterior to the angle of the mandible. (B) CT scan shows a type IB first branchial cleft sinus in continuity with the EAC. There is a cyst on the tympanic membrane (a), which was in continuity with the neck mass (c) via a dehiscence in the inferior portion of the bony canal (b). (C) At resection, the mass (a) traveled underneath the stretched and laterally-displaced facial nerve (b). The dissection revealed that the cyst traveled under the main branch of the facial nerve, which had itself been pushed laterally by the mass. The dissection was carried out medially until the sinus entered the EAC.

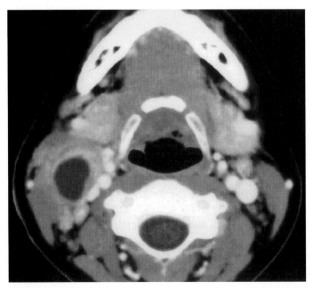

Figure 58–10: This CT scan of the neck shows a second branchial cleft cyst deep to the sternocleidomastoid muscle at the level of the hyoid bone.

may extend superiorly from the cyst between the internal and external carotid arteries and continue to the constrictor muscles, at which point it may be ligated as it inserts into the tonsillar fossa.

Second branchial cleft anomalies can present as sinuses or fistulous tracts connecting the skin to the mucosa of the tonsillar fossa. Typically, these anomalies present along the anterior border of the sternocleidomastoid muscle in its lower third as a stoma with intermittent discharge of mucoid material. The tract is treated surgically by complete excision, often via a stepped incision to allow identification of the tract to the level of the bifucation of the carotid artery (second branchial cleft sinus) and occasionally to the level of the pharyngeal wall (branchial cleft fistula) (Fig. 58-11). A second, higher incision is required almost always for a full dissection of a true fistula at the level of the carotid arteries and definitive excision of the upper portion of the tract.

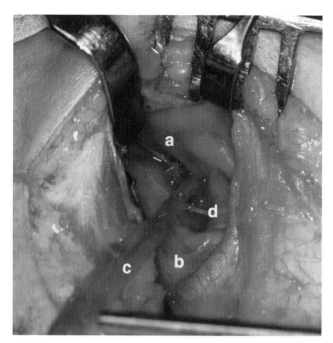

Figure 58–11: An excised second branchial cleft sinus tract (c) at the level of the carotid bifurcation (b) passing between the internal and external branches of the carotid artery. Notice the digastric muscle superiorly retracted (a) and the hypoglossal nerve inferomedial to the tract (d).

Third branchial cleft lesions are rare but can present as masses low in the anterior neck, most often on the left side.[47]. The proximal end exits the aerodigestive tract in the pyriform fossa, travels through the thyrohyoid membrane, and tracks under the glossopharyngeal nerve and internal carotid artery, but superficial to the vagus nerve (Fig. 58-12). Fourth arch masses exist theoretically, but clinically appear rarely.[48,49] (The literature defines third and fourth cleft anomalies inconsistently.) Treatment of these lesions is surgical excision often after resolution of a localized infection.

SPECIAL CONSIDERATION:

Third branchial cleft lesions often present with recurrent infections in the left lower lateral neck, which often have a minimal proximal tract at operation or on CT/MRI. These lesions often track adjacent to or through the upper pole of the thyroid, and a hemithyroidectomy is required sometimes for complete resection, especially when the surgeon is faced with recurrent infections after seemingly-adequate initial resection.

AT A GLANCE . . .
Branchial Cleft Lesions

Pathogenesis: these developmental lesions are persistent structures arising from the embryonic branchial clefts and pouches. Instead of disappearing, these lesions retain their epithelial surface and develop into sinuses, fistulae, or cysts in the region of the ear (type I) and the neck (types II and III)

Adverse Effects: may become inflamed and enlarged with URI

Symptoms and Signs: varies from a nonresolving mass in the neck to a persistently-discharging lesion in the EAC or anterior neck

Diagnosis: clinically diagnosed with confirmation on CT/MRI

Treatment: elective resection

Thyroglossal Duct Cyst

The thyroid gland develops from primordial tissue at the foramen cecum on the floor of the embryologic pharynx just caudal to the tuberculum impar.[41] This thyroid diverticulum descends to the anterior neck via a tract in close approximation to the developing hyoid bone and with a persistent connection to the foramen cecum. This connection, the *thyroglossal duct,* usually disappears, but persistence of the tract at any point between the pyramidal lobe of the thyroid and the foramen cecum can present as a thyroglossal duct cyst. A thyroglossal duct sinus opening anteriorly onto the surface of the neck is invariably secondary to rupture of the cyst after infection and rapid expansion or surgical drainage of the neck.

The *thyroglossal duct cyst* is the most common benign cervical mass after cervical lymphadenopathy in children.[50] Most often these masses present before the age of 5 years, and clinically are diagnosed by their position and the mobility of the mass with protrusion of the tongue.[51] The location of the mass is most commonly at the level of the hyoid bone, but can be anywhere along the tract of the thyroid gland's descent (but not below it) (Fig. 58-13).

Histologic examination reveals ductal architecture lines of either squamous or ciliated squamous pseudostratified epithelium. Occasionally, mucous glands or ectopic thyroid may be present in the cyst

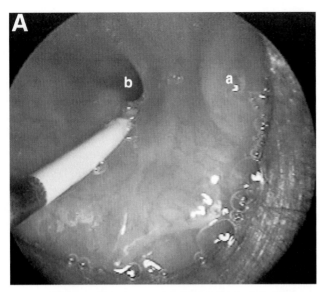
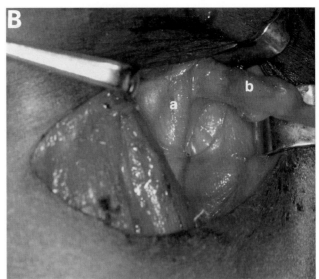

Figure 58–12: A third branchial cleft sinus tract. (A) An endoscopic view of the proximal end of the tract in the left pyriform fossa. The posterior portion of the left arytenoid joint (a) is shown and the sinus tract (b) is seen with a uretheral catheter entering it. (B) The dissection in the neck revealed a sinus tract (b) that passed behind and medial to the common carotid artery (a).

wall. Ultrasonography aids in delineating the extent of the cyst, but is most useful in confirming the presence of the normal thyroid lower in the neck.[52] In rare instances where the thyroid is not visualized on ultrasonography, a technicium scan of the neck is imperative as the mass my represent the only functioning thyroid tissue in the patient. (Fig. 58-13).

Treatment is surgical and recurrence can be minimized by excising the entire tract, including the central portion of the hyoid bone[53] and a generous portion of the tongue base around the foramen cecum.[54] Carcinoma can occur exceptionally rarely in the thyroglossal duct tract and usually is papillary thyroid carcinoma.[55,56] In malignancy, treatment is complete excision of the tract (with or without excision of the thyroid gland) followed by thyroid suppression therapy.

SPECIAL CONSIDERATION:

Infantile neck masses (branchial cleft cysts, thyroglossal duct cysts, and lymphangiomas) commonly present secondary to URIs, and this, rather than any physiologic or anatomic factor, differentiates them from neonatal neck masses. Lymphagiom commonly present in infants and children, but their appearance in this age group usually follows trauma or URI.

AT A GLANCE . . .

Thyroglossal Duct Cyst

Pathogenesis: congenital lesion representing the embryologic tract of the thyroid's descent into the lower anterior neck that has failed to be obliterated. This tract retains epithelial structures and is capable of developing cysts.

Adverse Effects: cosmetic lesion that can rupture and discharge onto the surface of the neck; rarely, can harbour malignancy of thyroid origin.

Symptoms and Signs: midline swelling in the neck, usually at the level of the hyoid bone. May elevate with swallowing.

Diagnosis: ultrasound confirms the cystic structure and confirms clinical suspicion. Must identify normal thyroid gland on ultrasound or proceed with radioisotope scan to identify location of functioning thyroid prior to resection.

Treatment: elective resection to the base of the tongue, including the central portion of the hyoid bone, is curative.

Dermoid Cysts

Dermoid cysts commonly are considered in the differential diagnosis of midline neck masses.[57] Clinically, they are firm mobile masses that do not rise with tongue protrusion and may blanch when the

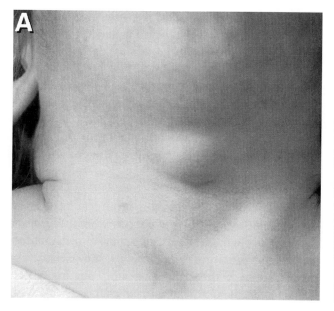

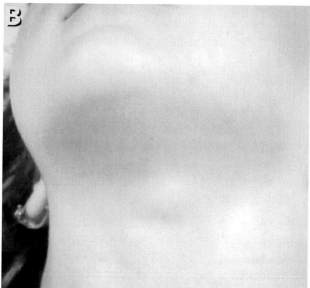

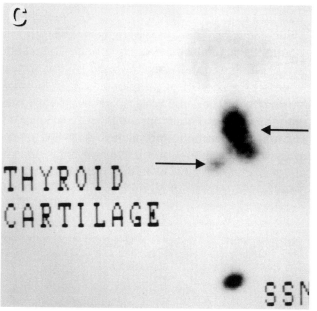

Figure 58–13:   This child presented with a firm, mobile mass in the neck just off the midline that moved with swallowing. (A) a common presentation of a thyroglossal duct cyst. (B) A similarly-appearing lesion in a 3-year-old girl. Ultrasonography failed to show a normal positioned thyroid gland, and (C) subsequent technicium scan shows that the mass contains the only functioning thyroid tissue in this child. Note the position of the suprasternal notch, the thyroid notch (left arrow), and the mass (right arrow).

overlying skin is stretched. Usually, ultrasonography can not differentiate these cysts from thyroglossal duct cysts, and differentiation of these two lesions is based on clinical findings. A midline cyst of the neck that is caudal to a palpable thyroid isthmus is most likely a dermoid cyst. A dermoid cyst consists of tissue from all three germinal layers and can contain skin appendages, including sweat glands and sebaceous glands. Total surgical excision is required to remove the enlarging mass and prevent its recurrence.

Thymic Cysts

Thymic masses usually present in the lower aspect of the neck, but may occur anywhere from the level of the pyriform sinus to the chest. They are firm, rounded lesions that are occasionally associated with respiratory symptoms, including cough and respiratory compromise rarely. Initial evaluation usually includes a radiograph of the chest that reveals a mass of smooth density filling the anterior mediastinum. Histology can reveal a thymic cyst, thymic hyperplasia, thymoma, or rarely a thymic lymphosarcoma.[58]

Laryngoceles

Laryngoceles are found rarely in the neck of a child. They occur as a result of abnormal dilatation of the laryngeal saccule, which becomes filled and distended with air. The laryngocele is lined with respi-

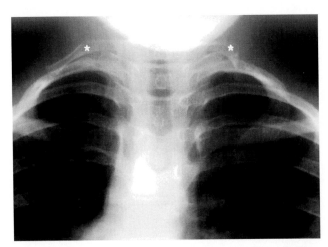

Figure 58–14: This 2-year-old girl presented with bilateral firm lateral neck masses that were found on radiologic examination to be accessory cervical ribs (*).

ratory epithelium and has the ability to secrete mucus.[59] If the opening of the laryngocele becomes obstructed, the mass may fill with inspissated mucus (saccular cyst) (Fig. 58–14) or alternatively can become infected and result in a *laryngopyocele.*

The mass initially extends within the larynx posterosuperiorly between the thyroid cartilage and the false vocal cord, and is termed an *internal laryngocele.* If it extends above the level of the thyroid ala, it often extends out through the thyrohyoid membrane in a region through which the superior laryngeal nerve enters the larynx. Such a laryngocele is termed an *external laryngocele* and may exist alone or in continuity with the internal component. An external laryngocele manifests clinically as a soft swelling that is noted to one side of the midline over the thyroid ala. Saccular cysts are more common in children and are thought to arise from obstruction of the saccule at the level of the ventricle.

Laryngoceles are symptomatic as they expand and may cause hoarseness and possibly airway compromise with continued growth. They are diagnosed on endoscopic exam, and CT or MRI delineate the mass precisely, which aids in planning surgical resection. Internal laryngoceles can be excised endoscopically, or alternatively, they can be unroofed widely and marsupialized. External or combined lesions often require an external approach to completely remove the lesion.

Plunging Ranula

A simple *ranula* is a retention cyst (*mucocele*) that is caused by obstruction of the sublingual or another major salivary gland duct.[60] A *plunging ranula,* a rarer type of sublingual gland mucocele, describes a lesion in which the intraoral mass extends through the floor of the mouth and appears in the anterior neck.[61,62] The mass presents typically as a soft, painless, gradually-expanding mass that begins in the submandibular region and extends inferiorly. Though far more common as a complication of salivary gland surgery,[63] some congenital ranula occur.[64]

A plunging ranula is a pseudocyst having no epithelial lining. The lining is composed of compressed, fibrous connective tissue containing fibroblasts, vascular channels, and other inflammatory cells. Extension into the neck is a result of extravasation of mucin through or around the mylohyoid muscle into the deep fascial planes of the neck. Aspiration of cystic contents reveals a high amylase content and electrolyte, protein, enzyme, and glucose values similar to those of sublingual mucin, differentiating the ranula from cystic hygroma. The diagnosis of plunging ranula is confirmed by the appearance on CT or MRI of a uniloculated, cystic mass arising from the sublingual space with extension into the submandibular or parapharyngeal spaces.[65]

Multiple treatment approaches including marsupialization, simple sublingual gland excision, and cervical excision have been described with variable results. The preferred method is intraoral excision

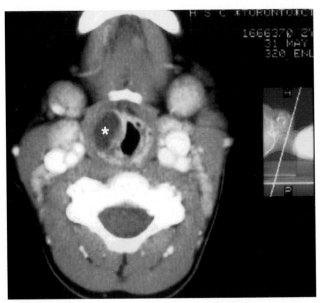

Figure 58–15: This 2-year-old boy presented with a palpable anterior neck mass and hoarseness. A saccular cyst (*) was identified on the CT scan. Complete excision via a laryngofissure was carried out.

Practice Pathway 58–3 INFANTILE NECK MASS

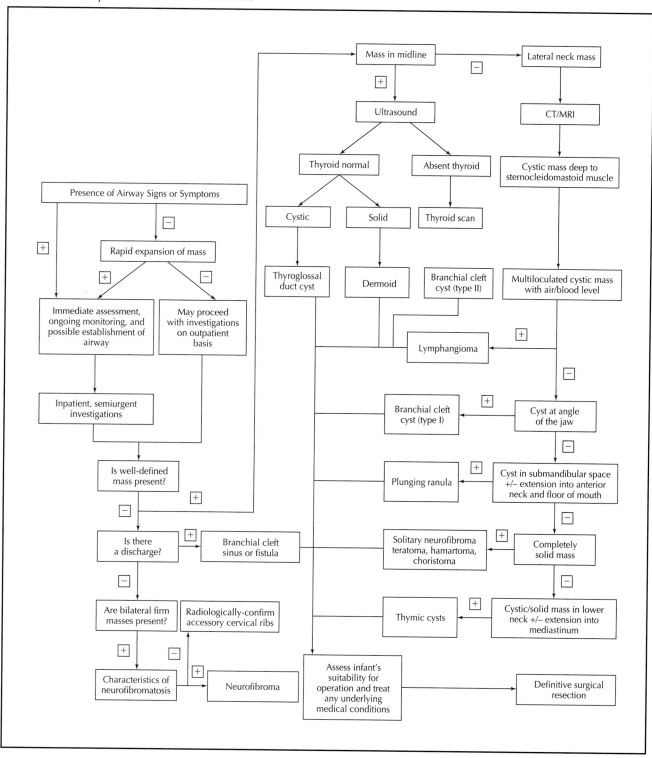

of the sublingual gland and evacuation of the cyst without the need for cervical dissection.[64] Care must be taken to preserve the hypoglossal and lingual nerves, the submandibular duct, and the sublingual artery.

Other Lesions

Though rare, a number of other lesions must be included because they should be considered in the differential diagnosis of congenital neck masses in children. *Accessory first cervical ribs* can present with an asymptomatic lateral neck mass deep to the sternocleidomastoid muscle. An important finding is that this mass is not mobile and is exceptionally firm. Plain radiographs of the neck confirm the presence of accessory first cervical ribs (Fig. 58–15).

Neurogenic tumors (e.g., neurilemoma, neurofibroma) are discussed elsewhere but also must be considered in the differential diagnosis of neck masses in the child. These firm and slowly-growing lesions can present as lateral neck masses usually arising from the vagus nerve within the neurovascular bundle. Neurilemomas (Schwannomas) are unusual in children, but most commonly present in the lateral neck.[66] Of importance, these lesions typically grow on the surface of the peripheral nerve and theoretically are encapsulated, allowing dissection with preservation of the nerve.

As part of von Recklinghausen's disease, neurofibromas may present as multiple neck masses, but sporadic tumors (solitary neurofibromas) can occur also.[66] In contrast to neurilemomas, these lesions typically are infiltrative, and resection without damage to the nerve is more difficult.[67,68]

Practice Pathway

Practice Pathway 58–3 is very straightforward, despite looking complex. As with neonatal neck masses, the rapidity of evaluation and therapy is first determined by the degree of airway compromise and the rate at which the mass is expanding. Next, discharging masses (branchial cleft sinuses) and firm masses (accessory ribs and neurofibromas) are diagnosed and treated appropriately. The body of the pathway divides the remaining masses into those in the lateral neck and those in the midline. Midline masses are first subjected to ultrasonographic evaluation with attention paid to the presence of a normal thyroid gland. Cystic midline masses (thyroglossal duct cysts) are differentiated

in this way from solid masses (dermoid cysts), although in reality the final confirmation is only possible at the time of surgery. In cases where the thyroid is not identified, nuclear scan is recommended prior to undertaking any surgical options.

The lateral neck mass is investigated with a CT or an MRI, and first and second branchial cleft cysts, plunging ranulas, and lymphangiomas usually are differentiated from one another based on their radiologic appearance and location. The remaining solid and cystic/solid masses are resected surgically. We rarely use needle biopsy in children.

REFERENCES

1. Meyer CM. Congenital masses in the neck. In: Papparella MM, Shumrick DA, Gluckman JL, et al, eds. *Otolaryngology, Vol 3.* Philadelphia: Saunders, 1991, p. 2535–2543.
2. Boyd PA, Anthony MY, Manning N, et al. Antenatal diagnosis of cystic hygroma or nuchal pad—report of 92 cases with follow up of survivors. Arch Dis Child 1996; 74:F38–F42.
3. Rothschild MA, Catalano P, Urken M, et al. Evaluation and management of congenital cervical teratoma. Arch Otolaryngol Head Neck Surg 1994;120: 444–448.
4. Holinger LD, Birnholz JC, Bruce DR, et al. Management of an infant with prenatal ultrasound diagnosis of upper airway obstruction. Int J Pediatr Otolaryngol 1985; 10:263–270.
5. Hedrick MH, Ferro MM, Filly RA, et al. Congenital high airway obstruction syndrome (CHAOS): A potential for perinatal intervention. J Pediatr Surg 1994; 29:271–274.
6. Catalano PJ, Urken ML, Alvarez M, et al. New approach in "high risk" neonates. Arch Otolaryngol Head Neck Surg 1992; 118:306–309.
7. Kennedy LT. Cystic hygroma—lymphangioma: A rare and still unclear entity. Laryngoscope 1989; 99: 1–10.
8. Emery PJ, Bailey CM, and Evana JNG. Cystic hygroma of the head and neck: A review of 37 cases. J Laryngol Otol 1984; 98:613–619.
9. Raveh E, deJong AL, Taylor GP, et al. Prognostic factors in the treatment of lymphatic malformations. Arch Otolaryngol Head Neck Surg 1997; 123(10): 1061–1065.
10. Groetach E. Hygroma colli cysticum and hygromae axillae. Arch Surg 1938; 36:394–479.
11. McClure CFW, Sylvester CF. A comparative study of the lymphatico-venous communication in adult mammals. Anat Rec 1909; 3:353–354.

12. Sabin FR. On the origin of the lymphatic system from the veins and the development of the lymph heart and thoracic duct in the pig. Am J Anat 1901; 1: 367–389.

13. Leipzig B, Rabuzzi DD. Recurrent massive cystic lymphangioma. Otolaryngology 1978; 86:758–760.

14. Batsakis JG. In: *Tumors of the Head and Neck, 2nd ed.* Baltimore: Williams and Wilkins, 1979, pp. 301–304.

15. Ravitch MM, and Rush BF. Cystic hygroma. In: Ravitch MM, Welch KJ, Benson CD, et al, eds. *Pediatric Surgery, Vol 1, 3rd ed.* Chicago: Year Book Medical Publisher, 1979, pp. 368–373.

16. Williams WT, Cole RR. Lymphangioma presenting as congenital stridor. Int J Pediatr Otorhinolaryngol 1993; 26:185–191.

17. Brock ME, Smith RJH, Parey SE, et al. Lymphangioma. An otolaryngologic perspective. Int J Pediatr Otorhinolaryngol 1987; 14:133–140.

18. Smith RJ, Burke DK, Sato Y, et al. OK-432 therapy for lymphangiomas. Arch Otolaryngol Head Neck Surg 1996; 122(11):1195–1199.

19. Papsin BC, Evans JNG. Isolated laryngeal lymphangioma: A rare cause of airway obstruction in infants. J Laryngol Otol 1996; 110:969–972.

20. Cohen SR, Thompson JW. Lymphangioma of the larynx in infants and children: A survey of pediatric lymphangioma. Ann Otol Rhinol Laryngol 1986; 95(6)(Supplement 27) 1–20.

21. Myer CM, Bratcher GO. Laryngeal cystic hygroma. Head Neck Surg 1983; 6:706–709.

22. Wright CC, Cohen DM, Vegunta RK, et al. Intrathoracic cystic hygroma: A report of three cases. J Pediatr Surg 1996; 31(10):1430–1432.

23. Stal S, Hamilton S, Spira M. Hemangiomas, lymphangiomas, and vascular malformations of the head and neck. Otolaryngol Clin North Am 1986; 19:769–796.

24. Folkman J, D'Amore PA. Blood vessel formation: What is its molecular basis? Cell 1996; 87(7): 1153–1155.

25. Garfinkle TJ, Handler SD. Hemangiomas of the head and neck in children—A guide to management. J Otolaryngol 1980; 9:439–450.

26. Burrows PE, Mulliken JB, Fellows KE, et al. Childhood hemangiomas and vascular malformation: Angiographic differentiation. AJR 1983; 141:483–488.

27. Chang E, Boyd A, Nelson CC, et al. Successful treatment of infantile hemangiomas with interferon-alpha-2b. J Pediatr Hematol Oncol 1997;9(3): 237–244.

28. Batsakis JG, Littler ER, Oberman HA. Teratomas of the neck: A clinicopathological appraisal. Arch Otolaryngol 1964; 76:619–624.

29. Batsakis JG, el-Naggar AK, Luna MA. Teratomas of the head and neck with emphasis on malignancy. Ann Otol Rhinol Laryngol 1995; 104(6):496–500.

30. Azizkhan RG, Haase GM, Applebaum H, et al. Diagnosis, management, and outcome of cervicofacial teratomas in neonates: A Children Cancer Group study. J Pediatr Surg 1995; 30(2):312–316.

31. Gundry SR, Wesley JR, Klein MD, et al. Cervical teratomas in the newborn. J Pediatr Surg 1983;18: 382–386.

32. Frech RS, McAlister WH. Teratoma of the nasopharynx producing depression of the posterior hard palate. J Can Assoc Radiol 1969; 20:204–205.

33. Nicklaus PJ, Forte V, Friedberg J. Congenital mid-line cervical cleft. J Otolaryngol 1992; 21(4):241–243.

34. Ayache D, Ducroz V, Roger G, et al. Midline cervical cleft. Int J Pediatr Otorhinolaryngol 1997; 40(2–3): 189–193.

35. Gargan TJ, McKinnon M, Mulliken JB. Midline cervical cleft. Plast Reconstr Surg 1985; 76:225–227.

36. Bergevin MA, Shefis S, Myer C, et al. Congenital midline cervical cleft. Pediatr Pathol 1989; 9:731–733.

37. Porter SB, Blount BW. Pseudotumor of infancy and congenital muscular torticollis. Am Fam Physician 1995; 52(6):1731–1736.

38. Walsh S. Torticollis in infancy. J Pediatr Health Care 1997; 11(3):151–152.

39. Blythe WR, Logan TC, Holmes DK, et al. Fibromatosis colli: A common cause of neonatal torticollis. Am Fam Physician 1996; 54(6):1965–1967.

40. Bharadwaj VK. Sternomastoid myoplasty: Surgical correction of congenital torticollis. J Otolaryngol 1997; 26(1):44–48.

41. Moore KL. The branchial apparatus and the head and neck. In: *The Developing Human: Clinically Oriented Embryology 3rd ed.* Toronto: Saunders, 1982, pp. 179–215.

42. Karmody CS. Anomalies of the first and second branchial arches. In: English GM, ed. *Otolaryngology.* Philadelphia; Harper and Row, 1983, pp. 1–18.

43. Work WP. Cysts and congenital lesions of the parotid glands. Otolaryngol Clin North Am 1977;10: 339–344.

44. Lambert PR, Dodson EE. Congenital malformations of the external auditory canal. Otolaryngol Clin North Am 1996; 29(5):741–760.

45. Ikarashi F, Nakano Y, Nonomura N, et al. Clinical features of first branchial cleft anomalies. Am J Otolaryngol 1996; 17(4):233–239.

46. Choi SS, Zalzal GH. Branchial anomalies: A review of 52 cases. Laryngoscope 1995; 105(9 Pt 1):909–913.

47. Edmonds JL, Girod DA, Woodroof JM, et al. Third branchial anomalies. Avoiding recurrences. Arch Otolaryngol Head Neck Surg 1997; 123(4):438–441.

48. Johnson IJ, Soames JV, Birchall JP. Fourth branchial arch fistula. J Laryngol Otol 1996; 110(4):391–393.

49. Murdoch MJ, Culham JA, Stringer DA. Pediatric case of the day. Infected fourth branchial pouch sinus with extensive complicating cervical and mediastinal

abscess and left-sided empyema. Radiographics 1995; 15(4):1027-1030.

50. Roback SA, Telander RL. Thyroglossal duct cysts and branchial cleft anomalies. Sem Pediatr Surg 1994; 3(3):142-146.

51. Noyek AM, Friedberg J. Thyroglossal duct and ectopic thyroid disorders. Otolaryngol Clin North Am 1981; 14:187-201.

52. Sturgis EM, Miller RH: Thyroglossal duct cysts. J La State Med Soc 1993; 145(11):459.

53. Schlange H. Uber die fistula colli congenita. Arch Klin Chir 1893; 46:390-399.

54. Sistrunk WE. The surgical treatment of cysts of the thyroglossal tract. Ann Surg 1920; 71:121-122.

55. Walton BR, Koch KE. Presentation and management of a thyroglossal duct cyst with a papillary carcinoma. South Med J 1997; 90(7):758-761.

56. Wigley TL, Chonkich GD, Wat BY. Papillary carcinoma arising in a thyroglossal duct cyst. Otolaryngol Head Neck Surg 1997; 116(3):386-388.

57. Davenport M. ABC of general surgery in children. Lumps and swellings of the head and neck. BMJ 1996; 312(7027):368-371.

58. Johnson CM III, Cantrell RW. Congenital neck masses. In: Gates GA ed. *Current Therapy in Otolaryngology—Head and Neck Surgery 3.* Toronto: Decker, 1987, pp. 218-220.

59. Rutka J, Birt D. Laryngocele: A case report and review. J Otolaryngol 1983; 12:389-392.

60. Morton RP, Bartley JR. Simple sublingual ranulas: Pathogenesis and management. J Otolaryngol 1995; 24(4):253-254.

61. Ichimura K, Ohta Y, Tayama N. Surgical management of the plunging ranula: A review of seven cases. J Laryngol Otol 1996; 110(6):554-556.

62. Tavill MA, Wetmore RF, Poje CP, et al. Plunging ranulas in children. Ann Otol Rhinol Laryngol 1995; 104(5):405-408.

63. Crysdale WS, White A. Submandibular duct relocation for drooling: A 10-year experience with 194 patients. Otolaryngol Head Neck Surg 1989; 101(1): 87-92.

64. Crysdale WS, Mendelsohn JD, Conley S. Ranulas-Mucoceles of the oral cavity: Experience in 26 children. Laryngoscope 1988; 98(3):296-298.

65. Coit WE, Harnsberger HR, Osborn AG, et al. Ranulas and their mimics: CT evaluation. Radiology 1987; 163:211-216.

66. Barnes L, Peel RL, Verbin RS. Tumors of the nervous system. In: Barnes L, ed. *Surgical Pathology of the Head and Neck.* New York: Marcel Dekker, 1985, pp. 660-668.

67. Franklin DJ, Moore GF, Fisch U. Jugular foramen peripheral nerve sheath tumors. Laryngoscope 1989; 99(10 Pt 1):1081-1087.

68. Green JD Jr, Olsen KD, DeSanto LW, et al. Neoplasms of the vagus nerve. Laryngoscope 1988; 98(6 Pt 1): 648-654.

59 Infectious and Inflammatory Disorders of the Neck

David W. Roberson and Daniel J. Kirse

Neck masses in children can be subdivided usefully into three groups: inflammatory, congenital, and neoplastic. Confronted with a child with a neck mass, the pediatric otolaryngologist's first task is to determine whether the mass represents a tumor, a congenital lesion, or an inflammatory process. This chapter is concerned with the differential diagnosis and treatment of inflammatory (including infectious) processes.

Children can be affected by many different infectious and inflammatory processes in the neck. A careful history and physical examination usually allows the physician to narrow the diagnostic possibilities considerably, and often establishes the diagnosis with reasonable certainty. In children with unusual presentations or rare disorders, further studies may be necessary to establish the diagnosis.

HISTORY, EXAMINATION, AND LABORATORY EVALUATION

History

The history usually is obtained before it is established definitively that the patient's disease is inflammatory in nature. Although this chapter is limited to inflammatory and infectious disorders of the neck, the clinician always must consider the possibility that the patient has a congenital lesion or a neoplasm, and the history obtained should be directed accordingly.

The child's age at the onset of the process, the exact location of the disease, and the time course of the disease should be determined. Probing questions should be used to determine the presence of any associated signs or symptoms in the head and neck region, as well as elsewhere in the body. Constitutional symptoms such as weight loss, fevers, chills, night sweats, and changes in the child's behavior are particularly important. Issues about which the parents should be questioned specifically include the child's vaccination history, history of neck trauma, history of ionizing radiation, any unusual travel, exposure to tuberculosis, and exposure to cats, farm animals, and ticks.

Past history of neck surgery, of any upper respiratory infections (URIs) and of any major medical problems should be ascertained. Particularly important are any history of immune or immune-mediated disease, any history of malignancy, and any history of other neck disease of any kind.

The family history should determine whether there is a family history of congenital lesions and any other major illnesses.

Social History

For young children, the most pertinent item in the social history is whether the child is in day care (or school), where he/she is much more likely to be exposed to community viruses. Adolescents should be questioned about their sexual history and intravenous drug use. In the subspecialist's office, with the parents present, it may be difficult to obtain an accurate social history. If a diagnosis of primary human immunodeficiency virus (HIV) or cytomegalovirus (CMV) infection is considered, it may be useful to call the primary pediatrician, who often has interviewed the adolescent alone and may be able to supply the pertinent information.

Physical Examination

It must again be stressed that the possibility of congenital or neoplastic lesions should always be on

Pediatric Otolaryngology, Edited by R.F. Wetmore, H.R. Muntz, and T.J. McGill. Thieme Medical Publishers, Inc., New York © 2000.

the physician's mind when performing the examination. A complete, meticulous head and neck examination therefore should be performed always. The exam should include a gross assessment of the patient's overall appearance and apparent health; the presence of any skin erythema and induration; the appearance of the ears, nose, and nasal mucosa; and the appearance of the oral cavity and its mucosa. The presence of any masses is obviously of paramount concern, and the mucosal integrity and health is evaluated also. Mirror exam of the nasopharynx, hypopharynx, and larynx is performed in the cooperative older child. In younger and uncooperative patients, fiberoptic nasopharyngoscopy and laryngoscopy usually should be performed, particularly if the child fails to improve rapidly or an initial diagnosis of a benign process subsequently is called into question. The neck should be examined meticulously and patiently. Range of motion in all directions is assessed and torticollis noted if present. The presenting lesion's location, size, shape, mobility, hardness, and character are assessed. Redness, swelling, warmth, and tenderness are noted if present. Any adjacent nodes or masses are examined carefully and the findings recorded. The remainder of the neck, both anterior and posterior, is examined carefully for additional masses or adenopathy. The thyroid and cricoid cartilages, the trachea, and the thyroid gland are palpated.

Except in mild viral adenitis, an appropriate multisystem exam usually should be performed. Vital signs should be noted. Fever frequently accompanies infection or inflammation. Tachycardia may be seen as a systemic response to infection even when the temperature is normal. The patient's heart, lungs, abdomen, skin, and axillary and inguinal lymph nodes should be examined. The presence or absence of hepatomegaly, splenomegaly, and adenopathy elsewhere in the body should be documented specifically. Although the pediatric otolaryngologist ideally will be proficient in every aspect of the pediatric physical examination, in practice one may not often examine patients with (for example) splenomegaly. If this is the case, it may be prudent to ensure that the patient is examined by a physician who performs the complete pediatric examination more commonly and who can detect or exclude pertinent findings outside of the head and neck region with more assurance.

Laboratory Evaluation

In all but the mildest cases of viral adenitis, a complete blood count and differential should be considered. This will be abnormal in the presence of some hematologic malignancies, and also may alert the physician to a serious infectious process.

Other laboratory evaluations that may be appropriate for specific patients include monospot testing, Epstein-Barr virus (EBV) immunoglobulin M and G (IgM and IgG) titers, CMV IgG and IgM titers, toxoplasmosis titers, throat culture, and a tuberculin skin test if there is any suspicion of mycobacterial disease. More specialized, specific, and in some case, experimental tests for specific disorders are discussed below in the sections on those disorders.

If drainage is present or if a lesion drained surgically, routine and anaerobic bacterial cultures, fungal stains and cultures, and acid-fast stains and cultures should be sent. Sensitivity is improved by sending as much material as possible. If a lesion is drained surgically, it is often wise to obtain a specimen for pathology to ensure that an apparently-infectious process does not actually represent infection around an underlying neoplasm. Pathologic examination is also very important for diagnosing tuberculosis and atypical mycobacterial infections, as the presence of granulomas and acid-fast organisms may be detected by pathologic exam days or weeks before these organisms grow in culture. If cat-scratch disease is suspected, a Warthin-Starry stain must be requested specifically. If an unusual process is suspected, it is often wise to have the pathology laboratory save a tissue sample for special testing that may be desired at a later date [e.g., polymerase chain reaction (PCR) to identify deoxyribonucleic acid (DNA) from specific microorganisms].

AT A GLANCE . . .

Laboratory Evaluation

- CBC with differential
- Monospot
- EBV IgM and IgG titers
- CMV IgM and IgG titers
- Toxoplasmosis titers
- Throat culture
- Tuberculin skin test

Radiologic Evaluation

A lateral neck film may help determine the presence of a retropharyngeal phlegmon or abscess. The retropharyngeal space may appear thickened if the child is crying, swallowing, or in flexion. In such cases, airway fluoroscopy can be obtained and usually clarifies whether the retropharyngeal thickening is real or artifactual.

Ultrasound may be helpful in determining whether a neck mass has a fluid center, but it does not assist in surgical planning. Neck abscesses can have loculations that extend superiorly, inferiorly, or deep to vital structures in the neck, which are not apparent on ultrasound. Therefore, if an abscess is suspected or surgical drainage or biopsy contemplated, contrast computed tomography (CT) scan is mandatory. Although CT cannot distinguish phlegmon from abscess with absolute accuracy, it does determine the extent of the disease reliably and allow accurate anatomic surgical planning.

Usually, magnetic resonance imaging (MRI) does not add useful information about the child in whom CT scanning suggests abscess or phlegmon. MRI may, however, be extremely helpful in the child who appears to have an unusual infectious or inflammatory process, or in whom a tumor, vascular malformation, or other lesion may be suspected.

When the cause of cervical adenopathy is unclear and a diagnostic workup is undertaken, a chest X-ray may be useful if there is a suspicion of sarcoid, tuberculosis, or malignancy.

In this chapter, specific infectious processes in the neck are grouped by pathogen (i.e., viral, bacterial, fungal, and parasitic). A discussion of noninfectious inflammatory processes follows. Table 59–1 summarizes some of the potential causes of inflammatory neck disorders.

AT A GLANCE . . .
Radiologic Evaluation

- Lateral and AP neck radiographs
- Computed tomography with contrast
- Chest radiograph
- Magnetic resonance imaging
- Ultrasound

VIRAL INFECTIONS

Viral Adenitis

Probably the most common infectious process in the neck is *viral adenitis*. It is the rare child who

TABLE 59–1: Some Causes of Neck Inflammation in Children

Infectious causes
Viral
  Viral adenitis
    rhinovirus
    adenovirus
    enterovirus
    measles
    mumps
    rubella
    varicella
  Mononucleosis
  CMV
  HIV infection
    acute initial infection
    chronic HIV lymphadenopathy
Bacterial
  Suppurative cervical lymphadenitis
    external (submandibular triangle, zone V)
    retropharyngeal/parapharyngeal
  Suppurative infections of deep neck spaces
    suppurative lymphadenitis that has spread beyond nodal confines
    direct inoculation of deep neck spaces
  Necrotizing fasciitis
  Septic large vein thrombosis
Mycobacterial
  Mycobacterium tuberculosis
  "Atypical" mycobacteria
Other bacterial
  Cat-scratch disease
  Bacillary angiomatosis
  Bubonic plague
  Tularemia
  Actinomycosis
  Brucellosis
  Syphilis
Fungal
  Histoplasmosis
  Uncommon fungal pathogens
    Candida
    Aspergillus
Parasitic
  Toxoplasmosis
  Filariasis
Inflammatory disorders
  Kawasaki syndrome
  Sarcoidosis
  Sinus histiocytosis with massive lymphadenopathy
  Kikuchi-Fujimoto disease
  PFAPA syndrome (Periodic *Fever*, *Aphthous stomatitis*, *Pharyngitis*, and cervical *Adenitis*)
  Focal myositis

does not have some enlargement of the cervical lymphatics during a viral infection at some time in their life. Common pathogens include rhinovirus, adenovirus, and enterovirus. Cervical adenopathy often is accompanied by upper respiratory symptomatology. Both are typically self-limited, and no specific diagnostic maneuvers or therapy is indicated.

Measles, mumps, rubella, and varicella can all cause cervical adenopathy. Diagnosis is usually made on clinical grounds, although sophisticated diagnostic testing (e.g., ELISA, latex agglutination, viral cultures) is available for the unusual case where it may be indicated. Treatment is supportive. Acyclovir may be indicated for varicella in the immunosuppressed or otherwise vulnerable child.

Infectious Mononucleosis

Infectious mononucleosis is caused by EBV. EBV is transmitted primarily by mucous membrane contact (e.g., kissing). Mononucleosis often causes a confluent, exudative, almost necrotic-appearing tonsillitis and very impressive cervical lymphadenopathy, as well as systemic symptoms of fever, fatigue, and malaise. Hepatosplenomegaly also may be present.[1]

Atypical lymphocytes on the peripheral blood smear suggest the diagnosis of mononucleosis. Heterophile antibodies (i.e., monospot testing) helps confirm the diagnosis, but may be negative early in the disease. Titers of anti-EBV IgG and IgM may be useful if monospot testing is negative and mononucleosis is suspected on clinical grounds. PCR for EBV is available as an experimental test, but may be useful in difficult situations.[2,3]

Treatment of mononucleosis is usually supportive. Full spontaneous recovery is expected. Cases with hepatosplenomegaly should be followed by a pediatrician or pediatric infectious disease specialist.

The pediatric otolaryngologist may become involved with children who have mononucleosis because of airway obstruction. The tonsillitis that accompanies mononucleosis, as well as enlargement of the lingual tonsils and adenoids, may cause acute airway insufficiency. If airway symptoms are emerging but the patient is not in acute danger, intravenous antibiotics are given to treat any secondary bacterial infection, high-dose steroids are administered, and the child is monitored closely. Ampicillin and amoxicillin should be avoided as they typically cause a rash in patients with mononucleosis.

If the child progresses to frank airway compromise, endotracheal or nasotracheal intubation should be performed in the operating room, with bronchoscopy and tracheotomy equipment immediately available. Tracheotomy is rarely necessary. Tonsillectomy can be performed acutely, and does not seem to carry an increased risk of bleeding. However, if there is no history of tonsillar enlargement prior to mononucleosis, the tonsils usually rapidly return to a more normal size; therefore acute tonsillectomy is not indicated usually except for airway compromise.

Cytomegalovirus

Cytomegalovirus (CMV) is ubiquitous, and it is transmitted primarily by mucous membrane contact (e.g., kissing). It also can be transmitted sexually and by blood products. In most populations, over 50% of adults show serologic evidence of past infection. The infection may be completely subclinical, or it may produce a mononucleosis-like illness characterized by malaise, fever, mild liver dysfunction, lymphocytosis with atypical lymphocytes, and adenopathy including cervical adenopathy. Acute CMV infection can be impossible to distinguish from mononucleosis or acute HIV infection on clinical grounds. Treatment is supportive.[4]

In immunocompromised patients or rarely in immunocompetent patients, CMV may cause a multisystem life-threatening illness. Treatment with ganciclovir or foscarnet should be discussed with a pediatric infectious disease specialist.

Acquired Immunodeficiency Syndrome

The *acquired immunodeficiency syndrome* (AIDS) is caused by infection with HIV. The virus is transmitted by sexual contact, exchange of blood (e.g., sharing needles, blood transfusion prior to universal screening), and vertically from mother to child. The majority of pediatric AIDS is acquired vertically, but adolescents may acquire the disease from sexual contact or intravenous drug use. Patients may harbor the HIV virus for years or decades before progressing to AIDS.

Acute HIV infection

Acute HIV infection presents as a flu-like illness several weeks after initial inoculation with the HIV virus. Patients commonly have fever, headache, diarrhea, malaise, and cervical as well as generalized lymphadenopathy. Acute HIV infection can be clinically indistinguishable from infectious mononucleosis, acute CMV infection, or a viral URI with cervical adenopathy.[5] Therefore a sexual and social history should be obtained in adolescents with this presentation. As noted above, the primary pediatrician may be able to supply this information if it is difficult to obtain from the child or parents.

Patients with HIV infection who are not diagnosed at their initial illness may not develop AIDS for years or decades. Many will, however, develop diffuse lymphadenopathy early after seroconversion. Lymph nodes are usually soft, symmetrically distributed, and in the posterior triangle. Generalized lymphadenopathy is also common.

It is now clear that patients with HIV infection obtain significant improvement in life expectancy with early antiretroviral treatment.[6] It is incumbent on all physicians who may encounter acute HIV infection or chronic HIV-associated lymphadenopathy to recognize it (or at least to include it on their differential diagnosis) so that the patient may be referred promptly to an infectious disease specialist for further evaluation and treatment if the diagnosis is confirmed.

Chronic HIV infection/AIDS

Children who acquire HIV vertically from their mothers usually are diagnosed early in life; almost always, when the pediatric otolaryngologist is involved, the diagnosis is known already. The diagnostic challenge that may be faced is determining whether cervical lymphadenopathy or a cervical mass represents HIV-associated lymphadenopathy or some other infectious process. Atypical infections (e.g., fungal, parasitic) may occur in children with AIDS and a high index of suspicion for unusual processes should be maintained. Children with AIDS and a suspected neck infection always should be evaluated in consultation with a pediatric infectious disease specialist.

BACTERIAL INFECTIONS

Suppurative Cervical Lymphadenitis

Bacterial cervical adenitis in the pediatric patient progresses through a series of stages in a predictable

order. Bacterial inoculation of the cervical nodes, most typically from the pharynx, causes an infectious adenitis, with swelling, tenderness, and systemic signs (e.g., malaise, fever). If untreated, the node may progress to seminecrotic tissue (phlegmon) and then suppurate to form a frank abscess. In early abscess formation, the pus is confined within the nodal capsule and the reactive abscess wall. Ultimately, however, the pus may rupture the nodal capsule. Depending on the space into which the pus ruptures, the abscess either necessitates (through the skin or into the pharynx) or the pus escapes the nodal capsule to spread freely in the deep fascial spaces of the neck. As long as the suppurative process is confined within the nodal capsule/abscess wall, it rarely produces systemic sepsis. If pus escapes the nodal capsule to dissect in the deep fascial spaces of the neck, a life-threatening sepsis often ensues. At any point in this sequence, the process may be halted and ultimately reversed by the patient's own immune system, by antibiotic therapy, by spontaneous abscess necessitation, or by surgical drainage.

The distinction between a suppurative process within a lymph node that is confined by the nodal capsule and the reactive abscess wall and an infection that has escaped the node and is dissecting freely in the deep spaces of the neck cannot be stressed too strongly. The former, although an urgent surgical disease, almost always can be successfully treated; the latter is a true life-threatening emergency that may have a catastrophic outcome despite the best available treatment.

Over the past few decades, pediatric health care access has improved, physicians' awareness of the problem of deep neck infection has increased, and newer imaging modalities (specifically, CT scan) have greatly facilitated the diagnosis of deep neck suppurative adenitis. The diagnosis typically is made much earlier in the disease course, and progression of suppurative adenitis to rapidly spreading deep neck space infection has become very rare. This epidemiologic difference must be understood when comparing literature from the preantibiotic era to current literature. When diagnosis and treatment was delayed, rapidly-spreading deep neck space infection was common and mortality was high; six large series published in the first half of this century reported mortality rates of 4 to 15%.[7] Understandably, in that era, more aggressive surgical therapy was often necessary. Today, these infections usually are diagnosed while still confined within an abscess wall, and more limited surgical procedures often are used successfully. Today's pediatric otolaryngologist, however, should never forget the natural history of this disorder, and must still be prepared to recognize and treat aggressively the occasional case of true unconfined deep neck infection.

Unconfined deep neck abscesses also can be caused by direct bacterial inoculation into the deep neck spaces (e.g., by trauma or by self-administered substance injections into the internal jugular vein) or by local spread from an adjacent site (e.g., dental infections). Pus collections that form initially in the deep fascial spaces of the neck (i.e., not within the capsule of a lymph node) typically dissect rapidly within those spaces, are not limited in their spread by a thickened nodal capsule, and are typically life-threatening infections demanding aggressive surgical drainage and debridement.

Typical causative organisms include Streptococcus species, *Staphylococcus aureus, Staphylococcus epidermidis,* Neisseria species, and anaerobes. The frequency of anaerobic isolates varies, but organisms reported include *Peptostreptococcus, Bacteroides,* and *Fusibacterium.* Polymicrobial infections are common. Uncommon infectious agents must be suspected in the immunocompromised patient, especially mycobacterial and fungal organisms.

Suppurative adenitis can occur in any cervical node, but most typically occurs in submandibular nodes, posterior triangle (zone V) nodes, or in nodes in the retropharyngeal/parapharyngeal junction in the nasopharynx, oropharynx, and hypopharynx. Infection of submandibular or posterior triangle nodes cause large abscesses that are obvious on examination and palpation. Infection of retropharyngeal/parapharyngeal nodes cause a much more insidious illness that may be very difficult to

diagnose unless a high index of suspicion is maintained.

AT A GLANCE . . .

Bacterial Agents Causing Suppurative Lymphadenitis

- Streptococcal species
- *Staphylococcus aureus*
- *Staphylococcus epidermidis*
- Neisseria species
- *Peptostreptococcus*
- *Bacteroides*
- *Fusibacterium*

Suppurative cervical lymphadenitis with external presentation

Suppurative cervical lymphadenitis in the submandibular region or posterior triangle causes an obvious external mass. The child may be recovering from a pharyngitis or other infection, often has a fever, an elevated white blood cell count, and erythema, and tenderness surrounding the neck mass. The child may present before the node has suppurated, in which case fluctuance is not present. Fluctuance may be difficult to appreciate through the thickened abscess wall, especially in the ill uncooperative child, but often a careful examination establishes whether pus is present.

If the node has not suppurated yet, the child should be admitted and placed on broad spectrum intravenous antibiotic coverage (e.g., ampicillin and sulbactam). In some cases, antibiotic therapy reverses the process before pus formation occurs. More often, the disease progresses to abscess formation over a few days. Antibiotic therapy often reduces the cellulitis, swelling and induration around the abscess; the child may appear clinically better despite the evolution of the abscess. It is important not to be misled by this phenomenon. The patient should be examined carefully daily and, should fluctuance develop, the abscess should be drained. Ultrasound is helpful in determining the presence of a liquid center, but is an inadequate study for surgical planning. Superficial suppurative adenitis may be accompanied by an unsuspected deep loculation that is only detected by CT. Therefore, contrast CT usually should be obtained prior to draining these lesions.

> ## SPECIAL CONSIDERATION:
>
> In cases of suppurative lymphadenitis, contrast CT should be obtained prior to surgical drainage to detect unsuspected deep loculations.

If detected early, these abscesses can be drained through a limited (i.e., 2–3 cm) incision, placed in a horizontal neck crease for best cosmetic result. Care should be taken to avoid injury to the marginal branch of the facial nerve, the accessory nerve, and to the great vessels. The wound should be left open and, if a cavity of any size is present, drained with a Penrose drain or a strip of gauze packing, which can be advanced over several days.

Treatment of cervical abscesses with needle aspiration or CT-guided needle aspiration with good success has been reported.[8] However, it is not clear that needle aspiration offers a significant reduction in morbidity or cost, particularly because general anesthesia may be required and a significant fraction of abscesses do not respond to needle drainage alone.

Retropharyngeal/Parapharyngeal Suppurative Lymphadenitis

Suppurative lymphadenitis of the retropharyngeal/parapharyngeal space presents most commonly in children <5 years of age. After that age, the lymph nodes in this space involute. Infections in this area are most commonly a result of infection involving sites that drain into these nodes which include the nasal cavity, paranasal sinuses, nasopharynx, and middle ear. The involved nodes almost always straddle the junction of the retropharyngeal and parapharyngeal spaces. Duration of symptoms prior to suppurative change in these nodes is highly variable, ranging from a few days to weeks. Because these infections commonly occur in preverbal children, a high index of suspicion must be maintained to make the diagnosis. Retropharyngeal/parapharyngeal suppurative lymphadenitis should be suspected in the ill-appearing child who presents with fever, drooling, malaise, decreased oral intake, fussiness, torticollis, and/or trismus. Physical findings are generally limited. Tachycardia and fever are often present, as is torticollis. Otherwise, the physical exam is often nonspecific. The classic bulge in the posterior or lateral pharyngeal wall is usually difficult, if not impossible to appreciate. Advanced disease, especially in the infant, occasionally may cause respiratory distress, but usually the diagnosis is made before that stage.

Lateral X-ray of the neck usually shows widening of the prevertebral soft tissues. False-positive results are common because of technical error. Flexion of the neck and expiration can both cause artifactual widening of the prevertebral soft tissues. Fluoroscopy of the neck is an excellent means of clarifying equivocal results seen on plain X-rays. If a retropharyngeal abscess is present, the prevertebral soft tissues stay widened throughout the respiratory cycle, regardless of neck position.

If the lateral radiograph is suspicious, or if there are other clinical grounds to suspect retropharyngeal abscess, contrast-enhanced CT is mandatory (Practice Pathway 59–1). Intravenous contrast increases sensitivity for abscess detection, and also allows precise localization of the abscess relative to the great vessels. If airway swelling is present, particularly if the child is ill or exhausted, sedation of the patient for CT may lead to airway obstruction. In children presenting with any degree of airway compromise, it may be wisest to intubate the child in the operating room prior to obtaining a CT scan.

Suppurative adenopathy of the retropharyngeal space produces a ring-enhancing, low-intensity signal that is situated between the pharynx and the great vessels (Fig. 59–1). The enlarging suppurative process causes lateral displacement of the major vessels of the neck. CT is not completely reliable in distinguishing phlegmon (presuppurative) from frank abscess. Ultrasound may be more reliable. However, due to the fact that these infections often occur high in the retropharyngeal space near the skull base, ultrasound can often be technically difficult to perform. Most importantly, ultrasound may not allow detection always of unsuspected loculations of pus extending in the deep neck spaces or the carotid sheath.

If CT shows a ring-enhancing abscess, surgical drainage should be performed. If CT findings are unclear, suggesting phlegmon with some possibility

Practice Pathway 59–1 DIAGNOSIS AND MANAGEMENT OF RETROPHARYNGEAL ABSCESS

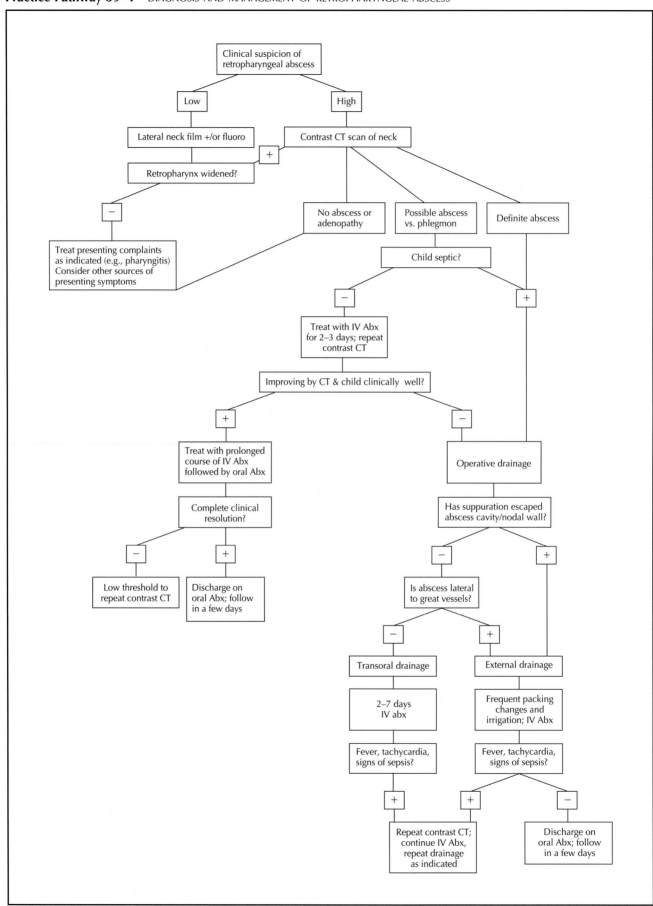

Abbreviations: IV Abx, Intravenous Antibiotics; P.O. Abx, Prolonged Oral Antibiotics.

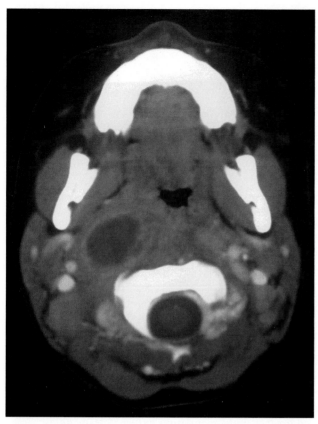

Figure 59–1: CT of suppurative node located in the retropharyngeal/parapharyngeal space. Hypodense center and ring enhancement are characteristic. Note location medial to great vessels.

of abscess, and if the child is not septic, intravenous antibiotic treatment should be instituted and repeat CT scan obtained in 2 to 3 days. Intravenous antibiotics, by reducing the periabscess swelling and cellulitis, often cause clinical improvement in the child's malaise and other symptoms even in the presence of an evolving abscess. Clinical improvement should therefore not lead to canceling the re-

---

AT A GLANCE . . .

Signs and Symptoms of Retropharyngeal/ Parapharyngeal Suppurative Lymphadenitis

Fever
Drooling
Malaise
Decreased oral intake
Irritability
Torticollis
Trismus

---

peat CT scan. If abscess is present on followup scan, drainage should be performed. If the phlegmon is resolving, treatment with a prolonged course of intravenous antibiotics followed by oral antibiotics is appropriate.

Surgical drainage of retropharyngeal/parapharyngeal abscesses.

When surgical drainage is planned, an approach (transoral vs. external) must be chosen. The route of choice has been a source of controversy for at least 80 years. Dean[9] unequivocally condemned the transoral approach, whereas Richards[7] and Grodinsky[10] both stated that the vast majority of these abscesses could be managed transorally. Disagreement about the best surgical approach persists to the present day.

As discussed above, as long as the purulent process remains confined within a nodal capsule/abscess wall, the child rarely is truly septic. In this case, the authors believe these abscesses can be drained safely transorally. We recently reviewed 50 consecutive cases of parapharyngeal/retropharyngeal abscess in children. Two that had extensions lateral to the great vessels required external drainage. The remaining 48 were all drained transorally, and all children recovered fully without any long-term morbidity. We propose that suppurative adenitis in the retropharyngeal/parapharyngeal space in the child can be drained transorally with a high degree of safety, provided that the abscess is confined within a nodal capsule and that there is no extension lateral or posterior to the great vessels.

Today, transoral drainage begins with careful management of the airway during induction of anesthesia and intubation. The airway usually is controlled by the skilled anesthesiologist, but bronchoscopy and tracheotomy equipment should be readily available and the pediatric otolaryngologist should be present during induction. The patient is then placed in the Rose position with a tonsil gag in place. The lateral and posterior pharyngeal walls are then palpated and clinical correlation is made with the CT images to assure that the abscess is approached at the proper level. Needle aspiration is performed to localize the abscess and to rule out carotid pseudoaneurysm. If purulence is encountered with needle aspiration, the aspirate is sent for culture and gram stain. In some patients, it is advantageous to perform a tonsillectomy first to enhance exposure of the lateral portions of the retropharyngeal space. A vertical incision is made through the lateral pharyngeal wall (or through the tonsillar fossa if a tonsillectomy has been performed). The tissue is then dissected bluntly until the abscess cavity is entered. The abscess cavity is then gently irrigated using copious amounts of saline. The abscess cavity can be explored digitally to assure that all loculations are opened. The incision is left open. A drain has not been found to be necessary in our experience. If significant postoperative swelling is present, particularly in the young infant, the patient may require postoperative endotracheal intubation until airway edema subsides. Intravenous antibiotics are then begun. The patient is discharged from the hospital on oral antibiotics once afebrile and clinically improving, usually in 3–4 days. Recurrence of the abscess is uncommon, but should be considered if the patient does not have rapid improvement in symptoms or if a persistent fever or tachycardia is present. Intravenous antibiotics may mask symptoms of abscess reaccumulation and therefore the pediatric otolaryngologist should not discharge the patient with fever, tachycardia, or any other worrisome signs or symptoms.

Of historical interest is the transoral procedure described by Richards as "the custom" in 1936.[7] No local or general anesthesia was given in order to maintain the patient's ability to protect their airway. The child was restrained in the sitting position by (presumably sturdy) assistants, and the abscess was approached by "reaching over the tongue with the left index finger, palpating the abscess, and then inserting a knife into the abscess wall blindly." The assistants then immediately turned the patient head down to prevent aspiration of septic secretions.

An external drainage procedure is indicated when a transoral approach is deemed unsafe or inadequate to drain the suppurative process. In general, external drainage is indicated when the suppurative process has ruptured the confines of the lymph node or abscess wall and has significant extension into the deep neck spaces. External drainage is mandatory if the abscess has spread laterally to the great vessels or is spreading freely in the carotid space (Fig. 59-2). Preoperative CT is of paramount importance for surgical planning. CT delineates the precise extent of the suppurative process, including unexpected extensions or loculations (Fig. 59-3).

The description of the external approach by Dean

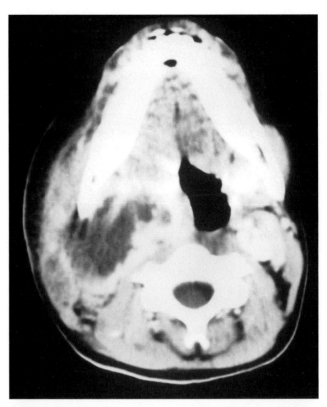

Figure 59–2: Deep abscess that has spread laterally to the great vessels, mandating external drainage.

in 1919 is still accurate.[9] One or more horizontal incisions that lead to the abscess most directly are created. As purulence around the carotid can cause carotid blowout, vascular control is essential. The superior and inferior limits of the carotid should be exposed early so that vascular control can be obtained early. Then the abscess is approached with blunt dissection, just anterior to the anterior edge of the sternocleidomastoid muscle and posterior to the carotid sheath. If the abscess has spread beyond the retropharyngeal/parapharyngeal space, dissection (preferably blunt) should be carried to all extensions of the abscess. The abscess is entered and all loculations are explored with a fingertip and broken up carefully. The cavity should be irrigated copiously. One or more drains are placed and advanced very slowly over several days. If the patient is toxic, the cavity should be irrigated at the bedside or in the operating room, daily if necessary, for several days postoperatively. For these life-threatening infections, intravenous antibiotics probably should be continued for 10 to 14 days or more. Many of these patients will be critically ill.

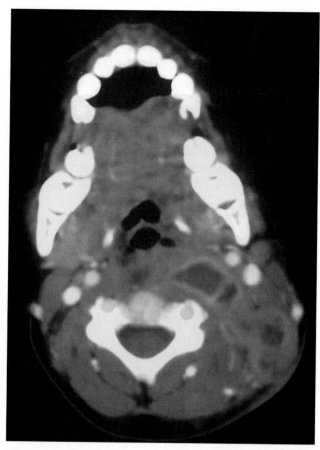

Figure 59–3: CT of a child with a zone V abscess. CT revealed unsuspected retropharyngeal/parapharyngeal abscess, which required separate drainage through a transoral approach. The possibility of such unsuspected extensions makes preoperative CT essential.

Nonoperative management of deep neck abscess

The advent of intravenous antibiotics has made it possible to treat small collections of pus nonsurgically, regardless of the location in the neck. One study has reported that 25% of cases of suppurative lymphadenitis can be treated successfully with antibiotics alone.[11] This conclusion is difficult to interpret because, without surgery, it is impossible to be certain whether the process treated was an abscess or a phlegmon. Some of the patients included are from the pre-CT era, which makes diagnostic certainty very difficult in the nonoperated patient. Nonetheless, it seems that some selected small retropharyngeal abscesses, preferably <1 cm in diameter, can be treated successfully with antibiotics alone. It is not clear that nonsurgical management results in less morbidity or lesser cost, particularly because it often requires prolonged home intravenous therapy.

If nonsurgical management is chosen, a course of intravenous antibiotics is given for a specified duration and followed by a course of antibiotics by mouth. There is no agreement on the optimal course of antibiotics, but in general, the intravenous antibiotics should be continued until the patient remains afebrile for at least 48 hours and clinical improvement is established clearly. Frequently, a prolonged course of intravenous antibiotics is given as an outpatient. Because antibiotic therapy reduces periabscess inflammation/cellulitis it may cause clinical improvement even in the presence of an evolving abscess; therefore, the patient should be followed closely for a prolonged period and treatment should not be shortened because of early improvement. A high index of suspicion should be maintained for residual infection and progression, and serial radiographic imaging should be considered to assure that the suppurative collection is treated adequately.

Complications of deep neck abscesses

Catastrophic complications of deep neck space infections include damage to the major neurovascular structures, septic venous thrombosis, airway compromise, sepsis, and spread of the infection within the involved fascial space. Descending infections can cause mediastinits. Rupture of a retropharyngeal abscess into the pharynx can cause aspiration and life-threatening pneumonitis. The widespread use of antibiotics and modern imaging techniques along with the increased knowledge of pathogenesis of these infections has made catastrophic complications of deep neck infections uncommon today. Nonetheless, these infections always must be taken extremely seriously if such complications are to be avoided. If improvements in the diagnosis and treatment of deep neck infections lead to a cavalier approach to these infections, we can expect to see increasing numbers of serious complications in the future.

Necrotizing Fasciitis

Necrotizing fasciitis of the head and neck can follow any infection in the region. A number of cases have been reported following scratching of varicella pustules. The infection is usually polymicrobial, spreads rapidly along fascial planes, and causes toxicity, airway compromise, and sepsis. Patients are usually very ill and subcutaneous crepitus is usually present. Treatment is with intravenous antibiotics and extremely-aggressive surgical debridement, repeated frequently if necessary.

Lemierre's Syndrome

Classic *Lemierre's syndrome,* or postanginal sepsis, is a septic thrombosis of the internal jugular (IJ) vein following tonsillitis and most often is caused by *Fusobacterium necrophorum.* (Why this particular organism has a propensity to migrate to and cause thrombosis of the IJ is unknown.) Lemierre's syndrome was common in the preantibiotic era and very large series were reported in the first half of this century. For uncertain reasons—probably due to the widespread use of antibiotics for severe tonsillitis—it is now rare.

The classic presentation is of a patient who presents a week after an episode of tonsillitis obviously ill or toxic, repeatedly spiking high fevers in a "picket fence" fashion, with tenderness and/or fullness in one side of the neck. Respiratory distress is uncommon, but subtle chest film findings suggestive of pulmonary emboli are often present. Untreated, the patient progresses to frank sepsis with a mortality of >90%.

Other veins beside the IJ may be involved—Lemierre's original paper includes cases involving the tonsillar or facial veins.[12] Other organisms may be involved occasionally. Thrombosis of large neck veins may follow essentially any infection in the head and neck, though tonsillitis and dental infections remain the most common causes.

If septic IJ thrombosis is suspected, contrast CT scan should be obtained and is usually diagnostic. In addition, contrast CT determines if any other deep neck process is underlying the IJ thrombosis. Once the diagnosis is made, the patients should be admitted, monitored closely, and treated with intravenous antibiotics. If an infectious source is present (e.g., dental infection, deep neck abscess), it should be drained urgently or removed if at all possible. The use of anticoagulants is controversial; good outcomes are reported with and without their use.[13] A fairly long course of intravenous antibiotics followed by prolonged oral antibiotics would seem advisable, although there are no controlled data supporting this. Surgical intervention is rarely necessary, but if repeated septic emboli occur and cause significant pulmonary compromise, the septic jugular vein should be ligated or excised. Survival now approaches or exceeds 95%.

Mycobacterial Infections

Lymphadenitis that is caused by mycobacterial infections is demanding renewed attention due to a resurgence of pulmonary tuberculosis. In the United Kingdom and certain parts of the United States, an increased incidence of mycobacterial lymphadenitis has been seen in recent years.[14,15] Mycobacterial infections fall into two groups based on the type of organism. The first is caused by *Mycobacterium tuberculosis* and the second category encompasses those infections that are caused by all other species of mycobacteria. This second group of bacteria are referred to collectively as 'atypical' mycobacteria or nontuberculous mycobacteria (NTM). The most common of these are *Mycobacterium avium-intracellulare, Mycobacterium scrofulaceum, Mycobacterium bovis,* and *Mycobacterium kansasii.* The term *scrofula* was used historically for cervical lymphadenitis caused by *Mycobacterium tuberculosis* and *Mycobacterium bovis,* but now it is used to describe any mycobacterial lymphadenitis.

The etiologic agent differs markedly with the age of the afflicted patient. In a large study, it was found that 80% of children with NTM infections were <5 years of age and that girls are more commonly afflicted than boys.[16] *Mycobacterium tuberculosis* is the more common cause of cervical adenitis in adults.

For infections caused by *Mycobacterium tuberculosis,* there is often a known family contact. NTM organisms are ubiquitous in the soil and water, but there is no established human to human communication of NTM infection. It is not known what predisposes some children to NTM infections. The patient with mycobacterial cervical adenitis is usually immunocompetent, although disseminated infections with NTM are seen in immunosuppressed patients.

Mycobacterial lymphadenitis generally presents as a nontender node that enlarges slowly over several weeks to months in the upper cervical or submandibular area. The preauricular, intraparotid, and posterior triangle nodes are involved less commonly. Single node involvement is classic, but synchronous nodal involvement is not uncommon. Fever and other systemic signs are rare in NTM. Later in the disease process, dermal involvement causes a characteristic violaceous appearance of the skin overlying the node (Fig. 59–4).

Chest X-ray should be obtained and may be posi-

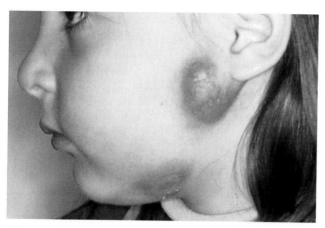

Figure 59–4: Atypical mycobacterial infection in the preauricular and submandibular areas. The submandibular infection has undergone incision and drainage and is somewhat decompressed compared to the preauricular lesion. Note the characteristic skin involvement and induration and the violaceous color of the involved skin.

tive in infections caused by *Mycobacterium tuberculosis*. Chest X-ray is usually normal in NTM. Purified protein derivative (PPD) testing is usually strongly positive in infections caused by *Mycobacterium tuberculosis*; NTM infections usually are associated with no reaction or an intermediate reaction (5–15 mm induration).

The clinical presentation of NTM, particularly when it progresses to violaceous skin involvement, is so classic that diagnosis often can be made with reasonable certainty on clinical grounds alone. However, establishing the laboratory diagnosis of NTM is frequently difficult. Fine-needle aspiration, surgical drainage, or excision of an involved node can yield material for culture and/or pathology. However, staining for acid-fast bacilli may be negative even in culture-positive specimens, and NTM is notoriously difficult to grow in culture. Even if culture results are positive, they may not return for several weeks. PCR is being used currently in some institutions, and is particularly helpful when DNA can be recovered from culture medium but not enough viable organisms are present for definitive identification.

The distinction between *Mycobacterium tuberculosis* and NTM organisms may be particularly difficult. Even if acid-fast bacilli are present in excised nodes, it is controversial as to whether pathology can distinguish the two categories of mycobacteria. Some suggest differing patterns of granuloma formation may be diagnostic,[17] whereas others disagree.[18] In the absence of a positive skin test or a history of

tuberculosis exposure, however, the vast majority of mycobacterial infections in the neck are caused by NTM.

Treatment of mycobacterial infections

The optimal modality for treatment depends on the mycobacteria involved. Lymphadenitis caused by *Mycobacterium tuberculosis* is best treated with combination chemotherapy once the proper diagnosis is made. Therapy is similar to pulmonary tuberculosis with combinations of isoniazid, ethambutol, rifampin, and streptomycin being mainstays of therapy. Surgical therapy is seldom needed.

Therapy for NTM, on the other hand, is controversial, difficult, and not always satisfying (Practice Pathway 59-2). If untreated, the node typically progresses to frank suppuration and formation of draining sinus tracts to the skin. The process often drains to the skin for many months before resolving spontaneously. There is often skin breakdown around the drainage tract and significant residual cosmetic deformity. However, these infections almost invariably resolve spontaneously in the immunocompetent patient. Therapy is not therefore lifesaving, but is directed at shortening the disease process and improving the cosmetic outcome.

Neither medical nor surgical therapy for NTM are entirely satisfactory. NTM are notoriously resistant to traditional antituberculosis agents. Therefore, surgical intervention has traditionally been recommended. If diagnosed early and confined within a lymph node, total excision is preferable and usually curative. Once the disease spreads beyond the confines of the originating lymph node, surgical therapy is often difficult as NTM typically spreads without regard for tissue boundaries, often wrapping around important structures (e.g., the marginal branch of the facial nerve). Total surgical excision often causes damage to these structures and thus unacceptable morbidity.

Needle aspiration, I & D alone, and I & D with surgical curettage have been advocated for NTM that is not amenable to total excision. In fact, some authors employ these techniques as the primary mode of intervention in all cases of NTM lymphadenitis and report good results.[19,20] In our hands, anything less than total excision has led on occasion, to a draining sinus tract, which is unsightly, unpleasant, and difficult for the family to care for.

In situations of problematic NTM lymphadenitis,

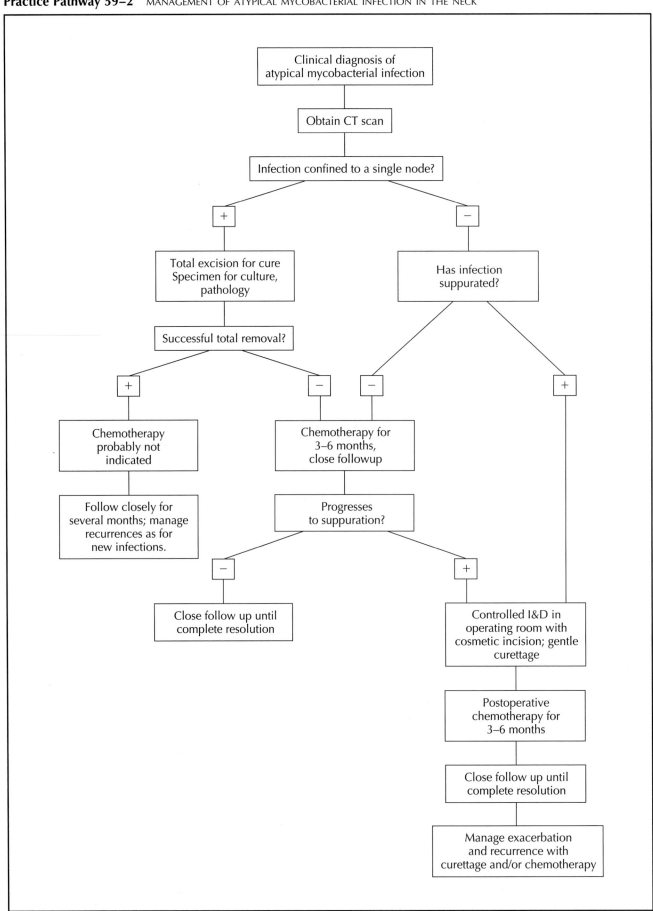

Abbreviations: I & D, incision and drainage.

chemotherapy has been used.[21-23] Historically, patients relegated to chemotherapy usually have failed primary surgical therapy and have residual disease that is not amenable to repeated surgical procedures. This usually entails prolonged courses of multiagent chemotherapy, combining traditional antituberculosis agents with some of the newer oral antibiotics. More experience has been gained in recent years using regimens including clarithromycin, azithromycin, clofazimine, and ciprofloxacin. In vitro studies of the newer macrolides have shown activity against NTM organisms.[24] Combination therapy currently is being used by the infectious disease division at our institution for many cases of NTM that might have been considered for surgical excision in the past. Definitive results from this modality have not been reported.

In summary, we believe the following to be a reasonable approach for treating pediatric cervical NTM at this time:

1. NTM that is limited to a single node and amenable to complete surgical excision should be excised. Cure rates are higher, and the cosmetic result is usually excellent.

2. As NTM is not a life-threatening disorder, radical excision of infections that involve important structures in the neck (most typically the branches of the facial nerve) is difficult to justify. Once CT shows extension beyond the initially-involved node, curative surgical therapy often is not an option.

3. If NTM has extended beyond the initially-involved node but has not suppurated or involved the skin, chemotherapy may be tried; because of the potential toxicity of some of the agents involved, chemotherapy usually should be administered by a pediatric infectious disease specialist.

4. If NTM has suppurated or goes on to suppuration despite chemotherapy, controlled drainage in the operating room that is followed by gentle curettage may yield a better cosmetic result than spontaneous drainage through the skin. Patients who are treated with drainage alone or curettage alone probably should receive chemotherapy as well.

5. At the first and subsequent visits, parents should be cautioned repeatedly that the disorder may not respond completely to either medical or surgical management and that it may need to "run its course" over several months. This will help to prevent disappointment and misunderstanding later. They should be reassured that it is a self-limited disorder, and that any residual cosmetic deformity can be addressed when the child is older.

Management of NTM is evolving and may change further as newer chemotherapeutic agents become available and as the results of patients treated with primary chemotherapy are published over the next few years. These suggestions should not be regarded as the last word on treatment of this frustrating disease.

Cat-Scratch Disease and Bacillary Angiomatosis

Cat-scratch disease (CSD) is now known to be caused by *Bartonella henselae* infection. Earlier reports implicating a new bacterial species, *Afipia felis,* have not been borne out by subsequent work. In the last decade, a great deal has been learned about the epidemiology and pathogenesis of CSD.

Bartonella henselae can be cultured from the blood of 30 to 60% of healthy domestic and wild cats; kittens <1 year old are affected more commonly. It appears to be transmitted from cat to cat by fleas, and from cat to human by cat scratches. It has not been shown whether fleas can transmit the organism directly to humans, but epidemiologic evidence suggests that, even if possible, this is an uncommon mode of transmission.

As CSD is not a reportable disease and causes little morbidity and essentially no mortality, the incidence data are sketchy. Annual incidence estimates range from 1.8 to 9.3 per 100,000.[25,26] CSD is more common in geographic areas where the cat population is higher and where the incidence of cat flea infestation is higher.

In the immunocompetent patient, the classic clinical picture of CSD is a self-limited, unilateral, regional lymphadenopathy following a cat scratch distal to the affected node. Most patients give a history of a cat scratch or contact with a cat. An inoculation papule at the site of the cat scratch is present in approximately half of all cases. The upper extremity nodes are affected most commonly followed by the cervical nodes. Systemic symptoms including a low-grade fever and malaise that are present in approximately half of cases. The disease usually resolves spontaneously over several months, but the nodes progress to suppuration and require drainage in about 10% of patients.

In immunocompetent patients, major complications are rare, but variants of the classic presentation may occur. *Oculoglandular syndrome,* which consists of preauricular adenopathy and unilateral conjunctivitis, is a well described manifestation of CSD. Retinitis, endocarditis, transient encephalopathy, and other neurologic complications have been described in a small percentage of cases.

As cervical adenopathy often persists for weeks or months, many of these children often come to surgical biopsy to rule out neoplasm. CSD is not diagnosed on routine tissue sections; a Warthin-Starry stain must be requested specifically. This shows small, pleomorphic gram-negative rods, the presence of which essentially confirms the diagnosis. The organism may be cultured, but is fastidious and may take several weeks to grow out. CSD skin testing with antigen prepared from infected individuals is a poorly-standardized test that is not readily available, not food-and-drug-administration (FDA) approved, and should not be used any longer.

The use of serologic testing appears to be increasingly promising. In earlier studies, sensitivity and specificity of serologic testing were less than ideal. In more recent studies, indirect fluorescent antibody testing, enzyme-linked immunofluorescent antibody testing for IgM (but not IgG), and PCR for *Bartonella* DNA have had sensitivity and specificity as high as 98%. Hopefully, more widespread availability and reliability of serologic testing will spare many children an open biopsy in the future. Testing is available from the Centers for Disease Control (CDC) at no charge, and commercial tests are beginning to become available. As these tests are new and still under study, it is impossible to recommend an "ideal" serologic test at this time. At this time, it seems wisest to consult with a laboratory-medicine or infectious-disease specialist when considering serologic testing for CSD.

Management usually has been supportive as the disease is usually self-limited and antibiotic therapy usually unrewarding. Anecdotal evidence has suggested a benefit from erythromycins, aminoglycosides, ciprofloxacin, rifampin, and sulfamethoxazole-trimethoprim in some patients.[27] A small, randomized, double-blind study has shown a modest improvement in the rate of resolution of lymphadenopathy following a 5 day course of azithro-

mycin.[28] As accurate diagnostic tests become available, more information on the benefit of treatment should accumulate over the next few years.

In immunosuppressed individuals, treatment of CSD seems more useful. A pediatric infectious disease specialist should be consulted to assist in choosing a treatment regimen for the immunosuppressed patient with CSD. *Bacillary angiomatosis* is a vasoproliferative disorder caused by *Bartonella henselae* that occurs almost entirely in severely immunocompromised patients (typically in AIDS patients, organ recipients, and chemotherapy patients). It causes brown to violaceous vascular tumors of the skin and subcutaneous tissue. Three distinct types of lesions have been described: (1) pyogenic granuloma-like; (2) subcutaneous-nodular; and (3) hyperpigmented, indurated plaque. Bacillary angiomatosis also may affect visceral organs, particularly the liver and spleen.

Bubonic Plague

Plague is caused by the bacillus *Yersinia pestis* (more correctly, *Yersinia pseudotuberculosis,* subspecies *pestis*). The major world-wide reservoir for *Yersinia pestis* is rats. In the United States, the important reservoirs are squirrels, prairie dogs, and other small mammals. Domestic animals (e.g., rabbits and cats) occasionally can be infected. The bacillus is transmitted to humans when they are bitten by a flea from an infected animal; occasionally, humans acquire the illness from handling contaminated animal tissue. Person-to-person transmission occurs only in the pneumonic form of the disease. In the United States, cases have been limited almost entirely to the southwestern states of New Mexico, Arizona, Colorado, Utah, and California. A history of contact with wild animals is present in some but not all cases. In the United States, 60% of patients are under 20 years of age.

In the most common manifestation, bubonic plague patients typically present 2 to 8 days following inoculation with the sudden onset of fever, chills, weakness, and headache, followed by the appearance of a bubo within the next 24 hours. The buboes of plague patients are oval, from 1 to 10 cm in length, and may be either solitary or an irregular cluster of several nodes. Pain and tenderness are typically very intense. The skin is often warm and edematous. Fluctuance is rare. Buboes are seen most often in the groin, axilla, or neck. Plague is unusual in that the extremely, sudden onset of fever, bubo with associated intense inflammation, and fulminant course can be fatal in 2 to 4 days if untreated.

Diagnosis of plague is made by stain of aspirated material from a bubo. Treatment is with streptomycin, tetracycline, or chloramphenicol. An infectious-disease specialist should be consulted.

Tularemia

Tularemia is caused by the gram-negative bacillus *Francisella tularensis.* It is a zoonosis transmitted by the bites of insects (including ticks, mosquitoes, deerflies), by handling infected animals (rabbits, muskrats), or by consuming infected meats (most commonly rabbit). Tick-borne transmission is now the most common mode of transmission in the United States, and a history of a tick bite can often be elicited. It may present in an ulceroglandular form (with a primary skin ulcer and lymphadenopathy), an oropharyngeal form (with a primary ulcer in the mouth), or a purely glandular form (lymphadenopathy without a primary ulcer). Although tularemia typically is described as causing a severe systemic febrile illness with an appreciable mortality (5–7%), a more benign self-limited variant also is recognized. Children may present with mild fever, headache, and cervical lymphadenopathy that is usually unilateral. A nonexudative pharyngitis also may be seen. It is likely that mild tularemia is underdiagnosed in the United States. Diagnosis may be quite difficult, but ideally is confirmed by a rise in tularemia agglutination titer from the acute to convalescent phase of the illness. Biopsy may be performed to rule out malignancy in some cases; pathologic findings (caseous necrosis with polymorphonuclear leukocyte infiltration) are not diagnostic but may raise the suspicion of tularemia. Treatment is with streptomycin, tetracycline, aminoglycosides, or chloramphenicol.

Actinomycosis

Actinomycosis is caused by gram-positive nonspore-forming bacteria. The most common human pathogen is *Actinomyces israelii,* but several other *Actinomyces* species rarely can be pathogenic as well. About 50% of cases are cervicofacial. *Actinomyces* are normal commensals in the oral cavity, and most cervicofacial infections are thought to be due to a violation of the oral mucosa. Often, infections follow dental extraction or oral injury, although in other cases no initial injury site can be identified.

The most typical presentation is a slow-growing, painless mass near the mandible. Lymph nodes may become involved by direct extension, but cervical lymphadenopathy is rare. About 10% of cases will have metastatic disease, usually of the liver or brain. Untreated, the mass progresses to chronic suppuration and fibrosis and often forms one or more draining sinuses. A less common presentation is the relatively-acute development of a warm, tender indurated mass (or masses) that is accompanied by fever and chills. Actinomycosis is most common in young and middle-aged adults, but a number of cases have been reported in children as young as 3 years.[29]

The presence of sulphur granules on pathologic specimen is suggestive, but not absolutely diagnostic, of actinomycosis. The organism is fastidious and can be cultured in anaerobic conditions less than 50% of the time. If actinomycosis is suspected, laboratory medicine should be notified in advance of surgery, as special swab and culture techniques can be used to improve yield.

Because <100 cases yearly are reported in the United States, it is difficult to make absolute statements about treatment. Most cases are treated by surgical removal followed by prolonged antibiotic therapy. If vital structures (e.g., the facial nerve) are involved, they probably should be spared because subtotal excision followed by prolonged antibiotic therapy is usually successful. Penicillin is the standard antibiotic, but clindamycin, erythromycin, and tetracycline have been used in patients allergic to penicillin. Prolonged courses (up to 6 months) typically are recommended, as recurrences after short courses of antibiotic therapy are common.

Brucellosis

Brucellosis is caused by several species of the genus *Brucella.* It can be acquired through working with infected livestock or through consumption of unpasteurized dairy products. It can affect any organ or system, but often causes an insidious nonspecific set of systemic symptoms including fever, sweats, anorexia, fatigue, depression, and mild lymphadenopathy. Diagnosis can be made presumptively by documenting rising titers of specific antibodies; definitive diagnosis is by culture of blood, bone marrow, or other affected tissue. Treatment is usually with a combination of tetracycline (older children only), streptomycin, gentamicin, and rifampin. Long courses of therapy are necessary as relapses are common after short course of antibiotics and after single-agent therapy.

Syphilis

Primary syphilis can cause a regional adenopathy or adenitis. The expected oral chancre may be difficult or impossible to demonstrate in some cases. Early presentation with a neck mass may be more common in patients with HIV.

FUNGAL INFECTIONS

Histoplasmosis

Histoplasmosis is caused by the fungus *Histoplasma capsulatum.* In the central United States, from 50 to 100% of the population has been infected. It is associated with bird droppings and acquired via inhaled airborne spores. Infections are typically asymptomatic. In immunocompromised, and occasionally in immunocompetent patients, histoplasmosis may cause a mild or rarely a severe pulmonary or systemic disease. Head and neck involvement is usually limited to lesions of the mucosa of the aerodigestive tract, which may mimic carcinoma and require biopsy. Rarely, histoplasmosis may present as an isolated neck mass. This may be a less rare presentation in those who have immigrated from or who have traveled in Africa because African histoplasmosis, caused by *Histoplasma dubosii,* more commonly presents with lymphadenopathy. Biopsy is necessary to establish the diagnosis and treatment is surgical excision. It is not known whether following excision there is any benefit to systemic antifungal treatment in the otherwise healthy host.

Other Fungal Infections of the Neck

Infections caused by *Candida* species and *Aspergillus* species have been reported to present as isolated neck masses. These presentations are extraordinarily rare, and are limited almost exclusively to immunocompromised patients. Biopsy probably is necessary to establish the diagnosis.

PARASITIC INFECTIONS

Toxoplasmosis

Toxoplasmosis causes a small but significant number of cases of cervical lymphadenopathy. Although the illness is typically self-limited, the adenopathy may persist for months and many patients require biopsy to rule out malignancy. Once the diagnosis is made in an immunocompetent patient, further therapy usually is not needed. In immunosuppressed patients, toxoplasmosis may cause significant systemic disease; in the pregnant female, toxoplasmosis may cause severe injury to the developing embryo or fetus.

Toxoplasma gondii is an obligate intracellular parasite. It is found in many animal species and is common worldwide. It reproduces asexually in many animal species, but sexual reproduction can take place only in the gastrointestinal tract of the cat. During a primary infection, cats shed millions of infectious oocysts daily for several weeks. These oocysts may remain infectious for up to 1 year, especially in moist environments. Humans may acquire toxoplasmosis through ingestion of oocysts following handling of cat litter or contaminated food sources (e.g., unwashed garden vegetables). Infection also can follow ingestion of undercooked meat (especially pork, mutton, and beef) or unpasteurized milk or vertical transmission from mother to embryo or fetus. In serologic studies, 30 to 50% of the U.S. population has been shown to be infected by age 50. The acute infection is usually asymptomatic, but occasionally may produce a flu-like illness. The parasites become encysted in host tissues and remain permanently. In immunocompetent patients, they usually cause no disease. In immunosuppressed patients, toxoplasmosis may reactivate and cause severe systemic, ocular, central nervous system (CNS), or disease.

In patients with symptomatic toxoplasmosis, 80 to 90% have painless cervical lymphadenopathy as the sole manifestation. The remainder of the examination and laboratory workup is almost always normal, although the IgM toxoplasma antibody titer may be high if obtained within a few weeks of onset of lymphadenopathy.

It is estimated that toxoplasmosis causes 3 to 7% of cervical lymphadenopathy that requires biopsy.[30,31] The disorder is almost always self-limited, but because the lymphadenopathy may persist for months, many patients require excisional biopsy to rule out malignancy. Whether serologic testing alone is adequate to rule out malignancy is unclear. The pathologic findings are usually diagnostic, but about 2% may be diagnosed initially as lymphoma. As well a small percentage of cases diagnosed initially as toxoplasmosis ultimately prove to be lymphoma, and in a few patients the two disorders apparently present simultaneously.

SPECIAL CONSIDERATION:

A small percentage of cases initially diagnosed as toxoplasmosis ultimately prove to be lymphoma, and vice versa.

In immunosuppressed patients, toxoplasmosis may cause severe systemic disease. It is a common cause of blindness and CNS lesions in the HIV-infected population. Systemic manifestations also should be sought if the diagnosis is considered in other immunosuppressed patients (e.g., patients undergoing aggressive chemotherapy).

If the diagnosis is considered in an adolescent female, it is important to inquire about the possibility of pregnancy. Congenital toxoplasmosis causes a spectrum of disorders in the developing fetus, ranging from mild ocular damage to severe CNS injury. Drug regimens are available that appear to reduce the rate of transmission to the fetus, and perhaps to minimize the injury if transmission does occur. If toxoplasmosis is diagnosed in the pregnant female, obstetrical and infectious-disease consultation should be obtained immediately.

Filariasis

Lymphatic filariasis is caused by roundworms. The larvae develop in mosquito vectors and are then transmitted to humans for the final stages of larval development. The parasites mature in humans over 6 to 24 months and then reproduce. The mature female may produce up to 50,000 larvae daily. The larvae are transmitted back to a mosquito vector when the human carrier is bitten.

The adult worms live in lymphatic channels and may survive a decade or more. The acute phase is characterized by acute localized lymphadenitis in a solitary node or a group or nodes that are large, firm, and discrete. Lymphangitis may ensue, and the patient may be systemically ill with fevers, chills, sweats, and malaise. Recurrent acute episodes are common. Over months or years, lymphatic channels scar and lymphedema (most classically, elephantiasis) may follow. The inguinal and axillary nodes are most commonly affected but cervical nodes can be involved.

Although filariasis is rare in the United States, approximately 2% of the world population is infected.[32] The disorder should be considered in immigrants from endemic areas.

INFLAMMATORY DISORDERS OF THE NECK

Kawasaki Syndrome

Kawasaki syndrome (KS) is an acute multisystem vasculitis. It was first described in Japan in 1967, and in the English literature in 1974. Its etiology is unknown. The clinical presentation (see below) is similar to that of many childhood infectious diseases, and epidemiologic features (e.g., the occurrence of community-wide outbreaks every 3–5 years) also have suggested that KS may be an infectious disease. However, despite exhaustive work by many labs, no specific etiologic agent has been identified. More recently, it has been suggested that KS might be caused by an immune response to a superantigen, such as the massive immune activation to a specific toxin that causes toxic shock syndrome. The precise cause of the illness remains a mystery.

KS is a disease of young childhood. Fifty percent of cases occur before age 2 years and 80% by age 4 years. It is almost unknown over the age of 8. The male: female ratio is 3:2, and it is more common in children of Asian ancestry. The diagnosis is clinical and usually should be made in children who have five of six principal diagnostic criteria, which are: high fever (38–41° C); conjunctival injection; erythema of the lips, oral mucosa, and/or tongue; polymorphous erythematous rash; cervical adenopathy; and changes in the hands and feet including firm edema, erythema, and convalescent desquamation. Cervical adenopathy occurs in up to 83% of patients[33] and is almost never suppurative. Some children, particularly those <6 to 12 months of age, may present with a more limited spectrum of symptoms and present a more challenging diagnostic problem.

Associated symptoms include CNS symptoms, principally extreme irritability and emotional lability, urethritis and sterile pyuria, abdominal pain, and cardiac symptoms that can range from a benign tachycardia to frank congestive failure and cardiogenic shock. Arthritis was common prior to the advent of early diagnosis and effective treatment. Because arthritis typically does not manifest until the second week of the illness and many patients are now treated before that point, it has become a less common manifestation.

Laboratory findings are nonspecific, and include an elevated white blood cell count with a left shift, elevation of markers for acute inflammation [e.g., erythrocyte sedimentation rate (ESR) and C-reactive protein] thrombocytosis, and elevated liver enzymes.

SPECIAL CONSIDERATION:

In the United States, Kawasaki syndrome has now passed rheumatic fever as the most common cause of acquired heart disease in children.

The vasculitis of KS is self-limited, but unfortunately causes permanent cardiac damage in about 20% of untreated patients. The most common lesions are coronary artery aneurysms. It appears that, in the United States, KS has now passed rheumatic fever as the most common cause of acquired heart disease in children. Because recognition and treatment reduces the incidence of permanent cardiac damage to <5%, it is crucial to make the diagnosis and institute appropriate treatment early.

KS is treated with high-dose immunoglobulin and aspirin. The mechanism of action of immune globulin is not clear, but it is postulated that immune globulin contains antibodies against the etiologic microbe or toxin. Aspirin is thought to reduce platelet aggregation and vasculitis. All patients with KS should have an initial echocardiogram and subsequent cardiac follow-up based on the severity of their illness and initial findings. Cardiac sequellae account for the mortality of 1 to 2% still associated with this disease.

Patients with KS initially may develop high fevers, oral cavity changes, and cervical adenopathy; they may present to the primary physician, or pediatric otolaryngologist, prior to developing other manifestations of KS. At a very early stage of the illness, it may be difficult to make the diagnosis. If patients are treated with antibiotics and subsequent rash is ascribed to an antibiotic reaction, diagnosis may be delayed further. The pediatric otolaryngologist always should consider KS as a potential diagnosis in the febrile child, and should be alert for the development of other symptoms of KS in the child who first presents with a more limited set of symptoms. This is particularly true in children <1 year who may never develop a "complete" picture, but who are at the highest risk for cardiac sequelae. If in doubt, a pediatric specialist experienced in treating KS should be asked to evaluate the child.

AT A GLANCE . . .

Diagnostic Criteria for Kawasaki Syndrome

1. High fever (38–41° C)
2. Conjunctival injection
3. Erythema of the lips, oral mucosa, and/or tongue
4. Polymorphous erythematous rash
5. Cervical adenopathy
6. Edema, erythema, and desquamation of the hands and feet

Sarcoidosis

Sarcoidosis is a chronic multisystem granulomatous disease with an unknown etiology. It can affect almost any organ system, but most commonly the lungs and intrathoracic lymph nodes. Systemic symptoms may include fever, weight loss, dyspnea on exertion, cough, chest pain, and other symptoms referable to affected organ systems. Fifteen to twenty-five percent of patients have eye involvement, which may include retinitis and uveitis. *Neurosarcoidosis* is usually a late manifestation, but occasionally neurologic involvement may be seen early in the disease course. Patients may remain asymptomatic indefinitely, may go into spontaneous remission, or may undergo chronic progression. When indicated, the mainstay of treatment is steroids, but other immunosuppressive agents also are used at times.

The most common otolaryngologic manifestations are neck masses, parotid masses, and facial nerve palsy, which may be reversible. Cervical nodes are the most commonly involved peripheral nodes. Cervical adenopathy is typically bilateral with mobile, nontender nodes.

Diagnosis is by biopsy and pathologic examination. If the initial disease presentation is solely in the neck and the patient does not have pulmonary symptoms, the diagnosis may not be considered strongly on clinical grounds prior to biopsy. If the diagnosis is considered preoperatively, a chest X-ray may show characteristic pulmonary findings and provide direction for the diagnostic work up.

Sinus Histiocytosis with Massive Lymphadenopathy (Rosai-Dorfman Disease)

Sinus histiocytosis with massive lymphadenopathy is an idiopathic benign histiocytic proliferation seen most often in the first two decades of life. Almost 90% of patients have involvement of the cervical nodes, which are typically painless and massively enlarged. Systemic manifestations typically include fever, leukocytosis with an elevated neutrophil count, and elevated ESR. Almost half of patients have extranodal involvement. Extranodal involvement is most commonly in the head and neck region, including the upper respiratory tract, the orbit, and the salivary glands.

Biopsy is almost always necessary to rule out malignancy. Occasionally, it may be difficult to distinguish sinus histiocytosis with massive lymphadenopathy from a malignant histiocytosis on pathologic examination.

Treatment is usually unnecessary because the disease appears to regress spontaneously in most cases. In a few cases, the disease takes a fulminant course and can be fatal. In fatal cases, the patients most often have some underlying immunologic abnormality, and there is systemic involvement of multiple organ systems.

Kikuchi-Fujimoto Disease

Kikuchi-Fujimoto disease was first described in Japan in 1972. Approximately 400 cases have been reported, of which about half have been reported in Japan. It is an idiopathic disorder, which has lymphadenopathy as its hallmark. Lymph gland enlarge-

ment may occur anywhere in the body, but is cervical in 80% of cases. Intraparotid nodes also may be involved. The nodes are often tender. Fever, chills, and weight loss are common. Other systemic symptoms, such as night sweats and nausea, also may be present. Women are affected in approximately 80% of cases. It can occur at any age, but is most common in young adults. Spontaneous regression over a period of months is the rule, although one death has been reported.[34]

Although the disease is self-limited, the patient often comes to biopsy to rule out a malignancy. Diagnosis only can be made by pathologic examination of excised nodal tissue. White blood cell count is often low and the ESR is often high, but other laboratory testing is typically normal. Although imaging is probably obtained in most cases as part of the workup, CT findings are nonspecific.

The disorder is significant in that, prior to its description, a number of cases were diagnosed as malignant lymphomas and in some cases received chemotherapy.[35] It is important to be aware of this entity to avoid treating these patients with cytotoxic agents.

PFAPA Syndrome

Marshall et al. first described a syndrome of periodic recurring fever, aphthous stomatitis, pharyngitis, and cervical adenitis, and they later applied the acronym PFAPA (*Periodic Fever, Aphthous stomatitis, Pharyngitis, and cervical Adenitis*).[36] The 12 children about whom they reported experienced attacks characterized by abrupt onset of fevers up to 40° C, chills, malaise, pharyngitis, aphthous stomatitis, and tender cervical lymphadenopathy. Episodes typically last several days and occur at regular intervals that are approximately monthly. The syndrome appears to resolve spontaneously over a period of several years. The attacks typically begin before age 5 years, and the duration of illness is reported to be from 1 to 15 years at the time of this report. White blood cell counts and ESR are typically elevated only during episodes. Extensive workup for infectious, autoimmune, idiopathic, and immunodeficiency disease is negative in most patients. Cyclic neutropenia and other periodic fever syndromes must be excluded specifically to make the diagnosis. Patients in whom this diagnosis is suspected should be evaluated in conjunction with a pediatric infectious-disease specialist.

One report has suggested a beneficial effect of

cimetidine treatment,[37] but as the disorder appears to be benign and self-limiting, it is likely that many children do not need specific treatment.

Focal Myositis

Focal myositis is an inflammatory pseudotumor of skeletal muscle. It most commonly presents in the extremities, but several cases have been reported in the sternocleidomastoid muscle.[38-40] It may be difficult to distinguish from an infectious process or abscess as it may present with fever, inflammation, and torticollis. It also may be difficult to distinguish from a muscle sarcoma. Incisional biopsy is often necessary to establish the diagnosis. Total excision is not necessary. Treatment is supportive and cases typically regress spontaneously over several months.

REFERENCES

1. Chetham MM, Roberts KB. Infectious mononucleosis in adolescents. Pediatr Ann 1991; 20:206-213.
2. Schuster V, Kreth HW. Epstein-Barr virus infection and associated diseases in children: I. Pathogenesis, epidemiology and clinical aspects. Eur J Pediatr 1992; 151:718-725.
3. Schuster V, Kreth HW. Epstein-Barr virus infection and associated diseases in children: II. Diagnostic and therapeutic strategies. Eur J Pediatr 1992; 151:794-798.
4. Zachariae H. Herpesvirus infection in man. Scand J Infect Dis 1985; 47(Supplement):44-50.
5. Levy JA. Pathogenesis of human immunodeficiency virus infection. Microbiol Rev 1993; 57:183-289.
6. McKinney RE Jr. Antiretroval therapy: Evaluating the new era in HIV treatment. Adv Pediatr Infect Dis 1996; 12:297-323.
7. Richards L. Retropharyngeal abscess. NEJM 1936; 215:1120-1130.
8. Brodsky L, Belles W, Brody A, et al. Needle aspiration of neck abscesses in children. Clin Pediatr 1992; 31:71-76.
9. Dean LW. The proper procedure for external drainage of retropharyngeal abscess secondary to caries of the vertebrae. Ann Otol Rhinol Laryngol 1919; 28:566-572.
10. Grodinsky M. Retropharyngeal and lateral pharyngeal abscesses: An anatomic and clinical study. Ann Surg 1939; 110:177-199.
11. Thompson JW, Cohen SR, Reddix P. Retropharyngeal abscess in children: A retrospective and historical analysis. Laryngoscope 1988; 98:589-592.
12. Lemierre A. On certain septicaemias due to anaerobic organisms. Lancet 1936; 2:701-703.
13. Goldhagen J, Alford BA, Prewitt LH, et al. Suppurative thrombophlebitis of the internal jugular vein: Report of three cases and review of the literature. Pediatr Infect Dis J 1988; 7:410-414.
14. Pransky SM, Reisman BK, Kearns DB, et al. Cervicofacial mycobacterial adenitis in children: Endemic to San Diego? Laryngoscope 1990; 100:920-925.
15. Yates MD, Grange JM. Bacteriological survey of tuberculous lymphadenitis in southeast England, 1981-1989. J Epidemiol Community Health 1992; 46:332-335.
16. Wolinsky E. Mycobacterial lymphadenitis in children: A prospective study of 105 nontuberculous cases with long-term follow-up. Clin Infect Dis 1995; 20:954-963.
17. Pinder SE, Colville A. Mycobacterial cervical lymphadenitis in children: Can histological assessment help differentiate infections caused by non-tuberculous mycobacteria from mycobacterium tuberculosis? Histopathology 1993; 22:59-64.
18. Benjamin DR. Granulomatous lymphadenitis in children. Arch Pathol Lab Med 1987; 111:750-753.
19. Aleesi DP, Dudley JP. Atypical Mycobacteria-induced cervical adenitis: Treatment by needle aspiration. Arch Otolaryngol Head Neck Surg 1988; 114:664-666.
20. Kennedy TL. Curettage of nontuberculous mycobacterial cervical lymphadenitis. Arch Otolaryngol Head Neck Surg 1992; 118:759-762.
21. Green PA, von Reyn CF, Smith RP. Mycobacterium avium complex parotid lymphadenitis: Successful therapy with clarithromycin and ethambutol. Pediatr Infect Dis J 1993; 12(7):615-616.
22. Berger C, Pfyffer GE, Nadal D. Treatment of nontuberculous mycobacterial lymphadenitis with clarithromycin plus rifabutin. J Pediatr 1996; 128(3):383-386.
23. Tessier HM, Amoric JC, Mechinaud F, et al. Clarithromycin for atypical mycobacterial lymphadenitis in non-immunocompromised children. Lancet 1994; 344:1778.
24. Rapp RP, McCraney SA, Goodman NL, et al. New macrolide antibiotics: Usefulness in infections caused by mycobacteria other than mycobacterium tuberculosis. Ann Pharmacother 1994; 28:1255-1263.
25. Zangwill KM, Hamilton DH, Perkins BA, et al. Cat scratch disease in Connecticut. NEJM 1993; 329:8-13.
26. Jackson LA, Perkins BA, Wenger JD. Cat scratch disease in the United States: An analysis of three national databases. Am J Public Health 1993; 83:1707-1711.
27. Maurin M, Birtles R, Raoult D. Current knowledge of

Bartonella species. Eur J Clin Microbiol Infect Dis 1997; 16:487-506.

28. Bass JM, Freitas BC, Freitas AD, et al. Prospective randomized double blind placebo-controlled evaluation of azitrhomycin for treatment of cat-scratch disease. Pediatr Infect Dis J 1998; 17:447-452.

29. Foster SV, Demmler GJ, Hawkins EP, et al. Pediatric cervicofacial actinomycosis. South Med J 1993; 86: 1147-1150.

30. McCabe RE, Brooks RG, Dorfman RF, et al. Clinical spectrum in 107 cases of toxoplasmic lymphadenopathy. Rev Infect Dis 1987; 9:754-774.

31. Engel JE, Lydiatt DD, Ruskin J. Toxoplasmosis appearing as an anterior neck mass. Ear Nose Throat J 1993; 72:584-586.

32. Michael E, Bundy DAP, Grenfell BT. Re-assessing the global prevalence and distribution of lymphatic filiariasis. Parasitology 1996; 112:409-428.

33. Seicshnaydre MA, Frable MA. Kawasaki disease: Early presentation to the Otolaryngologist. Otolaryngol Head Neck Surg 1993; 108:344-347.

34. Chan JKC, Wong KC, Ng CS. A fatal case of multicentric Kikuchi's histiocytic lymphadenitis. Cancer 1989; 63:1856-1862.

35. Garcia CE, Girdhar-Gopal HV, Dorfman DM. Kikuchi-Fujimoto disease of the neck update. Ann Otol Rhinol Laryngol 1993; 102:11-14.

36. Marshall GS, Edwards KM, Butler J, et al. Syndrome of periodic fever, pharyngitis, and aphthous stomatitis. J Pediatr 1987; 10:43-46.

37. Feder HM. Cimetidine treatment for periodic fever associated with aphthous stomatitis, pharyngitis and cervical adenitis. Pediatr Infect Dis 1992; 11: 318-321.

38. Isaacson G, Chan KH, Heffner RR. Focal myositis: A new cause for the pediatric neck mass. Arch Otolaryngol Head Neck Surg 1991; 117:103-105.

39. Josephson GD, de Blasi H, McCormick S, et al. Focal myositis of the sternocleidomastoid muscle: A case report and review of the literature. Am J Otolaryngol 1996; 17:215-217.

40. Rivest C, Miller FW, Love LA, et al. Focal myositis presenting as pseudothrombophlebitis of the neck in a patient with mixed connective tissue disease. Arthritis Rheum 1996; 39:1254-1258.

60 Pediatric Neck Neoplasms

John P. Bent, III, Richard L. Hebert, and Richard J.H. Smith

Pediatric neck neoplasms create an ironic challenge. Although they present as a neck mass, most pediatric neck masses are not neoplastic. Consequently, evaluation and treatment of the pediatric neck mass requires knowledge of multiple neoplastic, inflammatory, and congenital lesions. Whereas a neck mass in an adult should be considered malignant until proven otherwise, most pediatric neck masses represent benign disease. Nevertheless, because a pediatric neck mass may signal malignancy, the physician must maintain an awareness of all diagnostic possibilities. Proper execution of this work-up mandates an understanding of pediatric neck pathology and the studies available to arrive at the correct diagnosis.

Benign cervical lymph node hypertrophy represents the most common cause of a pediatric neck mass. A myriad of viral, bacterial, fungal, and protozoan infections cause lymph node hypertrophy, which may persist for several months even with appropriate treatment. In general, children < 12 years old normally have nodes < 1 cm in diameter, although any palpable node in a newborn is abnormal.[1] Children routinely experience idiopathic self-limiting episodes of lymph node enlargement to 2 to 3 cm in diameter.

An asymptomatic neck mass represents the most common presentation of a pediatric head and neck malignancy.[2] Masses require further investigation and consideration for open biopsy if they are located in the supraclavicular fossa, unusually large or remain enlarged beyond 6 weeks, progress in size after initial presentation, or are accompanied by other symptoms, such as pain, fever, or weight loss. In a series of 239 children who underwent peripheral lymph node biopsy for lymph node enlargement, 49% had idiopathic lymphoid hyperplasia,

37% had infectious hyperplasia, and only 13% had neoplasms.[3] Because most lymph nodes do not require excision, removed pediatric neck masses are most often congenital. Torsiglieri et al. reported 445 children who underwent excision of any neck mass (including lymph nodes) and found 55% congenital masses, 27% inflammatory lesions, 5% noninflammatory benign lesions, 3% benign neoplasms, and 11% malignancies.[4] These data confirm that most neck masses are not malignant, but also demonstrate that of neck neoplasms, malignancies outnumber benign tumors.

The majority of pediatric malignancies consist of lymphomas and leukemias (48%) and central nervous system (CNS) tumors (20%).[5] Lymphoma accounts for over half of pediatric neck malignancies,[3,4] whereas rhabdomyosarcomas represent the most common pediatric soft-tissue malignancy of the head and neck.[6] Thyroid malignancies formerly composed 50% of pediatric neck malignancies,[7] but the incidence has been reduced with judicious use of head and neck irradiation.

> ## SPECIAL CONSIDERATION:
>
> Lymphoma accounts for over half of pediatric neck malignancies, whereas rhabdomyosarcomas represent the most common pediatric soft-tissue malignancy of the head and neck.

Many pediatric malignancies, including those in the neck, show an age-related or sexual bias. It is rare for lymphoma to occur before 3 years of age or for thyroid cancer to appear during the first decade. Neuroblastoma represents the most common neck malignancy in children < 6 years of age.[8] Boys have a higher rate of malignancy than girls, with a notable

Pediatric Otolaryngology, Edited by R.F. Wetmore, H.R. Muntz, and T.J. McGill. Thieme Medical Publishers, Inc., New York © 2000.

exception being teratoma, which occurs primarily in females. Geography also plays a role, as exemplified by Burkitt's lymphoma (BL), which rarely occurs outside of the African "Burkitt's belt". Phenomenons such as this may be due to unique racial or genetic predispositions to malignancy or to the greater presence of oncogenic cofactors [such as Epstein-Barr Virus (EBV)] in certain regions.[5] Prenatal exposure to carcinogenic agents, as seen with the increased incidence of neuroblastoma in fetal alcohol-hydantoin syndrome, also demonstrates the susceptibility of the developing child.[5] Some genetic disorders carry increased risk of particular malignancies (e.g., leukemia in Down's syndrome and fibrosarcoma and rhabdomyosarcoma in von Recklinghausen's disease), whereas certain genetic immune disorders (e.g., Wiskott-Aldrich syndrome) predispose the affected individual to a greater risk for all malignancies.

History alone significantly narrows the differential. The presence of a lesion at birth suggests a congenital cyst or a benign neoplasm such as a teratoma, cystic hygroma, or a hemangioma. Symptoms such as rapid growth, pain, cranial nerve defects, and airway or vascular compression suggest the possibility of malignancy. Several weeks or more of fever, anorexia, weight loss, and other systemic complaints raise the likelihood of lymphoma. Children with human immunodeficiency virus (HIV) infection face an increased risk of lymphoma, but also may develop infectious adenopathy masquerading as a neoplasm. Occasionally, family history yields critical information about hereditary disease such as multiple endocrine neoplasias (MEN) or neurofibromatosis.

Physical exam allows further refinement of the diagnostic possibilities. The location of the mass has significant implications. Midline and cystic lesions are more likely to be congenital, whereas suprasternal masses suggest thyroid pathology. Supraclavicular and posterior triangle masses are more often malignant than anterior or midline masses. Characteristics such as large size, tissue infiltration, and lack of tenderness suggest malignancy, whereas fluctuance, erythema, and tenderness usually herald an inflammatory lesion. The presence of fluctuation implies a probable communication with the aerodigestive tract (ADT) and branchial cleft cysts and laryngoceles must be considered. Superficial midline lesions, such as dermoid cysts, usually do not move with swallowing, whereas thyroglossal duct cysts and deeper lesions within or attached to the strap

muscles do. A mass within the sternocleidomastoid muscle of a neonate suggests congenital torticollis.

> ## SPECIAL CONSIDERATION:
>
> Characteristics such as large size, tissue infiltration, and lack of tenderness suggest a malignant neck mass, whereas fluctuance, erythema, and tenderness usually herald an inflammatory lesion.

Exam outside the neck also may provide useful information. For example, nasopharyngoscopy may demonstrate a nasopharyngeal mass or vocal cord paralysis (VCP). Lisch nodules or axillary freckling are found with neurofibromatosis type I. Lytic calvarial lesions in an infant with atopic dermatitis suggests Langerhans' histiocytosis. The presence of a polymorphous rash, conjunctivitis, strawberry tongue, inflammation of the hands and feet, and a fever in a child with an acutely-enlarged, nonpurulent unilateral cervical lymph node is the mucocutaneous lymph node syndrome of Kawasaki.[9]

The history and physical examination therefore refine the diagnosis, enabling the clinician to plan additional studies carefully. An abnormal purified protein derivative (PPD) skin test or elevated antibody titers for toxoplasmosis, EBV, cytomegalovirus (CMV), or *Bartonella* suggest a nonneoplastic etiology. Leukocytosis supports inflammation, whereas leukopenia, anemia, or thrombocytopenia may be seen in lymphoma or HIV infection. With the exception of medullary thyroid cancers, pediatric neck neoplasms do not have serologic markers. A chest roentgenogram must be obtained to assess the hilum and mediastinum for involvement.

Magnetic resonance imaging (MRI) and/or computed tomography (CT) usually are warranted for extensive or deep masses, particularly those suspected of being malignant, but may not be necessary for isolated, superficial masses. Ultrasound accurately distinguishes cystic from solid mass, and its application in the neck has expanded beyond thyroid masses. It can differentiate cystic from solid, facilitate needle aspiration, and define the depth of a lesion, often obviating the need for an open biopsy or CT scan. More specialized radiologic procedures such as arteriography and nuclear scans may be useful for vascular and thyroid neoplasms, respectively.

Definitive diagnosis requires pathologic examination. Fine-needle aspiration biopsy (FNAB) plays a major role in the management of thyroid cancer and occasionally guides management of nonthyroid neck masses. Seven of 17 patients in Tunkel et al.'s series avoided open biopsy based on FNAB results.[10] Polymerase chain reaction (PCR) technology applied to the contents of aspirated cervical nodes can be used to identify atypical mycobacteria,[11] and may have a broader future application for neck neoplasms. Despite the utility of FNAB, its accuracy does not compare to excisional biopsy, which remains the diagnostic gold standard against which new technologies must be compared.

SPECIAL CONSIDERATION:

Despite the utility of fine needle aspiration biopsy, its accuracy does not compare to excisional biopsy, which remains the diagnostic gold standard.

Pediatric malignancies may present with atypical or indolent symptoms, but when suspected should be investigated aggressively (and occasionally emergently) because of their high potential for rapid growth and destruction. Prognostic information can be determined by stage, site, and extent of disease, and complemented in some instances by recent technological advances based on tumor histology, immunologic classification (i.e., the CD40 antigen present in Hodgkin's disease), or molecular evidence of genetic abnormalities. Treatment and prognosis vary widely based on the pathologic results, and in general, oncologists select more toxic and potent treatments for the most aggressive tumors.

The ensuing pages cover the diagnosis, treatment, and prognosis of each pathologically-distinct pediatric neoplasm known to present in the neck. Discussion excludes nonneoplastic neck masses, extremely rare pediatric neoplasms (such as parathyroid neoplasms), and primary neoplasms of the skull, mandible, parotid, nasopharynx, pharynx, clavicles, and chest.

PRIMARY NEOPLASMS

Congenital Neoplasms

Choristoma, hamartoma, and teratoma represent congenital neoplasms that may present in the head and neck. *Choristomas* contain normal tissue that is foreign to the site of involvement, and they very rarely present in the neck. *Hamartomas* consist of tissue that is indigenous to the area, but abnormal in quantity, arrangement, and differentiation. Like choristomas, hamartomas rarely occur in the neck. When they present at multiple sites, the clinician should suspect *Cowden's disease,* which is an autosomal dominant disease that is characterized by hamartomas of all three primordial germ-cell layers and a high rate of internal malignancy.[12]

Literally translated in Greek, *teratoma* means monstrous tumor. It includes a diverse group of neoplasms that contain tissue from all three germ-cell layers. Unlike hamartomas, teratomas contain tissue that is foreign to the location and grow progressively and unpredictably. They are most common in the sacrococcygeal region, however 3% originate in the neck.[13] Teratomas fall into 2 categories based on age of presentation and clinical behavior: (1) congenital or infantile masses that are benign but cause significant mortality secondary to their massive size and airway compression; and (2) those presenting in adolescence or adulthood, which are smaller but much more likely to be malignant.[14] Malignant teratomas may present in infants, but such cases are the exception.[15] In general, survival with malignant teratomas is < 2 years.[16]

Obstetricians now diagnose most large congenital teratomas prenatally via ultrasound. Sonograms show a characteristic mixed echogenicity with multiloculated areas,[17] allowing advanced preparations to establish an airway at birth before interrupting maternal–fetal circulation. Postpartum plain radiographs or CT may show intralesional calcifications, adding support to the diagnosis and rendering preoperative biopsy unnecessary. Despite the remarkable and grotesque appearance of some lesions, resection often occurs with greater ease than anticipated.[18] Consequently, most authorities advocate complete removal with preservation of normal anatomic structures.[19] Gundry's review of cervical teratomas, which demonstrated a mortality rate of 15% for surgical treatment and 80% for observation, justifies expeditious operative intervention.[20]

Submandibular Gland Neoplasms

Submandibular gland neoplasms may be confused with cervical adenopathy, but always should be considered with masses in the submandibular triangle. The small size of an infant's submandibular gland makes it difficult to identify by palpation, although in older children the gland can be identified manually and distinguished from nearby lymph nodes. When examining a patient with a submandibular mass, attention should be directed toward the facial nerve, particularly the marginal mandibular branch, which may be destroyed by aggressive neoplasms. Similarly, the hypoglossal nerve may manifest impairment in deeply-invasive lesions. CT scans are not always necessary, but can demonstrate the size and invasiveness of a lesion. There is no role for sialography, unless the physician suspects gland inflammation secondary to a Wharton's duct stone. Occasionally, a submandibular gland mucocele extends into the neck as a *plunging ranula,* imitating a cervical neoplasm. It also should be remembered that parotid tail neoplasms, which are not included in this chapter, commonly appear as masses immediately behind the mandibular angle.

SPECIAL CONSIDERATION:

Occasionally, a submandibular gland mucocele will extend into the neck as a plunging ranula, imitating a cervical neoplasm.

Congenital, benign, and malignant neoplasms all present infrequently in the submandibular gland. Congenital masses include teratomas, choristomas, and *sialoblastomas.* The latter are composed of benign basal cells with ductal or acinar cell differentiation or myoepithelial cells,[21] and like choristomas, they respond well to surgical excision. Submandibular gland teratomas are extremely rare.[22]

Of the benign neoplasms, the majority are *pleomorphic adenomas.*[23] A genetic translocation may be responsible for some of these tumors.[24] Successful treatment consists of a simple submandibular gland excision, being careful not to enucleate the lesion because of this technique's high recurrence rate.

The most common types of pediatric submandib-

ular gland cancer, in order of decreasing frequency, are *mucoepidermoid carcinoma, acinic cell carcinoma, undifferentiated carcinoma, adenocarcinoma,* and *adenoid cystic carcinoma.*[25] These tumors account for only 8% of all pediatric salivary cancers. The value of diagnostic FNAB is questionable, as accuracy is less than that for other neck neoplasms. Because multiple series have shown a higher rate of local recurrence and cervical lymph node involvement in children,[25] surgical excision requires removal of nonsalivary soft tissue to develop a clear surgical margin. A radical or modified neck dissection is indicated for confirmed cervical lymph node metastasis, but no role has been established for an elective neck dissection, regardless of histology. Similarly, no clear role exists for chemotherapy or radiation treatment.

Thyroid Neoplasms

Pediatric thyroid carcinoma comprises 0.5; to 3% of pediatric malignancies, and has a relatively favorable prognosis compared to other childhood malignancies.[26-28] Ten percent of thyroid carcinomas occur in patients < 21 years of age,[29] the majority being between 15 and 19 years of age.[30] However, cases have been reported at all stages of childhood, including the newborn period.[26,31] Girls outnumber boys by a 2:1 ratio (compared to 3.5:1 in adults).[30]

In comparison to their adult counterpart, pediatric thyroid malignancies manifest as larger, more locally-invasive, multicentric masses. Most commonly, they present as a painless anterior mass in the lower neck, with or without a palpable thyroid nodule (Fig. 60-1). Cervical lymphadenopathy occurs in 70 to 90% of patients on initial presentation,[30,32] with bilateral involvement in 26 to 38%,[33] and histologic examination reveals nearly 90% of these patients have cervical lymph node metastases.[30] Pulmonary metastases are found on initial presentation in 8 to 22%.[33] However, despite this aggressive behavior, survival rates exceed 90% in series with 15 and 20 year follow-up.[27,32,33]

Another significant difference between adult and pediatric thyroid carcinoma is the incidence of histologic types. Well-differentiated tumors (i.e., papillary, follicular, and mixed tumors) account for > 90% of childhood thyroid carcinomas.[33] *Papillary carcinoma* is the most common (> 70%), followed by *follicular* (15-20%), *medullary* (3-10%), and *anaplastic* (3%) carcinomas (Table 60-1).[30,34] In

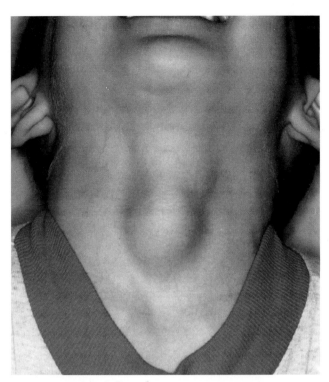

Figure 60–1: Midline thyroid mass.

adults the incidences are 50%, 20%, 10%, and 20%, respectively.[34]

History and physical exam

Pertinent facts in the history and physical examination include the rate of growth, the time of onset of the mass, and the presence of pain, hoarseness, dysphagia, and systemic symptoms of hypo/hyperthyroidism. Prior radiation exposure significantly increases the likelihood of malignancy, especially in

children, with the risk peaking 10 to 20 years following exposure.[30] Until the 1950s, low-dose radiation treatments were offered for benign diseases such as adenotonsillar hypertrophy, enlarged thymus, or acne. Today, exposure occurs from industrial nuclear accidents (e.g., Chernobyl, 1986), treatment of malignant diseases (e.g., Hodgkin's disease), radioactive iodine treatment (e.g., Grave's disease), and diagnostic X-rays.[35,36]

Some authorities suspect that certain illnesses, such as iodine deficiency, Hashimoto's thyroiditis, and Grave's disease, contribute to childhood thyroid carcinoma.[30,34] Other familial syndromes, such as Pendred's or Gardner's syndromes as well as MEN IIA and IIB, clearly increase thyroid carcinoma risks.[34,36] Recently, four oncogenes (ras, gsp, ret, and trk) have been linked with sporadic occurrences of papillary carcinoma.[30] A missense mutation on chromosome 10 involving the (ret) protooncogene in patients with MEN IIA also has been discovered.[30,37] These findings may presage reliable screening and earlier detection in children at risk for developing thyroid carcinoma.

Physical exam should include assessment for vocal cord mobility, cervical lymphadenopathy, and palpable thyroid nodules. Large, firm, and fixed lesions associated with lower cervical adenopathy suggests malignancy.

Laboratory and imaging

A solitary thyroid nodule is uncommon in the pediatric population, but represents malignancy in 10 to 24% of cases.[38] Therefore, all cervical masses, especially in the lower neck, should be investigated for malignant potential. The differential diagnosis of a solitary thyroid nodule is listed in Table 60–2. T3, T4, thyroid stimulating hormone (TSH), calcitonin, antithyroid antibody (ATA), and antimicrosomal an-

TABLE 60–1: Histopathologic Types of Thyroid Carcinoma

Incidence	Types	Histologic Findings	Metastases
>70%	Papillary Carcinoma	Psamomma bodies Multifocal Noninvasive No capsule	Lymphatic
15–20%	Follicular Carcinoma	Unifocal Vascular invasion Capsular invasion Capsule	Hematogenous
4–10%	Medullary Carcinoma	No capsule C-cell origin Whorling pattern	Lymphatic
2–5%	Anaplastic Carcinoma	Large or small cell	

TABLE 60–2: Solitary Thyroid Nodule Differential Diagnosis

Congenital anomolies
Thyroid cysts
Colloid Nodules
Thyroid infections
Thyroid abscesses
Hashimoto's thyroiditis
Thyroid adenomas
Benign neoplasms
Malignant neoplasms

tibody (AMA) levels should be determined. AMA and ATA elevations are associated with autoimmune inflammatory disorders such as thyroiditis.[30] Calcitonin is the only significant cancer screening tool; elevated levels are associated with medullary thyroid carcinoma (MTC).[30] Although most persons with thyroid carcinoma are euthyroid, elevated thyroid function tests can lead to an earlier diagnosis in children with other thyroid disorders and therefore assist in the initial evaluation.

Chest X-ray and lateral soft-tissue films of the neck may show the radiopaque psammoma bodies of papillary carcinoma.[36] Scintigraphy can distinguish between "cold" (hypofunctioning) and "hot" (hyperfunctioning) nodules based on isotope concentration and organification. Technetium 99 (Tc 99) is used first to demonstrate the uptake ability of a nodule because of its cost-effectiveness and efficiency. Iodine 123 (I 123), although more expensive and time consuming, demonstrates both uptake and organification. "Cold" nodules account for 40 to 70% of all thyroid nodules in children,[38] with 17 to 36% being malignant.[39] A Tc 99 "hot" nodule may be hyperfunctional (i.e., increased uptake with organification) or hypofunctional (i.e., increased uptake without organification), and it requires an I 123 scan to distinguish the two. "Hot" nodules comprise 5% of thyroid nodules in children and are most often toxic in nature, but several cases have been documented to have a carcinomatous component.[40] Multinodular goiters detected by thyroid scan or ultrasonography are treated medically with antithyroid medications and thyroid hormone suppression. Close observation is maintained to detect any suspicious changes to indicate malignancy.

Biopsy

Ultrasonography distinguishes cystic from solid thyroid masses and guides FNAB when indicated. Cystic thyroid lesions in children do not exclude malignancy.[30] FNAB has proven in adults to be an effective tool in diagnosing thyroid carcinomas (papillary, medullary, and anaplastic), when reviewed by an experienced cytopathologist.[40] Secondary to the need to confirm vascular or capsular invasion, the malignant potential of follicular or Hürthle cell neoplasms cannot be determined by FNAB; surgical frozen biopsies are required.[41] In the past, FNAB was bypassed enroute to open surgical biopsy of solitary thyroid nodules in children due to the malignant potential. Some now recommend

FNAB for adolescents and select sedated small children.[30,36]

Thyroid suppression

Thyroid suppression is no longer recommended for distinguishing between benign and malignant solitary nodules in children. Well-differentiated thyroid tumors in children have been found to be sensitive to thyroid-stimulating hormone (TSH) and therefore could decrease in size with hormone suppression causing a delay in diagnosis.[30,40]

> ## SPECIAL CONSIDERATION:
> Thyroid suppression is no longer recommended for distinguishing between benign and malignant solitary thyroid nodules in children.

Surgery

Surgical management represents the most controversial aspect of the pediatric solitary thyroid nodule. Children with a suspicious thyroid nodule and no histologic diagnosis undergo an open surgical biopsy consisting of an ipsilateral lobectomy and frozen section diagnosis.[36,41] If the frozen section reveals benign histology, the procedure ends. A diagnosis of well-differentiated thyroid carcinoma leads to a near-total or total thyroidectomy and appropriate neck dissection.[30,34,36,42] The recurrent laryngeal nerves (RLN) and parathyroid glands and vessels are identified, leaving minimal to no thyroid tissue. Injury to these structures is only 2% in experienced hands, diagnosis and ablation of occult disease with iodine 131 (I 131) is facilitated, and follow-up screening with thyroglobulin levels is possible. Therefore, although the trend is toward near-total or total thyroidectomy, some favor subtotal thyroidectomy.[43,44] This procedure removes the majority of both thyroid lobes, but leaves significant residual thyroid tissue and does not involve RLN or parathyroid gland identification.

Palpable cervical lymphadenopathy in the presence of thyroid carcinoma is addressed surgically based on the Tumor Node Metastases (TNM) stage of the neck. A negative neck exam (N0) does not require a prophylactic neck dissection. However, a neck with palpable lymphadenopathy (N1) requires a modified radical neck dissection. Radical neck dissections are indicated for surgically visible spread beyond the lymph node capsule.[27,30,34,36] Total laryngectomy, tracheoesophageal resection, or RLN excision are never indicated secondary to their morbidity, especially given the effectiveness of postoperative I 131 ablation for residual disease.[36]

Postoperative I 131 scanning and ablation is indicated following a near-total or total thyroidectomy to control residual disease and occult metastases. Scanning occurs 6 weeks after resection with the patient in a hypothyroid state. If a positive scan is detected, an ablative dose of I 131 is administered.[34] A baseline thyroglobulin level is obtained prior to ablation. I 131 complications include pulmonary fibrosis, bone marrow suppression, increased incidence of leukemia, and reversible spermatogenic damage.[34] Patients undergo a yearly physical exam, chest X-ray, TG level, and I 131 scan. They should take thyroid hormone replacement to maintain a euthyroid state and suppress TSH, which has been shown to have receptor sites on well-differentiated carcinomas.[36]

Other Thyroid Neoplasms

Medullary thyroid carcinoma (MTC) originates from the parafollicular C cells in the thyroid gland and accounts for 3% of pediatric thyroid malignancies.[30] C cells are of neural crest origin and secrete calcitonin, which contributes to serum calcium regulation. Elevated basal levels or pentagastrin stimulated levels can be early detectors of C cell hyperplasia or MTC.[45] Sporadic cases of MTC do occur, but are unifocal and present after 30 years of age.[30]

Multiple Endocrine Neoplasias (MEN IIA and IIB) are autosomal dominant, familial disorders diagnosed in 20 to 30% of MTC patients.[30] *MEN IIA* involves the adrenal gland (pheochromocytoma), parathyroid gland (hyperparathyroidism), and MTC. Onset is between 12 and 30 years of age and arises from bilateral multicentric C cell hyperplasia.[46] Recently, an association between missense mutations on chromosome 10, involving the ret oncogene, and MEN IIA have been discovered.[37] These genetic discoveries have allowed earlier screening, diagnosis, and surgical treatment of patients susceptible to MEN IIA. *MEN IIB* patients develop mucosal gangli-

oneuromatosis, Marfan's syndrome, atypical facies, pheochromocytomas, and MTC, but rarely parathyroid abnormalities. Age of onset is earlier (2 years old) and MTC is more aggressive in these patients.[30]

Treatment of MTC is total thyroidectomy with a central compartment lymph node dissection (hyoid bone to innominate artery). A modified radical neck dissection is indicated with palpable lymphadenopathy.[30,34] Calcitonin levels and chest radiographs are followed for recurrence. The overall mortality of MTC is 50% at 10 years.[30] Practice Pathways 60-1-60-4 demonstrate a treatment pathway for a solitary thyroid nodule.

Thyroglossal duct carcinoma (TDC) can be an incidental finding on removal of a thyroglossal duct cyst, especially if there is a predominately solid component to the cyst. Surgical treatment consists of TDC resection via the Sistrunk procedure.[47,48] Most authorities advocate thyroid suppression and close observation,[49] although others support prophylactic total thyroidectomy based on the pathology of a palpable thyroid nodule, if present.[50] There is a reported incidence of 25% for papillary carcinoma in the remaining thyroid gland.[47]

Lymph Node Neoplasms

Lymphoma

Lymphomas comprise the third largest group of pediatric and adolescent cancers in the United States, representing 11.5% of all childhood cancers and 13% of newly-diagnosed childhood cancers.[51,52] *Hodgkin's Disease* (HD), *Non-Hodgkin's Lymphoma* (NHL), *Burkitt's Lymphoma* (BL), and unspecified lymphomas make-up the major subsets of lymphoma and respectively comprise 5.1%, 3.8%, 1.5%, and 1.1% of all childhood cancers.[52] Of newly-diagnosed lymphomas, 60% are NHL.[51] Each subset varies in its epidemiology and clinical features, but most commonly presents to an otolaryngologist with painless cervical lymphadenopathy.[53]

Hodgkin's Disease. Childhood HD occurs most often in later adolescence ($\geq$ 15 years old) and rarely before the age of 10 years; the male to female incidence ratio is 3:1, but decreases to 1.4:1 after puberty.[54] Diagnosis depends on the classic histologic finding of Reed-Sternberg (RS) cells. Oncologists recognize four histologic subtypes (Table 60-3), which are: Lymphocyte Predominance (LP)

Practice Pathway 60–1   SOLITARY THYROID NODULE TREATMENT

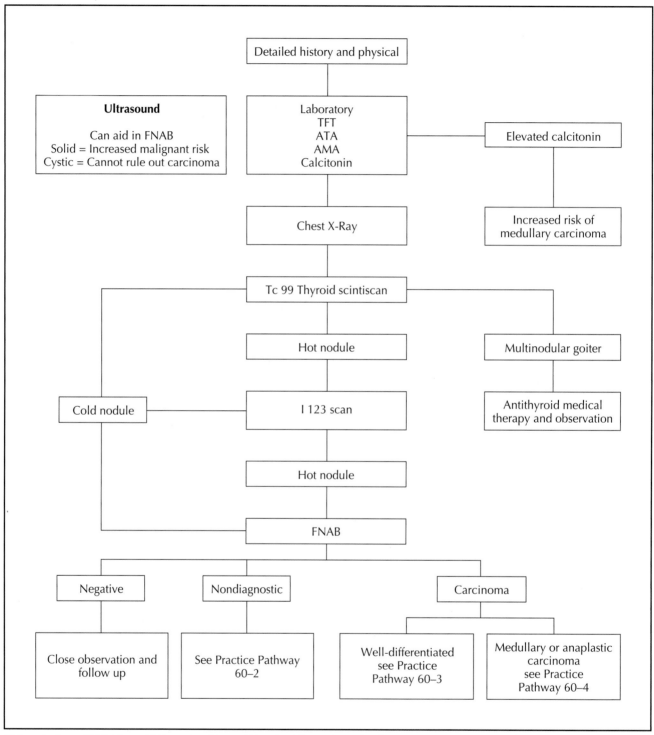

Abbreviations: TFT, Thyroid Function Tests; ATA, Antithyroid Antibody; AMA, Antimicrosomal Antibody; FNAB, Fine-Needle Aspiration Biopsy.

Practice Pathway 60–2   NONDIAGNOSTIC FNAB OF THY-
ROID

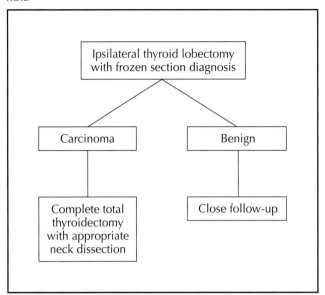

Practice Pathway 60–4   MEDULLARY AND ANAPLASTIC THY-
ROID CARCINOMA

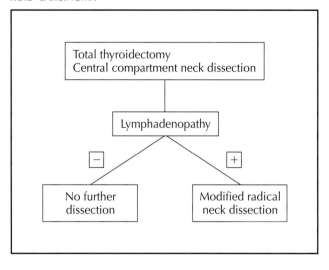

Practice Pathway 60–3   WELL-DIFFERENTIATED THYROID CARCINOMA

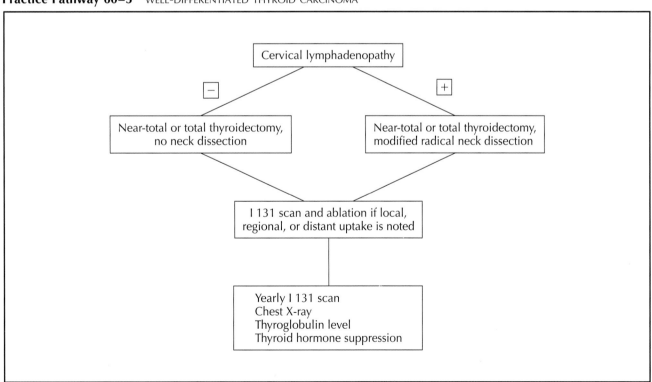

TABLE 60–3: Hodgkin's Disease

Histologic Subtype	% of Lymphomas
Lymphocyte Predominant	10-20%
Nodular Sclerosing	40-60%
Mixed Cellularity	20-50%
Lymphocyte Depleted	5-10%

(10-20%), Nodular Sclerosing (NS) (40-60%), Mixed Cellularity (MC) (20-50%), and Lymphocyte Depletion (LD) (5-10%), although most pediatric HD pathology consists of LP and NS.[54,55] The most common presenting signs of HD in children are cervical (LP) or mediastinal (NS) lymphadenopathy.[55] Systemic symptoms, consisting of fever, night sweats, and weight loss, are known as *B symptoms.*

HD has a documented association with HIV and EBV infections, but is not considered an acquired immunodeficiency virus (AIDS) defining condition.[55] Most AIDS patients with HD present at an earlier age, have B symptoms, higher presenting stages, and extranodal disease.[55] EBV association with HD has been confirmed by increased titers of EBV antibodies and increased risk of HD after mononucleosis infections. EBV exposure has been documented in 19% (by Southern Blot Hybridization) to 56% by (PCR) of patients with HD.[56]

AT A GLANCE . . .

Hodgkin's Disease Staging—Ann Arbor Classification

Stage I: involvement of a single lymph node region (I) or a single extralymphatic organ (IE)

Stage II: involvement of two or more lymph node regions on the same side of the diaphragm (II) or one lymph node region and one extralymphatic organ on the same side of the diaphragm (IIE)

Stage III: involvement of lymph node regions on both sides of the diaphragm (III) plus an extralymphatic organ (IIIE), the spleen (IIIS), or both (IIISE)

Stage IV: diffuse involvement of one or more extralymphatic organs with or without lymph node involvement (IV)

A: no systemic symptoms

B: weight loss, fever, or night sweats

Besides visualization of the RS cell on light microscopy, immunophenotyping has been explored as an aid to the diagnosis of HD. The surface antigen, CD40, has been shown to be expressed on RS cells in 100% of HD patients, regardless of histologic phenotype.[57] Although, a predominant B- or T-cell lineage has not been found. Staging determines the treatment plan (see **AT A GLANCE . . .** Hodgkin's Disease Staging).

HD treatment has become very successful (80-90% 5-year survival) with the advent of multiagent chemotherapy with concurrent localized radiation therapy.[54] Advanced HD requires radiation therapy in combination with longer and more aggressive chemotherapy, such as MOPP (nitrogen mustard, vinblastine, procarbazine and prednisone) or ABVD (adriamycin, bleomycin, vincristine, and dacarbazine). Radiation therapy consists of ≤ 20 Gray that is limited to the involved nodal fields. Higher doses put the child at increased risk of secondary malignancies, as do long-term and high-dose chemotherapy. The most common second malignancies are acute nonlymphoblastic leukemia, sarcomas, and breast carcinoma.[58]

Non-Hodgkin's Lymphoma. The incidence of NHL increases throughout life, but the peak incidence in the pediatric age group is between 7 and 11 years old.[59] There is a male to female bias of 3:1, with a Caucasian to African-American bias of 2:1.[51] Compared to adult NHL, the childhood form presents as a more malignant, poorly-differentiated, and clinically-aggressive tumor.[51,59] The majority of pediatric NHL are of the T-cell lineage and often resemble *acute lymphoblastic leukemia* (ALL).[59] A bone marrow biopsy demonstrating > 25% lymphoblasts confirms the diagnosis of ALL.

The risk of NHL is increased significantly in congenital immunodeficiency syndromes (e.g., Ataxia-Telangectasia, Wiskott-Aldrich syndrome, X-Linked Lymphoproliferative diseases), iatrogenically immunosuppressed patients (i.e., bone marrow or organ transplants), and AIDS patients.[51,60] A deficiency of T-cell function is suspected, but B-cell lymphomas are the predominant subtype in this population. Now, in HIV positive patients, a diagnosis of NHL is considered a presumptive criterion for the diagnosis of AIDS.[51,60]

NHLs can be subdivided into low, intermediate, or high grade categories based on clinical aggressiveness. *High-grade NHL* are the most malignant

TABLE 60–4:   Non-Hodgkin's Lymphoma

Low Grade
Small lymphocyte
Follicular, small cleaved
Follicular, small cleaved and large cell mixed
Intermediate Grade (Diffuse)
Small cleaved cell
Mixed small and large cell
Large cell +/− cleaved
High Grade
Large cell
Lymphoblastic
Small cell noncleaved, Burkitt's lymphoma

AT A GLANCE . . .

Non-Hodgkin's Lymphoma Staging—Murphy Classification

Stage I: single tumor (extranodal) or single anatomic area (nodal) without abdominal or mediastinal involvement

Stage II: single tumor (extranodal) with regional lymphadenopathy; two or more nodal areas on one side of the diaphragm; two single (extranodal) tumors with or without regional lymphadenopathy or one side of the diaphragm; primary gastrointestinal tract tumor (resectable) with or without mesenteric lymphadenopathy

Stage III: two single (extranodal) tumors on opposite sides of the diaphragm; two or more nodal areas above and below the diaphragm; primary intrathoracic tumor involvement; extensive primary intraabdominal involvement; any paraspinal or epidural involvement

Stage IV: any of the above findings with initial involvement of the CNS or bone marrow

---

and are further categorized into *Large Cell lymphoma* (LC), *Lymphoblastic lymphoma* (LL), *and small cell noncleaved lymphoma* (SCN), of which BL is the most common (Table 60-4).

LCNHL occurs in 27% of pediatric NHL, but rarely involves the lymph nodes of the head and neck region.

Nearly all Lymphoblastic NHL are immature T-cell derivatives (95%) and express surface antigen markers of intrathymic T-cells.[51] Twenty-nine percent of cases are lymphoblastic, and can involve translocations of chromosomes 7 or 14 that effect transcription factor genes such as TAL-1.[51] LLs usually present as a mediastinal mass that can cause respiratory distress by tracheal compression.[51] Treatment is dependent on clinical stage at time of presentation (see **AT A GLANCE . . .** Non-Hodgkin's Lymphoma Staging).

BL is a SCN and a B-cell derivative with surface antigen markers CD19, CD20, and CD45.[51,61] SCNs comprise 34% of all NHL cases in children.[51] In the United States clinical presentation usually occurs sporadically in the abdomen, head, or neck region, whereas in Africa it occurs endemically, particularly in the mandible or abdomen.

BL has been found to have a definitive relationship with EBV: 90% of endemic (African) BL and 20% of sporadic (American) BL patients having positive EBV titers.[51,61] A translocation on chromosome 8q24 involving the C-Myc oncogene to an immunoglobulin receptor subunit on chromosomes 2,14, or 22 leads to unchecked lymphoproliferation.[51] EBV infected cells are prone to this genetic alteration and therefore are more susceptible to BL. Treatment depends more on the clinical stage of disease than the histologic subtype.[51]

Treatment. The improved survival rates of pediatric high-grade NHL are secondary to the advancements in multidrug chemotherapeutic protocols initially developed for ALL.[51] The regimens vary somewhat depending on histologic grades of NHL, but the greatest difference is in the length of treatment. Lower clinically-staged patients receive shorter treatment periods in order to decrease toxic side effects and late complications of chemotherapy.

Patients with stage I and II BL and LC receive cyclophosphamide, vincristine and prednisone for 9 to 26 weeks, a protocol that is extended 33 weeks to 24 months for LL. The event free 3 to 5 year survival is 85 to 95%.[51] For patients with stage III and IV BL, the protocol includes the addition of methotrexate for 2 to 8 months; the long-term survival is 75 to 85%. Late stage (III/IV) LL has a 65 to 75% survival with vincristine, prednisone, and methotrexate for 3 to 24 months with a 3 to 5 year event free survival of 50 to 70%.[51]

These regimens are given in induction of remission, consolidation, and continuation phases. Patients with relapse are treated with a variety of other agents based on the histologic subtype of lymphoma. Bone marrow transplants are considered for patients who obtain a second remission.

Diagnostic Work-Up.   An enlarged painless cervical lymph node always should invite the possibility, no matter how remote, of lymphoma (Practice Pathway 60–5). The clinician should inquire about systemic symptoms such as fever, night sweats, and weight loss (i.e., B symptoms). In addition to routine physical exam and laboratory studies, anterior-posterior (AP) and lateral chest X-rays may be included to rule out pulmonary or mediastinal involvement. FNAB can be obtained to rule out other etiologies

Practice Pathway 60–5   CERVICAL LYMPHADENOPATHY

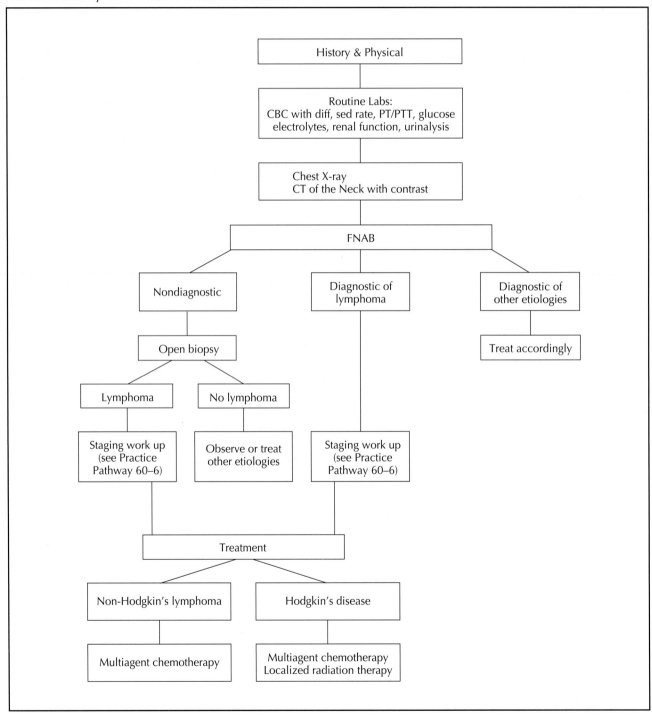

Abbreviations: CBC with diff, Complete Blood Count with differential; PT/PTT, Prothrombin Time/Partial Thromboplastin Time; Sed rate, Sedimentation rate; FNAB, Fine-Needle Aspiration Biopsy.

(oncologic, congenital, or infectious), but it does not aid significantly in the diagnosis of lymphoma.

An open surgical excisional or incisional biopsy is the gold standard. A high index of suspicion must be present in order to alert the pathologist of the suspected diagnosis and prepare fresh tissue correctly. The divided specimen undergoes a touch prep, frozen analysis, flow cytometry, immunohistiologic phenotyping, culture, formalin fixation, and electron microscopy, if indicated. Once the pathologist confirms lymphoma, a clinical staging work-up is completed to determine the best treatment regimen (Practice Pathway 60–6). A review of the preoperative labs in addition to lactate dehydrogenase level (indicates tumor burden), liver function tests (liver involvement), and HIV status (high risk for lymphoma) is performed. Bilateral bone marrow biopsies and lumbar puncture with cerebrospinal fluid (CSF) analysis are performed to assess the extent of disease. CT scans of the chest, abdomen, and pelvis are done to evaluate for lymphadenopathy,

and a radionucleotide bone scan detects bony involvement. Staging laparotomy is indicated in HD patients unless they already exhibit symptoms of diffuse spread (Stage III/IV). Thirty percent of patients are upgraded by this method when staging HD.[54] NHL patients do not require a staging laparotomy.

The appropriate clinical stage plays an important role in the correct treatment of the different histologic types of lymphoma. The goal is not to overtreat early stage disease due to the toxic affects of the chemotherapeutic regimens. Multiagent chemotherapeutic regimens are the most effective form of treatment for NHL. HD is treated in a similar manner, but with the addition of localized radiation therapy. The future goal of treatment is to maintain current survival rates while decreasing toxicity.

Lymphoproliferative disorders

Langerhans' cell histiocytosis (LCH) refers to the condition previously known as Histiocytosis X, which encompassed eosinophilic granuloma, Hand-Schuller-Christian Syndrome, and Letterer-Siwe disease. Whether it represents a neoplasm, a hyperactive immune response to an antigenic stimulus, or an unknown process remains a matter of conjecture.[62] The disease primarily affects children, most typically presenting in the head and neck, particularly the skull. Cervical lymph node involvement occurs in approximately 20% of LCH presenting to otolaryngologists.[63] Common signs and symptoms, in addition to adenopathy, include rashes, otorrhea, oral lesions, and hepatosplenomegaly.

Pathologic diagnosis requires identification of Langerhan's cells, which are pale eosinophilic histiocytes that evolve from T-cell immune regulating dendritic cells.[64] Electron microscopic evidence of Birbeck granules and immunohistochemistry positive for adenosine triphosphate, alpha-D-mannosidase, and S100 protein confirms the diagnosis.[65] Recommended initial studies include a complete blood count (CBC) liver function tests, chest and skeletal radiographs, and urine osmolality after water deprivation.[65] Treatment options include curettage, excision, intralesional steroids, systemic steroids, low-dose radiation therapy, and chemotherapy. Tempered by the disease's unpredictable course and the lack of evidence that aggressive treatment favorably impacts outcome, most authorities now recommend conservative medical treatment, with surgery limited to biopsy.[63] Overall survival

Practice Pathway 60–6 STAGING WORK-UP

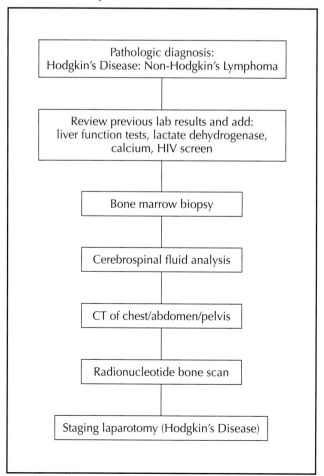

Pathologic diagnosis:
Hodgkin's Disease: Non-Hodgkin's Lymphoma

Review previous lab results and add:
liver function tests, lactate dehydrogenase,
calcium, HIV screen

Bone marrow biopsy

Cerebrospinal fluid analysis

CT of chest/abdomen/pelvis

Radionucleotide bone scan

Staging laparotomy (Hodgkin's Disease)

approximates 90% with follow-up between 3 to 15 years.[66] However, skeletal defects and endocrine problems such as diabetes insipidus frequently persist after recovery,[64,66,67] and the estimated event-free survival 15 years postdiagnosis is only 30%.[67] The youngest patients and those with multisystem involvement tend to have the worst outcomes.

LCH resembles *Rosai-Dorfman disease* which is another histiocyte proliferation disorder that also is known as sinus histiocytosis with massive lymphadenopathy. It generally involves bilateral cervical lymph nodes of children, although it may present in multiple locations including extranodal sites, 75% of which occur in the head and neck.[68] In addition to painless cervical lymph node hypertrophy, patients frequently experience systemic symptoms such as fever, weight loss, leukocytosis, and elevated sedimentation rates.[69] Adjacent vital structures may be compressed by soft-tissue expansion. Histology shows histiocytes that stain for S100 without the eosinophilia or characteristic cells of LCH.[8] The disease often remits spontaneously.[68] However, surgical excision combined with chemotherapy, radiotherapy, or steroids may be indicated for aggressive disease.[70] Wenig et al. reported long-term survival in 12 of 14 patients.[70]

An increasing number of patients are seen with head and neck manifestations of *posttransplant lymphoproliferative disorder* (PTLD), reflecting the improved survival and greater application of pediatric organ transplantation. PTLD occurs in approximately 2% of transplant patients, presumably because T-cell suppression permits EBV-associated B-cell proliferation.[71] The proliferation ranges from diffuse polyclonal proliferations resembling mononucleosis to malignant monoclonal lymphomas.[72] Rapid onset tonsilloadenoid or cervical lymph node hyperplasia are the most common head and neck signs. Early intervention, consisting of lowering immunosuppression in combination with systemic steroids and antiviral therapy, improves prognosis, but mortality still may be as high 25 to 50%.[73] Awareness of this disorder is critical in order to perform prompt diagnostic tonsillectomy or cervical lymph node biopsy in high-risk patients.

Soft Tissue Neoplasms

Neural neoplasms

Peripheral Nervous System. *Neurofibromas* (NF) are tumors of neural origin that may occur in

TABLE 60–5: Diagnostic Criteria for Neurofibromatosis Type 1

1. Six or more "Cafe-au-lait" spots that are >5mm (prepubertal) or >15mm (postpubertal)
2. Two or more neurofibromas of any type or one plexiform type
3. Distinctive osseous lesion with or without psuedoarthrosis
4. First-degree relative with neurofibromatosis type 1
5. Two or more Lisch nodules (iris hamartomas)
6. Inguinal or axillary freckling
7. Optic glioma

isolation or in association with genetic disorders like Neurofibromatosis type I (NF-1) (Von Recklinghausen's disease), Neurofibromatosis type II (NF-II) or six less common forms of disease (Neurofibromatosis types III–VIII). *Neurofibromatosis type I* (85% of NF patients) has an incidence of 1:4000 live births, and although inheritance is autosomal dominant, penetrance is variable (70–80%) and 50% of cases represent new mutations.[74] The NF-1 gene product, *neurofibromin*, is a tumor suppressor gene that has been mapped to chromosome 17. Approximately 33% of NF-1 patients have otolaryngologic manifestations[75] such as cervical skin discoloration, neck masses, sphenoid fibrous dysplasia, airway compression, or involvement of the larynx, parotid, periorbita or infratemporal fossa. A diagnosis of NF-1 requires 2 or more of the criteria listed in Table 60-5.[76]

Neurofibromatosis type 2 (NF-2) occurs in 1:50,000 live births. Characterized by tumors of the eighth cranial nerve (usually bilateral), meningiomas of the brain, and schwannomas of the dorsal roots of the spinal cord, it has few of the hallmarks of NF-1. Cataracts and discrete, well-circumscribed, slightly raised, roughened areas of pigmented skin can be found in one-third of affected persons. Diagnosis remains clinical, based on the criteria listed in Table 60-6.[76] The defective gene, schwannomon, maps to chromosome 22. Although hearing loss and

TABLE 60–6: Diagnostic Criteria for Neurofibromatosis Type 2

1. Bilateral eighth cranial nerve tumors diagnosed by biopsy, CT, or MRI; or
2. First-degree relative with Neurofibromatosis type 2 and either a unilateral eighth cranial nerve tumor or two of the following: neurofibroma, meningioma, schwannoma, glioma, or juvenile posterior subcapsular lenticular opacity.

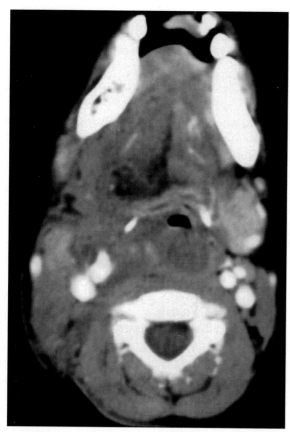

Figure 60–2: CT of a cervical plexiform neurofibroma infiltrating the tongue.

acoustic neuromas are prominent in NF-2, an acoustic neuroma has never been documented in NF-1.[77]

Four types of NF exist: cutaneous, subcutaneous, nodular plexiform, and diffuse plexiform. The most common is cutaneous. *Plexiform lesions* tend to infiltrate surrounding tissues (Fig. 60–2). Histopathologically, NF contain all components of a peripheral nerve (neurites, Schwann cells, and fibroblasts) and are not encapsulated. The potential for transformation to *neurofibrosarcoma* is 3 to 15%.[78] NF may be differentiated histologically from *schwannomas* (neurilemmomas), which also contain all components of a peripheral nerve but are encapsulated and usually solitary.

Extensive involvement of vital structures in the head and neck region creates a high risk of morbidity for surgical resection. CT and MRI assist with determining the extent of structural involvement. Chemotherapy and radiation therapy have not been proven as acceptable treatment options, leaving surgical resection as the mainstay of treatment. However, an extensive number or size of lesion(s) may justify observation as the best treatment. The overall goal is conservative management with complete or near-complete excision when possible to preserve function.

Neuroectodermal. *Neuroblastoma* (NB) is the second most common solid tumor of childhood, with approximately two-thirds occurring in children < 5 years old. Originating from neural crest cells in the adrenal medulla or sympathetic nervous system, NB most commonly presents as a painless mass or with bone pain from metastases. Up to 70% of newly-diagnosed patients have regional lymph nodes or bone metastases,[79] and a solitary cervical mass or lymphadenopathy may be the initial presentation. Additional otolaryngology manifestations include Horner's syndrome from a primary neck NB, proptosis with periorbital ecchymosis (retrobulbar metastasis), and nasal obstruction with epistaxis (esthesioneuroblastoma).

Diagnosis depends on pathologic confirmation of sympathetic neuronal differentiation in the tumor specimen by light microscopy, electron microscopy, or immunohistologic stains. Bone marrow biopsy or aspirates containing immunohistologically-proven cells or unequivocal tumor cells facilitates staging and diagnosis, as do increased levels of urine or serum catecholamines and metabolites [homovanillic acid (HVA), vanillymandelic acid (VMA), dopamine].[80]

Prognosis relates to patient age at diagnosis, clinical stage, regional lymph node involvement, aneuploidy of tumor DNA, and amplification of the N-Myc oncogene. Infants < 1 year of age with any stage of disease, as well as children of any age with localized disease, have an excellent likelihood of survival.[81,82] Conversely, adolescents and adults have a much worse long-term prognosis regardless of clinical stage.[83] Prognosis is improved by hyperdiploid DNA, but it worsens with amplification of the N-Myc oncogene.[84] VMA and HVA levels can detect tumors with characteristics that are favorable for spontaneous regression, but routine infant screening does not detect advanced stage disease with unfavorable characteristics and thus is not recommended.[85]

A metastatic work-up must be completed on each newly-diagnosed patient to assist in clinical staging (see **AT A GLANCE . . .** Children's Cancer Group Neuroblastoma Staging System) and treatment planning. Screening for metastatic disease requires bilateral bone marrow core biopsies and aspirates as well as a nuclear medicine (Tc 99) bone scan. Palpable lymph nodes require histologic evaluation by FNAB or excisional biopsy. CT scans assess for non-palpable adenopathy in regions suspicious for spread.

AT A GLANCE . . .

Children's Cancer Group Neuroblastoma Staging System

Stage I: confined to the organ or structure of origin

Stage II: extending in continuity beyond the structure of origin but not across midline; +/− ipsilateral regional lymph nodes

Stage III: invasively extending in continuity beyond the midline; +/− bilateral regional lymph nodes

Stage IV: remote disease involving the skeleton, soft tissue, parenchymatous organs or distant lymph nodes

Stage IV-S: patients who would be stage I or II but have distant metastases to the liver, skin, or bone with a negative radiologic skeletal survey

---

Clinical staging and prognostic variables determine the treatment regimen and prognosis. Disease is categorized as local-resectable, local-unresectable, regional, disseminated, or stage IV-S, and treatment is determined accordingly. Options include complete surgical excision alone, combined surgical excision and chemotherapy, surgical excision, chemotherapy and radiation, myeloablative chemotherapy and radiation with autologous bone marrow transplant, or observation (stage IV-S).[86-89] Survival can be as high as 90% for patients < 1 year with stage IV-S,[90] 50 to 80% with stage IV,[89] and as poor as 10 to 30% for patients > 1 year with stage IV.[91]

Ewing's sarcoma (ES) is a malignant tumor of neuroectodermal origin resembling other histologically-primitive round cell tumors of childhood (e.g., lymphoma, neuroblastoma, rhabdomyosarcoma) that consists of uniformly dense packed small round cells. The disease usually presents in the second decade of life, and although the pelvis and long bones are the most frequently reported primary sites, head and neck involvement can occur in the form of either a primary tumor or as a metastatic lesion to

the cervical lymph nodes. Ninety percent of newly-diagnosed patients have occult metastases,[92] most commonly to lung, bone, and bone marrow, respectively. In spite of this, 50% of persons without gross metastatic disease enjoy a long-term disease-free survival.[93]

The two most important prognostic variables are primary tumor site and presence of metastases. Primary tumors of the head and neck region and distal extremities fare better than disease of the pelvis, sacrum, or proximal extremities.[92,94-96] Distant metastases found at the time of diagnosis decrease the long-term survival.

Because all primitive round cell tumors of childhood share similar histologic findings by light microscopy, electron microscopy, immunocytochemistry, and cytogenetics have become essential in confirming the diagnosis.[97,98] ES cells express a surface antigen called p30/32 mic 2 or HBA71, which is used for immunohistologic diagnosis.[99] Translocations on chromosomes 22, 11, and 12 also have been described as ES-specific markers in cytogenetic testing (t11;22 and t21;22).[97,98] Adequate tissue for testing is essential and can be acquired by primary surgical excision or needle biopsy.

CT, MRI, and nuclear medicine bone scans assist in the metastatic work-up, with treatment dependent upon the primary site and presence or absence of metastases. Surgery and radiation therapy with multiagent chemotherapy comprise the mainstay of treatment. Complete surgical excision and radiation therapy are used for local control with equal success.[100] Choice often is determined by the attendant morbidity. The presence of occult metastases makes multiagent chemotherapy essential.[95,101] Patients who relapse do poorly, and although myeloablative chemotherapy and radiation followed by autologous bone marrow transplantation has not been effective in primary ES, it does play a role in recurrent disease.[102,103]

Peripheral primitive neuroectodermal tumors (PNET) are biologically indistinguishable from extraosseous ES. Even cytogenetic testing reveals identical translocations on chromosomes 11 and 22.[104] Consequently, treatment regimens are identical and consist of aggressive surgical excision with chemotherapy and radiation for progressive disease.[104]

Paragangliomas arise from small rests of neural crest cells that are closely associated with major neural and vascular structures that serve as chemoreceptors for the autonomic nervous system and are located along the paraaxial skeleton. Although histologically benign, paragangliomas often cause considerable morbidity. Carotid body tumors are the most frequently described (60–70%) followed by jugulotympanicum paragangliomas.[105] Multicentricity is not uncommon, with up to 10% of cases having secondary paragangliomas.[106] A familial pattern also is seen with autosomal dominant inheritance and variable penetrance. Initial presentation is as a slow-growing painless neck mass mobile in the horizontal but not the vertical planes of the neck, signifying attachment of the tumor in the carotid bifurcation. The rich vascular supply is of diagnostic importance for angiography, a study which also permits screening for smaller incidental paragangliomas, enabling preoperative embolization. CT scans of the neck with intravenous contrast or magnetic resonance angiography (MRA) can help to localize the mass and surrounding structures. Other preoperative screening tests should include urine studies for free catecholamines or their derivatives, which may be secreted by the tumor or an undiagnosed pheochromocytoma,[105] as elevated catecholamines during the operative procedure could lead to a fatality. Complete surgical excision is the treatment of choice, with chemotherapy reserved for metastatic disease.[105]

Muscle neoplasms

Rhabdomyoma arises infrequently from the soft tissue or mucosa of the head and neck of toddlers.[107,108] Fetal rhabdomyomas, composed of immature spindle and muscle cells in a myxoid matrix, usually present at birth or within the first year.[108] An intermediate or juvenile form that occurs in older children and adults features more abundant and differentiated muscle cells.[108,109] The relative lack of nuclear atypia allows differentiation of rhabdomyoma from rhabdomyosarcoma; simple excison is usually curative.[108]

Although it infrequently occurs, *rhabdomyosarcoma* (RMS) represents the most common pediatric head and neck soft-tissue malignancy. Primary cervical RMS is less common than orbital and skull base RMS; < 10% of those with primary head RMS develop cervical lymph node metastasis.[110] Prior to the 1970s, RMS was treated with surgery alone, with high recurrence and low survival rates. This poor outcome prompted a comprehensive undertaking known as the Intergroup Rhabdomyosarcoma Study (IRS). The associated trials employed a grouping system for staging (see **AT A GLANCE . . .** IRS Clinical

Grouping), with roughly one-third of cases having head and neck involvement.[111] With multimodal therapy using surgery, chemotherapy, and radiation therapy, outcomes have improved considerably.[111] Sercarz et al. reviewed 32 children with RMS of the head and neck origin and found multimodal therapy to yield a 72% 5-year survival, compared to a 14% cure rate with surgery alone.[110] Lyos et al.'s review of 56 children with head and neck RMS also support multimodal treatment.[112]

AT A GLANCE . . .

IRS-Clinical Grouping

Group I: localized, completely resected disease: (1) tumor confined to muscle or organ of origin; (2) infiltration outside this structure without regional lymph node involvement

Group II: regional, incompletely resected disease: (1) grossly resected with microscopic residual; (2) completely resected regional disease, in which nodes may be involved and/or extension of the tumor into an adjacent organ; or (3) regional disease with involved nodes grossly resected, but with evidence of microscopic residual

Group III: incomplete resection or biopsy with gross residual

Group IV: distant metastatic disease at diagnosis

Complete resection, if feasible, offers the best results. Group I IRS patients did not benefit from radiation treatments,[111] and therefore it is not currently recommended for these patients. Pathologically, embryonal RMS outnumbers alveolar,[113] and enjoys a slightly better prognosis.[111,114] Vincristine, dactinomycin, and cyclophosphamide (VAC) represent the most common chemotherapeutic regimen. Radiation doses range between 4500 to 600 cGy with generous ports.[110] Elective surgical or radiation treatment of the neck has not been recommended for primary head RMS. In children with nonorbital head and neck RMS with residual disease after initial nonsurgical cytoreductive therapy, Blatt et al. demonstrated improved outcomes by adding delayed cranial base surgery.[115] Thus, if the tumor is unresectable initially patients should be reevaluated as potential surgical candidates after chemotherapy and radiation. In general, children have a considerably better prognosis than adults,[116] with the exception being RMS of infancy, which behaves very aggressively.[117]

Leiomyoma and *leiomyosarcoma* are benign and malignant tumors of smooth muscle, respectively. Leiomyomas occur in buccal mucosa and esophageal smooth muscle, but not in the soft tissues of the neck. They have an association with Alport's syndrome. Leiomyosarcomas are exceedingly rare in children and present in the head and neck region with even less frequency. A confirmed tissue diagnosis of leiomyosarcoma warrants surgical excision and chemotherapy.[118] Local recurrences and distant metastases are common.

Fibrous neoplasms

Fibrous histiocytomas (FH) are soft tissue tumors that contain a biphasic population of fibroblasts and histiocytes, rarely presenting in the head and neck of children. *Benign fibrous histiocytomas* (BFH) can arise as slow growing painless masses in the cervical region, and follow an indolent noninvasive course. Surgical excision usually proves effective, with an 11% recurrence rate.[119] Of *malignant fibrous histiocytomas* (MFH), only 1 to 3% occur in the head and neck region,[120] and the prevalence is even lower in the pediatric population. The diagnosis is confirmed by light microscopy (pleomorphic sarcomatous cells, increased mitotic figures, and giant cells), immunohistologic staining, and electron microscopy, and requires aggressive multimodal therapy with radical surgery, chemotherapy, and radiation.

Dermatofibromas, also in the FH class, are benign tumors with ill-defined borders, hyperpigmentation, and hyperkeratosis. Regression is not common, and surgical excision is indicated for cosmetic reasons. *Dermatofibrosarcoma protuberans* is a rare tumor evolving from fibroblasts with a locally-invasive malignant nature. Although they grow slowly, recurrences are common unless microscopic margins are clear. Moh's micrographic surgery is the procedure of choice. The treatment of choice is aggressive surgical excision with radiation therapy for recurrences and positive margins.[121] *Desmoid tumors* (or *aggressive fibromatosis*) are another form of rare fibrous tumor, with an invasive, destructive nature, which must be differentiated histologically from fibrosarcoma. Treatment consists of complete surgical excision.

Fibrosarcomas are the second most common soft-tissue sarcoma in children.[122] They behave in a more benign fashion in children as compared to adults, and infants fare even better. The tumor usually presents as a slow-growing painless mass in the cervical region. Distant metastatic disease is uncommon, especially in young children or infants. Optimal management is complete surgical excision, and if the surgeon can maintain clear surgical margins, radiation therapy can be avoided. Grossly-positive margins require the addition of radiation and adjuvant chemotherapy. However, reexcision for positive margins should be considered to avoid radiation and its complications[121,123]

Mesenchymal neoplasms

Lipomatous tumors are of mesenchymal origin and include benign *lipoma, lipoblastoma* and malignant (*liposarcoma*) varieties. Lipomas rarely occur in children, and liposarcomas seldom arise from preexisting lipomas.[124] A histologically-confirmed liposarcoma requires complete surgical excision, which yields an 83% 5-year survival.[125] Uniform adipose cells, scattered lipoblasts, and primitive mesenchymal cells suggest the diagnosis of lipoblastoma. This tumor can be distinguished from a myxoid liposarcoma by the lack of abnormal number or appearing mitotic figures.[126]

Osteomas and *chondromas* are benign tumors of densely-sclerotic bone and hyaline cartilage, respectively. Malignant transformation rarely occurs except when associated with systemic syndromes and multiple tumors,[127] a finding that is more frequent with chondromas. *Osteogenic sarcoma* produces bone and is more commonly found in the bones of the face or skull than the neck.[128] *Chondrogenic sarcomas* are rarer and have a better prognosis. They are slow growing, less aggressive, and follow a more indolent course.[129] Neither of these tumors commonly cause a pediatric neck mass, but they should be included in an extended differential diagnosis. The treatment for both tumors is aggressive surgery and chemotherapy.

Chordoma arise from notochordal remnants, and typically present as skull base neoplasms. Extranotochordal chordomas presenting as neck masses have been reported,[130] although they are extremely rare. *Myxomas* are composed of benign primitive connective tissue cells and stroma. They resemble *mesenchymomas* which are tumors composed of two or more mesenchymal components and fibrous tissue. Both myxomas and mesenchymomas are unusual in children, and when present in the head and neck, tend to develop in the aerodigestive tract. Cervical and facial skin myxomas combined with cardiac myxomas occur in *Carney complex,* which is an autosomal dominant familial disease causing multiple neoplasia, including those that cause Cushing's syndrome and acromegaly.[131] Complete surgical excision leads to cure.

Synovial sarcoma (SS) is a highly-malignant and very uncommon tumor of mesenchymal origin. Rarely found in the head and neck region, only 80 cases have been reported between 1954 and 1993.[132] When found, it most commonly arises in the parapharyngeal or retropharyngeal spaces, and affects adolescents and young adults. Light microscopy and immunohistochemistry staining for type IV collagen, neural markers, S100, and neuron-specific enolase confirm the diagnosis.[133] Schmidt et al reported a 7-year survival of 63% with complete surgical excision.[133] Regional lymph node metastases and distant spread to bone and lung tissue are common findings that require adjuvant chemotherapy for the best possible outcome.[134]

Vascular neoplasms

Most vascular lesions, although histologically benign, create significant cosmetic and occasionally functional impairments. These neoplasms tend to present at birth or shortly thereafter. All have the potential for a high degree of morbidity if not managed correctly. Although physical exam usually makes the diagnosis readily apparent (Fig. 60–3),

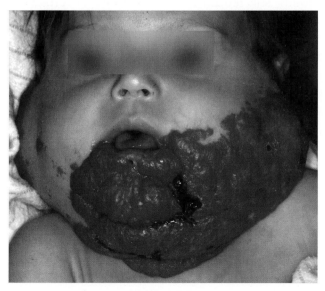

Figure 60–3:   Massive cervical hemangioma.

sometimes only subtle differences separate these tumors. High-flow *arteriovenous malformations* (AVMs) may be distinguished from low-flow lesions (i.e., *hemangiomas* or *lymphangiomas*) by arteriography. Distinct MRI findings, such as large signal voids in high-flow lesions and prominent enhancement on low-flow lesions, provide a less invasive alternative.[135] Because the prognosis and treatment of these tumors vary considerably, correct diagnosis is critical.

AVMs are much less common than low-flow vascular anomalies, but usually cause considerable difficulties when present in the head and neck. They manifest at birth and grow in parallel with the patient, producing pain, bleeding, skin erosion, airway or adjacent vascular compression, or high-output cardiac failure. Given the absence of any legitimate medical solutions, treatment depends upon interventional radiology, with or without surgery.

Conventional treatment consists of embolization followed by surgical resection when feasible. The proximity of AVMs to vital head and neck anatomy, such as the facial nerve, mandible, carotid sheath, mediastinal structures, or large dermal surface area, frequently makes surgery impractical or dangerous. Nonsurgical alternatives include stereotactic radiosurgery[136] or serial embolization. Chen et al. reported satisfactory results in 14 cases where major distal feeding arteries were ligated and the lesion then injected with 3% tetradecyl sulfate and excised.[137] Occasionally, if the feeding vessels have been closed by embolization or ligation, direct puncture of the AVM with embolization remains an option either as a treatment or a preoperative procedure.[138] However, because the surgical defect often includes a large area of soft tissue and skin, free tissue transfer may be required to achieve adequate reconstruction. Although this continues to be a challenging problem, advances in both neurovascular radiology and microvascular surgery have improved overall outcomes.

Hemangiomas affect 10% of white infants, typically presenting as an erythematous macule several weeks after birth.[139] The diagnosis is usually obvious, except with subdermal hemangiomas, which can be differentiated from AVMs and other nonvascular neoplasms by MRI. Unlike AVMs, hemangioma undergo a rapid proliferative growth phase, lasting 12 to 18 months, followed by gradual involution. Fifty percent resolve by age 5 years and 70% by age 7 years, justifying observation alone as treatment in the majority of cases. A small percentage of patients experience functional compromise of their eyes, ears, or airway; life-threatening thrombocytopenia; anemia; high-output cardiac failure; or chronic infection. These patients warrant treatment.[140] In the past, oral steroids provided the mainstay of medical therapy, but recent evidence suggests that only 30% respond significantly to high-dose oral corticosteroids (2–3 mg/kg/d).[141] Intralesional steroids are not indicated in smaller lesions and have not demonstrated efficacy in larger lesions. Alpha-2A interferon (IFN-2A or Roferon-A by Hoffan-La Roche) has demonstrated excellent potential for inhibiting vascular proliferation, and several initial series showed a response rate above 75% in the airway[142] and the head and neck.[143-145] Because of many potential side effects, including tardive dyskinesias,[143] a pediatric hematology consultation may facilitate initial administration. Although most neck hemangiomas do not require surgery, recent experience suggests that focal cervical hemangiomas, particularly those impinging upon the airway, may be excised safely via open excision.[146] Serial laser treatments with a variety of lasers including KTP, argon, Nd:YAG, yellow, and flashlamp lasers also can be used to decrease hemangioma size.[147] However, because lasers may cause scarring from thermal injury and deepithelialization that would not have occurred with spontaneous resolution, they should be used cautiously.

Lymphangiomas represent congenital lymphatic hamartomas that usually present before 2 years of age.[148] They can be classified as capillary, cavernous, or cystic (cystic hygroma), with the former often containing a vascular component that infiltrates surrounding tissue, negatively impacting prognosis. The usual differential includes branchial cleft cysts or thymic cysts[149] for macrocystic lesions, and hemangiomas or soft-tissue neoplasms for microcystic (capillary and cavernous) lymphangiomas. Aspiration of a macrocystic lesion reveals chylous fluid from a cystic hygroma but not a branchial cleft cyst. Ultrasound of microcystic lesions shows distinctive hypoechogenic cystic masses with septa, but does not define the extent of the lesion as well as a gadolinium-enhanced MRI.[150]

Cervical lymphatic malformations outnumber those of the face and oropharynx by approximately 2:1.[151] In classifying cervical lymphatic malformations, de Serres et al. proposed a staging system based on unilateral versus bilateral involvement, and location above, below, or on both sides of the hyoid.[152] They found that unilateral infrahyoid

lymphangiomas responded best to surgical treatment, and that complications and persistent disease was greatest in children with bilateral and/or suprahyoid lymphangiomas.[152] Lymphangiomas may flucuate in size, rarely resolve spontaneously, and should be expected to persist or expand without treatment.[153,154] It has long been recognized that incomplete excision does not equate necessarily with automatic recurrence.[155] Complete excision, although frequently impractical, usually does provide a cure. Raveh et al. reported a 22% recurrence rate in their series of 74 surgical excisions.[151] Motivated by similar high recurrence rates, many authorities have attempted percutaneous schlerotherapy, using such agents as bleomycin,[156] triamcinolone,[157] and doxycycline,[158] with good results and no lasting morbidity. However, persistent concerns about adjacent tissue reaction continues to limit the widespread use of these therapies. Smith et al. suggested percutaneous and fluoroscopically-guided injection of OK-432, which is a byproduct of lypholized group A *Streptococcus pyogenes.* It caused no adverse sequelae when injected in six children; led to complete remission in two macrocystic lymphangiomas; and no response in three microcystic lymphangiomas and 1 venous malformation (hemangioma).[159]

The options for studying and treating these tumors have expanded, but the standard therapy remains complete surgical excision, regardless of the age at diagnosis. However, it is often most appropriate to observe difficult surgical lesions. Unfortunately, microcystic suprahyoid lesions, particularly those that have infiltrated the tongue or floor of the mouth, still remain a common cause of refractory airway and swallowing difficulties as well as recurrent infection and cosmetic disfigurement. Ultimate decisions regarding surgery must be based on the degree of cosmetic and functional morbidity, the likelihood of complete excision, and the risks of operation.

Malignant vascular neoplasms rarely appear in children. Head and neck *angiosarcoma* primarily involves the scalp of elderly males. Pediatric cases are extremely rare, but when diagnosed, they should be treated with aggressive surgery followed by radiation and chemotherapy.[160] Head and neck *lymphangiosarcoma* has not been described in children.

The advent of HIV infections has led to a significant increase in *Kaposi's sarcoma* (KS). This increase has been particularly dramatic among children living in regions with epidemic AIDS.[161] Grossly, the lesion appears vascular and macular, often in clusters or multicentric. Authorities suspect that the tumor originates from vascular endothelium and in some cases may be incited by CMV infection.[162] Although KS frequently involves the head and neck, it manifests much less commonly in cervical skin, glands, and lymph nodes than the oral cavity and adjacent mucosa. Because the tumor grows slowly and rarely threatens life, treatment is directed at palliation of symptoms such as pain, bleeding, or airway compression. Therapy consists of individualized combinations of radiation, chemotherapy, and immune modulation.[163] Occasionally, tumor bulk requires laser reduction, but the high potential for bleeding should be a deterrent to surgical excision. Prognosis depends on the degree of underlying immunodeficiency.

Hemangiopericytoma may present as a congenital or acquired neck mass. It originates from vascular pericytes and generally poses a low malignant potential. Treatment consists of complete surgical excision. Unresectable or incompletely-excised tumors warrant chemotherapy.[164] Although spontaneous remission has been reported,[165] we advocate aggressive treatment and vigilant follow-up because metastasis and death are well-described possibilities.[166]

Dermal neoplasms

The incidence of dermal neoplasms occurring in the head and neck has increased dramatically in the last 2 decades. With the thinning of earth's ozone layer, younger ages of presentation for sun-induced neoplasms can be expected. Fortunately, pediatric presentation of *malignant melanoma, squamous cell carcinoma,* and *basal cell carcinoma* remains uncommon. Clinical management resembles that recommended for adults.

Dermal malignancies that present in childhood suggest the possibility of genetic disease. *Nevoid basal cell carcinoma syndrome,* also known as *Gorlin's syndrome,* features multiple nevi and basal cell carcinomas with a predisposition for palmal and plantar pits, jaw cysts, ovarian fibromas, medulloblastoma, and skeletal abnormalities of the skull, spine, and ribs.[167] Inheritance occurs via an autosomal dominant pattern, although 40% of cases represent new mutations.[168] A review of the National Institutes of Health (NIH) cases indicates that the first tumor occurs at a mean age of 23 years, and the

number of basal cell carcinomas per individual range from 1 to 1000 (median = 8).[167] The predisposition to basal cell carcinoma stems from a chromosome 9 aberration, which inactivates a tumor suppresser gene.[169]

In addition to facing risks of basal cell carcinoma, patients with *xeroderma pigmentosum* also have high rates of cutaneous squamous cell carcinoma and malignant melanoma. Affected individuals lack the normal capacity to repair radiation-induced DNA damage.[170] They often have coexisting central or peripheral neurologic problems because faulty DNA repair leads to premature neuron death.[171] Inheritance is autosomal recessive.[172] Avoidance of direct ultraviolet radiation diminishes, but does not eliminate, the risk of cutaneous neoplasms.

METASTATIC NEOPLASMS

Virtually any malignancy can metastasize to cervical lymph nodes. As mentioned previously, approximately 80% of pediatric thyroid carcinoma presents with a neck mass. Aerodigestive tract squamous cell carcinoma causes the vast majority of cervical lymph node metastasis in adults, but is much less common among children. Unfortunately, the infrequent pediatric mucosal squamous cell carcinoma tends to behave very aggressively with frequent cervical metastasis. Treatment protocols parallel those for adults. *Nasopharyngeal carcinoma* represents another leading cause of metastatic cervical adenopathy in adolescents. For this reason, the nasopharynx should be carefully examined in all teenagers with a neck mass.

SECONDARY MALIGNANCIES IN THE CURED CANCER PATIENT

With over two-thirds of all pediatric cancer patients now expected to survive beyond 5 years,[173] a new more ominous problem, which is the development of a second malignancy, has emerged. The risk of a second malignancy in long-term (5 years) survivors of all forms of childhood cancer appears to be 2 to 3%,[174] although longer follow-up and continued improvement in survival rates may raise this percentage. The mean time for presentation of a second neoplasms is 7 to 11 years post-treatment, but in many cases, over 20 years have lapsed.[173,175] These children already have demonstrated an oncogenic predisposition, and may suffer from defective immune surveillance systems. Regardless of underlying risk factors, the actual treatment of the initial primary neoplasm, in itself, increases the likelihood of a second primary. Malignancies such as squamous cell carcinoma, melanoma,[176] and soft-tissue sarcomas and osteosarcomas[173] may develop in radiation fields. Secondary leukemias and lymphomas, as well as soft-tissue neoplasms, may occur in patients initially treated with chemotherapy but not radiation. Relatively higher doses of radiation and chemotherapy appear to increase risks of secondary malignancies. In addition to concerns regarding second malignancies, surviving females also may experience problems with fertility and mutagenesis.[177] The head and neck surgeon can serve a useful role in counseling patients with no evidence of residual neoplasms to select appropriate dietary and exercise habits while avoiding alcohol, tobacco, and excessive sunlight.

TRENDS FOR THE TWENTY-FIRST CENTURY

The turning of the millenium will bring many new challenges, including the aforementioned diseases in cured cancer patients and the management of prenatally diagnosed neck masses. Rapidly-evolving technology also will deliver many rewarding advances, like molecular biology to improve diagnosis via less invasive techniques and PCR analysis of nucleotide sequences from FNAB biopsied neoplasms. Similar molecular diagnostic assays may detect subclinical, residual, or recurrent neoplasms. Advanced detection of chromosomal abnormalities may allow earlier diagnosis. Other potential directions for therapy include immune modulation and gene therapy via oncogenic manipulation.[178] These possibilities as well as less toxic, more efficacious medical treatment of neoplastic disease are exciting trends that can be expected in the twenty-first century.

REFERENCES

1. Barness LA. *Manual of Pediatric Physical Diagnosis, 4th ed.* Chicago: Yearbook Medical publishers, 1972, pp. 46–47.

2. Cunningham H, Myers E, Bluestone C. Malignant tumors of the head and neck in children: A twenty year review. Int J Pediatr Otorhinolaryngol 1987; 13:279–292.

3. Knight PJ, Mulne AF, Vassy LE. When is lymph node biopsy indicated in children with enlarged peripheral nodes? Pediatrics 1982; 69:391–396.

4. Torsiglieri AJ Jr, Tom LWC, Ross AJ III, et al. Pediatric neck masses: Guidelines for evaluation. Int J Pediatr Otorhinolaryngol 1988; 16:199–210.

5. Pizzo PA, Miser JS, Cassady JR, Filler RM. *Solid Tumors of Childhood in Cancer: Principles and Practice of Oncology, 2nd ed.* Devita VT Jr, Hellman S, Rosenberg SA, eds. Philadelphia: Lippincott, 1985, pp. 1511–1545.

6. Raney R, Handler S. Management of neoplasms of the head and neck in children, II. Malignant tumors. Head & Neck 1981; 3:500–507.

7. Putney F. The diagnosis of head and neck masses in children. Otolaryngol Clin North Am 1970; 3:277–294.

8. May M. Neck masses in children: Diagnosis and treatment. Ear Nose Throat J 1978; 57:12–54.

9. Waggoner-Fountain LA, Hayden GF, Hendley JO. Kawasaki syndrome masquerading as bacterial lymphadenitis. Clin Pediatr 1995; 34:185–189.

10. Tunkel DE, Baroody FM, Sherman ME. Fine-needle aspiration biopsy of cervicofacial masses in children. Arch Otolaryngol Head Neck Surg 1995; 121:533–536.

11. April MM, Garelick JM, Nuovo GJ. Reverse transcriptase in situ polymerase chain reaction in atypical mycobacterial adenitis. Arch Otolaryngol Head Neck Surg 1996; 122:1214–1218.

12. Yen BC, Kahn H, Schiller AL, et al. Multiple hamartoma syndrome with osteosarcoma. Arch Pathol Lab Med 1993; 117:1252–1254.

13. Jordan RB, Gauderer MWL. Cervical teratomas: An analysis, literature review, and proposed classification. J Pediatr Surg 1988; 23:583–591.

14. Abemayor E, Newman A, Dudley J, et al. Teratomas of the head and neck in childhood. Laryngoscope 1984; 94:1489–1493.

15. Azizkhan RG, Haase GM, Applebaum H, et al. Diagnosis, management, and outcome of cervicofacial teratomas in neonates: A Children's Cancer Group study. J Pediatr Surg 1995; 30:312–316.

16. Heffner DK, Hyams VJ. Teratocarcinoma (malignant teratoma?) on the nasal cavity and paranasal sinuses: A clinicopathologic study of 20 cases. Cancer 1984; 53:2140–2154.

17. Silberman R, Mendelsohn IR. Teratoma of the neck: Report of two cases and review of the literature. Arch Dis Child 1960; 35:159–170.

18. Rothschild MA, Catalano P, Urken M, et al. Evaluation and management of congenital cervical tera-

toma. Arch Otolaryngol Head Neck Surg 1994; 120:444–448.
19. Ward RF, April M. Teratomas of the head and neck. Otolaryngol Clin North Am 1989; 22:621–629.
20. Gundry SR, Wesley JR, Klein MD, et al. Cervical teratomas in the newborn. J Pediatr Surg 1983; 18:382–386.
21. Harris MD, McKeever P, Robertson JM. Congenital tumours of the salivary gland: A case report and review. Histopathology 1990; 17:155–157.
22. Mckiernan DC, Koay B, Vinayak B, et al. A case of submandibular teratoma. J Laryngol Otol 1995; 109:992–994.
23. Li Z, Yu G, Zhang Y. The diagnosis and treatment of the epithelial salivary gland tumors in children and adolescents. Chinese J Stomatology 1995; 30:137–139.
24. Kamaeyama J, Okumura T, Kawauchi S, et al. Pleomorphic adenoma with translocation (3;8) (p24;q13) in a child. Cancer Genet Cytogenet 1988; 35:281–282.
25. Rasp G, Permanetter W. Malignant salivary gland tumors: Squamous cell carcinoma of the submandibular gland in a child. Am J Otolaryngol 1992; 13:109–112.
26. Winship T, Rosvoll RV. Childhood thyroid carcinoma. Cancer 1961; 14:734–743.
27. Goepfert J, Dichtel WJ, Samaan NA. Thyroid cancer in children and teenagers. Arch Otolaryngol 1984; 110:72–75.
28. Desjardins JG, Kahn AH, Montupet P, et al. Management of thyroid nodules in children; A 20 year experience. J Pediatr Surg 1987; 22:736–739.
29. Buckwalter JA, Gurll NJ, Thomas CG Jr. Cancer of the thyroid in youth. World J Surg 1981; 5:15–25.
30. Geiger JD, Thompson NW. Thyroid tumors in children. Otolaryngol Clin North Am 1996; 4(29):711–719.
31. Saigal RK, Khanna SD. Carcinoma of the thyroid in a stillborn male child. Indian J Pediatr 1973; 40:224–226.
32. Gorlin JB, Sallan SE. Thyroid cancer in childhood. Endocrinol Metab Clin North Am 1990; 19:649–662.
33. Zohar Y, Strauss M, Laurian N. Adolescent versus adult thyroid carcinoma. Laryngoscope 1986; 96:555–559.
34. Millman B, Pellitteri PK. Thyroid carcinoma in children and adolescents. Arch Otolaryngol Head Neck Surg 1995; 121:1261–1264.
35. Baverstock K, Egloff B, Pinchera A, et al. Thyroid cancer after Chernobyl (letter). Nature 1992; 359:21–22.
36. Dekeyser LFM, Van Herle AJ. Differentiated thyroid cancer in children. Head Neck Surg 1985; 8:100–114.
37. Mulligan LM, Kwok JB, Healey CS, et al. Germ line mutations of the RET protooncogene in multiple endocrine neoplasia type 2A. Nature 1993; 363:458–460.
38. Hung W. Well differentiated thyroid carcinomas in children and adolescents: A review. Endocrinologist 1994; 4:117–126.
39. Hung W, Anderson KD, Chandra R. Solitary thyroid nodules in 71 children and adolescents. J Pediatr Surg 1992; 27:1407–1409.
40. Flannery TK, Bertuch AA, Lefkothea PK, et al. Papillary thyroid cancer: A pediatric perspective. Pediatrics 1996; 98(3 pt 1):464–466.
41. Gharib H, Goellner JR, Zinsmeister AR, et al. Fine needle aspiration biopsy of the thyroid: The problem of suspicious cytologic findings. Ann Intern Med 1984; 101:25–28.
42. Harness J, Thompson NW, McCleod MK, et al. Differentiated thyroid carcinoma in children and adolescents. World J Surg 1992; 16:547–554.
43. La Quaglia MP, Curbally MT, Heller G, et al. Recurrence and morbidity in differentiated thyroid carcinoma in children. Surgery 1988; 104:1149–1156.
44. Zimmerman D, Hay ID, Gough IR, et al. Papillary thyroid carcinoma in children and adults: Long-term follow-up of 1039 patients conservatively treated at one institution during three decades. Surgery 1988; 104:1157–1163.
45. Guilloteau D, Perdrisot R, Calmette SC, et al. Diagnosis of medullary carcinoma of the thyroid (MCT) by calcitonin assay using monoclonal antibodies: Criteria for the pentagastrin stimulation test in hereditary MCT. J Clin Endocrinol Metab 1990; 71:1064–1067.
46. Telander R, Moir C. Medullary thyroid carcinoma in children. J Pediatr Surg 1994; 3:188–193.
47. Silverberg E, Lubera J. Cancer statistics, 1987. CA Cancer J Clin 1987; 37:2–19.
48. Androulakis M, Johnson JT, Wagner RL. Thyroglossal duct and second branchial cleft anomalies in adults. Ear Nose Throat J 1990; 69:318–322.
49. Kristensen S, Juul A, Moesner J. Thyroglossal cyst carcinoma. J Laryngol Otol. 1984; 98:1277–1280.
50. Cote DN, Sturgis EM, Peterson T, et al. Thyroglossal duct cyst carcinoma: An unusual case of Hürthle cell carcinoma. Otolaryngol Head Neck Surg 1995; 113(1):153–156.
51. Sandlund JT, Downing JR, Crist WM. Non-Hodgkin's lymphoma in childhood. N Engl J Med 1996; 334(19):1238–1248.
52. Miller RW, Young JL, Novakovic B. Childhood cancer. Cancer 1995; 75(supplement 1):395–405.
53. Weisberger EC, Davidson DD. Unusual presentations of lymphoma of the head and neck in childhood. Laryngoscope 1990; 100(4):337–342.
54. Williams J, Thompson E, Smith K. Long-term results of treatment of childhood adolescents with Hodgkin's disease. Cancer 1980; 46:2123.

55. Carbone A, Gloghini A, Weiss LM, et al. Hodgkin's disease: Old and recent clinical concepts. Ann Otol Rhinol Laryngol 1996; 105:751–758.

56. Drexler HG. Recent results on the biology of Hodgkin and Reed-Sternberg cells I. Biopsy material. Leuk Lymphoma 1992; 8:283–313.

57. Carbone A, Gloghini A, Gattei V, et al. Expression of functional CD40 antigen on Reed-Sternberg cells and Hodgkin's disease cell lines. Blood 1995; 85:780–789.

58. Beaty O, Hudson MM, Greenwald C, et al. Subsequent malignancies in children and adolescents after treatment for Hodgkin's disease. J Clin Oncol 1995; 13:603–609.

59. Altman AJ. Pediatric oncology. Pediatr Clin North Am 1985; 32:541–862.

60. Wang MB, Strasnick B, Zimmerman MC. Extranodal American Burkitt's lymphoma of the head and neck. Arch Otolaryngol 1992; 118:193–199.

61. Wright D, Mckeevor P, Carter R. Childhood non-Hodgkins lymphoma in the United Kingdom: Findings from the UK children's cancer study group. J Clin Pathol 1997; 50:128–134.

62. Devaney KO, Putzi MJ, Ferlito A, et al. Head and neck Langerhans' cell histiocytosis. Ann Otol Rhinol Laryngol 1997; 106:526–532.

63. Irving RM, Broadbent V, Jones NS. Langerhans' cell histiocytosis in childhood: Management of head and neck manifestations. Laryngoscope 1994; 104:64–70.

64. Lieberman PH, Jones CR, Steinman RM, et al. Langerhans' cell (eosinophilic) granulomatosis. A clinicopathologic study encompassing 50 years. Am J Surg Path 1996; 20:519–552.

65. Angeli SI, Alcade J, Hoffman HT, Smith RJ. Langerhans' cell histiocytosis of the head and neck in children. Ann Otol Rhinol Laryngol 1995; 104:173–180.

66. Anonymous. A multicentre retrospective survey of Langerhans' cell histiocytosis: 348 cases observed between 1983 and 1993. The French Langerhans' Cell Histiocytosis Study Group. Arch Dis Child 1996; 75:17–24.

67. Willis B, Ablin A, Weinberg V, et al. Disease course and late sequelae of Langerhans' cell histiocytosis: 25-year experience at the University of California, San Francisco. J Clin Oncol 1996; 14:2073–2082.

68. Goodnight JW, Wang MB, Sercarz JA, et al. Extranodal Rosai-Dorfman disease of the head and neck. Laryngoscope 1996; 106:253–256.

69. Shaver EG, Rebsamen SL, Yachnis AT, et al. Isolated extranodal intracranial sinus histiocytosis in a 5-year-old boy. J Neurosurg 1993; 79:769–773.

70. Wenig BM, Abbondanzo SL, Childers EL, et al. Extranodal sinus histiocytosis with massive lymphadenopathy (Rosai-Dorfman disease) of the head and neck. Human Path 1993; 24:483–492.

71. Ho M, Jaffe R, Miller G, et al. The frequency of Epstein-Barr virus infection and associated lymphoproliferative syndrome after transplantation and its manifestation in children. Transplantation 1988; 45:719–727.

72. Deschler DG, Osorio R, Ascher NL, et al. Posttransplant lymphoproliferative disorder in patients under primary tacrolimus (FK 506) immunosuppression. Arch Otolaryngol Head Neck Surg 1995; 121:1037–1041.

73. Sculerati N, Arriaga M. Otolaryngologic management of post transplant lymphoproliferative disease in children. Ann Otol Rhinol Laryngol 1990; 99:445–450.

74. Riccardi VM. Genotype, malleotype, phenotype, and randomness: lessons from Nf-1. Am J Hum Genet 1993; 53:301–4.

75. Robbins SL, Cotran RS, Kumar V. Pathologic Basis of Disease, 3rd ed. Philadelphia: Saunders, 1984, pp. 138–139.

76. National Institutes of Health Consensus Development Conference. Neurofibromatosis. Arch Neurol 1988; 45:575–578.

77. Mulvihill JJ, Parry DM, Sherman JL, et al. NIH conference. Neurofibromatosis 1 (Recklinghausen disease) and neurofibromatosis 2 (bilateral acoustic neurofibromatosis). An update. Ann Intern Med 1990; 113(1):39–52.

78. Knight WA, Murphy WK, Gottlieb JA. Neurofibromatosis associated with malignant neurofibromas. Arch Dermatol 1973; 107:747–775.

79. Hayes FA, Green A, Husto HO, et al. Surgicopathologic staging of neuroblastoma: Prognostic significance of regional lymph node metastases. J Pediatr 1983; 102(1):59–62.

80. Brodeur GM, Pritchard J, Berthold F, et al. Revisions of the international criteria for neuroblastoma diagnosis, staging, and response to treatment. J Clin Oncol 1993; 11(8):1466–1477.

81. Adams GA, Shochat SJ, Smith EI, et al. Thoracic neuroblastoma: A pediatric oncology group study. J Pediatr Surg 1993; 28(3):372–378.

82. Brodeur GM, Azar C, Brother M, et al. Neuroblastoma: Effect of genetic factors on prognosis and treatment. Cancer 1992; 70(6, Supplement):1685–1694.

83. Franks LM, Bollen A, Seeger RC, et al. Neuroblastoma in adults and adolescents: An indolent course with poor survival. Cancer 1997; 79(10):2028–2035.

84. Look AT, Hayes FA, Shuster JJ, et al. Clinical relevance of tumor cell ploidy and n-myc gene amplification in childhood neuroblastoma: A pediatric oncology group study. J Clin Oncol 1991; 9(4):581–591.

85. Woods WG, Lemieux B, Leclerc JM, et al. Screening for neuroblastoma in North America: The Quebec

project. In: Evans AE, Bielder JL, Brodeur GM, et al, eds. *Advances in Neuroblastoma Research 4.* Wiley-liss (NY, NY), 1994, pp. 377–382.

86. Haase GM, O'Leary MC, Ramsay NK, et al. Aggressive surgery combined with intensive chemotherapy improves survival in poor-risk neuroblastoma: A single center analysis of prognostic factors. European J Cancer 1993; 29A(7):947–956.

87. Cheung NV, Heller G. Chemotherapy dose intensity correlates strongly with response, median survival, and median progression free survival in metastatic neuroblastoma. J Clin Oncol 1991; 9(6): 1050–1058.

88. McCowage GB, Vowels MR, Shaw PJ, et al. Autologous bone marrow transplantation for advanced neuroblastoma using teniposide, doxorubicin, melphan, cisplatin and total body irradiation. J Clin Oncol 1995; 13(11):2789–2795.

89. Paul SR, Tarbell NJ, Korf B, et al. Stage IV neuroblastoma in infants: Long-term survival. Cancer 1991; 67(6):1493–1497.

90. Nickman HJ, Nesbit ME, Grosfeld JL, et al. Comparison of stage IV and IV-S neuroblastoma in the first year of life. Med Pediatr Oncol 1985; 13(5): 261–268.

91. Phillips T, Zucker JM, Bernard JL, et al. Improved survival at 2 and 5 years in the LMCE1 unselected group of 72 children with stage IV neuroblastoma older than 1 year of age at diagnosis: Is a cure possible in a small subgroup? J Clin Oncol 1991; 9(6): 1037–1044.

92. Evans RG, Nesbit ME, Gehan EA, et al. Multimodal therapy for the management of localized Ewing's sarcoma of pelvic and sacral bones: A report from the second intergroup study. J Clin Oncol 1991; 9(7):1173–1180.

93. Grier H, Krailo M, Link M, et al. Improved outcome in non-metastatic Ewing's sarcoma and PNET of bone with the addition of ifosfamide and etoposide to vincristine, adriamycin, cyclophosphamide, and actinomycin: A childrens cancer group and pediatric oncology group report. Proceedings of the American Society of Clinical Oncology 1994; 13(30):A1443.

94. Siegal GP, Oliver WR, Reinus WR, et al. Primary Ewing's sarcoma involving the bones of the head and neck. Cancer 1987; 60(11):2829–2840.

95. Nesbit ME, Gehan EA, Burgert EO, et al. Multi-modal therapy for the management of primary non-metastatic Ewing's sarcoma of bone: A long-term follow-up of the first intergroup study. J Clin Oncol 1990; 8(10):1664–1674.

96. Gehan EA, Nesbit ME, Burgert EO, et al. Prognostic factors in children with Ewing's sarcoma. J Natl Cancer Inst 1981; Monograph 56:273–278.

97. Turc-Carel C, Aurias A, Mugneret F, et al. Chromosomes in Ewing's sarcoma: I. An evaluation of 85 cases and remarkable consistency of (t11;22) (q24; q12). Cancer Genet Cytogenet 1988; 32(2): 229–238.

98. Whang-Peng J, Triche TJ, Knutsen T, et al. Cytogenetic characterization of selected small round cell tumors of childhood. Cancer Genet Cytogenet 1986; 21:185–208.

99. Ambros IM, Ambros PF, Strehl S, et al. Mic 2 is a specific marker for Ewing's sarcoma and peripheral primitive neuroectodermal tumors. Cancer 1991; 67(7):1886–1893.

100. Dunst J, Jurgens H, Sauer R, et al. Radiation therapy in Ewing's sarcoma: An update of the CESS 86 trial. Int J Radiat Oncol Biol Phys 1995; 32(4):919–930.

101. Vietti TJ, Gehan EA, Nesbit ME, et al. Multimodal therapy in metastatic Ewing's sarcoma: An intergroup study. J Natl Cancer Inst 1981; Monograph 56:279–284.

102. Cornbleet MA, Corringham RE, Prentice HG, et al. Treatment of Ewing's sarcoma with high dose melphan and autologous bone marrow transplantation. Cancer Treat Rev 1981; 65(3/4):241–244.

103. Burdach S, Jurgens H, Peters C, et al. Myeloablative radio-chemotherapy and autologous bone marrow rescue in the treatment of twenty-two children with advanced tumors. Aust Pediatr J 1984; 209: 195–201.

104. Jones JE, McGill T. Peripheral primitive neuroectodermal tumors of the head and neck. Arch Otolaryngol head Neck Surg 1995; 121:1392–1395.

105. Sobol SM, Dailey JC. Familial multiple cervical paragangliomas: Report of a kindred and review of the literature. Otolaryngol Head Neck Surg 1990; 102: 382–390.

106. Shamblin WR, Remine WH, Sheps SG, et al. Carotid body tumor (chemodectoma). Am J Surg 1971; 122: 732–739.

107. al Rikabi AC, al Kharfy T, al Sohaibani MO, et al. Fetal rhabdomyoma. A case report with the diagnosis suggested by intraoperative cytology. Acta Cytologica 1996; 40:786–788.

108. Kapadia SB, Meis JM, Frisman DM, et al. Fetal rhabdomyoma of the head and neck: A clinocopathologic and immunophenotypic study of 24 cases. Human Path 1993; 24:754–765.

109. Crotty PL, Nakhleh RE, Dehner LP. Juvenile rhabdomyoma. An intermediate form of skeletal muscle tumor in children. Arch Path Lab Med 1993; 117: 43–47.

110. Sercarz JA, Mark RJ, Nasri S, et al. Pediatric rhabdomyosarcoma of the head and neck. Int J Pediatr Otorhinolaryngol 1995; 31:15–22.

111. Maurer HM, Ghehan EA, Beltangady M, et al. The Intergroup Rhabdomyosarcoma Study-II 1993; 71: 1904–1922.

112. Lyos AT, Goepfert H, Luna MA, et al. Soft tissue

sarcoma of the head and neck in children and adolescents. Cancer 1996; 77:193-200.

113. Lawrence W, Hays DM, Heyn R, et al. Lymphatic metastases with childhood rhabdomyosarcoma: A report from the Intergroup Rhabdomyosarcoma Study. Cancer 1987; 60:910-915.

114. Selch MT, Parker RG. Rhabdomyosarcoma of the head and neck in children. Am J Clin Oncol 1984; 7:291-303.

115. Blatt J, Snyderman C, Wollman MR, et al. Delayed resection in the management of non-orbital rhabdomyosarcoma of the head and neck in childhood. Med Ped Oncol 1997; 28:294-298.

116. La Quaglia MP, Heller G, Ghavimi F, et al. The effect of age at diagnosis on outcome in rhabdomyosarcoma. Cancer 1994; 73:109-117.

117. Dillon PW, Whalen TV, Azizhan RG, et al. Neonatal soft tissue sarcomas: The influence of pathology on treatment and survival. Children's Cancer Group Surgical Subcommittee. J Pediatr Surg 1995; 30:1038-1041.

118. Ragab AH, Maurer HM. Malignant tumors of soft tissues. In: Sutow WW, Ferbach DJ, Vietti TJ, eds. *Clinical Pediatric Oncology*, 3rd ed. St. Louis: Mosby, 1984, pp. 652-683.

119. Bielamowicz S, Daver MS, Chang B, et al. Noncutaneous benign fibrous histiocytoma of the head and neck. Otolaryngol Head Neck Surg 1995; 113(1):140-146.

120. Zapater E, Bag JV, Martorell M, et al. Malignant fibrous histiocytoma of the head and neck. Case report. Bull Group Int Rech Sci Stomatol Odontol 1995; 38:121-124.

121. Weber BD, Kempf HG, Lenz M, et al. Diagnosis and therapy of aggressive fibromatosis (extra-abdominal desmoid) in the head and neck area. Laryngorhinootologie 1991; 70(7):367-374.

122. Chabalko J, Creagan E, Fraumeni J Jr. Epidemiology of selected sarcomas in children. J Natl Cancer Inst 1974; 53:675-679.

123. Chung E, Enzinger F. Infantile fibrosarcoma. Cancer. 1976; 38:729-739.

124. Weiss SW. Lipomatous tumors. Monogr Pathol 1996; 38:207-239.

125. Golledge J, Fisher C, Rhys-Evans PH. Head and Neck Liposarcoma. Cancer 1995; 76(6):1051-1058.

126. Mentzel T, Calonje E, Fletcher CD. Lipoblastoma and lipoblastomatosis: A clinicopathological study of 14 cases. Histopathology 1993; 23(6):527-533.

127. Liu J, Hudkins PG, Swee RG, Unni KK. Bone sarcomas associated with Oillier's disease. Cancer 1987; 59:1376-1385.

128. Mark RJ, Sercarz JA, Tran L, et al. Osteogenic sarcoma of the head and neck. The UCLA experience. Arch Otolaryngol Head Neck Surg 1991; 117(7):761-766.

129. Kristensen IB, Sunde LM, Jensen OM. Chondrosarcoma. Increasing grade of malignancy and local recurrence. Acta Pathol Microbiol Immunol Scand 1986; 94:73-77.

130. Thakar A, Tandon DA, Bahadur S, et al. Extranotochordal chordoma presenting as multiple neck masses: Report of a case. J Laryngol Otol 1993; 107:942-945.

131. Stratakis CA, Jenkins RB, Pras E, et al. Cytogenic and microsatellite alterations in tumors from patients with the syndrome of myxomas, spotty skin pigmentation, and endoscrine overactivity (Carney complex). J Clin Endocrinol Metab 1996; 81:3607-3614.

132. Onerci M, Sarioglu T, Gedikoglu G, et al. Synovial sarcoma in the neck. Int J Pediatr Otorhinolaryngol 1993; 27(1):79-84.

133. Schmidt D, Thump P, Harms D, et al. Synovial sarcoma in children and adolescents. A report from the Kiel pediatric tumor registry. Cancer 1991; 67(6):1667-1672.

134. Pappo AS, Fontanesi J, Luo X, et al. Synovial sarcoma in children and adolescents: The St. Jude children's research hospital experience. J Clin Oncol 1994; 12(11):2360-2366.

135. Baker LL, Dillon WP, Hieshima GB, et al. Hemangioma and vascular malformations of the head and neck: MR characterization. AJNR 1993; 14:307-314.

136. Sellar RJ. Imaging blood vessels of the head and neck. J Neurol Neurosurg Psychiatry 1995; 59:225-237.

137. Chen MT, Horng SY, Yeong EK, et al. Treatment of high-flow vascular malformations of the head and neck with arterial ligation followed by sclerotherapy. Ann Plastic Surg 1996; 36:147-153.

138. Svedsen PA, Wikholm G, Fogdestam I, et al. Direct puncture of large arteriovenous malformations in head and neck for embolization and subsequent reconstructive surgery. Scand J Plast Reconstr Surg 1994; 28:131-135.

139. Jacobs AH, Walton RG. The incidence of birthmarks in the neonate. Pediatrics 1976; 58:218-222.

140. Miller SH, Raymond L, Smith MD, et al. Compression treatment of hemangiomas. Plast Reconstr Surg 1975; 58:573-579.

141. Enjolras O, Riche MC, Merland JJ, et al. Management of alarming hemangiomas in infancy: A review of 25 cases. Pediatrics 1990; 85:491-498.

142. Ohlms LA, Jones DT, McGill TJI, et al. Interferon alpha-2a therapy for airway hemangiomas. Ann Otol Rhinol Laryngol 1994; 103:1-8.

143. Bauman NM, Burke DK, Smith RJH. Treatment of massive or life-threatening hemangiomas with recombinant alpha-2a interferon. Otolaryngol Head Neck Surg 1997; 117:99-110.

144. Ezekowitz RAB. Interferon alpha-2a therapy for life-

threatening hemangiomas in infancy. N Engl J Med 1994; 330:300.

145. MacArthur CJ, Senders CW, Katy J. The use of interferon alpha-2a for life-threatening hemangiomas. Arch Otolaryngol Head Neck Surg 1995; 121: 690–693.

146. Wiatrak BJ, Reilly JS, Seid AB, et al. Open surgical excision of subglottic hemangioma in children. Int J Pediatr Otorhinolaryngol 1996; 34:191–206.

147. Ries WR, Speyer MT. Cutaneous application of lasers. Otolaryngol Clin North Am 1996; 29:915–929.

148. Brock ME, Smith RJH, Parey SE, et al. Lymphangioma: An otolaryngologic perspective. Int J Pediatr Otorhinolaryngol 1987; 14:133–140.

149. Nguyen Q, deTar M, Wells W, et al. Cervical thymic cysts: Case reports and review of the literature. Laryngoscope 1996; 106:247–252.

150. Borecky N, Gudinchet F, Laurini R, et al. Imaging of cervico-thoracic lymphangiomas in children. Pediatr Radiol 1995; 25:127–130.

151. Raveh E, deJong AL, Taylor GP, et al. Prognostic factors in the treatment of lymphatic malformations. Arch Otolaryngol Head Neck Surg 1997; 123: 1061–1065.

152. de Serres LM, Sie KC, Richardson MA. Lymphatic malformations of the head and neck. A proposal for staging. Arch Otol Head Neck Surg 1995; 121: 577–582.

153. Ninh TH, Ninh TX. Cystic hygroma in children: A report of 126 cases. J Pediatr Surg 1974; 9:191–195.

154. Emory PJ, Bailey CM, Evans JNG. Cystic hygroma of the neck: A review of 37 cases. J Laryngol Otol 1984; 98:613–619.

155. Proctor B, Proctor C. Congenital lesions of the head and neck. Otolaryngol Clin North Am 1970; 3: 221–248.

156. Orford J, Barker A, Thonell S, et al. Bleomycin therapy for cystic hygroma. J Pediatr Surg 1995; 30: 1282–1287.

157. Farmand M, Kuttenberger JJ. A new therapeutic concept for the treatment of cystic hygroma. Oral Surg Oral Med Oral Pathol Oral Radiol Endod 1996; 81:389–395.

158. Molitch HI, Unger EC, Witte CL, et al. Percutaneous sclerotherapy of lymphangiomas. Radiology 1995; 194:343–347.

159. Smith RJH, Burke DK, Sato Y, et al. OK-432 therapy for lymphangiomas. Arch Otolaryngol Head Neck Surg 1996; 122:1195–1199.

160. Mark RJ, Tran LM, Sercarz J, et al. Angiosarcoma of the head and neck. The UCLA experience 1955 through 1990. Arch Otolaryngol Head Neck Surg 1993; 119:973–978.

161. Chintu C, Athale UH, Patil PS. Childhood cancers in Zambia before and after the HIV epidemic. Arch Dis Child 1995; 73:100–104.

162. Siegal B, Levington-Kriss S, Schiffer A, et al. Kaposi's sarcoma in immunosuppression. Cancer 1990; 65: 492–498.

163. Goldberg AN. Kaposi's sarcoma of the head and neck in acquired immunodeficiency syndrome. Am J Otolaryngol 1993; 14:5–14.

164. del Rosario ML, Saleh A. Preoperative chemotherapy for congenital hemangiopericytoma and a review of the literature. J Pediatr Hematol Oncol 1997; 19:247–250.

165. Chung KC, Weiss SW, Kuzon WM. Multifocal congenital hemangiopericytomas associated with Kasabach-Merritt syndrome. Br J Plast Surg 1995; 48: 240–242.

166. Bailey PV, Weber TR, Tracy TF. Congenital hemangiopericytoma: An unusual vascular neoplasm of infancy. Surgery 1993; 114:936–941.

167. Kimonis VE, Goldstein AM, Pastakia B, et al. Clinical manifestations in 105 persons with nevoid basal cell carcinoma syndrome. Am J Med Genet 1997; 69: 299–308.

168. Gorlin RJ. Nevoid basal-cell carcinoma syndrome. Medicine 1987; 66:98–113.

169. Gailani MR, Bale SJ, Leffell DJ, et al. Developmental defects in Gorlin syndrome related to a putative tumor suppressor gene on chromosome 9. Cell 1992; 69:111–117.

170. Cleaver JE. Defective repair replication of DNA in xeroderma pigmentosum. Nature 1968; 218: 652–656.

171. Andrews AD, Barrett SF, Robbins JH. Xeroderma pigmentosum neurological abnormalities correlated with colony-forming ability after ultra-violet radiation. Proc Nat Acad Sci 1978; 75:1984–1988.

172. Leal-Khouri S, Hruza GJ, Hruza LL, et al. Management of a young patient with xeroderma pigmentosum. Pediatr Dermatol 1994; 11:72–75.

173. Rich DC, Corpron CA, Smith MB, et al. Second malignant neoplasms in children after treatment of soft tissue sarcoma. J Pediatr Surg 1997; 32:369–372.

174. Hudson MM, Jones D, Boyett J, et al. Late mortality of long-term survivors of childhood cancer. J Clin Oncol 1997; 15:2205–2213.

175. Kuttesch JF, Wexler LH, Marcus RB, et al. Second malignancies after Ewing's sarcoma: Radiation dose-dependency of second sarcomas. J Clin Oncol 1996; 14:2818–2825.

176. Corpron CA, Black CT, Ross MI, et al. Melanoma as a second malignant neoplasm after childhood cancer. Am J Surg 1996; 172:459–462.

177. Robison LL. Methodologic issues in the study of second malignant neoplasms and pregnancy outcomes. Med Pediatr Oncol Supplement 1996; 1: 41–44.

178. Rubnitz JE, Crist WM. Molecular genetics of childhood cancer: Implications for pathogenesis, diagnosis, and treatment. Pediatr 1997; 100:101–108.

Index

Page numbers followed by t indicates table, f indicates figure.